Adrenergic Activators and Inhibitors

Part II

Contributors

D. M. Aviado · W. C. Bowman · G. Burnstock · J. Greven
J. Hannappel · P. Juul · Á. Kahán · L. Kovács
M. S. Micozzi · H. Osswald · C. W. I. Owens · D. E. Potter
B. N. C. Prichard · K. H. Rahn · D. Robertshaw · M. Sas
A. J. Smith · H. A. J. Struyker-Boudier · G. T. Tucker
J. Tuckman · H. Wong

Editor

L. Szekeres

Springer-Verlag Berlin Heidelberg New York 1981

Professor Dr. LÁSZLO SZEKERES
Institute of Pharmacology, University Medical School of Szeged,
Dóm tér 12, H-6701 Szeged, Hungary

With 118 Figures

ISBN-13: 978-3-642-67586-7 e-ISBN-13: 978-3-642-67584-3
DOI: 10.1007/978-3-642-67584-3

Library of Congress Cataloging in Publication Data. Main entry under title: Adrenergic activators and inhibitors. (Handbook of experimental pharmacology; v. 54) Includes bibliographies and index. 1. Sympathomimetic agents. 2. Sympatholytic agents. 3. Neuropharmacology. I. Andén, N. E. II. Szekeres, L. III. Series: Handbuch der experimentellen Pharmakologie New series; v. 54. QP905.H3 vol. 54 [RM323.6] 615'.1 [615'.78]. 79-23866

Softcover reprint of the hardcover 1st edition 1981

Handbook of Experimental Pharmacology

Continuation of Handbuch der experimentellen Pharmakologie

Vol. 54/II

List of Contributors

Professor Dr. D. M. Aviado, New Jersey Medical School, P.O. Box 307, Short Hills, NJ 07078/USA

Professor Dr. W.C. Bowman, University of Strathclyde, Department of Physiology and Pharmacology, Royal College, 204 George Street, GB-Glasgow G1 1XW

Professor Dr. G. Burnstock, Department of Anatomy and Embryology, University College London, Gower Street, GB-London WC 1E 6BT

Professor Dr. J. Greven, Abteilung Pharmakologie der Medizinischen Fakultät der RWTH, Melatener Straße 213, D-5100 Aachen

Dr. J. Hannappel, Franzstraße 46, D-5100 Aachen

Professor Dr. P. Juul, Department of Pharmacology, Royal Danish School of Pharmacy, Universitetsparken 2, DK-2100 Copenhagen

Professor Dr. Á. Kahán, Clinic of Ophthalmology, Korányi Sándor rkp. 16, H-6701 Szeged

Dr. L. Kovács, Clinical Obstet. et Gynaec., Universitatis, Semmelweis μ. 1., H-6725 Szeged

Dr. M. S. Micozzi, Department of Research Medicine, University of Pennsylvania, Medical School, Department of Pathology, Pennsylvania Hospital, Philadelphia, PN/USA

Priv.-Doz. Dr. H. Osswald, Abteilung Pharmakologie der Medizinischen Fakultät der RWTH, Melatener Straße 213, D-5100 Aachen

Dr. C. W. I. Owens, University College Hospital, Medical School, University Street, GB-London WC1E 6JJ

Professor Dr. D. E. Potter, Department of Pharmacology and Therapeutics, School of Medicine, Texas Technical University, Health Sciences Center, P.O. Box 4569, Lubbock, TX 79409/USA

Dr. B. N. C. Prichard, Clinical Pharmacology, University College Hospital, Medical School, University Street, GB-London WC1E 6JJ

Professor Dr. K. H. Rahn, Department of Pharmacology, University of Limburg, P.O. Box 616, NL-6200 MD-Maastricht

Professor Dr. D. Robertshaw, Department of Physiology and Biophysics, Colorado State University, Fort Collings, CO 80523/USA

Professor Dr. M. Sas, Clinical Obstet. et Gynaec., Universitatis, Semmelweis μ. 1., H-6725 Szeged

Professor Dr. A. J. Smith, Clinical Pharmacology, Faculty of Medicine, Division of Clinical Investigation, The University of Newcastle, AUS-2308 New South Wales

Dr. H. A. J. Struyker-Boudier, Department of Pharmacology, University of Limburg, P.O. Box 616, NL-6200 MD-Maastricht

Dr. G.T. TUCKER, Clinical Pharmacology and Therapeutics, Department of Therapeutics, Hallamshire Hospital, Glossop Road, GB-Sheffield S10 2JF

Dr. J. TUCKMAN, Institute of Rehabilitation Medicine, New York University Medical Center, 400 East 34th Street, New York, NY 10016/USA

Dr. H. WONG, Department of Pharmacology, University of Melbourne, Parkville, AUS-3052 Victoria

Contents of Part II*

Section IV: Effects on Organ Systems Other Than the Nervous and the Cardiovascular System

CHAPTER 1

Systemic Pharmacology of Adrenergic Activators and Inhibitors: Effects on the Respiratory System. D. M. AVIADO and M. S. MICOZZI

* Contents of Part I, Section I to III see p. XXI

CHAPTER 2

Effects of Adrenergic Activators and Inhibitors on the Skeletal Muscles.
W.C. Bowman. With 14 Figures

CHAPTER 3

Systemic Pharmacology of Adrenergic Agonists and Antagonists: Effects on the Digestive System. G. Burnstock and H. Wong. With 1 Figure

CHAPTER 4

Effects of Adrenergic Activators and Inhibitors on the Endocrine System.
D.E. POTTER. With 6 Figures

CHAPTER 5

Systemic Pharmacology of Adrenergic Activators and Inhibitors: Effects on the Genital System. M. SAS and L. KOVÁCS. With 7 Figures

CHAPTER 6

Effects of Adrenergic Activators and Inhibitors on Kidney Function.
H. Osswald and J. Greven. With 6 Figures

CHAPTER 8

Miscellaneous Effects: Effects of Adrenergic Activators and Inhibitors on the Eye.
Á. KAHÁN. With 2 Figures

CHAPTER 9

Effects of Adrenergic Activators and Inhibitors on the Sweat Glands.
D. ROBERTSHAW. With 4 Figures

Section V: Kinetics, Biotransformation, Toxic Effects and Clinical Implications

CHAPTER 1

Kinetics and Biotransformation of Adrenergic Activators and Inhibitors: Adrenergic Alpha- and Beta-Receptor Activators. K.H. RAHN. With 7 Figures

CHAPTER 2

Kinetics and Biotransformation of Adrenergic Activators and Inhibitors: Adrenergic Transmitter Releasing Agents. H. A. J. STRUYKER-BOUDIER. With 3 Figures

CHAPTER 5

Clinical Features of Adrenergic Agonists and Antagonists.
B. N. C. PRICHARD, C. W. I. OWENS, and J. TUCKMAN

Contents
Part I: Activators and Inhibitors

Section I: General Considerations

Section II: Effects on the Autonomic and on the Central Nervous System

Section III: Effects on the Cardiovascular System

Section IV: Effects on Organ Systems Other Than the Nervous and the Cardiovascular System

CHAPTER 1

Systemic Pharmacology of Adrenergic Activators and Inhibitors: Effects on the Respiratory System

D. M. AVIADO and M. S. MICOZZI

A. Introduction

This chapter is written as a general guide for the interested reader in the pharmacology of the respiratory system; thus, there are topics that necessarily overlap with the pharmacology of organs covered in other chapters. For example, the general stimulatory effect on respiration resulting from administration of toxic doses of most adrenergic activators is related to their central nervous system effects, as discussed in Chap. Sec. II B. A change in resistance to breathing in the upper respiratory tract is mediated by the pharmacologic effects of adrenergic activators on nasal blood vessels. This vascular phenomenon is pharmacologically related to behavior of the peripheral blood vessels, as discussed in Chap. Sec. III, Chap. 5. Any discussion of the pharmacology of the pulmonary circulation must include consideration of pulmonary blood flow or cardiac output, which is, in turn, dependent upon cardiac performance, as discussed in Chap. Sec. III, Chap. 5. More than three-quarters of the total clinical use of adrenergic drugs is in the treatment of diseases of the respiratory system. The pharmacologic basis for antiasthmatic drugs and cold remedies discussed in this chapter should supplement the clinical usage discussed in Chap. Sec. 5, Chap. 5. The remaining one-quarter of the clinical use of adrenergic inhibitors and activators (e.g., vasopressors, antihypertensives, antiarrhythmics, anorexigenics, antispasmodics) is also discussed in this chapter but additional details appear in Chap. Sec. 5, Chap. 5. Thus, these drugs may engender adverse reactions involving the respiratory system.

Although there is much supplemental information contained elsewhere, this chapter is devoted to a consideration of the pharmacologic effects of adrenergic drugs upon the respiratory system. These effects can be documented in the following frames of reference: (a) a definitive analysis of the role and consequences of the autonomic nervous system in the regulation of bronchial smooth muscles, pulmonary arteries, pulmonary veins, bronchial arteries, bronchial veins, and bronchopulmonary anastomoses; (b) a current discussion of the manner in which adrenoceptors influence the regulation of ventilation, blood perfusion, and gas exchange of the lung; (c) a comprehensive explanation of the desired or therapeutically useful effects of adrenergic drugs, as well as their undesired or adverse reactions involving the respiratory system; and (d) a theoretical exposition of the distribution of α- and β-receptors for the respiratory system. This latter discussion is based upon extensive studies on the pharmacology of the various anatomic structures of the respiratory system, i.e., airways, pulmonary blood vessels, bronchial blood vessels, and bronchopulmonary anastomoses, as well as pulmonary blood flow dependent upon cardiac function.

The structural organization of this chapter is not based on the outline in the preceding paragraph; sections are segregated according to the nature of the pharmacologic effect on α- and β-adrenoceptors. These sections are illustrated by the following prototypes with characteristic pharmacologic actions such as *epinephrine* (direct α- and β-activation); *norepinephrine* (predominantly direct α-activation); *isoproterenol* (direct β-activation); *terbutaline* (direct bronchoselective effect); *ephedrine* (that also has releasing action of adrenergic transmitter); and *propranolol, phentolamine,* and *reserpine* (block or inhibit the activity of adrenergic receptors). The discussion of the eight prototypes will include a comparison with a further fifty drugs that resemble one of the selected categorical adrenergic drugs.

B. Epinephrine: A Unique Example of Direct Activator of Alpha- and Beta-Adrenoceptors

Within a historic perspective, this chapter devoted to the respiratory system must begin with a consideration of epinephrine, because it was the first drug available for the treatment of bronchial asthma, as well as for the experimental elucidation of the functional consequences of stimulation of the autonomic nerve supply to the respiratory system, and of the release of adrenal medullary hormones. Essential features of the respiratory effects of intravenous administration of epinephrine include bronchodilation, pulmonary hypertension, vasoconstriction, and vasodilation of pulmonary blood vessels, bronchial blood vessels, and bronchopulmonary anastomoses. Overall, the vasculature of the lung is less sensitive than the peripheral blood vessels, heart, and bronchial smooth muscles. With progressively increasing doses of epinephrine, the sequence of isolated pharmacologic actions are as follows: bronchodilation with tachycardia; coincidental rise followed by a fall in aortic blood pressure; and simultaneous rise followed by a fall in pulmonary blood pressure. The relative doses that elicit each of the three responses are approximately 0.5, 1.0, and 2.0 μg/kg intravenously in experimental dogs. In humans, there are no supportive observations relating to intravenous administration. However, since subcutaneous injections elicit only bronchodilation and tachycardia, whereas intravenous injections also influence the systemic and pulmonary blood pressures, it is reasonable to assume that the comparative sensitivities of components of the cardiopulmonary system in man are similar to those in the experimental dog.

As an introduction to the methodology for study of the respiratory system response to adrenergic activators and inhibitors, this section on epinephrine covers techniques which illustrate the similarities between the effects of sympathetic innervation to the lungs and those of the administration of epinephrine by intravenous, subcutaneous, and inhalational routes. Epinephrine simulates the pattern of sympathetic nervous activation of the respiratory system, whereas norepinephrine does not. The hypothesis that epinephrine is the neurohumoral transmitter in the lung is contrary to the concept advanced for other organs, in which norepinephrine is the accepted neurohumoral mediator for sympathetic nerve activity. Unlike the heart, there has been no demonstrated release of norepinephrine in the airways as a result of experimental stimulation of sympathetic nerves. The experimental complexities of the demonstration of neurohumoral transmitters for adrenoceptors are discussed below (p. 11).

I. Alpha- and Beta-Receptors in the Respiratory System

The uniqueness of epinephrine lies in its ability to activate both α- and β-receptors throughout the body, including the respiratory system. Only epinephrine is capable of duplicating the functional expression of stimulation of sympathetic nerves controlling the various components of the respiratory system. Epinephrine directly activates all α- and β-receptors, whereas all other direct activators have action limited to either α or β or to a combination of α and β_1 (cardiac) or β_2 (bronchial) receptors. Table 1 outlines the distribution of receptors in discrete anatomic areas of the respiratory system. The headings include examples of direct acting drugs in order to express the differences between epinephrine, which activates all adrenergic receptors, and norepinephrine, isoproterenol, and methoxamine, which activate some, but not all, receptors.

Table 1. Distribution of adrenergic α- and β-receptors in the respiratory system

Anatomic divisions of respiratory system	α-responses to epinephrine, norepinephrine, and methoxamine	β-responses to epinephrine and isoproterenol
Upper respiratory tract:		
Nasal and pharyngeal blood vessels	Vasoconstriction	Vasodilation
Lower respiratory tract		
Bronchial mucosa	Vasoconstriction	Vasolidation
Bronchial smooth muscles	Bronchoconstriction	Bronchodilation
Bronchial glands	Reduced secretion	Augmented secretion
Mucociliary transport	Decreased movement	Increased movement
Pulmonary circulation:		
Pulmonary arteries	Vasoconstriction	Vasodilation
Pulmonary veins	Vasoconstriction	Vasodilation
Pulmonary blood flow	(See text)	Increased cardiac output
Pulmonary arterial pressure	(See text)	Increased or decreased
Bronchial circulation:		
Bronchial arteries	Vasoconstriction	Vasodilation
Bronchial veins	Vasoconstriction	Vasodilation
Bronchopulmonary anastomoses	Increased bronchopulmonary flow and venous admixture	Decreased bronchopulmonary flow and venous admixture
Ventilation/perfusion:		
V/Q ratio	(See text)	Decreased
Oxygen content in peripheral arterial blood	(See text)	Reduced

1. Upper Respiratory Tract

The origins of the sympathetic nerves conveying impulses to nasal and pharyngeal mucosa include the T 1 and T 2 segments of the spinal cord, the superior cervical sympathetic ganglia and the plexus surrounding the carotid arteries and their nasal and pharyngeal branches. The major responses to sympathetic nerve stimulation are selective vasoconstriction and vasodilation. The latter effect is elicited with nerve stimulation in the presence of α-receptor inhibition by corresponding blockers. Congestion of the nasal and pharyngeal mucosa, resulting from allergic processes or viral infection, is caused by vasodilation and increased glandular secretion. Epinephrine administered topically causes vasoconstriction and decongestion with symptomatic relief. However, after the period of vasoconstriction or decongestion, a second phase of vasodilation is encountered. These two phases are seen following topical use of epinephrine and are identified respectively as α- and β-receptor activation, since they are blocked respectively by α- and β-blockers. Methoxamine and related pure α-activators are preferred for decongestion of the respiratory tract (AVIADO and DEBEER, 1959).

2. Lower Respiratory Tract

The sympathetic nerves to the lower respiratory tract, or tracheobronchial passages, originate from the T 2 to T 7 spinal segments, passing to their respective paravertebral ganglia, their pulmonary branches, and then to the tracheobronchial plexus. There are four reactive areas: (a) blood vessels of the bronchial mucosa containing α-receptors to mediate vasoconstriction, as well as β-receptors to mediate vasodilation; (b) bronchial smooth muscle, containing predominantly β-receptors for bronchodilation, and also under special circumstances, α-receptors for bronchoconstriction; (c) bronchial glands, where α-mediated vasoconstriction is probably responsible for reduction of secretion; and (d) mucociliary transport, with α-receptors that mediate decreased ciliary activity and β-receptors that increase mucociliary transport (see AVIADO, 1970). From the above pharmacologic actions, the following can be identified as desirable in the treatment of bronchial asthma: (a) α-vasoconstriction to reduce bronchial congestion; (b) β-bronchodilation to widen the internal diameter of the air passages; (c) α-reduction in bronchial secretion; and (d) β-increase in mucociliary transport. Only epinephrine is capable of eliciting all four therapeutically useful actions. Norepinephrine is devoid of the (b) and (d) components; isoproterenol lacks (a) and (c), and methoxamine lacks (b) and (d).

3. Pulmonary Circulation

The sympathetic innervation to the pulmonary blood vessels is identical to that of the lower respiratory tract. The basic pattern of response of the pulmonary vascular bed is similar to that of the systemic vascular beds, including the nasal, pharyngeal, and bronchial areas. α-Receptors mediate vasoconstriction and β-receptors control vasodilation. There is evidence from experiments in canine lungs that the postcapillary pulmonary venules are more reactive to α-activators than are the precapillary pulmonary arterioles. Postcapillary venular constriction may result in congestion of the pulmonary capillaries and lead to the development of pulmonary edema (see AVIADO, 1965).

The caliber of the pulmonary blood vessels is not the only determinant of pulmonary circulation. The blood pressure levels in the precapillary and postcapillary areas are also influenced by the cardiac output, or pulmonary blood flow. Accordingly, the β-receptors in the heart are activated by epinephrine, for example, which increases cardiac activity and pulmonary blood flow and elevates pulmonary arterial blood pressure. The extent of blood pressure elevation is determined by the heart activity as well as the coincidental changes in blood vessel caliber, i.e., vasoconstriction or vasodilation by epinephrine. For a predominant β-activator such as isoproterenol, the cardiac and pulmonary vascular actions are hemodynamically opposed. A β-mediated increase in cardiac activity or pulmonary blood flow would tend to elevate pulmonary arterial blood pressure, whereas the β-mediated vasodilation would tend to reduce it. The end result is an indeterminant rise or fall in pulmonary arterial blood pressure depending upon the net balance of the cardiac and vascular actions. The pulmonary hemodynamic consequences of norepinephrine and methoxamine are complex and are discussed elsewhere (p. 13, and 15).

4. Bronchial Circulation

As in the pulmonary circulation, the sympathetic innervation of the bronchial blood vessels is similar to that of the lower respiratory tract. The bronchial arteries supply blood to the bronchial mucosa and related tissues, but the venous drainage is divided into two distributions, i.e., the bronchial veins and the bronchopulmonary anastomoses (AVIADO et al., 1961). In canine experiments, α-activation by epinephrine is seen to cause constriction of the bronchial veins, thus favoring a shift of venous drainage to the bronchopulmonary anastomoses. Consequently, there is an increase of venous admixture into the oxygenated blood in the pulmonary veins with a reduction in the oxygen content of blood reaching the left heart for distribution to the systemic circulation. It should be stated for completeness that the bronchial arteries, like nasal, pharyngeal, and other peripheral arteries, are supplied from the aorta and manifest typical α-vasoconstriction and β-vasodilation (see AVIADO, 1965).

5. Ventilation–Perfusion Relationship

The overall consequences of α- and β-adrenoceptor activation in the lower respiratory tract and the pulmonary circulation can be covered by a discussion of ventilation–perfusion relationships. In simple terms, delivery of air to the lungs should maintain an ideal relationship to pulmonary blood flow of 4 l air/5 l blood per minute (80% V/Q ratio). Epinephrine increases both ventilation and perfusion; however, perfusion is augmented to a proportionately greater extent than ventilation, resulting in a ratio of approximately 5 l air/8 l blood per minute, or a reduction to approximately 60% V/Q ratio. The net result is insufficient blood oxygenation, i.e., reduction in the oxygen content of blood which can be collected from a peripheral artery. This decrease in oxygenation is an important consideration when epinephrine is used in the treatment of bronchial asthma. This adverse effect of epinephrine may be partially ameliorated with concurrent administration of oxygen.

II. Antiasthmatic Use and Airway Resistance

Epinephrine has been in clinical use for the treatment of bronchial asthma since the turn of the century. The pharmaceutical preparation was originally made from an extract of the adrenal medulla, but was eventually replaced by the synthetic form. At the present time, only the levo-rotatory form of epinephrine is used in therapeutics, and is administered subcutaneously and by inhalation of a nebulized solution or of the aerosol with a propellant.

The pharmacologic features of epinephrine are discussed in terms of the classic or physiologic, and the recent or biochemical, concepts of its antiasthmatic action. It is important to differentiate between the widely accepted explanations and the recently proposed hypotheses in the direction of research for the future. A discussion of tachyphylaxis, believed to be absent for epinephrine, is included below because of recent developments in the treatment of intractable bronchial asthma, resistant to epinephrine (referred to clinically as status asthmaticus).

1. Classic Physiologic Concept

It has generally been accepted that the primary action of epinephrine in the relaxation of bronchial smooth muscles is the most important explanation for its efficacy in the treatment of an acute asthmatic attack. This concept originated from the early observations that relief of bronchial wheezing is accompanied by a cessation of labored breathing and coughing, and a significant reduction in airway resistance. In the laboratory, the bronchodilator action of epinephrine could be readily demonstrated in the intact animal with measurements of airway resistance, and in the perfused lung with recordings of airway resistance. In vitro preparations of tracheal muscle ring chain show relaxation of the smooth muscle portion of the airways with administration of epinephrine (see AVIADO, 1970). The relief of coughing by epinephrine is believed to be an indirect outcome of its bronchodilator action rather than a direct influence on the cough receptors (see SALEM and AVIADO, 1964).

Laboratory experiments led to identification of the two groups of airway receptors discussed in the preceding section. Briefly, therapeutic doses of epinephrine activated β-receptors in bronchial smooth muscles and in the ciliated cells as well as α-receptors in the bronchial mucosa and bronchial glands. The end results are a decrease in airway resistance initiated by β-bronchodilation and α-vasoconstriction (bronchial decongestion), reduced bronchial secretion from α-activity in the bronchial glands and improved mucociliary transport from β-activity in the ciliated bronchial epithelium. Although each anatomic component of the airways contains both α- and β-receptors, it appears that β-receptors predominate in the bronchial muscles and ciliated cells, whereas α-receptors predominate in the bronchial blood vessels and bronchial glands. The existence of the alternate group of receptors is revealed when the appropriate blocking agents are given, and epinephrine administration is repeated.

Another approach to the demonstration of the existence of two sets of receptors is to compare epinephrine (which activates both groups of receptors) with drugs for α-receptors only and with drugs for β-receptors only. LIPPMANN et al. (1975) demonstrated an increase in mucociliary transport in human subjects for both epinephrine and isoproterenol (β-activator only). MELVILLE et al. (1976) showed similar effects for both drugs in increasing ciliary activity of airways in various animal species.

2. Recent Biochemical Concepts

During the past few years, three concepts have been introduced regarding the antiasthmatic mode of action of epinephrine and related drugs. The first maintains that antiasthmatic drugs, such as epinephrine and other β-activators, inhibit the release of histamine and other chemical bronchospastic agents from degranulation of mast cells. This hypothesis is based on observed reduction of the antigen-induced release of histamine, slow reacting substance of anaphylaxis (SRS-A), platelet activating factors (PAF), and prostaglandins from human lung tissue and from rat mast cells as a result of prior treatment with epinephrine (ORANGE and AUSTEN, 1971; SÖRENBY, 1975; STRANDBERG et al., 1977). A second hypothesis stresses the primary importance of cyclic adenosine-3′,5′-monophosphate (cAMP) as the intermediary agent in the bronchodilation brought about by epinephrine (DUNCAN et al., 1975). The third hypothesis shifts the site of action for the antiasthmatic effect of epinephrine from the lung parenchyma to circulating lymphocytes, which become abnormally deficient in β-receptor activity in asthmatic patients (SZENTIVANYI, 1968; CONOLLY and GREENACRE, 1977).

The above concepts are based entirely upon biochemical observations, which are difficult to make concurrently with the functional or physiologic measurements that form the basis of the classic explanation for antiasthmatic activity. The reduction in airway resistance is a dynamic measurement repeatedly performed in the asthmatic patient or animal, whereas detection of chemical mediators, cAMP and related enzymes are performed on excised lungs of experimental animals. Thus, it has been difficult to determine the relevance of biochemical observations to the asthmatic patient treated with epinephrine. Additional research is needed to identify which, if any, of these three biochemical concepts can be incorporated into the classic physiologic rationale for the treatment of bronchial asthma.

III. Adverse Effects on the Pulmonary Circulation

Tachycardia is the most frequent adverse reaction to epinephrine in the treatment of bronchial asthma. It is encountered following either subcutaneous or inhalational administration. The β-receptors in the airways are just as sensitive to epinephrine as those in the heart, so that the desired bronchodilator action is usually accompanied by the undesired tachycardia (see AVIADO, 1970). The pharmacologic activity of epinephrine is manifest in the pulmonary circulation by effects including transient increase in pulmonary blood flow and pulmonary arterial blood pressure, pulmonary arterial constriction, pulmonary venular constriction, and potentially fatal pulmonary edema.

1. Pulmonary Arterial Hypertension

Epinephrine has a biphasic action on pulmonary blood vessels, manifesting vasodilation in small doses and vasoconstriction in large doses. However, the vasodilation is usually accompanied by an increase in pulmonary blood flow, so that there is usually no net change in mean pulmonary arterial pressure. Doses sufficiently large to produce pulmonary vasoconstriction also cause an increase in pulmonary blood flow with a rise in mean pulmonary arterial pressure and increase in total pulmonary vascular resistance. These hemodynamic effects of epinephrine have been repeatedly demonstrated in human subjects and experimental animals by measurements of pulmonary blood flow or cardiac output, and also by measurements of blood pressure in the pulmonary artery, pulmonary vein, or left artium with catheterization (see AVIADO, 1965).

The relative sensitivities of the pulmonary and bronchial blood vessels to epinephrine have been examined in the canine lung. The pulmonary veins are more reactive to constriction than the pulmonary arteries; bronchial veins more sensitive than bronchial arteries; and there is an overall shift in bronchial venous drainage in favor of the bronchopulmonary anastomoses (ARAMENDIA et al., 1962a, b). The diversion of venous blood to the pulmonary veins would contribute to a decrease in oxygen content of the peripheral arterial blood.

The above-mentioned changes are unlikely to be harmful to the asthmatic patient if oxygen supply to the lung is supplemented. However, during an acute asthmatic attack, pulmonary arterial pressure is characteristically elevated (ZIMMERMAN, 1951). Further elevation in pulmonary arterial pressure by epinephrine may be dangerous if the asthmatic patient is also suffering from cor pulmonale due to the increased load on the right ventricle. An adrenergic bronchodilator with no pulmonary vasoconstrictor (such as isoproterenol) would be preferred in the treatment of such an asthmatic condition.

2. Acute Pulmonary Edema

Another adverse reaction to administration of epinephrine is acute pulmonary edema, which is potentially fatal. Deaths have occurred in children from epinephrine as a result of the injection of toxic doses miscalculated to be therapeutic as based upon adult use. The occurrence of pulmonary edema is explained by the intense systemic vasopressor action causing failure of a heart which may in some instances develop arrhythmia (see AVIADO, 1978). The pathogenesis of epinephrine induced pulmonary edema is more than that of the stated backward failure of the left ventricle arising from systemic hypertension. In experimental animals, the following additional mechanisms for pulmonary edema have been proposed: pulmonary venular constriction (ELIAKIM and AVIADO, 1961); stimulation of an edematogenic center in the medulla of the central nervous system (LUISADA, 1940); and increase in permeability of pulmonary capillaries (BARIETY and KOHLER, 1953). The last mentioned mechanism should not be confused with the inhibitory action of antiasthmatic doses of epinephrine on the release of histamine (p. 9). Toxic doses of epinephrine cause an opposite effect, i.e., release of histamine, which in turn increases the permeability of capillaries. Epinephrine alone is known to reduce permeability and is the only adrenergic drug that is useful in the treatment of serum sickness and acute anaphylaxis.

IV. Tachyphylaxis and Status Asthmaticus

In 1942, DE BURGH DALY et al. reported a paradoxical response of canine airways to epinephrine; instead of bronchodilation, there was bronchoconstriction. This phenomenon was observed in the canine lung after 2 h of perfusion. In 1962, CASTRO DE LA MATA et al. offered an explanation for this paradoxical response, viz, bronchial smooth muscles contain α-receptors which if activated by epinephrine cause bronchoconstriction. The presence of α-receptors is ordinarily masked by β-receptor activity and becomes apparent only with blockade of the β-receptors by drugs, with repeated injections of large doses of epinephrine, or with deterioration of the lung preparation. This explanation of α-mediated bronchoconstriction for epinephrine has subsequently been confirmed for other adrenergic activators (p. 12).

This phenomenon of epinephrine reversal for the airways may be similar to the clinical syndrome of status asthmaticus characterized by refractoriness to epinephrine. Testing the hypothesis by administration of an α-blocking drug in status asthmaticus is a subject for future clinical investigation (p. 30). There are complicating factors in the patient with status asthmaticus, such as hypercapnia, hypoxemia, and respiratory acidosis, which would reduce the sensitivity of β-bronchodilator receptors. However, epinephrine continues to be ineffective in spite of correction of the abnormalities in acid-base balance. The insensitivity of β-receptors to epinephrine is a complex phenomenon because other β-activators, such as isoproterenol, can still be effective (p. 17).

V. Epinephrine as Neurohumoral Transmitter of the Airways

This section is concluded by proposing that epinephrine is the most likely candidate for a neurohumoral transmitter in the airways. The similarities between the effects of sympathetic nerve stimulation to those of administered epinephrine are discussed above (p. 4). The activation of both α- and β-receptors by epinephrine has been demonstrated not only in vascular components of the lung but also in the airways.

The induction of an asthmatic attack by muscular exercise has defied explanation because the generalized increase in sympathetic activity is not accompanied by bronchodilation but instead by bronchoconstriction. Although BEIL et al. (1977) have failed to show an increase in circulating catecholamines in patients during exercise-induced asthma, the participation of epinephrine has not been completely excluded. It is still possible that epinephrine is released into the airways but could only be detected in the bronchial venous effluent. Since the effluent is less than 1% of the total venous return to the heart, any catecholamine released would be diluted 100-fold and would not be detected by current analytic methods applicable to the whole blood. MCFADDEN and INGRAM (1979) have proposed respiratory heat loss as the initiating stimulus for exercise-induced asthma but they overlooked the role of the sympathetic nerves.

The hypothesis that epinephrine is released into the airways as a result of sympathetic activity will require confirmatory investigation combining the collection of bronchial venous and bronchopulmonary anastomotic effluent, which is possible only in the isolated canine lung. The technique for binding of tritium-labeled epinephrine demonstrated in the rat lung by U'PRICHARD et al. (1978) could be modified and applied to the canine lung. In the same preparation, tagged epinephrine could also be examined as a potential neurohumoral transmitter. However, norepinephrine cannot be the accepted neurotransmitter for the airways because it fails to activate bronchial β-receptors and is not a bronchodilator. Norepinephrine is an α-activator and is discussed with all other such drugs in the next section.

C. Direct Activator of Alpha-Receptors

Drugs that directly activate α-receptors exert their primary effects on the respiratory tract as nasal vasoconstriction, bronchial decongestion, pulmonary vasoconstriction, and bronchial vasoconstriction. Based upon their systemic vasoconstrictor action, four drugs are used as vasopressor agents, but their effects on the respiratory system are of special interest for several reasons. Two α-activators (norepinephrine and dopamine) are naturally present in the lung and have been considered as candidates for airway neurohumoral transmitters. Three α-activators (norepinephrine, dopamine, and phenylephrine) are also β-stimulators but are dissimilar to epinephrine in that they activate the cardiac (β_1) but not the bronchial or vascular (β_2)-receptors. When these three α- and β_1-activators are used as vasopressor agents, there are potential effects on the pulmonary circulation associated in part with their cardiac action, and also with the indirect consequences of their vasopressor action. One α-activator (methoxamine) exerts a variable effect on the pulmonary blood vessels, unlike the other drugs. It has been possible to identify the structural features of methoxamine that correlate with a lack of pulmonary vasoconstriction, and even pulmonary vasodilation (AVIADO and SCHMIDT, 1957). There appears to be differences in adrenergic receptors between the pulmonary circulation and systemic circulation, which would lead to future consideration for synthesis of a selective pulmonary vasodilator.

I. Norepinephrine

In a previous section, a naturally occurring amine, epinephrine, was proposed as the neurohumoral transmitter for sympathetic innervation of the airways. This hypothesis was initiated because norepinephrine lacks β-bronchodilator action, and its only identifiable effect is α-mediated bronchoconstriction. In 1962, based upon observations that bronchoconstriction would be blocked by an α-blocker, CASTRO DE LA MATA et al. reported evidence that norepinephrine activated α-receptors in the canine lung. Evidence derived from the human lung was not available until 1978, when KNEUSSL and RICHARDSON examined the responses of human tracheal and bronchial smooth muscles obtained from postmortem bronchopulmonary specimens. In diseased human tissue, norepinephrine elicited bronchial muscle contraction that can be blocked with phentolamine. However, normal human tissue did not respond to norepinephrine unless pretreated with histamine or potassium chloride. These observations support the hypothesis that the airways contain α-receptors sensitive to norepinephrine, but that norepinephrine cannot be an acceptable neurohumoral transmitter in airways containing predominantly β-receptors.

There has been one successful detection of norepinephrine following electric stimulation of the sympathetic nerve supply to the perfused rabbit lung (MATHE et al., 1977). It should be noted that the origin of the released norepinephrine was from the pulmonary blood vessels, where the induced vasoconstriction simulates that of electric stimulation. If any catecholamine was released in the airways, it would appear in the bronchial circulation which was excluded in the preparation used by MATHE et al. (1977). The rabbit is rarely used for the study of bronchial circulation and for bronchomotor responses to norepinephrine. The preferred animal for investigation of catecholamine release is the dog (see SALEM and AVIADO, 1974).

1. Pulmonary Vasoconstriction and Pulmonary Edema

The primary clinical use of norepinephrine is in the treatment of systemic hypotension, developing from spinal anesthesia, trauma, or myocardial infarction. The intravenous infusion of norepinephrine, in doses that increase systemic arterial blood pressure, causes the following changes in the pulmonary circulation: reduction in pulmonary blood flow, rise in pulmonary arterial blood pressure, and increase in pulmonary vascular resistance (GOLDENBERG et al., 1948). Since norepinephrine is a known cardiac stimulant, the surprising reduction in cardiac output or pulmonary blood flow is an indirect consequence of the rise in systemic arterial blood pressure and reflex bradycardia.

The observed norepinephrine-induced fall in cardiac output in patients suffering from cardiogenic shock is caused not only by reflex bradycardia, but also by interference with ventricular function from elevated aortic blood pressure. The fact that some patients treated with norepinephrine develop pulmonary edema is explained by the inability of the infarcted heart to compensate for correction in aortic blood pressure from hypotensive to normotensive levels. This reaction to norepinephrine, as well as its arrhythmogenic property, have contributed to its de-emphasis in clinical use in favor of dopamine (ADELSON and GILBERT, 1959).

The pulmonary arterial hypertension seen following intravenous infusion of norepinephrine is entirely dependent upon vasoconstriction of the pulmonary blood vessels. The earlier experiments showing constriction of both arterioles and venules (see AVIADO, 1965) have been recently confirmed by JOINER et al. (1975), who observed contraction of isolated helical strips of intrapulmonary arteries and veins from human, canine, swine, and sheep lungs. There are also recently reported perfusion experiments of the canine lung indicating that norepinephrine is predominantly an arteriolar, rather than venular, constrictor (GRIMM et al., 1978). Use of epinephrine in the study would have proved an opportunity to verify its predominantly pulmonary venular constrictor nature, which was suggested on the basis of experiments performed in the 1960s (see AVIADO, 1965).

Although there is a suggested difference in the primary site of vasoconstriction in the pulmonary blood vessels for epinephrine and norepinephrine, both have similar vasoconstrictor action in the bronchial veins. In the bronchial arteries, norepinephrine is a pure vasoconstrictor agent, whereas epinephrine is both a vasoconstrictor and vasodilator (MARTINEZ L. DE LETONA et al., 1961). Thus, epinephrine is the adrenergic activator which most closely reflects the actions of sympathetic nervous innervation to the bronchial circulation.

2. Uptake of Norepinephrine in the Pulmonary Circulation

Until recently, the pulmonary circulation was regarded as an important metabolic organ for biogenic amines, including norepinephrine. However, the experiments in human subjects performed by STJÄRNE et al. (1975) indicate a different conclusion. Compared to the forearm circulation the pulmonary blood vessels do not remove tagged norepinephrine other than by a nonspecific filtration and diffusion. The subsequent fate of norepinephrine is dependent upon whether the extraluminal tissues of the lung possess specific concentration and/or inactivation mechanisms.

On the other hand, experiments using animal lungs show a definite uptake of norepinephrine in the endothelial lining of the pulmonary blood vessels. This uptake can be as much as 40% during a single pulmonary circulation of blood containing norepinephrine (JUNOD, 1975a).

Compared to almost complete uptake of serotonin, or 5-hydroxytryptamine, JUNOD (1975b) concluded that the limited uptake of norepinephrine justifies some skepticism about the importance of this process. The above-mentioned study on man questions the importance of pulmonary endothelium as the primary storage site of norepinephrine extracted from blood. Uncertainty over the fate of norepinephrine in the lung, together with the fact that epinephrine is not significantly retained in the lung (VANE, 1969), strengthens the hypothesis that epinephrine is more likely than norepinephrine to be the pulmonary neurohumoral transmitter. If epinephrine were retained in the lung, there would be excessive accumulation from intra- and extrapulmonary sources. Thus, epinephrine would be disqualified as a transmitter released with each sympathetic nerve impulse because the amine would persist in the neuroeffector junction site. This event is unlikely to occur because epinephrine is not retained in the lung (JUNOD and ODY, 1977).

II. Dopamine

Dopamine is an endogenous catecholamine and is the immediate metabolic precursor of norepinephrine. As a vasopressor agent, dopamine has almost effectively replaced norepinephrine for the treatment of shock (p. 13). Unlike norepinephrine, dopamine increases cardiac output. Therefore, there is less likelihood of the development of pulmonary edema in treated patients in cardiogenic shock. Another important difference is the overall systemic vasoconstriction by norepinephrine whereas dopamine induces systemic vasodilation. One advantage of dopamine over norepinephrine in the treatment of shock is the preservation of renal blood flow.

The difference between dopamine and norepinephrine can be explained by activation of α-receptors by norepinephrine, versus dopaminergic receptors by dopamine, in the systemic circulation. The net result is an increase in pulmonary blood flow with dopamine but a decrease with norepinephrine, as a result of reflex bradycardia from vasoconstrictor-induced systemic hypertension (see SCHWARZ and AVIADO, 1976). Similarities between dopamine and norepinephrine include activation of α-receptors in the airways and in the pulmonary blood vessels. Dopamine constricts the airways of most animal species. Dopamine constricts pulmonary blood vessels, both with intact preparations and perfused lungs (KAUFMAN and OCHOA, 1971; MENTZER et al., 1976). The vasoconstriction can be prevented by prior injection of α-blockers. Although there are no clinical reports of pulmonary edema or pulmonary insufficiency as complications of the use of dopamine, additional clinical studies are needed with special reference to measurement of ventilation and perfusion relationships. It is possible, as with epinephrine, that there may be a reduction in the oxygen content of arterial blood due to disproportionate increases in pulmonary blood flow from β-activation accompanied by reductions in ventilation from α-activation, with administration of dopamine.

III. Phenylephrine

Phenylephrine is a potent activator of α-receptors in the systemic and pulmonary vasculature. The hemodynamic consequences of intravenous phenylephrine in patients with mitral stenosis or pulmonary hypertension were reported by BECK et al.

(1961). There was a biphasic response consisting of an initial sharp rise in pulmonary arterial pressure with a fall in pulmonary arterial wedge or venous pressure; and later a rise in both parameters with a reduction in pulmonary blood flow and increase in pulmonary vascular resistance. The initial effect was attributed to local constriction of the pulmonary arteries proximal to the point of wedging of the catheter; the latter effect is explained by systemic vasoconstriction with resulting aortic hypertension, reflex bradycardia, and reduction in pulmonary blood flow. The hemodynamic changes are brought about by activation of α-receptors in the pulmonary and systemic blood vessels. Therapeutic doses of phenylephrine do not activate cardiac β-receptors; however, toxic doses cause stimulation as manifested by the appearance of tachycardia and cardiac arrhythmias. As with norepinephrine, the use of phenylephrine has been reported to cause pulmonary edema resulting from elevated blood pressure load on the left ventricle (RENAIS et al., 1957).

Until recently, phenylephrine was contained in aerosol bronchodilator preparation together with a β-activator. This combination was presumably intended to elicit β-mediated bronchodilation and α-mediated vasoconstriction of mucosal blood vessels, which combination of effects can be obtained by the use of epinephrine alone. A review of the literature has failed to document any reduction in airway resistance in asthmatic patients following inhalation of phenylephrine alone (BÜRKMANN et al., 1976). Possibly, α-receptors in the bronchial smooth muscles would also be activated, producing an increase in airway resistance. CHAND (1979) has demonstrated the existence of α-receptors sensitive to phenylephrine in lung strips of the rat. However, the observed shortening of lung strips with administration of phenylephrine is not entirely due to constriction of the airways but also to a response of the blood vessels.

IV. Methoxamine

A discussion of another α-activator, such as methoxamine, may supply an answer to the question raised by the actions of phenylephrine: What is the overall effect on airway resistance following the inhalation of a drug that can potentially produce α-mediated bronchoconstriction and α-mediated contraction of vascular components of the bronchial mucosa? ANTHRACITE et al. (1971) observed that inhalation of a nebulized methoxamine solution caused an increase in resistance (decrease in conductance) in normal subjects. The observations support the existence of α-receptors in the bronchial airways. However, the primary bronchomotor effect seen with normal airways, may not be applicable to congested or asthmatic airways. Recent studies by SNASHALL et al. (1978) in asthmatic patients showed a definite increase in airway resistance following the administration of methoxamine. With an α-activator, bronchial mucosal vasoconstriction is therefore masked by bronchial muscle constriction.

As with norepinephrine and phenylephrine, the hemodynamic consequence of the systemic vasopressor effect of methoxamine is a reduction in pulmonary blood flow (STANFIELD and YU, 1960). Pulmonary blood vessels do not consistently constrict in response to methoxamine and may even dilate (AVIADO and SCHMIDT, 1957). Several derivatives of methoxamine have been tested and some show consistent dilation of pulmonary blood vessels but constriction of the systemic vasculature. These results suggest the existence of basic differences between the receptors in the two groups of blood vessels.

V. Nasal Decongestants

Those α-activators whose clinical usage has been limited to nasal decongestion include naphazoline, tetrahydrozoline, and oxymetazoline. Although there is some information on their systemic toxicity, the lungs are rarely affected in cases of abuse of nasal decongestants (see AVIADO, 1970). Most of these nasal decongestants are predominantly α-activators and do not manifest the after-congestion phenomenon seen with epinephrine (CARRILLO et al., 1969). The development of tolerance with repeated use of certain compounds has been reported. The use of an animal model to differentiate the sensitivity of nasal vessels relative to extranasal branches of the common carotid artery has revealed a preference for nasal vessels with some α-activators (AVIADO et al., 1959). Chronic abuse of epinephrine-containing formulations may result in permanent dilation of the mucosal vascular beds of the nose, due to selective β-activation, resulting in dependence.

D. Direct Activators of Beta-Receptors

So far in this chapter, adrenergic drugs that influence α-receptors have been discussed. Differences among α-activator drugs lie in varying degrees of stimulation of β-receptors as well. The α-activator drugs can be arranged in the following order of consistent

Table 2. Extent of activity of adrenergic activators[a]

	α-bronchoconstriction vasoconstriction	β-$_1$-cardiac stimulation	β_2-bronchodilation vasodilation
Direct activators of α- and β-receptor:			
Epinephrine	+	+	+
Norepinephrine	+	+	0
Dopamine	+	+	0
Phenylephrine	+	0	0
Methoxamine	+	0	0
Direct activators of β-receptors:			
Isoproterenol	0	+	+
Protokylol	0	+	+
Ethylnorepinephrine	0	+	+
Bronchoselective β_2-activators:			
Isoetharine	0	0+	+
Metaproterenol	0	0+	+
Terbutaline	0	0+	+
Salbutamol	0	0+	+
Carbuterol	0	0+	+
Pirbuterol	0	0+	+
Albuterol	0	0+	+
Hexaprenaline	0	0+	+
Ibuterol	0	0+	+
Rimiterol	0	0+	+
Zinterol	0	0+	+

[a] + present; 0 absent; 0+ dose-dependent, i.e. present in large doses

α-stimulation but with increasing involvement of β-receptors: (a) methoxamine: no β-activation; (b) phenylephrine: toxic doses activate cardiac (β_1)-receptors; (c) norepinephrine: therapeutic doses activate cardiac (β_1)-receptors; and (d) epinephrine: therapeutic doses activate both cardiac (β_1)- and bronchial (β_2)-receptors.

The group of drugs discussed in this section have no α-activity, and instead are stimulants of β-receptors, both cardiac (β_1) and bronchial (β_2). In other words, the pattern of activity of the group of β-activators is similar to epinephrine minus the α-component (Table 2).

I. Isoproterenol

Like epinephrine, isoproterenol is widely used in the treatment of acute asthmatic attack and is administered by subcutaneous injection or aerosol inhalation. There is sufficient documentation for the effectiveness of isoproterenol in relieving the symptoms of asthma, as well as improving functional tests of airway resistance. However, there has been no properly designed study comparing the efficacy, and incidence of adverse reactions, of epinephrine and isoproterenol. Thus, any relative advantage or disadvantage of the specific α-properties of epinephrine, as distinct from β-activation, had not been identified. For instance, occurrence of the locked-lung syndrome (p. 18) although documented for isoproterenol, has not been encountered with epinephrine. Specific α-activation by epinephrine may possibly prevent occurrence of the syndrome. The pulmonary vascular effects are diametrically opposite, i.e., vasoconstriction and vasodilation by epinephrine but vasodilation only by isoproterenol. In the treatment of pulmonary hypertension, only a pure β-activator such as isoproterenol is useful.

1. Antiasthmatic Use and Airway Resistance

There have been elaborate studies on lung function changes following the inhalation of isoproterenol aerosol in asthmatic patients (ENGEL et al., 1976; BENSON, 1978; SIEGLER et al., 1976). The most recent developments in measurement of regional ventilation and airway closure indicate a general improvement with isoproterenol administration. The essence of all of the observed effects is that isoproterenol significantly improves pulmonary function in patients and experimental animals (AVIADO et al., 1969).

Like epinephrine, isoproterenol elicits biochemical changes in the lung such as an increase in the rate of cAMP formation (TRINER et al., 1977), inhibition of the release of bronchospastic humoral agents (ORANGE and AUSTEN, 1971) and inhibition of granulocytic release of lysosomal enzymes (BUSSE, 1977). As with epinephrine, it is not possible to evaluate the relative merits of these biochemical changes and their potential bronchodilator effect in explaining the antiasthmatic use of isoproterenol.

Also like epinephrine, isoproterenol improves mucociliary transport in man (FOSTER et al., 1976). Experiments in rat reveal some potentially harmful effects of isoproterenol which have not been seen with epinephrine. BOLDUC and REID (1978) observed an increase in mitotic index and goblet cell number at most airway levels of the rat. BASKERVILLE (1976) detected bronchial gland hypertrophy and goblet-cell hyperplasia in pigs after repeated administration of isoproterenol for 6 consecutive days. There has been no reported comprehensive search for similar lesions of postmortem lungs of asthmatic patients treated with isoproterenol for extended period of time.

2. Paradoxical Bronchospasm

During the 1960s, there was a reported increase in mortality from bronchial asthma in Great Britain, Scandinavia, and Australia (see AVIADO, 1975). Circumstances surrounding some of the fatalities indicated excessive use and abuse of aerosol units containing isoproterenol. From the United States, VAN METRE (1968) reported 29 fatalities from asthma in patients who had been resistant to isoproterenol and had actually showed improvement when they stopped using the aerosol. Other clinicians reported the occurrence of paradoxical bronchospasm from isoproterenol, also referred to as the locked-lung syndrome or iatrogenic asthma (see AVIADO, 1975; TRAUTLEIN et al., 1976).

A review of the earlier literature on asthmatics who do not succumb to the disease, indicates that there have been reports of ineffectiveness of isoproterenol. KEIGHLEY (1966) reported three patients who developed protracted airway obstruction following repeated use of isoproterenol aerosol. He proposed two explanations for the paradoxical response, namely: (a) hyperactivity to aerosol particulates; and (b) altered response to isoproterenol, such as mucosal congestion. The former explanation was rendered less probable by the observations that aerosols containing aqueous propylene glycol did not provoke bronchospasm. Experiments in dogs showed that repeated inhalation of isoproterenol causes a paradoxical increase in airway resistance that can be reversed subsequently by inhalation of an α-vasoconstrictor agent (CHO et al., 1968). These observations strengthen the credibility of explanation (b), since isoproterenol causes congestion of bronchial mucosa by β-mediated vasodilation.

Subsequent publications reiterated the potential development of the locked-lung syndrome in patients using isoproterenol aerosol. CAPLIN and HAYNES (1969) reported three asthmatic patients who experienced relief after use of the aerosol was discontinued. VAN METRE (1969) and REISMAN (1970) contributed reports of additional cases of iatrogenic asthma from the use of isoproterenol aerosol.

Meanwhile, the number of explanations for the syndrome has been increasing beyond the two proposed (KEIGHLEY, 1966). CHAPMAN (1976) suggested (c) increased bronchial secretion, supported by animal experimentation. The late AREND BOUHUYS (1978) reviewed the pharmacologic basis for refractoriness to isoproterenol, and the following can be added to the list: (d) decrease in the number of specific binding sites in the cell membrane for isoproterenol leading to decreased formation of cAMP. However, BOUHUYS discussed experimental findings that are not consistent with explanation (d). The authors of this chapter favor explanation (b) relating to the vascular effects of isoproterenol, which is the subject of the next paragraph.

3. Pulmonary Vasodilation and Venous Admixture

The effects of isoproterenol on ventilation – perfusion relationships are similar to those of epinephrine (p. 7). There is a reduction in oxygen content of systemic arterial blood resulting from disproportionate increase in pulmonary perfusion relative to ventilation (TAI and READ, 1967a, b; STONE et al., 1970).

Catheterization studies in human subjects have consistently shown that isoproterenol dilates pulmonary blood vessels. The initial report of KAUFMAN et al. (1951)

dealt with normal subjects, showing an increase in pulmonary blood flow with no fall in pulmonary arterial blood pressure even though the vessels were dilated, following the injection of isoproterenol. However, in patients suffering from pulmonary hypertension, there was a definite reduction in pulmonary arterial pressure following isoproterenol inhalation (BUHR, 1953). In patients with pulmonary hypertension secondary to emphysema, there was a fall in pulmonary arterial pressure, increase in pulmonary blood flow, and reduction in pulmonary vascular resistance (WILLIAMS et al., 1963).

Lung perfusion experiments have uniformly demonstrated vasodilation of pulmonary and bronchial blood vessels (see AVIADO, 1965). Although vasodilation is a desired effect in the treatment of pulmonary hypertension, it is undesired in the treatment of acute pulmonary insufficiency. This belief is based on laboratory experiments showing that isoproterenol inhalation exaggerates the pulmonary edema induced in rats by phenylthiourea (COMBS and JONES, 1975). The intravenous infusion of isoproterenol in anesthetized dogs caused increased pulmonary shunting of blood and other signs of pulmonary insufficiency (BERK et al., 1976). These observations reflect a dual action of isoproterenol on the pulmonary circulation, viz, pulmonary vasodilation and increased pulmonary blood flow, both mediated by receptors in the pulmonary blood vessels and in the heart.

4. Toxicity of Aerosol Propellants

Although fatalities associated with the misuse and abuse of isoproterenol have been reported (p. 18), the initial reaction of drug manufacturers was to underemphasize the hazards of the propellants used. There were two reasons for this estimation: (a) the propellants were "known" to be inert and nontoxic; and (b) the amount of propellant contained in the inspired aerosol was small, and little was absorbed into the blood. PHILLIPS (1967) questioned the nontoxicity of the propellants, since the only available information was based upon topical skin testing of animals, without inhalation studies. The subsequent investigation of propellant inhalation in animals revealed that the most frequently used aerosol propellant (trichlorofluoromethane) is also the most toxic to the heart and lungs among commercially available fluorocarbons. Trichlorofluoromethane depresses the myocardium, sensitizes the heart to arrhythmic actions of epinephrine, causes bronchospasm, and is a respiratory irritant. The aerosol per se also stimulates vagal and sympathetic afferent receptors in the upper and lower respiratory tract with consequent increases in vagal influence on the heart. It was reasonable to hypothesize that the misuse or abuse of isoproterenol aerosols can be fatal because the propellant sensitizes the heart to actions of the administered isoproterenol as well as the vagal reflex induced by the respiratory irritant properties of the propellant (see AVIADO, 1975). Although some manufacturers continue to use this toxic fluorocarbon to propel isoproterenol aerosols, others are dispensing isoproterenol in mechanical units free of the propellant.

II. Protokylol

Protokylol was synthesized by BIEL et al. (1954) as an orally administered bronchodilator. The pharmacologic action of protokylol appears to be similar to that of isoproterenol. There is no determination of the relative potency of both drugs in man, since protokylol is administered orally, whereas isoproterenol is not. Both drugs are available for inhalation by nebulization, but there are no comparative reports. In order to obtain identical effects upon blood pressure in anesthetized dogs, it is necessary to administer 16 times as much protokylol as isoproterenol, and to increase the heart rate by an increment of over forty times as much. There are no corresponding observations on bronchodilator potency in animals (see MARION LABORATORIES, 1974).

III. Ethylnorepinephrine

The ethyl analog of norepinephrine was first synthesized by TAINTER (1933). As compared with epinephrine, ethylnorepinephrine is a more potent bronchodilator, and is devoid of the vasopressor effect of α-activation (SLY, 1969). Ethylnorepinephrine is weaker than isoproterenol in regard to its cardiovascular and bronchodilator effects; the subcutaneous therapeutic dose of ethylnorepinephrine is four times that of isoproterenol (CHRISTENSEN et al., 1958).

E. Bronchoselective Beta-Activators

The most frequent adverse reactions encountered in the clinical use of epinephrine and isoproterenol, as discussed in the preceding sections, are tachycardia and arrhythmias, which have proven fatal in some asthmatic patients with coronary heart disease. These drugs are administered by inhalation in aerosol form in order to reduce the occurrence of the undesired cardiac effects. Unfortunately, these cardiac reactions cannot be completely avoided because the sensitivities of the airways and of the heart are approximately the same.

The subclassification of β-receptors into two types, viz, β_1 and β_2, was suggested by LANDS et al. in 1967. This distinction was made on the basis of in vitro studies using catecholamines. With respect to isoproterenol, there exist two distinct orders of relative potency for pharmacologic responses, namely: β_1-mediated positive chronotropic and inotropic cardiac responses, relaxation of intestinal smooth muscle, and lipolysis; and β_2-receptor mediated relaxation of bronchial, uterine and vascular smooth muscle, glycogenolysis, glycolysis, skeletal muscle tremor, and lymphocytic changes in cAMP (CONOLLY and GREENACRE, 1977). The therapeutic consequence of Lands' hypothesis was the introduction of the first bronchoselective β-activator, isoetharine which is approximately ten times more active on bronchial smooth muscle than on heart muscle in the guinea pig. This selectivity for bronchial muscles is not absolute with respect to isoetharine since tachycardia was still encountered with therapeutic doses in man. At about the same time, the pharmacology of metaproterenol was being investigated in animals and asthmatic patients and it became apparent that isoetharine and metaproterenol were similar in the degree of bronchoselectivity as compared to isoproterenol.

At present there are available many bronchoselective β-activators, both commercially distributed and under clinical study. Most of them have a better index of bronchoselectivity than isoetharine and metaproterenol. However, it is not possible to formulate a definitive list of increasing order of selectivity because the studies have been performed on different species (guinea pig, rat, cat, and dog). Furthermore, human studies do not confirm the intensity of bronchoselectivity derived from animal experiments (HARMS, 1976; BURNS and DOE, 1978; HARMS and SPOELSTRA, 1978). In their assessment of animal models, BOWMAN and RAPER (1976) concluded that the sensitivities of bronchial and vascular smooth muscle and slow-contracting skeletal muscles (β_2-receptors) to a given bronchodilator drug seem to be about the same in different species. However, the sensitivity of the heart (β_1-receptors) differs widely according to species. Results from human studies indicate that the cat most closely resembles man in the degree of bronchoselectivity of adrenergic β-activators.

The differences in sensitivity of bronchial smooth muscles and systemic blood vessels are currently under investigation. Most comparisons consist of in vitro or in vivo studies of the airways and the systemic blood vessels showing no differences in sensitivity (O'DONNELL and WANSTALL, 1976; HOOKER et al., 1977; WEISSBERG et al., 1977). Studies relating to binding sites for tritium labeled [^{3}H]dihydroalprenolol (a specific β-adrenoceptor ligand) indicate the presence of β_1- and β_2-adrenoceptors on the cell membranes of the rat lung, without differentiation between bronchi and blood vessels (BARNETT et al., 1978). The distribution of the two groups of β-receptors is not absolute and there is a certain degree of cross distribution between the cardiac and bronchial receptors, i.e., β_1 also appearing in the airways.

The bronchoselective β-activators are presented in a manner which differentiates those that are available commercially from those that are still under clinical investigation. The discussion of the former group is preceded by a table of bronchoselectivity index based on a value of 1 for isoproterenol. The index is derived from the effective concentration of the drug that causes significant cardiac acceleration, divided by the effective concentration that causes bronchodilation. The highest calculated index of bronchoselectivity is 1755 for pirbuterol (p. 25).

I. Isoetharine

Effective concentrations referred to isoproterenol (1)

	Broncho-dilation	Cardiac acceleration	Selectivity index	
Guinea pigs	7.2	570	79	(MARDEL et al., 1974)
Cats	10.0	24.3	2.14	(RODGER, 1973)

Isoetharine was initially reported by LANDS et al. (1967) to have a bronchoselective index of approximately 10, but subsequent studies show diametrically opposite magnitude of indices; i.e., 2.14 and 79 respectively in cats and guinea pigs. When isoetharine was introduced as an aerosol inhalant, phenylephrine was added to the preparation for its topical or mucosal decongestive action, and also for prolongation of bronchodilation. However, SPECTOR et al. (1977) could not detect any differential effect on airway responses, or on oxygen saturation of the peripheral blood, following the addition of phenylephrine to isoetharine. Subsequently, the α-activator was omitted and isoetharine alone is dispensed as an aerosol inhalant.

II. Metaproterenol

Effective concentrations referred to isoproterenol (1)

	Broncho-dilation	Cardiac acceleration	Selectivity index	
Guinea pigs	4.0	4.0	10	(BOEHRINGER INGELHEIM, 1975)
Cats	5.0	6.3	12.6	(BOEHRINGER INGELHEIM, 1975)

Metaproterenol was first synthesized by ENGELHARDT et al. (1961) with bronchodilator activity approximately four to five times less than that of isoproterenol but longer in duration. The antiasthmatic action can be elicited by oral administration and inhalation. SCHWITTER et al. (1975) reported the superiority of aerosol inhalation of metaproterenol as compared to the oral route. Vasodilation of the pulmonary blood vessels in man has been demonstrated by catheterization studies.

III. Terbutaline

Effective concentrations referred to isoproterenol (1)

	Broncho-dilation	Cardiac acceleration	Selectivity index	
Guinea pigs	17.0	126.0	7.4	(PERSSON and OLSSON, 1970)
Cats	16.8	38.2	2.4	(BRITTAIN and JACK, 1976)

Development of terbutaline as a bronchoselective β-receptor activator started with in vitro testing of guinea pig trachea and isolated guinea pig heart (PERSSON and OLSSON, 1970). Although the effects were qualitatively similar to those of isoproterenol, there was a significant difference in the relative potency, viz, isoproterenol was 17 times more effective than terbutaline in relaxing the spirally cut trachea, 126 times in exerting inotropism, and 165 times in exerting chronotropism, in the isolated heart. It is the difference in potency ratio that forms the basis for concluding that terbutaline is a bronchoselective β-receptor activator, relative to isoproterenol. Other in vitro and in vivo tests performed in experimental animals have confirmed the differences in sensitivity between bronchial and cardiac adrenergic receptors, and the participation of β-receptors was suggested by blockade of responses with propranolol.

1. Bronchomotor System

The efficacy of terbutaline in treatment of asthmatic patients was initially reported by ARNER et al. (1970). A subcutaneous injection of 0.25 mg terbutaline caused an increase in peak expiratory flow rate, accompanied by tachycardia. Subjective improvement in dyspnea was accompanied by palpitation and slight trembling in 7 out of 72 experimental injections of terbutaline ranging from 0.125 to 0.50 mg.

During the past decade, there has been a growing literature on the clinical use of terbutaline administered subcutaneously at the usual dose of 0.25 mg; orally at a dose of 5 mg three times daily; and by inhalation at a dose of 0.5 mg. It can be noted immediately that the potency ratio for terbutaline and isoproterenol, as based upon the recommended antiasthmatic dose, is as follows: inhalation of 0.75–0.150 mg for isoproterenol, which suggests 3.3–6.7 times higher potency relative to terbutaline. The comparison reflects not only the results of in vitro experiments as above, but also the susceptibility of isoproterenol (a catecholamine) to enzymatic breakdown in contrast to terbutaline (not a catecholamine). The extensive clinical studies on terbutaline include double-blind comparisons with a placebo, and detailed studies of large and small airway resistance (see LARSSON, 1977).

Tremor of the extremities and palpitation continue to be encountered as side effects to the clinical use of terbutaline. The incidence of tremor is unrelated to the route of administration, but tachycardia occurs progressively with increasing incidence by the inhalation route, by oral administration, and by subcutaneous injection. It has been suggested that the adrenergic receptors in the skeletal muscle are pharmacologically similar to the bronchomotor receptors. If terbutaline is accepted as a tool for mapping β-receptors associated with bronchodilation, it is pertinent to recall the observations of MOSSBERG et al. (1976). They observed that subcutaneous injection of terbutaline improved tracheobronchial clearance in patients with bronchial asthma. This effect, although therapeutically desirable, has not been found to occur in the course of oral or inhalational administration of terbutaline. The enhancement of mucociliary clearance is not unique for terbutaline, but is also seen with most other adrenergic drugs (p. 6).

2. Pulmonary Circulation

The coincidental changes in the pulmonary circulation which occur in the course of treatment of the bronchial asthmatic patient remain unknown. However, STOCKLEY et al. (1977) examined patients with chronic bronchitis and cor pulmonale following intravenous injection of 0.25 mg terbutaline. Although mean pulmonary arterial pressure remained unaltered, there was a rise in cardiac index associated with a fall in calculated pulmonary vascular resistance. Coincidentally, there was a significant increase in venous admixture. Despite this increase, there was no alteration in arterial oxygen tension, which was explained by the investigators as a reflection of increased mixed venous oxygen saturation. The influence of terbutaline on the bronchopulmonary anastomoses has not been considered in suppression of an anticipated reduction in arterial oxygen tension. Animal experiments, similar to those described for epinephrine, are required in order to determine the possible vasodilator action of terbutaline on pulmonary and bronchial blood vessels.

IV. Salbutamol

Salbutamol was synthesized by HARTLEY et al. (1968) with a bronchoselectivity index of 2.7–55. The drug has been shown to be an effective bronchodilator when administered by inhalation in bronchial asthma (PALMER and DIEMANT, 1969), chronic bronchitis (MINETTE et al., 1976), and left ventricular disease (COLLINS et al., 1975). Tachycardia is a frequent reaction seen with salbutamol aerosol use.

Effective concentrations referred to isoproterenol (1)

	Broncho-dilation	Cardiac acceleration	Selectivity index	
Guinea pig	10	200	20.0	(HARTLEY et al., 1968)
Guinea pig	1.8	101	55.0	(WARDELL et al., 1974)
Dog	24.9	224	9.0	(BRITTAIN and JACK, 1976)
Cat	8.6	28.6	3.4	(BRITTAIN and JACK, 1976)
Cat	6.8	20.0	3.0	(RODGER, 1973)
Dog	3.9	10.4	2.7	(WARDELL et al., 1974)

V. Carbuterol

Effective concentrations referred to isoproterenol (1)

	Broncho-dilation	Cardiac acceleration	Selectivity index	
Guinea pig	3.6	230	74	(WARDELL et al., 1974)
Dog	6.2	30.8	5.0	(WARDELL et al., 1974)

WARDELL and his collaborators (1974) evaluated the bronchodilator and cardiovascular actions of carbuterol in several animal species. In guinea pig trachea, the effective concentration for relaxation by carbuterol was 3.6 times that of isoproterenol, with no significant difference in potency between carbuterol and salbutamol. Pretreatment with reserpine in the same preparation did not offset the tracheal relaxant activity, whereas propranolol blocked the activity, thus establishing direct activation of β-receptors. The corresponding potency ratios in the isolated guinea pig heart were as follows: isoproterenol was 230 times more potent than carbuterol in increasing atrial rate and 400 times in increasing left atrial contractile force. Additional experiments in anesthetized cats and dogs, and conscious dogs, indicate bronchoselectivity of carbuterol as compared to isoproterenol. Although carbuterol was similar in bronchodilator potency to isoproterenol in the anesthetized dog, its relative vasodepressor potency was much lower, thereby demonstrating selectivity of action between bronchial and vascular smooth muscles.

Oral administration of carbuterol causes a reduction in airway resistance in human subjects. An oral dose of 4 mg caused a more significant increase in forced expiratory volume than did an equivalent dose of salbutamol (CHAPMAN, 1970). However, like other bronchoselective β-stimulants, carbuterol caused palpitation and tremors in some subjects. In a double-blind study of adult and childhood asthmatics, the inhalation of 0.200 mg carbuterol produced equivalent or slightly more significant bronchodilator action than 0.150 mg isoproterenol (RHOADES et al., 1976). There are no reported studies on the effects of injections of carbuterol on the airways or on the pulmonary circulation.

VI. Pirbuterol

Effective concentrations referred to isoproterenol (1)

	Broncho-dilation	Cardiac acceleration	Selectivity index	
Guinea pig	2.98	4 519	1 755	(MOORE et al., 1978)

MOORE et al. (1978) have recently reported initial animal studies on pirbuterol. The bronchoselectivity for β-receptors is based on the observation that isoproterenol is 2.98 times the potency of pirbuterol in relaxing isolated guinea pig trachea, and 4,519 times in stimulating the rate of isolated guinea pig atria. In the same group of experiments, salbutamol was more potent than pirbuterol in relaxing the tracheal muscle (2.98 times) and in accelerating the heart rate (11.7 times). The difference in bronchodilating potency in the in vitro test is reflected by the difference in oral doses needed to produce bronchodilation. In a double-blind trial in asthmatics, WILLEY et al. (1976) observed that 15 mg oral pirbuterol and 4 mg oral salbutamol produced equal peak increases of forced expiratory volume, with similar intensity of tachycardia and incidence of tremors. Pirbuterol inhaled in doses of 0.1–0.4 mg caused a reduction in airway resistance, but there are no comparative measurement with other drugs in the same group of patients (STEEN et al., 1974).

VII. Bronchoselective Drugs Under Clinical Investigation

APPERLEY et al. (1976) have completed a comprehensive comparison of 15 β-activators, including the 5 listed below. Their report can also be used to identify additional references relating to animal experimentation. Only clinical studies are discussed below. The bronchoselective drugs, bitolterol and clenbuterol, have no published results on clinical studies and are omitted from the following discussion.

1. Albuterol

SPECTOR and GARZA (1977) observed a dose-related improvement in pulmonary function in asthmatic patients treated with albuterol aerosol. Compared with isoproterenol, there were minimal side effects on the heart, and the bronchodilation persisted for a longer time. Other studies showed reduced response or subsensitivity to the bronchodilator action after 2 weeks of oral use of albuterol (NELSON et al., 1977). Maximal decrease in response occurred after 2 weeks of treatment, and no further reduction occurred after prolonged treatment with the same dose for periods as long as 1 year. It should be noted that the subsensitivity to albuterol is similar to that seen with ephedrine (p. 27). Therefore, the possibility that albuterol is also an adrenergic transmitter releasing agent should be examined.

2. Hexoprenaline

The bronchodilator effects of hexoprenaline aerosol were compared with those of isoproterenol in patients with bronchial asthma or chronic bronchitis. Increased forced expiratory volume elicited by both drugs were similar. The doses used did not elicit tachycardia or cardiac arrhythmia (SCHONELL et al., 1977).

3. Ibuterol

Oral administration of ibuterol (2 mg) produced a bronchodilator effect equivalent to that of terbutaline (4 mg) in asthmatic patients (ARNER and MAGNUSSON, 1976). There were no significant changes in heart rate or pulse amplitude.

4. Rimiterol

Rimiterol aerosol has been compared with metered doses of salbutamol and isoproterenol (BIANCO et al., 1975; ERIKSSON and LINDGREN, 1978). Although there was a reduction in airway resistance brought about by all three aerosols, the incidence of tachycardia was less for rimiterol and salbutamol than for isoproterenol. Intravenous injections of isoproterenol, rimiterol, and salbutamol elicited tachycardia, with similar increases in pulse pressure and skeletal muscle tremor. Isoproterenol was approximately 8 and 5 times as potent in bronchodilator action as rimiterol and salbutamol respectively, and isoproterenol 16 and 12 times as potent in eliciting tachycardia. In other words, for an equal bronchodilator action, isoproterenol increased the heart rate 2 and 2.5 times more than rimiterol and salbutamol. These indices of selectivity are approximately similar to those reported for the cat and lower than those for guinea pigs, again supporting the greater applicability of the cat model to the human heart and airways (MARLIN and TURNER, 1975).

5. Zimterol

In a double-blind crossover study including placebo, VAN DER STRAETON et al. (1978) observed bronchodilation following the oral intake of zimterol. Tachycardia was seen in some patients with chronic obstructive pulmonary disease.

F. Adrenergic Transmitter Releasing Agents

The presentation of this section is difficult because the concept of adrenergic transmitter release by drugs has not been proved to be applicable to the respiratory system. This concept that some drugs do not directly activate the adrenergic receptors, but instead cause their actions indirectly by releasing adrenergic transmitters, is based upon experimental observations on the heart and systemic vasculature. Briefly, pretreatment with transmitter depleting agents (such as reserpine or guanethidine) reduced or completely prevented the cardiac stimulatory and vasopressor effects of the releasing agent. The first example of a so-called adrenergic transmitter releasing agent was ephedrine, and although it continues to be popular in the treatment of bronchial asthma, there is no proof that pretreatment with a depleting agent interferes with the bronchodilating action.

The deficiency in basic information relating to the bronchodilator activity of ephedrine also applies to other releasing drugs used as nasal decongestants (pseudoephedrine and phenylpropanolamine), systemic vasopressors (mephentermine and metaraminol), and anorexigenics (aminorex and chlorphentermine). With the exception of other bronchodilators and nasal decongestants used for the treatment of respiratory tract diseases, the systemic vasopressors and anorexigenics have their desired therapeutic effect on the systemic circulation and the central nervous system. However, the pulmonary circulation suffers adversely from the clinical use of these drugs, with the appearance of pulmonary edema from the use of vasopressors and pulmonary hypertension from anorexigenics.

I. Ephedrine as an Antiasthmatic Drug

If the current concept of adrenergic releasing agents is correct, then the bronchodilator effect of ephedrine should be simulated by norepinephrine. Since norepinephrine is not a bronchodilator but is even a bronchoconstrictor (p. 12), another transmitter must be considered. Epinephrine is more acceptable because it is a bronchodilator. The similarities between ephedrine and epinephrine can be added to the list of reasons supporting the role of epinephrine as a neurotransmitter for the airways (p. 11).

There is a considerable amount of literature supporting the bronchodilator effect of ephedrine as used in the treatment of bronchial asthma. The pattern of effect in the pulmonary circulation consists of an increase in pulmonary blood flow, rise in pulmonary arterial blood pressure, and elevation in pulmonary vascular resistance (see AVIADO, 1965). Thus, the similarities between ephedrine and epinephrine extend to the pulmonary circulation.

NELSON et al. (1975) have observed a reduction in sensitivity to epinephrine in normal subjects, after a 1-week administration of ephedrine. The phenomenon was interpreted by the investigators as an adaptive response to prolonged excessive stimulation by ephedrine. If this interpretation is correct, the adaptation to ephedrine raises the question of possible adaptation to norepinephrine. It is conceivable that if the study were extended to compare both epinephrine and norepinephrine, and include measurements of airway resistance before and after ephedrine, the results would help show that epinephrine, instead of norepinephrine, is indeed being constantly released by ephedrine in the airways, thus explaining the reduction in sensitivity.

The clinical observations of TASHKIN et al. (1975) on oral use of ephedrine in asthmatics are as follows: with reduction in airway resistance, there was an increase in arterial blood oxygen tension, indicating an improvement in ventilation – perfusion ratios. Since epinephrine causes a decrease in arterial oxygenation by changes in ventilation – perfusion relationships, epinephrine may be disqualified as the adrenergic transmitter agent. However, the effects of epinephrine were noted when the drug was injected and caused a significant increase in pulmonary blood flow. In the study of TASHKIN et al. (1975), ephedrine was administered orally causing minimal tachycardia. The route of administration should be the same, i.e., subcutaneous or intravenous infusion, in order to make a meaningful comparison of the two drugs.

II. Pseudephedrine and Phenylpropanolamine as Oral-Nasal Decongestants

The two drugs, pseudephedrine and phenylpropanolamine are classified as adrenergic transmitter releasing agents on the basis of the experiments of BURN and RAND (1958) showing that pretreatment with a depleting agent (reserpine) reduced their effect. As for ephedrine, there are no supportive studies that show that pseudephedrine and phenylpropanolamine release norepinephrine, or that epinephrine may be the adrenergic transmitting agent responsible for this relatively weak bronchodilator effect seen in animal experiments (AVIADO et al., 1958). The clinical use of pseudephedrine and phenylpropanolamine is limited to nasal decongestion by oral administration.

III. Mephentermine and Metaraminol as Vasopressor Agents

The vasopressor effect of mephentermine is believed to be mediated entirely by the release of norepinephrine, because pretreatment with reserpine inhibits the vasoconstrictor component of the observed rise in systemic blood pressure. However, the bronchodilator effect seen in human subjects and experimental animals cannot be simulated by norepinephrine release, so that the role of epinephrine as a transmitter can be explored by future research. The overall effect of mephentermine on the pulmonary circulation is a reduction in pulmonary vascular resistance, but the influence of reserpine has not been studied (see AVIADO 1965, 1970).

Another systemic vasopressor agent, metaraminol, belongs to a special category that is partly direct activator, partly releaser of adrenergic transmitter, and also replaces norepinephrine as a false transmitter. Metaraminol, initially a vasopressor, becomes a vasodepressor agent after continuous administration because it replaces norepinephrine in the adrenergic nerve ending. These events have been considered only for the systemic circulation and have not been examined in the airways and pulmonary blood vessels. The bronchomotor effects are unknown for man and pulmonary vasoconstriction has been reported only in the anesthetized dog (see AVIADO, 1965, 1970). Recent studies on the rat lung have been directed to the measurement of uptake of metaraminol (DAVILA and DAVILA, 1975).

IV. Aminorex and Chlorphentermine as Anorexigenics

Prior to the recent trend in discouraging prolonged use of anorexigenics, they were known to cause transient pulmonary hypertension when injected intravenously into experimental animals (AVIADO and SCHMIDT, 1957). In 1968, pulmonary hypertension was detected in a group of patients receiving aminorex. The hypertension was reversed by termination of the drug treatment. Since animal experimentation could not reproduce pulmonary hypertension induced by aminorex, and since its commercial distribution has been suspended, a causal relationship in unlikely to be examined by additional experimentation.

Chlorphentermine, another appetite suppressant, causes lipidosis in the lung, liver, and adrenal glands of rats (KARABELNIK and ZBINDEN, 1975; GLOSTER et al., 1976). The mechanism involved in the accumulation of phospholipid is not known, and is unlikely to be of increasing interest since the disease has not been reported to occur in patients undergoing therapy with anorexigenics.

G. Adrenergic Alpha-Receptor Blocking Agents

Agents that block adrenergic α-receptors have several pharmacologic actions. They (a) inhibit the respiratory tract effect of stimulation of sympathetic nerves mediated through α-receptors, viz, nasal vasoconstriction, bronchial mucosal vasoconstriction, bronchoconstriction, and pulmonary vasoconstriction; (b) prevent similar responses to α-receptor stimulation by direct activators (such as epinephrine, norepinephrine, and methoxamine) and to adrenergic transmitter releasing agents (such as ephedrine); (c) permit continued β-mediated responses to sympathetic nerve stimulation and to administration of direct β-activators (such as epinephrine, isoproterenol) and bronchoselective β-activators (such as terbutaline); (d) stimulate β-receptors throughout the body, manifested in the respiratory tract as bronchodilation, pulmonary vasodilation, and increased pulmonary blood flow. It should be noted from the list that pulmonary vasodilation and bronchodilation are the combined effect of (a) blockade of α-receptors and (d) stimulation of β-receptors. As a group, the α-blocking agents exert an opposite effect on β-receptors that is complimentary to their primary action on α-receptors. In the discussion that follows, each α-blocking agent is paired to a pulmonary disease, namely, phenoxybenzamine for acute pulmonary insufficiency, tolazoline for pulmonary hypertension, phentolamine for acute left ventricular failure, and thymoxamine for intractable bronchial asthma. The pairing is based on the available clinical studies and it is probable that all four drugs can be used interchangeably.

I. Phenoxybenzamine and Acute Pulmonary Insufficiency

Acute pulmonary insufficiency is a syndrome characterized by capillary bleeding, edema, and failure of gas exchange in the lung. It appears terminally in patients suffering from traumatic shock, hemorrhagic shock, thoracic injury, or poisoning from toxic inhalants . The pathogenesis of the syndrome is complex and is still undergoing clinical investigation. However, two pathogenic processes have been identified which can be corrected by α-blocking agents such as phenoxybenzamine (see AVIADO, 1965).

1. Correction of Pulmonary Vascular Consequences of Hypoxemia

Hypoxemia appears either as a contributory cause or as a consequence of acute pulmonary insufficiency. With a reduction in oxygen content in blood, there is significant vasoconstriction of the pulmonary blood vessels mediated by the pulmonary sympathetic nerves. Vasoconstriction is prevented either by surgical sympathectomy or by administration of phenoxybenzamine or related blocking agents (AVIADO et al., 1957). The blockade by phenoxybenzamine of pulmonary vasoconstriction induced by hypoxemia in experimental animals has recently been confirmed by PORCELLI et al. (1977a, 1977b). MALIK (1977) has also demonstrated that phenoxybenzamine blocks pulmonary vasoconstriction following elevation of intracranial pressure in dogs. Although there are documented cases of the therapeutic effectiveness of phenoxybenzamine in patients in shock (NICKERSON and GOURZIS, 1962), it is not certain whether the desired action is based upon blockade of neurogenic vasoconstriction from hypoxemia, or upon inhibition of catecholamine-induced vasoconstriction discussed in the next paragraph.

2. Blockade of Pulmonary Vasoconstriction Induced by Catecholamines

Elevation of blood levels of circulating catecholamines has been demonstrated in patients suffering from acute pulmonary insufficiency. Experimental induction of the syndrome in animals has also caused elevation in blood levels, and the syndrome was reversed by administration of phenoxybenzamine (GOURZIS et al., 1963). The pulmonary lesions can be duplicated by intravenous infusion of epinephrine, and prevented by prior injection of phenoxybenzamine (BERK et al., 1977). However, there are experimental studies showing (a) therapeutic failure of phenoxybenzamine alone and

(b) the effectiveness of combined α-blockade and β-blockade, which can be logically explained by dual action of epinephrine on both receptors. It is the opinion of the authors that the beneficial action of phenoxybenzamine can be explained by blockade of humoral vasoconstriction as well as of that of neurogenic origin.

II. Tolazoline and Chronic Pulmonary Hypertension

DRESDALE and his collaborators (1954) were the first group of cardiologists to demonstrate the effectiveness of tolazoline in reducing the level of pulmonary arterial pressure in patients with pulmonary arterial hypertension. The desired reduction has been demonstrated, by several groups of investigators in patients suffering from pulmonary hypertension caused by mitral stenosis, congenital heart anomalies, pulmonary emphysema, or primary hypertensive disease of the pulmonary blood vessels (see AVIADO, 1965). The hemodynamic measurements show an increase in pulmonary blood flow as well as a reduction in pulmonary vascular resistance, attributable to α-blockade and β-activation, the characteristic pharmacologic actions of tolazoline (see ROCH-BESSER, 1950).

Relief of pulmonary hypertension by tolazoline is temporary and incomplete. The drug does not prevent or reverse the pathologic lesions responsible for the elevated arterial pressure, e.g., medial hypertrophy and endothelial proliferation. However, the neurogenic component of the hypertension is reversed by the administration of tolazoline or related drugs (see AVIADO, 1965).

III. Phentolamine and Acute Ventricular Failure

TADEI et al. (1975) have reported the efficacy of intravenous injections of phentolamine in relieving cardiac asthma arising from acute failure of the left ventricle. The observed reduction in pulmonary arterial pressure can be explained by known actions of phentolamine: (a) systemic vasodilation from blockade of α-receptors and consequent reduction of the load on the left ventricle; (b) cardiac stimulation from activation of β-receptors and the further improvement of left ventricular performance; (c) pulmonary vasodilation from activation of β-receptors, as well as blockade of α-receptors; and (d) bronchodilation from both groups of adrenergic receptors thus facilitating cessation of asthmatic attack. Each of the changes in hemodynamic parameters (a, b, c) has been demonstrated to occur in patients not suffering from acute left ventricular failure, but from other cardiopulmonary diseases such as aortic vascular disease, cor pulmonale, mitral stenosis, ventricular septal defect, or acute pulmonary edema (see AVIADO, 1965). The occurrence of bronchodilation has not been seen in man but is inferred from observations of the bronchodilator property of another α-receptor blocking agent, described in the next paragraph.

IV. Thymoxamine and Acute Bronchial Asthma

Some asthmatic patients who are nonresponsive to epinephrine or isoproterenol have been successfully treated with thymoxamine for relief of asthmatic attack (see PATEL, 1975). Thymoxamine has a dual action, α-blockade and β-activation, which serve to relax the bronchial smooth muscles. NOUSIAINEN et al. (1977) have supplied experimental support for this explanation by observing potentiation of the relaxing action of β-activators and α-blockers in the isolated human bronchus preparation. Their observations strengthen the concept of the existence of α-receptors in human bronchial muscle (p. 6, 12).

H. Adrenergic Beta-Receptor Blocking Agents

Although the adrenergic α-blocking agents are useful in the treatment of certain diseases of the respiratory system (p. 29) there is no corresponding therapeutic application for the adrenergic β-blocking agents. The respiratory effects of β-blocking agents have been entirely adverse in nature and have indirectly guided the search for an ideal drug to be primarily used in the treatment of cardiac arrhythmias and essential hypertension (see Sec. III, Chaps. 1, Sec. II, Chap. 4). Specifically, the use of nonselective β-blockers (β_1 and β_2) such as propranolol, is contraindicated in about 5% of patients suffering from disease of the heart and systemic circulation because the drug provokes an asthmatic attack. The development of β-blockers with cardioselective action (β_1 only) without broncho-blocking action (β_2) has been an important consideration in the improvement of nonselective β-blockers. There are several drugs, such as practolol, that are being considered for the treatment of cardiac disease and essential hypertension because they do not adversely block the β-receptors in the lungs, i.e., they do not induce bronchoconstriction.

This section covers the practical considerations in the use of nonselective and cardioselective β-blockers for the treatment of diseases external to the respiratory system, as well as a theoretical discussion of the importance of adrenergic β-receptors in the regulation of pulmonary circulation. Blockade of β-receptors is expected to influence the pulmonary circulation by opposite hemodynamic actions: pulmonary vasoconstriction by inhibition of β_2-receptors in the blood vessels and decrease in pulmonary blood flow or cardiac output via β_1-receptors in the heart. The analysis would have been a simple one except for the fact that the effects of some of the available β-blockers are not limited to their primary action, but also initially stimulate the cardiac β_1-receptors and even depress the myocardium (a quinidinelike or procainelike depression of the heart). Any reduction in pulmonary blood flow or cardiac output resulting from the administration of a β-blocker is the result of a combination of its primary action on β-receptors as well as secondary influence on the myocardium, unrelated to the adrenergic receptor inhibitory activity (see AVIADO, 1969, 1979). The occurrence of bronchospasm which appears with the use of β-blockers, such as propranolol, for the treatment of cardiovascular diseases, can be explained by the predominance of α-mediated bronchoconstriction as well as parasympathetic or vagal induced influences on the airways. Ibidomide, a unique blocker of α- and β-receptors, has been used to identify the causation of bronchospasm by propranolol as an unbalanced exaggeration of α-receptors in the airways in the absence of β-activity. SKINNER et al. (1975) compared the intravenous effects of propranolol and ibidomide and concluded that both drugs block β_1- and β_2-receptors. Only ibidomide did not provoke bronchospasm due to its α-inhibitory effect, absent from propranolol. The use of ibidomide has been examined in patients with essential hypertension, showing a definite reduction in pulmonary blood flow and pulmonary vascular resistance (KOCH, 1977). When both groups of adrenergic receptors are blocked, the predominant manifestation on the heart is an inhibition of β-receptors, on the pulmonary blood vessels an inhibition of α-receptors, and on the bronchial smooth muscles a depression of both.

The adrenergic β-blockers discussed below are summarized in Table 3. The examples given comprise half of the available drugs, commercially sold or undergoing clinical study. Such commercially available drugs as alprenolol, pondolol, and oxprenolol (DRIMAL and AVIADO, 1971) have been omitted from the table because there is no available information on their respiratory effects. However, it is reasonable to assume that all have effects on the airways similar to those of the drugs listed in Table 3 (see AVIADO, 1979). It is important to note that for nonselective and cardioselective β-blockers, there are representative examples of combined or unilateral manifestation of initial cardiac β_1-stimulation and/or quinidine or procainelike depression.

Table 3. Extent of activity of adrenergic β-blockers

	β_1 blockade	β_2 blockade	Cardiac stimulation	Cardiac depression
Nonselective adrenergic β-receptor blocking agents:				
Propranolol	+	+	−	+
Sotalol	+	+	−	−
Pindolol	+	+	+	+
Dichlorisoproterenol	+	+	+	−
Cardioselective β_1-receptor blocking agents:				
Practalol	+	−	+	−
Acebutol	+	−	+	+
Atenolol	+	−	−	−
Bunitrolol	+	−	−	+

I. Nonselective Adrenergic Beta-Receptor Blocking Agents

There are fundamental pharmacologic actions common to the five nonselective, adrenergic β-blockers listed in Table 3. They are: (a) bronchospasm by blockade of β-receptors and predominance of α-receptors (p. 5); and (b) pulmonary vasoconstriction, which may be masked by potential concurrent changes in pulmonary blood flow. Although a reduction in pulmonary blood flow is the usual accompaniment of pure β-blockade of cardiac receptors (as with sotalol), some blocking drugs also initially stimulate β-receptors and increase pulmonary blood flow (such as pindolol and dichloroisoproterenol). Still other blockers consistently reduce pulmonary blood flow by a quinidinelike or procainelike depression of myocardial contractility (e.g., propranolol). The hemodynamic consequences of administration of any one of the five nonselective β-blockers are unpredictable and are determined by the integrated effect of changes in pulmonary blood flow and pulmonary vascular resistance.

1. Propranolol

There is a considerable literature documenting the appearance of bronchospasm in patients suffering from cardiac arrhythmia or essential hypertension (see AVIADO, 1969, 1979). The clinical study of GAYRARD et al. (1975b) is noteworthy because it documents an increase in airway resistance following a single injection of propranolol, which was stronger in asthmatic patients than nonasthmatic subjects, although the intensity of cardioacceleration was similar in both groups. The results indicate that normal subjects have a weak bronchodilator adrenergic β-activity. In contrast, asthmatic patients have exaggerated β-activity, which does not support the view that airways of asthmatic patients suffer from a deficiency in β-receptors, as suggested by studies in lymphocytes (p. 9). The bronchoconstriction provoked by deep inspiration in asthmatics is exaggerated by the administration of propranolol (GAYARD et al., 1975a). Propranolol exaggerates the bronchoconstriction induced by injection of methacholine (TOWNLEY et al., 1976) as well as that of histamine (PLOY-SONG-SAND et al., 1978). In the latter situation there is a specific blockade of released catecholamines by the injection of histamine. Thus, there is an exaggeration of histamine-induced bronchospasm. In the former situation, the exaggeration of methacholine by propranolol is simply a shift in the balance from β-receptor control to exaggerated cholinergic bronchoconstriction.

Early cross-perfusion experiments by NIDEN and AVIADO (1956) of the canine lung showed pulmonary vasoconstriction of a nonembolized lobe as a result of embolization of another lobe. Recent perfusion experiments by KEALEY and BRODY (1977) indicate that reflex vasodilation occurs instead, which is blocked by propranolol. The differences in perfusion techniques suggest that the most recent group of experiments may have sacrificed some pulmonary nerves essential for vasoconstriction. The phenomenon of pulmonary embolization requires further investigation since the available results are conflicting and confusing. The necessity for treatment with α-blockers, or contraindication of β-blockers such as propranolol, would be suggested from a therapeutic standpoint.

2. Sotalol

The net effect of sotalol is variable or unchanged pulmonary arterial blood pressure in human subjects and experimental animals (FOLLE and AVIADO, 1965; AVIADO et al., 1967). There is coincident reduction in pulmonary blood flow from a pure blockade of cardiac β-receptors free of quinidinelike action, and a constriction of pulmonary blood vessels from blockade of vascular β-receptors. As for propranolol, there is documentation of bronchospasm occurring in the course of clinical use of sotalol for the treatment of cardiovascular diseases (ARESKOG et al., 1975; VANCROMBREUCQ et al., 1974).

3. Pindolol

Unlike propranolol and sotalol, pindolol exerts weak activation of cardiac β-receptors in addition to its persistent blocking action. There are other differences such as higher potency and prolonged duration of action of pindolol compared to propranolol. AEL-

LIG (1977), in a clinical study of normal volunteers, observed a less intense bronchodilation by pindolol than by propranolol using equivalent antihypertensive doses. He explained the difference by recalling the activating and blocking actions of pindolol as opposed to the exclusive blocking action of propranolol.

4. Dichloroisoproterenol

Dichloroisoproterenol was the first β-blocker tested in man, but was immediately discarded on account of its toxicity. However, it is included in this section because of its historical significance in the development of safer β-blockers. The discovery of the β-blocking action of dichloroisoproterenol started with the testing of isoprophenamine, a β-activator which relaxes isolated bronchial muscles, but unexpectedly blocks the relaxing action of epinephrine. The observation led to the testing of other chlorinated phenylethylamines, and dichloroisoproterenol proved to be the most active β-blocker with partial activation of β-receptors. There are no bronchomotor or pulmonary hemodynamic studies in man. In the laboratory, dichloroisoproterenol was used in the early discovery of the unaffected α-receptors in the airways of the dog (p. 5).

II. Cardioselective Beta-Receptor Blocking Agents

The development of β-blockers which are selective for the heart (β_1) and spare the airways (β_2) was prompted by the appearance of bronchospasm in some individuals being treated with propranolol and related drugs. The evolution of cardioselective β_1-blockers has been reviewed by WEETMAN (1977). In practice, although the cardioselectivity has been proven in animals, clinical testing is still necessary to prove that the margin of safety is sufficiently large to proceed with the use of the drug in patients with chronic obstructive pulmonary disease. JOHNSSON (1976) has cautioned cardiologists that the cardioselective β_1-blocker should be routinely administered concurrently with a bronchoselective β_2-activator to patients with chronic obstructive pulmonary disease and also suffering from cardiac disease. This combination will serve the dual purpose of alleviating the cardiac disease by cardioselective blockade, as well as dilating the airways by bronchoselective dilation.

1. Practalol

Practalol was the first cardioselective β_1-blocker and was introduced in 1968. The most conspicuous difference from propranolol was that practalol has minimal blocking action on β_2-receptors of the airways, demonstrated in animals as well as in humans (RYO and TOWNLEY, 1976). The occurrence of adverse reaction such as skin rash, ocular disturbances, and fatal sclerosing peritonitis led to practalol being withdrawn from commercial distribution in 1975. Prior to its withdrawal, there was a case report of chronic obstructive pulmonary disease in a patient who had been treated for hyperkinetic heart syndrome with practalol for 5 years (BARTSCH and REGINSTER, 1977). The causation of pulmonary disease should be further investigated and taken into consideration when other cardioselective β_1-blockers become used for extended periods of time.

2. Acebutol

Although the cardioselectivity of acebutol has been demonstrated in animals, the drug is not as selective as practalol in human volunteers. KUMANA et al. (1975) observed some reduction in exercising peak-flow rate and forced expiratory volume following equivalent doses of acebutol for blockade of cardiac β_1-receptors, which were less than that of propranolol, but more than that of practolol.

3. Atenolol

The cardioselectivity of atenolol is relative rather than absolute. Dosages of atenolol that reduce resting and exercising heart rate, also cause an increase in thoracic gas volume and a reduction in peak-flow rate, indicating some change in airways (MARLIN et al., 1975; BEIL and ULMER, 1977).

4. Bunitrolol

The clinical studies of KAIK (1976) show a lack of bronchomotor effects in resting subjects treated with bunitrolol. It will be necessary to examine patients during exercise for definitive evidence that lungs are not influenced by bunitrolol.

I. Adrenergic Neuron Blocking Agents

The last group of adrenergic inhibitors interfere with the function of the adrenergic neuron in contrast to the two preceding groups which block receptors. Briefly, the mechanisms of adrenergic neuron blockade are as follows: (a) interference with the release of norepinephrine from neuronal intragranular pool, as exemplified by *bretylium*; (b) depletion of neuronal intragranular content of norepinephrine by interruption of its uptake from the cytoplasmic pool, as with *reserpine*; (c) depletion of neuronal intragranular content of norepinephrine by its release to the extraneuronal space, as by *guanethidine*; and (d) competitive displacement of norepinephrine in the adrenergic nerve ending by a metabolite of the drug, such as *methyldopa*. The common feature of all four mechanisms is the inadequate amount of norepinephrine with which to transmit impulses across the neuroeffector junction. Thus, there is interference in sympathetic nervous control of all organs, possibly including the respiratory tract.

There is no information supporting the contention that norepinephrine is the transmitter for the adrenergic nerve endings in the respiratory tract (p. 11). Theories for the involvement of norepinephrine in the above stated actions of the four adrenergic neuron blocking agents are based upon observations from the study of the heart, peripheral blood vessels, and the central nervous system (p. 12). Direct proof is lacking for the depletion or inhibition of release of norepinephrine in the airways. As a matter of fact, there is not even information regarding the direct consequences of administration of neuron blockers on the bronchial smooth muscle. Since there have been no reported adverse effects on the respiratory tract (such as bronchospasm) when these drugs are used for the treatment of essential hypertension, it is safe to assume that the airways are not adversely affected by neuron blockers. This conclusion reinforces the suspicion that the properties of bronchial smooth muscles are distinct from those of other adrenergic innervated tissues.

The following discussion is almost entirely devoted to the effects of adrenergic neuron blockers on the pulmonary circulation. The changes in pulmonary blood flow and pulmonary vascular resistance are those expected, based upon the known pharmacologic effects of the drugs on the heart (Chap. Sec. III, Chaps. 1–4) and systemic blood vessels (Cap. Sec. III, Chap. 5). The one exception is that the efficacy of the neuron blockers in the treatment of essential hypertension does not extend to the management of pulmonary arterial hypertension. Possible reasons for this observation are discussed below.

I. Bretylium

Bretylium, when injected intravenously, has a biphasic effect on the pulmonary circulation. There is an initial epinephrinelike elevation in pulmonary blood flow, pulmonary arterial pressure and pulmonary vascular resistance, followed by a delayed reduction in pulmonary blood flow but continuous elevation in pulmonary vascular resistance (TAYLOR and DONALD, 1960). The initial phase is caused by release of catecholamines whereas the delayed phase is a manifestation of persistent blockade of adrenergic innervation, including the cardiac and pulmonary nerves. The changes in pulmonary blood flow are understandable, but the persistent increase in pulmonary vascular resistance is difficult to explain. Vasodilation would have been the expected response, based upon the assumption that the sympathetic vasoconstrictor nerves to the pulmonary blood vessels are blocked. Another available explanation is that bretylium sensitizes the drug induced denervated structures to circulating catecholamines, so that the pulmonary vascoconstriction is similar to sensitization by surgical denervation (AVIADO and DIL, 1960).

II. Reserpine

The administration of reserpine causes a variable effect on pulmonary blood flow and a decrease in pulmonary vascular resistance unlike bretylium. There is a significant fall in pulmonary arterial blood pressure in patients suffering from pulmonary hypertension, secondary to mitral disease, chronic obstructive pulmonary disease, sclerosis of the pulmonary artery, or pulmonary edema (see AVIADO, 1965). However, the relief of pulmonary hypertension is partial and temporary, indicating that only the neurogenic component of pulmonary hypertension is corrected by reserpine, and that the organic changes in the blood vessels continue to be unaffected by the drug.

III. Guanethidine

Like bretylium, the hemodynamic effects of guanethidine consist of two phases: an initial release of catecholamines and their persistent depletion in nerve endings. However, there is no persistent change in pulmonary vascular resistance, neither an increase like bretylium, nor a decrease like reserpine (see AVIADO, 1961, 1965). Since all three drugs block adrenergic neurons in general, the effect on pulmonary vascular nerves are probably dissimilar, and requires further investigation.

IV. Methyldopa

The available hemodynamic studies in patients with essential hypertension treated with methyldopa show variable effects on pulmonary blood flow and pulmonary vascular resistance (WILSON et al., 1962; SANNERSTEDT et al., 1962). The reasons for the variability are not known and may be another example of differences in sensitivity to neuron blockers between pulmonary and systemic sympathetic nerves. Additional research is needed to focus on differentiating features of adrenergic nerves to the lung, both in the vascular and bronchial smooth muscles.

J. Concluding Remarks

The organization of this chapter on the respiratory system, like those of other organ systems, is centered around groups of drugs, rather than pharmacologic actions. This final section emphasizes similarities in the influences of adrenergic activators and inhibitors upon the nasal cavity or upper respiratory tract, the lower respiratory tract including bronchial smooth muscle, the pulmonary circulation, and the bronchial circulation. The central theme of the concluding remarks is the necessity for additional investigation directed to the identification of adrenergic transmitters for the respiratory tract in general, and for the bronchial smooth muscles in particular.

1. Nasal Congestion and Decongestion

There is sufficient information supporting the role of α-adrenoceptors in mediating nasal vasoconstriction, and β-adrenoceptors in nasal vasodilation or congestion. A large group of drugs has been developed specifically for topical use to decongest the nasal mucosa in allergic or infectious rhinitis. Most of these drugs have not been studied for their actions in other parts of the respiratory tract. However, since all are α-activators, they would be expected to constrict most blood vessels in the lungs.

2. Bronchial Mucosal Decongestion

The swelling and shrinking of bronchial mucosa cannot be measured in man or in animals due to the difficulty in excluding the bronchial muscle. It is reasonable to assume that, like the nasal mucosa, adrenergic α-activators cause shrinkage of the bronchial mucosa. However, in patients with bronchial asthma, the inhalation of an α-activator (such as phenylephrine) does not cause a significant reduction in airway resistance. The lack of a change in resistance cannot exclude shrinkage of the bronchial mucosa because the neighboring smooth muscle contains α-receptors, which would produce an increase in airway resistance when activated. It is possible that α-mediated shrinkage of the bronchial mucosa is approximately equal in intensity to the α-mediated bronchoconstriction, and that the two balance each other. Observations that α-receptors in the vascular and in the muscular components of the airways are pharmacologically similar, and are identical in their affinity for tagged adrenergic drugs, support the explanation that the two groups of receptors are equal but diametrically opposite, in their intensity of response.

3. Bronchodilation

Since stimulation of sympathetic nerves to the lung causes bronchodilation, while norepinephrine causes bronchoconstriction, another adrenergic neurohumoral transmitter should be considered. The authors propose that epinephrine as a bronchodilator, is a more acceptable candidate for the adrenergic transmitter. There are numerous adrenergic drugs that are useful in the treatment of bronchial asthma; some of them are direct activators of both β- and α-receptors (such as epinephrine), others are β-activators of both bronchial (β_2) and cardiac (β_1)-receptors (such as isoproterenol), and still others are β_2 bronchoselective (such as terbutaline). The margin of safety for the bronchoselective drugs is wider in animals than in man; human bronchoselectivity is not absolute, but is a relative phenomenon, since tachycardia occurs as an adverse reaction.

Another group of bronchodilators useful for the treatment of bronchial asthma is the category of adrenergic transmitter releasing agents, such as ephedrine. The hypothesis that ephedrine releases norepinephrine in the airways has not been proven. Epinephrine, a known bronchodilator, is a more acceptable candidate for the transmitter released by ephedrine because of the similarities in their pharmacologic actions in the respiratory tract, viz, airways and pulmonary and bronchial circulations.

A third group of potentially useful bronchodilators is the category of adrenergic α-receptor blocking agents, such as thymoxanine. Since there is experimental evidence for the existence of α-receptors in the airways (responsive to norepinephrine), it is reasonable to explain the observed bronchodilation by α-receptor blockade. However, most adrenergic α-blockers, including thymoxamine, also stimulate β-adrenergic receptors, so that this activity would pose a second mechanism for the observed bronchodilation.

4. Bronchoconstriction

In recent years, there has been an increasing body of information supporting the existence of α-receptors in the airways, mediating bronchoconstriction. The experiments include administration of norepinephrine, methoxamine, and epinephrine preceded by a β-blocker. The participation of α-receptors has been suggested as a cause of refractoriness to the bronchodilator action of epinephrine. Reversal of the desired bronchodilator action of the isoproterenol is a more complex process and may relate to its vasodilator action, causing mucosal swelling and masking relaxation of bronchial smooth muscles. Bronchoconstriction appears as an adverse reaction in the clinical use of adrenergic β-receptor blockers (such as propranolol). This reaction is less likely to occur with the use of cardioselective β_1-blockers, which have been developed specifically to have lower affinity for β_2-receptors in the airways. The selectivity is not absolute, but is relative, since bronchospasm can still occur with the use of cardioselective β_1-blockers.

5. Pulmonary Vasodilation

The following categories of adrenergic drugs are known to reduce pulmonary arterial blood pressure in the treatment of pulmonary hypertension: adrenergic β-activators (such as isoproterenol), adrenergic α-blockers (such as tolazoline), and adrenergic transmitter depleting agents (such as reserpine). The reduction in pulmonary hypertensive level is not dramatic and permanent, because most patients with diagnosed hypertension are already in an advanced stage characterized by organic changes in the blood vessels, irreversible by any form of drug therapy.

6. Pulmonary Vasoconstriction, Congestion, and Edema

There have been reports of the occurrence of pulmonary edema in the course of treating shock with adrenergic vasopressors. The mechanisms are varied and include failure of the left ventricle, constriction of the pulmonary veins, and elevation of hydrostatic pressure in the pulmonary capillaries. The overloading of the ventricle is more likely to occur with α-activators that elicit vasoconstriction only (such as methoxamine) than with adrenergic drugs that activate β-receptors (such as dopamine).

7. Bronchial Circulation

Although the behavior of bronchial arteries is similar to that of the pulmonary and systemic arteries, in response to adrenergic drugs, presence of bronchopulmonary anastomoses complicates interpretation of the significance of the vascular changes. For example, norepinephrine constricts the bronchial veins leading to a shift of venous blood to the bronchopulmonary anastomoses, thus increasing venous admixture in the systemic arterial blood. In the same context, a reduction in oxygen content of the blood occurs with parenteral injection of epinephrine or isoproterenol in asthmatics. This undesired effect is precipitated by a disproportionate increase of perfusion relative to ventilation and can be overcome by supplementing the supply of oxygen to the lungs. As a final note, the bronchial venous blood effluent is an ideal site for the collecting of any released transmitter from the airways, before being diluted in the general circulation. Isolation of these vessels, although technically difficult, has been accomplished in the past. If properly collected, such blood samples may not only resolve the identity of the respiratory neurotransmitter, but will also help verify the existence of diverse biochemical events revealed by in vitro techniques. In the future, it is important to combine physiologic and biochemical approaches in the same experimental preparations, since the development of each of these sets of techniques has been proceeding in disparate directions. Attempts at a meaningful communication across the resultant hiatus may place stress on the use of scientific information for new initiatives in the treatment of diseases of the respiratory tract.

References

Adelson, B.H., Gilbert, R.P.: The effect of levarterenol on the dye-dilution curve in two patients with shock from acute infarction of the myocardium. Q. Bull. Northw. Univ. Med. Sch. *33*, 191–193 (1959)

Aellig, W.H.: Experiments with pindolol (Visken) in healthy volunteers. Med. J. Aust. *2* (Suppl. 2), 8–11 (1977)

Anthracite, R.F., Vachon, L., Knapp, P.H.: Alpha-adrenergic receptors in the human lung. Psychosom. Med. *23*, 481–489 (1971)

Apperley, G.H., Daly, M.J., Levy, G.P.: Selectivity of beta-adrenoceptor agonists and antagonists on bronchial, skeletal, vascular, and cardiac muscle in the anaesthetized cat. Br. J. Pharmacol. *57*, 235–246 (1976)
Aramendia, P., Martinez L. De Letona, J., Aviado, D.M.: Exchange of blood between pulmonary and systemic circulations via bronchopulmonary anastomoses. Circ. Res. *11*, 870–879 (1962a)
Aramendia, P., Martinez L. De Letona, J., Aviado, D.M.: Responses of the bronchial veins in a heart-lung bronchial preparation with special reference to a pulmonary bronchial shunt. Circ. Res. *10*, 3–10 (1962b)
Areskog, N.H., Cullhed, I., Ringqvist, I., Strom, G.: Cardiovascular and respiratory effects of the β-adrenoceptive antagonist sotalol. Studies in health, angina pectoris and obstructive lung disease. Eur. J. Clin. Pharmacol. *8*, 403–408 (1975)
Arner, B., Magnusson, P.O.: Comparison between ibuterol hydrochloride and terbutaline in asthma. Br. Med. J. *1*, 72–74 (1976)
Arner, B., Bertler, A., Karlefors, T., Westling, H.: Bronchodilator effect of a new sympathomimetic β-receptor-stimulating agent, terbutaline, given subcutaneously to asthmatic patients. Acta Med. Scand. [Suppl.] *512*, 41–43 (1970)
Aviado, D.M.: Sympathetic nerve blocking drugs for the treatment of hypertension. TM-10, Beta Tm-10, Bretylium and guanethidine. Am. J. Med. Sci. *244*, 650–661 (1961)
Aviado, D.M.: The lung circulation. Vol. 1. Physiology and pharmacology. Vol. 2. Pathological physiology and therapy of diseases. Vol. 1, pp. 1–590, Vol. 2, pp. 591–1405. Oxford: Pergamon Press 1965
Aviado, D.M.: Pharmacology of hypertension with special reference to the cardiovascular effects of beta-adrenergic blocking agents. In: Advances in cardiopulmonary diseases. Banyai, A.L., Gordon, B.L. (eds.), Vol. IV, pp. 129–143. Chicago: Yearbook Medical 1969
Aviado, D.M.: Sympathomimetic drugs, pp. 1–615. Springfield: Thomas 1970
Aviado, D.M.: Potential hazards of bronchodilator aerosols. Toxicity of aerosols. J. Clin. Pharmacol. *15*, 86–104 (1975)
Aviado, D.M.: Adrenergic agents in bronchial asthma, emphasizing undesirable reactions. In: Status asthmaticus. Weiss, E.B. (ed.), pp. 215–223. Baltimore: University Park Press 1978
Aviado, D.M.: Sotalol: A pure beta-adrenergic blocking agent for the treatment of essential hypertension and other cardiovascular diseases. J. Clin. Pharmacol. *19*, 497–504 (1979)
Aviado, D.M., De Beer, E.J.: A comparative study of nasal decongestion by sympathomimetic drugs. Arch. Otolaryngol. *69*, 598–605 (1959)
Aviado, D.M., Dil, A.H.: Effects of a new sympathetic blocking drug (Bretylium) on cardiovascular control. J. Pharmacol. Exp. Ther. *129*, 330–337 (1960)
Aviado, D.M., Schmidt, C.F.: Effects of sympathomimetic drugs on pulmonary circulation with special reference to a new pulmonary vasodilator. J. Pharmacol. Exp. Ther. *120*, 512–527 (1957)
Aviado, D.M., Ling, J.S., Schmidt, C.F.: Effects of anoxia on pulmonary circulation: Reflex pulmonary vasoconstriction. Am. J. Physiol. *189*, 253–262 (1957)
Aviado, D.M., Wnuck, A.L., De Beer, E.J.: Cardiovascular effects of sympathomimetic bronchodilators: Epinephrine, ephedrine, pseudoephedrine, isoproterenol, methoxyphenamine, and isoprophenamine. J. Pharmacol. Exp. Ther. *122*, 406–417 (1958)
Aviado, D.M., De Burgh Daly, M., Lee, C.Y., Schmidt, C.F.: The contribution of the bronchial circulation to the venous admixture in pulmonary venous blood. J. Physiol. (Lond.) *155*, 602–622 (1961)
Aviado, D.M., Folle, L.E., Pisanty, J.: The influence of a new adrenergic beta-receptor (MJ 1999) blocking drug on the pulmonary circulation. Arch. Int. Pharmacodyn. Ther. *168*, 323–338 (1967)
Aviado, D.M., Kishimoto, T., Kneidinger, H.J.: Bronchopulmonary effects of pentaerythrityl tetranitrate and isoproterenol. J. Pharmacol. Exp. Ther. *165*, 274–285 (1969)
Aviado, D.M., Wnuck, A.L., De Beer, E.J.: A comparative study of nasal decongestion by sympathomimetic drugs. Arch. Otolaryngol. *69*, 598–605 (1959)
Bariety, M., Kohler, D.: Sur l'existence d'un facteur histaminique dans le determinisme de l'oedeme pulmonaire aigu adrenalinque chez le lapin. C. R. Acad. Sci. (Paris) *236*, 1389–1391 (1953)

Barnett, D.B., Rugg, E.L., Nahorski, S.R.: Direct evidence of two types of beta adrenoceptor binding site in lung tissue. Nature *273*, 166–168 (1978)
Bartsch, P., Reginster, M.: Chronic obstructive lung disease after practolol. Lancet *1*, 908–909 (1977)
Baskerville, A.: The development and persistence of bronchial gland hypertrophy and goblet-cell hyperplasia in the pig after injection of isoprenaline. J. Pathol. *119*, 35–47 (1976)
Beck, W., Schrire, V., Vogelpoel, L., Nellen, M., Swanepoel, A.: Hemodynamic effects of amyl nitrite and phenylephrine on the normal human circulation and their relation to changes in cardiac murmurs. Am. J. Cardiol. *8*, 241–349 (1961)
Beil, M., Ulmer, W.T.: Effects of a new cardioselective beta-adrenergic blocker (atenolol) on airway resistance in chronic obstructive disease. Arzneim. Forsch. *27*, 419–422 (1977)
Beil, M., Brecht, H.M., Rasche, B.: Plasma catecholamines in exercise induced bronchoconstriction. Klin. Wochenschr. *55*, 577–581 (1977)
Benson, M.K.: Bronchial responsiveness to inhaled histamine and isoprenaline in patients with airway obstruction. Thorax *33*, 211–213 (1978)
Berk, J.L., Hagen, J.F., Koo, R., Maly, G.: Pulmonary insufficiency produced by isoproterenol. Surg. Gynecol. Obstet. *143*, 725–726 (1976)
Berk, J.L., Hagen, J.F., Tong, R.K., Levy, M.L., Martin, P.J.: The role of adrenergic stimulation in the pathogenesis of pulmonary insufficiency. Surgery *82*, 366–372 (1977)
Bianco, S., Kamburoff, P.L., Prime, F.J.: Comparison between the bronchodilator and cardiovascular effects of inhaling 0.5 mg. rimiterol ("Pulmadil") and 0.2 mgs salbutamol. Curr. Med. Res. Opin. *3*, 30–35 (1975)
Biel, J.H., Schwartz, E.G., Sprengeler, E.P., Leiser, H.A., Friedman, H.L.: Bronchodilators, N-substituted derivatives of 1-(3′4′-Dihydroxyphenyl)-2-aminoethanol (Arterenol). J. Am. Chem. Soc. *76*, 3149–3153 (1954)
Boehringer Ingelhein Ltd.: Alupent brand of metaproterenol sulfate. Tablets of 20 ng metered dose inhaler. AL-448, pp. 1–72. Elmsford, N.Y.: Boehringer Ingelheim 1975
Bolduc, P., Reid, L.: The effect of isoprenaline and pilocarpine on mitotic index and goblet cell number in rat respiratory epithelium. Br. J. Exp. Pathol. *59*, 311–318 (1978)
Bouhuys, A.: Pharmacological basis for refractoriness. In: Status asthmaticus. Weiss, E.B. (ed.), pp. 49–58. Baltimore: University Park Press 1978
Bowman, W.C., Raper, C.: Sympathomimetic bronchodilators and animal models for assessing their potential value in asthma. J. Pharm. Pharmacol. *28* (Suppl. 4), 369–374 (1976)
Brittain, R.T., Jack, D.: Recent work on selective beta-adrenoceptor stimulants. In: Mechanisms and therapeutics. Weiss, E.B., Segal, M.S. (eds.). Boston: Little, Brown and Co. 1976
Bürkmann, I., Heberling, J.H., Herold, B., Kling, K.: Ventilation, gas-exchange, and pulmonary arterial pressure during aerosol inhalation of sympathicomimetics. Z. Erkr. Atmungsorgane *145*, 350–353 (1976)
Buhr, G.: Über den Einfluß der Aludrin-Aerosol-Inhalation auf die Druckverhältnisse in der Arteria pulmonalis beim Menschen. Z. Kreisl. Forsch. *42*, 669–683 (1953)
Burn, J.H., Rand, M.J.: The action of sympathomimetic amines in animals treated with reserpine. J. Physiol. (Lond.) *144*, 314–336 (1958)
Burns, J.W., Doe, J.E.: A comparison of drug-induced responses on rat tracheal, bronchial, and lung strip in vitro preparations. Br. J. Pharmacol. *64*, 71–74 (1978)
Busse, W.W.: Decreased granulocyte response to isoproterenol in asthma during upper respiratory infections. Am. Rev. Respir. Dis. *115*, 783–791 (1977)
Caplin, I., Haynes, J.T.: Complications of aerosol therapy in asthma. Ann. Allergy *27*, 65 (1969)
Carrillo, L., Kishimoto, T., Aviado, D.M.: The nasal and bronchopulmonary effects of xylometazoline and KB 227. Ann. Otol. Rhinol. Laryngol. *78*, 415–420 (1969)
Castro de la Mata, R., Penna, M., Aviado, D.M.: Reversal of sympathomimetic bronchodilation by dichloroisoproterenol. J. Pharmacol. Exp. Ther. *135*, 197–203 (1962)
Chand, N.: Evidence for the existence of α-adrenoceptors in the rat lung. Res. Commun. Chem. Pathol. Pharmacol. *25*, 215–225 (1979)
Chapman, T.T.: Comparison of Carbuterol, a new selective bronchodilator agent, with salbutamol in a single dose cross-over trial. J. Irish Med. Assoc. *69*, 113–116 (1976)
Chapman, T.T.: Spasm and secretion in asthma. Br. Med. J. *2*, 50 (1970)

Cho, Y.W., Lish, P.M., Aviado, D.M.: Efficacy of a new bronchodilator, soterenol, on experimental locked-lung syndrome in dogs. J. Allergy. *42*, 36–48 (1968)
Christensen, J.M., Valasek, F.E., Tainter, M.L.: Ethylnorepinephrine: A unique bronchodilator. American Productioner *9*, 916–921 (1958)
Collins, J.V., Clark, T.J., Brown, D.J.: Airway function in healthy subjects and patients with left heart disease. Clin. Sci. Mol. Med. *49*, 217–228 (1975)
Combs, A.B., Jones, J.: The action of isoproterenol on phenylthiourea induced pulmonary edema. Res. Conmun. Chem. Pathol. Pharmacol. *12*, 177–180 (1975)
Conolly, M.E., Greenacre, J.K.: The beta-adrenoceptor of the human lymphocyte and human lung parenchyma. Br. J. Pharmacol. *59*, 17–23 (1977)
Davila, D., Davila, T.: Uptake and release of 3-H-metaraminol by rat lung. Basic aspects, ionic and energy requirements. Arch. Int. Pharmacodyn. Ther. *214*, 53–61 (1975)
De Burgh Daly, I., Hebb, C.O., Petrovskaia, B.: Adrenaline bronchoconstriction in isolated blood-perfused lungs. Q. J. Exp. Physiol. *31*, 129–159 (1942)
Dresdale, D.T., Michtom, R.J., Schultz, M.: Recent studies in primary pulmonary hypertension including pharmacodynamic observations on pulmonary vascular resistance. Bull. N.Y. Acad. Med. *30*, 195–207 (1954)
Drimal, J., Aviado, D.M.: Effects of oxprenolol on coronary circulation and cardiac metabolism. J. Pharmacol. Exp. Ther. *176*, 312–319 (1971)
Duncan, P.E., Griffin, J.P., Solomon, S.S.: Bronchodilator drug efficacy via cyclic AMP. Thorax *30*, 192–196 (1975)
Eliakim, M., Aviado, D.M.: Effects of nerve stimulation and drugs on the extra-pulmonary portion of the pulmonary vein. J. Pharmacol. Exp. Ther. *133*, 304–312 (1961)
Engel, L.A., Landau, L., Taussig, L., Martin, R.R., Sybrecht, G.: Influence of bronchomotor tone on regional ventilation distribution at residual volume. J. Appl. Physiol. *40*, 411–416 (1976)
Engelhardt, A., Hoefke, W., Wick, H.: Zur Pharmakologie des sympathomimeticums 1-(3,5-dihydroxyphenyl)-1-hydroxy-2-isopropylaminoäthan. Arzneim. Forsch. *11*, 521–525 (1961)
Eriksson, N.E., Lindgren, S.B.: The rapidity of bronchodilation. A comparison of isoprenaline, terbutaline, and rimiterol. Scand. J. Respir. Dis. *59*, 30–36 (1978)
Folle, L.E., Aviado, D.M.: Cardiovascular effects of anoxia and the influence of a new beta adrenergic receptor blocking drug. J. Pharmacol. Exp. Ther. *149*, 79–90 (1965)
Foster, W.M., Bergofsky, E.H., Bohning, D.E., Lippmann, M., Albert, R.E.: Effect of adrenergic agents and their mode of action on mucociliary clearance in man. J. Appl. Physiol. *41*, 146–152 (1976)
Gayrard, P., Orehek, J., Grimaud, C., Charpin, J.: Bronchoconstrictor effects of a deep inspiration in patients with asthma. Am. Rev. Respir. Dis. *111*, 433–439 (1975a)
Gayrard, P., Orehek, J., Grimaud, C., Charpin, J.: Beta-adrenergic function in airways of healthy and asthmatic subjects. Thorax *30*, 657–662 (1975b)
Gloster, J., Heath, D., Hasleton, P., Harris, P.: Effect of chlorphentermine on the lipids of rat lungs. Thorax *31*, 558–564 (1976)
Goldenberg, M., Pines, K.L., Baldwin, E. de F., Greene, D.G., Roh, C.E.: The hemodynamic response of man to norepinephrine and epinephrine and its relation to the problem of hypertension. Am. J. Med. *5*, 792–805 (1948)
Gourzis, J.T., Roque, N., Nickerson, M.: Chemical structure and antishock activity among compounds related to phenoxybenzamine (dibenzyline). J. Pharmacol. Exp. Ther. *141*, 314–320 (1963)
Grimm, D.J., Dawson, C.A., Hakin, T.S., Linehan, J.H.: Pulmonary vasomotion and the distribution of vascular resistance in a dog lung lobe. J. Appl. Physiol. *45*, 545–550 (1978)
Harms, H.H.: Isoproterenol antagonism of cardioselective beta adrenergic receptor blocking agents: A comparative study of human and guinea-pig cardiac and bronchial beta adrenergic receptors. J. Pharmacol. Exp. Ther. *199*, 329–335 (1976)
Harms, H.H., Spoelstra, A.J.: Cardiac and bronchial beta-adrenoceptor antagonistic potencies of atenolol, metoprolol, acebutolol, practolol, propranolol, and pindolol in the anaesthetized dog. Clin. Exp. Pharmacol. Physiol. *5*, 53–59 (1978)
Hartley, D., Jack, D., Lunts, L.H.C., Ritchie, A.C.: New class of selective stimulants of β adrenergic receptors. Nature *219*, 861–862 (1968)

Hooker, C.S., Calkins, P.J., Fleisch, J.H.: On the measurement of vascular and respiratory smooth muscle responses in vitro. Blood Vessels *14*, 1–11 (1977)
Johnsson, G.: Use of beta-adrenoreceptor blockers in combination with beta-stimulators in patients with obstructive lung disease. Drugs *1* (Suppl. 11), 171–177 (1976)
Joiner, P.D., Kadowitz, P.J., Hughes, J.P., Hyman, A.L.: NE and ACh responses of intrapulmonary vessels from dog, swine, sheep, and man. Am. J. Physiol. *228*, 1821–1827 (1975)
Junod, A.F.: Mechanism of uptake of biogenic amines in the pulmonary circulation. In: Lung metabolism. Junod, A.F., de Haller, R. (eds.), pp. 387–398. New York: Academic Press 1975a
Junod, A.F.: The lung and the metabolism of vasoactive substances. Schweiz. Med. Wochenschr. *105*, 1656–1658 (1975b)
Junod, A.F., Ody, C.: Anine uptake and metabolism by endothelium of pig pulmonary artery and aorta. Am. J. Physiol. *232*, C88–94 (1977)
Kaik, G.: Study of the influence of the beta-sympatholytic drug KÖ 1366 (Bunitrolol on lung function). Wien. Klin. Wochenschr. *88*, 68–71 (1976)
Karabelnik, D., Zbinden, G.: Drug-induced foam cell reactions in rats. II. Chemical analysis of lipids stored in lungs and foam cells after treatment with chlorphentermine, 5-(p-(fluoren-9-ylidenemethyl)phenyl)-2-piperidineethanol (RMI 10.393) and 1-chloramitriptyline. Hoppe Seylers Z. Physiol. Chem. *356*, 1151–1160 (1975)
Kaufman, A.J., Ochoa, E.: Similar receptors mediating the norepinephrine and dopamine contraction in the main pulmonary artery of the dog. Acta Physiol. Lat. Am. *20*, 451–463 (1971)
Kaufman, A.J., Iglauer, A., Herwitz, G.K.: Effect of isuprel (isopropyl-epinephrine) on circulation of normal man. Am. J. Med. *11*, 442–447 (1951)
Kealey, G.P., Brody, M.J.: Studies on the mechanism of pulmonary vascular responses to miliary pulmonary embolism. Circ. Res. *41*, 807–814 (1977)
Keighley, J.F.: Iatrogenic asthma associated with adrenergic aerosols. Ann. Intern. Med. *65*, 985 (1966)
Kneussl, M.P., Richardson, J.B.: Alpha-adrenergic receptors in human and canine tracheal and bronchial smooth muscle. J. Appl. Physiol. *45*, 307–311 (1978)
Koch, G.: Acute hemodynamic effects of an alpha- and beta-receptor blocking agent (AH 5158) on the systemic and pulmonary circulation at rest and during exercise in hypertensive patients. Am. Heart J. *93*, 585–591 (1977)
Kumana, C.R., Kaye, C.M., Leighton, M., Turner, P., Hamer, J.: Cardiac and pulmonary effects of acebutolol. Lancet *2*, 89–93 (1975)
Lands, A.M., Arnold, A., McAuliff, J.P., Luduena, F.P., Brown, T.G.: Differentiation of receptor systems activated by sumpathomimetic amines. Nature *214*, 597–599 (1967)
Larsson, S.: Long-term treatment with β_2-adrenostimulants in asthma. Side-effects, selectivity, tolerance, and routes of administration. Acta Med. Scand. [Suppl] *608*, 1–40 (1977)
Lippmann, M., Albert, R.E., Yeates, D.B., Berger, J.M., Foster, W.M., Bohning, D.E.: Factors affecting tracheobronchial mucociliary transport. Inhaled Part. *1*, 305–319 (1975)
Luisada, A.A.: The pathogenesis of paroxysmal pulmonary edema. Medicine (Baltimore) *19*, 475–504 (1940)
Malik, A.B.: Pulmonary vascular response to increase in intracranial pressure: Role of sympathetic mechanisms. J. Appl. Physiol. *42*, 335–343 (1977)
Mardel, M.J., Smith, H., Spicer, B.A.: Bronchodilators giving reduced cardiovascular effects. Relative biological activities of the four isomers of 1-(3,4-dihydroxyphenyl)-2-isopropylaminobutanol. J. Med. Chem. *17*, 513–516 (1974)
Marion Laboratories. Ventair. 2 mg Tablets (protokylol HCl) Marion. A drug monograph, pp. 1–54. Kansas City: Marion Laboratories 1974
Marlin, G.E., Turner, P.: The relative potencies and beta 2-selectivities of intravenous rimiterol, salbutamol, and isoprenaline in asthmatic patients. Int. J. Clin. Pharmacol. Biopharm. *12*, 158–169 (1975)
Marlin, G.E., Kumana, C.R., Kaye, C.M., Smith, D.M., Turner, P.: An investigation into the cardiac and pulmonary beta-adrenoceptor blocking activity of ICI 66,082 in man. Br. J. Clin. Pharmacol. *2*, 151–157 (1975)
Martinez L. De Letona, J., Castro de la Mata, R., Aviado, D.M.: Local and reflex effects of bronchial arterial injection of drugs. J. Pharmacol. Exp. Ther. *133*, 295–303 (1961)

Mathé, A.A., Tong, E.Y., Tisher, P.W.: Norepinephrine release from the lung by sympathetic nerve stimulation inhibition by vagus and methacholine. Life Sci. *20*, 1425–1430 (1977)
McFadden, E.R. Jr., Ingram, R.H. Jr.: Exercise-induced asthma; observations on the initiating stimulus. N. England J. Med. *301*, 763–769 (1979)
Melville, G.N., Horstmann, G., Iravani, J.: Adrenergic compounds and the respiratory tract. A physiological and electron-microscopical study. Respiration *33*, 261–269 (1976)
Mentzer, R.M., Alegre, C.A., Nolan, S.P.: The effects of dopamine and isoproterenol on the pulmonary circulation. J. Thorac. Cardiovasc. Surg. *71*, 807–814 (1976)
Minette, A., Marcq, M., Gepts, L.: Carbuterol, fenoterol, orciprenaline, salbutamol, and terbutaline per os in reversible obstructive chronic bronchitis. Bull. Eur. Physiopathol. Respir. *12*, 545–553 (1976)
Moore, P.F., Constantine, J.W., Barth, W.E.: Pirbuterol, a selective $Beta_2$ Adrenergic bronchodilator. J. Pharmacol. Exp. Ther. *2*, 410–418 (1978)
Mossberg, B., Strandberg, K., Philipson, K., Camner, P.: Tracheobronchial clearance in bronchial asthma: Response to beta-adrenoceptor stimulation. Scand. J. Respir. Dis. *57*, 119–128 (1976)
Nelson, H.S., Black, J.W., Branch, L.B., Pfuetze, B., Spaulding, H., Summers, R., Wood, D.: Subsensitivity to epinephrine following the administration of epinephrine and ephedrine to normal individuals. J. Allergy Clin. Immunol. *55*, 299–309 (1975)
Nelson, H.S., Raine, D., Jr., Doner, H.C., Posey, W.C.: Subsensitivity to the bronchodilator action of albuterol produced by chronic administration. Am. Rev. Respir. Dis. *116*, 871–878 (1977)
Nickerson, M., Gourzis, J.T.: Blockade of sympathetic vasoconstriction in the treatment of shock. J. Trauma *2*, 399–411 (1962)
Niden, A.H., Aviado, D.M.: Effects of pulmonary embolism on the pulmonary circulation with special reference to arteriovenous shunts in the lung. Circ. Res. *4*, 67–73 (1956)
Nousiainen, O.T., Arnala, I., Airaksinen, M.M., Kokkola, K.: Potentiation of beta-sympathomimetics with alpha-adrenoceptor blocking drugs in guinea pig trachea and human bronchus preparations. Pharmacology *15*, 469–477 (1977)
O'Donnell, S.R., Wanstall, J.C.: The contribution of extraneuronal uptake to the trachea-blood vessel selectivity of β-adrenoceptor stimulants in vitro in guinea-pigs. Br. J. Pharmacol. *57*, 369–373 (1976)
Orange, R.P., Austen, K.F.: Immunological release of the chemical mediators of anaphylaxis, identification of asthma. Ciba Foundation Study Group No. 38. Porter, R., Birch, J. (eds.), pp. 99–110. Edinburgh: Churchill Livingstone 1971
Palmer, K.N.V., Diemant, M.L.: Effect of salbutamol on spirometry and blood-gas tensions in bronchial asthma. Br. Med. J. *1*, 31–32 (1969)
Patel, K.R.: Atropine, sodium cromoglycate, and thymoxamine in PGF_2 alpha-induced bronchoconstriction in extrinsic asthma. Br. Med. J. *2*, 360–362 (1975)
Persson, H., Olsson, T.: Some pharmacological properties of terbutaline (INN), 1-(3.5-Dihydroxyphenyl)-2-(T-Butylamino)-ethanol. A new sympathomimetic β-receptor-stimulating agent. Acta Med. Scand. [Suppl.] *512*, 11–19 (1970)
Phillips, M.A.: Bronchodilator aerosols. Lancet *2*, 677 (1967)
Ploy-Song-Sand, Y., Corbin, R.P., Engel, L.A.: Effects of intravenous histamine on lung mechanics in man after beta-blockage. J. Appl. Physiol. *44*, 690–695 (1978)
Porcelli, R.J., Viau, A.T., Naftchi, N.E., Bergofsky, E.H.: Beta-receptor influence on lung vasoconstrictor responses to hypoxia and humoral agents. J. Appl. Physiol. *43*, 612–616 (1977a)
Porcelli, R.J., Viau, A., Demeny, M., Naftchi, N.E., Bergofsky, E.H.: Relation between hypoxic pulmonary vasoconstriction, its humoral mediators and alpha-beta adrenergic receptors. Chest *71* (Suppl. 2), 249–251 (1977b)
Reisman, R.E.: Asthma induced by adrenergic aerosols. J. Allergy *46*, 102 (1970)
Renais, J., Scebat, L., Lenegre, J.: Oèdeme pulmonaire expérimental par insuffisance ventriculaire gauche aigue. Arch. Mal. Coeur. *50*, 715–719 (1957)
Rhoades, R.B., Leifer, K.N., Bloom, F.L., Wittig, H.J.: Spirometric comparison of carbuterol and isoproterenol aerosol therapy in bronchial asthma. A double blind, matched-pair study of 28 adults and a double blind crossover study of 18 children. Am. Rev. Respir. Dis. *114*, 79–86 (1976)

Roch-Besser, B.: La Benzyl-inidazoline (priscol). Etude pharmacodynamique et applications cliniques. Helv. Med. Acta *17*, Suppl. 27, 1–175 (1950)

Rodger, I.W.: Effect of isoetharine on airways resistance, heart rate, and contractions of the soleus muscle of the anaesthetised cat. Eur. J. Pharmacol. *24*, 211–217 (1973)

Ryo, U.Y., Townley, R.G.: Comparison of respiratory and cardiovascular effects of isoproterenol, propranolol, and practolol in asthmatic and normal subjects. J. Allergy Clin. Immunol. *57*, 12–24 (1976)

Salem, H., Aviado, D.M.: Antitussive drugs with special reference to a new theory for the initiation of the cough reflex and the influence of bronchodilators. Am. J. Med. Sci. *247*, 585–600 (1964)

Salem, H., Aviado, D.M.: Preclinical and clinical investigation of drugs. I. Bronchodilators and antiasthmatic drugs. Drug. Inform. Bull. *8*, 14–19 (1974)

Sannerstedt, R., Varnauskas, E., Werko, L.: Hemodynamic effects of methyldopa (Aldomet), at rest and during exercise in patients with arterial hypertension. Acta Med. Scand. *171*, 75–82 (1962)

Schonell, M., Harris, M., McMiken, D., Jenne, H., Evers, R.: Bronchodilator effect of hexoprenaline aerosol in bronchial asthma and chronic bronchitis. Med. J. Aust. *2*, 828–831 (1977)

Schwarz, R.H., Aviado, D.M.: Drug action, reaction, and interaction. III. Dopamine for endotoxic shock. J. Clin. Pharmacol. *16*, 88–98 (1976)

Schwitter, E., Février, D., Bachofen, H.: The inhalation of beta stimulators. Effect of the inhaled aerosol deposited in the oropharynx and in the bronchial tree. Schweiz. Med. Wochenschr. *105*, 497–499 (1975)

Siegler, D., Fukuchi, Y., Engel, L.: Influence of bronchomotor tone on ventilation distribution and airway closure in asymptomatic asthma. Am. Rev. Respir. Dis. *114*, 123–130 (1976)

Skinner, C., Gaddie, J., Palmer, K.N.V.: Comparison of intravenous AH 5158 (ibidomide) and propranolol in asthma. Br. Med. J. *2*, 59–61 (1975)

Sly, R.M.: Comparison of bronkephrine and epinephrine in the treatment of acute asthmatic attacks in children. Ann. Allergy *27*, 384–389 (1969)

Snashall, P.D., Boother, F.A., Sterling, G.M.: The effect of alpha-adrenoceptor stimulation on the airways of normal and asthmatic man. Clin. Sci. Mol. Med. *54*, 283–289 (1978)

Sörenby, L.: The beta-adrenoceptors of the lung mediating inhibition of antigen-induced histamine release. Eur. J. Pharmacol. *30*, 140–147 (1975)

Spector, S.L., Garza, G.M.: Dose-response effects of albuterol aerosol compared with isoproterenol and placebo aerosols: Response to albuterol, isoproterenol, and placebo aerosols. J. Allergy Clin. Immunol. *59*, 280–286 (1977)

Spector, S.L., Hudson, L., Petty, T.L.: Effect of bronkosol and its components on cardiopulmonary parameters in asthmatic patients. J. Allergy Clin. Immunol. *59*, 371–376 (1977)

Stanfield, C.A., Yu, P.N.: Hemodynamic effects of methoxamine in mitral valve disease. Circ. Res. *8*, 859–864 (1960)

Steen, S.N., Ziment, I., Smith, R., Kuo, J.: Effect of aerosolized pirbuterol on airway conductance. Res. Clin. Pharmacol. Ther. Res. System *2*, 1623 (1974)

Stjärne, L., Kaijser, L., Mathé, A., Birke, G.: Specific and unspecific removal of circulating noradrenaline in pulmonary and systemic vascular beds in man. Acta Physiol. Scand. *95*, 46–53 (1975)

Stone, D.J., Zaldivar, C., Keltz, H.: The effects of very low doses of nebulized isoproterenol, nebulized saline, and intravenous isoproterenol on blood gases in patients with chronic bronchitis. Am. Rev. Respir. Dis. *101*, 511 (1970)

Strandberg, K., Mathe, A.A., Yen, S.S.: Release of histamine and formation of prostaglandins in human lung tissue and rat mast cells. Int. Arch. Allergy Appl. Immunol. *53*, 520–529 (1977)

Stockley, R.A., Finnegan, P., Bishop, J.M.: Effect of intravenous terbutaline on arterial blood gas tensions, ventilation, and pulmonary circulation in patients with chronic bronchitis and cor pulmonale. Thorax *32*, 601–605 (1977)

Szentivanyi, A.: β-adrenergic theory of the atopic abnormality in bronchial asthma. J. Allergy *42*, 203 (1968)

Tadei, A., Geslin, P., Delhumeau, A., Victor, J., Le Douarin, L., Richard, M.: Phentolamine in treatment of acute left ventricular insufficiencies. Arch. Mal. Coeur *68*, 877–885 (1975)

Tai, E., Read, J.: Blood-gas tensions in bronchial asthma. Lancet *1*, 644 (1967a)
Tai, E., Read, J.: Response of blood gas tensions to aminophyline and isoprenaline in patients with asthma. Thorax *22*, 543 (1967b)
Tainter, M.L.: Comparative actions of sympathomimetic compounds phenyl and substituted phenyl derivatives, non-phenylic ring compounds and aliphatic amines. Arch. Int. Pharmacodyn. Ther. *46*, 192–232 (1933)
Tashkin, D.P., Meth, R., Simmons, D.H., Lee, Y.E.: Double-blind comparison of acute bronchial and cardiovascular effects of oral terbutaline and ephedrine. Chest *68*, 155–161 (1975)
Taylor, S.H., Donald, K.W.: The circulatory effects of bretylium tosylate and guanethidine. Lancet *2*, 389–394 (1960)
Townley, R.G., McGeady, S., Bewtra, A.: The effect of beta adrenergic blockage on bronchial sensitivity to acetyl-beta-methacholine in normal and allergic rhinitis subjects. J. Allergy Clin. Immunol. *57*, 358–366 (1976)
Trautlein, J., Allegra, J., Field, J., Gillin, M.: Paradoxic bronchospasm after inhalation of isoproterenol. Chest *70*, 711–714 (1976)
Triner, L., Vulliemoz, Y., Verosky, M.: Cyclic 3′5′-adenosine monophosphate and bronchial tone. Eur. J. Pharmacol. *4*, 37–46 (1977)
U'Prichard, D.C., Bylund, D.B., Snyder, S.H.: (+/−)-(3H)Epinephrine and (−) (3H) dihydroalprenolol binding to beta 1- and beta 2-noradrenergic receptors in brain, heart, and lung membranes. J. Biol. Chem. *253*, 5090–5102 (1978)
Vancrombreucq, J.C., Etien, J.L.: Effect of sotalol on the pulmonary function of cardiac and pulmonary patients. In: Advances in beta-adrenergic blocking therapy. Sotalol. Snart, A.G. (ed.), pp. 33–37. Rome: Excerpta Medica 1974
Van der Straeton, M., Lamont, H., Pauwels, R.: Studies on the effects of MJ-9184-1 in man. Arzneim. Forsch. (Drug Res.) *28*, 1191–1194 (1978)
Vane, J.R.: The release and fate of vasoactive in the pulmonary circulation. Br. J. Pharmacol. *35*, 209–242 (1969)
Van Metre, T.E., Jr.: Possible adverse effects of excessive nebulized isoproterenol in status asthmatics. Trans. Am. Clin. Clinatol. Assoc. *79*, 139 (1968)
Van Metre, T.E., Jr.: Adverse effects of inhalation of excessive amounts of nebulized isoproterenol in status asthmaticus. J. Allergy *43*, 191 (1969)
Wardell, J.R., Jr., Colella, D.F., Shetzline, A., Fowler, P.J.: Studies on carbuterol (SK F 40383-A), a new selective bronchodilator agent. J. Pharmacol. Exp. Ther. *189*, 167–183 (1974)
Weetman, D.F.: A review of the actions and clinical uses of β-adrenoceptor blocking drugs. Drugs Today *7*, 261–305 (1977)
Weissberg, R.M., Marian, J., Bradshaw, J., Alvarez, R.: Differences in pulmonary and cardiovascular beta receptors in the guinea pig and rabbit. J. Pharmacol. Exp. Ther. *202*, 337–345 (1977)
Willey, R.F., Grant, I.W.B.: Effects of oral salbutamol and pirbuterol on FEV_1, heart rate and blood pressure in asthmatics. Br. J. Clin. Pharmacol. *3*, 595–600 (1976)
Williams, J.F., Jr., White, D.H., Jr., Behnke, R.H.: Changes in pulmonary hemodynamics produced by isoproterenol infusion in emphysematous patients. Circulation *28*, 396–401 (1963)
Wilson, W.R., Fisher, F.D., Kirkendall, W.M.: The acute hemodynamic effects of alpha-methyldopa in man. J. Chronic. Dis. *15*, 907–913 (1962)
Zimmerman, H.A.: A study of the pulmonary circulation in man. Dis. Chest *20*, 46–74 (1951)

CHAPTER 2

Effects of Adrenergic Activators and Inhibitors on the Skeletal Muscles

W.C. BOWMAN

A. Introduction

Sympathomimetic amines affect the functioning of skeletal muscles in several different ways and through a number of different peripheral mechanisms and sites of action. Depending to some extent on the species and the conditions of the experiment, they can be shown to influence the extrafusal muscle fibres themselves, the muscle spindles, the process of neuromuscular transmission, and conduction in the motor nerve. The compounds also affect the tone and spontaneous fibrillatory activity of chronically denervated muscles. Even in the same animal, different types of muscle respond differently, and in some muscles the response obtained may differ, at least quantitatively, according to the age of the animal and to the condition of the muscle (that is, whether or not it is fatigued). In addition to the peripheral actions, central noradrenergic and dopaminergic mechanisms play important roles in the control of skeletal muscle function, but central mechanisms are outside the scope of this chapter.

The diversity of peripheral actions led to early confusion in the literature, because attempts were made to attribute the different effects to a common cause. Much of the early literature was referred to in a series of papers by GRUBER (1913, 1914a, b, 1917a, b, 1919, 1922a, b, 1924), and more recent work has been reviewed by GOFFART (1952), BOWMAN and RAPER (1967), and BOWMAN and NOTT (1969). In a recent article, BÜLBRING (1976) engagingly confesses that in the past she and her co-workers had contributed to the confusion by publishing apparently contradictory papers relating to the site of action of adrenaline. However, subsequent events had clearly demonstrated that adrenaline does have multiple sites of action, and she points out "that in the end, after many years of controversy, nobody has been wrong and everybody right."

It has generally been accepted for many years that, with the possible exception of the extraocular muscles, non cardiac striated muscles do not receive a direct sympathetic innervation (see, e.g., reviews by HINES, 1927; HINSEY, 1934; and TIEGS, 1953). Any influence of the sympathetic nervous system on these muscles, other than that which is secondary to vascular changes, is therefore considered to be due to an adrenergic transmitter from the abundant vascular sympathetics which diffuses to the muscle fibres, or to circulating catecholamines released from the adrenal medullae. Drugs whose main action is exerted on adrenergic neurones would therefore not be expected to influence skeletal muscle activity other than through side-effects or toxic effects, and this is found to be so.

The extraocular muscles may be a special case, since, in the cat at least, they take up considerable amounts of noradrenaline and this uptake is reduced after section and degeneration of the postganglionic cervical sympathetic trunk (HERTTING et al., 1961).

Furthermore, adrenaline or stimulation of the cervical sympathetic produces contraction of the superior rectus muscle of the eye, a response which is mediated by α-adrenoceptors (BROWN, 1951; EAKINS and KATZ, 1967; SANGHVI, 1967). It may therefore be that the extraocular muscles are exceptional in that they do receive a direct sympathetic innervation.

This chapter deals with the peripheral effects of sympathomimetic amines and their antagonists on skeletal muscle activity. Adrenergic neurone blocking drugs and other agents that modify adrenergic mechanisms are dealt with only in so far as they produce side-effects on skeletal muscle.

B. Direct Action on Contractions of Nonfatigued Muscles

With few exceptions, notably the extraocular muscles (HESS and PILAR, 1963; BACH-Y-RITA and ITO, 1966), the internal ear muscle and, in some species, the striated muscle of the oesophagus (CSILLIK, 1965) that contain many densely multiply-innervated tonic fibres, mammalian muscles are composed almost entirely of focally-innervated twitch fibres. On both morphological and histochemical grounds, mammalian twitch fibres can be classified into three groups that have been variously termed by different authors. CLOSE (1972) summarises the different properties of the three groups and advances logical reasons for describing them as fast-twitch white fibres, fast-twitch red fibres, and slow-twitch intermediate fibres, a classification originally proposed by BARNARD et al. (1971). Both the red and the intermediate fibres have a high myoglobin content and are therefore red in colour. However, the red fibres resemble the white fibres in their rapid rates of contraction and relaxation, whereas the intermediate fibres are relatively slow in contracting and relaxing. The speed of the muscle as a whole depends on the proportions of the fibre types of which it is composed. Fast-contracting muscles contain a higher proportion of white or red fibres or both, whereas slow-contracting muscles contain a high proportion of intermediate fibres. Fast-twitch white fibres are adapted for short-term powerful phasic activity and predominate in flexor muscles such as the tibialis anterior and the flexor digitorum longus, and in superficial extensor muscles such as the extensor digitorum longus and the gastrocnemius. Fast-twitch red fibres are adapted for sustained phasic activity and predominate in muscles such as the diaphragm. Slow-twitch intermediate fibres are adapated for economical, low-speed, sustained tonic activity. They predominate in deep extensor muscles, such as the soleus and the cruraeus, that are mainly involved in the maintenance of posture. The time from the start of the contraction to peak tension in an isometric twitch of a fast-contracting muscle of a medium sized mammal, such as the cat, is around 20 ms. Slow-contracting limb muscles in the cat have contraction times of around 75 ms. Muscles composed of comparable proportions of fast-contracting and slow-contracting fibres have intermediate contraction speeds. The smaller the animal species, the faster the speeds of contraction of all their muscles, but the ratio of the contraction times for the slowest and the fastest limb muscles is approximately constant at about 3.5:1 for all mammalian species (BULLER, 1970). In the early stages of development, all limb muscles are slow-contracting, and differentiation into fast or slow types occurs over a few weeks, the time from the onset to the completion of the change being shorter in small species than in large ones. In different species, the differentiation takes place at different times during ontogeny; for example, it is mainly prenatal in the guinea pig, mainly postnatal in the rat, and partly prenatal and partly postnatal in the cat (BANU, 1922; DENNY-BROWN, 1929a; BULLER et al., 1960; CLOSE, 1964, 1965a, b, 1972; BULLER and LEWIS, 1965; CLOSE and HOH, 1967). There is clear evidence from definitive experiments, including those in which muscles have been surgically cross-innervated, that differences in the contraction speeds of fast- and slow-contracting muscles are dependent to a large extent on a specific neural influence from the motor nerve that operates throughout life. The nature of the neural influence, whether it be simply the pattern of activation by nerve impulses or some specific trophic chemical elaborated and released by the nerve, has not yet been unequivocally solved. For reviews of the relevant literature, articles by GUTH (1968), BULLER (1970), GUTMANN (1970), and CLOSE (1971, 1972) may be consulted.

The effects of sympathomimetic amines on muscle contractions differ according to the contraction speed of the muscle. The contractions of fast-contracting muscles are increased, whereas those of slow-contracting muscles are decreased. The data in Table 1 are culled partly from the literature and partly from previously unpublished experiments carried out by the author. Where a correlation is possible, the data indicate that an increase in twitch tension produced by adrenaline is associated with a high proportion of fast white or fast red fibres in the muscle, whereas the opposite response is associated with a high proportion of slow intermediate fibres. The pig constitutes a possible exception to this generalisation; thus, Cruickshank and Zaimis (personal communication) were unable to detect any histological difference in the fibre contents of the tibialis anterior and the soleus muscle of this species, yet, as usual, the former muscle is fast-contracting and responded to sympathomimetic amines by an increase in twitch tension, and the soleus muscle is slow-contracting and responded in the opposite way.

I. Fast-Contracting Muscles

In 1895 OLIVER and SCHÄFER showed that extracts of the adrenal medulla increase the tension and the duration of twitches of the nonfatigued gastrocnemius muscle of the anaesthetised dog. Adrenaline was isolated from the adrenal medulla in 1901 (ALDRICH, 1901; TAKAMINE, 1901) but it was not until 1922 that GRUBER (1922a, b) confirmed, with adrenaline, OLIVER and SCHÄFER's earlier work with adrenal medulla extracts. GRUBER also showed that stimulation of the splanchnic nerves to the adrenal medullae produced effects similar to those produced by adrenaline. In the intervening years most attention had been directed towards the effects of adrenaline on fatigued muscles, an action which is briefly described in Sect. G. Since 1922, many workers have confirmed that adrenaline or splanchnic stimulation produces a small increase (10%–20%) in the tension of isometric or partially isometric contractions of nonfatigued fast-contracting mammalian skeletal muscles (GOFFART and BROWN, 1947; WEST and ZAIMIS, 1949; BROWN et al., 1950; GOFFART, 1952; GOFFART and RITCHIE, 1952; HUIDOBRO et al., 1952; BOWMAN and ZAIMIS, 1955, 1958; MONTAGU, 1955; BOWMAN et al., 1962; BOWMAN and RAPER, 1962, 1964a, 1967; JURNA and RUMMEL, 1962; BLECKMAN et al., 1963; JURNA et al., 1963; LEWIS and WEBB, 1976).

In the adult cat, the smallest effective dose of (−)-adrenaline necessary to increase the tension of maximal isometric twitches of the tibialis anterior muscle is of the order of 3 μg/kg intravenously or 0.2 μg close-arterially (BOWMAN and ZAIMIS, 1958; BOW-

Table 1. Fibre composition of, twitch speed of, and effect of adrenaline on some mammalian muscles[a]

Muscle	Approximate % of total number of fibres			Reference to data at left	Mean (±SD) Time to peak Twitch tension (*n*=6 or 7)	Muscle speed	Effect of adrenaline on maximal twitch
	Fast white	Fast red	Slow intermediate				
Cat							
Flexor digitorum longus	41.6	30.4	28.0	OLSON and SWETT (1966)	19.3 (±1.5)	Fast	+
Flexor hallucis longus	50.2	35.8	14.0	OLSON and SWETT (1966)	18.6 (±1.0)	Fast	+
Tibialis anterior	—	—	—	—	20.5 (±1.3)	Fast	+
Medial gastrocnemius	50.9	27.8	21.3	HENNEMAN and OLSON (1965)	21.9 (±1.8)	Fast	+
Soleus	0	0	95–100	GUTH and SAMAHA (1969), HENNEMAN and OLSON (1965), KARPATI and ENGEL (1967), MCPHEDRAN et al. (1965)	76.5 (±2.2)	Slow	—
Cruraeus	—	—	—	—	71.2 (±3.5)	Slow	—
Rabbit							
Tibialis anterior	—	—	—	—	15.9 (±0.7)	Fast	+
Soleus	—	—	—	—	51.0 (±5.2)	Slow	–
Dog (mongrel)							
Tibialis anterior	—	—	—	—	22.7 (±3.4)	Fast	+
Plantaris	—	—	—	—	78.3 (±5.4)	Slow	–
Guinea Pig							
Tibialis anterior	—	—	—	—	16.1 (±0.8)	Fast	+
Flexor digitorum longus	53.8	35.5	10.7	BARNARD et al. (1971)	14.0 (±1.1)	Fast	+
Medial gastrocnemius	38.6	50.2	11.7	BARNARD et al. (1971)	20.1 (±2.2)	Fast	+
Soleus	0	0	100	BARNARD et al. (1971), BROOKE and KAISER (1969)	48.7 (±4.3)	Slow	—
Rat							
Diaphragm (isolated)	20	60	20	GAUTHIER (1969)	21.1 (±2.2)	Fast	+
Tibialis anterior	41	41	·18	KUGELBERG and EDSTRÖM (1968)	15.6 (±2.1)	Fast	+
Extensor digitorum longus	60	45	3.8	EDGERTON and SIMPSON (1969, 1971)	11.9 (±0.9)	Fast	+
Soleus	0	13	85	KARPATI and ENGEL (1967), EDGERTON and SIMPSON (1969), FEX and SONESSON (1970)	38.0 (±3.2)	Slow	–

[a] The data relating to muscle composition are from those compiled by CLOSE (1972). Under "Effect of adrenaline", + indicates increases in peak tension and in twitch duration; – indicates decreases in these parameters. All animals were anaesthetised with α-chloralose to which a small amount of sodium pentobarbitone was added. The resting tension on the muscle was that giving the greatest evoked twitch tension. Muscle temperature was maintained at 36–38 °C.

MAN and RAPER, 1967). After a dose of 10 μg/kg intravenously, the onset of the increase in twitch tension occurs in 20–40 s and reaches its peak in 100–180 s; the whole effect lasts about 15 min. Other fast-contracting muscles of the cat and other mammals listed in Table 1 show a similar sensitivity. In kittens shortly after birth, adrenaline produces effects on the contractions of the tibialis anterior muscle that are qualitatively similar to those produced in the adult, but the effective doses, on a body-weight basis, are 2–3 times larger. The adult sensitivity is reached within 1–2 months after birth (BOWMAN and RAPER, 1962).

The increase in isometric twitch tension produced by adrenaline is associated with proportionate prolongations of the time from the start of each contraction to its peak tension, and of the time from peak tension to half-relaxation (GOFFART and RITCHIE, 1952; BOWMAN and ZAIMIS, 1958; LEWIS and WEBB, 1976), the rate of rise of tension is unaffected (cat tibialis anterior – BOWMAN and ZAIMIS, 1958; rabbit tibialis anterior – BOWMAN and RAPER, 1967; cat flexor digitorum longus – LEWIS and WEBB, 1976) or is initially slightly slowed (rat diaphragm – GOFFART and RITCHIE, 1952). Figure 1 a illustrates the effects of adrenaline on the tension and time course of maximal twitches of the tibialis anterior muscle of a rabbit.

The same effects on the maximal twitches are produced by adrenaline whether the stimulation is applied to the motor nerve or directly to the fully curarized or chronically denervated muscles (GOFFART, 1952; GOFFART and RITCHIE, 1952; BOWMAN and ZAIMIS, 1958; BOWMAN et al., 1962) showing that they are exerted directly on the muscle fibres and are independent of neuromuscular transmission. Results of experiments in which muscle blood flow was recorded simultaneously with the contractions (BOWMAN and ZAIMIS, 1958) and of experiments on isolated muscles (GOFFART, 1947, 1952; GOFFART and BROWN, 1947; GOFFART and RITCHIE, 1952; MONTAGU, 1955; BOWMAN and RAPER, 1964 a) have shown that the effects of adrenaline on contractions are not a consequence of changes in muscle blood flow.

The fact that the twitches are prolonged by adrenaline, as well as increased in tension, means that fusion of responses is increased in incomplete tetanic contractions (Fig. 1 c). The effects on incomplete tetanic contractions are therefore somewhat more pronounced than those on twitches (BOWMAN and ZAIMIS, 1958; BOWMAN et al., 1962; BOWMAN and RAPER, 1967). Maximal tetanic tension is not increased by adrenaline but may be slightly decreased if the concomitant vasoconstriction is intense (GOFFART and RITCHIE, 1952; BOWMAN and ZAIMIS, 1958). The rate of rise of tension in a maximal tetanus is unchanged by adrenaline, but the rate of decline in tension at the end of the tetanus is slowed (JURNA and RUMMEL, 1962; JURNA et al., 1963; LEWIS and WEBB, 1976). In isotonic contractions, the velocity of shortening is also unaffected by adrenaline (LEWIS and WEBB, 1976).

The doses of adrenaline (3 μg/kg i.v.) and the frequency of splanchnic stimulation (20 Hz) necessary to increase the twitch tension of the cat tibialis anterior muscle are high, and BOWMAN and ZAIMIS (1958) concluded that it is unlikely that the effect of adrenaline on fast-contracting muscles has any physiological significance, since the effective blood concentrations are probably in excess of any that occur even under conditions of extreme stress. This conclusion was reached in relation to the effect of adrenaline on peak twitch tension. However, the smallest effective doses of adrenaline affect twitch duration without altering peak isometric tension (BOWMAN and RAPER, 1967), and prolongation of the unit response can itself increase the fusion, and therefore the tension, of incomplete tetanic contractions. In some more recent, unpublished experiments it has been found that single doses of adrenaline around 0.5 μg/kg intravenously or intravenous infusions of 0.25–0.5 $\mu g \cdot kg^{-1} \cdot min^{-1}$ are sufficient to produce a detectable increase in the time from peak tension to half-relaxation, and in the degree of fusion and tension of incomplete tetanic contractions of the cat flexor digitorum longus muscle stimulated at a frequency of 40 Hz for 0.25 s every 20 s. The effects on both twitches and on incomplete tetanic contractions were more clearly evident when the contraction record was electronically integrated with respect to time. A roughly similar effect was produced by stimulation of the left splanchnic nerve at a frequency of 5–10 Hz, which has been estimated to be within the discharge frequency occurring during severe stress (CELANDER, 1954; FOLKOW, 1955). These results must therefore modify the earlier view, since they suggest that adrenaline output from the adrenal medullae may play some part in improving the performance of fast-contracting muscles during severe stress.

Stimulation of the lumbar sympathetic chain for prolonged periods at frequencies up to 20 Hz is without effect on the tension and time course of isometric twitches of the cat tibialis anterior muscle (GOFFART, 1952; BOWMAN and ZAIMIS, 1958); presumably the amount of noradrenaline that is released from the vascular sympathetics and that reaches the skeletal muscle fibres is inadequate to affect their contractility.

II. Slow-Contracting Muscles

BOWMAN and ZAIMIS (1955, 1958) first showed that not all skeletal muscles of the cat are alike in their reaction to the direct effect of adrenaline. In fact, the slow-contracting soleus muscle of the cat was found to react in a completely opposite way to fast-contracting muscles (Fig. 1 b). Thus, adrenaline reduces, by up to 20%–25%, the peak isometric twitch tension, the time from the onset of contraction to peak tension, and the time from peak tension to half-relaxation of the cat soleus muscle. The rate of rise of tension, as in fast-contracting muscles, is unaffected. The smallest effective doses of adrenaline affect the time course of the twitch rather than the peak tension. The effects are independent of neuromuscular transmission, being the same whether the stimulation is applied to the motor nerve or directly to the fully curarized or chronically denervated muscle. Muscle blood flow recording shows that the effect is not a consequence of concomitant vascular changes.

The decrease in the duration of the unit responses produced by adrenaline results in a pronounced decrease in the degree of fusion and therefore of the tension of incomplete tetanic contractions of the cat soleus muscle; any decrese in the peak tension of the unit responses adds to the depressant effects on the tension of the clonic contractions (Fig. 1 d). The depressant effect on incomplete tetanic contractions of the soleus is more striking than the augmenting effect on those of a fast-contracting muscle. At the optimum stimulation frequency for demonstrating the effect on the soleus, the contractions may be depressed by over 60%. The peak tension and the rate of rise of tension of a maximum tetanus of the cat soleus muscle are not affected by adrenaline, but the rate of relaxation on cessation of stimulation is enhanced. In isotonic contractions, the velocity of shortening is unaltered by adrenaline (LEWIS and WEBB, 1976). The results relating to isometric contractions of the cat soleus muscle have been repeatedly confirmed and have been extended to other slow-contracting

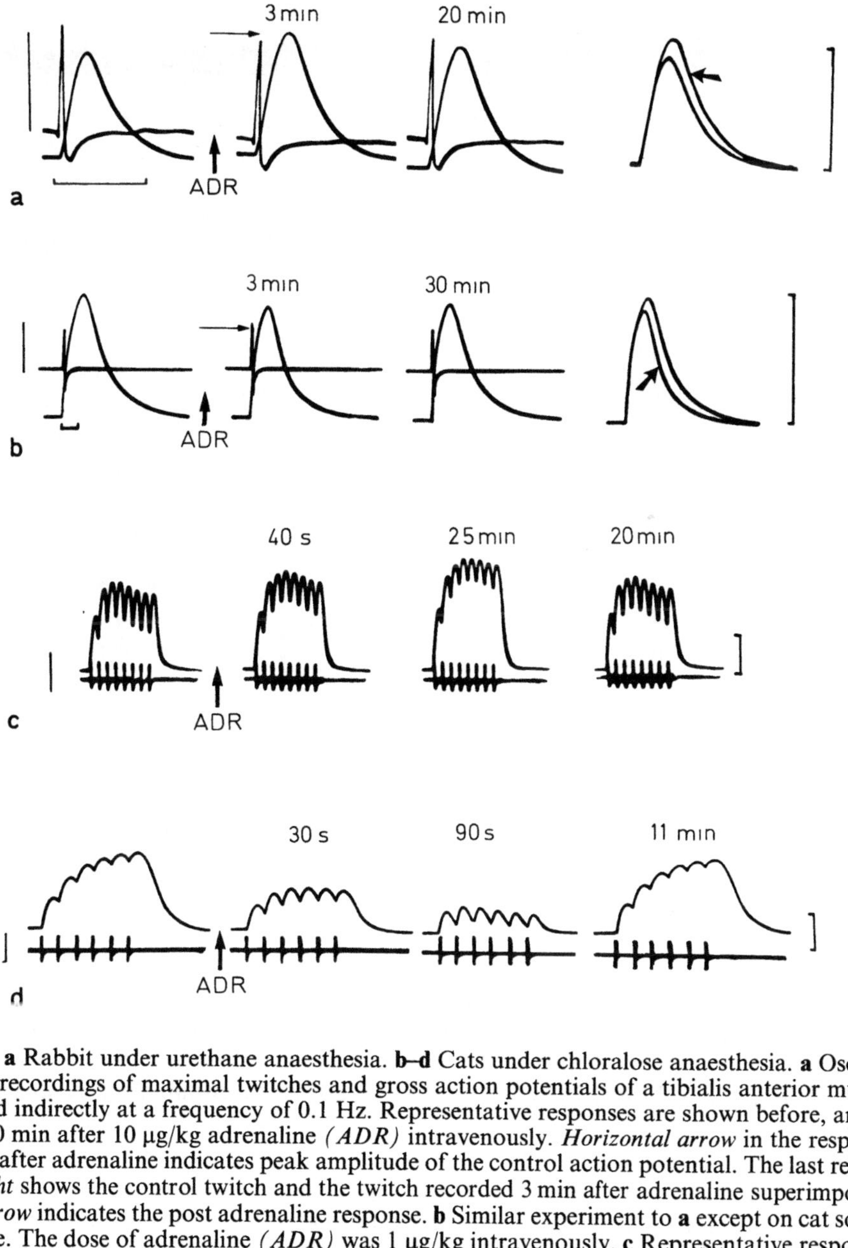

Fig. 1. a Rabbit under urethane anaesthesia. **b–d** Cats under chloralose anaesthesia. **a** Oscilloscope recordings of maximal twitches and gross action potentials of a tibialis anterior muscle elicited indirectly at a frequency of 0.1 Hz. Representative responses are shown before, and 3, and 20 min after 10 μg/kg adrenaline *(ADR)* intravenously. *Horizontal arrow* in the response 3 min after adrenaline indicates peak amplitude of the control action potential. The last record on *right* shows the control twitch and the twitch recorded 3 min after adrenaline superimposed; the *arrow* indicates the post adrenaline response. **b** Similar experiment to **a** except on cat soleus muscle. The dose of adrenaline *(ADR)* was 1 μg/kg intravenously. **c** Representative responses of a tibialis anterior muscle stimulated indirectly at 32 Hz for 0.25 s every 10 s; tension above, gross muscle action potentials below. Responses before, and 40 s, 2.5 min, and 20 min after 8 μg/kg adrenaline *(ADR)* intravenously are shown. **d** Similar experiment to **c** except that soleus muscle was stimulated at 6 Hz for 1 s every 10 s. The dose of adrenaline *(ADR)* was 2 μg/kg intravenously. *Calibrations: vertical lines* on *left* apply to action potentials and are equal to 20 mV; *vertical lines* on *right* apply to contractions and are equal to 5 N; *horizontal lines* below *a* and *b* are each equal to 50 ms. Note that the sweep speed for *a* was much slower than that for *b*. (Composite figure from Bowman et al., 1962; the action potentials shown in *d* had been removed from the original published figure)

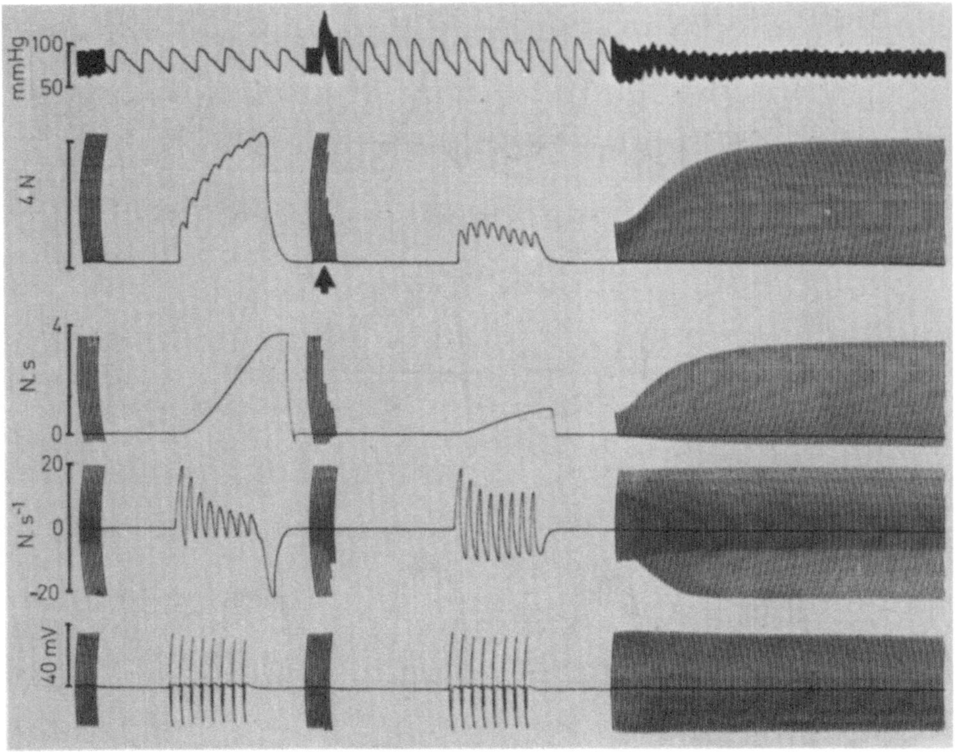

Fig. 2 a–e. Cat under chloralose anaesthesia. Adrenaline (1 µg/kg) was injected intravenously at the *arrow* below the tension record. **a** Arterial blood pressure. **b** Incomplete tetanic contractions of the soleus muscle evoked by stimulating the muscle nerve at a frequency of 8 Hz for 1 s every 10 s (2 contractions were recorded on fast moving paper). **c** Tension-time integral of soleus muscle contractions. **d** Differentiated soleus muscle contractions with respect to time. **e** Gross muscle action potentials

muscles, not only in the cat but also in the other mammals listed in Table 1 (BOWMAN et al., 1962; BOWMAN and RAPER, 1962, 1967; JURNA and RUMMEL, 1962; JURNA et al., 1963; RAPER, 1965; NOTT, 1973; LEWIS and WEBB, 1976; unpublished results of the author).

In unpublished experiments by NOTT, RAPER, and the author, the tension responses of the cat soleus muscle were electronically integrated with respect to time, since this allows more accurate determinations of minimal effective doses. The type of record obtained is illustrated in Fig. 2. The smallest effective doses of adrenaline necessary to decrease the tension-time integral of incomplete tetanic contractions recorded under the optimal conditions described by BOWMAN and NOTT (1970) were around 0.002 µg close-arterially, 0.04 µg/kg intravenously, or 0.02 $\mu g \cdot kg^{-1} \cdot min^{-1}$ as an intravenous infusion. After an intravenous dose of 1 µg/kg, the onset of the effect on the cat soleus muscle occurs in 20–40 s and reaches its peak in 60–100 s; the whole effect lasts about 12 min. The effects on peripherally evoked muscle contractions always outlast the cardiovascular changes, presumably because reflex compensatory mechanisms play no part in recovery from the muscle effects.

Stimulation of the lumbar sympathetic chain of the cat at frequencies up to 20 Hz for several minutes is without effect on soleus muscle contractions. BOWMAN and ZAIMIS (1958) did record a slight effect in one out of five cats, but in many subsequent experiments in which the adrenals were excluded from the circulation, no effect was produced by lumbar sympathetic stimulation on soleus muscle contractions. With the adrenals intact, stimulation of the left splanchnic nerve at frequencies of 10 or 20 Hz was effective in decreasing soleus muscle contractions in the experiments of BOWMAN and ZAIMIS (1958), and in more recent experiments stimulation at frequencies as low as 1–2 Hz has produced an obvious effect. Stimulation at frequencies of 10–20 Hz produced effects equivalent to the maximum obtainable with injected adrenaline (i.e., with 2–3 μg/kg intravenously).

The concentration of catecholamines reflexly released from the adrenal medullae in response to hypoxia induced by occluding the trachea for 10–20 s, or in response to the depressor effects produced by small doses (0.5 μg/kg i.v.) of methacholine or histamine, are sufficient to produce a clear depressant effect on incomplete tetanic contractions of the cat soleus muscle. A similar effect is produced by pressor doses of nicotine or dimethylphenylpiperazinium. These reflex effects, and the effects of nicotinic stimulants are abolished by excluding the adrenal glands from the circulation (NOTT, unpublished experiments).

Slow-contracting adult muscles are thus considerably more sensitive to the action of adrenaline than are fast-contracting muscles, and there seems little doubt that the effects of adrenaline on these muscles reflect some physiological role, especially in view of the fact that the optimum frequency of soleus muscle stimulation for demonstrating the effects (i.e., around 10 Hz at the optimal resting muscle length; BOWMAN and NOTT, 1970) is within the range at which soleus motoneurones fire in maintaining postural tone (DENNY-BROWN, 1929 b). However, the nature of the survival value, assuming the effect to be advantageous to the organism, is not obvious. In a voluntary contraction, the various muscle units within a muscle contract asynchronously and intermittently at subtetanic frequencies, but the pattern of activity is so integrated at central level that the algebraic sum of the contractions and relaxations of the units gives an almost smooth contraction of the whole muscle. Possibly, as was suggested by BOWMAN and ZAIMIS (1958), in a mixed muscle, a decrease in the duration of slow motor unit responses, perhaps coupled with an increase in the duration of fast motor unit responses, can improve muscle performance by increasing the synchrony of the contractions. Any reduction in the degree of fusion should then presumably be counteracted by reflex adjustment of the firing frequency.

On the other hand, the feeling of weakness in the back and knees and the tremor associated with sudden extreme fright and anxiety are well known. That these effects are produced in man by adrenaline infusions was demonstrated by BARCROFT and SWAN (1953); they are also associated with phaeochromocytoma (PICKERING, 1955). It is possible that the postural weakness is the result of abruptly produced high concentrations of adrenal medullary adrenaline acting on the slow-contracting units in the postural muscles (BOWMAN and ZAIMIS, 1958). Furthermore, in a mixed muscle, a marked decrease in fusion of the slow-contracting units produced by a sudden high concentration of adrenaline might disorganise the integrated contraction in such a way that it contributes to the characteristic coarse tremor of the extremities. It seems likely that effects on the muscle spindles also contribute to this effect, which is discussed in Sect. D.II.

In kittens, a few days after birth, the effects of adrenaline on soleus muscle contractions are variable and unpronounced, and require large doses to elicit them. The sensitivity and type of response characteristic of the adult muscle is gained at about the age of 1 month (BOWMAN and RAPER, 1962).

III. Other Sympathomimetic Amines and Adrenoceptor Blocking Drugs

(−)-Noradrenaline is considerably less potent than (−)-adrenaline in its actions on both fast-contracting and slow-contracting muscles, whereas isoprenaline is somewhat more potent (WEST and ZAIMIS, 1949; BROWN et al., 1950; GOFFART, 1952, 1954; HUIDOBRO et al., 1952; BOWMAN and ZAIMIS, 1955, 1958; BOWMAN et al., 1962; BOWMAN and RAPER, 1964a; WALDECK, 1977; HOLMBERG and WALDECK, 1977). In earlier work, relative potency determinations were usually made on the basis of the doses necessary to affect peak twitch tension. Since the maximum change in twitch tension is small, such determinations are difficult to make accurately. More recently, NOTT (1973) compared the doses necessary to alter the tension-time integral of the contractions; a parameter which can be more accurately measured and which is affected by a wider range of doses. He found in the cat that, at threshold level, (−)-noradrenaline was about 10 times less potent than (−)-adrenaline in increasing the tension-time integral of twitches of the tibialis anterior muscle, and about 250 times less potent than (−)-adrenaline in decreasing the tension-time integral of the soleus muscle. Although the potency of noradrenaline is always low, the relative potency of adrenaline and noradrenaline tends to vary widely in different cats, presumably at least partly according to the efficiency of the inactivating mechanisms, including the uptake processes. Relative potencies of synthetic compounds are generally more constant from animal to animal. The relative inactivity of noradrenaline accounts for the fact that stimulation of the lumbar sympathetic chain, even at high frequencies, is without effect on the contractions of nonfatigued muscles.

Several other sympathomimetic amines, especially those that are used as bronchodilators, have been tested on skeletal muscles of the cat. In most cases, the soleus muscle has been studied because the effect on this muscle is believed to reflect the tremorgenic effect that sympathomimetic bronchodilators often produce as an unwanted side-effect in man (see Subsect. D.II.1). The abilities of the compounds to decrease tension and fusion of incomplete tetanic contractions of the soleus muscle have usually been measured and compared with the effects of isoprenaline or its more potent laevoisomer [(−)-isoprenaline, laevoisoprenaline]. The approximate relative potencies of a range of sympathomimetic amines compared with laevoisoprenaline on the cat soleus muscle are summarised in Table 2, which includes references to the original work. The structures of most of the compounds included are given in Fig. 3. Long-acting sympathomimetic amines can be conveniently compared by injecting the doses cumulatively and constructing cumulative log dose-response curves (NOTT and RAPER, 1972). Some of the newer drugs have also been tested on the soleus muscle of the anaesthetised guinea pig (APPERLEY and LEVY, 1975; BOHMER and RAPER, 1976, 1977; BOHMER and O'DONNELL, 1977); results essentially similar to those produced in the cat were obtained.

TASHIRO (1973) showed that isoprenaline produces its characteristic effects on the isometric twitches of the isolated extensor digitorum longus and soleus muscles of the

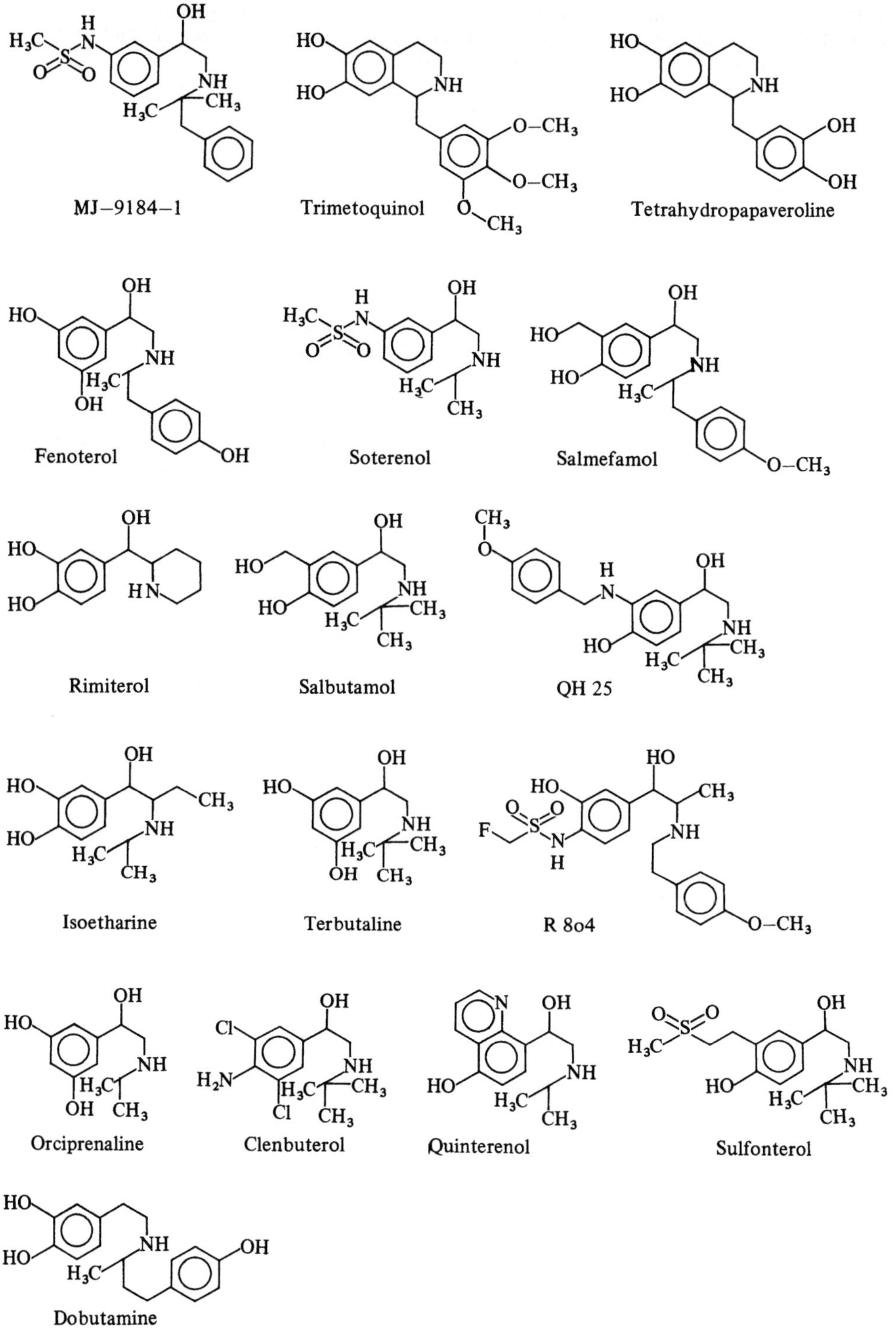

Fig. 3. Structures of some of the sympathomimetic amines referred to in the text and in Table 2

Table 2. Approximate intravenous dose ratios (molar basis; laevoisoprenaline = 1) of some sympathomimetic amines with respect to their effect in decreasing tension and fusion of incomplete tetanic contractions of the cat soleus muscle

Sympathomimetic amines	Approximate molar dose ratio (i.v.)	References
Laevoisoprenaline	1 (0.04 μg/kg i.v.)	
MJ 9184-1	1.5	GWEE et al. (1972)
(±)-Isoprenaline	1.8	RODGER (1973)
Trimetoquinol	2	HOUSTON and RODGER (1974); APPERLEY et al. (1976)
Fenoterol	2	APPERLEY et al. (1976)
Soterenol	6	APPERLEY et al. (1976)
Salmefamol	7	APPERLEY et al. (1976)
Rimiterol	7	BOWMAN and RODGER (1972)
(−)-Adrenaline	7.5	BOWMAN and NOTT (1978)
Salbutamol	8	BOWMAN and NOTT (1970), APPERLEY and DALY (1972), BOWMAN and RODGER (1972), APPERLEY et al. (1976), von ENGELHARDT (1976)
QH 25	9	LARSEN and HERMANSEN (1977)
Isoetharine	11	RODGER (1973)
Terbutaline	20	RODGER (1974), APPERLEY et al. (1976), MALTA and RAPER (1976)
R 804	26	RODGER (1974)
Clenbuterol	30	von ENGELHARDT (1976)
Quinterenol	35	BOWMAN and NOTT (1970)
Tetrahydropapaveroline	36	NOTT and HEAD (1978)
Sulfonterol	38	KAISER et al. (1975)
Orciprenaline	50	BOWMAN and NOTT (1970), APPERLEY and DALY (1972), ZAIMIS (1973), APPERLEY et al. (1976), MALTA and RAPER (1976)
(−)-Noradrenaline	1,000	BOWMAN and NOTT (1978), NOTT (1973)
Dobutamine	3,000	RODGER, I.W. (personal communication)
Dopamine	4,600	BOWMAN and NOTT (1978)

The dose in μg/kg given for laevoisoprenaline is the approximate dose producing 50% of the maximum effect. On the cat soleus muscle, the dose response curves for the above drugs are parallel and the drugs are full agonists. The approximate relative molar potencies of the drugs compared with laevoisoprenaline are the reciprocals of the dose ratios in the Table. Information about the time courses of the drug effects is given in the references quoted. The structures of many of the drugs are given in Fig. 3

guinea pig studied in vitro (Fig. 4a), thus providing further evidence that the effects are independent of blood flow changes. TASHIRO found that whereas isoprenaline characteristically decreased the tension of soleus muscle twitches evoked by stimulation with narrow pulse widths (0.5 ms or 1 ms), it slightly increased the tension when wide pulse widths (5 ms or 10 ms) were used. Since the wide pulse widths must greatly exceed the refractory period of the muscle fibres, the contractions evoked by them were presumably brief high-frequency tetani rather than true twitches, but it is not clear why isoprenaline should increase their tension: in vivo, isoprenaline is without effect on maximal tetanic tension. Whatever the parameters of the stimuli, TASHIRO found that isoprenaline always increased the time to peak and to half-relaxation of

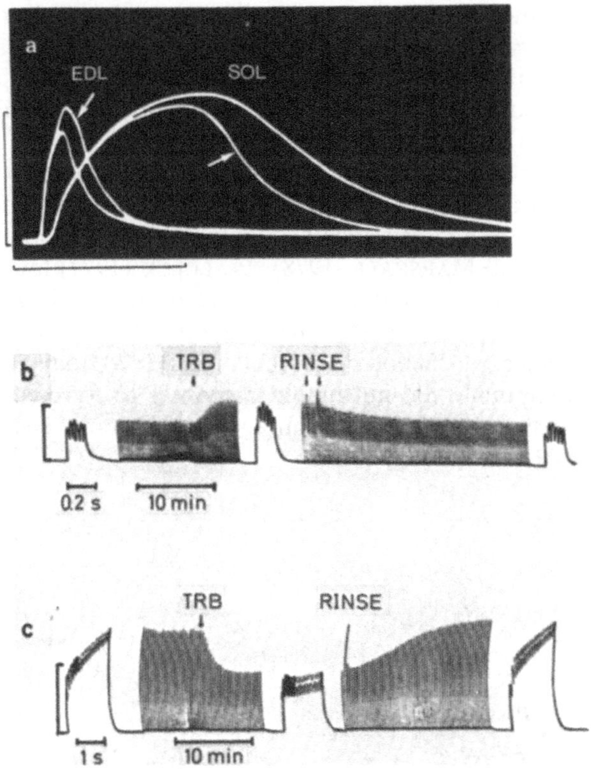

Fig. 4 a–c. Isolated muscles of the guinea pig. **a** Effects of isoprenaline (at 33 °C) on the extensor digitorum longus muscle *(EDL)* and soleus muscle *(SOL)*. Superimposed oscilloscope records of twitches elicited by 1 ms pulses before and 20 min after the application of 1 μg/ml of isoprenaline. *Arrows* indicate the response after isoprenaline in each case. *Calibrations: vertical line,* 0.1 N for *EDL,* 0.05 N for SOL; *horizontal line,* 50 ms (Part of a figure from TASHIRO, 1973). **b** Effect of terbutaline (*TRB,* 0.57 μg/ml) on incomplete tetanic contractions of the extensor digitorum longus muscle (40 Hz for 150 ms every 15 s). Tension calibration, 0.1 N (from HOLMBERG and WALDECK, 1977). **c** Effects of terbutaline (0.57 μg/ml) on incomplete tetanic contractions of the soleus muscle (14 Hz for 1.5 s every 22 s). Tension calibration, 0.05 N. In **b** and **c**, 3 contractions have been spread out on faster moving paper. (From WALDECK, 1976)

the extensor digitorum longus muscle, and decreased these values in the soleus muscle. WALDECK (1976, 1977, 1979), HOLMBERG et al. (1977), HOLMBERG and WALDECK (1977), and AL-JEBOORY and MARSHALL (1978) also experimented on the isolated guinea pig soleus and extensor digitorum longus muscles, and showed that they could be used to demonstrate the effects of sympathomimetic amines on incomplete tetanic contractions (Fig. 4 b, c).

In recent years, relatively few experiments with sympathomimetic bronchodilators have been carried out on fast-contracting muscles. However, salbutamol (NOTT, 1973) and rimiterol (unpublished experiments) have been examined on the tibialis anterior of the cat; on a molar basis, each was found to be 4–6 times less potent than (−)-isoprenaline in increasing the tension of incomplete tetanic contractions. HOLMBERG and

WALDECK (1977) studied the effect of terbutaline on the isolated extensor digitorum longus muscle of the guinea pig. They found it to be about 15 times less potent than racemic isoprenaline in increasing the incomplete tetanic contractions. In the same preparation, AL-JEBOORY and MARSHALL (1978) found salbutamol to be about six times less potent than racemic isoprenaline.

Although the isolated muscles of the guinea pig respond well to non-selective adrenoceptor agonists or to selective β_2-adrenoceptor agonists, they fail to respond to selective β_1-adrenoceptor agonists such as tazolol, H 80/62 (WALDECK, 1977), or H 133/22 (AL-JEBOORY and MARSHALL, 1978). WALDECK (1977) found that, although they are without effect per se, both tazolol and H 80/62 inhibited responses to subsequently applied β_2-receptor agonists. The compound H 80/62 is a racemate, and H 133/22 is its (−)-isomer. AL-JEBOORY and MARSHALL (1978) found that H 133/22, unlike the racemic compound, did not inhibit responses to β_2-receptor agonists; they therefore concluded that the whole of the antagonistic action of H 80/62 (and possibly of tazolol also) resides in the (+)-isomer.

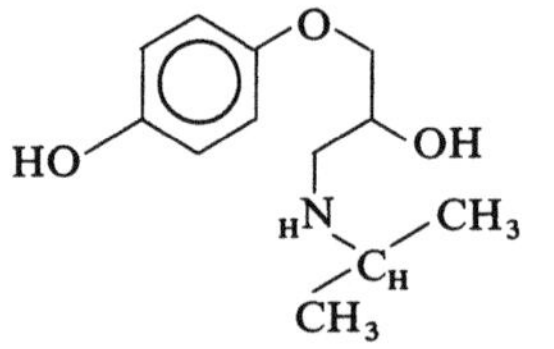

H 133/22 (H 80/62 is the racemate)

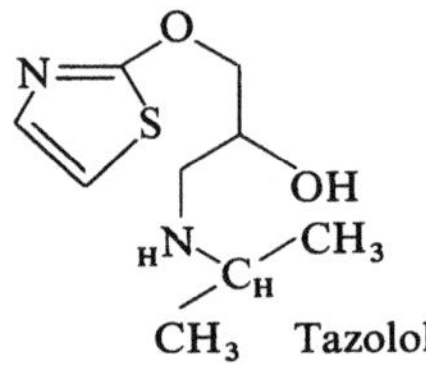

Tazolol

AL-JEBOORY and MARSHALL (1978) found that racemic isoprenaline and salbutamol (which is also a racemate) produced smaller maximal responses in isolated guinea pig muscle than did laevoisoprenaline. They concluded that, at least in the case of isoprenaline, the (+)-isomer exerts β_2-receptor blocking activity. Although they did not interpret it in this way, the evidence of HOLMBERG and WALDECK (1977) is compatible with the same explanation, for they found that the racemic compounds terbutaline and (±)-isoprenaline produced smaller maximal effects than did the (−)-isomers of adrenaline or noradrenaline. A blocking action of the nonagonist isomer [usually the (+)-isomer] in a racemate puts in doubt some of the reports that some sympathomimetic bronchodilators behave as partial agonists in some guinea pig tissues, and the whole question therefore requires to be re-examined. The problem does not appear to be relevant to cat tissues, for although differing in potency, racemic isoprenaline and other racemic compounds, produce the same maximal responses as do laevoisoprenaline and (−)-adrenaline in the cat (for references see Table 2), indicating that the (+)-isomers have neither agonistic nor antagonistic activity in this species.

The direct effects of sympathomimetic amines on the nonfatigued contractions of both fast- and slow-contracting muscles of cats and guinea pigs are unaffected or even enhanced by α-adrenoceptor blocking drugs, such as ergotoxine, ergotamine, tolazoline, 933 F, dibenamine, phenoxybenzamine and phentolamine (BROWN et al., 1950; GOFFART, 1952; BOWMAN and ZAIMIS, 1958; WALDECK, 1977; HOLMBERG and WALDECK, 1977). They are blocked by the β-receptor blocking drugs dichloroisoprenaline, pronethalol, propranolol, H 56/28, H 35/25, methoxamine, and butoxamine, but not by practolol or atenolol in doses that abolish the effects of sympathomimetics on the heart (BOWMAN and RAPER, 1964a, 1967; BOWMAN and NOTT, 1969, 1970, and unpublished observations; APPERLEY and DALY, 1972; TASHIRO, 1973; APPERLEY and LEVY, 1975; APPERLEY et al., 1976; BOHMER and RAPER, 1976; WALDECK, 1977; HOLMBERG and WALDECK, 1977; AL-JEBOORY and MARSHALL, 1978).

IV. Adrenoceptors

The observations described above with agonists and antagonists make it clear that the adrenoceptors that mediate the direct effects on contractility in nonfatigued muscles of fast- and slow-contracting types belong to the β_2 subclassification as defined by LANDS et al. (1967). Several workers have previously reached this same conclusion (BOWMAN and NOTT, 1969, 1970; BRITTAIN et al., 1970; APPERLEY and DALY, 1972; BOWMAN and RAPER, 1976; APPERLEY et al., 1976; BOHMER and RAPER, 1976; WALDECK, 1977; HOLMBERG and WALDECK, 1977; AL-JEBOORY and MARSHALL, 1978). In general it appears that whereas β_1-adrenoceptors (e.g., in the heart) are usually directly innervated by noradrenergic fibres, β_2-adrenoceptors (e.g., in blood vessels and the airways), which in most species are characteristically insensitive to noradrenaline, do not usually receive a direct innervation, and respond physiologically only to adrenaline released from the adrenal medullae. Thus, for example, the sympathetic noradrenergic fibres to blood vessels impinge on α-adrenoceptors which mediate vasoconstriction, and any sympathetic vasodilator fibres are usually cholinergic. The smooth muscle of the airways contains β_2-adrenoceptors, but evidence is accumulating to show that the sympathetic noradrenergic fibres end, not on the smooth muscle cells, but rather on the parasympathetic neuronal plexus where they act by a mechanism resembling presynaptic inhibition to inhibit parasympathetic constrictor tone (see, for example, KOELLE, 1975). The observation that the skeletal muscle β-adrenoceptors are of the β_2 type is thus compatible with the absence of a sympathetic innervation of this tissue and with the lack of effect of lumbar sympathetic stimulation, but with the pronounced effect of splanchnic stimulation.

Relative lack of responsiveness to noradrenaline is one of the characteristics of the β_2-adrenoceptors; this is so in both fast- and slow-contracting skeletal muscles. The smallest effective doses of noradrenaline are large and about equal in size in both types of muscle. However, the effective doses of (−)-isoprenaline or adrenaline are not the same in the two types of muscle, being much smaller in slow-contracting than in fast-contracting muscles in vivo; this accounts for the relative potencies [(−)-isoprenaline:noradrenaline] of 1:60 for the cat tibialis anterior and 1:1,000 for the cat soleus muscle (Table 2). ÅBLAD et al. (1975) presented evidence that while the majority of cardiac β-receptors are of the β_1 type, there is a small proportion of β_2-receptors also present. Furthermore, the proportion of β_2-receptors appears to differ in the hearts of different species, with the result that the relative activity of selective β_2-receptor agonists compared with that of isoprenaline differs from species to species. A similar explanation involving different proportions of β_1-receptors might account for the widely different relative potencies of isoprenaline to noradrenaline in fast- and slow-contracting muscles. However, if any β_1-receptors are present in skeletal muscle, the proportion must be very small and similar in size in the two types of muscle, since the same large doses of noradrenaline are required to affect the evoked tension. A more likely explanation appears to be that there are no β_1-receptors present, and the weak action of noradrenaline simply reflects its relative inactivity on β_2-receptors. The different ratios of effectiveness of isoprenaline to noradrenaline in the two types of muscle may then indicate different efficacies, different numbers of β_2-receptors, or different types of isoreceptor within the broad β_2-receptor classification.

Surprisingly, although they had found a similar difference in ratios of effectiveness between fast- and slow-contracting muscles in the cat and the guinea pig in vivo, Holmberg and Waldeck (1977) and Holmberg et al. (1977) found that the difference in sensitivity between the two types of muscle of the guinea pig disappeared when the contractions were recorded in vitro. Al-Jeboory and Marshall (1978), however, were unable to confirm this observation. They found that the isolated guinea pig soleus in vitro remained much more sensitive than the extensor digitorum longus muscle under the same conditions.

V. Electrical and Ionic Changes

1. Resting Membrane Potential

Brown et al. (1950) showed that isoprenaline, adrenaline, and noradrenaline consistently produced a small increase in the demarcation potential recorded between an injured and an uninjured part of the tibialis anterior muscle of the cat. Bowman and Raper (1965, 1966) confirmed this observation and also showed that a similar effect occurred in the slow-contracting soleus muscle of the cat even though the contractions of the two muscles are affected in opposite ways by the same compounds. They further showed (Raper and Bowman, 1968) that the demarcation potential of the gastrocnemius muscle of the domestic fowl was increased by the sympathomimetic amines, yet the contractions of this muscle were not directly affected.

In cat muscles, the changes in the tensions of the twitches matched, in their time course, the changes in demarcation potential. Isoprenaline was the most potent and noradrenaline the least potent in both respects. Brown et al. (1950) found that the increase in demarcation potential that they recorded in the tibialis anterior muscle was followed by a decrease of longer duration and greater magnitude. They also found that a small secondary decrease in twitch tension followed the initial augmentation. Tachyphylaxis was evident both in the electrical response and in the twitch tension response when injections were made at intervals of less than an hour. Secondary changes in twitch tension and demarcation potential were not evident in the experiments of Bowman and Raper (1965, 1966), who used smaller doses of the catecholamines; nor was tachyphylaxis a feature of the responses.

Brown et al. (1950), Bowman and Raper (1965, 1966), and Raper and Bowman (1968) interpreted the increases in demarcation potential that they recorded as evidence of hyperpolarization of the muscle fibre membranes.

Krnjević and Miledi (1958), who recorded from single muscle fibres of the isolated diaphragm of the rat and of the gracilis muscle of the anaesthetised rat with intracellular microelectrodes, were unable to detect any significant effect of adrenaline on the resting membrane potential. Bray et al. (1976) obtained similar negative results with adrenaline, noradrenaline, and isoprenaline in the innervated isolated rat diaphragm preparation. More recently, Lewis et al. (1977) failed to record any significant effect of adrenaline on the resting membrane potentials of fibres of the flexor digitorum longus or the soleus muscles of cats under pentobarbitone sodium anaesthesia. In the experiments of LEWIS et al., the pre-adrenaline control measurements and the measurements after adrenaline were made from different muscle fibres, and, since any hyperpolarization is likely to be small, it is possible that it was undetectable within the range of resting membrane potentials in a population of fibres.

It seems likely that a small degree of hyperpolarization is in fact produced. This was clearly evident in responses to adrenaline and isoprenaline in the experiments of KUBA (1970), who recorded intracellularly from the endplate regions of fibres of the isolated diaphragm of the rat (Fig. 11); also, in response to adrenaline in the experiments of KENDIG and BUNKER (1972), who recorded intracellularly from the gastrocnemius muscle of the anaesthetised rat; in response to isoprenaline in the experiments of TASHIRO (1973), who recorded intracellularly from fibres of the isolated flexor digitorum longus and soleus muscles of the guinea pig; in response to isoprenaline in the experiments of SMITH and THESLEFF (1976), who recorded intracellularly from fibres of the isolated diaphragm of the rat; in response to adrenaline or noradrenaline in the experiments of CLAUSEN and FLATMAN (1977), who recorded intracellularly from isolated rat soleus muscles; and finally, in response to adrenaline or salbutamol in further experiments by the last named authors (personal communication), who recorded intracellularly from the soleus muscle of the anaesthetised rat. Furthermore, DOCKRY et al. (1966) provided circumstantial evidence of a hyperpolarizing action of isoprenaline on rat soleus muscle fibres; the depressant action of catecholamines on neuromuscular transmission (described later) is difficult to explain other than by a postjunctional hyperpolarizing action. It is difficult therefore to account for the absence of this effect in the experiments of some authors, although it appears from the literature that the occurrence of hyperpolarization may be influenced by the composition of the bathing fluid for in vitro experiments (BRESSLER et al., 1975), or the anaesthetic used for in vivo experiments (KENDIG and BUNKER, 1972; and see Sect. B.VI); factors of this type might have played a part.

Huge concentrations of noradrenaline (10^{-2} *M;* 1.5 mg/ml) have been shown to produce hyperpolarization of frog sartorius muscle fibre membranes bathed in normal (K^+, 2.5 m*M*) Ringer's solution, to be without effect in K^+-free solution, and to produce depolarization in high K^+ (7 m*M*) solution (BRESSLER et al., 1975). The observations thus provide further evidence of a hyperpolarizing action of catecholamines at normal potassium ion concentrations, although it is not clear why such large concentrations of noradrenaline were used nor whether they were in fact necessary. KENDIG and BUNKER (1972) provided evidence consistent with the view that in mammalian muscle (rat gastrocnemius) physiological concentrations of catecholamines exert a tonic effect in maintaining the resting membrane potential, and a detailed analysis by CLAUSEN and FLATMAN (1977) supports this view (rat soleus).

GOFFART and PERRY (1951) showed that in cat fast-contracting muscle preloaded with $^{42}K^+$, isoprenaline, adrenaline and noradrenaline produced an initial decrease followed by an increase in potassium loss. These changes parallelled the changes in demarcation potential and twitch tension produced in the experiments of BROWN et al. (1950). The initial decrease in K^+ efflux matched, in its time course, the increase in twitch tension, and since the latter effect is the only one produced by lower doses of adrenaline, the decrease in K^+ efflux is presumably the more relevant effect. CLAUSEN and FLATMAN (1977) suggest that the inhibitory effect of the amines on the washout of isotopic K^+, as reported by GOFFART and PERRY (1951), does not necessarily indicate a direct effect on K^+ efflux. Because of the diffusional delay in the washout of labelled K^+, stimulation of K^+ influx might give rise to reaccumulation of $^{42}K^+$ that had been released into the interstitial space, so that less would gain access to the perfusion fluid in which it was measured. Several workers, among them VICK et al. (1972), HAYS et al. (1974), COSTIN et al. (1976), and CLAUSEN and FLATMAN (1977) have in fact shown that catecholamines increase K^+ uptake into skeletal muscle. According to COSTIN et al. (1976), this effect is several times greater shortly after contraction than in a muscle remaining at rest.

The resting membrane potential of skeletal muscle has a cardiac glycoside-sensitive component (LOCKE and SOLOMON, 1967; BOLTE and LÜDERITZ, 1969; SOMLYO and SOMLYO, 1969; TASHIRO, 1973, HAYS et al., 1974; CLAUSEN and FLATMAN, 1977; CLAUSEN and HANSEN, 1977; see also the results on chronically denervated muscle of SMITH and THESLEFF, 1976; described under Sect. E.II) which is the result of electrogenic activity of the Na^+–K^+ pump (CLAUSEN and FLATMAN, 1977). The magnitude of the electrogenic component differs in different muscles. The cardiac glycoside-sensitive electrogenic component of the Na^+–K^+ pump is stimulated by catecholamines (DOCKRY et al., 1966; TASHIRO, 1973; HAYS et al., 1974; BRESSLER et al., 1975; CLAUSEN and FLATMAN, 1977; CLAUSEN and HANSEN, 1977) and some other agents (e.g., chloride-deficiency – TASHIRO, 1973; insulin and veratrine – CLAUSEN and HANSEN, 1977). Stimulation of the electrogenic component of the pump by catecholamines increases Na^+ efflux to a greater extent than K^+ influx (CLAUSEN and FLATMAN, 1977), and is responsible for hyperpolarizing the membrane. Stimulation of the pump enhances the rate of ouabain binding without increasing the total number of ouabain binding sites, thus further suggesting that the hyperpolarizing action of catecholamines is the result of stimulation of Na^+–K^+-activated ATPase in the plasma membrane (CLAUSEN and HANSEN, 1977).

The stimulant action of sympathomimetic amines on the membrane Na^+–K^+ pump and the consequent hyperpolarizing action exhibit the characteristics of effects mediated by β-adrenoceptors in that isoprenaline is more potent than adrenaline, and noradrenaline is the least potent, and the effect is blocked by propranolol but not by α-adrenoceptor blocking drugs (see BOWMAN and NOTT, 1969 for review, and the more recent references quoted above). CLAUSEN and FLATMAN (1980) have extended the observations to show that, like the receptors that mediate the changes in evoked contractions, those that mediate stimulation of the Na^+–K^+ pump can be further subclassified as belonging to the β_2 subgroup. Thus, the specific β_2-receptor agonist salbutamol was potent in stimulating the pump and producing hyperpolarization of rat soleus muscle fibres, and adrenaline was at least 100 times more potent than the specific β_1-receptor agonist H 133/22. The nonspecific β-receptor blocking drug propranolol was at least 10 times more potent than the relatively selective β_1-receptor antagonist metoprolol in blocking the action of adrenaline.

COSTIN et al. (1976) suggest that the effect of propranolol in blocking the action of adrenaline on pump activity, especially after exercise, may be the basis of the muscle fatigue associated with propranolol therapy.

2. Action Potentials

The decreases in the twitch or incomplete tetanic tensions of the cat soleus muscle produced by catecholamines are associated with slight increases in the amplitudes of the

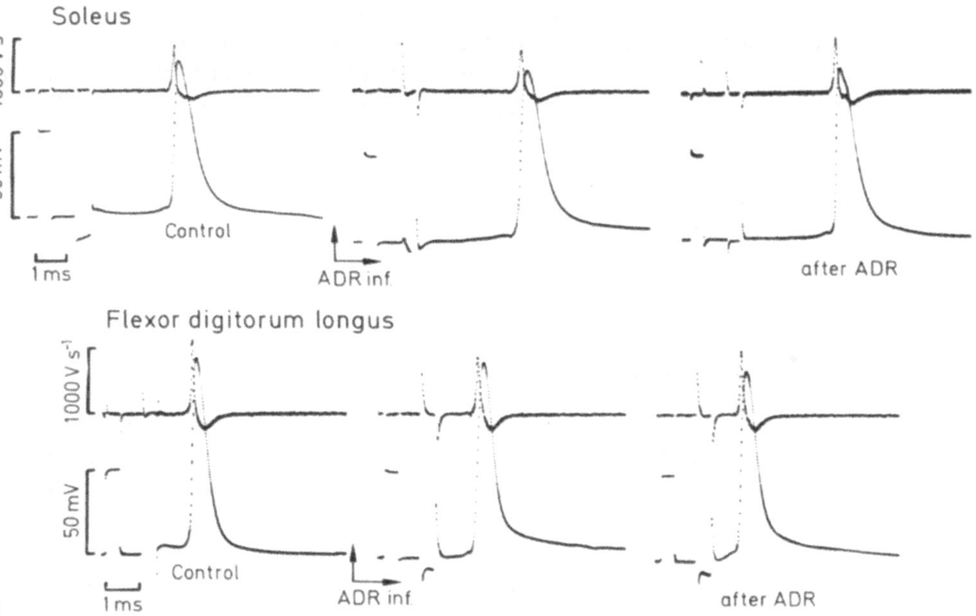

a

b	Control	FDL ADR 5 µg · kg⁻¹ · min⁻¹	Post-ADR control	Control	Soleus ADR 1 µg · kg⁻¹ · min⁻¹	Post-ADR control
No. of fibres	118	111	98	129	90	90
Resting potential (mv)	84.0 (0.79)	82.0 (0.65)	83.9 (0.81)	82.9 (0.49)	79.3 (0.83)	77.1 (0.64)
Overshoot (mv)	33.1 (0.86)	33.9 (0.81)	34.4 (0.95)	20.2 (0.57)	23.3 (0.95)	21.7 (0.88)
Tine above 0 mv (µs)	382.7 (0.91)	442.9 (0.61)	422.5 (0.68)	457.7 (0.51)	476.5 (0.82)	453.5 (0.80)
Time above −50 mv (µs)	807.6 (1.69)	866.3 (0.93)	834.6 (1.23)	1066.1 (0.95)	1156.4 (1.75)	1085.7 (1.24)
Time to peak (µs)	382.1 (0.65)	397.5 (0.55)	375.4 (0.64)	507.2 (0.79)	464.9 (0.76)	432.2 (1.18)
Rate of rise ($v.s.^{-1}$)	1062.2 (18.5)	912.8 (19.4)	976.1 (22.8)	630.1 (9.8)	622.5 (16.5)	719.1 (18.5)

Figures in brackets are s.e. mean.

Fig. 5a. Small bundles of fibres in the soleus and flexor digitorum longus muscles of cats under sodium pentobarbitone anaesthesia were stimulated with concentric needle electrodes before, during, and 1–1.5 h after a 40 min intravenous infusion of adrenaline (1 µg · kg^{-1} · min^{-1}) for soleus and 5 µg · kg^{-1} · min^{-1} for FDL). Representative intracellularly recorded action potentials shown with corresponding first differentials. (Lewis, D.M., Pardoe, M.J., and Webb, S.N.). **b** Measured parameters from experiments on 4 soleus muscles and on 4 flexor digitorum longus muscles (Lewis et al., 1977)

compound gross muscle action potentials recorded with belly-tendon leads, whereas the increases in contractility produced in the tibialis anterior muscle are associated with slight diminutions in the gross muscle action potentials (Goffart, 1952; Bowman et al., 1962; and see Fig. 1). The explanation of these opposite effects is not clear. Brown et al. (1947, 1948) found that adrenaline produced an increase in the duration, but not in the amplitude, of the action potential of the fast-contracting isolated diaphragm muscle of the rat recorded extracellularly; they concluded that this effect was due to retardation of the spread of the excitation wave along the fibre.

LEWIS et al. (1977) made the first detailed study of intracellularly recorded action potentials under the influence of adrenaline, and their results are illustrated in Fig. 5. They found that adrenaline was without significant effects on any on the action potential parameters measured in fibres of the fast-contracting flexor digitorum longus muscle and of the slow-contracting soleus muscle of the cat under sodium pentobarbitone anaesthesia. TASHIRO (1973) mentioned that in preliminary experiments, he also found that the action potential was little affected in the isolated soleus and extensor digitorum longus muscles of the guinea pig.

VI. Effect of Anaesthetics

The anaesthetic used may modify the effects of adrenaline on muscle contractions. Fast- and slow-contracting muscles respond in the characteristic ways described above in the nonanaesthetised decerebrate cat, and in all species tested when the anaesthetic used is α-chloralose. However, under urethane anaesthesia, BOWMAN et al. (1962) were unable to detect any effect of adrenaline on the contractions of the soleus muscle of the rabbit, although the fast-contracting tibialis anterior muscle responded normally. They attributed the absence of effect on the soleus muscle to the fact that urethane causes the discharge of catecholamines from the adrenal medullae (ELLIOT, 1912; HÖKFELT and MCLEAN, 1950; SPRIGGS and STOCKHAM, 1964); these might already have maximally affected the sensitive soleus muscle. Chloralose does not cause a discharge of adrenaline from the adrenals (EMMELIN and STRÖMBLAD, 1951), and under chloralose anaesthesia the rabbit soleus muscle responded well to adrenaline.

Small amounts of sodium pentobarbitone mixed with α-chloralose to quell its initial central stimulant action do not appear to affect the responses to adrenaline. However, in unpublished experiments, BOWMAN and RAPER found that when sodium pentobarbitone was the sole anaesthetic used, the tension responses of both the tibialis anterior and the soleus muscle of the cat to adrenaline were less pronounced than they were under chloralose anaesthesia or in the decerebrate animal. Pentobarbitone has been shown to inhibit the uptake of Ca^{2+} by mitochondria isolated from muscle (DRANSFELD et al., 1969), but it is not known whether this effect is relevant to the weaker effect of catecholamines on skeletal muscles in vivo when pentobarbitone is the anaesthetic used.

KENDIG and BUNKER (1972) found that halothane, which itself slightly depressed the resting membrane potential of rat gastrocnemius muscle fibres, also prevented the hyperpolarizing action of adrenaline. In contrast, cyclopropane itself produced hyperpolarization of the fibre membranes, and this effect was diminished by depletion of catecholamines produced by prior reserpine treatment. KENDIG and BUNKER (1972) postulated that halothane reduces the resting membrane potential because it both diminishes the release of endogenous catecholamines and blocks their tonic action on the electrogenic component of the Na^+–K^+ pump, whereas cyclopropane hyperpolarizes the membrane because it enhances the release of catecholamines (PRICE et al., 1959).

In view of KENDIG and BUNKER's (1972) proposals, it would be of interest to know whether the depolarizing action of halothane is a contributary factor in its liability to produce malignant hyperpyrexia in susceptible individuals, and whether pretreatment with a β_2-receptor agonist, such as salbutamol, would exert any protective action. This last suggestion is related to the use by ZAIMIS and coworkers of β-receptor agonists in other types of muscle spasticity (see Sect. D.III).

VII. Mechanism of Action

The catecholamine-induced increase in twitch tension, in time to peak, and in time to half-decay in fast-contracting muscles, and the decrease in these parameters in slow-contracting muscles, coupled with the absence of any effect on rate of rise of tension, on velocity of isotonic shortening, or on maximal tetanic tension in either type of muscle are compatible with a prolongation (in fast-contracting muscles) and a curtailment (in slow-contracting muscles) of the plateaus of the active states (HILL, 1949) of the stimulated muscles. GOFFART and RITCHIE (1952) reached this conclusion with respect to the fast-contracting tibialis anterior muscle of the cat and BOWMAN and RAPER (1962) with respect to the slow-contracting soleus muscle of the same species. JURNA and his co-workers (JURNA and RUMMEL, 1962; JURNA et al., 1963; BLECKMAN et al., 1963) made detailed measurements and concluded that it is the decaying phases of the active state curves that are affected rather than the durations of the plateaus; that is to say, the rate of decline from the plateau of full activity is slowed in fast-contracting muscles and hastened in slow-contracting muscles.

The question arises as to whether the mechanical changes are secondary to membrane changes. GOFFART (1950) considered the possibility that the slowed conduction of the extracellularly recorded action potential, which BROWN et al. (1947, 1948) had observed in the fast-contracting, isolated rat diaphragm muscle, might allow more time for the contractile component to stretch the series elastic component in an isometric twitch, so that an increase in peak tension resulted. However, GOFFART and RITCHIE (1952) ruled out this explanation by showing that adrenaline was just as effective in increasing twitch tension when a muscle was stimulated simultaneously at many points by a multi-electrode assembly, as it was when it was stimulated only at one end. Propagation time is obviously unimportant when the stimulation is applied all over the muscle fibre membranes. The more recent observations of LEWIS et al. (1977) that there are no significant changes in the intracellularly recorded single fibre action potentials during adrenaline infusions confirms the belief that the changes in contractility in both fast and slow muscles are not consequences of changes in the propagated electrical responses.

BOWMAN and NOTT (1969) felt that the weight of the evidence was against the possibility that the mechanical changes were secondary to any membrane hyperpolarization produced by β-adrenoceptor agonists; they considered that these were independent changes that occurred in parallel but that were not causally related. TASHIRO (1973) agreed that the effects of catecholamines on the relaxation phases of twitches were unrelated to the increases in resting membrane potential produced. However, he found that procedures that prevented the hyperpolarizing action of isoprenaline also reduced its effects on the peak twitch tension, and he therefore concluded that the changes in peak tension, although not those in time course, were at least related to the hyperpolarizing action. He suggested that stimulation of the Na^+–K^+ pump by isoprenaline at the same time as it increases the resting membrane potential, might, as a secondary consequence of the membrane ionic shifts, increase the release of Ca^{2+} from internal stores during a twitch of a fast-contracting muscle, thereby augmenting the peak tension. He further suggested that the decrease in twitch tension in the soleus muscle might be a consequence of a reduction in the number of muscle fibres contributing, owing to the increase in excitability threshold caused by the hyperpolarization. Hyperpolarization was always more marked in the soleus than in the extensor digitorum longus muscle in TASHIRO's experiments. It seems unlikely, however, that the decrease in twitch tension of the soleus muscle could be the result of a reduced number of contributing fibres, since the compound gross muscle action potential is always slightly increased during this effect, at least in the cat, yet the amplitudes of the individual fibre action potentials are unchanged.

The changes in the shapes of the contractions are incompatible with any changes in the rates of activation of the contractile mechanisms or in their intrinsic strengths. Whether or not the changes in peak twitch tension and the changes in rate of relaxation are separate events, as TASHIRO's (1973) results suggest, the most important effect is that on rate of relaxation, since it is this parameter that modifies fusion in incomplete tetanic contractions. The latter have more physiological relevance than have twitches, since they mimic the activity of the motor units within a muscle during physiological contractions. The question then is why β-adrenoceptor agonists should affect the relaxation phases in opposite ways in fast- and slow-contracting muscles, and the answer must presumably lie in one or other of the biochemical differences that exist in the contraction-relaxation mechanisms of the two types of muscle.

β-Adrenoceptor agonists are not the only factors that give rise to such opposite responses. Thus, the effects of a previous tetanus on subsequent twitches, although not completely identical with the effects of a β-adrenoceptor agonist, are sufficiently similar to suggest that overlapping mechanisms are involved. In fast-contracting muscles, there is a posttetanic augmentation of contractility and in slow-contracting muscles a posttetanic diminution of contractility, both effects being independent of the simultaneously occurring facilitatory actions of a tetanus on neuromuscular transmission. Fast-contracting muscles exhibit a positive staircase *(Treppe)* effect, whereas slow-contracting muscles exhibit a negative staircase effect. The extent of the similarity between the effects of a β-adrenoceptor agonist and the after-effects of a tetanus may be judged from the articles by BROWN and von EULER (1938), BROWN et al. (1950), ELLIS (1959), BOWMAN et al. (1962), CLOSE and HOH (1968), BOWMAN and NOTT (1969), and SMITH (1970). Cooling also affects the two types of muscle differently, the twitch tension of fast-contracting muscles being increased and that of slow-contracting muscles decreased by a fall in temperature; in both types of muscle, however, the times to peak tension and to half-decay are prolonged by cooling (BULLER et al., 1968a, b).

One important difference between fast- and slow-contracting twitch muscles is the higher myosin ATPase activity of the former (BÁRÁNY et al., 1965; BÁRÁNY, 1967; BULLER et al., 1969; GOLDSPINK et al., 1970). Myosins from fast- and slow-contracting muscles differ in their contents of low molecular weight proteins, and this difference appears to reflect the different myosin ATPase activities (PERRIE and PERRY, 1970). The maximum rate at which thick and thin filaments slide past one another during contraction is limited by the rate of hydrolysis of ATP by myosin ATPase, the activity of which is therefore the main determinant of contraction speed. The higher activity of myosin ATPase in fast muscle compared with slow muscle is supported by a higher affinity of fast muscle troponin for calcium ions which activate the enzyme (EBASHI et al., 1969). There is a clear relationship between myosin ATPase activity and contraction speed on the one hand and the duration of the active state on the other; that is to say that the intrinsic speed of shortening of the contractile component and the time course of the active state are coupled in some way, the faster the contraction speed, the shorter the duration of the plateau of full activity in a twitch (for references see CLOSE, 1972). However, it is unlikely that the effects of β-adrenoceptor agonists on muscle contractions involve myosin ATPase, since, if they did, changes in the rates of rise of tension would be expected to accompany the changes in the rates of decay of the active states, and in fact the rates of rise of tension are not altered.

A second important difference between fast- and slow-contracting muscles lies in the content and properties of the sarcoplasmic reticulum and mitochondria. Not only is there more sarcoplasmic reticulum in fast than in slow muscle fibres, but also the fast muscle sarcoplasmic reticulum takes up calcium ions at a faster rate (HARIGAYA et al., 1968; SRÉTER, 1969, 1970; YAMAMOTO et al., 1970; FIEHN and PETER, 1971; LUFF and ATWOOD, 1971). Mitochondria are also responsible for taking up some calcium ions (WEBER, 1966; CARAFOLI et al., 1969; DRANSFIELD et al., 1969; BORYS and KARLER, 1971; BATRA, 1972, 1973). Mitochondria are most numerous in fast-contracting red muscle fibres and least numerous in fast-contracting pale muscle fibres; slow-contracting intermediate fibres lie between the two extremes with respect to mitochondrial content (for references see CLOSE, 1972). ZAIMIS et al. (personal communication) have shown that the mitochondria of the slow-contracting cat soleus muscle take up calcium ions more avidly than do those of the fast-contracting tibialis anterior muscle of the same species. It might be supposed, therefore, that whereas the sarcoplasmic reticulum plays the most important role in calcium sequestration in fast-contracting fibres, the mitochondria assume relatively greater importance in slow-contracting fibres.

Sequestration of calcium ions is not the only factor determining the time course of the active state, but it is clearly an important one, and one that has been shown to differ correspondingly in fast- and slow-contracting muscles. BOWMAN and NOTT (1969) therefore postulated that β-adrenoceptor agonists affect the relaxation mechanisms by altering (in opposite ways in fast and slow muscle fibres) the rates of resequestration of activator calcium ions into intracellular binding sites, especially the sarcoplasmic reticulum. However, in view of the results of ZAIMIS et al. referred to above, this last suggestion should probably be modified. It may rather be that whereas adrenaline may slow the re-uptake of Ca^{2+} by sarcoplasmic reticulum of fast-contracting muscles, it hastens re-uptake into the mitochondria of slow-contracting muscles, and that these effects are the main determinants of the opposite changes produced by adrenaline in the rates of relaxation of the two types of muscle.

Many effects that are evoked by stimulation of β-adrenoceptors are thought to be mediated by stimulation of adenylate cyclase and the production of cyclic adenosine-3′,5′-monophosphate (cyclic AMP) from ATP (for reviews see ROBISON et al., 1968, 1971 a, b). Adrenaline, isoprenaline, salbutamol or terbutaline increases the content of cyclic AMP in both fast-contracting muscles (POSNER et al., 1965; SULLIVAN and ZAIMIS, 1973; LEFKOWITZ and DURHAM, 1974; AL-JEBOORY and MARSHALL, 1978; FELLENIUS et al, 1980) and slow-contracting muscles (SULLIVAN and ZAIMIS, 1973; AL-JE-

BOORY and MARSHALL, 1978; FELLENIUS et al, 1980). Adenylate cyclase stimulation in muscle appears to be mediated by β_2-adrenoceptors in that it is produced by the relatively selective β_2-adrenoceptor agonist salbutamol (AL-JEBOORY and MARSHALL, 1978) and blocked by the relatively selective β_2-receptor antagonist butoxamine, but not by the β_1-adrenoceptor antagonist practolol (LEFKOWITZ and DURHAM, 1974). In the experiments of AL-JEBOORY and MARSHALL (1978) on the isolated guinea pig soleus and extensor digitorum longus muscles, salbutamol produced mechanical changes and increased cyclic AMP content in the same concentration range; in both mechanical and biochemical responses the soleus was more sensitive than the extensor digitorum longus. Studies by Reddy et al. (1979) showed that, although there were more β-adrenoceptors present in the membranes of the fast-contracting extensor digitorum longus muscle fibres of the rat than in those of the slow-contracting soleus muscle fibres, the adenylate cyclase of the slow muscle was more effectively stimulated by β-adrenoceptor agonists. These results indicate that the coupling of the receptors to the enzyme differs in the two muscles. The more efficient coupling in the slow muscle may underlie the greater sensitivity of slow muscles to β-adrenoceptor agonists.

NOTT (1971) and BOWMAN and NOTT (1974) found that the effects of isoprenaline and salbutamol on contractions of the slow-contracting soleus and fast-contracting tibialis anterior and flexor digitorum longus muscles are potentiated by the previous administration of drugs that inhibit cyclic nucleotide phosphodiesterase and which thereby prolong the existence of cyclic AMP; the rank orders of potency of the phosphodiesterase inhibitors in potentiating the sympathomimetic amines in vivo and in inhibiting the enzyme in vitro were broadly similar. Although cyclic AMP itself and its dibutyryl derivative were without any consistent effect on contractions in the experiments of BOWMAN and NOTT (1974), the results on the whole support the idea that the mechanical effects of β-adrenoceptor agonists are mediated by the nucleotide. In fast-contracting muscles, adenylate cyclase is located in the mitochondrial and microsomal fractions of homogenates (RABINOWITZ et al., 1965; BUTCHER and ROBISON, personal communication), whereas in slow-contracting muscle (cat soleus) it is located in the surface membranes of the fibres BUTCHER and ROBISON, personal communication). The different locations of the enzyme might be another factor accounting for the greater sensitivity of slow-contracting muscles of the cat to β-adrenoceptor agonists.

BOWMAN and NOTT (1974) suggested the alternative possibility that β-adrenoceptor agonists enhance calcium uptake in both fast- and slow-contracting fibres, rather than affecting its sequestration in opposite ways. The difference between the contractile responses of the two would lie in the greater calcium-sequestering ability of the fast fibres and the possibility that fast fibres are less fully activated in a twitch than are slow fibres. If the rate of calcium uptake during relaxation of a fast fibre is already maximal, then no enhancement of relaxation rate could be produced by a β-receptor agonist. However, an increased amount of calcium ions sequestered during the intervals between contractions might result in more being available for release by a subsequent stimulus; hence, there would be greater activation during a twitch, and prolongations of the times to peak twitch tension and to half-relaxation. On the assumption that the mechanism involves the adenylate cyclase-cyclic AMP system, this suggestion for fast-contracting fibres is compatible with the observations of TOMLINSON et al. (1976), who showed that a cyclic AMP-protein kinase augmented the ability of calcium ions to activate a Ca^{2+}-stimulated, Mg^{2+}-dependent ATPase obtained from the sarcotubular system of rabbit limb muscle (mostly fast-contracting). This enzyme is believed to catalyse the active removal of Ca^{2+} from the sarcoplasm into the sarcoplasmic reticulum. SCHWARTZ et al. (1976) found that a cyclic AMP-protein kinase enhanced Ca^{+2} uptake into sarcoplasmic reticulum of both fast- and slow-contracting muscles. Possibly a different cyclic AMP-dependent protein kinase enhances the sequestration of Ca^{2+} by mitochondria of slow-contracting fibres. However, an alternative possibility that enhanced Ca^{2+} uptake into slow fibre mitochondria is indirect, or at least partly so, is worth considering. CLAUSEN and FLATMAN (1977) showed that the effect of adrenaline in enhancing the activity of the electrogenic component of the (Na^+–K^+)-pump, thereby producing an increase in the intracellular K^+/Na^+ ratio and in E_m, was mimicked by a combination of dibutyryl cyclic AMPand theophylline. They therefore postulated, as BRAY et al. (1976) had earlier done for denervated muscle, that the effects of adrenaline on pump activity are mediated by cyclic AMP. Mitochondrial uptake of Ca^{2+} in red breast muscle of pigeons (DRANSFELD et al., 1969) and in frog muscle (BATRA, 1972) is enhanced by an increased K^+/Na^+ ratio, whereas that of white back muscle of rabbits (DRANSFELD et al., 1969) is unaffected. Pigeon breast muscle and frog muscle mitochondria do not necessarily share the same properties as those of mammalian slow-contracting fibres. However, it is possible that in intact muscle fibres, a raised intracellular K^+/Na^+ ratio induced by β-adrenoceptor agonists acting via the adenylate cyclase-cyclic AMP system contributes to enhanced uptake of Ca^{2+} by mitochondria and to a consequently faster rate of relaxation of slow-contracting fibres.

At the present time, consideration of the mechanisms of action of β-adrenoceptor agonists at the molecular level in the two types of muscle is still largely speculative. It is to be hoped that the development of the technique for studying isolated fast- and slow-contracting muscles of the guinea pig by TASHIRO (1973), WALDECK (1976, 1977), and HOLMBERG and WALDECK (1977) will provide a suitable model for more detailed and fruitful studies.

C. Muscle Spindles

There is a long-standing controversy as to whether the intrafusal fibres of the muscle spindles receive a direct sympathetic innervation, or whether the abundant adrenergic terminals present are confined solely to the smooth muscle of the rich blood supply to the spindle capsule and to that of the sparser vessels supplying the extracapsular parts of the intrafusal fibres. Much of the earlier work was reviewed by HINSEY (1934) and TIEGS (1953), both of whom concluded that there is no direct adrenergic innervation of intrafusal muscle fibres; this is the currently accepted view of most workers (see, e.g., BOYD, 1962; BARKER, 1974; MCINNES, 1980), although there are exceptions (e.g., SANTINI and IBATA, 1971). Irrespective of whether the muscle spindles are directly innervated by the sympathetic, their various components may possess adrenoceptors and be influenced by circulating sympathomimetic amines. The spindle capsule possesses properties resembling those of the blood-brain barrier; catecholamines do not penetrate it (MCINNES, 1980). Since there are few or no capillaries within the capsule (CORVAJA et al., 1969; MCINNES, 1980), any action of injected catecholamines might arise from an action on the capsule itself (e.g., possibly on transport mechanisms through it, thus modifying the composition of the fluid within it), or indirectly, on the blood flow to the spindle; noradrenaline released from vascular sympathetics might spill over and act in similar ways.

Several workers have reported that the primary afferent discharge from muscle spindles is increased by "moderate" doses of adrenaline or noradrenaline but depressed by larger doses, whereas intermediate doses produce a biphasic effect (PAINTAL, 1959; HUNT, 1960; ELDRED et al., 1960; CALMA and KIDD, 1962; BHOOLA et al., 1962). Similar effects have been described in response to sympathetic stimulation at frequencies as low as 2 Hz (HUNT, 1960) and above (HUNT, 1960; ELDRED et al., 1960). PERUZZI et al. (1961) found that adrenaline produced various degrees of alternating enhancement and depression of the stretch reflex, depending upon the dose. Some workers have concluded that the effects on the spindles are secondary to the vasoconstrictor effects of the sympathomimetic amines or of sympathetic stimulation, and it is likely that this is to some extent so, since several of the workers quoted used huge doses of adrenaline and frequencies of stimulation well above the physiological range. Furthermore, arterial occlusion has been shown to produce effects that to some extent resemble those of adrenaline and sympathetic stimulation MATTHEWS, 1933; PAINTAL, 1959; ELDRED et al., 1960). However, vasoconstriction and consequent hypoxia are clearly not the sole cause of all the changes in discharge frequency, as some of the effects of adrenaline have been reproduced in isolated frog muscle preparations (PERUZZI and CORDA, 1961) and in cat tenuissimus muscles devoid of circulation (CORDA and STADERINI, 1962), although not all workers have been able to detect effects in isolated muscle (BHOOLA et al., 1962); for reviews see SMITH (1963, 1965). GROSSIE and YONAS (1969) found that prolonged intravenous infusions of quite low doses of adrenaline ($0.5\ \mu g \cdot kg^{-1} \cdot min^{-1}$) for several minutes produced increased primary afferent spindle activity coupled with an increased muscle blood flow in anaesthetised cats when the arterial oxygen tension was maintained within normal limits. A much larger dose ($5\ \mu g \cdot kg^{-1} \cdot min^{-1}$) produced vasoconstriction, but still increased primary afferent discharge when arterial oxygen tension was maintained within normal limits by artificial ventilation. An induced arterial hyperoxia enhanced the stimulant effect of adrenaline, whereas an induced hypoxia inhibited it. It thus seems clear that adrenaline does increase the primary afferent discharge from the muscle spindles by a mechanism independent of vascular changes, and the possibility has been contemplated that it plays a physiological role in maintaining spindle excitability (SMITH, 1965).

HODGSON et al. (1969) showed that intravenously or local intra-arterially injected adrenaline increased the tension of tonic contractions of human calf muscles evoked by vibrating the Achilles tendon. This evoked response is known to be generated by activity in the primary afferent endings of the muscle spindles (MATTHEWS, 1972). Adrenaline did not increase the amplitude of equivalent tetanic contractions evoked by direct electrical stimulation of spindle afferent nerve fibres, and HODGSON et al. (1969) therefore concluded that the adrenaline effect must be exerted on the spindles. They went on to show that the enhancing effect of adrenaline exhibited the characteristics of an effect mediated by β-adrenoceptors, being mimicked by isoprenaline, but not by noradrenaline, and blocked by racemic propranolol but not by the dextro isomer. HALE and KIDD (1974) have provided confirmatory evidence from experiments on rats that the muscle spindles or their associated structures contain β-adrenoceptors. Some of the earlier workers found that the changes in afferent discharge that they observed with larger doses of adrenaline, and the depressant effect on the knee jerk, were blocked by the α-adrenoceptor blocking drug phenoxybenzamine, but not by the β-adrenoceptor blocking drug, dichloroisoprenaline (ELDRED et al., 1960; MCLENNAN, 1961). It seems likely that this α-adrenoceptor-mediated component is that which is secondary to vasoconstriction and hypoxia. As already mentioned, HODGSON et al. (1969) found that noradrenaline did not mimic the effect of adrenaline and isoprenaline in increasing the tension evoked by vibrating the muscle tendon. This implies that the β-receptors present on the spindles belong to the β_2 subgroup; they probably contribute to the muscle tremor that accompanies the use of β_2-adrenoceptor agonists. This point is discussed in more detail in Subsect. D.II.1. Since noradrenaline is inactive, the results of HODGSON et al. (1969) also imply that, while adrenal medullary adrenaline may directly affect spindle excitability, the transmitter of sympathetic nerves (presumably noradrenaline) can do so only indirectly as a consequence of vascular changes. On these theoretical grounds therefore it is unlikely that the spindles receive a direct noradrenergic innervation other than that to their blood vessels.

The mechanism of action of β-adrenoceptor agonists in increasing primary afferent excitability is not known, although it seems likely that it will involve an effect or effects similar to one or more of those exerted on the extrafusal muscle fibres.

D. Human Muscles

I. Evoked Contractions

Human muscles contain fast- and slow-contracting fibres resembling those of other mammals, but there is no human muscle like the cat soleus that is composed entirely of slow-contracting fibres. However, since slow-contracting fibres are more sensitive to β-adrenoceptor agonists than are fast-contracting fibres, it might be expected that the action of these drugs in the smallest effective doses would be manifested selectively on the slow motor units, and that the extent of the effect would be related to the proportion of slow motor units in the muscle. MARSDEN and MEADOWS (1968, 1970) demonstrated that this is in fact so. They showed that adrenaline and isoprenaline in man increased the rate of relaxation of certain limb muscle twitches and decreased fusion in incomplete tetanic contractions evoked at a frequency of 10 Hz. The effects of the drugs were more marked, the greater the proportion of slow-contracting fibres present, as judged from the twitch duration. Thus, the effect on the triceps surae group (twitch time, 186 ms) was more pronounced than that on the tibialis anterior group (twitch time, 135 ms); in the doses used, the catecholamines were without effect on the adductor pollicis (twitch time, 123 ms). MARSDEN and MEADOWS (1970) found that the effects of adrenaline and isoprenaline were blocked by racemic propranolol but not by (+)-propranolol, showing that β-adrenoceptors were involved. Propranolol was effective as an antagonist whether given intravenously or by local intra-arterial injection to the appropriate muscle; the β-adrenoceptors are therefore located peripherally, presumably in the muscles themselves. ZAIMIS (1973) confirmed the conclusion that β-adrenoceptors mediate the effect; she showed that the β-adrenoceptor-selective drug orciprenaline reduced twitch duration and decreased subtetanic fusion in human calf muscles. In the experiments of MARSDEN and MEADOWS (1970) noradrenaline was ineffective at the dose level used, and this result suggests that, as in animals, the β-adrenoceptors involved belong to the β_2 subgroup. In fact, there is no reason to suppose that the effects recorded by MARSDEN and MEADOWS (1968, 1970) and by ZAIMIS (1973) from slow-contracting units in human muscles are in any way different from those produced, e.g., in the cat soleus muscle.

II. Tremor

1. Unwanted Effect of Sympathomimetic Bronchodilators

A so-called physiological tremor can be recorded (e.g., in the fingers of the outstretched arm) in any healthy individual. It has usually been considered to arise as the result of an inherant delay in a hunting mechanism in the muscle length servomechanism; i.e. in the stretch reflex that contributes to the control of muscle activity (HALLIDAY and REDFEARN, 1956; HAMMOND et al., 1956; LIPPOLD et al., 1957; STUART et al., 1966; LIPPOLD, 1971). However, MARSDEN et al. (1967b) found in a patient whose right arm had previously been totally deafferented surgically that physiological tremor was still present on the operated side with the same peak (9.5 Hz) in the spectral analysis curve as was present in that for the normal side, although the curve for the operated side was somewhat broader and smaller. These results, albeit on only one patient, suggest that, while the stretch reflex may modulate physiological tremor, the origin of the tremor must be independent of sensory feed-back from the muscle spindles; presumably it arises instead in a servo loop at spinal or supraspinal level (see e.g., MARSDEN et al., 1972).

Emotional disturbance (GRAHAM, 1945; REDFEARN, 1957), adrenaline (BARCROFT et al., 1952; BARCROFT and SWAN, 1953; LANDAU et al., 1966; MARSDEN et al., 1967a; FRANKENHAUSER, 1971) or isoprenaline (GAY and LONG, 1949; MARSDEN et al., 1967a) give rise to a pronounced tremor in man, the spectrum of which shows the same frequency peak (8–12 Hz) as physiological tremor but is greater in amplitude; it is regarded as augmented physiological tremor (MARSDEN et al., 1967a). Adrenaline does not penetrate the blood-brain barrier in appreciable quantities (AXELROD et al., 1959; DRASKOCI et al., 1960; BERTHLER et al., 1963; HAMBERGER and HAMBERGER, 1966). Hence, its effect must be peripheral. Peripheral enhancement of a centrally originating tremor would not be expected to modify the frequency but only the amplitude, as is found to be the case. MARSDEN et al. (1967a) confirmed the peripheral site of action of intravenously injected adrenaline by unilaterally preventing the tremor in one limb by intra-arterial injection of propranolol.

The accumulated evidence indicates that the adrenoceptors mediating the increase in tremor are β-adrenoceptors (MARSDEN et al., 1967a). Furthermore, careful analysis by MARLIN and TURNER (1975), THIRINGER and SVEDMYR (1976b), and LARSSON and SVEDMYR (1977) has shown that they can be further subclassified as of the β_2-type. They therefore belong to the same subgroup as those mediating effects on evoked muscle contractions (Sects. B.IV and D.I) and increased muscle spindle sensitivity (Sect. C).

As mentioned earlier (Sect. B.II) BOWMAN and ZAIMIS (1958) first suggested that the action of adrenaline in decreasing fusion of incomplete tetanic contractions of slow motor units within a mixed muscle might underly the tremor produced in man by adrenaline. Since they found that adrenaline still increased physiological tremor by a peripheral action in the deafferented limb of an operated patient, MARSDEN et al. (1967b) and MARSDEN and MEADOWS (1970) supported the suggestion of BOWMAN and ZAIMIS (1958), although they felt that an effect on the muscle spindles must also contribute, because the effect of adrenaline on the normal limb of their patient was proportionately slightly greater than that on the deafferented limb.

Sympathomimetic bronchodilators that are relatively selective for β_2-adrenoceptors are now widely used as bronchodilators, especially in asthma. Many of these are listed in Table 2 and their structures are given in Fig. 3. A satisfactory degree of selectivity for the bronchi can be achieved with these drugs when they are administered by aerosol, but after systemic absorption muscle tremor is a common and unpleasant side-effect (KENNEDY and SIMPSON, 1969; FREEDMAN, 1971; LEGGE et al., 1971; PATERSON et al., 1971; BEUMER, 1971; GIESSEN and ILLIG, 1972; WATSON and RICHENS, 1974; MARLIN and TURNER, 1975; FORMGREN, 1975; THIRINGER and SVEDMYR, 1975, 1976a; LARSSON, 1977), although it tends to disappear with long-term treatment (SVEDMYR et al., 1974; LARSSON et al., 1977), presumably because the central nervous system learns to compensate by adjusting the firing frequency of the motoneurones (BOWMAN and RODGER, 1972). LARSSON and SVEDMYR (1977) recommend starting treatment with low doses (e.g., of terbutaline) and gradually increasing the dose as resistance to the tremorgenic effect (but not the bronchodilator effect) develops.

Since both the bronchial and the skeletal muscle β-adrenoceptors belong to the β_2 subgroup and the receptors involved appear to be closely similar, the opinion has been expressed (BOWMAN and NOTT, 1969; BOWMAN and RODGER, 1972; APPERLEY et al., 1976; BOWMAN and RAPER, 1976; LARSSON and SVEDMYR, 1977) that it may be impossible to synthesize a sympathomimetic bronchodilator that does not carry with it the possibility of producing skeletal muscle tremor as an unwanted side-effect. From a comparison of selectivity ratios in man and animals (for references and discussion see BOWMAN and RAPER, 1976), it has been proposed that the cat provides the best animal model for forecasting adrenoceptor specificity in man (lungs, heart, blood vessels, and skeletal muscle). The ability of the compound to decrease tension and fusion of incomplete tetanic contractions of the cat soleus muscle is used to forecast tremorgenic action in man. The method appears to be reliable even though part of the human tremor effect may be evoked through the muscle spindles. Presumably the β_2-adrenoceptors in the extrafusal slow-contracting fibres are closely similar to those in the muscle spindles, and the one serves as a model for both.

According to KAISER et al. (1975) and LARSEN and HERMANSEN (1977) who used the cat model, the compounds sulfonterol and QH 25 [3-(methoxybenzylamino)-4-hydroxy-α-(tert. butylaminomethyl)-benzyl-alcohol] are each more potent on the bronchi than they are on the soleus muscle, the heart or the blood vessels. If these results are confirmed, they will indicate that the β_2-adrenoceptors of the lungs and skeletal muscle are not in fact absolutely identical, and they will encourage the hope that bronchodilators with minimal side-effects might be developed. However, both groups of authors used methods for recording bronchodilatation that differed from that used by BOWMAN and RODGER (1972) when they drew attention to the validity of their model for forecasting effects in man. KAISER et al. (1975), for example, assessed bronchodilatation against a background of bronchoconstriction produced by histamine, whereas BOWMAN and RODGER (1972) used 5-hydroxytryptamine. Sympathomimetic amines may be more potent in opposing the actions of some bronchoconstrictors than of others (Farmer and Lehrer, 1966), thus apparently enhancing their bronchodilator action in comparison with their actions on other tissues. Before it is finally concluded that the lung and muscle β-adrenoceptors differ, it is therefore important to study the actions of sulfonterol and QH 25 in tests on cats that are identical with those that have failed with other bronchodilators to differentiate the lung and muscle β-adrenoceptors and ultimately, of course, to demonstrate relative lack of tremorgenic activity of these drugs in man.

2. Parkinsonian Tremor

Tremor, arising from impairments in certain subcortical and mesencephalic neuronal circuits (see, e.g., Poirier et al., 1972) is one of the symptoms of Parkinson's disease. It is manifested mainly in the muscles of the distal extremities, but also in the muscles of the face and tongue. In most cases it is evident only when the patient is at rest, but occasionally there is also an action tremor which may be a consequence of an additional central lesion. (For a description and discussion of parkinsonian tremor, see Struppler et al., 1976). Whereas the frequency spectrum of physiological tremor shows a small peak at around 10 Hz, that of parkinsonian tremor has a pronounced peak at around 5 Hz; the amplitude of parkinsonian tremor is much greater than that of physiological tremor (Dietz et al., 1976).

Emotional stress or the administration of adrenaline (Barcroft et al., 1952; Constas, 1962; Owen and Marsden, 1965; Marshall and Schnieden, 1966) increases parkinsonian tremor. Part, although not necessarily all, of the stress-induced enhancement of tremor is probably produced by adrenal medullary adrenaline (but see Marsden and Owen, 1967). Owen and Marsden (1965) clearly showed that the enhancement of parkinsonian tremor produced by adrenaline was abolished by pronethalol or propranolol. The enhancement of parkinsonian tremor is presumably due to the same peripheral mechanism, mediated by β_2-adrenoceptors, as that giving rise to enhancement of physiological tremor.

β-Adrenoceptor blocking drugs are less effective in reducing the basic tremor of parkinsonism that has not been enhanced by adrenaline. Vas (1966) found that propranolol had no significant effect on alternating tremor, and, in an uncontrolled trial, Strang (1965) was unable to detect any benefit in most of his patients. He concluded that propranolol was not a very effective anti-parkinsonian drug. On the other hand, several workers have been able to show improvement in tremor with β-adrenoceptor blocking drugs in a substantial number of their patients. Herring (1964) first demonstrated improvement with pronethalol, and this was confirmed by Owen and Marsden (1965) with both pronethalol and propranolol, and by Gilligan (1972) and Rajput et al. (1973) with propranolol. Oxprenolol has also been used with some benefit (Jackson et al., 1971; Thompson, 1972; Dowzenko et al., 1976). On no occasion however did all the patients in the groups respond, nor was tremor totally abolished in any individual. The action of β-adrenoceptor blocking drugs in reducing the basic parkinsonian tremor exhibits a different time course and a different optimal dose from that responsible for blocking the augmentation of tremor produced by adrenaline, and it is less consistently present. It therefore appears that the two effects are consequences of different actions of the β-adrenoceptor blocking drugs. Since the basic lesion giving rise to parkinsonian tremor is within the central nervous system and there is no evidence for any peripheral adrenergic component, it is generally believed that the anti-parkinsonian tremor action of β-adrenoceptor blocking drugs is centrally mediated. Only drugs that pass the blood-brain barrier would therefore be expected to be effective. It is not yet known whether the anti-tremor action is exerted by blockade of central β-adrenoceptors, or whether some other action is responsible.

Since 1967 the main treatment of parkinsonism has been with levodopa. The initial stimulus for dopa therapy came chiefly from the discovery that there are abnormally small concentrations of dopamine in the basal ganglia of parkinsonian patients (EHRINGER and HORNYKIEWICZ, 1960). Since dopamine fails to cross the blood-brain barrier, its precursor amino acid, dopa, was the logical candidate for clinical trials, and its efficacy in parkinsonism is most simply explained in terms of its conversion to dopamine in the striatum (BIRKMAYER and HORNYKIEWICZ, 1961; BARBEAU et al., 1962).

It is generally agreed that the akinesia and rigidity of parkinsonism respond best to levodopa therapy, while the tremor is less satisfactorily treated. Nevertheless, in many patients who exhibit all three symptoms there is often a valuable improvement in tremor, as well as in other symptoms (CALNE et al., 1969; MAWDSLEY, 1970; HUGHES et al., 1971; COX et al., 1973; TEYCHENNE et al., 1975; YUILL, 1976). Unfortunately, there are some patients in whom levodopa has little or no effect on tremor (GODWIN-AUSTEN et al., 1969; MARKS, 1974) or even aggravates this symptom (MUENTER, 1971), while at the same time relieving rigidity and akinesia. Stereotactic thalamotomy to relieve the tremor may be considered for such patients. However, many workers have demonstrated a substantial extra improvement in tremor (but not in other symptoms) when propranolol was administered concurrently with levodopa (ABRAMSKY et al., 1971; KISSEL et al., 1972, 1974; GILLIGAN et al., 1972; JULIEN and VALLAT, 1973; KISSEL, 1974; TRIDON et al., 1975). On the other hand, MARSDEN et al. (1974) failed to obtain any benefit over levodopa alone when propranolol was added, and CLAVERIA et al. (1975) and SANDLER et al. (1975) obtained similar negative results with oxprenolol.

Viewed overall, it seems that some patients do obtain a clear extra relief of tremor when propranolol is added to the levodopa therapy. Furthermore, judging from the published reports, it seems that in the patients who do respond, the relief of tremor produced by a combination of levodopa and propranolol is greater than that produced by propranolol alone. In animal experiments, evidence has been obtained that levodopa is metabolised to catecholamines, especially dopamine, to a greater extent in the periphery than in the brain (BUTCHER and ENGEL, 1969; LOUIS et al., 1974), and SANDLER et al. (1973), NOTT (1975), and BOWMAN and NOTT (1978) have suggested that levodopa metabolites may act peripherally in skeletal muscle, as does adrenaline, to enhance tremor, thereby in some patients masking or even reversing any central relief produced by centrally formed dopamine. Levodopa produces a slowly developing decrease in the tension and degree of fusion of incomplete tetanic contractions of the cat soleus muscle (NOTT, 1975; BOWMAN and NOTT, 1978), an effect that is prevented by previous administration of a peripheral dopa decarboxylase inhibitor (benserazide) or by propranolol. If this animal model is accepted as valid for forecasting tremorgenic effects in man, the results imply that levodopa metabolites can produce tremor by a peripheral mechanism. The active metabolites might be dopamine, the much more potent adrenaline or noradrenaline, or tetrahydropapaveroline or salsolinol. The last two have been shown to be metabolites of levodopa in man (SANDLER et al.,

1973), and one of them, tetrahydropapaveroline, has been tested on the cat soleus muscle and shown to exert an adrenaline-like effect (NOTT and HEAD, 1978). Tetrahydropapaveroline is about 20 times less potent than adrenaline (on a molar basis) in this respect, but this is probably compatible with the large effective dose of levodopa that is necessary both in the cat and in man. Dopamine itself is even less active, being over a thousand times less potent than adrenaline in decreasing fusion in incomplete tetanic contractions of the cat soleus muscle (BOWMAN and NOTT, 1978). In fast-contracting mammalian muscles, huge doses of dopamine, especially when injected intra-arterially, exert depressant effects on contractility and complex facilitatory and depressant effects on neuromuscular transmission (BLUM, 1969; FERKO and CALESNICK, 1971; GALLAGHER and KARCZMAR, 1973; FERKO, 1976). These effects on fast-contracting muscle are probably not mediated by α- or β-adrenoceptors, but the depressant effect on contractility may involve dopamine receptors (FERKO, 1976). In view of the relatively large doses required to affect slow-contracting muscles, and the huge doses required to affect fast-contracting muscles, it is unlikely that these effects of dopamine itself have any relevance to the therapeutic use of levodopa.

KISSEL et al. (1974) and KISSEL (1974) concluded that the improvement in tremor produced by propranolol in conjunction with levodopa was due to a central action of the β-adrenoceptor antagonist. They based this conclusion mainly on the fact that practolol, which penetrates the blood-brain barrier poorly, did not produce an anti-tremor effect. However, an alternative explanation of the inactivity of practolol is that it is a selective β_1-adrenoceptor blocking drug, and the muscle receptors mediating tremor belong to the β_2 subgroup. Practolol does not block the effects of levodopa, or of catecholamines, on the cat soleus muscle (BOWMAN and NOTT, 1970, 1978). The inactivity of practolol cannot therefore be used as evidence for a central action of propranolol, although such an action is not excluded.

Evidence that does point to a central action of propranolol comes from results obtained in man when levodopa is administered concurrently with an extracerebral decarboxylase inhibitor. This practice increases the amount of circulating levodopa available for cerebral metabolism and allows therapeutic benefit with a much smaller dose of levodopa (MARSDEN et al., 1973). According to TRIDON et al. (1975), combination with a peripheral decarboxylase inhibitor, such as benserazide, reduced the dose of levodopa required but did not modify the therapeutic effect on akinesia, rigidity, or tremor in his group of patients; propranolol still produced an improvement in tremor. If the persistent tremor were due to peripheral levodopa metabolites, it would be expected that benserazide alone would abolish it. At the present time further work is necessary clearly to establish the site of action of propranolol in reducing tremor when given in conjunction with levodopa. The peripheral action of β-adrenoceptor agonists in producing tremor is such a powerful effect that it seems unlikely that it would never be involved after the administration of large doses of a catecholamine precursor, and it may well be that propranolol exerts actions both centrally and peripherally in those patients whose tremor is benefited by it.

3. Some Other Types of Tremor

A number of other types of tremor has been treated with β-adrenoceptor blocking drugs, mainly propranolol, with varying degrees of success. The types of tremor so treated include anxiety tremor, the tremor of thyrotoxicosis, lithium-induced tremor, alcohol-withdrawal tremor, senile tremor, intension tremor, and essential tremor. Tremor may not be the only symptom that is relieved by propranolol, but it is the only one that is relevant here. It seems clear that propranolol may inhibit tremor as results both of central and of peripheral mechanisms, but the relative importance of each is not always clear. What does appear to be clear is that propranolol is most consistently effective when there is a large peripheral adrenaline-induced component in the tremor. Thus, propranolol, sotalol and alprenolol, all nonselective β-adrenoceptor blocking drugs, have been found to be consistently effective in reducing the tremor associated with anxiety (TYRER and LADER, 1973, 1974; LINDEN and GOTTFRIED, 1974), an effect which appears to be mainly peripheral in origin (TYRER and LADER, 1974) and presumably largely caused by adrenal medullary adrenaline.

Most authors have found propranolol to be very effective in controlling the tremors associated with thyrotoxicosis (PEPINE et al., 1972; HAVARD, 1974; REES, 1976; MURCHISON et al., 1976), although PINTO et al. (1972) failed to obtain any benefit. There is a long-standing controversy as to whether some of the symptoms of thyrotoxicosis are a consequence of sensitization of the tissues to endogenous catecholamines by thyroid hormones. It is not pertinent to enter into this controversy here; for a brief review of current opinion, an Editorial in the *British Medical Journal* (1977) may be consulted. HAVARD (1974) found oxprenolol to be ineffective in controlling the tremor of thyrotoxicosis, whereas propranolol was very effective; MURCHISON et al. (1976) found practolol to be only marginally less effective than propranolol. Both practolol and oxprenolol are alike in possessing intrinsic sympathomimetic activity, so the inactivity of oxprenolol in tremor seems unlikely to be attributed to this property. Oxprenolol (nonselective) is effective in blocking the skeletal muscle effects of adrenaline, whereas practolol (β_1-selective) has very little activity in this respect. Results with these two drugs in the tremor of thyrotoxicosis, if confirmed, may therefore indicate that the tremor of thyrotoxicosis is not mediated by an adrenergic mechanism, and that the action of propranolol may therefore be independent of β-adrenoceptor blockade. Whatever the mechanism is, it is unlikely to be central in origin, since practolol penetrates the blood-brain barrier poorly; nor is it likely to depend on the membrane stabilising activity of propranolol, since practolol is virtually devoid of this activity.

Tremor is a common side-effect of treatment with lithium salts, and also frequently occurs following withdrawal of alcohol from alcoholics. The origin of these tremors is unknown, but they probably arise from a central disturbance of monoamine metabolism. Without exception, propranolol, presumably through a central action, has been found effective in relieving both lithium-induced (FLORU, 1971; KIRK et al., 1972, 1973) and alcohol-withdrawal-induced tremor (DREW et al., 1973; ZILM et al., 1975; LAPIERRE, 1976; SELLERS et al., 1975, 1976). Pindolol (FLORU et al., 1974) is also effective in lithium-induced tremor, whereas practolol is only weakly active.

A beneficial effect of propranolol in a high proportion of patients with essential tremor has been reported by many workers (MURRAY, 1972, 1976; FAHN, 1972; EASTON, 1972; PAKKENBERG, 1972; MORGAN et al., 1973; BARBEAU, 1973; SWEET et al., 1974; SEVITT, 1974; YOUNG et al., 1975; HERAUT and PERTJISET, 1975; TOLOSA and LOEWENSON, 1975; DAVIS et al., 1976; RAUTAKORPI et al., 1976; MCALLISTER et al., 1976; TERAVAINAN et al., 1976). The beneficial effect is slow in onset (several days) and requires large doses. Oxprenolol and sotalol are similarly effective (RAUTAKORPI et al., 1976). Workers who have failed to observe a beneficial effect (e.g., FOSTER et al., 1973) possibly failed to continue treatment long enough. There is clear evidence that the beneficial effect in essential tremor is the result of a central action (YOUNG et al., 1975; KOCH-WESER, 1975).

Propranolol has also been found useful in controlling action tremor (YOUNG and WINKLER, 1973; WINKLER and YOUNG, 1974) and intention tremor (DAVIES, 1976), and oxprenolol has proved beneficial in senile tremor (THOMPSON, 1975).

III. Therapy of Spasticity

ZAIMIS (1973) described preliminary trials with orciprenaline in a group of 6 patients suffering from the muscular hypertonia characteristic of the spastic state. Chronic treatment with orciprenaline (20 mg four times daily) resulted in a valuable degree of improvement in the patients' freedom of movement and in lessening of the spasticity. Tremor (Sect. D.II.1) was often an early unwanted side-effect but tended to diminish with continued treatment. Extension of the trial (ZAIMIS, personal communication) has confirmed the important beneficial effect of orciprenaline treatment. Figure 6 illustrates the improvement in muscular performance produced by orciprenaline (20 mg four times daily) in 3 patients who had originally been treated with dantrolene sodium.

The precise mechanism of action of orciprenaline in relieving spasticity and improving muscular performance is not fully understood, although ZAIMIS believes, as seems likely, that the action of the β-adrenoceptor agonist in enhancing the rate of relaxation of the slow units within the spastic muscles plays an important part. Further tests are in progress to study the mechanism of action more fully and to ascertain the types of spasticity against which β-adrenoceptor agonists are most effective. When

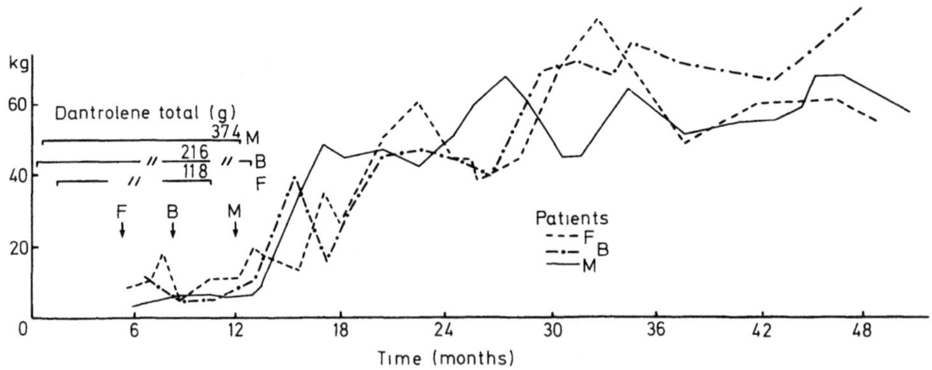

Fig. 6. Isometric contractions of calf muscle in 3 spastic patients who had previously been given dantrolene sodium for 6–11 months. Dantrolene reduced markedly the force of muscle contraction but did not diminish spasticity. In contrast orciprenaline treatment (starting at *arrows*) progressively reduced muscular stiffness characteristic of the "spastic" state and improved strength of muscle contraction. The improvement was maintained for years. For objective assessment of muscle performance, specially built calipers were used and contractions were evoked by electrical stimulation of the medial popliteal nerve delivered via surface electrodes (ZAIMIS, 1973). (Data presented by Prof. E. ZAIMIS and Drs. M. WILKINSON and N. E. GILCHRIST

these details are more precisely defined, long-acting β-adrenoceptor agonists, such as quinprenaline (quinterenol – SCRIABINE et al., 1968; BOWMAN and NOTT, 1970), may find a special place in therapeutics; a drug of this type with a relatively selective action on skeletal muscle, if it could be found, would be of especial value.

IV. Therapy of Hyperkalaemic Familial Periodic Paralysis

Hyperkalaemic familial periodic paralysis is a rare disease with an autosomal dominant mode of inheritance. Periods of flaccid paralysis, associated with pronounced hyperkalaemia and depolarization of the muscle fibre membranes, occur after exercise; the capacity to accumulate intracellular K^+ is apparently deficient (SAGILD and HELWEG-LARSEN, 1955; GAMSTORP, 1956; MCARDLE, 1962; BROOKS, 1969). Attacks are provoked by the ingestion of potassium chloride, and this forms the basis of the preferred diagnostic test (GAMSTORP et al., 1957).

β-Adrenoceptor agonists have been found to alleviate the attacks (KLEIN et al., 1960; WANG and CLAUSEN, 1976; WANG et al., 1978), apparently through their ability to stimulate the membrane Na^+–K^+ pump, thereby causing intracellular accumulation of K^+ and raising E_m, as described in Sect. B.V.1. WANG and CLAUSEN (1976) and WANG et al. (1978) studied the effects in a group of 15 related patients who suffer from the condition. They found that 2–4 inhalations of salbutamol at the beginning of an attack completely suppressed both the hyperkalaemia and the paralysis and provided a convenient and simple method of treatment.

E. Effects on Chronically Denervated Muscles

Twitches and tetani evoked by direct electrical stimulation of chronically denervated muscles exhibit the same changes in amplitude, time course, and degree of fusion in response to sympathomimetic amines as do indirectly stimulated muscles or directly stimulated fully curarized muscles. These observations have already been referred to under Sect. B. Chronically denervated muscles exhibit spontaneous myogenic activity and other changes, some of which are modified by sympathomimetic amines, and it is these, occurring in nonstimulated muscles, that are the subjects of this section. Changes in evoked contractions of chronically denervated muscles are superimposed on the changes in the background spontaneous activity.

I. Fibrillation

Among several changes that occur when a skeletal muscle is chronically deprived of its motor innervation (see, e.g., GUTMANN, 1962) is the onset of spontaneous fibrillations in many of its muscle fibres (LANGLEY and KATO, 1915; TOWER, 1939). The fibrillations are triggered by propagated action potentials that resemble those of a normally innervated fibre in amplitude but the rising phase is steeper and the declining phase is longer than normal, and the spike is followed by a pronounced positive after potential; conduction velocity is somewhat reduced (BROWN, 1937; JARCHO et al., 1954; LI et al., 1957; LÜLLMANN, 1960; THESLEFF, 1963). According to THESLEFF (1963) the propagating fibrillary potentials originate not only from the original endplate zone but also from elsewhere on the fibre membrane. BELMAR and EYZAGUIRRE (1966), on the other hand, reported that the fibrillary potentials originated only from

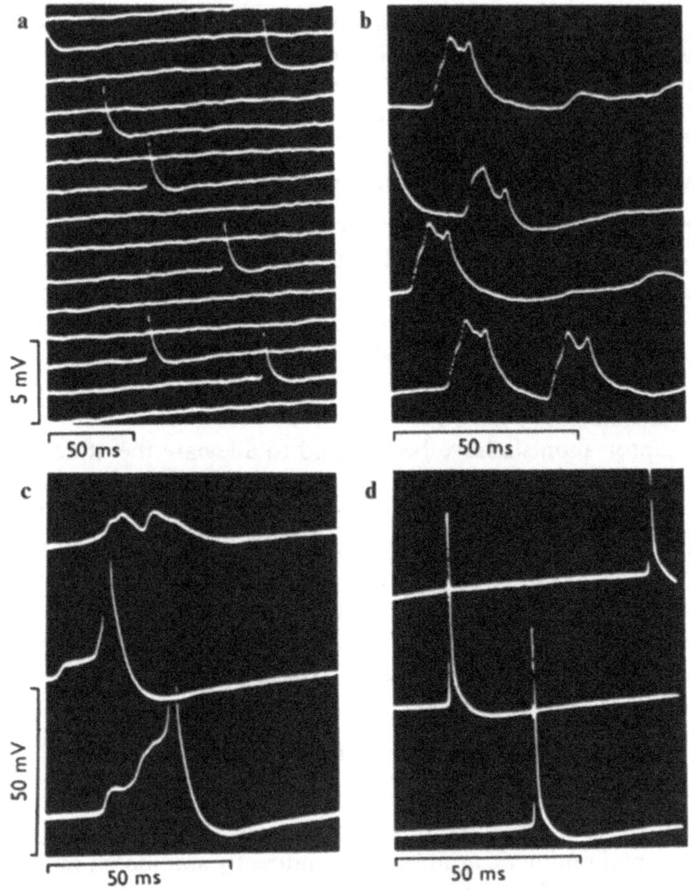

Fig. 7 a–d. Mouse, isolated denervated hemidiaphragm. Representative spontaneous potentials recorded in 9–10 days denervated muscles. **a** Discrete subthreshold depolarizations. **b** Depolarizations of complex appearance. **c** Subthreshold depolarizations recorded in the former endplate region summating to give rise to action potentials. **d** Fibrillation potentials lacking a prepotential, as recorded in the region of the tendon. (From SMITH and THESLEFF, 1976)

the former endplates which therefore acted as pacemakers. Two types of fibrillation have been described: one is generated by spontaneous rhythmic membrane potential oscillations, involving a mechanism similar to anode break excitation (THESLEFF, 1963; PURVES and SAKMANN, 1974; THESLEFF and WARD, 1975); the other arises from discrete, spontaneous and randomly occurring membrane depolarizations that trigger action potentials (PURVES and SAKMANN, 1974; SMITH and THESLEFF, 1976).

Under appropriate conditions in thin relatively easily oxygenated fibres, spontaneous activity can be demonstrated in isolated denervated muscles in vitro (PURVES and SAKMANN, 1974; SMITH and THESLEFF, 1976), showing that it is generated within the muscle and is not due to heightened sensitivity to an endogenous circulating chemical. Records of spontaneous electrical activity in the isolated denervated mouse diaphragm, from experiments of SMITH and THESLEFF (1976), are illustrated in Fig. 7.

The potentials sometimes had a sharp rising phase followed by an exponential decay, or they had a plateau-like appearance, frequently with either irregular or regular inflexions indicating a complex composition. The frequency of the spontaneous potentials, though relatively constant for any one fibre, varied from 0.1 to 25 Hz among the fibres in a muscle. In the isolated mouse diaphragm the spontaneous activity was exclusively of the second type mentioned above, that is, it arose from randomly occurring discrete depolarizations that occurred only in the region of the endplates. PURVES and SAKMAN (1974) suggested that the discrete depolarizations, which they showed to be blocked by tetrodotoxin, represent regenerative sodium conductance changes within the transverse tubules of the fibre. SMITH and THESLEFF (1976) added support to this suggestion by showing that glycerol treatment, which selectively disrupts transverse tubules (ZACHAR et al., 1972), abolished spontaneous activity, although such treatment does not abolish action potential conduction around the plasma membrane.

The denervated muscle exhibits a background tone arising at least partly from the fibrillary contractions of its component fibres, and which is therefore dependent on the frequency of the fibrillations (BOWMAN and RAPER, 1964b; BOWMAN and WEBB, 1972). In the cat, the spontaneous activity of the denervated slow-contracting soleus muscle is more vigorous than that of denervated fast-contracting muscles, such as the tibialis anterior (BOWMAN and RAPER, 1964b, 1965).

MENDEZ et al. (1970) reported that, after section of its motor nerve, reinnervation of the denervated striated muscle of the tongue by postganglionic adrenergic sympathetic fibres prevented the onset of fibrillation. LUCO and LUCO (1971) added support to this observation by showing that chronic sympathectomy of the denervated tongue removed a suppressant influence and thereby significantly increased its fibrillatory activity. Both groups of authors concluded that not only the normal motor nerve fibres but also vascular sympathetic adrenergic fibres continuously release a hypothetical trophic chemical (which is neither acetylcholine nor noradrenaline), the long-term effect of which is to control the excitability of the striated muscle fibre membranes so that fibrillation is supressed. Under normal circumstances, this chemical factor released from the vascular sympathetics presumably diffuses to the striated muscle fibres. These interesting observations are worthy of a great deal of further study, especially in relation to the work of BRAY et al. (1976) (referred to in Sect. E.II) on the effects of chronic denervation on the resting membrane potential.

Chronically denervated muscles are extrasensitive to acetylcholine and related agents (BROWN, 1937; CANNON and ROSENBLUETH, 1949) and this is associated, at least in mammalian muscle, with a spread of the acetylcholine-sensitive area to include the entire surface of the fibre membrane (GINETZINSKY and SHAMARINA, 1942; AXELSSON and THESLEFF, 1959). The spread of acetylcholine sensitivity is inhibited by drugs that inhibit protein synthesis and therefore seems to be the result of unrestrained synthesis of new protein receptors (GRAMPP et al., 1972). Small concentrations of acetylcholine augment the fibrillation frequency and produce contraction (BROWN, 1937), and it has been suggested that increased sensitivity to acetylcholine is the main factor giving rise to the spontaneous fibrillations (DENNY-BROWN and PENNYBACKER, 1938; MAGLADERY and SOLANDT, 1942; BERGAMINI et al., 1955). However, there is convincing evidence against this possibility (ROSENBLUETH and LUCO, 1937; HINES, 1942; MEAD, 1947; THESLEFF, 1960a, b, 1963; BOWMAN and RAPER, 1964b, 1965; LUCO and LUCO, 1971; PURVES and SAKMANN, 1974). Large concentrations of acetylcholine abolish all propagated electrical activity as a result of overall membrane depolarization (Brown, 1937; Rosenblueth and Luco, 1937), and the associated contraction then fulfils Gasser's (1930) definition of a contracture: viz., muscle contraction "in which tension, heat, and lactic acid are produced and the active portion of the muscle becomes negative. Only conduction of the mechanical response and a wave-like action potential are missing." Contracture tension is directly proportional to the degree of acetylcholine-elicited depolarization (Turkanis, 1969). Belmar and Eyzaguirre's (1966) results suggest that the increase in frequency of fibrillary potentials arises from the depolarizing action of acetylcholine selectively on the former endplate, whereas the contractural phase is a consequence of depolarization of the whole membrane.

Sympathomimetic amines also increase the frequency of the spontaneous fibrillary potentials of denervated muscles both in vivo (Luco and Sanchez, 1956; Bowman and Zaimis, 1961; Bowman and Raper, 1965; Raper and Bowman, 1968; Turkanis, 1969; Luco and Luco, 1971; Yamada, 1974) and in vitro (Smith and Thesleff, 1976). Figure 8a illustrates this effect of adrenaline on the denervated gastrocnemius muscle of the domestic fowl. The same response also occurs in denervated human muscles and has been used as a diagnostic aid for the detection of small amounts of denervation (Rushworth, 1963). Measurements from individual fibres show that sympathomimetic amines increase the number of spontaneously active fibres as well as the frequency of firing (Smith and Thesleff, 1976). There is clear evidence from the use of specific blocking drugs and other agents, that the increase in fibrillary activity produced by sympathomimetic amines is neither due to the release of acetylcholine nor to stimulation of acetylcholine receptors (Bowman and Raper, 1965; Turkanis, 1969; Luco and Luco, 1971; Smith and Thesleff, 1976). The increase in the frequency of fibrillary potentials is accompanied by an increase in the tone of the muscle or by isotonic shortening. The contractile response in vivo, at least in the cat, being accompanied by propagated fibrillary potentials, is therefore not a "contracture" in the terms defined by Gasser (1930). Several workers who did not make simultaneous electrical recordings have also demonstrated contractions of chronically denervated skeletal muscles in vivo and in vitro in response to sympathomimetic amines (von Euler and Gaddum, 1931; Montagu, 1955; Bhoola and Schachter, 1961; Cambridge, 1961; Paterson, 1963; Bhoola et al., 1972; Evans and Smith, 1976; Yamada and Harigaya, 1974; Bohmer and Raper, 1975), and some have gone on to show that the response is quite different from that produced by acetylcholine (Bhoola and Schachter, 1961; Bhoola et al., 1972; Evans and Smith, 1976).

Although the evoked contractions of fast-contracting and slow-contracting muscles are affected in opposite ways by sympathomimetic amines, the two types of muscle, as exemplified by the cat tibialis anterior and soleus muscles respectively, respond qualitatively similarly in so far as the effects on spontaneously-occurring fibrillary potentials and background tone are concerned, although the soleus muscle is more sensitive and responds more pronouncedly than does the tibialis anterior muscle (Bowman and Raper, 1965; Bohmer and Raper, 1975).

Bhoola et al. (1972) found that development of the responsiveness of the denervated mouse diaphragm to sympathomimetic amines was prevented by injecting the animals with the protein synthesis inhibitor actinomycin D within the first 2 days after nerve section. This result suggests that the adrenoceptors involved are protein in nature and that their synthesis occurs after denervation. If this is so, the implication is

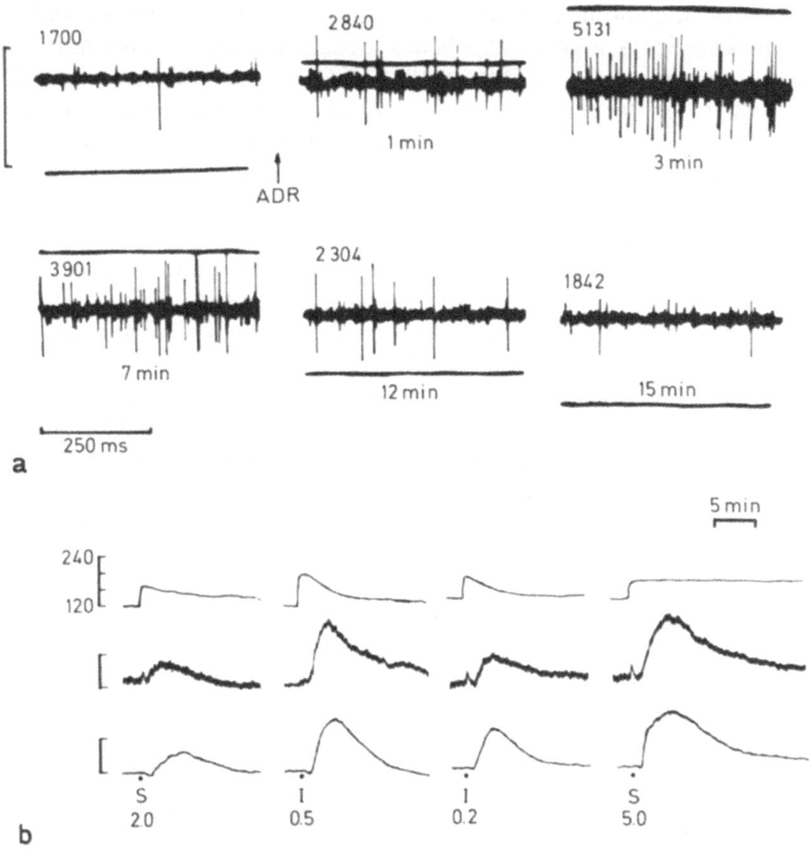

Fig. 8a. Domestic fowl under chloralose anaesthesia. Isometric tension and fibrillary potentials recorded simultaneously on an oscilloscope from the lateral head of a gastrocnemius muscle denervated for 14 days. *Arrow* indicates intravenous injection of 1 μg/kg adrenaline *(ADR)*. The following frames were taken at 1, 3, 7, 12, and 15 min afterwards. The numbers at *upper left* of each record of fibrillary potentials are the frequencies of potentials/min. (From RAPER and BOWMAN, 1968). **b** Cat under chloralose anaesthesia. Records from the top downwards: heart rate calibrated in beats/min; tension of the chronically denervated tibialis anterior muscle; tension of the chronically (14 days) denervated soleus muscle. *S* and *I* denote intravenous injections of salbutamol and isoprenaline respectively. (From BOHMER and RAPER, 1975)

that the population of adrenoceptors concerned with increasing fibrillation is a different one from the one that mediates effects on evoked contractions, since the latter are clearly present before denervation as well as afterwards. It would therefore be of interest to find out whether evoked contractions of denervated muscle are still modified by sympathomimetic amines in the usual ways after their effects on fibrillation have been prevented by protein synthesis inhibitors.

In most muscles studied, the adrenoceptors involved in mediating the effects on spontaneous fibrillation and tension exhibit the characteristics of β-receptors: isoprenaline is more potent than adrenaline, whereas noradrenaline is less potent; the effects are blocked by the β-receptor blocking drugs dichloroisoprenaline, propranolol, pronethalol, sotalol, and methoxamine and its derivatives, but not reduced by the α-receptor blocking drugs, ergotoxine, phenoxybenzamine and phentolamine (BOWMAN and ZAIMIS, 1961; BOWMAN and RAPER, 1965, 1967; RAPER and JOWETT, 1967; RAPER and BOWMAN, 1968; BHOOLA et al., 1972; EVANS and SMITH, 1976; SMITH and THESLEFF, 1976). In cat limb muscles, additional experiments with a range of selective agonists and antagonists have shown that, like those that mediate the effects on evoked contractions, the β-adrenoceptors involved in increasing fibrillation and tone can be subclassified as of the β_2-type (BOHMER and RAPER, 1975). Figure 8b illustrates part of an experiment of the last named authors in which the effects of the β_2-adrenoceptor-selective agonist salbutamol were compared with those of isoprenaline on heart rate and on the tension of the chronically denervated tibialis anterior and soleus muscles of a cat.

Rat muscles appear to be an exception in that at least part of the response to sympathomimetic amines is mediated by α-adrenoceptors. PATERSON (1963) found that the response of the chronically denervated isolated diaphragm of the rat to adrenaline was blocked most effectively by α-adrenoceptor blocking drugs. YAMADA (1974) obtained similar results with denervated limb muscles of the rat in vivo, whereas YAMADA and HARIGAYA (1974), who studied denervated rat limb muscles in vitro, described a biphasic response to adrenaline: an initial rapid contraction mediated by α-adrenoceptors was followed by a slower, more prolonged contraction mediated by β-adrenoceptors. Another exception appears to be the denervated striated muscle of the tongue of the cat. Fibrillation in this muscle was increased both by injected noradrenaline and by noradrenaline released upon stimulating the vascular sympathetic fibres to the tongue (5–10 Hz for 1 min), suggesting the involvement of α- or β_1-adrenoceptors or both. The response was in fact blocked totally by any one of a number of α-adrenoceptor blocking drugs (phenoxybenzamine, phentolamine, dibozane) or of the β-adrenoceptor blocking drug propranolol (LUCO and LUCO, 1971). Had the response been blocked partially by either type and totally by a combination of both, it could be concluded that both types of receptor are present; but the observation that either type alone was completely effective suggests a different type of receptor altogether. However, further study of the responsiveness of this muscle is advisable before jumping to such a conclusion.

Since sympathomimetic amines produce increased fibrillation and contraction in isolated muscles bathed in physiological salt solution, these responses are clearly not a consequence of concomitant vascular changes. Furthermore, in cats in vivo, similar increases in fibrillation and tension can occur in the presence of vasodilatation or vasoconstriction in the muscle (BOWMAN and RAPER, 1965). However, with large doses of adrenaline or noradrenaline that produce intense vasoconstriction, the increase in fibrillation and tension may be temporarily interrupted by a depression of both responses. That this effect is a consequence of the vasoconstriction is evidenced by the fact that it occurs only with vasoconstrictor doses and is blocked by doses of α-adrenoceptor blocking drugs that block the vasoconstriction (BOWMAN and RAPER, 1965). Fibrillation is very sensitive to a decrease in blood supply (LANGLEY and KATO, 1915; TOWER, 1939; HNÍK and SKORPIL, 1959). Vasoconstriction may account for the α-adrenoceptor-mediated component of the fall in the resting tension of chronically denervated rabbit muscle recorded by YAMADA (1974). Although sympathomimetic amines, including noradrenaline, can increase blood flow through cat muscles (Bow-

MAN and ZAIMIS, 1958; BOWMAN, 1959), the blood vessels of rabbit muscles rarely respond by vasodilatation (HARTMAN et al., 1918; GIRLING, 1951).

The presence and the amount of spontaneous fibrillary activity determine the response to sympathomimetic amines. Thus, in general, agents or procedures that enhance spontaneous activity (e.g., physostigmine, or, within limits, increase in temperature or resting tension) enhance the responses to sympathomimetic amines (BOWMAN and RAPER, 1964; BOWMAN and NOTT, 1969), whereas those that decrease or abolish spontaneous activity (e.g., long-acting depolarizing drugs; BOWMAN and RAPER, 1965; or tetrodotoxin, 2,4-dinitrophenol, KCN, oubain, strophanthin-K, Li^+ substituted for Na^+, glycerol treatment, hypertonic bath fluids, or low temperature; BHOOLA et al., 1972; EVANS and SMITH, 1976; SMITH and THESLEFF, 1976) decrease or abolish the response to sympathomimetic amines. It therefore appears that sympathomimetic amines enhance whatever process gives rise to the spontaneous background activity of denervated muscle. Calcium ions are a special case: calcium deficiency increases membrane excitability and enhances spontaneous fibrillary activity (SMITH and THESLEFF, 1976), but it diminishes the contractions produced by sympathomimetic amines (BHOOLA and SCHACHTER, 1961; EVANS and SMITH, 1976). Presumably extracellular calcium ions enter the fibres and play a role in the contractions produced by sympathomimetic amines, although they are less important for contractions evoked by electrical stimulation (EVANS and SMITH, 1976). Sympathomimetic amines have been shown to enhance the entry of calcium ions into denervated muscle fibres, this effect being essential to support the contractor effect: they do not have this action on calcium influx in innervated muscles (EVANS and SMITH, 1976). It is not known whether sympathomimetic amines enhance the frequency of fibrillary potentials in calcium-deficient solutions at the same time as their ability to produce contractions is diminished.

In chronically denervated muscle, but not in innervated muscle, isoprenaline increased the maximum rate of rise of the action potential and the overshoot and decreased the duration of the spike. Thus, the drug enhanced regenerative sodium conductance across the membrane (SMITH and THESLEFF, 1976). Several treatments mentioned elsewhere (e.g., metabolic inhibitors, K^+-lack, Li^+, cardiac glycosides, tetrodotoxin, glycerol) have been found to abolish the effects of sympathomimetic amines. However, these substances also abolish the spontaneous fibrillations, and it is not possible to determine whether any of them additionally act specifically to interfere with the sympathomimetic-stimulated mechanism or whether their effect is simply the result of blocking the spontaneous activity which is a prerequisite for the sympathomimetic effect. Nevertheless, a pronounced action of β-adrenoceptor agonists, such as isoprenaline, is stimulation of the Na^+–K^+ pump in chronically denervated skeletal muscle fibres (EVANS and SMITH, 1973; SMITH, 1974; BRAY et al., 1976), as in innervated muscles (Subsect. B.V.1), and SMITH and THESLEFF (1976) have suggested the possibility that catecholamine-induced stimulation of this pump may enhance the excitability of the transverse tubular system to the extent that spontaneous activity is augmented. More recent work by SHARMA et al. (1977) supports this possibility and suggests that the background fibrillatory activity may itself be at least partly due to enhanced Na^+–K^+ pump activity. They showed, by the use of ^3H-ouabain binding to cat muscles, that denervation increases the number of accessible Na^+–K^+ ATPase molecules in the muscle cell membrane.

At the same time the important observations of EVANS and SMITH (1973, 1976) that the influx of Ca^{2+} into denervated muscle fibres is a great deal faster than that into innervated fibres, and that isoprenaline initially enhances the influx about four-fold, cannot be ignored. It may be that, as suggested by these authors, the enhanced calcium influx is a secondary consequence of increased Na^+–K^+ pump activity. The sarcoplasmic reticulum of denervated muscle has an enhanced Ca^{2+}-sequestering ability as determined by the amount of Ca^{2+} binding to microsomes (BRODY, 1966). Possibly it is enhanced to the extent that Ca^{2+} is removed from the plasma membrane and transverse tubules, thereby further increasing their excitability and facilitating the spontaneous fibrillatory activity as suggested by BOWMAN and NOTT (1969). Removal of membrane Ca^{2+} together with spontaneous membrane activity may be the factors that enhance Ca^{2+} influx. The extra Ca^{2+} may be temporarily available to support excitation-contraction coupling before being bound in mitochondria and the sarcoplasmic reticulum. Slow-contracting muscles, with their sparser sarcoplasmic reticulum, would be expected, as is found to be the case, to bind the extra Ca^{2+} more slowly and therefore to exhibit more vigorous spontaneous movements and greater contractions in response to sympathomimetic amines.

Whether the effects of sympathomimetic amines on spontaneous fibrillatory activity are primarily mediated by the adenylate cyclase-cyclic AMP system is not known. EVANS and SMITH (1976) found cyclic AMP and its dibutyryl derivative to be without effect on the tension of denervated muscles. However, this negative result is not necessarily conclusive; cyclic AMP itself is not likely to be effective since it penetrates membranes poorly, and in some experiments (e.g., those of BRAY et al., 1976) a phosphodiesterase inhibitor given concurrently with dibutyryl cyclic AMP was found to be necessary before its effects were manifested.

II. Membrane Potential

Although a few workers (NICHOLLS, 1956; LI et al., 1957) have been unable to detect any change in the resting membrane potential of a muscle fibre as a consequence of its denervation, the majority has demonstrated a clear fall (WARE et al., 1951, 1954; LÜLLMANN and PRACHT, 1957; LÜLLMANN, 1958, 1960; KLAUS et al., 1960; LOCKE and SOLOMON, 1967; ALBUQUERQUE and THESLEFF, 1968; ALBUQUERQUE and MCISAAC, 1970; ALBUQUERQUE et al., 1971, 1974; REDFERN and THESLEFF, 1971; THESLEFF, 1974; BRAY et al., 1976). Indeed the fall in resting membrane potential is probably the first sign of denervation (ALBUQUERQUE et al., 1974; THESLEFF, 1974). Muscle fibres nearest to the site of nerve section are first affected; after the phrenic nerve innervating the rat diaphragm is sectioned at its point of entry into the muscle, resting membrane potential of fibres within 2.5 mm of the site of nerve section have already fallen significantly within 3 h (BRAY et al., 1976). The fall in membrane potential starts at the endplate region of the fibre and spreads out from there towards the tendons (LOCKE and SOLOMON, 1967; ALBUQUERQUE et al., 1971; BRAY et al., 1976). The fall in fibres of the rat diaphragm is not prevented by inhibitors of protein synthesis (BRAY et al., 1976), indicating that it is not a consequence of intracellular sequestration of K^+ by newly formed protein, as had been suggested by ALBUQUERQUE et al. (1971) and GUTH (1974). Denervation is known to induce increased protein synthesis in some muscles, including the rat diaphragm (HARRIS and MANCHESTER, 1966).

The resting membrane potential of normally innervated rat muscle fibres in vivo falls, within a few minutes, from about 80 mV to about 60 mV on topical application of ouabain. The resting membrane potental of denervated muscle on the other hand has already fallen to about 60 mV and is not further affected by ouabain (LOCKE and SOLOMON, 1967). These observations led the authors to suggest that about a quarter of the resting membrane potential of innervated fibres is derived from an electrogenic sodium pump, the activity of which is impaired by denervation or by ouabain. If this is so, the fact that the resting membrane potential is in agreement with the expected value derived from the calculated potassium equilibrium potential can only be coincidence. As BRAY et al. (1976) point out, such results assume an intracellular K^+ activity coefficient of 1, but there is accumulating evidence that in fact it is less than 1. LÜLLMANN (1958) had earlier reported a divergence between the measured resting membrane potential in rat muscle in vitro and the value calculated from the ionic gradients. It was then assumed that changes in membrane permeability to K^+ could explain the results. However, it is now known that such changes do not occur until 72 h after denervation (ALBUQUERQUE et al., 1971); the fall in membrane potential is present much earlier.

Isoprenaline, adrenaline, and noradrenaline increase the demarcation potential of denervated muscles (BROWN et al., 1950; BOWMAN and RAPER, 1965, 1966). More sensitive recordings with intracellular electrodes showed that the increase in membrane potential produced by these sympathomimetic amines in chronically denervated rat diaphragms is considerably greater than the effect in the innervated preparation (BRAY et al., 1976). Adrenaline is known to raise the cyclic AMP content of the isolated rat diaphragm (CRAIG et al., 1969). BRAY et al. (1976) showed that the hyperpolarizing action of dibutyryl cyclic AMP was antagonised by ouabain, indicating that the effect is dependent on stimulation of a sodium pump. The authors postulate that upon denervation, an electrogenic action of a sodium pump is blocked so that part of the membrane potential that is dependent on the pump (about 20%) disappears. Isoprenaline, adrenaline, and noradrenaline stimulate the formation of cyclic AMP in an appropriate compartment of the cell, and this reinstates the activity of the pump so that the membrane potential is restored. This is an attractive hypothesis but it has to be reconciled both with their own apparently paradoxical observation (BRAY et al., 1976) that denervation itself produces a pronounced increase in the cellular content of cyclic AMP, and with the observation of SHARMA et al. (1977) that denervation also increases the number of accessible Na^+–K^+ ATPase molecules in the muscle cell membrane. BRAY et al. (1976) suggest that the increased cyclic AMP content that arises from denervation alone need not necessarily be located at a site where it can stimulate the activity of the membrane sodium pump to maintain the membrane potential. Similarly, the fact that, from the results of SHARMA et al. (1977), there are apparently more sites of pump activity in denervated muscle does not necessarily mean that they are active, although their observation could explain the increased sensitivity of denervated muscle to agents that stimulate pump activity.

In contrast to the results of most other workers, TURKANIS (1969) found that intra-arterial injection of 1–15 μg/kg of isoprenaline, adrenaline, or noradrenaline produced depolarization and contracture of the chronically denervated anterior gracilis muscle of the rat. These doses, given intra-arterially, are larger than most workers have used and it is possible, though perhaps unlikely, that the size of the doses accounts for the difference in the results. When the sympathomimetic amines were applied directly to the surface of the muscle by a microdrop technique, they increased the frequency of the fibrillary potentials and occasionally caused a small hyperpolarization, but they did not increase the muscle tension. The increase in tension is in any case small, and it may be that the technique of micro application used did not activate sufficient of the muscle to produce a detectable effect of this type.

Although there are some discrepancies and some of the observations require further testing, the evidence summarized in this section as a whole suggests that activation of a sodium pump may be a common mechanism contributing to membrane hyperpolarization and to increased fibrillary activity produced by sympathomimetic amines. The former may arise from pump activity all over the membrane; if the hyperpolarization is large it may stabilise the membrane to the extent that fibrillation is temporarily depressed (BOWMAN and RAPER, 1965). Increased fibrillary activity, as discussed under Sect. E.1, may be initiated by stimulated pump activity specifically in the transverse tubules and contributed to by increased Ca^{2+} influx and possibly by hyperexcitability of the membrane, consequent upon removal of Ca^{2+} from it as a result of the increased Ca^{2+}-sequestering activity of the sarcoplasmic reticulum.

F. Actions on Neuromuscular Transmission

Adrenaline exerts a biphasic effect on neuromuscular transmission in mammals, an initial facilitatory action of relatively rapid onset being followed by a more slowly developing and more protracted depressant action. These effects on neuromuscular transmission are not powerful; they produce little or no change in the tension of indirectly evoked twitches unless the transmission process is in a vulnerable state because of fatigue (Sect. G) or disease or because of the presence of other drugs such as neuromuscular blocking drugs or anticholinesterases.

Both phases of the action on neuromuscular transmission are clearly seen (Fig. 9 a) during stimulation of the motor nerve at a frequency of 1 Hz when the transmission process is partially blocked by a continuous intravenous infusion of tubocurarine (BOWMAN and RAPER, 1966, 1967). Simultaneous recording of the gross muscle action potentials and the twitches (Fig. 9 b) shows that the two phases of the effect on twitch tension are associated with corresponding changes in the amplitudes of the action potentials (BOWMAN and RAPER, 1966, 1967). The "anticurare" effect of adrenaline is therefore a true antagonism of the neuromuscular block in the sense that it is chiefly the result of recruitment of formerly blocked muscle fibres, whereas the "curare-potentiating" effect arises mainly from a decrease in the number of fibres responding to each nerve impulse. The changes in twitch tension are thus only to a very small extent a consequence of those changes in contractility of the individual muscle fibres that are discussed in previous sections of this chapter. Both phases of the effect on transmission are independent of concomitant blood flow changes (BOWMAN and RAPER, 1966).

Noradrenaline is somewhat less potent than adrenaline in its anticurare action in the cat but considerably less potent in its curare-potentiating activity; racemic isoprenaline is without anticurare action, but is at least as powerful as (−)-adrenaline in its curare-potentiating action (Fig. 9 a). The anticurare actions of adrenaline and noradrenaline are blocked by α-adrenoceptor blocking drugs such as dibenamine (MAD-

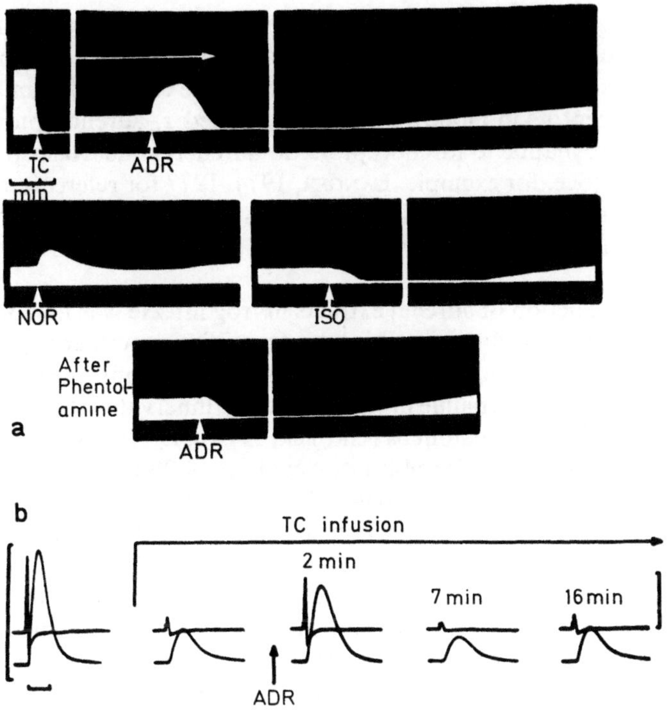

Fig. 9 a, b. Cats under chloralose anaesthesia. **a** Maximal twitches of a tibialis anterior muscle elicited indirectly once every second. At *TC* a single intravenous injection of tubocurarine (0.3 mg/kg) was given. During recovery from this dose, an intravenous infusion of tubocurarine *(TC inf)* was startet and adjusted to give a constant degree of partial block. The infusion ($0.58\ \text{mg}\cdot\text{kg}^{-1}\cdot\text{h}^{-1}$) was then maintained constant for the remainder of the experiment. At *ADR*, *NOR*, and *ISO*, 10 µg/kg of adrenaline, noradrenaline, and isoprenaline were injected intravenously. The second response to adrenaline was recorded after the intravenous injection of phentolamine (2 mg/kg). The gaps in the responses to adrenaline and isoprenaline each correspond to 10 min. **b** As for **a** but twitches and gross muscle action potentials were recorded on an oscilloscope. In this experiments the dose of adrenaline *(ADR)* was again 10 µg/kg intravenously. Responses are shown at 2, 7, and 16 min after injection of adrenaline. Note that the changes in twitch tension are accompanied by corresponding changes in the amplitude of the gross muscle action potentials.

Calibrations: tension on the *left*, 10 N; time *below*, 30 ms; action potential on the *right*, 20 mV. (From Bowman and Raper, 1966)

dock et al., 1948; Brown et al., 1950), phenoxybenzamine and phentolamine (Bowman and Raper, 1966, 1967); the curare-potentiating action is unaffected. In the presence of phentolamine, the effect of adrenaline resembles that of isoprenaline (Fig. 9 a). More recent unpublished experiments have shown that the curare-potentiating action (but not the anticurare action) is reproduced by salbutamol and rimiterol; it is blocked by (±)-propranolol but not by (+)-propranolol, nor by practolol in doses that completely abolish the action of adrenaline on the heart. These results demonstrate that the anticurare actions of adrenaline and noradrenaline are mediated by α-adrenoceptors, whereas the curare-potentiating actions of the amines are mediated by β_2-adrenoceptors. Experiments on cats (Malta et al., 1979) in which clonidine, methoxamine, oxymetazoline, adrenaline and phenylephrine were used as agonists, and phentolamine, tolazoline and thymoxamine as antagonists, indicate that the prejunctional α-adrenoceptors involved in the anticurare action are essentially similar to postjunctional α-adrenoceptors in blood vessels (i.e. so-called α_1-adrenoceptors), they do not resemble the presynaptic α-adrenoceptors on adrenergic neurones (i.e. so-called α_2-adrenoceptors). (See, for example, Langer, 1974, 1977 for reference to the two types of α-adrenoceptor in autonomically-innervated structures). However, further work on the anticurare action is necessary before the α-adrenoceptors involved can be fully characterized.

An anticurare action of adrenal extracts in frog muscle was first demonstrated by Panella, in 1907. A facilitatory action on transmission, either expressed as an anticurare action or by some other means, has since been confirmed by many workers with adrenaline or noradrenaline in cholinergically-innervated striated muscles of amphibians, avians, fish and mammals (Gruber, 1914b; Da Fonseca, 1919; Okushima, 1919; Rosenblueth et al., 1936; Maddock et al., 1948; Brown et al., 1950; Huidobro et al., 1952; Hutter and Loewenstein, 1955; Krnjević and Miledi, 1958; Bowman and Raper, 1966, 1967; Raper and Bowman, 1968; Jenkinson et al., 1968; Hidaka and Kuriyama, 1969; Kuba, 1970; Kuba and Tomita, 1971). Some workers (Brown et al., 1948; Beckett and Ellis, 1955; Ellis and Beckett, 1955) have been unable to detect any relief of tubocurarine paralysis in the isolated diaphragm muscle of the rat, although others have succeeded in demonstrating a facilitatory action on transmission in this preparation (Brand, 1952; Montagu, 1955; Krnjević and Miledi, 1958; Kuba, 1970; Kuba and Tomita, 1971, 1972). It does appear that the anticurare action is less obvious and more unpredictable in isolated muscle. One of the factors that may determine its presence is the ionic composition of the bathing fluid (Montagu, 1955). According to Miyamoto and Breckenridge (1974), adrenaline affects transmission in the isolated rat diaphragm only in the presence of high $[K^+]_0$.

It is clear from the above discussion that several observations indicate that the anticurare effect of adrenaline is the result of an entirely different mechanism of action from that underlying its direct effects on nonfatigued, noncurarized muscles. In summary, these observations are as follow. (1) The anticurare effect is mediated by α-adrenoceptors whereas the direct effects on contractility are mediated by β-adrenoceptors. (2) The anticurare effect occurs similarly in fast- and slow-contracting mammalian muscles (Bowman and Raper, 1966), but the direct actions on contractility give rise to opposite effects in the two types of muscle. (3) The anticurare effect occurs in the frog and the fowl as well as in mammals, whereas the direct action on contractility is not detected in nonfatigued amphibian muscle (Kuno, 1915; Guglielmetti, 1922; Corkill and Tiegs, 1933; Brown et al., 1950; Hutter and Loewenstein, 1955) or fowl muscle (Raper and Bowman, 1968).

The anticurare action of adrenaline in the cat is more pronounced during stimulation at 1 Hz than at 0.1 Hz (Bowman and Raper, 1966). When adrenaline is injected during a partial neuromuscular block produced by a single injection (rather than an infusion) of tubocurarine, the anticurare effect is obvious but the secondary curare-potentiating effect merges with and to a large extent is masked by the spontaneous recovery curve as the tubocurarine is removed from the biophase. The curare-potentiating action is, however, evident as a prolongation of the total duration of the block which is clearly observed when comparisons are made with the blocks produced

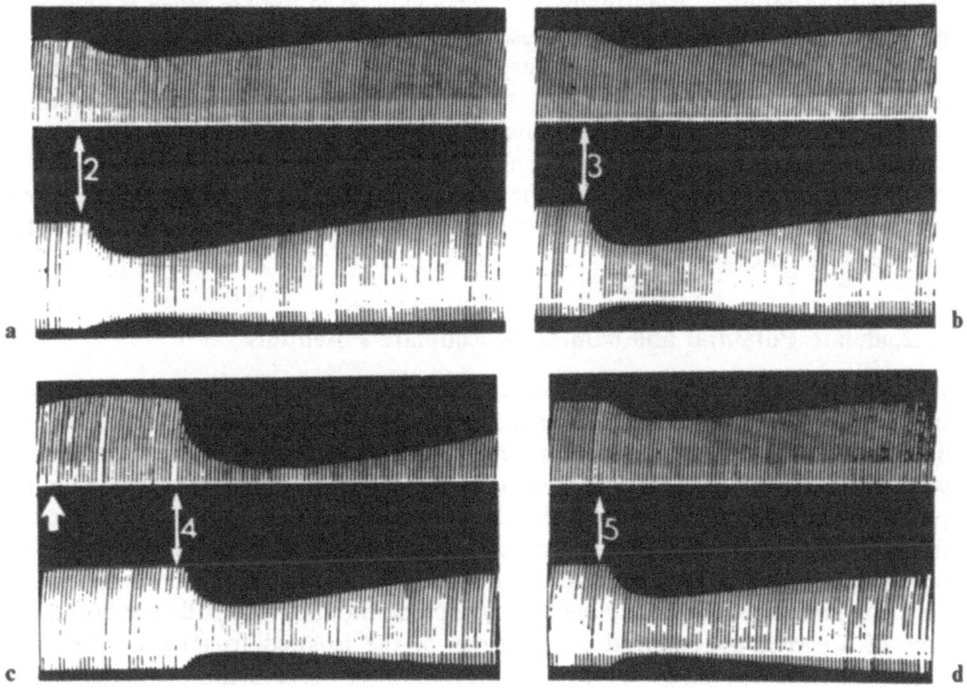

Fig. 10 a–d. Cat under chloralose anaesthesia. Indirectly excited maximal twitches of left (upper traces) and right (lower traces) tibialis anterior muscles recorded simultaneously once very 10 s. The four panels show responses to the second, third, fourth and fifth of a series of 6 doses of tubocurarine (0.15 mg/kg) injected intravenously at the *double headed numbered arrows* at intervals of 1 h. At the *large arrow* in **c**, 3 μg adrenaline was injected close-arterially to the left tibialis anterior muscle. The block of this muscle produced by the subsequent injection of tubocurarine was enhanced. (From BOWMAN and RAPER, 1966)

by tubocurarine alone both before and after that during which adrenaline is administered.

Some workers have considered that the curare-potentiating action of adrenaline is the more prominent feature of the interaction between the two drugs (NAESS and SIRNES, 1953; ELLIS and BECKETT, 1955). Indeed when adrenaline is injected before tubocurarine, the potentiating effect is the only effect seen (PATON and ZAIMIS, 1950; BOWMAN and RAPER, 1966). This effect is illustrated in Fig. 10. In this experiment, maximal indirectly-evoked twitches of both tibialis anterior muscles of the same cat were recorded simultaneously. A constant small dose of tubocurarine was injected intravenously at long but constant intervals to minimise cumulative effects. The tubocurarine produced partial block in both muscles. Adrenaline (3 μg) was injected close-arterially to one muscle only, 5 min before one of the intravenous doses of tubocurarine. The subsequent tubocurarine block in the adrenaline-treated muscle was increased from about 17% in the control response in that muscle to about 83% and was considerably prolonged. The tubocurarine block in the contralateral muscle was not affected. PATON and ZAIMIS (1950) made the point that because of this action of adrenaline, sensitivity to tubocurarine will be greater in a patient in whom adrenal medullary secretion is abnormally high. This may be so but the effect is unlikely to be of much importance, since the dose of adrenaline necessary (e.g., 3 μg close-arterially in Fig. 10) corresponds to a very large blood concentration that would be unlikely to be achieved even in the severest stress or disease. It is possible that asthmatic patients who have been chronically treated with long-acting sympathomimetic bronchodilators might be extrasensitive to nondepolarizing neuromuscular blocking drugs of the tubocurarine type, but again the potential interaction, although worth bearing in mind, is unlikely to be clinically important or it would have been noted in the clinical literature before now.

I. Endplate Potential and Miniature Endplate Potentials

Hutter and Loewenstein (1955) concluded that in frog muscle the facilitation of transmission produced by noradrenaline was the result of a postjunctional action, because in their experiments both endplate depolarizations evoked by acetylcholine added to the bathing fluid and epps evoked by nerve stimulation were increased in amplitude by noradrenaline. Jenkinson et al. (1968), who also studied frog muscle, confirmed Hutter and Loewenstein's observation that noradrenaline added to the bathing fluid for relatively long periods augments depolarizations elicited by acetylcholine. This postjunctional effect may underly the potentiation, by adrenaline or noradrenaline, of acetylcholine-induced contractures of the isolated frog rectus abdominis muscle described by Burn (1945). However, the slow onset of this postjunctional effect in frog muscle makes it unlikely that it accounts for the rapidly occurring facilitatory effect on transmission. Jenkinson et al. (1968) in fact found in the frog sartorius and extensor longus digitorum IV muscles that noradrenaline neither changed the amplitude of the mepps nor changed that of the depolarizations produced by iontophoretically applied acetylcholine, but that the frequency of the miniature endplate potentials (mepps) and the amplitude of endplate potentials (epps) evoked by nerve impulses in the presence of high $[Mg^{2+}]_0$ were increased; they concluded that the facilitatory action of noradrenaline on transmission is due to a prejunctional action through which the quantal content of the epp is increased. Hidaka and Kuriyama (1969) obtained similar results to those of Jenkinson et al. (1968) with noradrenaline on the cholinergic neuromuscular junctions of the fin muscles of the silver carp. They also concluded that noradrenaline acts on the nerve endings to increse the spontaneous and the evoked release of acetylcholine. According to Hidaka and Kuriyama (1969), adrenaline acts rather differently from noradrenaline in the fish muscle. They found that, unlike noradrenaline, adrenaline enhanced the amplitude of the miniature junctional potentials as well as those of the larger depolarizations evoked either by iontophoretic application of acetylcholine or by nerve stimulation; adrenaline also increased both the input resistance and the resting membrane potential of the muscle fibres. Although adrenaline slightly increased the frequency of the miniature junctional potentials, its main effects appeared to be exterted postjunctionally.

Work of this type on mammalian muscle appears so far to have been confined to the rat. Krnjević and Miledi (1958) found that adrenaline relieved the presynaptic failure of transmission that occurs in rapidly stimulated nerve muscle preparations, and their evidence was indicative of an action on the nerve endings. Kuba (1970) found that the amplitude and half-decay time of the epp of the rat diaphragm were increased by noradrenaline, adrenaline, and isoprenaline, the effect of noradrenaline on the epp amplitude being the most pronounced. Noradrenaline increased the frequency of the mepps but not their amplitude, whereas isoprenaline increased their amplitude but not their frequency. Adrenaline produced both effects. Adrenaline and isoprenaline, but not noradrenaline, increased the resting membrane potential of the muscle membrane and its input resistance, and also increased the depolarizations evoked by iontophoretically applied acetylcholine. The effects of noradrenaline were blocked by phentolamine, those of isoprenaline by propranolol, and those of adrenaline by one or the other. KUBA (1970) concluded that noradrenaline acts through α-adrenoceptors on the nerve endings to increase transmitter release, that isoprenaline acts through β-adrenoceptors in the muscle fibre membrane to hyperpolarize it and

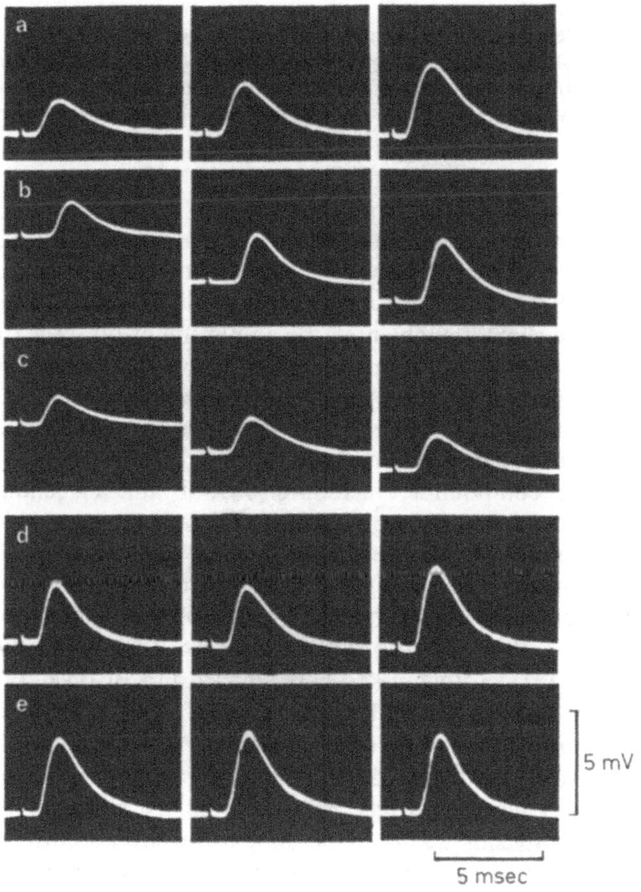

Fig. 11 a–e. Rat, phrenic nerve-diaphragm. Effects of catecholamines and of their antagonists on endplate potentials in a solution containing tubocurarine 1×10^{-6} g/ml in five different preparations. **a** Noradrenaline 1×10^{-6} g/ml; **b** adrenaline 1×10^{-6} g/ml; **c** isoprenaline 1×10^{-6} g/ml; **d** phentolamine 2×10^{-6} g/ml; **e** pronethalol 2×10^{-6} g/ml. First record in each horizontal row is a control; the second is 5 min and the third 10 min after application of drugs. The responses in each horizontal row were recorded from the same endplate. (From KUBA, 1970)

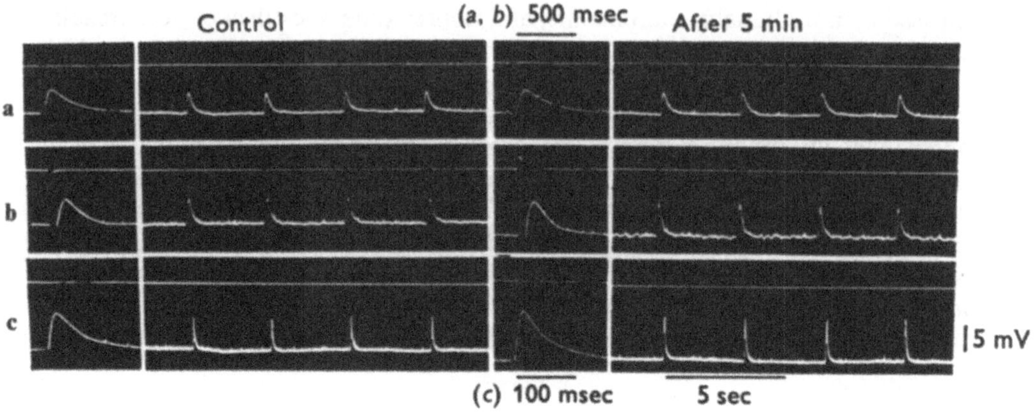

Fig. 12a–c. Rat, phrenic-nerve diaphragm. Effects of catecholamines on acetylcholine potentials evoked by iontophoretically applied acetylcholine. **a** Noradrenaline 5×10^{-6} g/ml; **b** adrenaline 5×10^{-6} g/ml; **c** isoprenaline 5×10^{-6} g/ml. Intensity of current pulses was 1×10^{-7} A and the duration was (a) 5 ms, (b) 8 ms, and (c) 1 ms. Three different preparations. (From KUBA, 1970)

increase the input resistance, and that adrenaline produces both types of action. The effects of adrenaline, noradrenaline, and isoprenaline on epps and on acetylcholine potentials in two of KUBA's (1970) experiments are illustrated in Figs. 11 and 12. Although isoprenaline slightly augmented the amplitude of the epps (through its postjunctional action) the peak of the epp remained below that of the control because of the simultaneous increase in the background hyperpolarization (Fig. 11c). Consequently, isoprenaline would not be expected to relieve but only to enhance tubocurarine paralysis, as illustrated in Figure 9a.

Other phenolic compounds, including phenol and catechol, also facilitate neuromuscular transmission by a prejunctional action through which acetylcholine release by nerve impulses is enhanced. They increase the frequency of mepps without altering their amplitude or time course; they augment epps evoked by nerve impulses but not endplate depolarizations produced by iontophoretically-applied acetylcholine (MOGEY and YOUNG, 1949; OTSUKO and NONOMURA, 1963; KUBA, 1969; BLABER and GALLAGHER, 1971; GALLAGHER, 1972; GALLAGHER and BLABER, 1973). Despite the similarity between the prejunctional effects of catechol and phenol on the one hand, and those of noradrenaline on the other, different mechanisms, or at least different receptors, appear to be involved since the effects of catechol and phenol are not modified by adrenoceptor blocking drugs. However, the last named authors suggest the possibility that in catechol we have the simplest α-adrenoceptor activating agent which is purely prejunctional in its activity. In order to explain the lack of effects of α-adrenoceptor blocking drugs on the action of catechol, they put forward the suggestion that the prejunctional α-adrenoceptor might be composed of 2 sites, one occupied by the catechol group and the other by the amine group, and that the antagonists occupy only the latter group. Hence, catechol would still stimulate the receptor in the presence of the antagonist, but a catecholamine would not. An argument against their suggestion is that catecholamines such as adrenaline are much more potent than catechol itself in terms of the size of the effective anticurare doses, but catechol is much more powerful than adrenaline in terms of the extent of its anticurare action. Nevertheless, the proposal of GALLAGHER and BLABER (1973) is worthy of further consideration.

II. Mechanisms of Action

The simplest explanation of the secondary curare-potentiating action of β-adrenoceptor agonists is that it is a consequence of their postjunctional membrane hyperpolarizing action illustrated in Fig. 11 and described and discussed under Sect. B.V.1 and B.VII.

The mechanism through which α-adrenoceptor agonists enhance acetylcholine release in response to nerve impulses has not yet been fully elucidated. KUBA and TOMITA (1971, 1972) have provided evidence that noradrenaline increases the probability of release of transmitter quanta from the resting nerve terminals and that this action is intensified by first raising the probability of release by some other means such as depolarization of the nerve terminals by current, either externally applied or from an action potential, by increasing $[Ca^{2+}]_0$, or by decreasing $[Na^+]_0$ or $[Mg^{2+}]_0$. They propose a kinetic model in which transmitter release is modified by the binding of Ca^{2+} to a specific site in the nerve terminal. According to their model, α-adrenoceptor agonists (such as noradrenaline) do not change the dissociation constant of the reaction between Ca^{2+} and the specific binding site, but they increase the rate constant of the calcium complex for releasing acetylcholine. The effect of noradrenaline is in fact similar to that of excess Ca^{2+}. KUBA (1970) found noradrenaline, in concentrations that augmented epps, to be without any detectable effect on the action current of the nerve terminal, thus indicating that the membrane potential of the nerve terminals is not modified by noradrenaline.

Since both excitation-contraction coupling in muscle and excitation-transmitter release coupling in nerve are strongly dependent on calcium ions, it is tempting to suppose that adrenaline exerts similar calcium-related actions on the two, the former being mediated by β- and the latter by α-adrenoceptors. Evidence has accumulated to suggest that the adenylate cyclase-cyclic AMP system, and possibly the guanylate cyclase-cyclic GMP system, play important roles in the activity of nervous tissue, including neuronal metabolism, microtubule function, axoplasmic transport, the synthesis, mobilization, storage, and possibly the release of transmitters, and the trophic influence of one neurone upon another or upon a neuroeffector cell (GREENGARD and COSTA, 1970; GOODMAN et al., 1970; RASMUSSEN, 1970; ROBISON et al., 1971b; GREENGARD et al., 1972; JOHNSON et al., 1973; VAPAATALO, 1974; COSTA et al., 1974; SLOBODA et al., 1975; BOEGMAN and WOOD, 1976). Since adrenaline stimulates adenylate cyclase, thereby increasing cyclic AMP concentrations in many cells, it was natural to consider the possibility that the sympathomimetic-induced increase in transmitter release at the neuromuscular junction is brought about by raised cyclic nucleotide concentrations within the terminal axoplasm. Circumstantial evidence that this might be so was first supplied by BRECKENRIDGE et al. (1967), who showed that theophylline, one action of which is to inhibit phosphodiesterase and thereby increase cyclic AMP concentrations, enhanced the ability of adrenaline to potentiate neostigmine at the neuromuscular junction. There is no doubt that theophylline and some other drugs with phosphodiesterase inhibiting activity do facilitate neuromuscular transmission by a prejunctional action (see, for example, GOLDBERG and SINGER, 1969; HOFMANN, 1969; VAPAATALO and ANTTILA, 1972; SINGER and GOLDBERG, 1970; WILSON, 1974; MIYAMOTO and BRECKENRIDGE, 1974); some of them have been proposed for use in myasthenia gravis (HOKKANEN et al., 1972). However, there is some doubt as to whether the effect is a consequence of the phosphodiesterase inhibiting activity of the drugs, since they do possess additional actions; caffeine, for example, mobilizes calcium ions in muscle (BIANCHI, 1961; LÜLLMANN and HOLLAND, 1962; WEBER, 1968; BLINKS et al., 1972) by an action that is probably unrelated to its phosphodiesterase inhibiting activity. A similar calcium-mobilizing action in nerve might account for, or contribute to, its facilitatory effects on transmitter release. Dibutyryl cyclic AMP (a derivative that more readily penetrates cell membranes and that is more stable than the parent nucleotide) has also been reported to facilitate transmitter release at the neuromuscular junction in vitro (GOLDBERG and SINGER, 1969); in addition it gives rise to antidromic repetitive firing in motor axons in vivo (DRETCHEN et al., 1976). The results of GOLDBERG and SINGER (1969) with dibutyryl cyclic AMP have been criticised by MIYAMOTO and BRECKENRIDGE (1974) on the grounds that their technique of adding the nucleotide to the preparation was likely to give rise to nonspecific osmotic effects on transmitter release. It is, however, more difficult to dismiss the results of DRETCHEN et al. (1976) who demonstrated a facilitatory action of dibutyryl cyclic AMP in vivo; antidromic repetitive firing of the type they observed is generally considered to reflect a prejunctional action on the transmission process.

MIYAMOTO and BRECKENRIDGE (1974) point out that there has been a tendency to confuse two not necessarily related questions: first, whether cyclic AMP plays an *obligatory* role in normal transmitter release, and secondly whether the nucleotide mediates the facilitatory effect of adrenaline on transmission without necessarily modifying normal background transmission. Kinetic studies by QUASTEL and HACKETT (1971) have provided strong evidence that cyclic AMP is not directly involved in the physiological mechanism underlying transmitter release, and the results of MIYAMOTO and BRECKENRIDGE (1974) and WILSON (1974) tend to confirm this conclusion. MIYAMOTO and BRECKENRIDGE found dibutyryl cyclic AMP (unlike theophylline) to be without effect on mepp frequency in normal nerve muscle preparations. Surprisingly, they also found adrenaline and noradrenaline to be similarly without effect on normal preparations, and it is difficult to explain this divergence from the results of other workers. When neuromuscular transmission was impaired by excess $[K^+]_o$, then both catecholamines and dibutyryl cyclic AMP increased the frequency of mepps. WILSON (1974) used the isolated phrenic nerve diaphragm preparation of the rat in which the muscle fibres were transversely cut to prevent muscle action potentials and contractions. Under these conditions, neither tubocurarine nor excess $[Mg^{2+}]_o$ is necessary to immobilize the preparation. He found that either theophylline or dibutyryl cyclic AMP produced increases in the quantum content of the first epp of a train, in the transmitter mobilization rate, and in the size of the releasable store of transmitter, but that neither had a significant effect on the probability of release. In contrast, the main action of noradrenaline (KUBA and TOMITA, 1971) like that of excess $[Ca^{2+}]_o$ (HUBBARD et al., 1968, 1971) is to increase the probability of release. WILSON (1974) interpreted his results to indicate that cyclic AMP is involved in regulating the metabolic activity of the neurone associated with the synthesis, storage, and mobilization of transmitter in the nerve terminal; but, unlike noradrenaline, the nucleotide does not directly stimulate the release mechanism. The results of MIYAMOTO and BRECKENRIDGE (1974) and of WILSON (1974) suggest that catecholamines, acting through the adenylate cyclase-cyclic AMP mechanism, may have an additional prejunctional role to play in conditions in which the transmission mechanism is fatigued; this possibility is discussed in Sect. G.

On the whole, the combined published results indicate that noradrenaline and adrenaline probably do not act through nerve terminal cyclic AMP to facilitate neuromuscular transmission and antagonise tubocurarine in normal, nonfatigued nerve-muscle preparations. Two additional pieces of evidence that support this view are as follow. First, adenosine and adenine nucleotides (AMP, ADP, ATP) which increase the cyclic AMP content of cerebral cortical slices (SATTIN and RALL, 1970) and therefore presumably of peripheral motor nerves, depress rather than facilitate neuromuscular transmission (GINSBORG and HIRST, 1972; GINSBORG et al., 1973; RIBEIRO and WALKER, 1975; GINSBORG and JENKINSON, 1976). Second, and perhaps the most difficult to reconcile with any evidence to the contrary, the facilitatory action of adrenaline and noradrenaline on neuromuscular transmission in normal, nonfatigued, nerve-muscle preparations is mediated by α-adrenoceptors as described above. Although there is evidence that some α-adrenoceptor-mediated effects depend on cyclic AMP production (ROBISON et al., 1971 b; SCHORDERET et al., 1972), it is generally β-adrenoceptor-mediated effects that are so dependent. In frog sciatic nerve, β-adrenoceptor specific concentrations of isoprenaline produced an increase in cyclic AMP concentration (HORN and MCAFEE, 1977), indicating that, unless a species difference is involved, motor nerves follow the usual pattern in that it is β-adrenoceptor activation that results in elevation of cyclic AMP concentrations.

The concept of regulation of transmitter release from nerve endings by changes in the activity of specific membrane-bound ATPases has been proposed (PATON et al., 1971; VIZI, 1972), and evidence in support of the idea has accumulated from the work of GILBERT et al. (e.g., GILBERT et al., 1975; GILBERT and WYLLIE, 1975). GILBERT et al. (1975) showed that noradrenaline, acting through α-adrenoceptors, stimulates a Na^+-ATPase and a (Na^+, K^+) ATPase in synaptosomes from guinea pig cerebral cortex, and they considered this in the light of evidence that noradrenaline inhibits its own release from noradrenergic nerve endings (for a review, see LANGER, 1977); noradrenaline also inhibits the release of acetylcholine from cholinergic endings in the intestine (KOSTERLITZ and WATT, 1965). These effects presumably arise through restriction of the availability of Ca^{2+} to the excitation-release mechanism. Motor nerve endings in skeletal muscle have not yet been studied from these points of view, but the possibility that α-adrenoceptor agonists directly or indirectly, inhibit a specific terminal membrane ATPase at this site, and that this results in an increased availability of Ca^{2+} to the release mechanism is worthy of further consideration.

G. Effects on Fatigued Muscles

DESSY and GRANDIS (1904) first showed that adrenaline temporarily restored the contractions of frog skeletal muscle that had been depressed by prolonged stimulation of its motor nerve. Similar results on fast-contracting mammalian muscles were subsequently recorded by CANNON and NICE (1911, 1913), and since that time numerous workers have confirmed that adrenaline, and, to a lesser extent, noradrenaline, markedly increase both the twitch and tetanic tensions of fatigued frog and fast-contracting mammalian muscles both in vivo and in vitro (GRUBER, 1913, 1914a, b, 1917a, b, 1919, 1922a, b, 1924; CANNON and GRUBER, 1916; GRUBER and FELLOWS, 1918; GUGLIELMETTI, 1918, 1922; DA FONSECA, 1919; OKUSHIMA, 1919; CAMPOS et al., 1929; KUSCHINSKY and VIAUD, 1933; ROSENBLUETH et al., 1936; LUCO, 1939; BÜLBRING and BURN, 1940; BÜLBRING, 1946; BROWN et al., 1947, 1948; BOWMAN, 1956). Stimulation of the splanchnic nerves produces similar effects to those of adrenaline on fatigued muscle contractions (CANNON and NICE, 1911, 1913). The effect on contractions of fatigued fast-contracting muscle is much greater than that in nonfatigued muscle.

ORBELI showed in 1923 that when the gastrocnemiums muscle of the frog was fatigued by prolonged stimulation of the motor roots, simultaneous stimulation of the lumbar sympathetic chain then partially restored the contractions. This effect of sympathetic stimulation became known as the "Orbeli effect": it is presumably due to transmitter released from the vascular sympathetics spilling over to affect the striated muscle, as first suggested by TIEGS (1934). The Orbeli effect has since been confirmed in both frog and mammalian fast-contracting muscles (MAIBACH, 1928; LABHART, 1929; CHARLET, 1930; BAETJER, 1930; CORKILL and TIEGS, 1933; WOLFF and CATTELL, 1934; WEBER, 1934; TIEGS, 1934, BÜLBRING and BURN, 1939). Mammalian muscle is more susceptible to impaired blood flow than is frog muscle at room temperature, and if the frequency of motor nerve stimulation is high and vasoconstriction pronounced, a common effect of adrenaline, noradrenaline, or sympathetic stimulation is depression of the fatigued contractions in the mammal. However, enhancement of contractions can occur accompanied by a moderate degree of vasoconstriction (Fig. 13), and since the effect also occurs in isolated muscles and in muscles perfused at a constant rate, it is clear that it is not simply a consequence of vascular changes, although it may be modified by them.

Slow-contracting mammalian muscles, such as the cat soleus, are difficult to fatigue by high frequency stimulation. When a degree of fatigue is achieved, adrenaline produces only weak and variable effects on the twitches (BOWMAN, 1956). During sustained high frequency tetanic contractions of the cat soleus muscle, changes in tension produced by adrenaline (and some other vasoactive substances) simply mirror the blood flow changes, an increase in flow being accompanied by an increase in tension and vice versa (BOWMAN, 1956). The soleus primarily utilises oxidative metabolism (ROMANUL, 1964, 1965) and its oxygen utilisation and blood flow are normally higher than those of fast-contracting muscles (BEATTY and PETERSON, 1963; HILTON et al., 1970). During sustained contractions evoked by nonphysiologically high frequencies of stimulation this muscle is therefore in a more vulnerable position with regard to its blood supply; hence the effects of changes in blood flow tend to mask any concomitant effects of catecholamines occurring on contractility or transmission.

In recent years little work has been done on the effects of sympathetic stimulation or of catecholamines on fatigued muscle, largely because the relevance of the type of fatigue produced by high frequency motor nerve stimulation to physiological fatigue is doubtful, and it is by no means certain that "physiological" frequencies of sympathetic nerve stimulation, or "physiological" concentrations of adrenaline and noradrenaline have any effect. Most of the early workers used high frequencies of sympathetic nerve stimulation and large doses of catecholamines. Much of the earlier work was reviewed by BOWMAN and NOTT (1969), and there appears to be little to add.

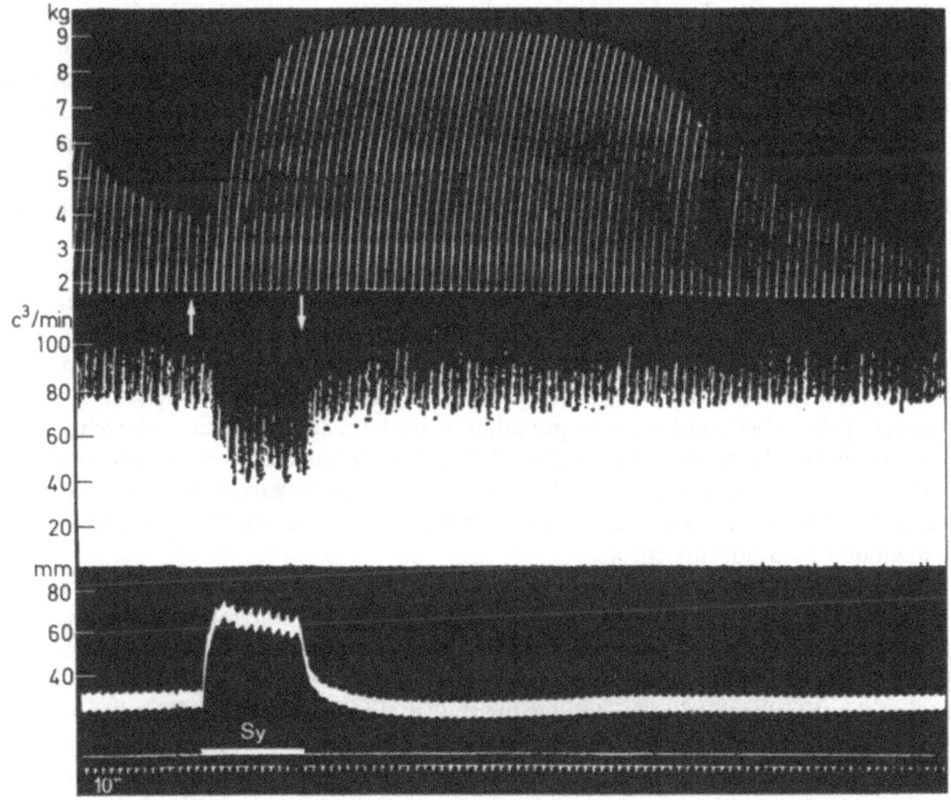

Fig. 13. Dog, perfused hindleg. The uppermost record shows tension produced by the gastrocnemius muscle in response to single shocks applied to the motor roots. The middle record shows venous outflow. The lowest record shows perfusion pressure. Between the *arrows* the lumbar sympathetic chain was stimulated for 2 min causing a prolonged increase in the muscle response. (From BÜLBRING and BURN, 1939)

In general it seems that the sympathomimetic amines produce essentially the same effects in fatigued and nonfatigued fast-contracting muscles, but that particular effects in fatigued muscles may be exaggerated depending upon which part of the system is fatigued. BÜLBRING and WHITTERIDGE (1941) found that adrenaline lowered the threshold of motor nerve, with the result that the amplitude of the compound action potential evoked by submaximal stimulation was increased. The effect was much greater in fatigued than in fresh nerve. KRNJEVIĆ and MILEDI (1958) found that adrenaline relieved the presynaptic failure of transmission that occurs in rapidly stimulated nerve-muscle preparations and, in a later paper, the same authors (KRNJEVIĆ and MILEDI, 1959) reported that hyperpolarization of the nerve endings by anodal currents produced a similar effect. Presynaptic failure is associated with nerve terminal depolarization, and the two papers by KRNJEVIĆ and MILEDI suggest that adrenaline may act to restore transmission by means of a hyperpolarizing action which is unmasked when the terminals are depolarized; adrenaline does not hyperpolarize the terminals at nonfatigued junctions (KUBA, 1970). MIYAMOTO and BRECKENRIDGE (1974) found that adrenaline and noradrenaline increased the frequency of mepps in the rat diaphragm only when the terminals were depolarized by treatment with excess $[K^+]_0$, a situation which they considered to be analogous to fatigue or to presynaptic failure. Under the same conditions dibutyryl cyclic AMP had a similar effect. As described earlier, WILSON (1974) reached the conclusion that cyclic AMP in the nerve terminal increased metabolic activity associated with the synthesis, storage, and mobilization of the transmitter but that, unlike noradrenaline, it does not directly stimulate the release mechanism. It may therefore be that when there is junctional fatigue, adrenaline exerts three actions on the terminals: (1) a hyperpolarizing action that counteracts the depolarization associated with presynaptic failure; (2) stimulation of metabolic activity and consequent enhancement of synthesis and mobilization of transmitter; (3) a direct calcium ion-like stimulation of the release mechanism that increases evoked release and therefore the quantum content of the epp. Actions (1) and (2) may be detectable only at fatigued junctions. Since they are mimicked by dibutyryl cyclic AMP, and since isoprenaline stimulates the formation of cyclic AMP in nerve, it may be tentatively concluded that they are mediated by β-adrenoceptors and the adenylate cyclase-cyclic AMP system. Action (3) is detectable at both fatigued and nonfatigued junctions; it accounts for the anticurare action of noradrenaline and is mediated by α-adrenoceptors.

Presynaptic failure is more pronounced in rapidly stimulated isolated muscles or in perfused muscles when the circulation is inadequate, and under these circumstances the defatiguing action of adrenaline is also more pronounced (BÜLBRING and BURN, 1939). It seems unlikely that junctional failure plays a part in physiological fatigue, so that the three prejunctional actions mentioned above may be irrelevant to any action of sympathomimetic amines on fatigued voluntary movements. All three may however contribute to the relatively weak beneficial effect on transmission that ephedrine produces in patients with myasthenia gravis. Ephedrine, acting both directly and indirectly, stimulates both α- and β-adrenoceptors.

Fatigue induced by high frequency motor nerve stimulation does not always involve or is not always confined to the neuromuscular junction (BROWN and BURNS, 1949; MERTON, 1954, 1956; MASCHIMA et al., 1962; EBERSTEIN and SANDOW, 1963; SMITH, 1974). It may be the result of a failure in excitation-contraction coupling in which the undiminished muscle fibre action potential fails to trigger full-sized contractions. Fatigue of voluntary movements may be partly central in origin, but the peripheral component seems to be entirely postjunctional at the level of excitation-contraction coupling failure (MERTON, 1956). Hence, any defatiguing effect of the sympathetic nervous system, especially of the adrenal medullae, on voluntary movements of fast-contracting units must be looked for at this site. Again there may be three contributory actions, all of which appear to be mediated by β-adrenoceptors and the adenylate cyclase-cyclic AMP system. They are as follow. (1) The proposed action on the sarcoplasmic reticulum of fast-contracting muscles through which the storage of Ca^{2+} is enhanced (see Sect. B.VII). (2) Restoration of normal transmembrane ionic distribution and membrane potential: in mouse diaphragms stimulated to fatigue in vitro, SMITH (1974) found that sodium concentrations were increased and potassium concentrations were decreased so that the membranes were depolarized; adrenaline and isoprenaline, by stimulating the membrane Na^+–K^+ pump, restored the ionic balance and the membrane potential. (3) Stimulation of glycogenolysis by activation of phosphorylase. Activation of phosphorylase is impaired in fatigued muscle, and adrenaline restores it towards normal (CORI and ILLINGWORTH, 1956; HELMREICH and CORI, 1966). It is not known to what extent these three actions are interrelated.

The different possible sites of fatigue and the multiple possible sites of drug action account for the variation in the responses to catecholamines which is a common feature of experiments on fatigued muscle. They also account for the early controversy as to whether the site of action was pre- or postjunctional and whether it involved α- or β-adrenoceptor. As BÜLBRING (1976) points out, everyone was correct.

H. Summary of Effects of Adrenaline

The postulated multiple sites of action of adrenaline on the neuromuscular system are summarised in Fig. 14.

The most pronounced effect, and probably the one with the major physiological, pathological, and therapeutic relevance is that on the contractility of slow-contracting mammalian twitch fibres. This effect is produced by the same blood concentrations of adrenaline as those that affect the cardiovascular system. In anaesthetised animals, in which the muscle or its motor nerve are stimulated electrically, the effect on contractility is considerably longer lasting than the cardiovascular effects, presumably because reflex compensatory mechanisms cannot be brought into play. The effect on the contractility of slow fibres, together with that on the muscle spindles, appears to be responsible for the tremor associated with the use of sympathomimetic bronchodilators. The same effect produced by β_2-adrenoceptor agonists may also be responsible for the improved muscular performance and relief of muscular hypertonia in patients with spasticity.

A second important action from both therapeutic and physiological points of view is that which stimulates the electrogenic component of membrane Na^+–K^+ pump activity. This action, for example of salbutamol, provides a simple and convenient method for the therapy of hyperkalaemic familial periodic paralysis. The possibility that the electrogenic component of the membrane potential is normally maintained by the action of circulating endogenous adrenal medullary adrenaline is worthy of further study.

A further action of physiological concentrations of adrenaline that has not been mentioned elsewhere in this review is that demonstrated by GARBER et al. (1976) on rat skeletal muscle. These authors showed that stimulation of β-adrenoceptors reduced the synthesis and release of amino acids (alanine and glutamine) from the muscle; the effect appeared to be mediated by cyclic AMP.

I. Effects Unrelated to Adrenergic Mechanisms

Some drugs whose therapeutic effects depend upon their ability to interfere in one way or another with adrenergic mechanisms produce unwanted effects on skeletal muscle that are probably unrelated to the sympathetic nervous system. An action involving this system would imply that skeletal muscle function is continually modulated by sympathetic nerves, and most evidence indicates that this is not so. Since these unwanted effects lie outside the main theme of this chapter they have been left to the end to be summarised here in this final section.

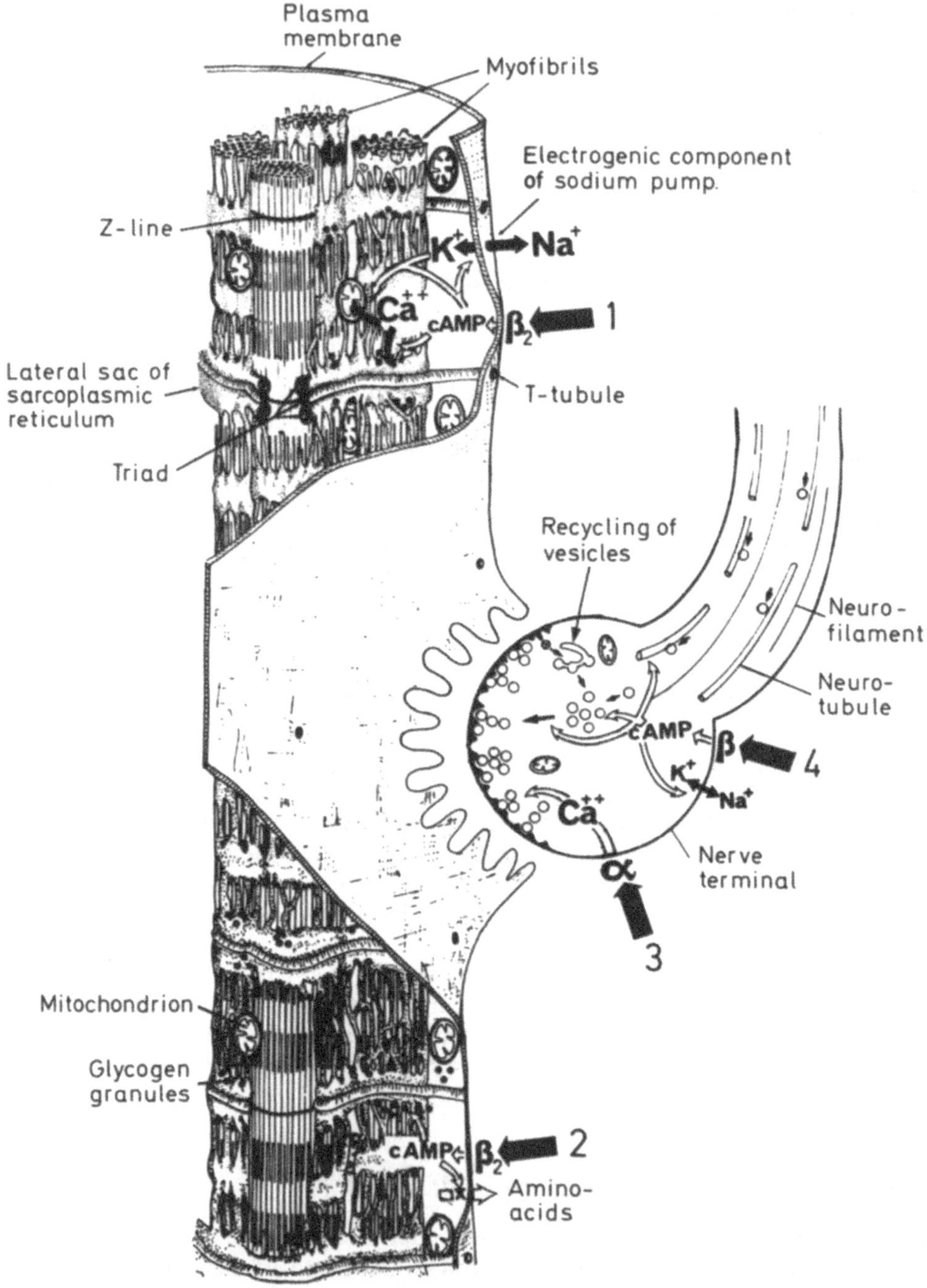
Plasma membrane
Myofibrils
Electrogenic component of sodium pump.
Z-line
K+
Na+
Ca++
cAMP
β2
1
Lateral sac of sarcoplasmic reticulum
T-tubule
Triad
Recycling of vesicles
Neuro-filament
Neuro-tubule
cAMP
β
4
K+
Na+
Ca++
Nerve terminal
α
3
Mitochondrion
Glycogen granules
cAMP
β2
2
Amino-acids

I. Adrenergic Neurone Blocking Drugs

Bretylium (an obsolete antihypertensive drug which is occasionally used as an antidysrhythmic agent) and guanethidine, a commonly used antihypertensive drug, have often been reported to produce muscle weakness in a small percentage of patients during prolonged therapeutic use (CAMPBELL and MONTUSCHI, 1960; EVANSON and SEARS, 1960; DOLLERY, 1961; PAGE, 1961; HOFMANN and SPIVAK, 1963). The explanation of the muscle weakness is not certain; it is not necessarily due to a single cause; nor do the two drugs necessarily act in the same way in this respect. Experiments on nerve-muscle preparations of animals in vivo and in vitro have demonstrated inhibitory effects on motor nerve endings, on the postjunctional membrane of the motor endplate, and on the muscle fibres elsewhere.

Bretylium, which may be considered to be an analogue of choline, produces a hemicholinium-like transmission failure in nerve-muscle preparations; that is to say, it exhibits the characteristics of a drug that impairs the synthesis of acetylcholine by inhibiting choline transport into the nerve endings (GREEN and HUGHES, 1966; BOWMAN et al., 1967; CHANG et al., 1967). Bretylium has in fact been shown to inhibit acetylcholine synthesis by rabbit brain homogenates, an effect which is reversed by excess choline (BOWMAN et al., 1967). The inhibitory effect on acetylcholine synthesis is not shared by guanethidine (GREEN and HUGHES, 1966), although DIXIT et al. (1961) and GOKHALE et al. (1963) were of the opinion that in high concentrations both drugs inhibited the release of acetylcholine from motor nerve endings, possibly as a result of their membrane stabilising activity.

Both drugs in high concentrations acutely impair contractile responses to nerve stimulation and to acetylcholine or other depolarizing agents (EDGE et al., 1957; BOURA and GREEN, 1959; RAND and WILSON, 1967; CHANG et al., 1967). The concen-

◄ **Fig. 14.** Diagrammatic representation of part of a nerve ending (showing neurotubules, neurofilaments, and the recycling of acetylcholine vesicles) impinging on part of a muscle fibre at the motor endplate. The numerals *1–4* indicate the postulated sites of action of adrenaline. *1* and *2:* Adrenaline stimulates β_2-adrenoceptors in the muscle fibre membrane, thereby activating adenylate cyclase and increasing the sarcoplasmic concentration of cyclic AMP. The raised cyclic AMP concentrations have the following effects. (i) The electrogenic component of the sodium pump is stimulated so that the muscle fibre membrane is hyperpolarized; this effect in denervated muscle may enhance the excitability of the T-tubules, thereby increasing fibrillary frequency, and as a secondary consequence may increase the uptake of Ca^{2+} through the plasma membrane. (ii) The uptake of Ca^{2+} by the sarcoplasmic reticulum and by mitochondria (the latter especially in slow-contracting muscles) is enhanced; the latter may also be facilitated by the increased intracellular potassium concentration arising from increased pump activity. (iii) The synthesis of amino acids by and their release from the muscle is inhibited. (iv) Glycogenolysis is stimulated through activation of phosphorylase. *3:* Adrenaline stimulates α-adrenoceptors in the nerve terminals resulting in an increased probability of release of acetylcholine quanta; the effect resembles that of raised $[Ca^{2+}]$ and may involve increased availability of these ions. *4:* Adrenaline stimulates β-adrenoceptors in the membrane of the nerve ending, thereby activating adenylate cyclase and increasing the axoplasmic concentration of cyclic AMP. The raised cyclic AMP concentration may enhance the synthesis, storage, and mobilization of transmitter, and stimulate the sodium pump so that the terminals are hyperpolarized. The prejunctional effects mediated by β-adrenoceptors are probably more pronounced in nerve-muscle preparations that have been fatigued by prolonged stimulation of the nerve. In addition to the effects illustrated in the diagram, adrenaline also increases the excitability of the muscle spindles, possibly through actions related to those on the extrafusal fibres and their nerve endings tration of bretylium necessary to produce this effect is greater than that necessary to produce hemicholinium-like activity. Depression of muscle contractions evoked by nerve stimulation or by acetylcholine may be due to an effect on the chemosensitive area of the postjunctional motor endplate membrane, or to any other postjunctional mechanism through which contractility might be impaired. In fact, HOFMANN and SPIVAK (1963) showed that guanethidine depressed the mepps of single muscle fibres of mouse intercostal muscles, and CHANG et al. (1967), in rat diaphragm and frog sartorius, found that both bretylium and guanethidine reduced the amplitude of epps and mepps without affecting the action potential in the nerve terminals. Although guanethidine inhibited the action of acetylcholine on the postjunctional membrane, there is no reason to suppose that this action is the result of competitive blockade of cholinoceptors. Indeed GYÖRGY et al. (1968) found that, in contrast to the effect of tubocurarine, guanethidine-induced blockade of responses of the frog rectus abdominis muscle to carbachol was noncompetitive in nature. Despite their evidence that these drugs can impair neuromuscular transmission by inhibiting the action of acetylcholine, CHANG et al. (1967) were of the opinion that this is not their main action on the neuromuscular system. They considered that bretylium acts chiefly to impair acetylcholine synthesis, as described above, whereas guanethidine acts mainly on the membrane of the muscle fibres themselves outside the endplate region. As a result of this action of guanethidine, the muscle fibre action potential in the experiments of CHANG et al. (1967) was depressed in amplitude, its rate of rise was slowed, and its rate of decay was prolonged. This conclusion relating to guanethidine supported that of VERNIKOS-DANELLIS and ZAIMIS (1960), who had earlier shown in cats that, in doses too small to block neuromuscular transmission, guanethidine produced a reduction in the number of functioning muscle fibres and gave rise to a myopathic-type pattern in the electromyogram in which the motor unit action potentials were reduced in duration. In their experiments bretylium acted similarly and, if anything, was more effective than guanethidine in producing myopathic patterns. KRONEBERG and STOEPEL (1962) also found that guanethidine depressed muscle responses to direct stimulation in curarized cats and isolated rat diaphragm preparations.

Any or all of the effects described might contribute to the muscle weakness produced in man by bretylium and guanethidine. It is not easy to relate effects produced by particular concentrations of drugs acutely administered in vivo or in vitro in animal experiments to effects produced in man by chronically administered therapeutic concentrations, especially when the effects produced in man occur in only a small proportion of patients.

Other adrenergic neurone blocking drugs, including xylocholine and bethanidine, have also been shown to depress neuromuscular transmission in animal experiments (EDGE et al., 1957; BOURA and GREEN, 1963), but they have not been studied to the same extent as have bretylium and guanethidine. Xylocholine has not been used clinically, and complaints of muscle weakness following the use of bethanidine in man appear to be less common than with guanethidine.

II. Beta-Adrenoceptor Blocking Drugs

Some β-adrenoceptor blocking drugs have been shown to exert effects on skeletal muscle that are independent of β-adrenoceptor blockade. Such effects can be broadly classified into those exerted on the plasma membrane including that of the motor endplate and those exerted on the sarcoplasmic reticulum. It is not unlikely that most of the effects at both sites are the results of the well-known membrane stabilising action possessed by some members of this group of drugs, but as yet an insufficient number of drugs in this class has been tested in order that a clear correlation can be established. Most experiments have been performed with propranolol, which is known to possess pronounced membrane stabilising activity (MORALES-AGUILERA and VAUGHAN WILLIAMS, 1965), although other drugs have also been used. It is possible that actions of this type on skeletal muscle contribute to the fatigue and reduced work capacity produced by at least some of these drugs in patients, healthy volunteers, and animals (EPSTEIN et al., 1965; EKBLOM et al., 1972; NAZAR et al., 1972; GREENBLATT and KOCH-WESER, 1974; FRISHMAN et al., 1975). Similar effects of propranolol on the membrane and sarcoplasmic reticulum of cardiac muscle have been described, and it has been proposed that they are responsible for the myocardial depressant action of some of these drugs (see, for example, NAYLOR and CHANG, 1973). It is possible that fatigue in man is at least partly attributable to the cardiovascular effects of the drugs, including their myocardial depressant action, combined with inhibition of adrenaline-induced glycogenolysis in most tissues.

1. Plasma Membrane

The membrane stabilising activity of β-adrenoceptor blocking drugs is evidenced by their ability to depress the spontaneously-occurring fibrillary potentials of chronically denervated skeletal muscles, an action which requires larger doses than their effect in blocking the actions of β-adrenoceptor agonists on this tissue and which is easily distinguished from it (RAPER and JOWETT, 1967; BOWMAN and RAPER, 1967).

The membrane stabilising action of pronethalol was first demonstrated by GILL and VAUGHAN WILLIAMS (1964). Its depressant action on the motor endplate membrane was clearly evident in the records of BOWMAN and RAPER (1966, 1967; see their Figs. 10 and 4b respectively) in which it slightly depressed the depolarization produced by succinylcholine. In the same doses, however, it was without depressant effect on the contractions evoked by nerve stimulation (BOWMAN et al., 1962), presumably because of the safety factor that normally exists in neuromuscular transmission.

Large doses of propranolol depress mepps, depress twitches and epps evoked by nerve stimulation, antagonise acetylcholine, and potentiate neuromuscular blocking drugs in frog or mammalian muscle (TURKER and KIRAN, 1965; WISLICKI and ROSENBLUM, 1967a, b; USUBIAGA, 1968; HARRAH et al., 1970; WERMAN and WISLICKI, 1971; SAINI and SHARMA, 1971; WISLICKI, 1973; MORALES-AGUILERA and VALLE, 1974; KHETARPAL and SHARMA, 1975; GANGULY, 1976). Two cases of unexpectedly prolonged curarization in man associated with the concurrent use of propranolol and tubocurarine have been reported (ROZEN and WHAN, 1972). These effects are clearly independent of β-adrenoceptor blockade, and most evidence indicates that they are a consequence of membrane stabilization. However, there are some discrepancies in the literature that are difficult to reconcile with this explanation. Thus, sotalol (MJ 1999), which is generally thought to lack membrane stabilising activity, has also been shown to depress neuromuscular transmission (WISLICKI, 1969; PATEL et al., 1971). There is, however, controversy as to whether sotalol does or does not posses membrane stabilising activity; the presence of the effect depends not only on the dose but also on the preparation used to test for it. Jindal et al. (1975) found that the ability of practolol, inpea, and a newer drug in the same class (given the code number JSVC 6524) blocked neuromuscular transmission in a rank order that did not correlate with their membrane stabilising activities. They were of the opinion that the depressant action on neuromuscular transmission was largely due to a specific block of acetylcholine receptors.

In frog sartorius muscle, huge concentrations of propranolol depolarize the plasma membrane, and produce irreversible contracture after chronic denervation (Wislicki, 1970).

In recent experiments, Myhre et al. (1977) have confirmed in the rabbit in vivo the results of earlier experiments from the same laboratory that were carried out in vitro (Lilleheil and Røed, 1971; Røed, 1973). Myhre et al. (1977) showed that in β-adrenoceptor blocking doses that did not affect indirectly evoked twitches, propranolol produced waning of tetanic tension and of muscle action potentials, including those of the diaphragm that accompanied the increased respiratory drive induced by partial tracheal obstruction. The muscle effect was not a consequence of β-adrenoceptor blockade, and it was not reproducible by atenolol, which lacks membrane stabilising activity (Barrett et al., 1973). The authors concluded that the depressant effect produced by propranolol on high frequency tetanic contractions was the result of its membrane stabilising activity.

Since tetanic contractions more closely resemble voluntary movements than do twitches, it seems likely that an effect of this sort could contribute to muscle weakness produced in patients by large doses of propranolol administered chronically. Although it does not appear yet to have been tested, a similar stabilising effect exerted on the muscle spindles and their associated nerve endings might also contribute.

2. Sarcoplasmic Reticulum

Propranolol and some other β-adrenoceptor blocking drugs inhibit the uptake and the release of calcium ions into and from isolated sarcoplasmic reticulum of skeletal (and cardiac) muscle (Scales and McIntosh, 1968; Temple et al., 1974; Tomlinson et al., 1976; Noack and Inesi, 1976). The effect is unrelated to β-adrenoceptor blockade, and it is by no means certain that it is a consequence of their membrane stabilising activity, even though other membrane stabilisers, such as some local anaesthetics, also influence Ca^{2+} exchange (Bianchi and Bolton, 1967).

Whether those β-adrenoceptor blocking drugs that affect Ca^{2+} movements in isolated systems can penetrate muscle cell membranes and influence the sarcoplasmic reticulum in vivo is not known. However, Bowman and Nott (1974) found that propranolol and sotalol blocked the adrenaline-like effect of high doses of phosphodiesterase inhibitors on the cat soleus muscle, under conditions in which it was unlikely that these drugs could have been acting by releasing catecholamines. They suggested the possibility that the antagonistic action against phosphodiesterase inhibitors might be independent of β-adrenoceptors, but rather due to interference with Ca^{2+} sequestration by internal storage sites.

References

Åblad, B., Borg, K.O., Carlsson, E., Ek, L., Johnsson, G., Malmfors, T., Regårdh, C.-G.: A survey of the pharmacological properties of metoprolol in animals and man. Acta Pharmacol. Toxicol. *36*, (Suppl. V) 7–23 (1975)

Abramsky, O., Carmon, A., Levy, S.: Combined treatment of parkinsonian tremor with propranolol and levodopa. J. Neurol. Sci. *14*, 491–494 (1971)

Albuquerque, E.X., McIsaac, R.J.: Fast and slow mammalian muscles after denervation. Exp. Neurol. *26*, 183–202 (1970)

Albuquerque, E.X., Thesleff, S.: A comparative study of membrane properties of innervated and chronically denervated fast and slow skeletal muscles of the rat. Acta Physiol. Scand. *73*, 471–481 (1968)

Albuquerque, E.X., Schuh, F.T., Kauffman, F.C.: Early membrane depolarization of the fast mammalian muscle after denervation. Pflügers Arch. Ges. Physiol. *328*, 36–50 (1971)

Albuquerque, E.X., Warnick, J.E., Sansone, F.M., Onur, R.: The effect of vinblastine and colchicine on neural regulation of muscle. Ann. N.Y. Acad. Sci. *228*, 224–243 (1974)

Aldrich, T.B.: A preliminary report on the active principle of the suprarenal gland. Am. J. Physiol. *5*, 457–461 (1901)

Al-Jeboory, A.A., Marshall, R.J.: Correlation between the effects of salbutamol on contractions and on cyclic AMP content of isolated fast- and slow-contracting muscles of the guinea-pig. Naunyn-Schmiedeberg's Arch. Pharmacol. *305*, 201–206 (1978)

Apperley, G.H., Daly, M.J.: Simultaneous measurement of skeletal muscle, pulmonary mechanical and vascular responses to bronchodilators in the cat. J. Pharm. Pharmacol. *24*, 152–153 (1972)

Apperley, G.H., Levy, G.P.: Characterisation of the β-adrenoceptors of guinea-pig tracheobronchial, skeletal and cardiac muscle. Br. J. Pharmacol. *54*, 260–261 P (1975)

Apperley, G.H., Daly, M.J., Levy, G.P.: Selectivity of β-adrenoceptor agonists and antagonists on bronchial, skeletal, vascular and cardiac muscle in the anaesthetised cat. Br. J. Pharmacol. *57*, 235–246 (1976)

Axelrod, J., Weil-Malherbe, H., Tomchick, R.: Physiological disposition of H^3 epinephrine and its metabolite metanephrine. J. Pharm. Exp. Ther. *127*, 251–256 (1959)

Axelsson, J., Thesleff, S.: A study of supersensitivity in denervated mammalian skeletal muscle. J. Physiol. (Lond.) *147*, 178–193 (1959)

Bach-y-Rita, P., Ito, F.: In vivo studies on fast and slow muscle fibres in extracular muscles. J. Gen. Physiol. *49*, 117–1198 (1966)

Baetjer, A.M.: The relation of the sympathetic nervous system to the contractions and fatigue of skeletal muscle in mammals. Am. J. Physiol. *93*, 41–56 (1930)

Banu, G.: Recherches physiologiques sur le developpement neuromusculaire chez l'homme et l'animal. Paris: Maretheux, 1922

Bárány, M.: ATPase of myosin correlated with speed of shortening. J. Gen. Physiol. *50*, 197–216 (1967)

Bárány, M., Bárány, K., Reckard, T., Volpe, A.: Myosin of fast and slow muscles of the rabbit. Arch. Biochem. Biophys. *109*, 185–191 (1965)

Barbeau, A.: Traitement du tremblement essentiel familiar par le propranolol. Union Med. Can. *102*, 899–902 (1973)

Barbeau, A., Sourkes, T.L., Murphy, G.F.: Les catécholamines de la Maladie de Parkinson. In: Monoamines et Système Nerveux Centrale. Ajuriaguerra, De, Masson, J. (Eds.). Paris, 1962, pp. 247–262

Barcroft, H., Swan, H.J.C.: Sympathetic Control of Human Blood Vessels. London: Arnold, 1953, pp. 88–89

Barcroft, H., Peterson, E., Schwab, R.S.: Action of adrenaline and noradrenaline on the tremor in Parkinson's disease. Neurology *2*, 154–160 (1952)

Barker, D.: The morphology of muscle receptors. In: Handbook of Sensory Physiology. Vol. III 2 Muscle Receptors. Hunt, C.C. (Ed.). Berlin-Heidelberg-New York: Springer, 1974, pp. 1–190

Barnard, R.J., Edgerton, V.R., Furukawa, T., Peter, J.B.: Histochemical, biochemical and contractile properties of red, white and intermediate fibres. Am. J. Physiol. *220*, 410–414 (1971)

Barrett, A.M., Carter, J., Fitzgerald, J.D., Hull, R., Le Count, D.: A new type of cardioselective adrenoceptive blocking drug. Br. J. Pharmacol. *48*, 340P (1973)
Batra, S.: The effect of sodium and potassium on calcium uptake by frog skeletal muscle mitochondria and vesicles. Can. J. Physiol. Pharmacol. *50*, 1157–1161 (1972)
Batra, S.: The effects of zinc and lanthanum on calcium uptake by mitochondria and fragmented sarcoplasmic reticulum of frog skeletal muscle. J. Cell. Physiol. *82*, 246–256 (1973)
Beatty, C.H., Peterson, R.D.: Metabolism of red and white muscle fiber groups. Am. J. Physiol. *204*, 939–942 (1963)
Beckett, S.B., Ellis, S.: Antagonistic and synergistic actions of neuromuscular blocking agents, acetylcholine and epinephrine. J. Pharmacol. Exp. Ther. *113*, 4 (1955)
Belmar, J., Eyzaguirre, C.: Pacemaker sites of fibrillation potentials in denervated mammalian muscle. J. Neurophysiol. *29*, 425–441 (1966)
Bergamini, V., Ferro, M.F., Rovizza, L.: Azione di alcuni farmaci su l'attività fibrillare spontanea del muscolo denervato. Arch. Fisiol. *55*, 254–262 (1955)
Berthler, A., Falck, B., Rosengren, E.: The direct demonstration of a barrier mechanism in brain capillaries. Acta Pharmacol. Toxicol. *20*, 317–321 (1963)
Beumer, H.M.: Comparative studies of the protective effect of Alupent and Th 1165a against histamine in man. Respiration *28*, 148–153 (1971)
Bhoola, K.D., Schachter, M.: Contracture of the denervated rat diaphragm by adrenaline. J. Physiol. *157*, 20–21P (1961)
Bhoola, K.D., Diette-Spiff, K., Webster, R.D.: Effect of adrenaline on mammalian muscle spindles. J. Physiol. (Lond.) *164*, 16P (1962)
Bhoola, K.D., Evans, R.H., Smith, J.W.: Catecholamine induced contractures of denervated muscle. Br. J. Pharmacol. *46*, 513–532P (1972)
Bianchi, C.P.: The effect of caffeine on radiocalcium movement in frog sartorius. J. Gen. Physiol. *44*, 848–858 (1961)
Bianchi, C.P., Bolton, T.C.: Action of local anesthetics on coupling systems in muscle. J. Pharmacol. Exp. Ther. *157*, 388–405 (1967)
Birkmayer, W., Hornykiewicz, O.: Der L-Dioxyphenylalanin (=L-DOPA)-Effekt bei Parkinson-Akinese. Klin. Wochenschr. *73*, 787–788 (1961)
Blaber, L.C., Gallagher, J.P.: The facilitatory effects of catechol and phenol at the neuromuscular junction of the cat. Neuropharmacology *10*, 153–159 (1971)
Bleckman, I., Jurna, I., Rummel, W.: Vergleichende Untersuchungen von Methoden zur Bestimmung der Plateaudauer des aktiven Zustandes am Warmblüter-Muskel. Pflügers Arch. Ges. Physiol. Menschen Tiere *277*, 422–433 (1963)
Blinks, J.R., Olson, C.B., Jewell, B.R., Braveny, P.: Influence of caffeine and other methylxanthines on mechanical properties of isolated mammalian heart muscle. Circ. Res. *30*, 367–392 (1972)
Blum, K.: The effect of dopamine and other catecholamines on neuromuscular transmission. Arch. Int. Pharmacodyn. *181*, 297–306 (1969)
Boegman, R.J., Wood, P.L.: Monoamine as possible mediators in the regulation of fast axoplasmic flow. J. Neurochem. *26*, 737–740 (1976)
Bohmer, K., Raper, C.: β-Adrenoreceptors in denervated skeletal muscles of the cat. Clin. Exp. Pharmacol. Physiol. *2*, 239–248 (1975)
Bohmer, K., Raper, C.: Sympathomimetic-induced effects in the soleus muscle of the guinea-pig. Arch. Int. Pharmacodyn. *221*, 60–65 (1976)
Bohmer, K., Raper, C.: Species difference in the β_1/β_2-adrenoceptor selectivity of Sm 220 Cl in the cat and guinea-pig. Clin. Exp. Pharmacol. Physiol. *4*, 349–358 (1977)
Bohmer, K., O'Donnell, S.R.: Beta-adrenoreceptor-mediated effects of clenbuterol (NAB 365) on trachea, heart and skeletal muscle in anaesthetized guinea-pigs. Clin. Exp. Pharmacol. Physiol. *4*, 383–390 (1977)
Bolte, H.D., Lüderitz, B.: Intra-extacellularer Kaliumkonzentrationsgradient und g-Strophanthinwirkung (Ouabain) bei Kaliummangel-Untersuchungen an Skeletmuskelzellen. Klin. Wochenschr. *47*, 889–891 (1969)
Borys, H.K., Karler, R.: Effects of caffeine on the intracellular distribution of calcium in frog sartorius muscle. J. Cell. Physiol. *78*, 387–404 (1971)
Boura, A.L., Green, A.F.: The actions of bretylium: adrenergic neurone blocking and other effects. Br. J. Pharmacol. Chemother. *14*, 536–548 (1959)

Boura, A.L., Green, A.F.: Adrenergic neurone blockade and other acute effects caused by *N*-benzyl-*N*¹*N*¹¹-dimethylguanidine and its ortho chloro derivative. Br. J. Pharmacol. Chemother. *20*, 36–55 (1963)
Bowman, W.C.: Blood flow in relation to the effects of adrenaline on skeletal muscle. Ph. D. Thesis, University of London (1956)
Bowman, W.C.: A comparison between the vascular responses to adrenaline and noradrenaline in individual skeletal muscles of the cat. J. Pharm. Pharmacol. *11*, 104–119 (1959)
Bowman, W.C., Nott, M.W.: Actions of sympathomimetic amines and their antagonists on skeletal muscle. Pharmacol. Rev. *21*, 27–72 (1969)
Bowman, W.C., Nott, M.W.: Actions of some sympathomimetic bronchodilator and beta-adrenoceptor blocking drugs on contractions of the cat soleus muscle. Br. J. Pharmacol. *38*, 37–49 (1970)
Bowman, W.C., Nott, M.W.: Effects of catecholamines, cyclic nucleotides and phosphodiesterase inhibitors on contractions of skeletal muscles in anaesthetized cats. Clin. Exp. Pharmacol. Physiol. *1*, 309–323 (1974)
Bowman, W.C., Nott, M.W.: Peripheral muscle effects of levodopa in the anaesthetized cat. Clin. Exp. Pharmacol. Physiol. *5*, 305–312 (1978)
Bowman, W.C., Raper, C.: Adrenaline and slow-contracting skeletal muscle. Nature (London) *193*, 41–43 (1962)
Bowman, W.C., Raper, C.: The effect of adrenaline and other drugs affecting carbohydrate metabolism in contractions of the rat diaphragm. Br. J. Pharmacol. Chemother. *23*, 184–200 (1964a)
Bowman, W.C., Raper, C.: Spontaneous fibrillary activity of denervated muscle. Nature (London) *201*, 160–162 (1964b)
Bowman, W.C., Raper, C.: The effects of sympathomimetic amines on chronically denervated skeletal muscles. Br. J. Pharmacol. *24*, 98–109 (1965)
Bowman, W.C., Raper, C.: Effects of sympathomimetic amines on neuromuscular transmission. Br. J. Pharmacol. Chemother. *27*, 313–331 (1966)
Bowman, W.C., Raper, C.: Adrenotropic receptors in skeletal muscle. Ann. N.Y. Acad. Sci. *139*, 741–753 (1967)
Bowman, W.C., Raper, C.: Sympathomimetic bronchodilators and animal models for assessing their potential value in asthma. J. Pharm. Pharmacol. *28*, 369–374 (1976)
Bowman, W.C., Rodger, I.W.: Actions of the sympathomimetic bronchodilator, Rimiterol (R 798), on the cardiovascular, respiratory and skeletal muscle systems of the anaesthetised cat. Br. J. Pharmacol. *45*, 574–583 (1972)
Bowman, W.C., Webb, S.N.: Acetylcholine and Anticholinesterase Drugs. In: Int. Encycl. Pharmac. Ther. Section 14 Vol 2 Chapter 16; Cheymol, J. (Ed.). Oxford: Pergamon Press 1972, pp. 427–502
Bowman, W.C., Zaimis, E.: A comparison between the responses of the tibialis anterior and the soleus muscles in the cat to adrenaline, noradrenaline and isoprenaline. J. Physiol. (Lond.) *128*, 14–15 P (1955)
Bowman, W.C., Zaimis, E.: The effects of adrenaline, noradrenaline and isoprenaline on skeletal muscle contractions in the cat. J. Physiol. (Lond.) *144*, 92–107 (1958)
Bowman, W.C., Zaimis, E.: The actions of adrenaline, noradrenaline and isoprenaline on the denervated mammalian muscle. J. Physiol. (Lond.) *158*, 24–25 P (1961)
Bowman, W.C., Goldberg, A.A.J., Raper, C.: A comparison between the effects of a tetanus and the effects of sympathomimetic amines on fast- and slow-contracting mammalian muscles. Brit. J. Pharmacol. Chemother. *19*, 464–484 (1962)
Bowman, W.C., Hemsworth, B.A., Rand, M.J.: Effects of analogues of choline on neuromuscular transmission. Ann. N.Y. Acad. Sci. *144*, 471–482 (1967)
Boyd, I.A.: The structure and innervation of the nuclear bag muscle fibre system and nuclear chain muscle fibre system in mammalian muscle spindles. Philos. Trans. R. Soc. B. *245*, 81–136 (1962)
Brand, H.: A propos du mode d'action du décaméthonium et de l'amyltriméthylammonium sur le préparation isoleé nerf phrénique-diaphragme du rat. Experientia *8*, 273 (1952)
Bray, J.J., Hawken, M.J., Hubbard, J.I., Pockett, S., Wilson, L.: The membrane potential of rat diaphragm muscle fibres and the effect of denervation. J. Physiol. (Lond.) *255*, 651–667 (1976)

Breckenridge, B.M., Burn, J.H., Matschinsky, F.M.: Theophylline, epinephrine and neostigmine facilitation of neuromuscular transmission. Proc. Natl. Acad. Sci. U.S.A. *57*, 1893–1897 (1967)

Bressler, B.H., Phillis, J.W., Kozachuk, W.: Noradrenaline stimulation of a membrane pump in frog skeletal muscle. Eur. J. Pharmacol. *33*, 201–204 (1975)

Brittain, R.T., Jack, D., Ritchie, A.C.: Recent β-adrenoreceptor stimulants. Adv. Drug Res. *5*, 197–253 (1970)

Brody, I.W.: Relaxing factor in denervated muscle: a possible explanation for fibrillation. Am. J. Physiol. *211*, 1277–1280 (1966)

Brooke, M.H., Kaiser, K.K.: Some comments on the histochemical characterization of muscle adenosine triphosphatase. J. Histochem. *17*, 431–432 (1969)

Brooks, J.E.: Hyperkalaemic periodic paralysis. Arch. Neurol. *20*, 13–18 (1969)

Brown, G.L.: The action of acetylcholine on denervated mammalian and frog's muscle. J. Physiol. *89*, 439–461 (1937)

Brown, G.L.: The sympathetic innervation of the extrinsic ocular muscles. J. Physiol. (Lond.) *112*, 211–214 (1951)

Brown, G.L., Burns, B.D.: Fatigue and neuromuscular block in mammalian skeletal muscle. Proc. R. Soc. B. Biol. Sci. *136*, 182–195 (1949)

Brown, G.L., von Euler, U.S.: The after effects of a tetanus on mammalian muscle. J. Physiol. (Lond.) *93*, 285–300 (1938)

Brown, G.L., Bülbring, E., Burns, B.D.: The effect of adrenaline upon striated muscle. J. Physiol. (Lond.) *106*, 15–16P (1947)

Brown, G.L., Bülbring, E., Burns, B.D.: The action of adrenaline on mammalian skeletal muscle. J. Physiol. (Lond.) *107*, 115–128 (1948)

Brown, G.L., Goffart, M., Vianna Dias, M.: The effects of adrenaline and of sympathetic stimulation on the demarcation potential of mammalian skeletal muscle. J. Physiol. (Lond.) *111*, 184–194 (1950)

Bülbring, E.: Observations on the isolated phrenic nerve diaphragm preparation of the rat. Br. J. Pharmacol. Chemother. *1*, 38–61 (1946)

Bülbring, E.: Catecholamines then and now. J. Pharm. Pharmacol. *28*, 345–355 (1976)

Bülbring, E., Burn, J.H.: Blood flow during muscle contraction and the Orbeli phenomenon in the dog. J. Physiol. (Lond.) *95*, 203–225 (1939)

Bülbring, E., Burn, J.H.: The effect of sympathomimetic and other substances on the contraction of skeletal muscle. J. Pharmacol. Exp. Ther. *68*, 150–172 (1940)

Bülbring, E., Whitteridge, D.: The effect of adrenaline on nerve action potentials. J. Physiol. (Lond.) *99*, 201–207 (1941)

Buller, A.J.: The neural control of the contractile mechanism in skeletal muscle. Endeavour *29*, 107–111 (1970)

Buller, A.J., Lewis, D.M.: Further observations on the differentiation of skeletal muscles in the kitten hind limb. J. Physiol. (Lond.) *176*, 355–370 (1965)

Buller, A.J., Eccles, J.C., Eccles, R.M.: Interactions between motoneurones and muscles in respect of the characteristic species of their responses. J. Physiol. (Lond.) *150*, 417–439 (1960)

Buller, A.J., Ranatunga, K.W., Smith, J.M.: The influence of temperature on the contractile characteristics of mammalian fast and slow twitch muscles. J. Physiol. (Lond.) *196*, 82P (1968a)

Buller, A.J., Ranatunga, K.W., Smith, J.M.: Influence of temperature on the isometric myograms of cross-innervated mammalian fast twitch and slow twitch skeletal muscles. Nature (London) *218*, 877–878 (1968b)

Buller, A.J., Mommaerts, W.F.H.M., Seraydarian, K.: Enzymic properties of myosin in fast and slow twitch muscles of the cat following cross-innervation. J. Physiol. (Lond.) *205*, 581–597 (1969)

Burn, J.H.: The relation of adrenaline to acetylcholine in the nervous system. Physiol. Rev. *25*, 377–394 (1945)

Butcher, L.L., Engel, J.: Peripheral factors in the mediation of the effects of L-dopa on locomotor activity. J. Pharm. Pharmacol. *21*, 614–616 (1969)

Calma, I., Kidd, G.L.: Effect of adrenaline on muscle spindles in cat. Arch. Ital. Biol. *100*, 381–393 (1962)

Calne, D.B., Spiers, A.S.D., Stern, G.M., Laurence, D.R., Armitage, P.: L-Dopa in idiopathic parkinsonism. Lancet *II*, 973–976 (1969)
Cambridge, G.W.: Comparison of the properties of denervated rat diaphragm muscle and an invertebrate smooth muscle. J. Physiol. (Lond.) *158*, 25–26P (1961)
Campbell, E.D.R., Montuschi, E.: Muscle weakness caused by bretylium tosylate. Lancet *II*, 789 (1960)
Campos, F.A.DeM., Cannon, W.B., Lundin, H., Walker, T.T.: Some conditions affecting the capacity for prolonged muscular work. Am. J. Physiol. *87*, 680–701 (1929)
Cannon, W.B., Gruber, C.M.: Oscillatory variations in the contractions of rhythmically stimulated muscle. Am. J. Physiol. *42*, 36–45 (1916)
Cannon, W.B., Nice, L.B.: The effect of splanchnic stimulation on muscular fatigue. Am. J. Physiol. *29*, xxiv–xxv (1911)
Cannon, W.B., Nice, L.B.: The effect of adrenaline secretion on muscular fatigue. Am. J. Physiol. *32*, 44–60 (1913)
Cannon, W.B., Rosenblueth, A.: The Supersensitivity of Denervated Structures. New York: Macmillan Company, 1949
Carafoli, E., Patriarca, P., Rossi, C.S.: A comparative study of the role of mitochondria and the sarcoplasmic reticulum in the uptake and release of Ca^{++} by the rat diaphragm. J. Cell. Physiol. *74*, 17–30 (1969)
Celander, O.: The range of control exercised by the sympathoadrenal system. Acta Physiol. Scand. *32*, (Suppl.) 116 (1954)
Chang, C.C., Chen, T.F., Cheng, H.C.: On the mechanism of neuromuscular blocking action of bretylium and guanethidine. J. Pharmacol. Exp. Ther. *158*, 89–98 (1967)
Charlet, H.: Fortgesetzte Untersuchungen über den Einfluß des Sympathikus auf den Kontraktionsablauf ermüdeter Skelettmuskeln. Z. Biol. *90*, 299–312 (1930)
Clausen, T., Flatman, J.A.: The effect of catecholamines on Na-K transport and membrane potential in rat soleus muscle. J. Physiol. (Lond.) *270*, 383–414 (1977)
Clausen, T., Flatman, J.A.: β_2-Adrenoceptors mediate the stimulating effect of adrenaline on active eletrogenic Na^+–K^+-transport in rat solens muscle. Br. J. Pharmacol. in press (1980).
Clausen, T., Hansen, O.: Active Na-K transport and the rate of ouabain binding. The effect of insulin and other stimuli on skeletal muscle and adipocytes. J. Physiol. (Lond.) *270*, 415–430 (1977)
Claveria, L.E., Vakil, S.D., George, C.F., Reid, J.L., Calne, D.B., Petrie, A.: Oxprenolol in parkinsonism. J. Clin. Pharmacol. *18*, 66–68 (1975)
Close, R.: Dynamic properties of fast and slow skeletal muscles of the rat during development. J. Physiol. (Lond.) *173*, 74–95 (1964)
Close, R.: The relation between intrinsic speed of shortening and duration of the active state of muscle. J. Physiol. (Lond.) *180*, 542–559 (1965a)
Close, R.: Force: velocity properties of mouse muscles. Nature (London) *206*, 718–719 (1965b)
Close, R.: Neural influences on physiological properties of fast and slow limb muscles. In: Contractility of Muscle Cells and Related Processes. Podolsky, R.J. (Ed.) Prentice-Hall, Inc., 1971
Close, R.: Dynamic properties of mammalian skeletal muscles. Physiol. Rev. *52*, 129–197 (1972)
Close, R., Hoh, J.F.Y.: Force; velocity properties of kitten muscles. J. Physiol. (Lond.) *192*, 815–822 (1967)
Close, R., Hoh, J.F.Y.: The after-effects of repetitive stimulation on the isometric twitch contraction of rat fast skeletal muscle. J. Physiol. (Lond.) *197*, 461–477 (1968)
Constas, C.: The effects of adrenaline, noradrenaline and isoprenaline on parkinsonian tremor. J. Neurol. Neurosurg. Psychiatr. *25*, 116–121 (1962)
Corda, M., Staderini, G.: Effeti dell'adrenaline et della noradrenalina sulle terminazione fusali primare e secundarie de mucuto tenvissimo suppavivente in vitro. Arch. Fisiol. *62*, 165–171 (1962)
Cori, G.T., Illingworth, B.: The effect of epinephrine and other glycogenolytic agents on the phosphorylase *a* content of muscle. Biochim. Biophys. Acta *21*, 105–110 (1956)
Corkill, A.B., Tiegs, O.W.: The effect of sympathetic nerve stimulation on the power of contraction of skeletal muscle. J. Physiol. (Lond.) *78*, 161–185 (1933)
Corvaja, N., Marinozzi, V., Pompeiano, O.: Muscle spindles in the lumbrical muscles of the cat. Arch. Ital. Biol. *107*, 365–543 (1969)

Costa, E., Guidotti, A., Handbauer, L.: Do cyclic nucleotides promote the trans-synaptic induction of tyrosine hydroxylase? Life Sci. *14*, 1169–1188 (1974)
Costin, J.C., Cohen, L.S., Zaret, B.L.: Effect of the beta receptor upon potassium uptake in skeletal muscle. Am. J. Cardiol. *37*, 129 (1976)
Cox, B., Danta, G., Schnieden, H., Yuill, G.M.: Interactions of L-dopa and amantadine in patients with Parkinsonism. J. Neurol. Neurosurg. Psychiatr. *36*, 354–361 (1973)
Craig, J.W., Rall, T.W., Larner, J.: The influence of insulin and epinephrine on adenosine 3′,5′-phosphate and glycogen transferase in muscle. Biochim. Biophys. Acta *177*, 213–219 (1969)
Csillik, B.: Functional structure of the post-synaptic membrane in the myoneural junction. Budapest: Akademiai Kiado, 1965
Davies, J.N.: Intention tremor. Practitioner *216*, 371 (1976)
Davis, D.A., Landstrom, D.L., Thong, N.N.: Essential tremor: a common and treatable disorder. J. Oklahoma State Med. Assoc. *69*, 35–37 (1976)
Denny-Brown, D.E.: The histological features of striped muscle in relation to its functional activity. Proc. R. Soc. Ser. B. Biol. Sci. *104*, 371–411 (1929a)
Denny-Brown, D.E.: On the nature of postural reflexes. Proc. R. Soc. Ser. B Biol. Sci. *104*, 252–310 (1929b)
Denny-Brown, D., Pennybacker, J.B.: Fibrillation and fasciculation in voluntary muscle. Brain *61*, 311–334 (1938)
Dessy, S., Grandis, V.: Contribution à l'étude de la fatigue. Action de l'adrénaline sur la fonction du muscle. Arch. Ital. Biol. *41*, 225–233 (1904)
Dietz, V., Freund, H.-J., Allum, J.H.J.: Parkinsonian tremor during rest and voluntary contraction and its correlation with single motor unit activity. In: Advances in Parkinsonism. Birkmayer, W., Hornykiewicz, O. (Eds.). Basel: Hoffmann-La Roche and Co. Ltd. 1976, pp. 244–250
Dixit, B.N., Gulati, O.D., Gokhale, S.D.: Action of bretylium and guanethidine at the neuromuscular junction. Br. J. Pharmacol. *17*, 372–379 (1961)
Dockry, M., Kernan, R.P., Tangney, A.: Active transport of sodium and potassium in mammalian skeletal muscle and its modification by nerve and by cholinergic and adrenergic agents. J. Physiol. (Lond.) *186*, 187–200 (1966)
Dollery, C.T.: The use of bretylium tosylate (Darenthine) in hypertension. Med. Clin. North Am. *45*, 429–439 (1961)
Dowzenko, A., Buksowicz, C., Kuran, W.: The effect of coretalpolfa (oxprenolol) on parkinsonian tremor and benign essential tremor. Neurol. Neurochir. Pol. *26*, 49–53 (1976)
Dransfield, H., Greef, K., Schorn, A., Ting, B.T.: Calcium uptake in mitochondria and vesicles of heart and skeletal muscle in the presence of potassium, sodium, K-strophanthin and pentobarbital. Biochem. Pharmacol. *18*, 1335–1345 (1969)
Draskoci, N., Feldberg, W., Haramath, P.S.R.K.: Passage of circulating adrenaline into perfused cerebral ventricles and subarachnoid space. J. Physiol. (Lond.) *150*, 34–49 (1960)
Dretchen, K.L., Standaert, F.G., Skirboll, L.R., Morgenroth III, V.H.: Evidence for a prejunctional role of cyclic nucleotides in neuromuscular transmission. Nature (London) *264*, 79–81 (1976)
Drew, L.R., Moon, J.R., Buchanan, F.H.: Inderal in the treatment of alcoholism. Med. J. Aust. *2*, 282–285 (1973)
Eakins, K.E., Katz, R.L.: The effect of sympathetic stimulation and epinephrine on the superior rectus muscle of the cat. J. Pharmacol. Exp. Ther. *151*, 524–531 (1967)
Easton, J.D.: Propranolol in neurology. Calif. Med. *117*, 63 (1972)
Ebashi, S., Endo, M., Ohtsuki, I.: Control of muscle contraction. Q. Rev. Biophys. *2*, 351–384 (1969)
Eberstein, A., Sandow, A.: Fatigue mechanisms in muscle fibres. In: The Effect of Use and Disuse on Neuromuscular Functions. Proceedings of a Symposium held at Liblice near Prague. Gutman, E., Hnik, P. (Eds.). Prague: Publishing House of the Czechoslovak Academy of Sciences. 1963, pp. 515–526
Edge, N.D., Mason, D.F.J., Wyllie, J.H.: Some actions of substituted choline phenyl ethers, particularly of choline 2:6 xylyl ether. Br. J. Pharmacol. Chemother. *12*, 312–318 (1957)
Edgerton, V.R., Simpson, D.R.: The intermediate muscle fibre of rats and guinea pigs. J. Histochem. Cytochem. *17*, 828–838 (1969)

Edgerton, V.R., Simpson, D.R.: Dynamic and metabolic relationships in the rat extensor digitorium longus muscle. Exp. Neurol. *30*, 374–376 (1971)
Editorial: Beta-adrenergic blocking drugs and thyroid function. Br. Med. J. *II*, 1039–1040 (1977)
Ehringer, H., Hornykiewicz, O.: Verteilung von Noradrenalin und Dopamin (3-Hydroxytyramin) im Gehirn des Menschen und ihr Verhalten bei Erkrankungen des extrapyramidalen Systems. Klin. Wochenschr. *38*, 1236–1239 (1960)
Ekblom, B., Goldbarg, A.N., Kilbom, A. Åstrand, P.O.: Effects of atropine and propranolol on the oxygen transport system during exercise in man. Scand. J. clin. Lab. Invest. *30*, 35–42 (1972)
Eldred, E., Schnitzlein, H.N., Buchwald, J.: Response of muscle spindles to stimulation of the sympathetic trunk. J. Exp. Neurol. *2*, 13–25 (1960)
Elliot, T.R.: The control of suprarenal glands by the splanchnic nerves. J. Physiol. (Lond.) *44*, 374–409 (1912)
Ellis, S.: Relaxation of biochemical effects of epinephrine to its muscular effects. Pharmacol. Rev. *11*, 469–479 (1959)
Ellis, S., Beckett, S.B.: Depression of neuromuscular transmission by epinephrine. Fed. Proc. *14*, 336 (1955)
Emmelin, N., Strömblad, R.: Adrenaline and noradrenaline content of the suprarenals of cats in chloralose and morphine-ether anaesthesia. Acta Physiol. Scand. *24*, 261–266 (1951)
Engelhardt, von, D.: Pharmakologisches Wirkungsprofil von NAB 365 (Clenbuterol), einem neuen Broncholytikum mit einer selektiven Wirkung auf die β_2-Rezeptoren. Arzneim.-Forsch. (Drug Res.) *26*, 1404–1420 (1976)
Epstein, S.E., Robinson, B.F., Kahler, R.L., Braunwald, E.: Effects of β-adrenergic blockade on the cardiac response to maximal and submaximal exercise in man. J. Clin. Invest. *44*, 1745–1753 (1965)
Euler, von, U.S., Gaddum, J.H.: Pseudomotor contractures after degeneration of the facial nerve. J. Physiol. (Lond.) *73*, 54–66 (1931)
Evans, R.H., Smith, J.W.: Mode of action of catecholamines on skeletal muscle. J. Physiol. (Lond.) *232*, 81–82P (1973)
Evans, R.H., Smith, J.W.: The effect of catecholamines on the influx of calcium and the development of tension in denervated mouse diaphragm muscle. Br. J. Pharmacol. *58*, 109–116 (1976)
Evanson, J.M., Sears, H.T.N.: Comparison of bretylium tosylate with guanethidine in the treatment of severe hypertension. Lancet *II*, 387–389 (1960)
Fahn, S.: Differential diagnosis of tremors. Med. Clin. North *56*, 1363–1375 (1972)
Farmer, J.B., Lehrer, D.N.: The effect of isoprenaline on the contraction of smooth muscle produced by histamine, acetylcholine or other agents. J. Pharm. Pharmacol. *18*, 649–656 (1966)
Fellenius, F., Hedberg, R., Holmberg, E., Waldeck, B.: Functional and metabolic effects of terbutaline and propranolol in fast- and slow-contracting skeletal muscle *in vitro*. Acta physiol. scand. in the press (1980)
Ferko, A.P.: The inhibitory action of dopamine on the anterior tibialis muscle preparation antagonised by pimozide and chlor promazine. Arch. Int. Pharmacodyn. *221*, 66–74 (1976)
Ferko, A.P., Calesnick, B.: L-Dopa and dopamine on skeletal muscle. Res. Commun. Chem. Pathol. Pharmacol. *2*, 146–153 (1971)
Fex, S., Sonesson, B.: Histochemical observation after implantation of a 'fast' nerve into an innervated mammalian 'slow' skeletal muscle. Acta Anat. *77*, 1–10 (1970)
Fiehn, W., Peter, J.B.: Properties of the fragmented sarcoplasmic reticulum from fast-twitch and slow-twitch muscles. J. Clin. Invest. *50*, 570–573 (1971)
Floru, L.: Klinische Behandlungsversuche des lithiumbedingten Tremors durch einen Beta-Rezeptorenantagonisten (Propranolol). Int. Pharmacopsychiatr. *6*, 197–222 (1971)
Floru, L., Floru, L., Tegeler, J.: Wirkung von Beta-Rezeptorenblockern (Pinduloc und Practolol) auf den lithiumbedingten Tremor-klinischen Versuch und theoretische Erwägungen. Arzneimittelforschung *24*, 1122–1125 (1974)
Folkow, B.: Nervous control of blood vessels. Physiol. Rev. *35*, 629–663 (1955)
Fonseca, Da, J.M.: Da asthenia suprarenal. Arq. Bras. Med. *9*, 149–163 (1919)
Formgren, H.: The therapeutic value of oral long-term treatment with terbutaline (Bricanyl®) in asthma. Scand. J. Respir. Dis. *56*, 321–328 (1975)

Foster, J.B., Longley, B.P., Stewart-Wynne, E.G.: Propranolol in essential tremor. Lancet *I*, 1455 (1973)
Frankenhauser, M.: Behaviour and circulating catecholamines. Brain. Res. *31*, 241–262 (1971)
Freedman, B.J.: Trial of new bronchodilator terbutaline, in asthma. Br. Med. J. *1*, 633–636 (1971)
Frishman, W., Smithen, C., Befler, B., Kligfield, P., Killip, T.: Noninvasive assessment of clinical response to oral propranolol therapy. Am. J. Cardiol. *35*, 635–644 (1975)
Gallagher, J.P.: An analysis of the facilitatory action of catechol and phenol at the neuromuscular junction of the cat. Ph. D. Thesis, Loyola University Medical Center, Maywood, Illinois, U.S.A. (1972)
Gallagher, J.P., Blaber, L.C.: Catechol, a facilitatory drug that demonstrates only in prejunctional site of action. J. Pharmacol. Exp. Ther. *184*, 129–135 (1973)
Gallagher, J.P., Karczmar, A.G.: A direct facilitatory action for dopamine at the neuromuscular junction. Neuropharmacology *12*, 783–791 (1973)
Gamstorp, I.: Adynamia episodica hereditaria. Acta Paediatr. (Suppl.) *45*, 108, 1–126 (1956)
Gamstorp, I., Hauge, M., Helweg-Larsen, H.F., Mjönes, H., Sagild, U.: Adynamia episodica hereditaria. Am. J. Med. *23*, 385–390 (1957)
Ganguly, D.K.: Antioxotremorine action of propranolol. Br. J. Pharmacol. *56*, 21–24 (1976)
Garber, A.J., Karli, I.E., Kipnis, D.M.: Alanine and glutamine synthesis and release from skeletal muscle. IV Beta-adrenergic inhibition of amino acid release. J. Biol. Chem. *251*, 851–857 (1976)
Gasser, H.S.: Contractures of skeletal muscle. Physiol. Rev. *10*, 35–109 (1930)
Gauthier, G.F.: On the relationship of ultrastructural and cytochemical features to color in mammalian skeletal muscle. J. Zellforsch. Mikroskop. Anat. *95*, 462–482 (1969)
Gay, L.N., Long, J.W.: Clinical evaluation of isopropylnorepinephrine in management of bronchial asthma. J. Am. Med. Assoc. *139*, 452–457 (1949)
Giessen, H.K., Illig, H.: Tremor nach Gabe eines neuen beta-Rezeptoren-Stimulators. Med. Klin. *67*, 1045–1047 (1972)
Gilbert, J.C., Wyllie, M.G.: Effects of prostaglandins on the ATPase activities of synaptosomes. Biochem. Pharmacol. *24*, 551–556 (1975)
Gilbert, J.C., Wyllie, M.G., Davison, D.V.: Nerve terminal ATPase as possible trigger for neurotransmitter release. Nature (London) *255*, 237–238 (1975)
Gill, E.W., Vaughan Williams, E.M.: Local anaesthetic activity of the beta-receptor antagonist, pronethalol. Nature (London) *201*, 199 (1964)
Gilligan, B.: Propranolol in essential tremor. Lancet *II*, 980 (1972)
Gilligan, B.S., Veale, J.L., Wodak, J.: Propranolol in the treatment of tremor. Med. J. Aust. *1*, 320–322 (1972)
Ginetzinsky, A.G., Shamarina, H.M.: Tonomotor phenomena in denervated muscle. Usp. Sovrem. Biol. *15*, 283–294 (1942)
Ginsborg, B.L., Hirst, G.D.S.: The effect of adenosine on the release of the transmitter from the phrenic nerve of the rat. J. Physiol. (Lond.) *224*, 629–645 (1972)
Ginsborg, B.L., Jenkinson, D.H.: Transmission of impulses from nerve to muscle. Chapter 3 In: The Neuromuscular Junction. Handbook of Pharmacology. (Ed.) Zaimis, E. Berlin-Heidelberg-New York: Springer, 1976, Vol. 42
Ginsborg, B.L., Hirst, G.D.S., Maizels, J.V., Walker, J.: Specificity of adenosine on transmitter output at the neuromuscular junction. Br. J. Pharmacol. *47*, 637P (1973)
Girling, F.: Effects of intravenous and intra-arterial adrenaline and of adrenaline after priscoline, in hind limb of intact rabbit. Am. J. Physiol. *164*, 400–406 (1951)
Godwin-Austen, R.B., Tomlinson, E.B., Frears, C.C., Kok, H.W.L.: Effects of L-Dopa in Parkinson's disease. Lancet *II*, 165–168 (1969)
Goffart, M.: Inversion d'action de l'adrénaline sur le muscle strié et taux du K^+ musculaire. C.R. Séances Soc. Biol. *141*, 1278–1279 (1947)
Goffart, M.: Mode of action of adrenaline on unfatigued mammalian muscle. Abstracts of communications, XVIII International Physiological Congress. Copenhagen, 1950, pp. 222–224
Goffart, M.: Recherches relatives a l'action de l'adrénaline sur le muscle strié de mammifere. I. Potentiation par l'adrénaline de la contraction maximale du muscle non fatigué. Arch. Int. Physiol. *60*, 318–366 (1952)

Goffart, M.: The action of *l*-noradrenaline and adrenochrone on unfatigued mammalian muscle. Pharmacol. Rev. *6*, 33–34 (1954)
Goffart, M., Brown, G.L.: Relation entre le potassium du milieu extracellulaire et l'action de l'adrénaline sur le muscle strié non fatigué du rat. C.R. Séances Soc. Biol. *141*, 958–959 (1947)
Goffart, M., Perry, W.L.M.: The action of adrenaline on the rate of loss of potassium ions from unfatigued striated muscle. J. Physiol. (Lond.) *112*, 95–101 (1951)
Goffart, M., Ritchie, J.M.: The effect of adrenaline on the contractions of mammalian skeletal muscle. J. Physiol. (Lond.) *116*, 357–371 (1952)
Gokhale, S.D., Gulati, O.D., Kelkar, V.V., Joshi, N.Y.: Effects of bretylium and guanethidine on some cholinergic effectors. Arch. Int. Pharmacodyn. Ther. *145*, 243–253 (1963)
Goldberg, A.L., Singer, J.J.: Evidence for a role of cyclic AMP in neuromuscular transmission. Proc. Natl. Acad. Sci. U.S.A. *64*, 134–141 (1969)
Goldspink, G., Larson, R.E., Davies, R.E.: The immediate energy supply and the cost of maintenance of isometric tension for different muscles in the hamster. Z. Vergl. Physiol. *66*, 389–397 (1970)
Goodman, D.B.P., Rasmussen, H., Di Bella, F., Guthrow, C.F.: Cyclic adenosine 3′,5′-monophosphate-stimulated phosphorylation of isolated neurotubule subunits. Proc. Natl. Acad. Sci. U.S.A. *67*, 652–659 (1970)
Graham, J.D.P.: Static tremor in anxiety states. J. Neurol. Neurosurg. Psychiatr. *8*, 57–60 (1945)
Grampp, W., Harris, J.B., Thesleff, S.: Inhibition of denervation changes in skeletal muscle by blockers of protein synthesis. J. Physiol. (Lond.) *221*, 743–754 (1972)
Green, A.F., Hughes, R.: Effects of adrenergic neurone blocking agents on voluntary muscle stimulated at different frequencies. Br. J. Pharmacol. Chemother. *27*, 164–176 (1966)
Greenblatt, D.J., Koch-Weser, J.: Adverse reactions to *β*-adrenergic receptor blocking drugs: a report from the Boston collaborative drug surveillance program. Drugs *7*, 118–129 (1974)
Greengard, P., Costa, E. (Eds.): Role of Cyclic AMP in Cell Function. New York: Raven Press, 1970
Greengard, P., Paoletti, R., Robison, G.A. (Eds.): Advances in Cyclic Nucleotide Research. New York: Raven Press, 1972, Vol. 1
Grossie, J., Yonas, H.: Response of primary spindle afferents with epinephrine during arterial decreased oxygen tension and partial asphyxia. Arch. Int. Pharmacodyn. *181*, 287–296 (1969)
Gruber, C.M.: Studies in fatigue. I. Fatigue as affected by changes of arterial pressure. Am. J. Physiol. *32*, 221–229 (1913)
Gruber, C.M.: Studies in fatigue. III. The fatigue threshold as affected by adrenalin and by increased arterial pressure. Am. J. Physiol. *33*, 335–355 (1914a)
Gruber, C.M.: Studies in fatigue. IV. The relation of adrenalin to curare and fatigue in normal and denervated muscle. Am. J. Physiol. *34*, 89–96 (1914b)
Gruber, C.M.: Further studies on the effect of adrenalin upon muscular fatigue and limb circulation. Am. J. Physiol. *42*, 610 (1917a)
Gruber, C.M.: Further studies on the effect of adrenalin upon muscular fatigue. Am. J. Physiol. *43*, 530–544 (1917b)
Gruber, C.M.: The significance of epinephrin in muscular activity. Endocrinology *3*, 145–153 (1919)
Gruber, C.M.: Studies in fatigue. XI. The effects of intravenous injections of massive doses of adrenalin upon skeletal muscle at rest and undergoing fatigue. Am. J. Physiol. *61*, 475–492 (1922a)
Gruber, C.M.: Studies in fatigue. XII. The effect of adrenal secretion on non-fatigued and fatigued skeletal muscle. Am. J. Physiol. *62*, 438–441 (1922b)
Gruber, C.M.: Studies in fatigue. XIV. The effect of adrenalin on the duration of the latent, the contraction and the relaxation periods of skeletal muscle at rest and undergoing fatigue. J. Pharmacol. Exp. Ther. *23*, 335–351 (1924)
Gruber, C.M., Fellows, A.P.: Studies on fatigue. VII. The effect of adrenalin on the irratability and contractility of mammalian nerve-muscle preparations after death. Am. J. Physiol. *46*, 472–477 (1918)

Guglielmetti, J.: The effect of adrenalin on muscular fatigue in *Leptodactylus ocellatus* (L. gir) and in *Bufo marinus*. Q. J. Exp. Physiol. Cog. Med. Sci. *12*, 139–151 (1918)
Guglielmetti, J.: Action de l'adrénaline sur le systèm musculaire strié. C.R. Séances, Soc. Biol. *87*, 692–694 (1922)
Guth, L.: 'Trophic' influences of nerve on muscle. Physiol. Rev. *48*, 645–687 (1968)
Guth, L.: 'Trophic' functions. In: The Peripheral Nervous System. Hubbard, J.L. (Ed.). New York: Plenum Press, 1974, pp. 329–343
Guth, L., Samaha, F.J.: Qualitative differences between actomyosin ATPase of slow and fast mammalian muscle. Exp. Neurol. *25*, 138–152 (1969)
Gutmann, E. (Ed.): The Denervated Muscle. Prague: Publishing House of the Czechoslovak Academy of Science, 1962
Gutmann, E.: Open questions in the study of the 'tropic' function of the nerve cell. In: Current Research in Neurosciences, Topical Problems in Psychiatry and Neurology. Wycis, H.T. (Ed.). Basel: Karger, 1970, Vol 10, pp. 54–64
Gwee, M.C.E., Nott, M.W., Raper, C., Rodger, I.W.: Pharmacological actions of a new β-adrenoceptor agonist, MJ-9184-1, in anaesthetised cats. Br. J. Pharmacol. *46*, 375–385 (1972)
György, L., Doda, M., Bite, A.: Guanethidine and carbachol on frog rectus: a non-competitive interaction. J. Pharm. Pharmacol. *20*, 575–576 (1968)
Hale, E.G., Kidd, G.L.: Evidence for a direct sympathetic reflex modification of muscle spindle excitability in the rat. In: Muscle Spindle Symposium, Paper 18. Anat. Soc. Great Britain Ireland (1974)
Halliday, A.M., Redfearn, J.W.T.: An analysis of the frequencies of finger tremor in healthy subjects. J. Physiol. (Lond.) *134*, 600–611 (1956)
Hamberger, A., Hamberger, B.: Uptake of catecholamines and penetration of trypan blue by the blood brain barrier. Z. Zellforsch. Mikrosk. Anat. *70*, 386–392 (1966)
Hammond, P.H., Merton, P.A., Sutton, G.G.: Nervous gradation of muscular contraction. Br. Med. Bull. *12*, 214–218 (1956)
Harigaya, S., Ogawa, Y., Sugita, H.: Calcium binding activity of microsomal fraction of rabbit red muscle. J. Biochem. *63*, 324–331 (1968)
Harrah, M.D., Way, W.L., Katzung, B.G.: The interaction of d-tubocurarine with antiarrhythmic drugs. Anesthesiology *33*, 406–410 (1970)
Harris, E.J., Manchester, K.L.: The effects of potassium ions and denervation on protein synthesis and the transport of amino acids in muscle. Biochem. J. *101*, 135–145 (1966)
Hartman, F.A., Kilborn, L.G., Lang, R.S.: Vascular changes produced by adrenalin in vertebrates. Endocrinology *2*, 122–142 (1918)
Havard, C.W.H.: The management of thyrotoxicosis. Br. J. Hosp. Med. *11*, 893–908 (1974)
Hays, E.T., Dwyer, T.M., Horowicz, P., Swift, J.G.: Epinephrine action on sodium fluxes in frog striated muscle. Am. J. Physiol. *227*, 1340–1347 (1974)
Helmreich, E., Cori, C.F.: The activation of glycolysis in frog sartorius muscle by epinephrine. Pharmacol. Rev. *18*, 189–196 (1966)
Henneman, E., Olson, C.B.: Relations between structure and function in the design of skeletal muscle. J. Neurophysiol. *28*, 581–598 (1965)
Heraut, L.A., Pertjiset, B.F.: Neurologie: Les beta-bloquers en neurologie et en psychiatrie. Med. Arm. *4*, 47–49 (1975)
Herring, A.B.: Action of pronethalol in parkinsonian tremor. Lancet *II*, 383–385 (1964)
Hertting, G., Axelrod, J., Kopin, I.J., Whitby, L.G.: Lack of uptake of catecholamines after chronic denervation of sympathetic nerves. Nature (London) *189*, 66 (1961)
Hess, A., Pilar, G.: Slow fibres in the extra-ocular muscles of the cat. J. Physiol. (Lond.) *169*, 780–798 (1963)
Hidaka, T., Kuriyama, H.: Effects of catecholamines on the cholinergic neuromuscular transmission in fish red muscle. J. Physiol. (Lond.) *201*, 61–72 (1969)
Hill, A.V.: The abrupt transition from rest to activity in muscle. Proc. R. Soc. Ser. B. Biol. Sci. *136*, 399–420 (1949)
Hilton, S.M., Jeffries, M.G., Vrbova, G.: Functional specialisations of the vascular bed of soleus. J. Physiol. (Lond.) *206*, 543–562 (1970)
Hines, M.: Nerve and muscle. Q. Rev. Biol. *2*, 149–180 (1927)
Hines, H.M.: Effects of immobilization and activity on neuromuscular regeneration. J. Am. Med. Assoc. *120*, 515–517 (1942)

Hinsey, J.C.: The innervation of skeletal muscle. Physiol. Rev. *14*, 514–585 (1934)

Hnik, P., Škorpil, V.: The significance of blood circulation for fibrillation activity in denervated muscles of the rat. Physiol. Bohemoslov. *8*, 81–86 (1959)

Hodgson, H.J.F., Marsden, C.D., Meadows, J.C.: The effect of adrenaline on the response to muscle vibration in man. J. Physiol. (Lond.) *202*, 98 P (1969)

Hofmann, W.W.: Caffeine effects on transmitter depletion and mobilization at motor nerve terminals. Am. J. Physiol. *216*, 621–629 (1969)

Hofmann, W.W., Spivack, A.P.: The effects of guanethidine on skeletal neuromuscular transmission. Am. J. Med. Sci. *244*, 64–69 (1963)

Hökfelt, B., McLean, J.: The adrenaline and noradrenaline content of the suprarenal glands of the rabbit under normal conditions and after various forms of stimulation. Acta Physiol. Scand. *21*, 258–270 (1950)

Hokkanen, E., Vapaatalo, H., Anttilo, P.: On the possible role of cyclic AMP in the neuromuscular transmission and in the treatment of myasthenia gravis. Acta Neurol. Scand. (Suppl.) *51*, 375–376 (1972)

Holmberg, E., Waldeck, B.: Analysis of the β-receptor mediated effect on fast-contracting skeletal muscle in vitro. Naunyn-Schmiedeberg's Arch. Pharmacol. *301*, 109–113 (1977)

Holmberg, E., Svedinger, I., Waldeck, B.: A comparison between the sympathomimetic induced effects on fast- and slow-contracting skeletal muscles in vitro. Acta Pharmacol. Toxicol. *41*, (Suppl. IV)

Horn, J.P., McAfee, D.A.: Modulation of cyclic nucleotide levels in peripheral nerve without effect on resting or compound action potentials. J. Physiol. (Lond.) *269*, 753–766 (1977)

Houston, J., Rodger, I.W.: Actions of the sympathomimetic bronchodilator, trimetoquinol (AQL 208) on the cardiac, respiratory and skeletal muscle systems in the anaesthetised cat, and on cat isolated atrial and tracheal preparations. Clin. Exp. Pharmacol. Physiol. *1*, 401–413 (1974)

Hubbard, J.I., Jones, S., Landau, E.M.: On the mechanism by which calcium and magnesium affect the release of transmitter by nerve impulses. J. Physiol. (Lond.) *196*, 75–87 (1968)

Hubbard, J.I., Jones, S.F., Landau, E.M.: The effect of temperature change upon transmitter release, facilitation and post tetanic potentiation. J. Physiol. (Lond.) *216*, 591–609 (1971)

Hughes, R.C., Polgar, J.G., Weightman, D., Walton, J.N.: L-Dopa in parkinsonism and the influence of previous thalamotomy. Br. Med. J. *I*, 7–13 (1971)

Huidobro, F., Cubillos, L., Eyzaguirre, C.: Effect of aromatic amines on neuromuscular function. Acta Physiol. Lat. *2*, 107–118 (1952)

Hunt, C.C.: The effect of sympathetic stimulation on mammalian muscle spindles. J. Physiol. (Lond.) *151*, 332–341 (1960)

Hutter, O.F., Loewenstein, W.R.: Nature of neuromuscular facilitation by sympathetic stimulation in the frog. J. Physiol. (Lond.) *130*, 559–571 (1955)

Jackson, R., Crawford, C.O., Peel, J.S.: Oxprenolol in Parkinson's disease. N.Z. Med. J. *74*, 246–247 (1971)

Jarcho, L.W., Berman, B., Dowben, R.M., Lilienthal, J.L.: Site of origin and velocity of conduction of fibrillary potentials in denervated skeletal muscle. Am. J. Physiol. *178*, 129–134 (1954)

Jenkinson, D.H., Stamenovie, B.A., Whittaker, B.D.L.: The effect of noradrenaline on the end-plate potential in twitch fibres of the frog. J. Physiol. (Lond.) *195*, 743–754 (1968)

Jindal, M.N., Shah, U.H., Patel, V.K., Kelkar, V.V.: A study of some beta-adrenoceptor blocking agents on skeletal muscle. Arzneimittelforschung *25*, 52–55 (1975)

Johnson, G.A., Boukma, S.J., Lahti, R.A., Mathews, J.: Cyclic AMP and phosphodiesterase in synaptic vesicles from the mouse brain. J. Neurochem. *20*, 1387–1392 (1973)

Julien, J., Vallat, J.-M.: Propranolol la traitment de la maladie de Parkinson. Bordeaux Med. *6*, 1957–1959 (1973)

Jurna, I., Rummel, W.: Die Wirkung von Adrenalin und Noradrenalin auf die Spannungswicklung vom Soleus und Tibialis anterior der Katze. Pflügers Arch. Ges. Physiol. *275*, 137–151 (1962)

Jurna, I., Rummel, W., Schäfer, H.: Die abfallende Phase des aktiven Zustandes des Tibialis anterior, Gastrocnemius und Soleus der Katze und ihre Beeinflussung durch Dehnung und Sympathicomimetica. Pflügers Arch. Ges. Physiol. *277*, 513–522 (1963)

Kaiser, C., Schwartz, M.S., Colella, D.F., Wardell, J.R.: Adrenergic agents. 3. Synthesis and adrenergic activity of some catechol amine analogs bearing a substituted sulfonyl or sulfonylalkyl group in the meta position. J. Med. Chem. *18*, 674–683 (1975)
Karpati, G., Engel, W.K.: Neuronal trophic function. Arch. Neurol. *17*, 542–545 (1967)
Kendig, J.J., Bunker, J.P.: Alterations in muscle resting potentials and electrolytes during halothane and cyclopropane anesthesia. Anesthesiology, *36*, 128–131 (1972)
Kennedy, M.C.S., Simpson, W.T.: Human pharmacological and clinical studies on salbutamol: a specific β-adrenergic bronchodilator. Br. J. Dis. Chest *63*, 165–174 (1969)
Khetarpal, V.K., Sharma, P.L.: Comparative effects of (+)- and (−)-isomers of propranolol and inpea on (+)-tubocurarine- and succinylcholine-induced neuromuscular blockade. Eur. J. Pharmacol. *33*, 325–335 (1975)
Kirk, L., Baastrup, P.C., Mogens, S.: Propranolol in lithium tremor. Lancet *I*, 839 (1972)
Kirk, L., Baastrup, P.C., Schou, M.: Propranolol treatment of lithium-induced tremor. Lancet *II*, 1086–1087 (1973)
Kissel, P.: Traitment du treblement parkinsonien par l'association L-Dopa-DL-propranolol. Bull. Acad. Nat. Med. (Paris) *158*, 292–296 (1974)
Kissel, P., Tridon, P., Masingue, M., André, J.M.: Association L-Dopa-propranolol et tremblement parkinsonien. Nouv. Presse Med. *I*, 1943 (1972)
Kissel, P., Tridon, P., André, J.M.: Levodopa-propranolol therapy in parkinsonian tremor. Lancet *I*, 403–404 (1974)
Klaus, W., Lüllmann, H., Muscholl, E.: Der Kalium-Flux des normalen und denervierten Rattenzwerchfells. Pflügers Arch. Ges. Physiol. *271*, 761–775 (1960)
Klein, R., Egan, T., Usher, P.: Changes in sodium, potassium and water in hyperkalemic familial periodic paralysis. Metabolism *9*, 1005–1024 (1960)
Koch-Weser, J.: Non-beta blocking actions of propranolol. New Eng. J. Med. *293*, 988–990 (1975)
Koelle, G.B.: Cholinergic and non-cholinergic pharmacology of the bronchioles. Postgrad. Med. J. *51*, (Suppl. 7) 63–66 (1975)
Kosterlitz, H.W., Watt, A.J.: Adrenergic receptors in the guinea-pig ileum. J. Physiol. (Lond.) *117*, 11–12P (1965)
Krnjević, K., Miledi, R.: Some effects produced by adrenaline upon neuromuscular propagation in rats. J. Physiol. (Lond.) *141*, 291–304 (1958)
Krnjević, K., Miledi, R.: Presynaptic failure of neuromuscular propagation in rats. J. Physiol. (Lond.) *149*, 1–22 (1959)
Kroneberg, G., Stoepe, K.: Über eine Wirkung von Guanethidin auf Skeletmuskulatur und Rückenmarkreflexe. Naunyn-Schmiedeberg's Arch. Exp. Pathol. Pharmacol. *243*, 36–43 (1962)
Kuba, K.: The action of phenol on neuromuscular transmission in red muscle of the fish. Jpn. J. Physiol. *19*, 762–774 (1969)
Kuba, K.: Effects of catecholamines on the neuromuscular junction in the rat diaphragm. J. Physiol. (Lond.) *211*, 551–570 (1970)
Kuba, K., Tomita, T.: Noradrenaline action on nerve terminal in rat diaphragm. J. Physiol. (Lond.) *217*, 19–31 (1971)
Kuba, K., Tomita, T.: Effects of noradrenaline on miniature endplate potentials and on endplate potentials. J. Theor. Biol. *36*, 81–88 (1972)
Kugelberg, E., Edström, L.: Differential histochemical effects of muscle contraction on phosphorylase and glycogen in various types of fibres: relation to fatigue. J. Neurol. Neurosurg. Psychiat. *31*, 415–423 (1968)
Kuno, Y.: On the alleged influence of adrenaline and of the sympathetic nervous system on the tonus of skeletal muscle. J. Physiol. (Lond.) *49*, 139–146 (1915)
Kuschinsky, G., Viaud, P.: Über die Wirkung des Adrenalins auf die Funktion des Skeletmuskels am nebennierenlosen Tier. Naunyn-Schmiedebergs Arch. Exp. Pathol. Pharmacol. *170*, 492–499 (1933)
Labhart, F.: Fortgesetzte Untersuchungen über den Einfluß des Nervus Sympathikus auf die Ermüdung des quergestreiften Muskels. Z. Biol. *89*, 217–236 (1929)
Landau, W.M., Struppler, A., Mehls, O.: A comparative electromyographic study of the reactions to passive movement in Parkinsonism and in normal subjects. Neurology *16*, 34–38 (1966)

Lands, A.M., Luduena, F.P., Buzzo, H.J.: Differentiation of receptors responsive to isoproterenol, Lif. Sci. (part 1) *6,* 2241–2249 (1967)

Langer, S.Z.: Presynaptic regulation of catecholamine release. Biochem. Pharmacol. *23,* 1793–1800 (1974)

Langer, S.Z.: Presynaptic receptors and their role in the regulation of transmitter release. Br. J. Pharmacol. *60,* 481–497 (1977)

Langley, J.N., Kato, T.: The physiological action of physostigmine and its action on denervated skeletal muscle. J. Physiol. (Lond.) *49,* 410–430 (1915)

Lapierre, Y. D.: Control of lithium tremor with propranolol. Can. Med. Assoc. J. *114,* 619–620 (1976)

Larsen, J.-J., Hermansen, K.: Pharmacodynamics of a new selective Beta$_2$-adrenergic bronchodilator 3-(4-methoxybenzylamino)-4-hydroxy-α-(tert. butylaminomethyl)-benzyl-alcohol, HCl (QH25). Acta Pharmacol. Toxiol. *40,* 42–64 (1977)

Larsson, S.: Long-term treatment with β_2-adrenostimulants in asthma. Acta Med. Scand. (Suppl) 608 (1977)

Larsson, S., Svedmyr, N.: Tremor caused by sympathomimetics is mediated by Beta$_2$-adrenoceptors. Scand. J. Respir. Dis. *58,* 5–10 (1977)

Lefkowitz, R.J., Durham, N.C.: Beta adrenergic “isoreceptors” and adenylate cyclase. J. Clin. Invest. *53,* 44A Abstract 165 (1974)

Legge, J.S., Gaddie, J., Palmer, K.N.V.: Comparison of two oral selective β_2-adrenergic stimulant drugs in bronchial asthma. Br. Med. J. *i,* 637–639 (1971)

Lewis, D.M., Webb, S.N.: Adrenaline on isotonic contractions of mammalian skeletal muscle. Br. J. Pharmacol. *58,* 467P (1976)

Lewis, D.M., Pardoe, M.J., Webb, S.N.: Effect of adrenaline on intracellularly recorded action potentials of mammalian skeletal muscles. Br. J. Pharmacol. *60,* 299P (1977)

Li, C.-L., Shy, G.M., Wells, J.: Some properties of mammalian skeletal muscle fibres with particular reference to fibrillation potentials. J. Physiol. (Lond.) *135,* 522–535 (1957)

Lilleheil, G., Røed, A.: Antitetanic effect of propranolol on mammalian motor nerve and skeletal muscle, and combined action of propranolol and neostigmine on the neuromuscular transmission. Arch. Int. Pharmacodyn. *194,* 129–140 (1971)

Linden, S., Gottfried, C.G.: Beta-blocking agents in the treatment of catecholamine-induced symptoms in musicians. Lancet *II,* 529 (1974)

Lippold, O.: Physiological tremor. Sci. Am. *224,* 65–73 (1971)

Lippold, O.C.J., Redfearn, J.W.T., Vučo, J.: The rhythmical activity of groups of motor units in the voluntary contraction of muscle. J. Physiol. (Lond.) *137,* 473–487 (1957)

Locke, S., Solomon, H.C.: Relation of resting potential of rat gastrocnemius and soleus muscles to innervation, activity and the Na-K pump. J. Exp. Zool. *166,* 377–386 (1967)

Louis, W.J., Doyle, A.E., Sampson, R.G.: The metabolic fate of levodopa in man and animals. Clin. Exp. Pharmacol. Physiol. *1,* 341–346 (1974)

Luco, J.V.: The defatiguing effect of adrenaline. Am. J. Physiol. *125,* 196–204 (1939)

Luco, C.F., Luco, J.V.: Sympathetic effects on fibrillary activity of denervated striated muscle. J. Neurophysiol. *34,* 1066–1071 (1971)

Luco, J.V., Sanchez, P.: Spontaneous activity and contractile responses to adrenaline of denervated auricular muscles. Acta Physiol. Lat. *6,* 171–172 (1956)

Luff, A.R., Atwood, H.L.: Developmental changes in the sarco plasmic reticulum and transverse tubular system in skeletal muscles of the mouse. J. Gen. Physiol. *57,* 243–244 (1971)

Lullman, H.: Über die Konstanz des Membranpotentials bei spontanen Änderungen der Ionengradienten am normalen und denervierten Rattenzwerchfell. Pflügers Arch. Ges. Physiol. *267,* 188–199 (1958)

Lüllmann, H.: Über die Ursache spontanen Fibrillationen denervierten Skeletmuskulatur. Klin. Wochenschr. *38,* 1169–1171 (1960)

Lüllmann, H., Holland, W.: Influence of ouabain on an exchangeable calcium fraction, contractile force, and resting tension of guinea-pig atria. J. Pharmacol. Exp. Ther. *137,* 186–192 (1962)

Lüllmann, H., Pracht, W.: Über den Einfluß von Acetylcholin auf das Membranpotential denervierten Rattenzwerchfelle. Experientia *13,* 288–289 (1957)

Maddock, W.O., Rankin, V.M., Youmans, W.B.: Prevention of the anti-curare action of epinephrine by dibenamine. Proc. Soc. Exp. Biol. Med. *67,* 151–153 (1948)

Magladery, J.W., Solandt, D.Y.: Relation of fibrillation to acetyl choline and potassium sensitivity in denervated skeletal muscle. J. Neurophysiol. *5*, 357–362 (1942)
Maibach, C.: Untersuchungen zur Frage des Einflusses des Sympathikus auf die Ermüdung der quergestreiften Muskulatur. Z. Biol. *88*, 207–226 (1928)
Malta, E., Raper, C.: Comparison of the effects of (−)-isoprenaline, orciprenaline, terbutaline and Me 506 on heart rate, soleus muscle, contractility and pulmonary resistance of anaesthetized cats. Clin. Exp. Pharmacol. Physiol. *3*, 49–58 (1976)
Malta, E., McPherson, G.A., Raper, C.: Comparison of pre-junctional α-adrenoceptors at the neuromuscular junction with vascular postjunctional α-adrenoceptors in cat skeletal muscle. Br. J. Pharmacol. *65*, 249–256 (1979)
Marks, J.: The Treatment of Parkinsonism with L-dopa. Lancaster, England: Medical and Technical Publishing Co. Ltd. 1974, p. 82
Marlin, G.E., Turner, P.: Comparison of the β_2-adrenoceptor selectivity of rimiterol, salbutamol, and isoprenaline by the intravenous route in man. Br. J. Clin. Pharmacol. *2*, 41–48 (1975)
Marsden, C.D., Meadows, J.C.: The effect of adrenaline on the contraction of human muscle – one mechanism whereby adrenaline increases the amplitude of physiological tremor. J. Physiol. (Lond.) *194*, 70P (1968)
Marsden, C.D., Meadows, J.C.: The effect of adrenaline on the contraction of human muscle. J. Physiol. (Lond.) *207*, 429–448 (1970)
Marsden, C.D., Owen, D.A.L.: Mechanisms underlying emotional variation in Parkinsonian tremor. Neurology *17*, 711–715 (1967)
Marsden, C.D., Foley, T.H., Owen, D.A.L., McAllister, R.C.: Peripheral β-adrenergic receptors associated with tremor. Clin. Sci. *33*, 53–65 (1967a)
Marsden, C.D., Meadows, J.C., Lange, J.W., Watson, R.S.: Effect of deafferentation on human physiological tremor. Lancet *II*, 700–706 (1967b)
Marsden, C.D., Merton, P.A., Morton, H.B.: Servo action in human voluntary movement. Nature (London) *238*, 140–143 (1972)
Marsden, C.D., Parkes, J.D., Rees, J.R.: A year's comparison of treatment of patients with Parkinson's disease with levodopa combined with carbidopa versus treatment with levodopa alone. Lancet *29*, 1459–1462 (1973)
Marsden, C.S., Parkes, J.D., Rees, J.E.: Propranolol in Parkinson's disease. Lancet *II*, 410 (1974)
Marshall, J., Schnieden, H.: Effect of adrenaline, noradrenaline, atropine, and nicotine on some types of human tremor. J. Neurol. Neurosurg. Psychiatr. *29*, 214–218 (1966)
Maschima, H., Matsumura, M., Nakayama, Y.: On the coupling relation between action potential and mechanical response during repetitive stimulation in frog sartorius muscle. Jpn. J. Physiol. *12*, 324–336 (1962)
Matthews, B.H.C.: Nerve endings in mammalian muscle. J. Physiol. (Lond.) *78*, 1–53 (1933)
Matthews, P.B.C.: Mammalian Muscle Receptors and their Central Actions. London: E. Arnold, 1972
Mawdsley, C.: Treatment of Parkinsonism with laeva-dopa. Br. Med. J. *I*, 331–337 (1970)
McAllister, R.G., Ware, R.W., Markesbery, W.R., Howell, S.M.: Correlation of propranolol plasma level with effect in patients with essential tremor. Clin. Res. *24*, 257A (1976)
McArdle, B.: Adynamia episodica hereditoria and its treatment. Brain *85*, 121–148 (1962)
McInnes, A.: The muscle spindle, its blood supply and the sympathetic nervous system. Ph. D. Thesis, University of Glasgow (1980)
McLennan, H.: The effect of some catecholamines upon a monosynaptic reflex pathway in the spinal cord. J. Physiol. (Lond.) *158*, 411–425 (1961)
McPhedran, A.M., Wuerker, R.B., Henneman, E.: Properties of motor units in a homogeneous red muscle (soleus) of the cat. J. Neurophysiol. *28*, 71–84 (1965)
Mead, S.: Some properties of denervated muscle. Arch. Phys. Med. Rehabil. *28*, 93–99 (1947)
Mendez, J., Aranda, L.C., Luco, J.V.: Antifibrillary effect of adrenergic fibres in denervated striated muscles. J. Neurophysiol. *33*, 882–890 (1970)
Merton, P.A.: Voluntary strength and fatigue. J. Physiol. (Lond.) *123*, 553–564 (1954)
Merton, P.A.: Problems of muscular fatigue. Br. Med. Bull. *12*, 219–221 (1956)
Miyamoto, M.D., Breckenridge, B.M.: A cyclic adenosine monophos phate link in the catecholamine enhancement of transmitter release at the neuromuscular junction. J. Gen. Physiol. *63*, 609–624 (1974)

Mogey, G.A., Young, P.A.: The antagonism of curarising activity by phenolic substances. Br. J. Pharmacol. Chemother. *4,* 359–365 (1949)

Montagu, K.A.: On the mechanism of action of adrenaline in skeletal nerve-muscle. J. Physiol. (Lond.) *128,* 619–628 (1955)

Morales-Aguilerá, A., Valle, J.R.: Neuromuscular transmission blockade produced by propranolol and by 2,3-*cis*-1,2,3,4-tetrahydro-5-(2-hydroxy-3-(tert-butylaminopropoxy)-2,3-naphthalenediol (SQ 11725). Fed. Proc. *33,* 579 (Abs 2074) (1974)

Morales-Aguilerá, A., Vaughan Williams, E.M.: The effects on cardiac muscle of β-receptor antagonists in relation to their activity as local anaesthetics. Br. J. Pharmacol. *24,* 332–338 (1965)

Morgan, M.H., Hewer, R.L., Cooper, R.: Effect of the beta adrenergic blocking agent propranolol on essential tremor. J. Neurol. Neurosurg. Psychiatr. *36,* 618–624 (1973)

Muenter, M.D.: Levodopa. Ann. Int. Med. *75,* 795–797 (1971)

Murchison, L.E., Bewsher, P.D., Chesters, M.I., Ferrier, W.R.: Comparison of propranolol and practolol in the management of hyperthyroidism. Br. J. clin. Pharmac. *3,* 273–277 (1976)

Murray, T.J.: Treatment of essential tremor with propranolol. Can. Med. Assoc. J. *107,* 984–986 (1972)

Murray, T.J.: Long term therapy of essential tremor with propranolol. Can. Med. Assoc. J. *115,* 892–894 (1976)

Myhre, L., Röed, A., Aars, H.: Inhibitory effect of propranolol on tetanic contractions in rabbit. Eur. J. Pharmacol. *42,* 355–361 (1977)

Naess, K., Sirnes, T.B.: A synergistic effect of adrenaline and α-tubocurarine on the neuromuscular transmission. Acta Physiol. Scand. *29,* 293–306 (1953)

Naylor, W.G., Chang, A.: Cellular pharmacology of beta-blocking drugs. In: New perspectives in beta blockade. Burley, D.M., Frier, J.H., Rondel, R.K., Taylor, S.H. (Eds.) Horsham, England: Ciba Laboratories Publication, 1973, pp. 41–71

Nazar, K., Brezińska, Z.M., Kowalski, W.: Mechanism of impaired capacity for prolonged muscular work following beta-adrenergic blockade in dogs. Pflügers Arch. *336,* 72–78 (1972)

Nicholls, J.G.: The electrical properties of denervated skeletal muscle. J. Physiol. (Lond.) *131,* 1–12 (1956)

Noack, E., Inesi, G.: Action of propranolol on active calcium transport in sarcoplasmic membranes of skeletal and cardiac muscle. Int. Res. Commun. Syst. Med. Sci.: Cardiovascular System, *4,* 149 (1976)

Nott, M.W.: Interaction between phosphodiesterase inhibitors and catecholamines on contractions of the cat soleus. Br. J. Pharmacol. *42,* 666–668P (1971)

Nott, M.W.: Actions of sympathomimetic amines and phosphodiesterase inhibitors on skeletal muscle. Ph. D. Thesis. University of Strathclyde (1973)

Nott, M.W.: Actions of levodopa on the cat soleus muscle. Clin. Exp. Pharmacol. Physiol. *2,* 413 (1975)

Nott, M.W., Head, G.A.: Actions of tetrahydropapaveroline on the cardiovascular system and skeletal muscles of the anaesthetized cat and on the guinea-pig soleus muscle in vitro. Clin. Exp. Pharmacol. Physiol. *5,* 313–323 (1978)

Nott, M.W., Raper, C.: Use of cumulative dose-response curves in potency comparisons of sympathomimetic amines on the cat soleus muscle. Br. J. Pharmacol. *44,* 589–591 (1972)

Okushima, K.: Über die Wirkung des Adrenalins, der aromatischen Amines und der Aminosäuren auf den Skelettmuskel. Acta Sch. Med. Univ. Kioto *3,* 261–276 (1919)

Oliver, G., Schäfer, E.A.: The physiological effects of extracts of the suprarenal capsules. J. Physiol. (Lond.) *18,* 230–276 (1895)

Olson, C.B., Swett, C.P.: A functional and histochemical characterization of motor units in a heterogeneous muscle (flexor digitorum longus of the cat). J. Comp. Neurol. *128,* 475–497 (1966)

Orbeli, L.A.: Die Sympathische Innervation der Skelettmuskeln. Izv. Petrog. Inst. P.F. Lesgafta *6,* 187–197 (1923)

Otsuko, M., Nonomura, Y.: The action of phenolic substances on motor nerve endings. J. Pharmacol. Exp. Ther. *140,* 41–45 (1963)

Owen, D.A.L., Marsden, C.D.: Effects of adrenergic β-blockade on parkinsonian tremor. Lancet *II,* 1259–1262 (1965)

Paintal, A.S.: Facilitation and depression of muscle stretch receptors by repetitive antidromic stimulation, adrenaline and asphyxia. J. Physiol. (Lond.) *148*, 252–266 (1959)
Page, I.H.: The prolonged use of guanethidine. Med. Clin. North Amer. *45*, 417–420 (1961)
Pakkenberg, H.: Propranolol in essential tremor. Lancet *I*, *633* (1972)
Panella, A.: Action du principe actif surrénal sur la fatigue musculaire. Arch. Ital. Biol. *48*, 430–463 (1907)
Patel, V.K., Kelkar, V.V., Jindal, M.N.: Mechanism of MJ 1999-induced blockade of neuromuscular transmission. J. Pharm. Pharmacol. *23*, 209–213 (1971)
Paterson, G.: The dual action of adrenaline on denervated skeletal muscle. Biochem. Pharmacol. *12*, 85 (1963)
Paterson, J.W., Courtenay Evans, R.J., Prime, F.J.: Selectivity of bronchodilator action of salbutamol in asthmatic patients. Br. J. Dis. Chest *65*, 21–38 (1971)
Paton, W.D.M., Vizi, E.S., Zar, M.A.: The mechanism of acetylcholine release from parasympathetic nerves. J. Physiol. (Lond.) *215*, 819–848 (1971)
Paton, W.D.M., Zaimis, E.J.: Actions and clinical assessment of drugs which produce neuromuscular block. Lancet *II*, 568–570 (1950)
Pepine, C.J., Wiener, L., Stout, B.: Management of hyperthyroidism with combined alpha and beta sympathetic blockade. Med. Times. *100*, 114–132 (1972)
Perrie, W.T., Perry, S.V.: An electrophoretic study of the low-molecular weight components of myosin. Biochem. J. *119*, 31–38 (1970)
Peruzzi, P., Corda, M.: Variazioni mella sacria fusale del muscolo ext. 1. IV dig. isolato di *Rana Esculenta* endotte da fattori stagionali e fattori neuroumorali. Arch. Fisiol. *61*, 80–96 (1961)
Peruzzi, P., Staderini, G., Procacci, P.: Comportamento della scarica afferente muscolare sotto l'azione dell 'adrenalina e della noradrenalina e suo significato nella variazione del reflessor miotatico. Arch. Fisiol. *61*, 115–144 (1961)
Pickering, G.W.: High Blood Pressure. London: Churchill, 1955, pp. 400–401
Pinto, O.Q., Cremer, G., Torres, A.P., Aranda, E.C., Caso, L.F.: Efectos del chlorhidrato de propranolol en la tirotoxicosis. Rev. Med. H.C.E. (Lima) *12*, 62–67 (1972)
Poirier, L.-J., Bédard, P., Langelier, P., Larochelle, L., Parent, A., Roberge, A.G.: Les circuits neuronaux impliques dans la physiopathologie des syndromes parkinsoniens. Rev. Neurol. *127*, 37–50 (1972)
Posner, J.B., Stern, R., Krebs, E.G.: Effects of electrical stimulation and epinephrine on muscle phosphorylase, phosphorylase b kinase and adenosine 3',5'-phosphate. J. Biol. Chem. *240*, 982–985 (1965)
Price, H.L., Linde, H.W., Jones, R.E.: Sympatho-adrenal responses to general anesthesia in man and their relation to hemodynamics. Anesthesiology *20*, 563–575 (1959)
Purves, D., Sakmann, B.: Membrane properties underlying spontaneous activity of denervated muscle fibres. J. Physiol. (Lond.) *239*, 125–153 (1974)
Quastel, D.M.J., Hackett, J.T.: Quantal release of acetylcholine at the neuromuscular junction is not mediated by cyclic 3',5'-adenosine monophosphate. Fed. Proc. *30*, 557 (1971)
Rabinowitz, M., Desalles, L., Meisler, J., Lorand, L.: Distribution of adenyl cyclase in rabbit skeletal muscle fractions. Biochem. Biophys. Acta *97*, 29–36 (1965)
Rajput, A.H., Jamieson, H., Hirsh, S.: Specificity of tremorilytic effects of alcohol and propranolol. Clin. Res. *21*, 1018 (Abstract) (1973)
Rand, M.J., Wilson, J.: The actions of some adrenergic neurone blocking drugs at cholinergic junctions. Eur. J. Pharmacol. *1*, 210–221 (1967)
Raper, C.: Studies on the mechanism of action of adrenaline on fast- and slow-contracting skeletal muscles. Ph. D. Thesis, University of London (1965)
Raper, C., Bowman, W.C.: Effects of catecholamines on the gastrocnemius muscle of the domestic fowl. Eur. J. Pharmacol. *4*, 309–316 (1968)
Raper, C., Jowett, A.: Antifibrillary and antiadrenaline activity of β-receptor blocking drugs. Eur. J. Pharmacol. *1*, 353–362 (1967)
Rasmussen, H.: Cell communication, calcium ion and cyclic adenosine monophosphate. Science *170*, 404–412 (1970)
Rautakorpi, I., Marttila, R., Rinne, U.K.: Essentiaali vapina. Duodecim *92*, 1225–1233 (1976)
Reddy, N.B., Oliver, K.L., Engel, W.K.: Differences in catecholamine-sensitive adenylate cyclase and β-adrenergic receptor binding between fast-twitch and slow-twitch skeletal muscle membranes. Life Sci. *24*, 1765–1772 (1979)

Redfearn, J.W.T.: Frequency analysis of physiological and neurotic tremor. J. Neurol. Neurosurg. Psychiatr. *20,* 302–313 (1957)

Redfern, P., Thesleff, S.: Action potential generation in denervated rat skeletal muscle. I. Quantitative aspects. Acta Physiol. Scand. *81,* 557–564 (1971)

Rees, L.H.: Clinical management of thyrotixicosis and hypothyroidism. Update *12,* 459–470 (1976)

Ribeiro, J.A., Walker, J.: The effects of ATP and ADP on transmission at the rat and frog neuromuscular junctions. Br. J. Pharmacol. *54,* 213–218 (1975)

Robison, G.A., Butcher, R.W., Sutherland, E.W.: Cyclic AMP. Ann. Rev. Biochem. *37,* 149–174 (1968)

Robison, G.A., Butcher, R.W., Sutherland, E.W.: Cyclic AMP. London: Academic Press, (1971 a)

Robison, G.A., Nahas, G.G., Triner, L. (Eds.): Cyclic AMP and Cell function. Ann. N.Y. Acad. Sci. *185,* (1971 b)

Rodger, I.W.: Effects of isoetharine on airways resistance, heart rate, and contractions of the soleus muscle of the anaesthetised cat. Eur. J. Pharmacol. *24,* 211–217 (1973)

Rodger, I.W.: Studies on sympathomimetic bronchodilators. Ph. D. Thesis, University of Strathclyde, Glasgow (1974)

Røed, A.: High frequency inhibition of the sarcolemma by propranolol. Acta Physiol. Scand. *III,* (Suppl.) 396 (Abstr. 180) (1973)

Romanul, F.C.A.: Enzymes in muscle: 1. Histochemical studies of enzymes in individual muscle fibres. Arch. Neurol. Psychiatr. *II,* 355–368 (1964)

Romanul, F.C.A.: Capillary supply and metabolism of muscle fibres. Arch. Neurol. Psychiatr. *12,* 497–509 (1965)

Rosenblueth, A., Luco, J.V.: A study of denervated memmalian skeletal muscle. Am. J. Physiol. *120,* 781–797 (1937)

Rosenblueth, A., Lindsley, D.B., Morison, R.S.: A study of some decurarising substances. Am. J. Physiol. *115,* 53–68 (1936)

Rozen, M.S., Whan, F. McK.: Prolonged curarization associated with propranolol. Med. J. Aust. *i,* 467–469 (1972)

Rushworth, G.: Some effects of catecholamines on the electrical activity of human denervated muscle. Communication to International EMG Meeting, Copenhagen, 1963, Electronmyography *3,* 154 (title only) (1963) and personal communication

Sagild, U., Helweg-Larsen, H.F.: Clinical picture of hereditary transitory muscular paralysis; periodic adynamia and periodic paralysis. Nord. Med. *53,* 981–985 (1955)

Saini, R.K., Sharma, P.L.: Effect of some adrenergic beta receptor antagonists on the action of D-tubocurarine and pancuronium bromide. Indian J. Med. Res. *59,* 1104–1108 (1971)

Sandler, M., Bonham Carter, S., Hunter, K.R., Stern, G.M.: Tetrahydroisoquinoline alkaloids: in vivo metabolites of L-dopa in man. Nature (London) *241,* 439–443 (1973)

Sandler, M., Fellows, L.E., Calne, D.B., Findley, L.J.: Oxprenolol and levodopa in parkinsonian patients. Lancet *I,* 168 (1975)

Sanghvi, I.: Effects of cholinergic and adrenergic agents and their antagonists at the neuromuscular junction of the cat extraocular muscles. Invest. Ophthalmol. *6,* 269–276 (1967)

Santini, M., Ibata, Y.: The fine structure of thin unmyelinated axons within muscle spindles. Brain. Res. *33,* 289–302 (1971)

Sattin, A., Rall, T.W.: The effect of adenosine and adenine nucleotides on the cyclic adenosine 3′,5′-phosphate content of guinea-pig cerebral cortex slices. Mol. Pharmacol. *6,* 13–23 (1970)

Scales, B., McIntosh, D.A.D.: Effects of propranolol and its optical isomers on the radiocalcium uptake and the adenosine triphosphatases of skeletal and cardiac sarcoplasmic reticulum fractions (SRF). J. Pharmacol. Exp. Ther. *160,* 261–267(1968)

Schorderet, M., McAfee, D.A., Greengard, P.: Muscarinic and α-adrenergic blockade of cAMP increase in stimulated ganglia. Experientia *28,* 743 (1972)

Schwartz, A., Entman, M.L., Kaniike, K., Lane, L.K., van Winkle, W.B., Borner, E.P.: The rate calcium uptake into sarcoplasmic reticulum of cardiac muscle and skeletal muscle. Effects of cyclic AMP-dependent protein kinase and phosphorylase b kinase. Biochim. Biophys. Acta *426*, 57–72 (1976)

Scriabine, A., Moore, P.F., Iorio, L.C., Goldman, I.M., McShane, W.K., Booker, K.F.: Quinterenol, a new beta adrenergic stimulant. J. Pharmacol. Exp. Ther. *162*, 60–69 (1968)
Sellers, E.M., Zilm, D.H., Macleod, S.M., Degani, N., Giles, H.G.: Chlordiazepoxide and propranolol treatment of alcoholic withdrawal. Clin. Res. *23*, 610A (1975)
Sellers, E.M., Zilm, D.H., Degani, N., Macleoud, S.M.: Propranolol in alcohol withdrawal. Clin. Pharmacol. Ther. *19*, 115 (1976)
Sevitt, I.: A comparison of propranolol and benzhexol in essential tremor. Practitioner *213*, 91–96 (1974)
Sharma, V.K., Dasgupta, S.R., Banerjee, S.P.: [^{3}H]-Ouabain binding to denervated and innervated skeletal muscle. Eur. J. Pharmacol. *43*, 273–276 (1977)
Singer, J.J., Goldberg, A.L.: Cyclic AMP and transmission at the neuromuscular junction. In Advances in Biochemical Psychopharmacology. (Eds.) Greengard, P., Costa, E. New York: Raven Press 1970, Vol 3, pp. 335–348
Sloboda, R.D., Rudolph, S.A., Rosenbaum, J.L., Greengard, P.: Cyclic AMP-dependent endogenous phosphorylation of a microtubule-associated protein. Proc. Natl. Acad. Sci. U.S.A. *72*, 177–181 (1975)
Smith, C.M.: Neuromuscular pharmacology: drugs and muscle spindles. Ann. Rev. Pharmacol. *3*, 223–242 (1963)
Smith, C.M.: Relaxants of skeletal muscle. In: Physiological Pharmacology, Vol II, The nervous system, part B. Root, W.S., Hofmann, F.G. (Eds.) New York: Academic Press 1965, pp. 1–96
Smith, J.M.: A comparison of the mechanical responses of cat fast and slow twitch skeletal muscle following repetitive stimulation. Ph.D. Thesis, University of Bristol (1970)
Smith, J.W.: On the mode of action of catecholamines on skeletal muscle. Ph.D. Thesis, University of Bristol (1974)
Smith, J.W., Thesleff, S.: Spontaneous activity in denervated mouse diaphragm muscle. J. Physiol. (Lond.) *257*, 171–186 (1976)
Somlyo, A.P., Somlyo, A.V.: Pharmacology of excitation-contraction coupling in vascular smooth muscle and in avian slow muscle. Fed. Proc. *28*, 1634–1642 (1969)
Spriggs, T.L.B., Stockham, M.A.: Urethane anaesthesia and pituitary-adrenal function in the rat. J. Pharm. Pharmacol. *16*, 603–610 (1964)
Sréter, F.A.: Temperature, pH and seasonal dependence of Ca-uptake and ATPase activity of white and red muscle microsomes. Arch. Biochem. Biophys. *134*, 25–33 (1969)
Sréter, F.A.: Effect of denervation on fragmented sarcoplasmic reticulum of white and red muscle. Exp. Neurol. *29*, 52–64 (1970)
Strang, R.R.: Clinical trial with a beta-receptor antagonist (propranolol in parkinsonism). J. Neurol. Neurosurg. Psychiatr. *28*, 404–406 (1965)
Struppler, A., Velho-Groneberg, P., Claussen, M.: Clinic and pathophysiology of tremor. In: Advances in Parkinsonism. Birkmayer, W., Hornykiewicz, O. (Eds.) Basel: Hoffmann-LaRoche and Co. Ltd. 1976, pp. 287–302
Stuart, D., Ott, K., Ishikawa, K., Eldred, E.: The rhythm of shivering. I. General sensory contributions. Am. J. Phys. Med. *45*, 61–74 (1966)
Sullivan, A., Zaimis, E.: The effect of isoprenaline on cyclic AMP concentrations in skeletal muscle. J. Physiol. (Lond.) *231*, 102–103P (1973)
Svedmyr, N., Larsson, S., Thiringer, G.: Studies on resistance to long-acting adrenergic beta-stimulants in asthmatic patients. Br. Med. J. *2*, 668–669 (1974)
Sweet, R.D., Blumberg, J., Lee, J.E., McDowell, F.H.: Propranolol treatment of essential tremor. Neurology *24*, 64–67 (1974)
Takamine, J.: The isolation of the active principle of the suprarenal gland. J. Physiol. (Lond.) *27*, xxix–xxx (1901)
Tashiro, N.: Effects of isoprenaline on contractions of directly stimulated fast and slow muscles of the guinea pig. Br. J. Pharmacol. *48*, 121–131 (1973)
Temple, D.M., Hasselbach, W., Makinose, M.: The inhibition by beta-adrenoceptor blocking agents of calcium uptake into and efflux from isolated sarcoplasmic vesicles. Naunyn-Schmiedeberg's Arch. Pharmacol. *282*, 187–194 (1974)
Teravainan, H., Fogelholm, R., Larson, A.: Effect of propranolol on essential tremor. Neurology *26*, 27–30 (1976)
Teychenne, P.F., Calne, D.B., Leigh, P.N., Greenacre, J.K., Reid, J.L., Petrie, A., Bamji, A.N.: Idiopathic parkinsonism treated with bromocriptine. Lancet *II*, 473–476 (1975)

Thesleff, S.: Effects of motor innervation on the chemical sensitivity of skeletal muscle. Physiol. Rev. *40*, 734–752 (1960a)
Thesleff, S.: Supersensitivity of skeletal muscle produced by botulinum toxin. J. Physiol. (Lond.) *151*, 598–607 (1960b)
Thesleff, S.: Spontaneous electrical activity in denervated rat skeletal muscle. In: The Effect of Use and Disuse on Neuromuscular Functions. Gutmann, E., Hnik, P. (Eds.) Prague: Czechoslovak Academy of Sciences, 1963, pp. 41–51
Thesleff, S.: Physiological effects of denervation of muscle. Ann. N.Y. Acad. Sci. *228*, 89–104 (1974)
Thesleff, S., Ward, M.R.: Studies on the mechanism of fibrillation potentials in denervates muscle. J. Physiol. (Lond.) *244*, 313–323 (1975)
Thiringer, G., Svedmyr, N.: Evaluation of skeletal muscle tremor due to bronchodilator agents. Scand. J. Respir. Dis. *56*, 93–102 (1975)
Thiringer, G., Svedmyr, N.: Comparison of infused and inhaled terbutaline in patients with asthma. Scand. J. Respir. Dis. *57*, 17–24 (1976a)
Thiringer, G., Svedmyr, N.: Interaction of orally administered metoprolol, practolol and propranolol with isoprenaline in asthmatics. Eur. J. Clin. Pharmacol. *10*, 163–170 (1976b)
Thompson, M.K.: Effect of oxprenolol on parkinsonian tremor. Lancet *II*, 388 (1972)
Thompson, M.K.: Oxprenolol in senile tremor. Scott. Med. J. *20*, 291–292 (1975)
Tiegs, O.W.: The function of sympathetic nerves in relation to skeletal muscle-evidence for humoral action. Proc. Roy. Soc. Ser. B. Biol. Sci. *116*, 351–375 (1934)
Tiegs, O.W.: Innervation of voluntary muscle. Physiol. Rev. *33*, 90–144 (1953)
Tolosa, E.S., Loewenson, R.B.: Essential tremor: treatment with propranolol. Neurology *25*, 1041–1044 (1975)
Tomlinson, C.W., Bernatsky, A.M., Dhalla, N.S.: Modification of skeletal muscle sarcotubular calcium-stimulated adenosine triphosphate activity by various agents. Biochem. Pharmacol. *25*, 2271–2274 (1976)
Tower, S.S.: Persistence of fibrillation in denervated skeletal muscle and its nonoccurrence in muscle after tenotomy. Arch. Neurol. Psychiatr. *42*, 219–223 (1939)
Tridon, P., André, J.M., Arnould, A.G.: Resultats thérapeutiques chez 42 parkinsoniens traités par l'association levodopa-inhibiteur de décarboxylase. Ann. Med. Nancy *14*, 657–660 (1975)
Turkanis, S.A.: Some properties of the denervated anterior gracilis muscle of the rat. Br. J. Pharmacol. *37*, 414–424 (1969)
Turker, K., Kiran, B.: Action of pronethalol on neuromuscular activity. Arch. Int. Pharmacodyn. *155*, 356–364 (1965)
Tyrer, P.J., Lader, M.H.: Effects of beta adrenergic blockade with sotalol in chronic anxiety. Clin. Pharmacol. Ther. *14*, 418–426 (1973)
Tyrer, P.J., Lader, M.H.: Physiological response to propranolol and diazepam in chronic anxiety. Br. J. Clin. Pharmacol. *1*, 387–390 (1974)
Usubiaga, J.E.: Neuromuscular effects of beta-adrenergic blockers and their interaction with skeletal muscle relaxants. Anesthesiology *29*, 484–492 (1968)
Vapaatalo, H.: Role of cyclic nucleotides in the nervous system. Med. Biol. *52*, 200–207 (1974)
Vapaatalo, H., Anttila, P.: Effects of some inhibitors of phosphodiesterase on neuromuscular transmission. Naunyn-Schmiedeberg's Arch. Pharmacol. *275*, 227–232 (1972)
Vas, C.J.: Propranolol in parkinsonian tremor. Lancet *I*, 182–183 (1966)
Vernikos-Danellis, J., Zaimis, E.: Some pharmacological actions of bretylium and guanethidine. Lancet *II*, 787–788 (1960)
Vick, R.L., Todd, E.P., Luedke, D.W.: Epinephrine-induced hypokalemia: relation to liver and skeletal muscle. J. Pharmacol. Exp. Ther. *181*, 139–146 (1972)
Vizi, E.S.: Stimulation of acetylcholine release from cortical slices of rat brain by inhibition of $Na^{+}K^{+}Mg^{++}$-ATPase. J. Physiol. (Lond.) *226*, 95–117 (1972)
Waldeck, B.: An in vitro method for the study of β-receptor mediated effects on slow-contracting skeletal muscle. J. Pharm. Pharmacol. *28*, 434–436 (1976)
Waldeck, B.: Analysis of the β-receptor mediated effect on slow-contracting skeletal muscle in vitro. J. Pharm. Pharmacol. *29*, 550–554 (1977)
Waldeck, B.: β-Adrenoceptors in skeletal muscle. Acta Pharmacol. Tox. *44*, Suppl. II, 28–30 (1979)
Wang, P., Clausen, T.: Treatment of attacks of hyperkalaemic familial periodic paralysis by inhalation of salbutamol. Lancet *I*, 221–223 (1976)

Wang, P., Clausen, T., Ørskov, H.: Salbutamol inhalations suppress attacks of hyperkalemia in familial periodic paralysis. Monographs in Human Genetics Vol. 10. S. Karger AG, Basel (1978), pp 62–65
Ware, F., Bennett, A.L., McIntyre, A.R.: Membrane resting potential of denervated mammalian skeletal muscle measured in vivo. Am. J. Physiol. *173*, 115–118 (1951)
Ware, F., Bennett, A.L., McIntyre, A.R.: Membrane resting potential of denervated skeletal muscle measured in vitro. Am. J. Physiol. *177*, 115–118 (1954)
Watson, J.M., Richens, A.: The effects of salbutamol and terbutaline on physiological tremor, bronchial tone and heart rate. Br. J. Clin. Pharmacol. *1*, 223–227 (1974)
Weber, A.: Energised calcium transport and relaxing factor. Curr. Top. Bioenerget. *1*, 203–254 (1966)
Weber, A.: The mechanism of action of caffeine on sarcoplasmic reticulum. J. Gen. Physiol. *52*, 760–772 (1968)
Weber, K.: Fortgesetzte Untersuchungen über die Wirkungsweise des Sympathikus auf die ermüdeten Muskeln. Z. Biol. *95*, 454–466 (1934)
Werman, R., Wislicki, L.: Propranolol, a curariform and cholinomimetic agent at the frog neuromuscular junction. Comp. Gen. Pharmacol. *2*, 69–81 (1971)
West, G.B., Zaimis, E.J.: A comparison of adrenaline and noradrenaline on mammalian muscle. J. Physiol. (Lond.) *110*, 18–19P (1949)
Wilson, D.F.: The effects of dibutyryl cyclic adenosine 3′,5′-monophosphate, theophylline and aminophylline on neuromuscular transmission in the rat. J. Pharmacol. Exp. Ther. *188*, 447–452 (1974)
Winkler, G.F., Young, R.R.: Efficacy of chronic propranolol therapy in action tremors of the familial, senile or essential varieties. N. Engl. J. Med. *290*, 984–988 (1974)
Wislicki, L.: Excitatory and depressant effects of β-adrenoceptor blocking agents on skeletal muscle. Arch. Int. Pharmacodyn. *182*, 310–317 (1969)
Wislicki, L.: Frog muscle responses to catecholamine beta-receptor blocking agents. Isr. J. Med. Sci. *6*, 224–227 (1970)
Wislicki, L.: Interactions of beta-adrenoceptor blocking agents with curarizing drugs-mechanisms of action. Eleventh Cong. scand. Soc. Anaesthesiologists. Abstracts of Communications. Paper 18, 1973, p. 54
Wislicki, L., Rosenblum, I.: The effects of propranolol on normal and denervated muscle. Arch. Int. Pharmacodyn. *170*, 117–123 (1967a)
Wislicki, L., Rosenblum, I.: Effects of propranolol on the action of neuromuscular blocking drugs. Br. J. Anaesth. *39*, 932–942 (1967b)
Wolff, H.G., Cattel, McK.: Effects of stimulation of sympathetic and dorsal roots on contractions of skeletal muscle. Arch. Neurol. Psychiatr. *32*, 81–117 (1934)
Yamada, K.: Species difference in denervated muscle response to epinephrine between rabbit and rat. Jpn. J. Vet. Sci. *36*, 19–26 (1974)
Yamada, K., Harigaya, S.: Contractile response to sympathomimetic amines in isolated rat muscles after chronic denervation. Jpn. J. Pharmacol. *24*, 487–490 (1974)
Yamamoto, T., Takauji, M., Nagai, T.: Some properties of relaxing factor system and calcium sensitivity of myofibrils of rabbit red muscle. Jpn. J. Physiol. *20*, 52–60 (1970)
Young, R.R., Growdon, J.H., Shahani, B.T.: Beta-Adrenergic mechanisms in action tremor. N. Engl. J. Med. *293*, 950–953 (1975)
Young, R.W., Winkler, G.F.: Documentation of the control of action tremor by propranolol. Electroencephalogr. clin. Neurophysiol. *34*, *820* (1973)
Yuill, G.M.: Effect of levodopa on Parkinsonian tremor. Br. Med. J. *I*, 283–284 (1976)
Zachar, J. Zacharova, D., Adrian, R.H.: Observations on "detubulated" muscle fibres. Nature (London) *239*, 153–155 (1972)
Zaimis, E.: Spasticity alleviation by drugs acting directly on skeletal muscle. Lancet *I*, 403–405 (1973)
Zaimis, E.: A technique for recording muscle contractions in spastic patients. J. Physiol. (Lond.) *246*, 8P. (1974)
Zilm, D.H., Sellers, E.M., Frecker, R., Macleod, S.M.: Propranolol and ethanol decreased normal and alcoholic withdrawal tremors. Clin. Res. *23*, 611A (1975)

CHAPTER 3

Systemic Pharmacology of Adrenergic Agonists and Antagonists: Effects on the Digestive System

G. BURNSTOCK and H. WONG

A. Introduction

The inhibitory effect of secretions of the adrenal glands on the tone and motility of the gastro-intestinal tract was originally observed by JACOBJ (1892). The similarity of this effect to that of adrenaline (A) and sympathetic nerve stimulation on gastro-intestinal smooth muscle led to the suggestion by several workers that A, or a similar substance, was being released as a neurotransmitter from sympathetic nerve endings (DALE, 1938; ELLIOTT, 1904; FINKLEMAN, 1930). The relaxation of the intestine by mesenteric nerve stimulation and adrenoceptor activation was reinvestigated by ÅSTROM (1949), and together with the results of biochemical assays, which showed that there was 12–15 times more noradrenaline (NA) than A in mesenteric nerves, it was suggested that NA was the neurotransmitter involved (VON EULER, 1951). Measurement of the concentrations of different catecholamines (CA) with bioassay and chromatographic techniques in the effluent form cat (MANN and WEST, 1951; MIRKIN and BONNYCASTLE, 1954) and rabbit (MIRKIN and BONNYCASTLE, 1954) intestine during mesenteric nerve stimulation provided confirmatory evidence. Of the CA released, 95% was shown to be NA in the rabbit, and 90% in the cat. High levels of NA were also found in intestinal homogenates of rabbit (SHORE, 1959), rat (BRODIE et al., 1964) and guinea pig (BAUMGARTEN et al., 1970; GOVIER et al., 1969).

BARGER and DALE (1910) studied the pharmacological activity of a large number of synthetic amines related to A and termed their action sympathomimetic. The effect of a sympathomimetic drug depends on the type of adrenoreceptor with which it interacts. In 1948, AHLQUIST classified adrenoceptors into two types, α and β, on the basis of their responsiveness to a series of sympathomimetic amines. The order of potency for α-adrenoceptors was A $\gg$ NA $\gg$ isoprenaline; while for β-adrenoceptors, the order was reversed. Evidence concerning the possible structure of these receptor types and their mechanism of action has been reviewed by TRIGGLE (1972) and BELLEAU (1966). The development of specific α- and β-adrenoceptor blocking agents has enabled more precise classification of these receptors: α-adrenoceptors are blocked by low concentrations of phentolamine, *N*(2-Chloroethyl)dibenzylamine (Dibenamine) or phenoxybenzamine; while β-adrenoceptors are blocked by low concentrations of propranolol and pronethalol (FURCHGOTT, 1972). Recently, several subtypes of β-adrenoceptors have been differentiated (see FURCHGOTT, 1972; JENKINSON, 1973; LANDS et al., 1967).

B. Alpha- and Beta-Adrenoceptor Agonists

I. Effect on Motility

1. Introduction

Adrenoceptor agonists exert their effect on gastro-intestinal smooth muscle either by a *direct* action of α- and β-adrenoceptors present on smooth muscle cells or by various *indirect* actions such as (a) inhibition of acetylcholine (ACh) release through α-adrenoceptors present on the enteric neurones, (b) inhibition of NA release from adrenergic neurones and (c) actions on ganglion cell bodies and terminals of interneurones, (d) vasomotor actions on blood vessels leading to hypoxia. These possible sites of action of adrenoceptor agonists are diagrammatically represented in Fig. 1.

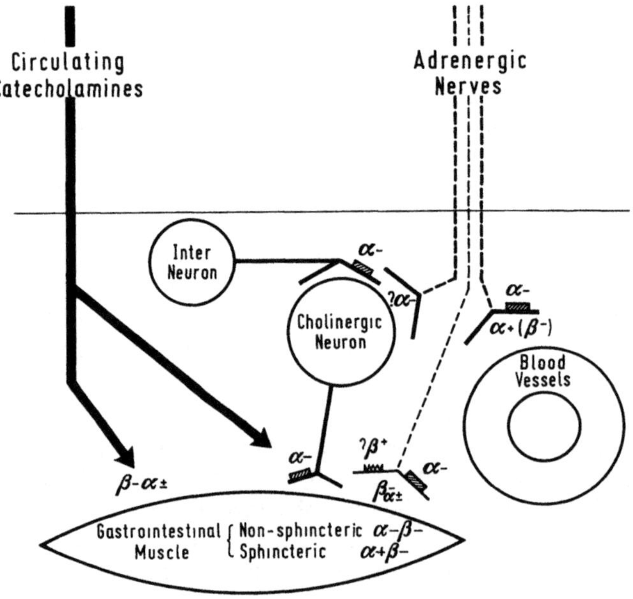

Fig. 1. A simplified diagrammatic representation of the arrangement of adrenergic receptors in the gastro-intestinal tract and of their major modes of activation. Positions of α- and β-receptors and the types of effect they mediate, either excitatory (+) or inhibitory (−), are indicated. Modified from FURNESS and BURNSTOCK (1975)

2. Effect on Non-Sphincteric Smooth Muscle

Studies on the inhibition of spontaneous activity and lowering of the tone of non-sphincteric smooth muscle by α- and β-adrenoceptor agonists are well documented (see FURNESS and BURNSTOCK, 1975; FURNESS and COSTA, 1974; LEE, 1970). Based on the relative potency of A, NA and isoprenaline in inhibiting the canine ileum, AHLQUIST (1948) had originally designated the adrenoceptors in the gastro-intestinal tract to be of the α-type. However, this conclusion was revised when it was found that a combination of α- and β-adrenoceptors antagonists were necessary to abolish the inhibitory effect of CA on the canine ileum in vivo (AHLQUIST and LEVY, 1959). It is now widely accepted that sympathomimetic amines may exert their inhibitory effects on non-sphincteric smooth muscle by an action on either α- or β-adrenoceptors or a combination of both. These results have been confirmed in vitro with isolated rabbit intestine (FURCHGOTT, 1967; LEE, 1970; VAN ROSSUM and MUJIC, 1965; WARREN and DAY, 1968), guinea pig taenia coli and the longitudinal muscle of the ileum (BRODY and DIAMOND, 1967; BÜLBRING and TOMITA, 1969a, b; JENKINSON and MORTON, 1967a, b; KOSTERLITZ et al., 1970; LEE, 1970), taenia of the human colon (BUCKNELL and WHITNEY, 1964) and kitten ileum, (WARREN and DAY, 1968). However, a number of exceptions to the inhibitory effects of adrenoceptor agonists on non-sphincteric smooth muscle have been reported. For example, contraction rather than relaxation has been reported in the oesophagus of guinea pig, cat and man (BAILEY, 1965; BURNSTOCK, 1960; CHRISTENSEN, 1970; CHRISTENSEN and DANIEL, 1966), the terminal ileum of the guinea pig, cat and dog (GAZET and JARRETT, 1974; JARRETT and GAZET, 1966; HENRICKSEN and IVY, 1931; MUNRO, 1951, 1952) and stomach of the guinea pig (GREEFF and HOLTZ, 1955; GREEFF et al., 1962; GUIMARAES, 1969; SMITH, 1918), dog (DALE, 1906; KURODA, 1924; MUREN, 1957a, b; NAKAZATO et al., 1970; SMITH, 1918; THOMAS, 1926), rabbit (BROWN and MCSWINEY, 1926; FURCHGOTT, 1967; KURODA, 1924; SMITH, 1918), man (ANDERSON and MORRIS, 1943; BENNETT and WHITNEY, 1966; DANIELOPULU and CARNIOL, 1922; GRAHAM, 1949; HAFFNER et al., 1969; SMITH, 1918; WOLF and WOLFF, 1943), ruminants (TITCHEN, 1968) and horse (ALEXANDER, 1949; BRUNARD and LABROUCHE, 1947; TANAKA and OHKUHO, 1940). The excitatory effect of adrenoceptor agonists in the oesophagus (BAILEY, 1965; BURNSTOCK, 1960), stomach (FURCHGOTT, 1967) and the terminal ileum (MUNRO, 1951; 1952; 1953), have been shown to be due to the presence of excitatory α-adrenoceptors. This effect can be reversed to inhibition in the presence of an α-adrenoceptor blocking agent.

3. Effect on Sphincteric Smooth Muscle

In contrast to their effects on non-sphincteric smooth muscle, adrenoceptor agonists usually cause contraction of sphincteric smooth muscle due to the presence of excitatory α-adrenoceptors (see FURNESS and BURNSTOCK, 1975; FURNESS and COSTA, 1974; LEE, 1970). This was first reported by ELLIOTT (1904) and DALE (1906) and has since been confirmed in a large number of species. However β-adrenoceptor agonists such as isoprenaline cause inhibition. Relaxation rather than contraction of sphincteric smooth muscle in response to CA has been reported in the cardiac sphincter of the rabbit (LANGLEY, 1901), in the pyloric sphincter of the rat (ARMITAGE and DEAN, 1966), dog (BASS et al., 1968; BROWN et al., 1930), rabbit (BROWN and MCSWINEY, 1926) and man (BASS et al., 1968; 1970; BENNETT and WHITNEY, 1966; HAFFNER et al., 1969; SHIPLEY and BLACKFAN, 1922; TEZNER and TUROLT, 1921), in the ileo-caecal sphincter of man (BUIRGE, 1944; WHITE et al., 1934), and the internal anal sphincter of the rabbit (LANGLEY, 1901), cat and man (KERREMANS and PENNINCKX, 1970; PARKS et al., 1969). This is probably due to the predominance of β-adrenoceptors in these preparations.

4. Effect on Acetylcholine Release from Enteric Neurones

Apart from their direct action on α- and β-adrenoceptors on smooth muscle, α-adrenoceptor agonists, in particular NA released form sympathetic nerves, inhibit the release of transmitter from cholinergic neurones in Auerbach's plexus. This mode of action of A and NA was first suggested by JACOBJ (1892), who found that sympathoadrenal discharge blocked the excitatory influence of the vagus on gastro-intestinal smooth muscle by an action separate from the direct muscle effect of the released amines, implying that A and NA might be exerting their action indirectly by inhibiting the excitatory neurones of the gut. Similar suggestions were made by MCDOUGAL and WEST (1954) and OBERDORF and KRONEBERG (1970) who found that the peristaltic reflex of the guinea pig ileum was inhibited by concentrations of A and NA which had no direct effect on the musculature and which did not alter the responses of the ileum to exogenous ACh. Further support came from histochemical techniques, which demonstrated extensive ramification of adrenergic fibres in the ganglia of Auerbach's plexus while few adrenergic fibres run in the musculature of the gut wall (JACOBOWITZ, 1965; NORBERG, 1964; NORBERG and SJÖQVIST, 1966; READ and BURNSTOCK, 1969, 1970).

There is now considerable evidence from transmitter release experiments using techniques for radioactive labelling of transmitter precursors, that α-adrenoceptor agonists like A, NA and phenylephrine can reduce ACh output from intrinsic neurones in intestinal tissue both at rest and during parasympathetic nerve stimulation in vitro (see VIZI, 1979). This has been shown in the guinea pig ileum and colon (BEANI et al., 1969; KAZIC, 1971; KNOLL and VIZI, 1971; KOSTERLITZ et al., 1970; PATON and VIZI, 1969; SCHAUMANN, 1958; KRONEBERG and OBERDORF, 1974), rabbit jejunum (VIZI, 1968) and human taeni coli (DELTACCA et al., 1970). The reduction in ACh output caused by A and NA was found to be greatest during low frequency parasympathetic nerve stimulation when the transmitter output per pulse was high, but was also apparent during high-frequency parasympathetic nerve stimulation (BEANI et al., 1969; KAZIC, 1971; KNOLL and VIZI, 1971; PATON and VIZI, 1969). The inhibition of ACh output produced by A was found to be four times as great as that caused by NA. This higher potency of A was attributed to its lower rate of uptake into adrenergic neurones (IVERSEN, 1967) and therefore its greater availability in the synaptic region (PATON and VIZI, 1969).

Evidence has been presented that the receptors mediating the inhibition of ACh release are α-adrenoceptors. In experiments using radioactively labelled ACh, exogenously administered A, NA and phenylephrine were found to reduce ACh output in both resting and stimulated intestine while the specific β-adrenoceptor agonist isoprenaline, and also dopamine were ineffective (KOSTERLITZ et al., 1970; PATON and VIZI, 1969). Data from experiments using specific α-adrenoceptor antagonists provide further evidence that α-adrenoceptors are involved in the inhibition of ACh release from enteric neurones (see Sect. C.). Evidence has been presented to suggest that inhibitory α-adrenoceptors are located prejunctionally on the cholinergic neurones (LUM et al., 1966; 1967; SALIMI et al., 1970; GILLESPIE and KHOYI, 1977). It seems likely that NA exerts its effects by reducing the release of ACh from the terminals of cholinergic interneurones (GILLESPIE and KHOYI, 1977). Adrenoceptor agonists action on the cell body appears unlikely, since NA has been found not to affect the sensitivity of ganglion cells to iontophoretically applied ACh (NISHI and NORTH, 1973). However, it is possible that the site of action of NA is located on another part of the cell soma, where action potentials are generated.

Sympathetic control of ACh output by a presynaptic rather than a post-synaptic mechanism has the advantage of transmitter economy compared to post-synaptic antagonism. In vivo experiments have shown that adrenergic modulation of ACh output may be the major physiological mechanism by which adrenergic nerve activation leads to smooth muscle inhibition (Furness and Costa, 1974). However, attempts to demonstrate that activation in vitro of the sympathetic nerves supplying Auerbach's plexus can cause a decrease in ACh output from cholinergic neurones have not been as successful and there is still some controversy concerning the role of adrenergic nerve stimulation on ACh output (Furness and Costa, 1974). The direct inhibitory effect of NA on smooth muscle becomes apparent during high-frequency nerve stimulation of the myenteric nerve plexus or vasoconstrictor nerve endings, when there is overflow of transmitter from the synaptic region onto the adjoining muscle (Gershon, 1967; Celander, 1959; Kock, 1959) or when there are CA circulating from the adrenal medulla (see Furness and Burnstock, 1975).

In the cat oesophagus, exogenous NA causes contraction rather than relaxation. Christensen and Daniel (1966) found that this contraction could be antagonized by the cholinergic antagonist atropine and at the same time potentiated by the acetylcholinesterase inhibitor physostigmine. Furthermore, pretreatment of the tissue with hemicholinium, which inhibits uptake of choline and thereby leads to depletion of ACh in cholinergic nerves, inhibits the responsiveness of the tissue to NA. This effect of hemicholinium could be reversed by administration of the ACh precursor choline. These results suggest that in this tissue, CA act on α-adrenoceptors present on cholinergic neurones to facilitate rather than inhibit ACh output.

5. Effect on Noradrenaline Release from Adrenergic Neurones

Evidence has accumulated showing that neurally released NA exerts a negative feedback effect on receptors located on adrenergic varicosities to cause a reduction of further transmitter release. These presynaptic receptors have been shown to be of the α-type; and their blockade results in a large increase in transmitter release during adrenergic nerve stimulation. This adrenergic autoregulatory system has been shown to be present in a large variety of tissues and species (see reviews by Stjärne, 1975; Westfall, 1977; Vizi, 1979).

Exogenously administered or neurally released NA and other α-adrenoceptor agonists may therefore affect gastro-intestinal motility by an inhibition of spontaneous or stimulation-induced release of NA from adrenergic nerves.

It has also been claimed that CA acting on presynaptic β-adrenoceptors can lead to an *increase* in NA release from sympathetic nerve terminals (see Story et al., 1975).

6. Mechanism of Action

Catecholamines cause inhibition of the activity of intestinal smooth muscle by hyperpolarizing the smooth muscle membrane, and thus causing a decrease or cessation of spike activity; excitation is elicited by a depolarization of the smooth muscle membrane, which results in initiation or increase of spike activity (Bülbring, 1954; Burnstock, 1958; Bülbring and Kuriyama, 1963; see Burnstock and Costa, 1975). There is still considerable controversy about the mechanism by which CA produce hyperpolarization (Axelsson, 1971; Bülbring and Tomita, 1969a, b, c,; Burnstock et al., 1963; Kuriyama, 1970; Setekleiv, 1970; Tomita, 1970; Shuba et al., 1976). Decrease in membrane Na conductance (Bülbring and Kuriyama, 1963) and stimulation of an electrogenic Na pump (Burnstock, 1958) were early proposals.

The effects of CA may be mediated by either α- or β-adrenoceptors located on the smooth muscle membrane. During the inhibition of intestinal smooth muscle activity by CA acting on α-adrenoceptors, there is an increased conductivity of the membrane to K^+ and Cl^- ions (TOMITA and WATANABE, 1973). This process is calciuim-dependent as it is potentiated by excess and abolished by the removal of calcium. (AXELSSON, 1971; BÜLBRING and TOMITA, 1969c, 1977a, b; FURNESS and COSTA, 1974; JENKINSON and MORTON, 1967a, b; SHUBA, 1977a, b). The excitatory effects of CA acting on α-adrenoceptors are also calcium dependent and may be due to an increased conductivity to Na^+, K^+ and other ions (BURNSTOCK, 1960; BOLTON, 1972; BURNSTOCK and COSTA, 1975).

Inhibition of smooth muscle activity by the action of CA on β-adrenoceptors involves an energy-requiring process which results in the formation of cAMP (see AXELSSON, 1971; BÜLBRING and HERTOG, 1977; FURCHGOTT, 1972; ROBISON et al., 1970; TRIGGLE, 1972). It is generally accepted that an increase in the sequestration or extrusion of Ca^{++} is the main mechanism underlying the effect of β-adrenoceptor activation (BÜLBRING and HERTOG, 1977).

It seems likely that the depolarization associated with the excitatory action of CA on smooth muscle of the alimentary tract is due to a general increase in membrane conductance to K^+, Na^+, Cl^-, and Ca^{2+} (BURNSTOCK, 1960; SHUBA et al., 1976).

II. Effect on Gastro-Intestinal Vasculature

The blood vessels of the gastro-intestinal area contain both excitatory α-adrenoceptors and inhibitory β-adrenoceptors (BÜLBRING and BURN, 1936; CLARK, 1930; GREEN et al., 1967; see FURNESS and BURNSTOCK, 1975; FURNESS and COSTA, 1974). Catecholamines cause vasoconstriction of isolated portal veins (HUGHES and VANE, 1967, 1970) and mesenteric arteries and veins (CAMPBELL, 1911; CONNET, 1920; EDMUNDS, 1915; FRANKLIN, 1925; GUNN and CHEVASSE, 1913; HOLMAN et al., 1968; JOHANSSON and LJUNG, 1967; MALIK and LING, 1969; MCGREGOR, 1965; SPEDEN, 1970). This action is reversed to vasodilatation in the presence of α-adrenoceptor inhibitors (FRANKLIN, 1925; HOLMAN et al., 1968; HUGHES and VANE, 1967, 1970; JOHANSSON and LJUNG, 1967; ROSS, 1970). The β-adrenoceptors appear to be more easily acitivated by low concentrations of CA causing dilatation, whereas higher concentrations of CA cause constriction (BÜLBRING and BURN, 1936; NICOLOFF et al., 1964; OGAWA, 1912; THOMPSON and VANE, 1953).

Infusion of CA into the splanchnic vasculature causes decreased blood flow by arterial constriction and a decreased blood volume in the circuit by constriction of large capacitance vessels (see reviews BRADLEY, 1963; GRAYSON and MENDEL, 1965; GREEN and KEPCHAR, 1959; GRIM, 1963; LACROIX, 1960). Although there is an overall decrease in blood volume in this area, redistribution may occur causing an actual increase in some areas. There is some evidence that blanching of the mucosa during CA infusion is accompanied by a preferential shunting of blood into submucosal vessels. DELANY and GRIM (1965) have shown that in the dog, NA causes a decreased total gastric blood flow but an increased muscle blood flow, i.e. a diversion away from the mucosa. However, these authors have also shown that the effects of CA in this preparation varied with the secretory activity of the gastric mucosa; when it was low, A caused an increased mucosal blood flow, whereas during high secretory activity, the mucosal flow was decreased.

The initial constriction of gastro-intestinal blood vessels by CA is not sustained and gives way to vasodilatation after 1 to 3 min. This phenomenon is known as autoregulatory escape (CLARK, 1930; DRESEL and WALLENTIN, 1966; FOLKOW et al., 1964; GOETZ, 1939; GREEN et al., 1955; HULTEN et al., 1969; MACLEAN et al., 1956; ROSS, 1970; WOODS et al., 1932). It has been suggested that autoregulatory escape may be partially due to a shift from activation of α-adrenoceptors to activation of β-adrenoceptors (HEINRICH and LUTZ, 1971; RICHARDSON and JOHNSON, 1970; ROSS, 1970; SHANBOUR and JACOBSON, 1971), but this is only a partial explanation for the observed phenomenon. Autoregulatory escape is observed in isolated vascular segments in vitro as well as in vivo and therefore is unlikely to be the consequence of accumulation of vasoactive metabolites. The escape is not specific to sympathetic nerve stimulation and CA but occurs with a variety of vasoconstrictor agents such as vasopressin, angiotensin and prostaglandin $F_{2\alpha}$; the degree of escape depends on the species, drug, method of administration and concentration (DRESEL and WALLENTIN, 1966; HEINRICH and LUTZ, 1971; ROSS, 1970, 1971; SHEHADEH et al., 1969).

During autoregulatory escape there is evidence of increased blood flow in the submucosa of the gut but the mucosa remains ischaemic throughout (COWLEY and CODE, 1970; DRESEL et al., 1966; FOLKOW et al., 1964). At the same time, the large veins maintain their constrictor responses to CA and thus maintain a decreased blood flow in this circuit. (COBBOLD et al., 1964; MELLANDER and JOHANSSON, 1968; ÖBERG, 1964). FOLKOW et al. (1964), using the distribution of indian ink in the mucosa, submucosa, external muscle and serosa of the cat intestine, showed that there is a marked decrease in blood flow in all layers during the constrictor responses to CA. During autoregulatory escape, blood flow only partially recovered in the mucosa, but substantially increased in the submucosa. The flow in the muscle and the serosa remained decreased. FOLKOW et al. (1964) concluded that there was a well sustained and important diversion of blood flow from the mucosa during autoregulatory escape. Similar conclusions were drawn by DRESEL and WALLENTIN (1966), who showed that there was substantial underperfusion of the mucosa during autoregulatory escape from sustained infusions of NA.

III. Effect on Gastric and Intestinal Secretion

Results of earlier studies on the effect of α- and β-adrenoceptor agonists on gastric secretion were contradictory, showing no effect on secretion in some cases, and enhancement of secretion in others (GALLONE and CONSOLO, 1961; IVY and MCILWAIN, 1923; KARVINEN and KARVONEN, 1952; LIM, 1922; LINDE, 1950; LOEPER and VERPY, 1971; ROTHSCHILD, 1925; VON SIROTININ, 1924). Later experiments showed that α- and β-adrenoceptor agonists were in fact largely antisecretory. These discrepancies may have been due to the low basal gastric secretion of the stomachs used in earlier experiments as a result of anaesthesia and operative conditions.

1. Action of Alpha- and Beta-Adrenoceptor Agonists

In general, both α- and β-adrenoceptor agonists decrease gastric acid secretion in conscious animals. The first convincing evidence of this effect came from the experiments of HESS and GUNDLACH (1920), who demonstrated that A markedly decreased the amount of gastric juice secreted in response to food in the dog. FORREST and CODE

(1954), also showed that A and NA administered intravenously into dogs decreased histamine-induced gastric acid secretion, and that A was more effective than NA. The antisecretory effects of A and NA have since been confirmed in rats (MISHER et al., 1969), monkeys (SMITH and JACOBSON, 1964) and dogs (NICOLOFF et al., 1964; GRECHISHKIN, 1970; HOLTON et al., 1969; JACOBSON et al., 1966, 1967; JACOBSON, 1970; PRADHAN and WINGATE, 1962). Inhibition of acid secretion in the resting stomach of man has also been reported (BERNSTEIN, 1952; DEMAND et al., 1968; WOLF and WOLFF, 1947), as well as inhibition of food and histamine-induced gastric secretion (LEONSINS and WADDELL, 1958; MOLL and FLINT, 1928).

The action of phenylephrine, a specific α-adrenoceptor agonist, has been studied by MISHER et al. (1969) who found that in small doses (0.25 mg/kg), it potentiated spontaneous gastric secretion in rats with gastric fistulae. Larger doses (0.5–1 mg/kg) caused a potentiation followed by a fall in secretion. CURWAIN et al. (1974) has suggested that the potentiation may be due to the ability of phenylephrine to increase histamine formation.

Isoprenaline, a relatively specific β-adrenoceptor agonist was shown to be the most potent of a series of CA in inhibiting gastric secretion in the dog (JACOBSON, 1970; JACOBSON et al., 1966, 1967; PRADHAN and WINGATE, 1962) and rat (BASS and PATTERSON, 1967; FJALLAND, 1972; MISHER et al., 1969; YAMAGUCHI et al., 1977). Infusion of isoprenaline in very small doses has been reported to enhance rather than inhibit histamine-induced secretion in the dog. Higher doses of isoprenaline reverse this enhancement to inhibition in conscious dogs. Enhancement with low doses of isoprenaline was not observed with either food or pentagastrin-induced secretion. Pentagastrin-induced acid secretion was very sensitive to inhibition by even low doses of isoprenaline in both conscious and anaesthetized dogs (CURWAIN et al., 1974; CURWAIN and HOLTON, 1972). The relatively selective β_2-adrenoceptor agonists salbutamol and terbutaline were also potent inhibitors of pentagastrin-induced, but not histamine-induced, gastric secretion. These effects were blocked by propranolol, are not secondary to a fall in mucosal blood flow.

It was first reported by HARRIES (1957) that histamine-induced gastric secretion was more difficult to suppress with CA than pentagastrin-induced secretion; this was confirmed in later experiments (CURWAIN and HOLTON, 1972; PRADHAN and WINGATE, 1962). About 40 times more isoprenaline was required to inhibit histamine-induced secretion compared to pentagastrin-induced secretion in conscious dogs.

In acute experiments using anaesthetized animals, the responses obtained with α-adrenoceptor agonists were essentially the same as in conscious animals, but some difference occurred with β-adrenoceptor agonists. In the anaesthetized dog, enhancement of acid secretion with A was frequently observed (PARROT and VERLIAC, 1941 a, b; THOMPSON and VANE, 1953; ZEPPA et al., 1968). However, other workers reported no effect or a decrease in secretion (CUMMING et al., 1963; HAIGH et al., 1967; PETERS and WOMACK, 1958; NICOLOFF et al., 1964).

2. Mechanism of Action

The mechanisms of action of α- and β-adrenoceptor agonists on gastric secretion are becoming clearer. One route for the inhibitory actions of A and NA on gastric secretion is via their α-adrenoceptor effects in constricting blood vessels (FORREST and Co-

DE, 1954; CURWAIN and HOLTON, 1972). In acute experiments using the innervated cat's stomach, THOMPSON and VANE (1953) showed that histamine-induced gastric secretion was inhibited by large doses of A but increased by small doses; this inhibition and enhancement was accompanied by increases and decreases in blood flow and could therefore be secondary to these changes. However, other workers reported no correlation between the haemodynamic effects of CA and their action on gastric secretion (CUMMING et al., 1963; PETERS and WOMACK, 1958; WALZ and VAN ZWIETEN, 1970). HARRIES (1956) suggested that the long lasting effects of CA could not be due to their effects on the circulation alone. Furthermore, isoprenaline, which has been shown by various workers to be a potent antisecretory agent, is vasodilatory, and is effective at doses lower than that necessary to have a haemodynamic effect (BASS and PATTERSON, 1967; MISHER et al., 1969; PRADHAN and WINGATE, 1962; YAMAGUCHI et al., 1977). Also, other vasoconstrictor substances such as vasopressin, angiotensin, and DL-Dopa are without effect on secretion (BASS and PATTERSON, 1967).

Another route for NA reduction of gastric secretion is via presynaptic α-adrenoceptors on cholinergic nerve terminals leading to inhibition of ACh release (PATON and VIZI 1969; KRONEBERG and OBERDORF, 1974, and see Sect. B.I.4.).

A third route for the action of β-adrenoceptor agonists is their powerful direct inhibitory action on gastric secretion (JACOBSON, 1970). NA released from sympathetic nerves appears to act via β_1-adrenoceptors (ABLAD et al., 1975) and under conditions of stress when circulatory blood levels of A are enhanced (CALLINGHAM, 1967), inhibition of gastric secretion via β_2-adrenoceptors is also evident (DALY et al., 1978).

It has been suggested that the difference in the effects of β-adrenoceptor agonists in conscious and anaesthetized animals may be due to the effects of laparotomy and associated surgical procedures in preparing animals for acute experiments, which cause an increase in sympathetic tone to the stomach. Although β-adrenoceptor agonists have a direct inhibitory action on the secretory process, in conditions of high sympathetic tone, where secretion may be limited by a restricted blood flow, the vasodilatory effect of β-adrenoceptor agonists may cause an increase in mucosal blood flow and thus an apparent enhancement of gastric secretion (HOLTON, 1973; COWLEY and CODE, 1970).

Isoprenaline in small doses increases histamine-induced gastric secretion (CURWAIN and HOLTON, 1972). The mechanism of this effect is not fully understood, and the possibility of a primary vascular action of isoprenaline has not been excluded. CURWAIN et al. (1974) suggested that it may be due to the abilitiy of isoprenaline to increase histamine formation.

Histamine-induced gastric secretion is more difficult to suppress with CA than pentagastrin-induced secretion. This has led to the suggestion that histamine may be the final secretagogue that stimulates the oxyntic cells, while pentagastrin and other stimuli initiate a longer chain of events, leading to the final secretory step, so that there are a series of points where secretion may be inhibited (CODE ,1956; CURWAIN et al., 1974; KAHLSON et al., 1973). The involvement of histamine in gastrin induced secretion has been confirmed by BLACK et al. (1972), who showed that burimamide, a specific H_2-receptor antagonist, blocks the actions of gastrin, pentagastrin, as well as histamine.

In general, CA do not have a strong action on mucous secretion. There is usually a slight decrease of mucous secretion in the presense of CA (MOLL and FLINT, 1928;

NICOLOFF et al., 1964; ROGERS et al., 1919; WOLF and WOLFF, 1943) and this may be due to changes in mucosal blood flow or a *direct effect of the CA* on mucous-secreting cells. Exceptions occur, and increased mucous secretion by CA has been reported in the oesophagus of the cat (LANGLEY, 1901), in the stomach of the cat and dog (BABKIN, 1950; BAXTER, 1934) and in the duodenum of the dog (HARTIOLA and TOIVENEN, 1954).

IV. Effect on Absorption

Early studies suggested that the action of CA on absorption appeared to be largely an indirect result of its action on blood flow (GUTHRIE and QUASTEL, 1956; JOSKE et al., 1958; REID, 1896; SHAW and MAYNARD, 1958; WINNE, 1966), and that only during extreme depression of blood flow was absorption inhibited. Active absorption appeared to be more readily affected than passive absorption; passive absorption was not substantially diminished if blood flow to the intestine was halved, but active absorption was reduced by 30–40% (SCHANKER et al., 1957; VARRO et al., 1965).

More recent studies, however, have shown that NA enhances intestinal absorption of Na^+, Cl^- and H_2O and reduces secretion of bicarbonate (FIELD and MCCOLL, 1973; FIELD et al., 1975; BRASITUS et al., 1976; HUBEL, 1976).

V. Summary

α- and β-adrenoceptor agonists such as A and NA cause inhibition of the tone and motility of most non-sphincteric intestinal smooth muscle preparations. Excitatory responses, however, have been reported in the oesophagus, terminal ileum and stomach of different species, and are due to the presence of excitatory α-adrenoceptors.

The inhibitory effects of α- and β-adrenoceptor agonists on non-sphincteric smooth muscle are mediated by inhibitory α- and β-adrenoceptors present on the smooth muscle membrane, and inhibitory α-adrenoceptors in cholinergic nerve terminals, which lead to inhibition of ACh release. α-Adrenoceptor agonists may also act presynaptically to modulate the release of NA from adrenergic nerve terminals.

α-Adrenoceptor agonists cause excitation of sphincteric smooth muscle, while β-adrenoceptor agonists such as isoprenaline cause relaxation.

Blood vessels in the gastro-intestinal area have both excitatory α-adrenoceptors and inhibitory β-adrenoceptors. Activation of α-adrenoceptors by CA infusions causes arterial and venous constriction, thus decreasing the blood volume in the intestinal circuit. The initial vasoconstriction is not sustained and is followed, after 1–2 min, by vasodilatation. This phenomenon is known as autoregulatory escape, and is not due to the accumulation of metabolites in the system. During autoregulatory escape, the total blood flow in the area remains decreased, but there is a redistribution of blood flow between the different layers of the gut wall; the flow in the submucosa recovers partially while that in the mucosa, muscle and serosa remains decreased.

It seems likely that under normal conditions, gastric acid secretion can be reduced by NA released from sympathetic nerves acting in three different ways: on post-synaptic α-adrenoceptors to reduce mucosal blood flow, on presynaptic α-adrenoceptors to inhibit ACh release and a direct antisecretory action on β_1-adrenoceptors. Under conditions of stress the circulating blood levels of A are enhanced by release from the adrenal glands. In these circumstances the inhibitory actions of the sympathetic nervous system described above would be augmented by an action of A on β_2-adrenoceptors as well as α-adrenoceptors. NA enhances intestinal absorption of Na^+ and K^+ ions and H_2O and reduces secretion of bicarbonate.

C. Adrenergic Transmitter Releasing Agents

I. Introduction

Substances which mimic the effects of adrenergic transmitters, as described in the previous section, do so by acting directly on adrenoceptors. A similar effect may be produced by compounds acting on adrenergic neurones to release stored transmitter which then acts on adrenoceptors. Compounds with this action are known as adrenergic transmitter releasing agents, or indirectly acting sympathomimetic amines. They usually resemble NA structurally but lack the chemical groups required for attachment to adrenoceptors. However, they retain the basic amino group in their structure, and thus have a greater affinity for NA storage sites than for adrenoceptors (BOWMAN et al., 1971). Amphetamine and tyramine are adrenergic transmitter releasing agents; probably acting by releasing vesicular stores of NA (see MUSCHOLL, 1966; CHUBB et al., 1972). The action of these drugs depends on the presence of transmitter stores; they are therefore ineffective in tissues that have been reserpinized or sympathectomized, but their effect is restored by the administration of NA or its precursors (BOWMAN et al., 1971).

II. Effect on Motility

Adrenergic transmitter releasing agents inhibit gastro-intestinal motility and lower the tone by releasing endogenous NA, which then acts on one or a combination of the adrenoceptor sites on smooth muscle cells and neural elements present in the gut wall.

An important site of action of NA in inhibiting gastro-intestinal motility is on the prejunctional α-adrenoceptors on cholinergic neurones in the gut wall. Activation of these adrenoceptors cause inhibition of ACh release (see Sect. A.I.4.). KNOLL and VIZI (1971) showed that the adrenergic transmitter releasing agents amphetamine and methylamphetamine reduced the output of ACh from enteric neurones in the guinea pig ileum.

High concentrations of guanethidine, an adrenergic neurone blocking agent (see Sect. E) have been shown to release NA (CASS et al., 1960; CASS and SPRIGGS, 1961; SHEPPARD and ZIMMERMAN, 1959). In isolated guinea pig ileum, guanethidine was found to reduce both basal and nerve-stimulated release of ACh (PATON and VIZI, 1969; VIZI and KNOLL, 1971) and since the effect was not observed in reserpinized preparations, this action was considered to be due to its transmitter releasing action.

Adrenergic transmitter releasing agents may interfere with the action of adrenergic neurone blocking agents (DAY, 1962; DAY and RAND, 1963; GERKENS et al., 1969; ATKINSON et al., 1972; RAND and WILSON, 1967). For example, in the isolated rabbit intestine the blocking effect of guanethidine persists for long periods, but this effect can be reversed by the addition of adrenergic transmitter releasing agents such as tyramine, dexamphetamine, methylamphetamine, ephedrine or dopamine (DAY, 1962; DAY and RAND, 1963; GERKENS et al., 1969; Atkinson et al., 1972; RAND and WILSON, 1967).

Other substances that have been shown to release CA from stores in intestinal tissue include nicotine and dimethylphenyl-piperazinium (DMPP) (HOLLANDS and VANOV, 1965). Bradykinin has been shown to inhibit contractions of the canine ileum (LEVY, 1963). Part of this action may be due to release of CA by bradykinin since the effect is absent after reserpinization (TÜRKER et al., 1964).

III. Effect on Gastric Secretion

In general, adrenergic transmitter releasing agents do not have any significant effect on gastric secretion. Guanethidine, which has been shown to release CA from adrenergic nerve endings at high-doses (SHEPPARD and ZIMMERMAN, 1959; CASS et al., 1960; CASS and SPRIGGS, 1961), did not markedly affect gastric secretory volume in pylorus-ligated rats (BASS and PATTERSON, 1967). The indirectly acting sympathomimetic amines tyramine, phenylethylamine and ephedrine were found to be weakly antisecretory (BASS and PATTERSON, 1967). Both bradykinin and angiotensin have been shown to release CA from the adrenals (FELDBURG and LEWIS, 1964), and DMPP has been shown to release CA from tissues (LINDMAR and MUSCHOLL, 1961). However these substances did not show any antisecretory activity in the rat (BASS and PATTERSON, 1967).

BASS and PATTERSON (1967) have suggested that since tissue CA are present in two or more pools with different turn over rates, the transmitter releasing agents may either fail to affect the pool that is responsible for antisecretory activity, or that the release of transmitter is so transient that no chance in secretory activity is noticeable.

IV. Summary

Adrenergic transmitter releasing agents act by displacing NA from its storage sites and thus have a similar effect on gastro-intestinal functions to that of exogenous NA. Gastro-intestinal tone and motility are decreased by inhibition of ACh release from enteric neurones by the released NA, as well as a post-synaptic action on α- and β-adrenoceptors present. Adrenergic transmitter releasing agents can also reverse the action of adrenergic neurone blocking agents. Their effect on gastric secretion is negligible.

D. Alpha- and Beta-Adrenoceptor Antagonists

I. Introduction

Since the original work of AHLQUIST and LEVY (1959), the presence of both α- and β-adrenoceptors on gastro-intestinal smooth muscle cells has been confirmed in many species. Thus, in most gastro-intestinal preparations, a combination of α- and β-adrenoceptor antagonists are necessary to block the responses to A and NA. Adrenoceptor sites on both adrenergic and cholinergic nerve terminals that mediate reduced release of transmitter, however, are all of the α-type. In general then, α- and β-adrenoceptor antagonists reverse the actions of α- and β-agonists described in detail in Sect. B.

II. Effect on Motility

There is evidence that in some parts of the gut, adrenoceptors present on the smooth muscle cells are predominantly of the β-tpye and that α-adrenoceptors are located predominantly on cholinergic neurones. KOSTERLITZ et al. (1970) showed that in the longitudinal muscle of the guinea pig ileum the inhibitory effect of A on the excitatory responses to electrical field stimulation were completely blocked by the α-adrenoceptor antagonists phentolamine or phenoxybenzamine; this inhibitory effect of A was associated with a reduction in labelled ACh output. In contrast inhibition by CA of the responses of the ileum to exogenous ACh was optimally antagonized by the β-adrenoceptor blocking agent propranolol. These authors concluded that adrenoceptors inhibit gastro-intestinal motility by acting on inhibitory β-receptors on the smooth muscle cells and inhibitory α-adrenoceptors on cholinergic neurones. WILSON (1964), who observed the relative potencies of four sympathomimetic amines in inhibiting histamine- and carbachol-induced contractions in the guinea pig ileum, claimed that adrenoceptors in this tissue were of the β-type. Further evidence that adrenoceptors on smooth muscle cells are predominantly of the β-type while α-adrenoceptors are located on neurones came from the experiments of GILLESPIE and KHOYI (1977). These workers reported that in the rabbit colon, the responses to cholinergic nerve stimulation are effectively inhibited by adrenergic nerve stimulation; and this inhibition can be blocked by phentolamine. In contrast, the response to exogenous ACh is inhibited equally by A, NA, isoprenaline and adrenergic nerve stimulation; this inhibition is blocked by propranolol.

The inhibitory effect of CA on the release of ACh from intestinal smooth muscle preparations both at rest and during cholinergic nerve stimulation is antagonized by α-adrenoceptor antagonists such as phentolamine, phenoxybenzamine and ergotamine, but not β-adrenoceptor antagonists such as propranolol (KOSTERLITZ et al., 1970; PATON and VIZI, 1969; KNOLL and VIZI, 1971; GILLESPIE and KHOYI, 1977).

In intact animals, α adrenoceptor antagonists such as phentolamine and tolazoline produce hyperperistalsis and diarrhoea. Since these effects are blocked by the muscarinic antagonist atropine they are probably due to parasympathetic predominance after blockade of adrenergic inhibition. In man, however, α-adrenoceptor blockade has little overall effect, i.e. dibenamine and phenoxybenzamine do not appreciably alter the rate of passage of barium salts along the gastro-intestinal tract (GOODMAN and GILMAN, 1975).

Sphincteric smooth muscle contracts in response to adrenoceptor agonists due to the presence of α-excitatory receptors. This was first demonstrated by DALE (1906), who found that the motor response of sphincters to sympathetic nerve stimulation and A is abolished by ergot alkaloids. Relaxations of sphincteric smooth muscle in response to CA have occasionally been reported and may be due to a predominance of inhibitory β-adrenoceptors in some preparations (BENZI et al., 1964; MORI et al., 1971; PERSSON, 1971). In all sphincters, contractions elicited by A and NA can be blocked by α-adrenoceptor antagonists, and the response is usually reversed to relaxation under these conditions.

III. Effect on Vasculature

The vasoconstriction of gastro-intestinal vasculature in response to adrenergic nerve stimulation or CA is either blocked or reversed to a slight dilatation by α-adrenoceptor antagonists such as ergotoxine, dibenamine and azapetine (DALE, 1913; WOODS et al., 1932; CLARK, 1934; BÜLBRING and BURN, 1936; FOLKOW et al., 1948; DEAL and GREEN, 1956). Conversely dilatation is reduced in the presence of β-adrenoceptor antagonists (GREEN et al., 1955; ROSS, 1967). It has been suggested (see Sect. B. II) that the phenomenon of autoregulatory escape is due to a shift from activation of α-adrenoceptors to activation of β-adrenoceptors. However, ROSS (1971) showed that autoregulatory escape is unaffected by the presence of β-adrenoceptor antagonists and may be due to non-adrenergic, non-cholinergic nerves (see BIBER, 1973; BURNSTOCK, 1980; FURNESS and COSTA, 1974; HULTEN, 1969).

IV. Effect on Gastric Secretion

In the stomach, the actions of α- and β-adrenoceptor agonists on gastric secretion indicate that they are predominantly antisecretory agents (see Sect. B. III). The actions of α- and β-adrenoceptor antagonists on gastric secretion are either direct or indirect via their effect on adrenergically mediated inhibition of secretion. Thus, α-adrenoceptor antagonists have been reported to increase (PRADHAN and WINGATE, 1966; WALZ and VAN ZWIETEN, 1970) and decrease gastric secretion (PRADHAN and WINGATE, 1966; BASS and PATTERSON, 1967; OKABE et al., 1970). Similarly, β-adrenoceptor antagonists have been reported to increase (EVANS and LIN, 1970; FJALLAND, 1972; DEBNATH et al., 1974; KONTIREK and OLEKSY, 1969), decrease (BASS and PATTERSON, 1967; PRADHAN and WINGATE, 1966; OKABE et al., 1970; GEUMEI et al., 1972a, b) or have no effect on gastric secretion MISHER et al., 1969).

1. Alpha-Adrenoceptor Antagonists

The 2-substituted imidazoline compounds, tolazoline (PRADHAN and WINGATE, 1966; NASIO, 1944) and phentolamine (PRADHAN and WINGATE, 1966) enhance gastric secretion in dogs in response to food, bethanechol or histamine. These stimulatory actions have been attributed to the structural similarity of the imidazoline nucleus of these compounds to histamine, which stimulates acid-secreting cells directly (PRADHAN and WINGATE, 1966; WALZ and VAN ZWIETEN, 1970). In anaesthetized rats, tolazoline and the structurally related compounds clonidine, naphazoline and xylometazoline also stimulated secretion. In these experiments, however, the effects of tolazoline could be abolished by atropine and appeared to be due to its parasympathetic actions (BARLOW, 1964). Clonidine also has a central site of action, and inhibition of gastric secretion rather than stimulation has been reported in conscious animals (BRODIE et al., 1969; WALZ and VAN ZWIETEN, 1970). Clinically, tolazoline increases the acidity of gastric juice and may activate gastric ulcers (DANIELL and BEAUMONT, 1964).

Other α-adrenoceptor antagonists tested, piperoxan, dibenamine, yohimbine, ergotamine and hydralazine, were found to be antisecretory (BASS and PATTERSON, 1967). Phenoxybenzamine caused marked inhibition of secretion induced by food, bethanechol or histamine in the dog (PRADHAN and WINGATE, 1966). Phenoxybenzamine is also antisecretory in the rat (JOW et al., 1960; BASS and PATTERSON, 1967), which may be due to its ability to increase blood CA levels (JOW et al., 1960).

The paradoxical finding that both adrenoceptor antagonists and adrenoceptor agonists have antisecretory actions, may be explained by the ability of the antagonists to prolong the biological half-life of CA (BASS and PATTERSON, 1967). The administration of α-adrenoceptor antagonists, regardless of their mechanism of action, has been shown to prolong the half-life of CA in blood and urine (BENFEY et al., 1959 a, b; MILLAR et al., 1959).

2. Beta-Adrenoceptor Antagonists

The β-adrenoceptor antagonist dichloroisoprenaline (DCI) has been reported to be antisecretory in dogs where gastric secretion has been stimulated by food, bethanechol or histamine (PRADHAN and WINGATE, 1966). Both DCI and pronethalol have been reported to be antisecretory in pylorus-ligated rats (BASS and PATTERSON, 1967). The antisecretory effects of these two compounds have been attributed to their sympathomimetic actions (BASS and PATTERSON, 1967).

Propranolol has been reported to have no effect on gastric secretion in rats (MISHER et al., 1969). Other workers have shown contradictory results. DANHOF and GEUMEI (1972) reported that in pylorus-ligated or cardiac-ligated rats, propranolol significantly decreased basal gastric secretion and inhibited formation of gastric secretion. Similar results in rats were reported by OKABE et al. (1970). An increase in gastric ulceration after propranolol has been demonstrated, and it has also been shown that propranolol decreases basal- and histamine-induced secretion in man (see GEUMEI et al., 1972 b) as well as histamine-induced secretion in pigeons (GEUMEI et al., 1972 a).

CURWAIN et al. (1974) have suggested that the large doses of propranolol used in the experiments above may have other actions, e.g. a local anaesthetic action (BOWMAN et al., 1971), and therefore they have looked at the effect of much smaller doses of drugs. Small doses of propranolol (0.3–0.5 mg/kg) were found to increase gastric secretion in conscious dogs (CURWIN et al., 1974; EVANS and LIN, 1970; LIN et al., 1973), spontaneous secretion in pylorus-ligated rats (ROSSOF and GOLDMAN, 1968) and pentagastrin-induced secretion in man (KONTUREK and OLEKSY, 1969). CURWAIN et al. (1974) have suggested that this effect may be due to the ability of propranolol to increase histamine formation, since practolol, also a β-adrenoceptor antagonist but one which has no effect on histamine formation, had no effect on gastric secretion.

V. Summary

A combination of α- and β-adrenoceptor antagonists is necessary to antagonize the post-synaptic inhibitory effects of A and NA on the tone and motility of most non-sphincteric smooth muscle preparations. The inhibition of ACh release from enteric neurones in the gut wall by A and NA is presynaptic, and blocked by α-adrenoceptor antagonists alone. Although it is generally accepted that both inhibitory α- and β-adrenoceptors are present on intestinal smooth muscle cells, it has been suggested that in some areas of the gut, e.g. longitudinal muscle of the guinea pig ileum and the rabbit colon, only inhibitory β-adrenoceptors are present. It was found that in these preparations, inhibition of the responses to cholinergic nerve stimulation by NA was most effectively antagonized by α-adrenoceptor blocking agents while the inhibition of the motor effects of exogenous ACh by NA were more effectively antagonized by β-adrenoceptor blocking agents.

After the blockade of excitatory α-adrenoceptors in sphincteric smooth muscle, the responses to A and NA were reversed to relaxation. This effect was antagonized by β-adrenoceptor blocking agents.

In general, the effects of α- and β-adrenoceptor antagonists on gastric acid secretion are small. Their effects are difficult to predict, as many of these agents have their own effects on gastric secretion unrelated to blockade of adrenoceptors. α-Adrenoceptor agents such as phentolamine, tolazoline and naphazoline stimulate gastric secretion in conscious dogs and rats. The stimulatory effect of these imidazoline compounds has been attributed to their similarity in structure to the histamine molecule, which directly stimulates the secretory cells. Clonidine, a related compound, has both central and peripheral actions on secretion. Many other α-adrenoceptor antagonists tested were found to be antisecretory, e.g. dibenamine, phenoxybenzamine, ergotamine, hydralazine, and this may be due to the ability of α-adrenoceptor antagonists to increase the biological half-life of CA in blood. The β-adrenoceptor antagonist dichloroisoprenaline was found to be antisecretory in both conscious dogs and rats. However, propranolol, another β-adrenoceptor antagonist has been reported to have variable actions on gastric secretion.

E. Adrenergic Neurone Blocking Agents and False Transmitters

I. Introduction

Adrenergic neurone blocking agents abolish the responses of effector cells to postganglionic adrenergic nerve stimulation by inhibiting the release of NA (HERTLING et al., 1962; BOURA and GREEN, 1965; CASS and SPRIGGS, 1961; COLLINS and WEST, 1968; KIRPEKAR et al., 1969). Responses to exogenous NA are unaffected. Guanethidine, debrisoquine, bethanidine and bretylium are the most widely used drugs of this group; their mechanism of action is unclear. It has been suggested that since the uptake of guanethidine into the nerves is a prerequisite for its action (THOENEN et al., 1966), it may block nerve conduction at the level of preterminal axons by an anaesthetic action (CAMPBELL, 1970). In high-doses, these drugs deplete NA from nerve endings by an action which seems unrelated to their blocking action (CASS and SPRIGGS, 1961; CHANG et al., 1965; KUNTZMAN et al., 1962; LUNDBORG and STITZEL, 1968). Chronic treatment of rats with guanethidine leads to long-lasting damage or, with high concentrations, destruction of adrenergic nerves (BURNSTOCK et al., 1971); this approach has given some new insights into the mechanism of action of adrenergic neurone blocking drugs (see BURNSTOCK, 1979).

Agents such as reserpine, prenylamine and tetrabenazine, deplete NA from nerve endings (see SHORE, 1966), probably by blockade of the ATP Mg^{++}-dependent neuronal uptake pump and subsequent binding of NA to granular vesicles (VON EULER and LISHAJKO, 1963; IVERSEN, 1967). The depletion is slow and the 'free' NA is deaminated in the cytoplasm by monoamine oxidase (SHORE, 1962; KOPIN, 1964; SMITH, 1966). Reserpine may sometimes produce short lasting sympathomimetic effects by releasing NA from the nerves (DOMINO and RECH, 1957; KRAYER and

FUENTES, 1958; BRIMIJOIN and TRENDELBURG, 1971). Depletion of NA by reserpine results in the loss of response from transmitter releasing agents such as tyramine. At the same time, neuronal uptake is impaired, leading to a greater availability of amines to act on the receptors, thus responses to exogenous A and NA are potentiated (KOSTERLITZ and LEES, 1961; MAXWELL et al., 1960).

A large number of chemicals are capable of substituting for NA precursors in its synthetic pathway, and the resultant "false transmitter" is stored and released in place of NA (see KOPIN, 1968; MUSCHOLL, 1972). Precursors of adrenergic false transmitters, including α-methyl-tyrosine, α-methyl-m-tyrosine and tyramine, are taken up by adrenergic nerves and converted to α-methyl-noradrenaline, metaraminol and octopamine respectively, which displace NA in the storage vesicles. Some of these drugs also have an inhibitory effect on the enzyme tyrosine hydroxylase, which is necessary for NA synthesis (KOPIN, 1968; MUSCHOLL, 1972; BURNSTOCK and COSTA, 1975). α-Methyl-noradrenaline is the false transmitter formed from methyl dopa. In some tissues, α-methyl-noradrenaline has the same potency as NA, while it is less potent in others, resulting in an impairment of adrenergic function (see MUSCHOLL, 1972; BURNSTOCK and COSTA, 1975). It is also very effective as an agonist on prejunctional α-receptors, probably acting like clonidine.

II. Effect on Motility

Adrenergic neurone blocking agents such as guanethidine (ATKINSON et al., 1972; BENTLEY, 1962; BOYD et al., 1962; DAY, 1962; DAY and RAND, 1961, 1963; DAY and WARREN, 1968; GERKENS and MCCULLOCH, 1969; RAND and WILSON, 1967), bretylium (BENTLEY, 1962; BOYD et al., 1962; GILLESPIE and MACKENNA, 1961; DAY, 1962; BOURA and GREEN, 1959; BÜLBRING and CREMA, 1958), xylocholine (BAIN, 1960; DAY, 1962; DAY and WARREN, 1968), dimethyphenylpiperazinium (BENTLEY, 1962) and phenyltrimethylammonium (BURN and FROEDE, 1963), block the inhibitory effect of periarterial sympathetic nerve stimulation on the intestine. As mentioned in Sect. C.II, blockade by adrenergic neurone blocking agents is reversed by adrenergic transmitter releasing agents such as tyramine, amphetamine and dexamphetamine (ATKINSON et al., 1972; GERKENS and MCCULLOCH, 1969; DAY and RAND, 1963; RAND and WILSON, 1967). Also, if these adrenergic transmitter releasing agents are given prior to adrenergic neurone blocking drugs, the latter are ineffective in blocking adrenergic nerves (DAY, 1962). These observations led to the suggestion that adrenergic neurone blockers act at the site of stored CA to prevent their release, and that adrenergic transmitter releasing agents reverse their action by displacing the blockers from these sites (DAY and RAND, 1963; RAND and WILSON, 1967). It has also been suggested that adrenergic transmitter releasing agents such as dexamphetamine may block the action of adrenergic neurone blocking agents by another mechanism, i.e. inhibiting their uptake into adrenergic neurones (GERKENS and MCCULLOCH, 1969).

Adrenergic neurone blocking agents not only block the inhibitory effect of periarterial nerve stimulation on the intestine, but can also reverse the relaxation to contraction (AKUBUE, 1966; BENTLEY, 1962; BOYD et al., 1962; DAY and RAND, 1961; GILLESPIE and MCKENNA, 1961). A similar effect is obtained after transmitter depletion with reserpine (GILLESPIE and MACKENNA, 1961; BOYD et al., 1962). It has been suggested that in the small intestine, this may be due to the presence of parasympathetic fibres in the periarterial nerve trunk, since the contraction can be blocked by hyoscine and hexamethonium (AKUBUE, 1966; BENTLEY, 1962; GILLESPIE and MACKENNA, 1961); further the reversal to contraction is more easily elicited with low-frequency nerve stimulation, which is characteristic of cholinergic rather than adrenergic nerves (BOYD et al., 1962). DAY and RAND (1961) however, found that the contractions of the rabbit ileum were not always blocked by hexamethonium. They suggested that this might be explicable in terms of a cholinergic link in sympathetic nerve transmission (BURN and RAND, 1959).

In the colon from rabbits pretreated with reserpine, it was found that the contractile responses to periarterial and pelvic nerve stimulation were similar. Both responses were blocked by atropine and hexamethonium (GILLESPIE and MCKENNA, 1961). However, after fatigue or degenerative section of the pelvic nerves, stimulation of perarterial nerves gave no response and it was suggested that the motor responses in the large intestine after reserpine treatment were not due to the presence of parasympathetic fibres in the periarterial nerves, but rather that sympathetic nerve stimulation may activate parasympathetic fibres. BOYD et al. (1962) showed that in the rabbit colon, periarterial nerve stimulation gave a smaller contraction in the presence of adrenergic neurone blocking agents than following treatment with the adrenergic transmitter depleting agent, reserpine. It was suggested that reserpine may have other actions unrelated to adrenergic transmitter depletion.

False transmitters have the same potency as NA in some tissues, but are less potent in others (KOPIN, 1968; BURNSTOCK and COSTA, 1975; MUSCHOLL, 1972). In the rabbit ileum, DAY and RAND (1964) showed that α-methydopa, α-methyl dopamine and α-methyl-noradrenaline had similar potencies to dopa, dopamine and NA in restoring inhibitory responses after reserpine.

III. Effect on Gastric Secretion

Adrenergic neurone blocking agents have little effect on gastric secretion in the rat (BASS and PATTERSON, 1967) and the cat (EMÅS, 1963, 1964). EMÅS (1964) concluded that adrenergic nerves innervating the stomach normally exert no effect on basal acid secretion or on the excitability of the parietal cells. Other adrenergic neurone blocking agents sucht as bretylium, trimethyl-[2-(2,6-xylyloxy)ethyl] ammonium bromide (TM-10) and trimethyl-[2-(2,6-xylyloxy)propyl] ammonium bromide (β-TM-10), also have no marked effect on gastric secretion (BASS and PATTERSON, 1967).

Neural transmitter depleting agents also have little effect on gastric acid secretion. In the unanaesthetized cat, with a gastric fistula, reserpine was found to increase basal acid secretion and to increase the secretory response to histamine and gastrin (EMÅS, 1963, 1964). These effects, however, seemed to be due to an action of reserpine unrelated to its transmitter depleting action since they were not abolished by sympathectomy (EMÅS, 1963, 1964).

IV. Summary

Adrenergic neurone blocking agents such as bretylium and guanethidine block the release of NA from adrenergic nerves and thus block the inhibitory action of sympathetic nerve stimulation on the gastro-intestinal tract. Their actions can be reversed or prevented by exposure to adrenergic transmitter releasing agents. Apart from blocking the inhibitory response of the gut to sympathetic nerve stimulation, adrenergic neurone blocking agents may reverse the response to contraction. This phenomenon is also observed in reserpinized tissues. The exact mechanism of action is unclear.

The effects of adrenergic transmitter depleting agents such as reserpine can be reversed by the administration of NA or its precursors. In some tissues, it can also be reversed by false transmitters such as α-methyldopa, α-methyldopamine or α-methylnoradrenaline.

Adrenergic neurone blocking agents do not have any significant effect on gastric acid secretion. Reserpine has been reported to increase gastric secretion, but by an action separate from its effects on adrenergic neurones since it was still observed in tissues that were sympathectomized.

References

Ablad, B., Borg, K.-O., Carlsson, E., Ek, L., Johnsson, G., Malmfors, T., Regardh, C.G.: A survey of the pharmacological properties of metoprolol in animals and man. Acta Pharmacol. Toxicol. [Suppl. V] (Kbh) *36*, 7–23 (1975)

Ahlquist, R.P.: A study of the adrenotropic receptors. Am. J. Physiol. *153*, 586–600 (1948)

Ahlquist, R.P., Levy, B.: Adrenergic receptor mechanism of canine ileum. J. Pharmacol. Exp. Ther. *127*, 146–149 (1959)

Akubue, P.I.: A periarterial nerve-circular muscle preparation from the caecum of the guinea-pig. J. Pharm. Pharmacol. *18*, 390–395 (1966)

Alexander, F.: The action of some humoral agents on the horse intestine. Q. J. Exp. Physiol. *35*, 11–24 (1949)

Anderson, W.F., Morris, N.: The effects of atropine, prostigmin, adrenaline and calcium on the movements of the fasting human stomach. J. Pharmacol. Exp. Ther. *77*, 258–265 (1943)

Armitage, A.K., Dean, A.C.B.: The effects of pressure and pharmacologically active substances on gastric peristalsis in a transmurally stimulated rat stomach-duodenum preparation. J. Physiol. (Lond.) *182*, 42–56 (1966)

Åström, A.: Anti-sympathetic action of sympathomimetic amines. Acta Physiol. Scand. *18*, 295–307 (1949)

Atkinson, R., Watkinson, B., Weetman, D.F.: The interaction between desmethylimipramine and guanethidine on the rabbit ileum. The importance of the noradrenaline uptake process in the reversal of guanethidine-induced adrenergic neurone blockade. Arch. Int. Pharmacodyn. Ther. *198*, 385–391 (1972)

Axelsson, J.: Catecholamine functions. Am. Rev. Physiol. *33*, 1–30 (1971)

Babkin, B.P.: Secretory mechanism of the digestive glands, 2nd ed. New York: Haeber 1950

Bailey, D.M.: The action of sympathomimetic amines on circular and longitudinal smooth muscle from the isolated oesophagus of the guinea pig. J. Pharm. Pharmacol. *17*, 782–787 (1965)

Bain, W.A.: Interference with the release of transmitter in response to nerve stimulation. In: Adrenergic mechanisms. Ciba Foundation Symposium: Vane, J.R., Wolsterholme, G.E.W., O'Connor, C.M. (eds.), pp. 131–147. London: Churchill 1960

Barger, G., Dale, H.H.: Chemical structure and sympathomimetic action of amines. J. Physiol. (Lond.) *41*, 19–59 (1910)

Barlow, R.B.: Introduction to chemical pharmacology, 2nd ed. London: Methuen 1964

Bass, P., Patterson, M.A.: Gastric secretory responses to drugs affecting adrenergic mechanisms in rats. J. Pharmacol. Exp. Ther. *156*, 142–149 (1967)

Bass, D.D., Ustach, T.J., Hambrecht, T., Schuster, M.M.: In vitro pharmacologic differentiation of sphincteric and non-sphincteric muscle. Clin. Res. *16*, 527 (1968)

Bass, D.D., Ustach, T.J., Schuster, M.M.: In vitro pharmacologic differentiation of sphincters and non-sphincter muscle. Johns Hopkins Med. J. *127*, 185–191 (1970)

Baumgarten, H.G., Holstein, A.-F., Owman, Ch.: Auerbach's plexus of mammals and man: Electron microscopic identification of 3 different types of neuronal processes in myenteric ganglia of the large intestine from rhesus monkeys, guinea-pigs and man. Z. Zellforsch. *106*, 376–397 (1970)
Baxter, S.G.: Sympathetic secretory innervation of the gastric mucosa. Am. J. Dig. Dis. *1*, 36–39 (1934)
Beani, L., Bianchi, C., Crema, A.: The effect of catecholamines and sympathetic stimulation on the release of acetylcholine from the guinea-pig colon. Br. J. Pharmacol. *36*, 1–17 (1969)
Belleau, B.: Steric effects in catecholamine interactions with enzymes and receptors. Pharmacol. Rev. *18*, 131–140 (1966)
Benfey, B.G., Ledoux, G., Melville, K.I.: Increased urinary excretion of adrenaline and noradrenaline after phenoxybenzamine. Br. J. Pharmacol. Chemother. *14*, 142–148 (1959a)
Benfey, B.G., Ledoux, G., Segal, M.: The action of antisympathomimetic drugs on the urinary excretion of adrenaline and noradrenaline. Br. J. Pharmacol. Chemother. *14*, 380–384 (1959b)
Bennett, A., Whitney, B.: A pharmacological investigation of human isolated stomach. Br. J. Pharmacol. *27*, 286–298 (1966)
Bentley, G.A.: Studies on sympathetic mechanisms in isolated intestinal and vas deferens preparations. Br. J. Pharmacol. *19*, 85–98 (1962)
Benzi, G., Berte, F., Crema, A., Frigo, G.M.: Actions of sympathomimetic drugs on the smooth muscle at the junction of the bile duct and duodenum studied *in sutu*. Br. J. Pharmacol. *23*, 101–114 (1964)
Bernstein, R.E.: The potassium, sodium and calcium content of gastric juice. J. Lab. Clin. Med. *40*, 707 (1952)
Biber, B.: Vasodilator mechanisms in the small intestine. An. experimental study in cat. Acta Physiol. Scand. [Suppl.] *401*, 5–31 (1973)
Black, J.W., Duncan, W.A.M., Durant, C.J., Granellin, C.R., Parsons, M.E.: Definition and antagonism of histamine H_2 receptors. Nature *236*, 385–390 (1972)
Bolton, T.B.: The depolarizing action of acetylcholine on carbachol in intestine smooth muscle. J. Physiol. (Lond.) *220*, 647–671 (1972)
Boura, A.L.A., Green, A.F.: The actions of bretylium: adrenergic neurone blocking and other effects. Br. J. Pharmacol. *14*, 536–548 (1959)
Boura, A.L.A., Green, A.F.: Adrenergic neurone blocking agents. Annu. Rev. Pharmacol. *5*, 183–212 (1965)
Bowman, W.C., Rand, M.J., West, G.B.: Textbook of Pharmacology, 4th ed. Oxford, Edinburgh: Blackwell Scientific Publications 1971
Boyd, G., Gillespie, J.S., Mackenna, B.R.: Origin of the cholinergic response of the rabbit intestine to stimulation of its extrinsic sympathetic nerves after exposure to sympathetic blocking agents. Br. J. Pharmacol. *19*, 258–270 (1962)
Bradley, S.E.: The hepatic circulation. In: Handbook of Physiology, Sect. 2, Vol. 2. Washington: American Physiology Society 1963
Brasitus, T.A., Field, M., Kimberg, D.V.: Intestinal mucosal cyclic GMP: Regulation and relation to ion transport. Am. J. Physiol. *231*, 275–282 (1976)
Brimijoin, S., Trendelburg, U.: Reserpine-induced release of norepinephrine from isolated spontaneously beating guinea-pig atria. J. Pharmacol. Exp. Ther. *176*, 149–159 (1971)
Brodie, B.B., Bogdanski, D.F., Bonomi, L.: Formature, storage and metabolism of serotonin (5-hydroxytryptamine) and catecholamines in lower vertebrates. In: Comparative neurochemistry. Richter, D. (ed.). Oxford: Pergamon Press 1964
Brodie, D.A., Lotti, V.J., Bauer, B.G.: Pharmacological separation of central nervous system sites controlling gastric secretion and stress induced gastric hemorrhage in the rat. Pharmacologist *11*, 264 (1969)
Brody, T.M., Diamond, J.: Blockade of the biochemical correlates of contraction and relaxation in uterine and intestinal smooth muscle. Ann. N.Y. Acad. Sci. *139*, 772–780 (1967)
Brown, G.L., McSwiney, B.A.: The movements and reaction to drugs of strips of the gastric musculature of the cat and dog. Q. J. Exp. Physiol. *16*, 9–39 (1926)
Brown, G.L., McSwiney, B.A., Wadge, W.J.: The sympathetic innervation of the stomach. 1. The effect on the stomach of stimulation of the thoracic sympathetic trunk. J. Physiol. (Lond.) *70*, 253–260 (1930)

Brunard, M., Labrouche, C.: L'adrénaline, agent contracturant des fibres longitudinals du duodenum du cheval. Compl. Rend. Soc. Biol. *141*, 167–169 (1947)

Bucknell, A., Whitney, B.: A preliminary investigation of the pharmacology of the human isolated taenia coli preparation. Br. J. Pharmacol. Chemother. *23*, 164–175 (1964)

Buirge, R.E.: Experimental observations on the human ileocaecal valve. Surgery *16*, 356–369 (1944)

Bülbring, E.: Membrane potentials of smooth muscle fibres of the taenia coli of the guinea-pig. J. Physiol. (Lond.) *125*, 302–315 (1954)

Bülbring, E., Burn, J.H.: Sympathetic vasodilation in skin and intestine of the dog. J. Physiol. (Lond.) *87*, 254–274 (1936)

Bülbring, E., Crema, A.: Observations concerning the action of 5-hydroxytryptamine on the peristaltic reflex. Br. J. Pharmacol. *13*, 444–457 (1958)

Bülbring, E., Hertog, A.D.: The beta action of catecholamines on the smooth muscle of guinea-pig taenia coli. J. Physiol. (Lond.) *268*, 29 P–30 P (1977)

Bülbring, E., Kuriyama, H.: Effects of changes in external sodium and calcium concentrations on spontaneous electrical activity in smooth muscle of guinea-pig taenia coli. J. Physiol. (Lond.) *166*, 29–58 (1963)

Bülbring, E., Tomita, T.: Increase of membrane conductance by adrenaline in the smooth muscle of guinea-pig taenia coli. Proc. R. Soc. Lond. [Ser. B] *172*, 89–102 (1969 a)

Bülbring, E., Tomita, T.: Suppression of spontaneous spike generation by catecholamines in the smooth muscle of the guinea-pig taenia coli. Proc. R. Soc. Lond. [Ser. B] *172*, 103–119 (1969 b)

Bülbring, E., Tomita, T.: Effect of calcium, barium and manganese on the action of adrenaline in the smooth muscle of the guinea-pig taenia coli. Proc. R. Soc. Lond. [Ser. B] *172*, 121–136 (1969 c)

Bülbring, E., Tomita, T.: The alpha-action of catecholamines on the guinea-pig taenia coli in K-free and Na-free solution and in the presence of ouabain. Proc. R. Soc. Lond. (Biol.) *197*, 255–269 (1977 a)

Bülbring, E., Tomita, T.: Calcium requirement for the alpha-action of catecholamines on guinea-pig taenia coli. Proc. R. Soc. Lond. [Biol.] *197*, 271–284 (1977 b)

Burn, J.H., Froede, H.: The action of substances which block sympathetic postganglionic nervous transmission. Br. J. Pharmacol. *20*, 378–387 (1963)

Burn, J.H., Rand, M.J.: Sympathetic postganglionic mechanisms. Nature *184*, 163–165 (1959)

Burnstock, G.: The action of adrenaline on excitability and membrane potential in the taenia coli of the guinea-pig and the effect of DNP on this action and on the action of acetylcholine. J. Physiol. (Lond.) *143*, 183–194 (1958)

Burnstock, G.: Membrane potential changes associated with stimulation of smooth muscle by adrenaline. Nature *186*, 727–728 (1960)

Burnstock, G.: Morphological changes produced by dugs acting on the autonomic nervous system. Pharmac. Ther. *5*, 49–53 (1979)

Burnstock, G.: Cholinergic and purinergic regulation of blood vessels. In: Vascular smooth muscle. Handbook of Physiology, Bohr, D., Somlyo, A.D., Sparks, H.W. (eds.). Baltimore: Williams & Wilkins in press (1980)

Burnstock, G., Costa, M.: Adrenergic neurons: Their organisation, function and development in the peripheral nervous system. London: Chapman & Hall 1975

Burnstock, G., Holman, M.E., Prosser, C.L.: Electrophysiology of smooth muscle. Physiol. Rev. *43*, 482–527 (1963)

Burnstock, G., Evans, B., Gannon, B.J., Heath, J.W., James, V.: A new method of destroying adrenergic nerves in adult animals using guanethidine. Br. J. Pharmacol. *43*, 295–301 (1971)

Callingham, B.A.: The catecholamines. Adrenaline, noradrenaline. In: Hormones in blood. Gray, Bacharach (eds.), Vol. 2, pp. 519–599. London: Academic Press 1967

Campbell, G.: Autonomic nervous supply to effector tissues. In: Smooth muscle. Bülbring, E., Brading, A., Jones, A., Tomita, T. (eds.), pp. 451–495. London: Arnold 1970

Campbell, J.A.: The effects of certain animal extracts upon the blood vessels. Q. J. Exp. Physiol. *4*, 1–17 (1911)

Carlsson, A., Fuxe, K., Hamberger, B., Lindqvist, M.: Biochemical and histochemical studies on the effects of imipramine-like drugs and (+) amphetamine on central and peripheral catecholamine neurons. Acta Physiol. Scand. *67*, 481–497 (1966)

Cass, R., Spriggs, T.L.B.: Tissue amine levels and sympathetic blockade after guanethidine and bretylium. Br. J. Pharmacol. *17*, 442–450 (1961)
Cass, R., Kuntzman, R., Brodie, B.B.: Norepinephrine depletion as a possible mechanism of action of guanethidine (SU 5864), a new hypotensive agent. Proc. Soc. Exp. Biol. Med. *103*, 871–872 (1960)
Celander, O.: Are there any centrally controlled sympathetic inhibitory fibres to the musculature of the intestine? Acta Physiol. Scand. *47*, 299–309 (1959)
Chang, C.C., Costa, E., Brodie, B.B.: Interaction of guanethidine with adrenergic neurons. J. Pharmacol. Exp. Ther. *147*, 303–312 (1965)
Christensen, J.: Pharmacologic identification of the lower esophageal sphincter. J. Clin. Invest. *49*, 681–691 (1970)
Christensen, J., Daniel, E.E.: Electric and motor effects of autonomic drugs on longitudinal oesophageal smooth muscle. Am. J. Physiol. *211*, 387–394 (1966)
Chubb, I.W., De Potter, W.P., De Schaepdryver, A.F.: Tyrmine does not release noradrenaline from splenic nerves by exocytosis. Arch. Exp. Pathol. Pharmakol. *274*, 281–286 (1972)
Clark, G.A.: The selective vaso-constrictor action of adrenaline. J. Physiol. (Lond.) *69*, 171–184 (1930)
Clark, G.A.: The vaso-dilator action of adrenaline. J. Physiol. (Lond.) *80*, 429–440 (1934)
Cobbold, A., Folkow, B., Lundgren, O., Wallentin, I.: Blood flow, capillary filtration coefficients and regional blood volume responses in the intestine of the cat during stimulation of the hypothalamic defence area. Acta. Physiol. Scand. *61*, 467–475 (1964)
Code, C.F.: In: Histamine and gastric secretion. Ciba Foundation. Wolstenholme, G.E.W., O'Connor, C.M. (eds.), pp. 189–219. London: Churchill 1956
Collins, G.G.S., West, G.B.: The release of ^{3}H-dopamine from the isolated rabbit ileum. Br. J. Pharmacol. *34*, 514–522 (1968)
Connet, H.: Effect of adrenaline on venous blood pressure. Am. J. Physiol. *54*, 96–121 (1920)
Cowley, D.J., Code, C.F.: Effects of secretory inhibitors on mucosal blood flow in nonsecreting stomach of conscious dogs. Am. J. Physiol. *218*, 270–274 (1970)
Cumming, J.D., Haigh, A.L., Harries, E.H.L., Nutt, M.E.: Gastric secretion and blood flow in the anaesthesized dog. J. Physiol. (Lond.) *168*, 219–233 (1963)
Curwain, B.P., Holton, P.: The effects of isoprenaline and noradrenaline on pentagastrin-stimulated gastric acid secretion and mucosal blood flow in the dog. Br. J. Pharmacol. *46*, 225–233 (1972)
Curwain, B.P., Holton, P., McIsaac, R.L., Spencer, J.: Can the actions of adrenoceptor agonists and antagonists on pentagastrin-induced gastric secretion be due to their effects on histamine formation. Br. J. Pharmacol. *51*, 217–223 (1974)
Dale, H.H.: On some physiological actions of ergot. J. Physiol. (Lond.) *34*, 163–206 (1906)
Dale, H.H.: On the action of ergotoxine: With special reference to the existence of sympathetic vasodilators. J. Physiol. (Lond.) *46*, 291–300 (1913)
Dale, H.H.: Natural chemical stimulators. Edin. Med. J. *45*, 461–480 (1938)
Daly, M.J., Long, J.M., Stables, R.: The role of β_1 and β_2-adrenoceptors in the inhibition of gastric acid secretion in the dog. Br. J. Pharmacol. *64*, 153–157 (1978)
Danhof, I.E., Geumei, A.: Effect of propranolol on gastric acid secretion in rats. Br. J. Pharmacol. *46*, 170–171 (1972)
Daniell, H.W., Beaumont, W.: Vasospastic reaction to methysergide malate simulating Leriche syndrome. Ineffective treatment with adrenergic blockade. Ann. Intern. Med. *60*, 881 (1964)
Danielopulu, D., Carniol, A.: Action de l'adrenaline sur l'estomac de l'homme. Voie intra veineuse et voie gastrique. Compt. Rend. Soc. Biol. *97*, 716–718 (1922)
Day, M.D.: Effect of sympathomimetic amines on the blocking action of guanethidine, bretylium and xylocholine. Br. J. Pharmacol. *18*, 421–439 (1962)
Day, M.D., Rand, M.J.: Effect of guanethidine in revealing cholinergic sympathetic fibres. Br. J. Pharmacol. *17*, 245–260 (1961)
Day, M.D., Rand, M.J.: Evidence for a competitive antagonism of guanethidine by dexamphetamine. Br. J. Pharmacol. *20*, 17–28 (1963)
Day, M.D., Rand, M.J.: Some observations on the pharmacology of α-methyl dopa. Br. J. Pharmacol. *22*, 72–86 (1964)

Day, M.D., Warren, P.R.: A pharmacological analysis of the responses to transmural stimulation in isolated intestinal preparations. Br. J. Pharmacol. Chemother. *32*, 227–240 (1968)
Deal, C.P., Green, H.D.: Comparison of change in mesenteric resistance following sphlanchnic nerve stimulation with responses to adrenaline and noradrenaline. Circ. Res. *4*, 38–44 (1956)
Debnath, P.K., Gode, K.D., Govinda Das, D., Sanyal, A.K.: Effects of propranolol on gastric secretion in albino rats. Br. J. Pharmacol. *51*, 213–216 (1974)
Delany, J.P., Grim, E.: Experimentally induced variations in canine gastric blood flow and its distribution. Am. J. Physiol. *208*, 353–358 (1965)
Deltacca, M., Soldani, G., Selli, M., Crema, A.: Action of catecholamines on release of acetylcholine from human taenia coli. Eur. J. Pharmacol. *9*, 80–84 (1970)
Demand, H.A., Weichmain, K., Berg, G.: Some effects of epinephrine on histamine-induced human gastric secretion. Gastroenterology *55*, 272–276 (1968)
Domino, E.F., Rech, R.H.: Observations on the initial hypertensive response to reserpine. J. Pharmacol. Exp. Ther. *121*, 171–182 (1957)
Dresel, P., Wallentin, I.: Effects of sympathetic vasoconstrictor fibres, noradrenaline and vasopressin on the intestinal vascular resistance during constant blood flow or blood pressure. Acta Physiol. Scand. *66*, 427–436 (1966)
Dresel, P., Folkow, B., Wallentin, I.: Rubidium^{86} clearance during neurogenic redistribution of intestinal blood flow. Acta Physiol. Scand. *67*, 173–184 (1966)
Edmunds, C.W.: Some vasomotor reactions of the liver, with special reference to the presence of vasomotor nerves to the portal vein. J. Pharm. Exp. Ther. *6*, 569–590 (1915)
Elliott, T.R.: On the action of adrenalin. J. Physiol. (Lond.) *31*, 20–21 (1904)
Emås, S.: Gastric acid secretion in gastric fistula cats during reserpine treatment. Acta Physiol. Scand. *59*, 169–183 (1963)
Emås, S.: Gastric acid secretion in sympathectomized gastric fistula cats before and during reserpine treatment and in gastric fistula cats during guanethidine treatment. Acta Physiol. Scand. *60*, 57–69 (1964)
Evans, D.C., Lin, T.M.: Effect of propranolol on steady state pentagastrin induced HCl secretion and gastric mucosal blood flow in dogs. Physiologist *13*, 190 (1970)
Feldburg, W., Lewis, G.P.: The action of peptides on the adrenal medulla. Release of adrenaline by bradykinin and angiotensin. J. Physiol. (Lond.) *171*, 98–108 (1964)
Field, M., McColl, I.: Ion transport in rabbit ileal mucosa. III. Effects of catecholamines. Am. J. Physiol. *225*, 852–857 (1973)
Field, M., Sheerin, H.E., Henderson, A., Smith, P.L.: Catecholamine effects on cyclic AMP levels and ion secretion in rabbit ileal mucosa. Am. J. Physiol. *229*, 86–92 (1975)
Finkleman, B.: On the nature of inhibition in the intestine. J. Physiol. (Lond.) *70*, 145–157 (1930)
Fjalland, B.: Biogenic amines and gastric secretion in rats. Acta. Pharmacol. Toxicol. [Suppl. 1] (Kbh) *31*, 48–49 (1972)
Folkow, B., Frost, J., Haeger, K., Uvnäs, B.: The sympathetic vasomotor innervation of the skin of dog. Acta Physiol. Scand. *17*, 195–200 (1948)
Folkow, B., Lewis, D.H., Lundgren, D., Mellander, S., Wallentin, I.: The effect of the sympathetic vasoconstrictor fibres on the distribution of capillary blood flow in the intestine. Acta. Physiol. Scand. *61*, 458–466 (1964)
Forrest, A.P.M., Code, C.F.: The inhibitory effect of epinephrine and norepinephrine on secretion induced by histamine in separated pouches of dogs. J. Pharmacol. Exp. Ther. *110*, 447–450 (1954)
Franklin, K.J.: The pharmacology of the isolated vein ring. J. Pharmacol. Exp. Ther. *26*, 215–225 (1925)
Furchgott, R.F.: The pharmacological differentiation of adrenergic receptors. Ann. N.Y. Acad. Sci. *139*, 553–570 (1967)
Furchgott, R.F.: A classification of adrenoceptors (adrenergic receptors). An evaluation from the stand-point of receptor theory. In: Catecholamines. Blaschko, H., Muscholl, J.E. (eds.), pp. 283–335. Berlin, Heidelberg, New York: Springer 1972
Furness, J.B., Burnstock, G.: Role of circulating catecholamines in the gastrointestinal tract. In: Handbook of Physiology, Sect. 7, Endocrinology VI, Adrenal gland, Chapt. 33. Blaschko, H., Smith, A.D. (eds.), pp. 515–536. Washington: American Physiological Society 1975

Furness, J.B., Costa, M.: The adrenergic innervation of the gastrointestinal tract. Ergeb. Physiol. *69*, 2–51 (1974)
Gallone, P., Consolo, F.: Studio comparativo degli effeti dell'adrenaline e della noradrenalina sulla secrezione gastrica. Boll. Soc. Ital. Biol. Sper. *37*, 74–76 (1961)
Gazet, J.C., Jarrett, R.J.: The ileocaeco-colic sphincter studies in vitro in man, monkey, cat, and dog. Br. J. Surg. *51*, 368–370 (1964)
Gerkens, J.F., McCulloch, M.W., Wilson, J.: Mechanism of the antagonism between guanethidine and dexamphetamine. Br. J. Pharmacol. *35*, 563–572 (1969)
Gershon, M.D.: Inhibition of gastrointestinal movements by sympathetic nerve stimulation: The site of action. J. Physiol. (Lond.) *189*, 317–327 (1967)
Geumei, A., Issa, I., Abd-el-Samie, Y.: Effects of β-adrenergic receptor stimulation and blockade on gastric acid secretion in pigeons. Pharmacology *7*, 29–35 (1972a)
Geumei, A., Issa, I., El-Gendi, M., Abd-el-Samie, Y.: Inhibitory effect of β-adrenergic blocking agent propranolol on histamine-stimulated gastric acid secretion in man. Am. J. Dig. Dis. *17*, 55–58 (1972b)
Gillespie, J.S., Khoyi, M.A.: The site and receptors responsible for the inhibition by sympathetic nerves of intestinal smooth muscle and its parasympathetic motor nerves. J. Physiol. (Lond.) *267*, 767–789 (1977)
Gillespie, J.S., MacKenna, B.R.: The inhibitory action of the sympathetic nerves on the smooth muscle of the rabbit gut, its reversal by reserpine and restoration by catecholamines and by dopa. J. Physiol. (Lond.) *156*, 17–34 (1961)
Goetz, R.H.: The control of the blood flow through the intestine as studied by the effect of adrenaline. Q. J. Exp. Physiol. *29*, 321–332 (1939)
Goodman, L.S., Gilman, A.: The pharmacological basis of therapeutics, 5th ed. London: MacMillan Press 1975
Govier, W.C., Sugrue, M.F., Shore, P.A.: On the inability to produce supersensitivity to catecholamines in intestinal smooth muscle. J. Pharmacol. Exp. Ther. *165*, 71–77 (1969)
Graham, J.D.P.: The effect of drugs on the motility of isolated strips of human stomach muscle. J. Pharm. Pharmacol. *1*, 95–102 (1949)
Grayson, J., Mendel, D.: Physiology of the splanchnic circulation. London: Arnold 1965
Grechishkin, L.L.: The effect of catecholamines on gastric secretion. Farmakol. Toksikol. *30*, 612–615 (1970)
Greeff, K., Holtz, P.: Untersuchungen am isolierten Vagusmagenpräparat. Arch. Exp. Pathol. Pharmakol. *227*, 427–435 (1955)
Greeff, K., Kasperat, H., Osswald, W.: Paradoxe Wirkung elektrischer Vagusreizung am isolierten Magen- und Herzvorhofpräparat. Arch. Exp. Pathol. Pharmakol. *243*, 528–545 (1962)
Green, H.D., Kepchar, J.H.: Control of peripheral resistance in major systemic vascular beds. Physiol. Rev. *39*, 617–686 (1959)
Green, H.D., Deal, C.P., Bardhanabaedya, S., Denison, A.B.: Effects of adrenergic substances and ischemia on blood flow and peripheral resistance of canine mesenteric vascular bed before and during adrenergic blockade. J. Pharmacol. Exp. Ther. *113*, 115–123 (1955)
Green, A.L., Fielden, R., Bartlett, D.C.: New norepinephrine-depleting agents. Beta-hydroxyphenethylguanidine and related compounds. J. Med. Chem. *10*, 1006–1008 (1967)
Grim, E.: The flow of blood in the mesenteric vessels. In: Handbook of Physiology, Vol. 2, Sect. 2. Washington: American Physiological Society 1963
Guimaraes, S.: Alpha-excitatory, alpha-inhibitory and beta inhibitory adrenergic receptors in the guinea-pig stomach. Arch. Int. Pharmacodyn. Ther. *179*, 188–201 (1969)
Gunn, J.A., Chevasse, F.B.: The action of adrenin on veins. Proc. Soc. Lond. [Ser. B] *86*, 192–197 (1913)
Guthrie, J.E., Quastel, J.H.: Absorption of sugars and amino acids from isolated surviving intestine after experimental shock. Arch. Biochem. Biophys. *62*, 485–496 (1956)
Haffner, J.F.W., Liavag, I., Setekliev, J.: Excitatory adrenergic receptors in the human stomach and pylorus. Scand. J. Gastroenterol. *4*, 145–150 (1969)
Haigh, A.L., Moffitt, J.A., Steedman, W.M.: The action of a synthetic gastroin-like peptide (ICI 50, 123) on gastric blood flow and acid secretion in the dog. J. Physiol. (Lond.) *191*, 45–46P (1967)

Harries, E.H.L.: The effect of noradrenaline on the gastric secretory response to histamine in the dog. J. Physiol. (Lond.) *133*, 498–505 (1956)
Harries, E.H.L.: The mode of action of sympathomimetic amines in inhibiting gastric secretion. J. Physiol. (Lond.) *138*, 48–50 P (1957)
Hartiola, K.J.V., Toivenen, T.: Studies on the effect of adrenaline and noradrenaline on the duodenal secretion in dog. Acta Physiol. Scand. *31*, 125–130 (1954)
Henricksen, J., Ivy, A.C.: Studies on the ileo-cecal sphincter of the dog. Am. J. Physiol. *96*, 494–507 (1931)
Henrich, H., Lutz, J.: Das vasculare Escape-Phänomen am Intestinalkreislauf und seine Auslösung durch unterschiedliche vasokonstruktorische Substanzen. Arch. Ges. Physiol. *329*, 82–94 (1971)
Hertling, G., Axelrod, J., Patrick, R.W.: Actions of bretylium and guanethidine on the uptake and release of (^{3}H)-noradrenaline. Br. J. Pharmacol. *18*, 161–166 (1962)
Hess, W.R., Gundlach, R.: Der Einfluß des Adrenalins auf die Sekretion des Magensaftes. Pfluegers Arch. *185*, 122–136 (1920)
Hollands, B.C.S., Vanov, S.: Localization of catecholamines in visceral organs and ganglia of the rat, guinea-pig and rabbit. Br. J. Pharmacol. *25*, 307–316 (1965)
Holman, M.E., Kasby, C.B., Suthers, M.B., Wilson, J.A.F.: Some properties of the smooth muscle of rabbit portal vein. J. Physiol. (Lond.) *196*, 111–132 (1968)
Holton, P.: Catecholamines and gastric secretion. In: The pharmacology of gastro intestinal motility and secretion. International Encyclopedia of Pharmacology and Therapeutics. Holton, P. (ed.), Sect. 39 a. Oxford: Pergamon Press 1973
Holton, P., Cumming, J.D., Putman, J.L., Charlton, K.: An analysis of the effect of adrenaline on histamine-induced gastric acid secretion in dogs. Proc. 4th Int. Congr. Pharmacol., 1969, pp. 105–106
Hubel, K.A.: Intestinal ion transport: Effect of norepinephrine, pilocarpine, and atropine. Am. J. Physiol. *231*, 252–257 (1976)
Hughes, J., Vane, J.R.: An analysis of the response of the isolated portal vein of the rabbit to electrical stimulation and to drugs. Br. J. Pharmacol. *30*, 46–66 (1967)
Hughes, J., Vane, J.R.: Relations of the isolated portal vein of the rabbit induced by nicotine and electrical stimulation. Br. J. Pharmacol. *39*, 476–489 (1970)
Hulten, L.: Extrinsic nervous control of colonic motility and blood flow. An experimental study in the cat. Acta Physiol. Scand. *335*, 1–116 (1969)
Hulten, L., Jodal, M., Lundgren, O.: Local and nervous control of the consecutive vascular sections of the colon. Acta Physiol. Scand. *335*, 51–64 (1969)
Iversen, L.L.: The uptake and storage of noradrenaline in sympathetic nerves. Cambridge: University Press 1967
Ivy, A.C., McIlwain, G.B.: The excitation of gastric secretion by application of substances to the duodenal and jejunal mucosa. Am. J. Physiol. *67*, 124–140 (1923)
Jacobj, C.: Beiträge zur physiologischen und pharmakologischen Kenntnis der Darmbewegungen mit besonderer Berücksichtigung der Beziehung der Nebenniere zur Denselben. Arch. Exp. Pathol. Pharmakol. *29*, 171–211 (1892)
Jacobowitz, D.: Histochemical studies of the autonomic innervation of the gut. J. Pharmacol. Exp. Ther. *149*, 358–364 (1965)
Jacobson, E.D.: Comparison of prostaglandin E_1 and norepinephrine on the gastric mucosal circulation. Proc. Soc. Exp. Biol. Med. *133*, 516–519 (1970)
Jacobson, E.D., Linford, R.H., Grossman, M.I.: Gastric secretion in relation to mucosal blood flow studied by a clearance technique. J. Clin. Invest. *45*, 1–13 (1966)
Jacobson, E.D., Swan, K.G., Grossman, M.I.: Blood flow and secretion in the stomach. Gastroenterology *52*, 414–420 (1967)
Jarrett, R.J., Gazet, J.C.: Studies in vivo of the ileocaeco-colic sphincter in the cat and dog. Gut *7*, 271–275 (1966)
Jenkinson, D.H.: Classification and properties of peripheral adrenergic receptors. Br. Med. Bull. *29*, 142–147 (1973)
Jenkinson, D.H., Morton, I.K.M.: Adrenergic blocking drugs as tools in the study of the actions of catecholamines on the smooth muscle membrane. Ann. N.Y. Acad. Sci. *139*, 762–771 (1967 a)

Jenkinson, D.H., Morton, I.K.M.: The role of α- and β-adrenergic receptors in some actions of catecholamines on intestinal smooth muscle. J. Physiol. (Lond.) *188*, 373–386 (1967b)
Johansson, B., Ljung, B.: Sympathetic control of rhythmically active vascular smooth muscle as studied by a nerve-muscle preparation of portal vein. Acta Physiol. Scand. *70*, 299–311 (1967)
Joske, R.A., Sharmag, M.H., Drummey, G.D.: Intestinal malabsorption following temporary occlusion of the superior mesenteric artery. Am. J. Med. *25*, 449–455 (1958)
Jow, E., Webster, D.R., Skoryna, S.C.: Effects of glucagon and insulin on gastric secretion in rats. Gastroenterology *38*, 732–739 (1960)
Kahlson, G., Rosengren, E., Svensson, S.E.: Histamine and gastric acid secretion with special reference to the rat. In: The Pharmacology of gastro-intestinal motility and secretion. International Encyclopedia of Pharmacology and Therapeutics. Holton, P. (ed.), Sect. 39a. Oxford: Pergamon Press 1973
Karvinen, E., Karvonen, M.J.: The effect of insulin hypoglycaemia on histamine-induced Hadenhain pouch secretion in the dog. Acta Physiol. Scand. *27*, 350–370 (1952)
Kažic, T.: Effect of adrenergic factors on peristalsis and acetylcholine release. Eur. J. Pharmacol. *16*, 367–373 (1971)
Keřremans, R., Penninckx, F.: A study in vitro of adrenergic receptors in the rectum and in the internal anal sphincter of the cat. Gut *11*, 709–714 (1970)
Kirpekar, S.M., Wakade, A.R., Dixon, W., Prat, J.C.: Effect of cocaine, phenoxybenzamine and calcium on the inhibition of norepinephrine output from the cat spleen by guanethidine. J. Pharmacol. Exp. Ther. *165*, 166–175 (1969)
Knoll, J., Vizi, E.S.: Effect of frequency of stimulation on the inhibition by noradrenaline of the acetylcholine output from parasympathetic nerve stimulation terminals. Br. J. Pharmacol. *42*, 263–272 (1971)
Kock, N.: An experimental analysis of mechanisms engaged in reflex inhibition of intestinal motility. Acta Physiol. Scand. *164*, 1–54 (1959)
Kontirek, S.J., Oleksy, J.: The effect of cholinergic and adrenergic blockade on basal and pentagastrin induced acid secretion. Scand. J. Gastroenterol. *4*, 13–16 (1969)
Kopin, I.J.: Storage and metabolism of catecholamines: The role of monoamine oxidase. Pharmacol. Rev. *16*, 179–191 (1964)
Kopin, I.J.: False adrenergic transmitters. Annu. Rev. Pharmacol. *8*, 377–394 (1968)
Kosterlitz, H.W., Lees, G.M.: Action of the bretylium on the isolated guinea-pig ileum. Br. J. Pharmacol. *17*, 82–86 (1961)
Kosterlitz, H.W., Lydon, R.J., Watt, A.J.: The effect of adrenaline, noradrenaline, and isoprenaline on inhibitory and α-adrenoreceptors in the longit muscle of the guinea-pig ileum. Br. J. Pharmacol. *39*, 398–414 (1970)
Krayer, O., Fuentes, T.: Changes of heart rate caused by direct cardiac action of reserpine. J. Pharmacol. Exp. Ther. *123*, 145–152 (1958)
Kroneberg, G., Oberdorf, A.: Inhibition of acetylcholine action in the guinea-pig ileum by sympathetic α- and β-receptor stimulation. In: 1st Congr. Hung. Pharmacol. Soc. Budapest. Knoll, E.J., Vizi, E.S. (eds.), pp. 39–48. Budapest: Akademiai Kiado 1974
Kuntzman, R., Costa, E., Gessa, G.L., Brodie, B.B.: Reserpine and guanethidine action on peripheral stores of catecholamines. Life Sci. *1*, 65–74 (1962)
Kuriyama, H.: Effects of ions and drugs on the electrical activity of smooth muscle. In: Smooth muscle. Bülbring, E., Brading, A., Jones, A., Tomita, T. (eds.), pp. 366–395. London: Arnold 1970
Kuroda, S.: Pharmakodynamische Studien zur Frage der Magenmotilität. Z. Ges. Exp. Med. *39*, 341–354 (1924)
Lacroix, E.: La circulation splanchnique. Acta Gastroenterol. Belg. *23*, 534–581 (1960)
Lands, A.M., Arnold, A., McAuliff, J.P., Luduena, F.P., Brown, T.G.: Differentiation of receptor systems activated by sympathiomimetic amines. Nature *214*, 597–598 (1967)
Langley, J.M.: Observations on the physiological action of extracts of the supra-renal bodies. J. Physiol. (Lond.) *27*, 237–256 (1901)
Lee, C.Y.: Adrenergic receptors in the intestine. In: Smooth muscle. Bülbring, E., Brading, A.F., Jones, A.W., Tomita, T. (eds.), pp. 549–557. London: Arnold 1970
Leonsins, A.J., Waddell, W.R.: Inhibiting effect of norepinephrine on gastric secretion in human subjects. J. Appl. Physiol. *12*, 334–338 (1958)

Levy, B.: The intestinal inhibitory response to oxytocin, vasopressin and bradykinin. J. Pharmacol. exp. Ther. *140*, 356–366 (1963)

Lim, R.K.S.: The question of a gastric hormone. Q. J. Exp. Physiol. *13*, 79–103 (1922)

Lin, T.M., Evans, D.C., Spray, G.F.: Mechanism studies of gastric inhibition by glucagon: Failure of KCl and adrenergic blocking agents to prevent its action. Arch. Int. Pharmacodyn. Ther. *202*, 314–324 (1973)

Linde, S.: Studies on the stimulation mechanism of gastric secretion. Acta Physiol. Scand. [Suppl. 74] *21*, 68 (1950)

Lindmar, R., Muscholl, E.: Die Wirkung von Cocain, Guanethidin, Reserpin, Hexamethonium, Tetracain und Psicain auf die Noradrenalinfreisetzung aus dem Herzen. Arch. Exp. Pathol. Pharmakol. *242*, 214–227 (1961)

Loeper, M., Verpy, G.: L'action de l'adrenaline sur le tractus digestif. Compt. Rend. Soc. Biol. *80*, 703–705 (1917)

Lum, B.K.B., Kermani, M.H., Heilman, R.D.: Intestinal relaxation produced by sympathomimetic amines in the isolated rabbit ileum: Selective inhibition by adrenergic blocking agents and by cold storage. J. Pharmacol. Exp. Ther. *154*, 463–471 (1966)

Lum, B.K.B., Heilman, R.D., Gaunt, M.A.: Selective loss of responsiveness to alpha-adrenergic receptor stimulation after cold storage. Eur. J. Pharmacol. *1*, 109–113 (1967)

Lundborg, P., Stitzel, R.E.: Studies on the dual action of guanethidine in sympathetic nerves. Acta Physiol. Scand. *72*, 100–107 (1968)

MacLean, L., Brackney, E., Visscher, M.: Effects of epinephrine, norepinephrine and histamine in canine intestine and liver weight continuously recorded in vivo. J. Appl. Physiol. *9*, 237–240 (1956)

Malik, K.U., Ling, G.M.: Modification by acetylcholine of the response of rat mesenteric arteries to sympathetic stimulation. Circ. Res. *25*, 1–10 (1969)

Mann, M., West, G.B.: The nature of uterine and intestinal sympathin. Br. J. Pharmacol. *6*, 79–82 (1951)

Maxwell, R.A., Plummer, A.J., Schneider, F., Poualski, H., Daniel, A.I.: Pharmacology of 2-(octahydro-1-azocinyl)-ethyl-guanidine-sulfate (SU-5864). J. Pharmacol. Exp. Ther. *128*, 22–29 (1960)

McDougal, M.D., West, G.B.: The inhibition of the peristaltic reflex by sympathomimetic amines. Br. J. Pharmacol. *9*, 131–137 (1954)

McGregor, D.D.: The effect of sympathetic nerve stimulation on vasoconstriction responses in perfused mesenteric blood vessels of the rat. J. Physiol. (Lond.) *177*, 21–30 (1965)

Mellander, S., Johansson, B.: Control of resistance, exchange and capacitance functions in the peripheral circulation. Pharmacol. Rev. *20*, 117–196 (1968)

Millar, R.A., Keener, E.B., Benfey, B.G.: Plasma adrenaline and noradrenaline after phenoxybenzamine administration and during haemorhagic hypotension in normal and adrenalectomized dogs. Br. J. Pharmacol. Chemother. *14*, 9–13 (1959)

Mirkin, B.L., Bonnycastle, D.D.: A pharmacological and chemical study of humoral mediators in the sympathetic nervous system. Am. J. Physiol. *178*, 529–534 (1954)

Misher, A., Pendleton, R.G., Staples, R.: Effects of adrenergic drugs upon gastric secretion in rats. Gastroenterology *57*, 294–299 (1969)

Moll, H., Flint, E.R.: The depressive influence of the sympathetic nerves on gastric acidity. Br. J. Surg. *16*, 283–306 (1928)

Mori, J., Azuma, H., Fujiwara, M.: Adrenergic innervation and receptors in the sphincter of Oddi. Eur. J. Pharmacol. *14*, 365–373 (1971)

Munro, A.F.: The effect of adrenaline on the guinea-pig ileum. J. Physiol. (Lond.) *112*, 84–94 (1951)

Munro, A.F.: Potentiation and reversal of the adrenaline motor response in the guinea-pig ileum by autonomic drugs. J. Physiol. (Lond.) *118*, 171–181 (1952)

Munro, A.F.: Effect of autonomic drugs on the responses of isolated preparations from the guinea-pig intestine to electrical stimulation. J. Physiol. (Lond.) *120*, 41–52 (1953)

Muren, A.: Influence of the vagal innervation on gastric motor responses to adrenaline and noradrenaline. Acta Physiol. Scand. *39*, 195–202 (1957a)

Muren, A.: Gastric motor responses to adrenaline and noradrenaline after treatment with a parasympathicolytic agent. Acta Physiol. Scand. *39*, 188–194 (1957b)

Muscholl, E.: Indirectly acting sympathomimetic amines. Pharmacol. Rev. *18*, 551–559 (1966)

Muscholl, E.: Adrenergic false transmitters. In: Catecholamines. Blaschko, H., Muscholl, E. (eds.), pp. 618–660. Berlin, Heidelberg, New York: Springer 1972
Nakazato, Y., Saito, K., Ohga, A.: Gastric motor and inhibitor response to stimulation of the sympathetic nerve in the dog. Jpn. J. Pharmacol. *20*, 131–141 (1970)
Nasio, J.: New text for gastric function. Am. J. Dig. Dis. *11*, 227–229 (1944)
Nicoloff, D.M., Peter, E.T., Stone, N.H., Wangensteen, O.H.: Effect of catecholamines on gastric secretion and blood flow. Ann. Surg. *159*, 32–36 (1964)
Nishi, S., North, R.A.: Intracellular recording from the myenteric plexus of the guinea-pig ileum. J. Physiol. (Lond.) *231*, 471–491 (1973)
Norberg, K.A.: Adrenergic innervation of the intestinal wall studied by fluorescence microscopy. Int. J. Neuropharmacol. *3*, 379–382 (1964)
Norberg, K.A., Sjöqvist, F.: New possibilities for adrenergic modulation of ganglionic transmission. Pharmacol. Rev. *18*, 743–751 (1966)
Oberdorf, A., Kroneberg, G.: Alpha- und beta-sympathicomimetische Wirkung am elektrisch gereizten isolierten Meerschweinchenileum. Arch. Exp. Pathol. Pharmakol. *267*, 195–207 (1970)
Öberg, B.: Effects of cardiovascular reflexes on net capillary fluid transfer. Acta Physiol. Scand. [Suppl.] *229*, 1–98 (1964)
Ogawa, S.: Beiträge zur Gefäßwirkung des Adrenalins. Arch. Exp. Pathol. Pharmakol. *67*, 89–110 (1912)
Okabe, S., Saziki, R., Takagi, K.: Effect of adrenergic blocking agents on gastric secretion and stress induced gastric ulcer in rats. Jpn. J. Pharmacol. *20*, 10–15 (1970)
Parks, A.G., Fishlock, D.J., Cameron, J.D.H., May, H.: Preliminary investigation of the pharmacology of the human internal anal sphincter. Gut *10*, 674–677 (1969)
Parrot, J.L., Verliac, F.: Sur les caractères de la sécrétion gastrique provoguée par l'adrenaline. C.R. Soc. Biol. (Paris) *135*, 1037–1041 (1941 a)
Parrot, J.L., Verliac, F.: Sur quelques modifications pharmacologiques de la sécrétion gastrique provoquée par l'adrénaline. C.R. Soc. Biol. (Paris) *135*, 1181–1184 (1941 b)
Paton, W.D.M., Vizi, E.S.: The inhibitory action of noradrenaline and adrenaline on acetylcholine output by guinea-pig ileum longitudinal muscle strip. Br. J. Pharmacol. *35*, 10–28 (1969)
Persson, C.G.A.: Adrenoceptor functions in the cat choledo-choduodenal junction in vitro. Br. J. Pharmacol. *42*, 447–461 (1971)
Peters, R.M., Womack, N.A.: Hemodynamics of gastric secretion. Am. Surg. *148*, 337–350 (1958)
Pradhan, S.N., Wingate, H.W.: Effects of adrenergic agents on gastric secretion in dogs. Arch. Int. Pharmacodyn. Ther. *140*, 399–408 (1962)
Pradhan, S.N., Wingate, H.W.: Effects of some adrenergic blocking agents on gastric secretion in dogs. Arch. Int. Pharmacodyn. Ther. *162*, 303–310 (1966)
Rand, M.J., Wilson, J.: The relationship between adrenergic neurone blocking activity and local anaesthetic activity in a series of guanethidine derivatives. Eur. J. Pharmacol. *1*, 200–209 (1967)
Read, J.B., Burnstock, G.: Adrenergic innervation of the gut musculature in vertebrates. Histochemie *17*, 263–272 (1969)
Read, J.B., Burnstock, G.: Development of the adrenergic innervation and chromaffin cells in the human fetal gut. Dev. Biol. *22*, 513–534 (1970)
Reid, E.W.: The influence of the mesenteric nerves on intestinal absorption. J. Physiol. (Lond.) *20*, 298–309 (1896)
Richardson, D.R., Johnson, P.C.: Changes in mesenteric capillary flow during norepinephrine infusion. Am. J. Physiol. *219*, 1317–1323 (1970)
Robison, G.A., Butcher, R.W., Sutherland, E.W.: The catecholamines. In: Biochemical actions of hormones, 2nd ed. Litwack, G. (ed.), pp. 81–111. New York: Academic Press 1970
Rogers, J., Rake, J.M., Ablahadain, E.: The stimulation and inhibition of gastric secretion which follows the subcutaneous administration of certain organ extracts. Am. J. Physiol. *48*, 79–92 (1919)
Ross, G.: Effects of epinephrine and norepinephrine on the mesenteric circulation of the cat. Am. J. Physiol. *212*, 1037–1042 (1967)

Ross, G.: Effects of catecholamines on splanchnic blood flow before and after beta adrenergic blockade. In: Cardiovascular beta adrenergic responses. Kattus, A.A., Ross, G., Hall, V.E. (eds.). Berkeley: University of California Press 1970

Ross, G.: Escape of mesenteric vessels from adrenergic and noradrenergic vasoconstriction. Am. J. Physiol. *221*, 1217–1222 (1971)

Rossoff, C.B., Goldman, H.: Effect of the intestinal bacterial flow on acute gastric stress ulceration. Gastroenterology *55*, 212–222 (1968)

Rothschild, F.: Die klinische Bedeutung der fraktionierten Magenausscheberung unter besonderer Berücksichtigung der Gesamtchloride und der Neutralchloride. Arch. Verdauungskr. *35*, 286–310 (1925)

Salimi, M., Kermani, R.Z., Djahansouz, B., Golshan, S.H.: Impairment of α-receptor activity induced by cold storage in the isolated of rabbit duodenum. Pharmacology *4*, 341–346 (1970)

Schanker, L.S., Shore, P.A., Brodie, B.B., Hogben, C.A.M.: Absorption of drugs from the stomach. 1. The rat. J. Pharmacol. Exp. Ther. *120*, 528–540 (1957)

Schaumann, W.: Zusammenhänge zwischen der Wirkung der Analgerita und Sympathicomimetic auf den Meerschweinchen-Dünndarm. Arch. Exp. Pathol. Pharmakol. *233*, 112–124 (1958)

Setekleiv, J.: Effects of drugs on ion distribution and flux in smooth muscle. In: Smooth muscle. Bülbring, E., Brading, A., Jones, A., Tomita, T. (eds.), pp. 343–365. London: Arnold 1970

Shanbour, L.L., Jacobson, E.D.: Autoregulatory escape in the gut. Gastroenterology *60*, 145–148 (1971)

Shaw, R.S., Maynard, E.P.: Acute and chronic thrombosis of mesenteric arteries associated with malabsorption. N. Engl. J. Med. *258*, 874–878 (1958)

Shehadeh, Z., Price, W.E., Jacobson, E.D.: Effects of vasoactive agents on intestinal blood flow and motility in the dog. Am. J. Physiol. *216*, 386–392 (1969)

Sheppard, H., Zimmerman, J.: Effect of guanethidine (SU-5864) on tissue catecholamines. Pharmacologist *1*, 69 (1959)

Shipley, P.G., Blackfan, K.D.: The pharmacological action of adrenaline on the sphincter pylori of the foetus. Bull. Johns Hopkins Hosp. *33*, 159–162 (1922)

Shore, P.A.: A simple technique involving solvent extraction for the estimation of norepinephrine and epinephrine in tissues. Pharmacol. Rev. *11*, 276–277 (1959)

Shore, P.A.: Release of serotonin and catecholamines by drugs. Pharmacol. Rev. *14*, 531–550 (1962)

Shore, P.A.: The mechanism of norepinephrine depletion by reserpine metaraminol and related agents. The role of monoamine oxidase. Pharmacol. Rev. *128*, 561–568 (1966)

Shuba, M.F.: The mechanism of the excitatory action of catecholamines and histamine on the smooth muscle of guinea-pig ureter. J. Physiol. (Lond.) *264*, 853–864 (1977a)

Shuba, M.F.: The effect of sodium-free and potassium-free solutions, ionic current inhibitors and ouabain on electrophysiological properties of smooth muscle of guinea-pig ureter. J. Physiol. (Lond.) *264*, 837–851 (1977b)

Shuba, M.F., Gurkovskaya, A.V., Klevetz, M.J., Kochemasova, N.G., Taranenko, V.M.: Mechanism of the excitatory and inhibitory actions of catecholamines on the membrane of smooth muscle cells. In: Physiology of smooth muscle. Bülbring, E., Shuba, M.F. (eds.), pp. 347–355. New York: Raven Press 1976

Smith, M.I.: The action of the autonomic drugs on the surviving stomach. A study of the innervation of the stomach. Am. J. Physiol. *96*, 232–243 (1918)

Smith, C.B.: The role of monoamine oxidase in the intraneuronal metabolism of norepinephrine released by indirectly-acting sympathomimetic amines or by adrenergic nerve stimulation. J. Pharmacol. Exp. Ther. *151*, 207–220 (1966)

Smith, G.P., Jacobson, E.D.: Effect of norepinephrine on gastric secretion in macaca mulatta. Fed. Proc. *23*, 213 (1964)

Speden, R.N.: Excitation of vascular smooth muscle. In: Smooth muscle. Bülbring, E., Brading, A., Jones, A., Tomita, T. (eds.), p. 558. London: Arnold 1970

Story, D.F., Allen, G.S., Glover, A.B., Hope, W., McCulloch, M.W., Rand, M.J., Sarantos, C.: Modulation of adrenergic transmission by acetylcholine. Clin. Exp. Pharmacol. Physiol. [Suppl.] *2*, 27–33 (1975)

Stjärne, L.: Basic mechanisms and local feedback control of secretion of adrenergic and cholinergic neurotransmitters. In: Handbook of Psychopharmacology, Iverson, L.L., Iversen, S.D., Snyder, S.H. (eds.), Vol. 6, pp. 179–233. New York: Plenum Press 1975

Tanaka, U., Ohkuho, Y.: Pharmacological studies on the autonomic nerves of the small intestine of the horse. 1. Sympathetic innervation of the small intestine. Jpn. J. Vet. Sci. *2*, 321–339 (1940)

Tezner, O., Turolt, M.: Studien über die Wirkung der Verschiebung der K- und Ca-Ionen auf den überlebenden menschlichen Magen. Z. Ges. Exp. Med. *24*, 1–10 (1921)

Thoenen, H., Hürlimann, A., Haefely, W.: Interactions of phenoxybenzamine with guanethidine and bretylium at the sympathetic nerve endings of the isolated perfused spleen of the cat. J. Pharmacol. Exp. Ther. *151*, 189–195 (1966)

Thomas, J.E.: The action of adrenaline on the pyloric sphincter. Proc. Soc. Exp. Biol. Med. *23*, 748–750 (1926)

Thompson, J.E., Vane, J.R.: Gastric secretion induced by histamine and its relationship to the rate of blood flow. J. Physiol. (Lond.) *121*, 433–444 (1953)

Titchen, D.A.: Nervous control of motility of the forestomach of ruminants. In: Handbook of Physiology, Code, C.F. (ed.), Sect. 6, Vol. V., pp. 2705–2724. Washington: American Physiological Society 1968

Tomita, T.: Electrical properties of mammalian smooth muscle. In: Smooth muscle. Bülbring, E., Brading, A., Jones, A., Tomita, T. (eds.), pp. 197–243. London: Arnold 1970

Tomita, T., Watanabe, H.: A comparison of the effects of adenosine triphosphate with noradrenaline and with the inhibitory potential of the guinea-pig taenia coli. J. Physiol. (Lond.) *231*, 167–177 (1973)

Triggle, D.J.: Adrenergic receptors. Annu. Rev. Pharmacol. *12*, 185–196 (1972)

Türker, K., Kiran, B.K., Kaymakcalan, S.: The effects of synthetic bradykinin on intestinal motility in different laboratory animals and its relation to catecholamines. Arch. Int. Pharmacodyn. Ther. *151*, 260–268 (1964)

Varro, V., Blaho, G., Csernay, L., Jung, I., Szarvas, F.: Effect of decreased local circulation on the absorptive capacity of a small intestine loop in the dog. Am. J. Dig. Dis. *10*, 170–177 (1965)

Vizi, E.S.: The inhibitory action of noradrenaline and adrenaline on release of acetylcholine from guinea-pig ileum longitudinal strips. Naunyn Schmiedebergs Arch. Exp. Pathol. Pharmakol. *259*, 199–200(1968)

Vizi, E.S.: Presynaptic modulation of neurochemical transmission. Prog. Neurob. *12*, 181–290 (1979)

Vizi, E.C., Knoll, J.: The effect of sympathetic nerve stimulation and guanethidine on parasympathetic neuroeffector transmission; the inhibition of acetylcholine release. J. Pharm. Pharmacol. *23*, 918–925 (1971)

Van Rossum, J.M., Mujić, M.: Classification of sympathomimetic drugs on the rabbit intestine. Arch. Int. Pharmacodyn. Ther. *155*, 418–431 (1965)

Von Euler, U.S.: The nature of adrenergic nerve mediators. Pharmacol. Rev. *3*, 247–277 (1951)

Von Euler, U.S., Lishajko, F.: Effect of reserpine on the uptake of catecholamines in isolated nerve storage granules. Int. J. Neuropharmacol. *2*, 127–134 (1963)

Von Sirotinin, G.W.: Über die Wirkung des Adrenalins auf die Sekretion des Magensaftes aus den nach Heidenhain isolierten kleinen Magen des Hundes. Z. Ges. Exp. Med. *40*, 90–97 (1924)

Walz, A., van Zwieten, P.A.: The influence of 2-(2,6-dichlorphenylamino)-2-imidazoline hydrochloride (Clonidine) and some related compounds on gastric secretion in the anesthetized rat. Eur. J. Pharmacol. *10*, 369–377 (1970)

Warren, P.R., Day, M.D.: A pharmacological analysis of the responses to transmural stimulation in isolated intestinal preparations. Br. J. Pharmacol. *32*, 227–240 (1968)

Westfall, T.C.: Local regulation of adrenergic neurotransmission. Physiol. Rev. *57*, 659–728 (1977)

White, H.L., Rainey, W.R., Monaghan, B., Harris, A.S.: Observation on the nervous control of the ileo caecal sphincter and on intestinal movements in an unanaesthetized human subject. Am. J. Physiol. *108*, 449–457 (1934)

Wilson, A.B.: Beta sympathetic inhibitory receptors in the small intestine of the guinea-pig. J. Pharm. Pharmacol. *16*, 834–835 (1964)

Winne, D.: Der Einfluß einiger Pharmaka auf die Darmdurchblutung und die Resorption tritiummarkierten Wassers aus dem Dünndarm der Ratte. Arch. Exp. Pathol. Pharmakol. *254*, 199–224 (1966)

Wolf, S.G., Wolff, H.G.: Human gastric function: An experimental study of a man and his stomach. New York, Oxford: 1943

Wolf, S., Wolff, H.G.: Human gastric function, 2nd ed. p. 79. London: Oxford University press 1947

Woods, G., Nelson, V., Nelson, E.: The effect of small amounts of ergotamine on the circulatory response to adrenaline. J. Pharmacol. Exp. Ther. *45*, 403–418 (1932)

Yamaguchi, I., Hiroi, J., Kumoda, S.: Central and peripheral adrenergic mechanisms regulating gastric secretion in the rat. J. Pharmacol. Exp. Ther. *203*, 125–131 (1977)

Zeppa, R., La Rosa, J.J., Bilbro, R.H.: Arteriovenous shunt mechanism in gastric secretion. Am. J. Surg. *115*, 185–190 (1968)

CHAPTER 4

Effects of Adrenergic Activators and Inhibitors on the Endocrine System*

D.E. POTTER

A. Introduction

The principle function of certain cells in the body (endocrine cells) is to produce chemical messengers (hormones) that convey information to other cells whose activity they regulate. These chemical messenger or endocrine cells can be classified as neuroendocrine, paracrine (secreted alongside), peptide-endocrine, and steroid-endocrine (GROSSMAN, 1976). The first three classes share several features including a related embryologic origin, common histochemical properties, and related hormone products. Neuroendocrine and paracrine transmitters can be either amines or peptides and in the latter case related to endocrine peptides. Examples of immunoreactive peptides found both in nerves and endocrine cells include somatostatin and substance P.

Adrenergic mechanisms provide an important link between the central and autonomic nervous systems and the secretory activity in the endocrine system. Catecholaminergic mechanisms are rarely if ever the sole factor regulating secretion of hormones, but these mechanisms are certainly one of the important inputs that modulate secretion.

Among the recent developments in endocrinology have been the discovery that the aminergic links are very widespread and that many endocrine tissues are possibly derived from elements of the neural crest and neural ridges (PEARSE, 1976). The adrenergic connections between the nervous and endocrine systems seem to be of two types: (1) those in the central nervous system, where dopamine and norepinephrine are synaptic mediators that affect the secretion of endocrine organs such as the pituitary, and (2) those in other parts of the body, where circulating catecholamines released from the adrenal medulla and/or catecholamines released locally from endings of sympathetic nerves alter the secretory pattern of various endocrine organs (GANONG, 1973).

The neuroendocrine link in the central nervous system is best exemplified by adrenergic modulation of anterior pituitary secretion. Numerous papers indicate that hypothalamic neural circuits which release either dopamine or norepinephrine can modulate pituitary hormone release either indirectly by way of hypothalamic-releasing hormones or by a direct action on the pituitary. Moreover, it has been observed that hormones, such as corticosteroids, may exert feedback effects at the pituitary level on ACTH release and may also act, in part, through an adrenergic mechanism in the central nervous system (DALLMAN and YATES, 1968; GANONG, 1972).

The influence of the sympathetic neurons on pancreatic endocrine secretion is an example of the second type of adrenergic-endocrine link. Both insulin and glucagon

* This review was completed in January 1978 and generally does not cover work published later than December 1977.

(and perhaps somatostatin) release are affected by changes in activity of sympathetic neurons to the pancreatic islets. The activation of the renin-angiotensin system by sympathetic postganglionic nerve fibers is another example of an endocrine organ that is controlled in part by the action of endogenous catecholamines.

The administration of drugs that alter the function of sympathetic nervous system by a central or peripheral mechanism of action is commonly used to investigate the relationship between the autonomic nervous system and the endocrine system. Moreover, a number of these drugs have proven to be therapeutically useful in treating and/or diagnosing endocrine disorders. For example, the dopaminergic agonist, bromergocryptine, has proven to be clinically useful in the treatment of hyperprolactinemia. Occasionally drugs that influence adrenergic function may produce bothersome secondary effects on endocrine organs. An example of this circumstance would be chlorpromazine-induced hyperprolactinemia, which leads to galactorrhea.

B. Embryologic Relationship of the Neural and the Endocrine Systems

The homeostasis of the mammalian organism is dependent upon the coordinated activity of the nervous system and the endocrine system. Until recently, these systems have been considered to be distinct from one another from a developmental point of view, although the functional significance of neurosecretory cells of the hypothalamus has been recognized for some time. The concept of a neuron's serving as a specialized glandular secretory unit was suggested by the work of SPEIDEL in 1919, who, while working with the spinal cord of fish, described giant neurons that had the appearance of secretory cells. More recently, a working hypothesis presented by PEARSE (1976) suggests a more general relationship between endocrine and neuronal cells in terms of development and function. Morphologic evidence strongly suggests that many endocrine cells are derived from neuroectodermal tissue and that it would therefore be more appropriate to consider many of them as neuroendocrine cells. Although originally considered to be nerve cells, cells of the neuroectoderm are believed to have undergone modification so that in addition to producing amines they evolved into polypeptide-producing cells as well.

The acronym APUD (amine content and/or amine precursor uptake and decarboxylation) is used to describe the following cytochemical properties of this cell line: normal amine content, high amine precursor uptake, high α-glycerophosphate dehydrogenase, and high esterase or cholinesterase content. This category of cells includes adrenal and extra-adrenal chromaffin cells, C-cells of the thyroid, and cells in the anterior pituitary, bronchi, and intestinal tract. A function common to all APUD cells appears to be the synthesis of peptide, polypeptide, or protein secretory products. This function may be accompanied by the synthesis of catecholamines or indolalkylamines. Moreover, peptide, polypeptide, and protein secretory products are present even in cells that secrete primarily amines. An example would be the granules in chromaffin tissue (including sympathetic neurons) that store the catecholamines in response to secretory stimuli. Similarly, although the endocrine cells of the gut were initially recognized because they synthesized and stored amines, present evidence suggests that the principal secretory products of enteric endocrine cells are polypeptides. Thus, neural crest cells of the APUD series are, to some extent, pluripotential before migration to their final location in the body. They remain so for some time after reaching their destination, but their final location is believed to provide the environment that determines their predominant secretory product. Furthermore, it is possible to demonstrate that some cells cultured from APUD tumors are electrically excitable.

From these findings, it seems possible that like amines, peptides can act either as hormones or as neurotransmitters.

Based upon the foregoing ideas, it seems that the nervous system and endocrine system not only interact functionally but also seem to have similar origins, at least in the case of the polypeptide-producing endocrine organs.

C. Role of Catecholamines in Modulating the Function of the Endocrine System

I. Mediators of Catecholamine-Induced Modulation of the Endocrine System

Calcium, the cyclic nucleotides (cyclic AMP and GMP), and prostaglandins are primary candidates for a role in the internal signaling system that regulates the activity of most cells, including those of the endocrine system (BERRIDGE, 1975; SILVER and SMITH, 1975). The primary function of these intracellular signals is to mediate the cell's response to a wide range of external stimuli. The plasma membrane usually serves as the receiver, transducer, and transformer, whereby incoming signals adjust cellular activity through alterations in one or more of the second messengers.

Calcium occupies the most prominent position and probably has a central role in directing cellular activity. In contrast to calcium, cyclic nucleotides and prostaglandins must be synthesized and released by the mammalian cells in response to catecholamines and other hormones. In such circumstances the cyclic nucleotides or prostaglandins formed may act as intracellular (second) messengers by directly affecting enzyme activity or by modulating levels of each other; that is, prostaglandins formed endogenously may influence substances like cyclic nucleotides or calcium ions, which then would become third messengers. For example, there is experimental evidence that prostaglandins can directly influence the activities of enzymes such as adenylyl cyclase (ABDULLA and MCFARLANE, 1971), phosphodiesterase (AMER and MARQUIS, 1972), and Na^+/K^+ activated ATPase (JOHNSON and RAMWELL, 1973), as well as influencing intracellular levels of calcium ions (RAMWELL and SHAW, 1970). The importance of the interactions between cyclic AMP and calcium during hormone action was determined on the basis of studies of the mode of action of parathyroid hormone and calcitonin (RASMUSSEN, 1970).

For a number of years, catecholamines were assumed to induce most, if not all of their effects by interaction with the adenylyl cyclase-cyclic AMP system of the cell. The three events of catecholamine action earliest recognized were a binding to the membrane, adenylyl cyclase stimulation, and protein kinase activation. However, some evidence suggests that while stimulation of β-adrenoceptors may lead to an increase in cyclic AMP levels, stimulation of α-adrenoceptors may sometimes cause a decrease in cyclic AMP levels (BILLING et al., 1969). In addition, it has been postulated that α-adrenoceptor stimulation may increase cyclic GMP levels, which are under some circumstances antagonistic to cyclic AMP functions (STEWART, 1975). Moreover, some α-adrenergic actions appear to be principally dependent upon calcium and independent of cyclic nucleotide generation (SZEGO, 1972).

The available information on the interaction between adrenergic drugs and the intracellular messengers (calcium, cyclic nucleotides, and possibly prostaglandins) in the endocrine system is very fragmentary in many areas of research and very contradictory in others. More often than not, research efforts have concentrated either on cyclic nucleotides, on prostaglandins, or on calcium as mediators of adrenergic drug effects; there have been few combined studies designed to unravel how adrenergic drugs may influence endocrine activity through an interaction with each second messenger system. Hopefully future studies will elucidate how adrenergic drugs influence endocrine function at the cellular level.

II. Adrenergic Drugs Used to Examine Hormone Secretion and Action

Seven classes of adrenergic drugs have been used to examine the secretion and action of hormones. These include: neutral amino acids and their analogs, enzyme inhibitors, inhibitors of catecholamine uptake, inhibitors of catecholamine storage, adrenoceptor agonists and antagonists, and neurotoxins.

1. Neutral Amino Acids

a) Tyrosine

This amino acid is the circulating precursor of all endogenous catecholamines. When injected, this amino acid can be considered a drug, i.e., the metabolic consequences of the injection of tyrosine can be quite different from those that follow its consumption as a constituent of dietary protein. Giving tyrosine can increase the synthesis of catecholamines within adrenergic neurons. Thus, this amino acid is probably among the most specific drugs currently used for modifying adrenergic transmitter synthesis and release. However, it should be appreciated that the specificity of tyrosine for adrenergic neurons is not complete; that is, tyrosine can inhibit the uptake of tryptophan by neurons and therefore may also suppress synthesis of serotonin.

b) L-Dopa and DOPS

Levodopa (L-Dopa) is the immediate precursor of catecholamines and is among the least specific that affect adrenergic neuron function in that the enzyme, L-aromatic-amino acid decarboxylase, exists in most cells of the body. Thus, administration of L-Dopa not only accelerates the release of dopamine but also norepinephrine and serotonin. This latter effect occurs because large amounts of dopamine are formed within serotonergic and noradrenergic nerve terminals and competes with the "normal" transmitters for storage sites. In addition, L-Dopa can produce a transient disruption of protein synthesis in neurons by disaggregating polyribosomes. With administration of L-Dopa, there is also depletion of the methyl donor, *S*-adenosylmethionine, and hence a slowing of the metabolism of other endogenous monoamines such as dopamine, norepinephrine, histamine, and other potential acceptors of methyl groups.

A synthetic amino acid L-threodihydroxyphenylserine (DOPS) is supposed to be decarboxylated to norepinephrine and thereby to enhance noradrenergic transmission. However, this precursor passes the pial-glial barrier poorly and also is a rather poor substrate for L-aromatic amino acid decarboxylase. Thus, if this drug does change neuroendocrine function, it could be due to peripheral activation of sympathetic synapses or from inhibition of the uptake of other neutral amino acids by neuronal tissue.

c) Alpha-Methyl-m-Tyrosine and Alpha-Methyldopa

These drugs are converted to α-methylated catecholamines by decarboxylation and hydroxylation. They are not readily metabolized by monoamine oxidase and therefore persist in the body for a relatively long period of time compared to naturally occurring catecholamines.

The products (substitute transmitters) of α-methyl-m-tyrosine are stored and released from noradrenergic neurons; their ability to activate adrenergic receptors is somewhat less than that of norepinephrine. In contrast, the product of α-methyldopa, α-methylnorepinephrine, is considered to have similar activity to norepinephrine in terms of stimulating adrenergic receptors. One biological effect of stimulating α-adrenoceptors in brainstem centers is, among other things, a fall in blood pressure. These drugs can also compete with tyrosine for neuronal uptake, inhibit the activity of L-aromatic amino acid decarboxylase to a limited extent, and deplete *S*-adenosylmethionine by serving as substrates for catechol-O-methyl transferase (COMT).

d) Alpha-Methyl-p-Tyrosine

α-Methyl-p-tyrosine is a potent inhibitor of the rate-limiting enzyme of catecholamine synthesis, tyrosine hydroxylase and causes major decreases in catecholamine stores. Unfortunately, the drug also tends to interfere with metabolism of tryptophan as well as tyrosine and can transiently affect serotonin levels as well.

2. Enzyme Inhibitors

a) Inhibitors of L-Aromatic Amino Acid Decarboxylase

Carbidopa was designed and is currently used to block peripheral decarboxylation of L-Dopa without modifying the conversion of dopa to dopamine in the brain. However, it should be noted that certain areas of the brain that have little or no pial-glial barrier may also be affected by carbidopa. Large doses of carbidopa (100 mg/kg in rats) also suppress the decarboxylation of endogenous dopa and hence modify sympathetic function. High doses (800 mg/kg) of other peripheral dopa decarboxylase inhibitors (R-4-4602) also inhibit catecholamine turnover in the brain and periphery. Thus, these agents can be used to determine the neuroendocrine effect of an amino acid analog, such as L-Dopa, on suppression of prolactin secretion.

Both of the dopa decarboxylase inhibitors mentioned above are hydrazines and thus bind pyridoxal phosphate. The metabolism of tyrosine to catecholamines is dependent in part on pyridoxal-dependent enzymes. Therefore, it is not surprising that plasma levels of tyrosine are elevated following administration of these drugs.

b) Monoamine Oxidase Inhibitors

Compounds which inhibit monoamine oxidase (MAO) also elevate tissue levels of catecholamines as a result. Oxidative deamination of catecholamines is not a major mechanism for inactivation of norepinephrine in vivo unless catecholamine storage is disturbed, such as by administration of reserpine, or unless COMT is inhibited. Re-uptake into presynaptic neuron terminals and, to a lesser extent, O-methylation are primarily responsible for catecholamine inactivation. MAO inhibitors can be classified according to chemical structure (that is, whether they are hydrazines or not) and by their spectrum of action on isozymes of MAO. Iproniazid, pheniprazine, nialamide, and isocarboxazid are hydrazine compounds; tranylcypromine and pargyline are not.

No MAO inhibitors are available that selectively block the oxidative deamination of only one amine without also affecting the fate of other amines as well.

c) Inhibitors of Dopamine Beta-Oxidase

Disulfiram is an example of a drug which can inhibit the conversion of dopamine to norepinephrine by chelating the copper needed for dopamine β-oxidase (DBH) activity. As a chelating agent, disulfiram also interferes with the activity of other enzymes such as aldehyde dehydrogenase. This nonspecificity complicates the interpretation of disulfiram and similar drugs on neuroendocrine function. Moreover, inhibiting DBH probably causes a build-up of dopamine that could be released instead of norepinephrine, thereby producing similar or differing effects. For example, dopamine will stimulate noradrenergic as well as dopaminergic receptors.

3. Inhibitors of Neuronal Uptake

Some agents interfere with catecholamine re-uptake by the presynaptic neuronal membrane and therefore tend to prolong and potentiate the effects of the neurotransmitter at the postsynaptic receptors. In addition, the build-up of neurotransmitter may augment feedback inhibition of transmitter release at a presynaptic site as well. Nisoxetine (Lilly 94939) appears to be relatively specific in terms of suppressing norepinephrine re-uptake. Drugs such as desmethylimipramine are somewhat less selective in that they block uptake of norepinephrine and serotonin. Imipramine seems to attenuate re-uptake of both catecholamines (norepinephrine and dopamine) as well as serotonin. Benztropine, an anticholinergic compound, and nomitensin inhibit dopamine re-uptake.

4. Receptor Agonists

Drugs can activate receptors either directly or indirectly by releasing neurotransmitter into the synaptic cleft. In the brain, apomorphine and piribidil are direct agonists for dopaminergic receptors, and clonidine is the same for noradrenergic α_2-receptors. It should be noted that receptor activation may occur at both presynaptic and postsynaptic sites. For example, the terminals of some dopaminergic and noradrenergic neurons contain presynaptic receptors that, when activated, inhibit the release of the catecholamine into the synapse. Thus, drugs may produce paradoxical effects: At low doses, apomorphine tends to act predominately on presynaptic receptors to suppress dopamine release and actually to decrease the activation of postsynaptic receptors. In contrast, at high doses, apomorphine stimulates postsynaptic receptors in the effector organ.

Indirect-acting agonists such as D-amphetamine and ephedrine not only release catecholamines but also inhibit re-uptake of catecholamines and antagonize MAO weakly. Amphetamine and ephedrine also have some direct agonist activity as well.

5. Receptor Antagonists

Antagonists of dopaminergic receptors such as pimozide, haloperidol, and butaclamol are fairly specific in their spectrum of action, but there is some evidence that pimozide may be a partial agonist. Although dibenzyline, phentolamine (α-receptor antagonists), prazosin (α_1-receptor antagonist) and propranolol (β_1- and β_2-receptor antagonist) have been clearly demonstrated to antagonize peripheral adrenergic receptors, there is a lack of rigorous evidence that these agents block central adrenoceptors in similar doses. The selective β_1-adrenoceptor antagonist, practolol, penetrates the pial-glial barrier to a lesser extent than propranolol. Thus, the neuroendocrinologist who uses these drugs should interpret the results conservatively.

6. Neurotoxins

Some drugs that are structural analogs of catecholamines can be taken up into noradrenergic and dopaminergic neurons. The adrenergic neurons concentrate 6-hydroxydopamine (6-OHDA) very effectively, and this compound or one of its metabolites damages the neuron terminal. Noradrenergic neurons are highly susceptible to this neurotoxin, as are dopaminergic neurons to a lesser extent. By giving MAO inhibitors along with 6-OHDA, one can accentuate the neurotoxicity; this occurs in part by slowing the metabolism of the drug. The specificity of 6-OHDA for dopaminergic neurons can be enhanced somewhat by coadministration of desmethylimipramine (which inhibits the uptake of 6-OHDA by noradrenergic neurons).

7. Inhibitors of Monoamine Storage and Release

Reserpine is the prototype of drugs that interfere with the granular storage of several monoamines, including norepinephrine, dopamine, and serotonin. The inability of the neuron to store catecholamines results in the intracellular degradation of the amines by MAO so that less neurotransmitter is released and more deaminated metabolites can be detected. Although reserpine can affect both central and peripheral noradrenergic neurons, there are other drugs, guanethidine and bretylium, which affect release and/or storage only in peripheral neurons. The early effect produced by guanethidine is inhibition of catecholamine release by the action potential, but chronic administration of guanethidine eventually leads to depletion of synaptic vesicles by interference with storage. Bretylium acts principally by inhibiting catecholamine release, but in large, repeated doses can produce depletion of norepinephrine. Since cholinergic neurons can influence neuroendocrine function, it should be recalled that suppression of sympathetic neuron function in an organ that is also innervated by parasympathetic (cholinergic) neurons may lead to signs of overactivity in the latter system.

D. Effects of Adrenergic Agents on the Endocrine System in Laboratory Animals and Man

I. Adrenergic Drugs and the Pituitary

1. Anterior Pituitary

The secretion of pituitary hormones, including synthesis and release, is under control of hypothalamic hormones, which in turn are controlled by neurotransmitters re-

Table 1. Actions of pharmacologic agents affecting adrenergic function

Drug	Mechanism of action	Effect on catecholamine(s)
Precursors		
Tyrosine and L-Dopa	Increases formation of catecholamines (CA)	Increased dopamine (DA) and norepinephrine (NE) levels in brain and peripheral sympathetic neurons
L-Threodihydroxyphenyl-serine (DOPS)	Increases formation of NE	Increased NE levels in peripheral sympathetic neurons and to a lesser degree in the brain
α-Methyldopa and α-Methyl-m-tyrosine	Synthesized and stored as substitute transmitter (methylated amine); also weak inhibitor of L-aromatic amino acid decarboxylase	Replaces stores of NE in brain and peripheral sympathetic neurons
Enzyme inhibitors		
α-Methyl-p-tyrosine	Inhibits the rate-limiting step of CA synthesis, tyrosine hydroxylase	Inhibits formation of DA and NE
Disulfiram	Inhibits dopamine-β-oxidase	Inhibits formation of NE
Carbidopa	Inhibits peripheral L-aromatic amino acid decarboxylase	Inhibits the conversion of dopa to DA
Pargyline	Inhibits monoamine oxidase	Increases levels of CA in neurons
Inhibitor of presynaptic uptake		
Imipramine	Inhibits re-uptake by nerve terminals	Prolongs and potentiates effects of CA at receptor; also may augment feedback inhibition of transmitting release
Inhibitors of storage		
Reserpine	Inhibits storage of CA by granules in central and peripheral neurons	Depletion of DA and NE from nerve endings
Guanethidine	Inhibits storage of CA by peripheral neurons	Depletion of NE from nerve endings
Inhibitors of release		
Guanethidine and bretylium (Clonidine?)	Inhibits release of CA by nerve action potential	Decreases availability of CA for release
Catecholaminergic nerve ending poisons		
6-Hydroxydopamine	Localizes in adrenergic nerve endings	Damages dopaminergic and noradrenergic nerve terminals
Receptor agonists (direct)		
Phenylephrine and clonidine	Stimulates α-adrenoceptor (post- and/or presynaptically)	Mimics α-receptor stimulation
Isoproterenol	Stimulates β_1- and β_2-adrenoceptors	Mimics β-receptor stimulation nonselectively
Salbutamol	Stimulates β_2-adrenoceptors predominately	Mimics β_2-receptor stimulation relatively selectively
Tazolol	Stimulates β_1-adrenoceptors predominately (partial-agonist)	Mimics β_1-receptor stimulation relatively selectively
Apomorphine and bromergocryptine	Stimulates dopaminergic receptors	Mimics dopamine receptor stimulation
Indirect and/or direct		
Amphetamines	Releases CA, blocks re-uptake	Increases NE and DA turnover; increases availability of NE and DA

leased from hypothalamic centers (DeWied and DeJong, 1974). Hypothalamic regulatory hormones (hypophysiotropes) are transported by the portal vessel to the anterior pituitary where they exert excitatory and inhibitory influences. Certain biogenic amines (in particular norepinephrine and dopamine) appear to play a crucial role in modulating secretion of anterior tropic hormones, although in some instances the biogenic amines (dopamine) may act directly on the pituitary itself (Fuxe and Hokfelt, 1969; McCann et al., 1972). The catecholamine neurotransmitters seem to exert their primary action at the hypothalamic level (median eminence) on the hypophysiotropic neurons to modulate the secretion of releasing hormone.

Changes in turnover of dopamine and norepinephrine in discrete hypothalamic nuclei after various endocrinologic and pharmacologic manipulations have given some insight concerning the role of these transmitters in endocrine function (Axelrod, 1975). Neuropharmacologic studies in experimental animals provide the most impressive support for the hypothesis that catecholamines play a fundamental role in neuroendocrine regulation.

The action of catecholamines on pituitary hormone release is still open to discussion due to indirect pharmacologic evidence. For example, dopamine has been reported both to inhibit (Müller, 1971) and stimulate (Collu et al., 1972) release of growth hormone (GH) in rats. In the dog and in the rat, dopamine appeared to inhibit release of adrenocorticotropic hormone (ACTH) (Ganong, 1972). Norepinephrine was postulated to facilitate FSH- and LH-release (Rubinstein and Sawyer, 1970), whereas dopamine inhibited LH- and FSH-release from the rat pituitary (Uemura and Kobayashi, 1974). Catecholamines are also involved in the neuroendocrine regulation of hypothalamic thyrotropin releasing factor (TRF) secretion (Grimm and Reichlin, 1973); the bulk of evidence favors participation of norepinephrine rather than dopamine in the neuroregulation of this releasing factor. Moreover, adrenergic terminals in the median eminence seem to participate in the feedback regulation of thyroxine (Kizer et al., 1974). By far the most compelling evidence for the involvement of a catecholamine in anterior pituitary hormone release is represented by the dopamine-prolactin interaction; dopamine exerts an inhibitory influence on prolactin release.

Depletion of catecholamines by reserpine in rats elevated the plasma levels of ACTH and corticosterone (Maickel et al., 1961), blocked ovulation and ovarian compensatory hypertrophy (Myerson and Sawyer, 1968; Müller et al., 1972), and prevented cold-induced elevations of plasma thyrotropin TSH (Kotani et al., 1973). Inhibition of catecholamine synthesis by α-methyl-p-tyrosine produced similar effects.

Adrenergic systems are also important in neuroendocrine regulation in man. Oral administration of L-Dopa, the precursor of both dopamine and norepinephrine, caused a prompt increase in plasma GH and inhibition of prolactin. These effects are so pronounced that L-Dopa has been used as a test agent for secretory reserve in pituitary failure. Administration of clonidine, a noradrenergic receptor stimulating agent, is also effective in releasing GH in both humans and subhuman primates.

a) Prolactin

Prolactin (PRL) is released in response to suckling (Gautvik et al., 1973), physical and emotional stress (Noel et al., 1972), arginine infusion (Frantz, 1973), hypoglycemia (Frantz, 1973), and estrogen administration (Macleod, 1975). Although many stimuli can release PRL, secretion is tonicly inhibited by the hypothalamus.

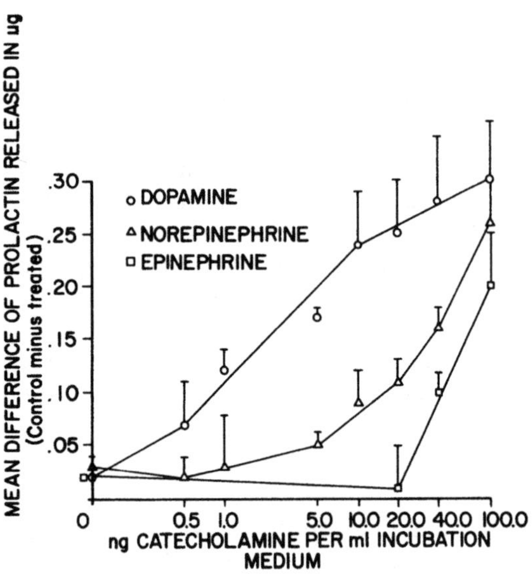

Fig. 1. Dose-response curves for the inhibition of prolactin secretion by catecholamines. Reproduced, with permission, from CLEMENS (1976)

Thus, PRL secretion is increased by any process that interferes with hypothalamus-pituitary continuity. Extensive evidence indicates that dopamine is important in the control of PRL in animals and in man (CLEMENS et al., 1974; MACLEOD, 1975; MEITES et al. 1972).

Neuropharmacologic studies have demonstrated that drugs which stimulate dopaminergic receptors generally inhibit PRL (LU and MEITES, 1973; OJEDA and MCCANN, 1973). One of the major controversies is whether dopamine acts directly to inhibit prolactin release or indirectly through the release of prolactin inhibitory factor (PIF). An infusion of dopamine or norepinephrine into the hypophysial portal vessels in the rat significantly suppressed serum PRL levels in a dose-related manner, which suggests that catecholamines can inhibit PRL release by a direct action (TAKAHARA et al., 1974). Pretreatment with L-Dopa effectively blocked the PRL response to suckling (MEITES, 1977) and to TRH, suggesting an effect also at the pituitary level (NOEL et al., 1973).

Other evidence is consistent with the suggestion that dopamine acts to release PIF. Injection of dopamine into the third ventricle of rats produced a lowering of plasma prolactin as did an injection of apomorphine, a relatively specific dopamine receptor stimulating agent. Implantation of the dopamine receptor blocking drug, pimozide, in the median eminence produced a rapid rise in PRL presumably by inhibiting the discharge of PIF. Thus, activation of dopaminergic receptors may inhibit PRL release directly as well as indirectly by releasing PIF.

As alluded to above, drugs that block dopamine receptors, such as pimozide, D-butaclamol, and lergotrile, tend to increase prolactin levels (DICKERMAN et al., 1972; CLEMENS et al., 1974). Large doses of neuroleptic drugs, such as chlorpromazine and haloperidol, which have dopamine receptor blocking activity, may induce excessive PRL release (FRANTZ and SUH, 1974). This can be a practical problem in the long-

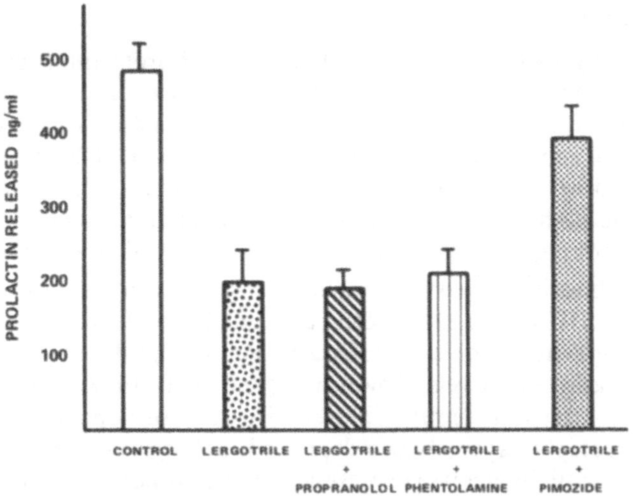

Fig. 2. Effects of various adrenoceptor antagonists on the ability of lergotrile mesylate (a dopaminergic receptor agonist) to inhibit prolactin release. Reproduced, with permission, from CLEMENS (1976)

term management of chronic schizophrenia. Moreover, drugs that depress levels of catecholamines in the brain, such as reserpine, tetrabenazine or α-methyl-p-tyrosine, facilitate the secretion of PRL (COPPOLA, 1965). Pretreatment of animals with an MAO inhibitor, such as iproniazid, which elevates brain catecholamine levels, protects against the effects of reserpine (LIPPMAN, 1967).

In humans, an oral dose of L-Dopa will produce a transient lowering of prolactin both in normal individuals and in many of those with pathological elevations of the hormone (KAMBERI et al., 1971; MALARKEY et al., 1971; FRIESEN et al., 1972). Chronic suppression of plasma PRL by L-Dopa has been tried in patients with metastatic breast cancer, but the effect is short-lived and the drug must be given every 3–4 h for optimum results (FRANTZ et al., 1972). Combinations of small doses of L-Dopa with peripheral dopa decarboxylase inhibitors, e.g., carbidopa, markedly lowered plasma PRL levels (FRANTZ and SUH, 1974). In contrast, carbidopa given alone elevated PRL levels in normal subjects presumably by blocking dopamine synthesis in neurons of the median eminence that lie outside the pial-glial barrier (GARFINKEL et al., 1977).

Suppression of PRL secretion by ergot derivatives has been demonstrated in rats (MEITES et al., 1972) and in humans (DEL POZO et al., 1972). Following an early observation that ergotamine inhibited luteotropic function in the rat, a number of derivatives were tested as inhibitors of lactation. A relatively new synthetic ergot derivative, 2-bromo-α-ergocryptine (bromoergocryptine) has been demonstrated to suppress abnormal PRL-induced lactation in humans (DEL POZO et al., 1972). This agent appears to act as a dopamine receptor stimulator and will lower plasma PRL within 1–2 months in almost all cases, including many patients with pituitary tumors. The suppressive effect of bromoergocryptine on PRL is more prolonged than that of L-Dopa, and therefore it has definite therapeutic potential. Bromoergocryptine is presently being used extensively to treat amenorrhea caused by excessive PRL secretion.

b) Growth Hormone

The secretion of growth hormone (GH), like that of prolactin, is precisely regulated by a complex interaction of excitatory and inhibitory neural influences (Krulich et al., 1972; Martin, 1972). Aminergic neurons control a dual system of hypothalamic hypophysiotropic hormones, one of which is inhibitory (GH-RIH, or SRIF, somatostatin) and the other, excitatory (GH-RH) for growth hormone release. At least three monoaminergic pathways are involved in GH regulation: noradrenergic, dopaminergic, and serotonergic. Only the adrenergic systems will be considered here.

Following the initial observation that ventricular injection of norepinephrine depleted pituitary GH content (Müller et al., 1968), evidence has accumulated that brain monoamines are involved in GH secretion; similar doses of dopamine were ineffective in elevating GH levels. However, Collu et al. (1972) reported that GH hormone levels fell after intraventricular administration of dopamine. Apomorphine, a dopaminergic receptor agonist, also depressed GH secretion in the rat. Kato et al. (1973) observed a slight increase in plasma GH after systemic administration of either phentolamine, methylamphetamine, isoproterenol, or chlorpromazine. No increase was detected in response to L-Dopa, the immediate precursor of dopamine, in rats. Müller et al. (1973) demonstrated that administration of FLA 63, a dopamine β-hydroxylase inhibitor, as well as L-Dopa into rats pretreated with α-methyl-p-tyrosine lowered immunoreactive GH. This led Müller to postulate that GH secretion is under dual aminergic control: an α-adrenergic component that stimulates and a dopaminergic component that inhibits the secretion of GH. Selective chemical destruction of noradrenergic and dopaminergic neuron endings by 6-OHDA was accompanied by a clear reduction in plasma GH (Müller et al., 1976). Likewise, functional blockade of noradrenergic and dopaminergic neuron function by α-methyl-p-tyrosine reduced plasma GH. These results suggest that both adrenergic neurotransmitters, norepinephrine and dopamine, are involved in GH secretion. In fact, protection of brain norepinephrine depletion by pretreatment with desmethylimipramine only partially counteracted but did not prevent the GH-lowering effect of 6-OHDA.

There is substantial evidence that norepinephrine is the principal mediator of L-Dopa-induced rises in GH level (Lovinger et al., 1976). This is based on several lines of evidence: (1) Clonidine and phenylephrine, both α-adrenoceptor agonists, stimulate GH release in the dog; (2) Intraventricular administration of α-adrenoceptor blocking drugs, phenoxybenzamine and phentolamine, inhibited the elevation in GH caused by L-Dopa and clonidine; (3) Blockade of central β-adrenoceptors with propranolol facilitated the GH response to L-Dopa.

Administration of α-methyl-p-tyrosine to rats resulted in marked suppression of episodic GH secretion (Durand et al., 1977). In the same study, clonidine, an agonist for α-adrenoceptors in the brain, produced marked elevation of GH levels whereas the dopaminergic agonist, apomorphine, had no effect. These data were interpreted as indicating a possible interaction between endogenous catecholamines and hypothalamic release and release-inhibiting factors for control of GH secretion.

In conscious cats, intravenous infusion of L-Dopa (20 mg/kg) increased plasma GH, hydrocortisone, and glucose (Ruch et al., 1977). Inhibition of peripheral aromatic amino acid decarboxylase by L-α-hydrazino-methyldopa abolished only L-Dopa-included hyperglycemia, indicating that CNS stimulation by newly synthesized catecholamines caused some of the endocrine changes. Since phenoxybenzamine but not pimozide pretreatment abolished GH release after L-Dopa, an α-adrenoceptor mechanism was implicated. Microinjection of norepinephrine into the preoptic anterior hypothalamus and medial hypothalamus raised GH levels, which is in agreement with α-adrenoceptor mediation. Amine depletion by administration of α-methyl-p-tyrosine did not alter basal GH levels but elevated hydrocortisone levels.

A role of α-adrenoceptors in secretory control of GH is supported by other experimental evidence in higher primates and humans. CHAMBERS and BROWN (1976) reported that systemic administration of clonidine and DL-DOPS (dihydroxyphenylserine, the immediate precursor of norepinephrine) induced an increase of plasma GH levels in rhesus monkeys. Moreover, microinjection of norepinephrine into or near the vicinity of the ventromedial nucleus of baboons induced a release of GH (TOIVOLA and GALE, 1972). This latter observation suggests the possibility that catecholamine receptor agonists and antagonists can act at a hypothalamic level to modulate excitatory or inhibitory releasing factors for GH. It seems, therefore, that the control of GH secretion in rats, dogs, and subhuman primates involves a mechanism that includes modulation by α-adrenoceptor activity. However, it is important to note that species do seem to differ with respect to GH release induced by some adrenergic drugs. For example, in the monkey and dog L-Dopa elevated GH levels, whereas in the rat GH levels were depressed by L-Dopa administration.

Reports from studies utilizing humans also indicate that many stimuli cause GH release via central α-adrenoceptors. In man, GH release evoked by insulin-induced hypoglycemia, arginine, exercise, ADH, L-Dopa, and stress, such as surgery, are all suppressed by phentolamine, an α-adrenoceptor antagonist (MARTIN, 1973; VIGAS et al., 1977). Moreover, GH release occurred after infusion of epinephrine and propranolol but not after epinephrine alone (MASSARA and STRUMIA, 1970). On the other hand, the β-adrenoceptor agonist, isoproterenol, has been reported to inhibit GH release (HEIDINGSFELDER and BLACKARD, 1968). Propranolol, a β-receptor blocker, enhanced GH release induced by glucagon, ADH, and L-Dopa. Pharmacologic blockade of GH release by chlorpromazine, pimozide, and haloperidol suggests that GH release in man is facilitated by activation of central dopaminergic receptors perhaps at the level of the hypothalamus. In fact, subemetic doses of the dopaminergic receptor agonist, apomorphine, also released GH, suggesting that there may be a dopaminergic control mechanism in man that is independent of norepinephrine (LAL et al., 1975).

In addition to serving as basic research tools, adrenergic drugs are also clinically useful. These agents can be used to diagnose and in some cases to treat disorders of GH secretion. Direct or indirect stimulants of dopaminergic receptors are capable of eliciting GH secretion in normal subjects, whereas these same drugs consistently inhibit high plasma GH levels in many acromegalic subjects. Dopaminergic drugs, L-Dopa (either alone or in combination with carbidopa) and apomorphine, have been used to test for GH secretory reserve, especially in children. Activation of dopaminergic receptors at the hypothalamic and/or pituitary level produces a "paradoxical" reduction in elevated levels of GH in the plasma of some acromegalics. For example, L-Dopa produced a short-lasting depression of GH in 19 out of 35 patients with acromegaly (MÜLLER et al., 1976). Likewise, apomorphine given in subemetic doses, also lowered GH in acromegalics. Bromoergocryptine, another dopaminergic receptor agonist, produced significant suppression of excessive GH and PRL secretion

(CAMANNI et al., 1977). Up to 60%–80% of acromegalics experience a dramatic fall in GH and improvement of clinical symptoms with bromoergocryptine. This drug is currently used in acromegalics in whom surgery or radiation has failed to produce definitive results. Thus, long-acting dopaminergic receptor stimulant drugs seem to provide a new, safe, and effective approach for the treatment of acromegaly.

c) Gonadotropins

Neural control of pituitary-gonad function has been demonstrated by basic research efforts and by the clinical effects of disease of the hypothalamus, emotional stress, psychopharmacologic drugs, and electroshock therapy. Two adrenergic neuronal systems arrive in the median eminence of the hypothalamic region: a noradrenergic system coming from the lower brain stem (ANDEN et al., 1966) to the rostral area and a dopaminergic tuberoinfundibular system to the caudal region (FUXE, 1965). Dopamine content in the hypothalamus seems to fluctuate during the estrous cycle (FUXE et al., 1967) and is diminished by castration in male and female animals (FUXE et al., 1976). Thus, both dopamine and norepinephrine seem to modulate secretion of gonadotropins. A third adrenergic system may also be present. Localization studies have indicated large numbers of nerve terminals containing epinephrine and phenylethylamine-*N*-methyl transferase (PNMT) in the median eminence, suggesting that epinephrine may also be involved in neuroendocrine control of gonadotropin secretion (HOKFELT et al., 1974).

The two hormones of the pituitary responsible for regulation of the gonads are follicle-stimulating hormone (FSH) and luteinizing hormone (LH) (MCCANN, 1974); together these hormones are refered to as gonadotropins. There are actually three groups of hormones involved in the pituitary-gonad relationship: (1) the hypothalamic hypophysiotropic hormones, such as luteinizing hormone-releasing hormone (LHRH); (2) the gonadotropins, LH and FSH; and (3) the gonadal hormones, estrogens, progestins, and androgens. Only the hypophysiotropic hormones and gonadotropins will be considered in this section.

Basal levels of gonadotropin secretion appear to be dependent on tonic hypothalamic influences from the medial tuberohypophysial system. There is considerable evidence obtained from laboratory animals that suggests that the hypophysiotropic neurons which release LHRH are in turn regulated by biogenic amines (MCCANN, 1974). SAWYER et al. (1947) demonstrated that the α-adrenoceptor antagonist, dibenamine, could inhibit ovulation; this was the pioneering work in adrenergic control of gonadotropin release. In recent studies it has been possible to measure the release of both FSH and LH in both in vivo and in vitro studies in order to determine more precisely the modulatory role of catecholamines.

In vitro incubation of catecholamines with pituitaries had very little effect on gonadotropins, but when ventral hypothalami were incubated together with anterior lobes of pituitary glands, dopamine was observed to increase both FSH (KAMBERI et al., 1970) and LH (SCHNEIDER and MCCANN, 1969a). These results suggest that catecholamines were probably producing their effect by way of gonadotropin-releasing factors from the ventral hypothalamic fragments. Dose-related gonadotropin release by dopamine was prevented by the α-receptor antagonist phentolamine, and by the dopamine receptor antagonist haloperidol. Moreover, the addition of the biogenic amine depleting agent reserpine to the in vitro system likewise suppressed the releasing effect of dopamine, which suggested that dopamine was active only after uptake and re-release from neurons (SCHNEIDER and MCCANN, 1969b). It is conceivable that dopamine itself was active or that it underwent conversion to norepinephrine, which served as the active agent.

In contrast, FUXE et al. (1976) have presented evidence of the existence of an inhibitory dopaminergic mechanism in the median eminence on LH secretion. The reduction in LH secretion and blockage of ovulation produced by a dopamine receptor agonist, ET-495[1-(2″-pyrimidyl)-4-piperonylpiperazine] and ergoconine, could be counteracted by pimozide, a dopamine receptor blocking agent. These results indicate the possibility that in rats there exists an inhibitory mechanism mediated by dopamine in the median eminence and a facilitatory norepinephrine mechanism in the hypothalamus for the control of LHRH secretion. In a recent study using rabbits, SAWYER et al. (1974) reported that intraventricular dopamine suppressed the increase in plasma LH produced by subsequent intraventricular injection of norepinephrine.

Catecholamines also may be involved in the negative feedback of estradiol on LH secretion. The releasing action of dopamine was blocked by estradiol in an in vitro system (SCHNEIDER and MCCANN, 1970b). Since the blockade could be prevented by inhibitors of protein synthesis, puromycin or cyclohexamide, this raises the possibility that at least part of the negative feedback of estrogens on gonadotropin secretion might be mediated by a system which attenuates the action of dopamine on the hormone-releasing neuron. On the other hand, FUXE et al. (1976) suggest that the inhibitory feedback control of LHRH by estrogens is at least partly exerted at the hypothalamic level by activation of the tuberoinfundibular dopaminergic neurons that inhibit LH secretion and by inactivation of the hypothalamic noradrenergic system that stimulates LH secretion. The effects of Fuxe's group were observed in castrated female rats and in prepubertal rats treated with pregnant mare serum.

The excitatory influence of dopamine on FSH, LH, and LHRH secretion in vitro reported by MCCANN's group (1969; 1970) was confirmed in vivo (SCHNEIDER and MCCANN, 1970). In the female, the hormonal condition appeared to modify the response to dopamine; i.e., the catecholamine was ineffective in ovariectomized rats and in rats in estrus. Thus estrogen and progesterone seem to determine the response to dopamine (SCHNEIDER and MCCANN, 1970). Reports of the relative activity of epinephrine, norepinephrine, and dopamine in releasing LH seem to vary. Once again the comparisons of activity were performed in female rats that were in differing stages of estrus (KAMBERI et al., 1969; RUBINSTEIN and SAWYER, 1970a) and this may account for the discordant results.

Of the adrenoceptor antagonists, the α-adrenoceptor antagonists produce the most consistent effects. In laboratory animals, such as the rat and monkey, phentolamine can inhibit the postcastration rise in gonadotropins (OJEDA and MCCANN, 1973) and the pulsatile release of LH in ovariectomized monkeys (BHATTACHARYA et al., 1972). These results are consistent with the first report by SAWYER et al. (1947).

Another approach used to examine the function of endogenous adrenergic mediators on gonadotripin secretion has been to alter catecholamine synthesis. Inhibition of the rate-limiting enzyme in catecholamine synthesis, tyrosine hydroxylase, attenuated the postcastration rise in gonadotropins. The suppression by α-methyl-p-tyrosine could be partially reversed by administration of the dopamine precursor, L-Dopa, and the norepinephrine precursor, dihydroxyphenylserine (DOPS) (OJEDA and

McCANN, 1973). Similarly, pretreatment with α-methyl-p-tyrosine inhibited the stimulatory effect of estrogen and progesterone on gonadotropin release in estrogen-primed rats (KALRA et al., 1972) and the preovulatory discharge of gonadotropins (KALRA and McCANN, 1974). Likewise, administration of a dopamine β-hydroxylase inhibitor, diethyldithiocarbamate, led to an interference with gonadotropin release in a variety of states (KALRA et al., 1972; OJEDA andMcCANN, 1973). Partial or complete restoration of gonadotropin release was attained by reinitiating norepinephrine production with DOPS, thereby circumventing the synthesis block.

Drugs, such as reserpine (a catecholamine-depleting agent) and chlorpromazine (a drug with complex effects on the autonomic and central nervous systems, including α- and dopaminergic receptor blockade) can interfere with ovulation (BARRACLOUGH and SAWYER, 1955), induce pseudopregnancy (BARRACLOUGH and SAWYER, 1957), and interfere in the sexual differentiation of the hypothalamus (LADOSKY et al., 1970).

Despite numerous observations in laboratory animals, some of which are controversial, there is little evidence available to indicate a role for catecholamines in control of FSH and LH secretion in man. Acute administration of L-Dopa, apomorphine, or clonidine has little or no effect on either hormone. However, LEBLANC et al. (1976) demonstrated recently that dopamine infusions (4 μg · kg · min) had an inhibitory effect on LH release. These results were interpreted as indicating that dopamine may normally serve to modulate the effect of LHRH at the level of the pituitary as well as inhibit the release of LHRH at the hypothalamic level.

In females, psychotropic drugs, such as the phenothiazines and reserpine (which produce their beneficial effects by altering adrenergic function in the brain), may also cause drug-induced amenorrhea. In general, any agent that interferes with central catecholamine function can have this effect. These drugs presumably alter control of LHRH and prolactin by virtue of a change in central adrenergic neuron function.

d) Adrenocorticotropic Hormone and Beta-Melanocyte Stimulating Hormone

Adrenocorticotropic hormone (ACTH) released from the anterior lobe of the pituitary gland is the primary governor of the adrenal cortex. The median eminence of the tuber cinereum is the final common pathway through which neural control of ACTH is exerted (FORTIER, 1966). Both excitatory and inhibitory control of ACTH secretion reside in the hypothalamus but probably in different areas. Total disconnection of the hypothalamus from the rest of the brain will eliminate some adrenal responses (e.g., diurnal rhythm and response to stress) but not the response to ether (KENDALL, 1971). This indicates that chemical agents and some forms of stress may act directly on the pituitary. Release of ACTH is strongly controlled by feedback effects. Removal or spontaneous degenerative disease of the adrenal glands leads to a marked rise in ACTH, whereas the administration of cortisol depresses ACTH secretion.

Corticotropin releasing factor (CRF) is released from peptidergic neurons and then acts on the pituitary to release ACTH. The secretion of CRF is regulated by a complex set of neurotransmitter neurons that includes three stimulatory components (cholinergic, adrenergic, and serotonergic) and another adrenergic component which is inhibitory (MARTIN et al., 1977). The pharmacologic analysis of neurotransmitter control of CRF-ACTH secretion has proven to be more difficult than the other anterior pituitary hormone systems. This is due in part to the number of different neuronal systems involved and to the participation of both excitatory and inhibitory adrenergic neurons in ACTH release (HIROSHIGE and ABE, 1973). The other complication exists within the control of the system itself; i.e., there are hypothalamic and extrahypothalamic influences on CRF secretion, and these are in turn influenced by "long-, short-, and ultrashort-loop" feedback systems.

Another problem is that some experiments are designed to study the effects of alteration in the content and biological actions of endogenous catecholamines whereas others have been directed towards studying the effects of administration of exogenous catecholamines. The administration of exogenous catecholamines stimulate ACTH release by central and perhaps even peripheral mechanisms (GANONG et al., 1971). On the other hand, hypothalamic catecholamines tonically inhibit CRF secretion. Administration of drugs that enhance catecholamine release or action (amphetamine or pargyline, a MAO inhibitor) inhibited stress-induced ACTH secretion (GANONG et al., 1971). Pretreatment with pargyline also prevented the effects of reserpine on both ACTH release and depletion of CRF that follows reserpine treatment (BHATTACHARYA and MARKS, 1969). Moreover, intraventricular administration of norepinephrine inhibited the ACTH hypersecretion produced by reserpine pretreatment (MARKS et al., 1970).

As with other pituitary hormones, there are species differences in the effects of various drugs on ACTH secretion. In the rat, a wide variety of adrenergic drugs blocked ACTH release in response to further stresses (BHATTACHARYA and MARKS, 1969). The dog differs from the rat in its response to chlorpromazine in that the dog responded to this neuroleptic drug by increasing ACTH and developing adrenal hypertrophy (BETZ and GANONG, 1963).

Infusion of epinephrine and norepinephrine directly into the basal hypothalamus caused prompt release of ACTH from the pituitary (KITAY et al., 1959; VERNIKOS-DANELLIS and MARKS, 1962). KRIEGER and KRIEGER (1970) showed that implantation of norepinephrine into certain areas of the rat brain acutely increased plasma levels of corticosteroids, thus demonstrating indirectly a stimulatory effect on ACTH secretion. Intravenous administration of L-Dopa clearly enhanced the response of plasma ACTH to metyrapone in monkeys (HSU et al., 1976).

On the other hand, suppression of endogenous catecholamine effects brought about by reserpine (a depletor), by chlorpromazine (an α-receptor antagonist), or by α-methyl-p-tyrosine (an inhibitor of catecholamine synthesis) also resulted in elevated ACTH and cortisol in rat and dog (VAN LOON, 1974). Maneuvers such as inhibition of dopamine-β-oxidase that deplete the hypothalamus of norepinephrine but not of dopamine caused a rise in plasma corticosterone in the rat, indicating that the inhibitory adrenergic pathway is probably noradrenergic. The inhibitory adrenergic effect appears related to stress responses rather than to control of resting (basal) output.

Evidence concerning the role of catecholamines in ACTH regulation in human subjects is inconclusive. In most studies ACTH release was unaffected by acute administration of L-Dopa. Likewise, L-Dopa was ineffective in treating elevated ACTH levels in Cushing's disease (KRIEGER, 1973). α-Adrenoceptor stimulants evoked an increase in plasma ACTH and cortisol in man. Blockade of β-adrenoceptors augmented the ACTH response to hypoglycemia. These results have been interpreted to mean that α-receptor stimulation elicits ACTH release whereas β-receptor activation is inhibitory in man (MARTIN et al., 1977).

At least one clinical study reports that the combination of long-term, large-dose reserpine treatment supplemented with pituitary irradication was very effective in treating Cushing's disease (MIURA et al., 1975). As indicated, the remission rate was high (18 out of 19 patients), and the remission was sufficient to allow the patients to return to their normal lives without further medication. Thus, the biogenic amine depleting agent reserpine appears to be a valuable component of a therapeutic measure for treatment of Cushing's disease.

Most ACTH-secreting cells also secrete melanophore-stimulating hormone or β-lipotropin. As with ACTH, the role of catecholamines in melanophore-stimulating hormone (MSH) release is contradictory. It has been reported that MSH release is inhibited by catecholamines (ITURRIZA and KASAL-ITURRIZA, 1972). However, a more recent report indicates that catecholamines can both stimulate and inhibit MSH from the rat and frog pituitary in vitro and do so through classical adrenoceptor mechanisms (BOWER et al., 1974). In this study, MSH release from the frog pituitary was completely inhibited by epinephrine, norepinephrine, and dopamine at 10^{-5} *M*, but at lower concentrations (10^{-6} to 10^{-7} *M*), epinephrine stimulated release of MSH. Phenylephrine at a high concentration (10^{-4} *M*) also inhibited MSH secretion from both frog and rat pituitaries. The β-adrenoceptor stimulant isoproterenol stimulated MSH release and counteracted the inhibitory effect of phenylephrine. Administration of the α-adrenoceptor blocking drugs dihydroergotamine and dibenamine antagonized the inhibition of MSH by epinephrine. Propranolol, a β-adrenoceptor antagonist, blocked the stimulation of MSH release by isoproterenol. Based upon this evidence, it was suggested that dopaminergic receptors and perhaps α-adrenoceptors may provide the mechanism for the primary inhibitory control of β-MSH release, but the precise role of β-adrenoceptors is unclear.

Thus, the role of catecholamines in the control of ACTH and MSH release in human subjects and laboratory animals is unresolved. Contradictory evidence indicates that catecholamines may have an inhibitory, an excitatory, or no role in ACTH secretion.

e) Thyroid-Stimulating Hormone

The pituitary-thyroid axis serves as the "textbook" example of a negative-feedback, self-regulatory system (HOSKINS, 1949). Three groups of hormones participate in controlling thyroid function: (1) Hypothalamic thyrotropin-releasing hormone (TRH) stimulates the synthesis and release of thyrotropin [thyroid-stimulating hormone, (TSH)] by the pituitary thyrotrope; (2) TSH, in turn, activates iodide uptake, hormonogenesis, and release of the thyroid hormones thyroxine (T4) and triiodothyronine (T3); (3) the circulating thyroid hormones T3 and T4 exert a negative-feedback effect at the pituitary level. The primary control of TSH secretion is determined by the stimulatory effects of TRH. Within the hypothalamus, bioaminergic neurons influence peptidergic neurons, which in turn release TRH (MARTIN et al., 1977). Thus, the hypothalamus tonically drives TSH secretion under basal conditions.

The present knowledge of the role of central adrenergic systems in the regulation of TRH and TSH secretion is still quite limited and controversial. GRIMM and REICHLIN (1973) observed that dopamine and norepinephrine released pulse-labeled TRH from mouse hypothalamic tissue in vitro and that dopamine-induced TRH was inhibited when conversion of dopamine to norepinephrine was blocked by disulfiram, an inhibitor of dopamine-β-oxidase. From these experiments it was concluded that adrenergic neurotransmitters may function in a regulatory manner to control synthesis and/or release of TRH.

COLEONI (1972) observed a decrease in thyroid activity in rats treated with high doses of α-methyl-p-tyrosine or α-methyldopa; however, guanethidine, a peripherally acting catecholamine depleting agent, produced a similar effect. Along these lines, TUOMISTO et al. (1975) have postulated a stimulatory role for the hypothalamic adrenergic system in cold-induced release of TSH. However, there are many unanswered questions regarding the pituitary-thyroid axis and thyroid hormone-catecholamine interaction in the adaptation to chronic cold.

More recent results have shown that TRH release from the hypothalamus, as reflected by changes in serum TSH, is linked with the activity of the central noradrenergic system (KRULICH et al., 1977). Central noradrenergic neurons appear to provide the drive for the tonic release of TRH in resting conditions as well as serving as the stimulus for the phasic release during exposure to cold. Inhibition of norepinephrine synthesis, which is followed by depletion of brain catecholamine levels, was associated with a decrease of serum TSH levels. Specific inhibitors of dopamine-β-oxidase, diethyldithiocarbamate, and bis(4-methyl-1-homopiperazinyl-thiocarbanyl) disulfite (FLA-63) depleted only norepinephrine and caused a striking decrease of serum TSH. Pretreatment with α-methyl-p-tyrosine produced a depletion of both norepinephrine and dopamine and a gradual decline in serum TSH levels. The centrally and peripherally acting α-adrenoceptor agonist clonidine increased serum TSH. Stimulation of dopamine receptors with apomorphine produced a dose-related and rapid decline in TSH secretion. L-Dopa also decreased the TSH response to cold. From these and

Table 2. Drugs affecting adrenergic function and anterior pituitary secretion[a]

Drug	Growth Hormone	Prolactin	Gonadotropin	TSH	ACTH
L-Dopa	↑	↓	→	Blocks response to TRH and cold stress	→
α-Methyl-p-tyrosine	↓	↑	Blocks ovulation	Cold stress ↓	↑
Carbidopa	→	↑	?	→	→
Disulfiram	↑	↓	?	?	?
Reserpine	↓	↑	Blocks ovulation	?	↑
Tricyclic antidepressants	↓	↑	→	→	→
Apomorphine ε Bromergocryptine	↑	↓	→	→	→
Clonidine	↑	→	→	→	→
Amphetamine	↑	↑	?	?	→
Isoproterenol	↓	→	?	?	?
Pimozide ε Haloperidol	↓	↑	Blocks ovulation ↓	→	→
Propranolol	↑	→	→	→	↑

[a] Key: ↑ (*increase*); ↓ (*decrease*); → (*no effect*); ? (*unknown*)

other data it was concluded that a central α-adrenoceptor system mediates an excitatory mechanism for TSH secretion, whereas the dopaminergic system is inhibitory.

The evidence for a role of catecholamines in the control of TRH and TSH secretion in man is tentative. Chronic L-Dopa administration is reported to interfere with TSH release induced by TRH, suggesting an effect of L-Dopa at the pituitary level (MARTIN et al., 1977). This effect of L-Dopa may be related to dopamine, the intravenous administration of which also interferes with TRH-induced TSH release. Bromoergocryptine, another dopaminergic receptor agonist, is reported to alter TSH release by TRH and to lower elevated basal TSH levels in some hypothyroid patients (MIYAI et al., 1974).

Administration of the dopaminergic receptor blocking drug metoclopramide has been reported to release TSH in hypothyroid patients; this is not evident in euthyroid subjects (SCANLON et al., 1977). These results were suggestive of inhibitory dopaminergic control of TSH release in man. Adrenoceptor blocking drugs, such as phentolamine (an α-adrenoceptor antagonist) and propranolol (a β-adrenoceptor antagonist), are reported to have no effect on TSH secretion induced by TRH administration.

2. Posterior Pituitary

Plasma osmolarity and effective circulating blood volume are regulated by homeostatic mechanisms, which regulate the excretion and intake of water and salt. The control of free-water clearance by the kidney is controlled in part by the secretion of antidiuretic hormone (ADH), vasopressin, from the posterior pituitary. ADH exerts its actions by influencing reabsorption of water in the distal tubule of the kidney. The function of the posterior pituitary (or neurohypophysis) is dependent upon the supraoptic-hypophysial and paraventricular-hypophysial nerve tracts (BISSET et al., 1971; HAYWARD, 1975), which originate in the hypothalamic area.

In addition to direct osmotic control of ADH by osmoceptors, there is evidence that cholinergic and adrenergic inputs to the magnocellular neurons influence cellular activity and mediate reflex control of secretion (BARKER et al., 1971: MOSS et al., 1971). Whereas cholinergic drugs stimulated ADH release, adrenergic drugs, e.g., norepinephrine, effectively caused inhibition of ADH release (MOSS et al., 1971). Systemic administration of epinephrine or norepinephrine may cause inhibition of ADH release predominately by effects mediated through peripheral baroceptor mechanisms. Central adrenergic mechanisms also seem to be important because centrally administered catecholamines also influence ADH release. Moreover, anatomic studies have shown that noradrenergic fibers terminate directly on neurons of supraoptic and paraventricular nuclei. Direct iontophoresis of putative adrenergic neurotransmitters upon cells of the supraoptic nuclei have provided additional evidence that dopamine and norepinephrine reduced the activity of these cells in the cat (BARKER et al., 1971). The inhibition of activity was blocked by β-adrenergic blocking drugs. In keeping with the suggestion that adrenergic control of ADH secretion is inhibitory, is the observation that chlorpromazine, a drug with adrenergic receptor blocking properties, can produce inappropriate ADH secretion (MARTIN et al., 1977). This possibility should be considered in patients with unexplained hyponatremia who are receiving neuroleptic drugs.

In contrast to the previous studies, others have reported that dopamine, in graded concentrations, caused dose-related increases in neurohypophysial hormone release from the hypothalamus in vitro (BRIDGES et al., 1976). The preparation used contained the supraoptic nuclei, paraventricular nuclei, median eminence, and proximal pituitary stalk. In similar doses, both dopamine and norepinephrine injected into the lateral cerebral ventricles of the brain of the anesthetized, hydrated, lactating rat caused the release of arginine-vasopressin and oxytocin. Apomorphine also released both hormones but was less potent and had less intrinsic activity than the catecholamines. Dopamine- and norepinephrine-induced hormone release could be suppressed by prior administration of their respective antagonists, haloperidol or phentolamine. In contrast, pimozide, a relatively more selective antagonist of dopamine receptors, completely inhibited the hormone release due to dopamine and apomorphine but not that due to norepinephrine. From these results it was concluded that release of neurohypophysial hormones can be stimulated by a dopaminergic pathway in addition to a cholinergic one. Moreover, it was suggested that the hormonal response to stimulation of osmoceptors may be modulated by a dopaminergic mechanism.

Intravenous infusion of norepinephrine increased renal excretion of water in human subjects (SMYTHE et al., 1952; BALDWIN et al., 1963; FISHER, 1968) and animals (LIBERMAN et al., 1970; KLEIN et al., 1971; SCHRIER and BERL, 1974). However, the mechanism of this renal effect of catecholamines is incompletely understood. Some studies suggested that norepinephrine can oppose the effect of ADH at the renal tubule whereas others suggested that water diuresis could be due to suppression of endogenous ADH as had been demonstrated in dogs. Recently it was demonstrated that infusion of norepinephrine at rates of 0.2 or 0.3 μg/kg·min suppressed ADH levels in human subjects (SHIMAMOTO and MIYAHARA, 1976). These authors proposed that norepinephrine-induced diuresis is related in part to the suppression of ADH release.

II. Adrenergic Drugs and the Pineal

The pineal organ synthesizes and releases melatonin and perhaps other hormones in response to norepinephrine, the postganglionic neurotransmitter released from sympathetic nerves. In this sense, the pineal organ is a neuroendocrine transducer like the adrenal medulla; i.e., both organs convert a neural input into an endocrine output (WURTMAN and AXELROD, 1965). Thus, the pineal is not a true endocrine organ like the adrenal cortex. Light activation of retinal photoceptors is a primary mechanism for control of pineal activity, and certain portions of the light spectrum inhibit pineal activity. The primary function of melatonin released from the pineal appears to be suppression of female and male gonadal function, presumably by an action on the brain. For example, melatonin can suppress LHRH-induced LH release.

Although environmental light is the major controlling factor in melatonin release, the major neuronal input controlling melatonin synthesis is norepinephrine released from postganglionic sympathetic nerves (TAYLOR and WILSON, 1970). Likewise any generalized stress (e.g., hypoglycemia or forced immobilization) that releases epinephrine will likewise activate the pineal. Increased sympathetic activity can override the inhibiting effect of light; this fact has led to the suggestion that perhaps melatonin is a stress hormone like ACTH, PRL, and ADH.

Norepinephrine and epinephrine are believed to activate pineal cells by way of the β-adrenoceptor and the adenylyl cyclase system. Drugs that activate noradrenergic receptors either directly or indirectly can also accelerate melatonin synthesis (KLEIN and WELLER, 1970). As one might expect, the activities of the melatonin-forming enzymes, SNAT (serotonin-*N*-acetyltransferase) and HIOMT (hydroxyindole-*O*-methyltransferase), are increased by norepinephrine and L-Dopa (DEGUCHI and AXELROD, 1972). Cocaine, an inhibitor of norepinephrine reuptake, also increased SNAT activity (HOLZ et al., 1972). It should be noted that in addition to stimulating melatonin synthesis, that synthesis of its precursor, serotonin, is also increased by L-norepinephrine in pineal culture systems (WURTMAN et al., 1971). Any number of compounds that are structurally related to L-norepinephrine—i.e., D-norepinephrine, L-epinephrine, dopamine, tyramine, octopamine, and amphetamine—can increase ^{14}C-tryptophan in cultured rat pineals (AXELROD et al., 1969; BACKSTROM and WETTERBERG, 1973). Moreover, since L-Dopa increases pineal melatonin release, it has been suggested that administration of this drug might serve the purpose of an in vivo "pineal function test" in humans (MINNEMAN and WURTMAN, 1976). MAO inhibitors also increase the synthesis of melatonin (KLEIN and ROWE, 1970).

Norepinephrine and the non-selective β-adrenoceptor agonist isoproterenol, are known to increase *N*-acetylserotonin in cultured rat pineals (KLEIN et al., 1970). The increase in cyclic AMP and melatonin synthesis evoked by administration of norepinephrine to cultured rat pineals can be blocked by propranolol and dichloroisoproterenol, but not by phenoxybenzamine and phentolamine (WEISS, 1969; WURTMAN et al., 1971). Selective β-adrenoceptor agonists have also been reported to stimulate the formation of *N*-acetylserotonin from serotonin (BACKSTROM, 1977). Whereas the β_2-adrenoceptor agonist terbutaline and the β_1-agonist KWD 2033 possessed similar intrinsic activity for the β-receptor, the β_1-agonist had greater affinity than the β_2-agonist terbutaline. These data were taken as evidence that the pineal β-adrenoceptors may be characterized as resembling the β_1 subgroup.

Stress-induced increases in pineal SNAT activity are produced by elevations of endogenous catecholamines from sympathetic nerve terminals in the pineal, sympathetic nerve terminals in other organs, and the adrenal medulla; propranolol blocks the effects from these endogenous sources (MINNEMAN and WURTMAN, 1976). Nocturnal rises in pineal SNAT activity are suppressed by catecholamine depletors such as reserpine (DEGUCHI and AXELROD, 1972). In general, drugs that modify the storage of norepinephrine within sympathetic nerve terminals elsewhere in the body act similarly in the pineal. For example, metaraminol, desmethylimipramine, 6-hydroxydopamine, and tyramine all modify pineal organ morphology and function to some degree (JAIM-ETCHVERRY and ZIEHER, 1971; ERANKO, 1971; PELLEGRINO DE IRALDI and SUBURO, 1972).

III. Adrenergic Drugs and the Thyroid and Parathyroid

1. Thyroxine and Triiodothyronine

Some years ago, MELANDER (1971) reported that exogenously administered catecholamines can induce secretion of thyroid hormone in vivo, presumably by a direct action of the thyroid follicle cells. The quantity of exogenous amines needed to induce secretion is large, and it is likely that circulating endogenous catecholamine levels are insufficient to stimulate continuously the thyroid gland. However, there is evidence that adrenergic nerve terminals end near thyroid follicles and that direct effects of endogenous catecholamines on thyroid function are possible (TICE and CREVELING, 1975). It has been observed that the frequency and distribution of sympathetic nerve fibers to the follicles are more numerous in some species (adult hamster, sheep, mouse, and man) than in others (adult rat, dog, and pig) (MELANDER et al., 1975). Moreover, the number of interfollicular sympathetic nerve fibers decline with increasing age (MELANDER, 1975). Thus, reliable information regarding the possible influence of the sympathetic nervous system on thyroid activity can be obtained only after thyroidal sympathetic innervation has been examined in the species being studied.

Adrenergic control of thyroid function has been the subject of much clinical and experimental interest since the description of hyperthyroidism and the suggestion that this disorder may be caused by overactivity in the cervical sympathetic nerves (HARRISON, 1964). Current treatment for hyperthyroidism both in preparing hyperthyroid patients for thyroidectomy and in managing thyrotoxic crises include drugs that suppress sympathetic neuron function (HAUSMANN, 1972; TURNER, 1974). The rationale behind the use of drugs that suppress adrenergic function is based upon the facts: (1) that adrenergic neuron function both centrally and peripherally can influence thyroid function; (2) that a sudden increase in sympathetic nervous activity might serve to initiate or accentuate hyperthyroidism; and (3) that adrenoceptor activation is enhanced by elevated thyroid hormone levels. Thus, it is important from both clinical and basic science points of view to ascertain whether or not the sympathetic nervous system can and does exert a significant influence on thyroid gland activity.

Not only can activation of the sympathetic nervous system induce secretion of thyroid hormone, it can also be mimicked by exogenous administration of norepinephrine; these effects can be counteracted by α-adrenoceptor blocking drugs (MELANDER et al., 1972; MELANDER et al., 1974). Moreover, secretion of thyroid hormone can be also induced by β-adrenoceptor stimulation with isoproterenol; this effect is suppressed completely by L-propranolol, but not by its weaker analog D-propranolol nor by α-adrenoceptor antagonists (MELANDER, 1970; ERICSON et al., 1970). Thus, evidence suggests that thyroid hormone secretion can be initiated through activation of β-adrenergic, as well as α-adrenergic receptors.

In a more recent study, the effect of isoproterenol was confirmed by demonstrating formation of colloid droplets accompanied by increased blood radioiodine levels, which indicates thyroid hormone secretion (MELANDER et al., 1975). The β_2-adrenoceptor stimulant terbutaline produced a similar response, whereas the β_1-adrenoceptor stimulant 1-isopropylamine-3-(2-thiazoloxy)-2-propanol was ineffective. L-Propranolol completely abolished terbutaline-induced thyroid hormone secretion. Thus, β-adrenergic stimulation of thyroid hormone secretion may be mediated by β_2-adrenoceptors in thyroid follicle cells.

It is frequently argued that the influence of exogenous catecholamines on glandular secretion is restricted to effects on glandular blood flow (MELANDER et al., 1975; SODERBERG, 1959). However, the fact that drugs producing vasoconstriction by α-adrenoceptor stimulation and those producing vasodilation by β-adrenoceptor stimulation both produce thyroid hormone secretion indicates that adrenergic drugs can act by mechanisms that are independent of their vascular effects. Thus, the overall effect of exogenous catecholamines on thyroid hormone secretion is probably a composite of effects on TSH secretion, on changes in thyroid blood flow, and on thyroid follicular cells.

It should be pointed out that exogenous catecholamines and TSH can exert either additive or mutually antagonistic effects on thyroid hormone secretion, depending on the timing of their administration relative to one another, and on the prevailing state of thyroid activity (MELANDER and SUNDLER, 1972). However, if one eliminates TSH secretion in order to avoid indirect effects and interactions alluded to above, electrical stimulation of sympathetic nerves, drug-induced release of norepinephrine, or administration of norepinephrine all induce secretion of thyroid hormone (MELANDER, 1971). Thus, the effect of norepinephrine seems to be mediated in part by a direct action on the follicular cell as demonstrated by the ability of the catecholamine to enhance incorporation of iodine and the synthesis of thyroid hormone in isolated calf thyroid cells (MAAYAN, 1968; MAAYAN and INGBAR, 1970).

Evidence would further suggest that adrenergic influences on thyroid gland function are of physiological, pharmacological, and clinical significance. In mice, sympathectomy evokes a moderate, short-lasting reduction in thyroid hormone secretion (MELANDER et al., 1974). Moreover, the administration of amphetamine to patients with mental disorders who otherwise are physically healthy produced a moderate rise of both T_3 (triiodothyronine) and T_4 (thyroxine) that parallels blood levels of drug (MELANDER et al., 1976). Plasma TSH levels in these patients declined. It is assumed that amphetamine-induced thyroid hormone secretion occurred primarily from release of norepinephrine from intrathyroidal sympathetic nerve endings.

Thyroid hormones can augment central and peripheral sympathomimetic effects that are not fully accounted for by increased catecholamine production or by enhanced adrenoceptor activity (AOKI et al., 1972). Contrariwise, many aspects of adrenergic nervous system activity are inversely correlated with the state of thyroid activity (CHRISTENSEN, 1972; GHIONE et al., 1974; LANDSBERG and AXELROD, 1968).

Drugs that suppress adrenergic activity have proven useful in the treatment of hyperthyroidism (MILLS, 1974). These agents are especially useful in the treatment of thyroid storm (thyrotoxicosis) presumably because there is increased tissue sensitivity to catecholamines induced by circulating thyroid hormone. Reserpine, which depletes central and peripheral sites of catecholamine stores and other biogenic amines, and guanethidine, which acts peripherally to inhibit adrenergic neurotransmitter release and to deplete norepinephrine storage, are of limited usefulness in treatment of thyrotoxicosis. Postjunctional adrenoceptor blocking agents, e.g., propranolol (a β-blocker) and phenoxybenzamine (an α-blocker) have been used in combination with good results (STOUT et al., 1969). Use of sympathetic suppressant drugs, particularly propranolol, has contributed greatly to the reduction in mortality. Propranolol is used to control symptoms while patients with suspected thyrotoxicosis are undergoing investigation, and it is also a useful adjunct to ^{131}I in the treatment of thyrotoxicosis, i.e., in alleviating symptoms until the radioiodine has a therapeutic effect (HADDEN et al., 1969). Recently, propranolol treatment was shown to lower plasma T_3 levels in individual hyperthyroid patients and in hypothyroid patients receiving L-thyroxine substitution therapy. It was postulated that the effect may be due to an effect of propranolol on peripheral conversion of T_4 to T_3 (WIERSINGA and TOUBER, 1977).

The ability of reserpine to ameliorate many of the hyperdynamic functions in hyperthyroid patients has been attributed to a reduction in sympathetic nervous system activity (CANARY et al., 1957). However, reserpine is also purported to reduce the concentration of $^{125}I–T_3$ concentration within sympathetically innervated tissue (DRATMAN et al., 1977).

2. Thyrocalcitonin and Parathyroid Hormone

Large doses of catecholamines (epinephrine and isoproterenol) raise blood calcium levels in parathyroidectomized rats but not in intact rats (KENNY, 1964). These results suggested that the effects on blood calcium levels may be mediated through stimulation of β-adrenoceptors. Others have shown that the hypocalcemia produced in rats by injection of thyrocalcitonin was antagonized by pretreatment with isoproterenol (WELLS and LLOYD, 1968). These authors suggested that β-adrenergic agonists might produce their calcium mobilizing effect through activation of adenylyl cyclase within bone cells. Recently other investigators have shown that epinephrine, an α- and β-adrenoceptor stimulant, can promote accumulation of cyclic AMP within isolated bone cells (PECK et al., 1974; RODAN and RODAN, 1974). However, other studies have suggested that catecholamines may act directly on the thyroid and parathyroid glands to stimulate the secretion of thyrocalcitonin and parathyroid hormone respectively (CARE et al., 1971; PHILLIPO et al., 1970; FISCHER et al., 1973; KUKREJA et al., 1975; WILLIAMS et al., 1973).

The recent study of HSU and COOPER (1975) has suggested the hypercalcemic effect of catecholamines can be produced in animals without the thyroid and parathyroid glands. However, in rats with intact thyroid glands the thyrocalcitonin levels rose rapidly following the injection of isoproterenol and salbutamol. These investigators did not determine, however, whether the promotion of thyrocalcitonin release by catecholamines was an action directly on the thyroid gland or whether it was produced by catecholamine-induced hypercalcemia. Nevertheless, the results from this study demonstrated that thyrocalcitonin levels can be increased by catecholamines and possibly explains the well-known ability of the thyroid-intact rat to resist catecholamine-induced hypercalcemia.

Studies in man have demonstrated that the β-adrenergic drugs isoproterenol and epinephrine in the usual therapeutic doses increase PTH secretion whereas the relatively pure α-adrenergic stimulant phenylephrine had no effect (KUKREJA et al., 1976). Moreover, propranolol appeared to depress basal levels of serum PTH, which suggests that β-adrenergic influences may play a role in PTH secretion and therefore in calcium homeostasis.

The fact that therapeutic doses of adrenergic drugs can influence PTH secretion and calcium homeostasis has some potentially important therapeutic implications. For example, one might predict an increased incidence of hyperparathyroidism in patients with asthma who are receiving β-adrenergic drugs for treatment of bronchial asthma. This possibility is further indicated by the finding that excessive catecholamines in patients with pheochromocytoma have been reported to produce elevated PTH levels and hypercalcemia that disappeared after removal of the tumor (KUKREJA et al., 1973).

IV. Adrenergic Drugs and the Gut

The gut is an endocrine organ that may well have the largest mass of endocrine-paracrine cells in the body. Moreover, the endocrine cells of the gut are of greater diversity than in any other endocrine organ of the body, being scattered throughout the mucosa of the gut rather than packaged in clusters as in other endocrine glands. The major neurophysiological control of gut hormone release appears to be cholinergic; i.e., control resides in the vagus nerves. Experiments in animals have demonstrated that the cephalic and gastric phase of gastric secretion is mediated predominately by cholinergic reflexes and that gastrin is considered to be a hormonal link in the neural chain (GROSSMAN, 1967). However, the finding that truncal vagotomy in man did not abolish the gastrin response to hypoglycemia suggested that factors other than cholinergic neurons may be functioning (STADIL, 1972).

Observations that patients with catecholamine-secreting tumors (pheochromocytoma) had elevated gastrin levels and that infusions of epinephrine in dogs also elevated immunoreactive plasma gastrin levels suggested that catecholamines are factors linking stress with gastrin-induced ulceration of the gut (HAYES et al., 1972). Doses of epinephrine as low as 0.25 μg·kg·min produced significant elevations of plasma gastrin in dogs. STADIL and REHFELD (1973) also demonstrated later that 25 ng·kg·min of epinephrine in human subjects increased serum gastrin levels. The gastrin response to epinephrine could be inhibited by the β-adrenoceptor blocking drug, pindolol. Moreover, KRONBORG et al. (1974) reported that another β-adrenoceptor antagonist, propranolol, had a small inhibitory effect on insulin-activated acid secretion before and 2–3 months after vagotomy. HAYES et al. (1972) found that α-adrenoceptor blockade with phenoxybenzamine as well as removal of pheochromocytomas reduced gastrin levels in two patients. Thus, it seems that both α- and β-adrenoceptor blockade can suppress effectively the gastrin response to circulating epinephrine.

As in the interaction of catecholamines with other endocrine organs, there is some controversy regarding catecholamine-induced gastrin release. For example, both stimulatory and inhibitory actions on gastric secretion have been ascribed to epinephrine (CODE, 1951; JACOBSON, 1965). Some of the controversy may be attributed to species differences and the different state of the experimental organ, i.e., whether the stomachs were intact or prepared as pouches.

A recent study in rats has indicated that catecholamine-induced increases in serum gastrin appear to be mediated by β-adrenoceptors (HSU and COOPER, 1977). Evidence supporting this suggestion was: (1) the demonstration that isoproterenol and epinephrine raised serum gastrin levels even in vagotomized rats with high basal gastrin levels, and (2) the demonstration that the β-adrenoceptor blocking agent propranolol inhibited the hypergastrinemic effect of isoproterenol feeding and acetylcholine gavage. In addition, an α-adrenoceptor antagonist phenoxybenzamine increased serum gastrin levels in rats, but the α-agonist phenylephrine did not. Several lines of evidence support a direct action of catecholamines on antral gastrin-producing cells: (1) isoproterenol increased blood gastrin levels after direct instillation into the stomachs of rats with pylorus ligation; and (2) interestingly, parenterally administered isoproterenol did not increase serum gastrin levels. These data indicate that β-adrenergic drugs can influence gastrin secretion in the rat.

V. Adrenergic Drugs and the Pancreas

In most species the principle components of the pancreatic islet are the A, B, and D cells. For some time it has been known that A (alpha) cells contain glucagon and that B (beta) cells contain insulin (LACY and GREIDER, 1972). More recently, it has been shown that D cells contain another hormone, somatostatin, which was originally isolated from the hypothalamus (DUBOIS, 1975; POLAK et al., 1975). This cytologic finding is one of the latest findings that suggest a close functional relationship between the pancreatic islets and the nervous system (PEARSE, 1969; see Sect. A).

The endocrine pancreas of most vertebrates is innervated by both the sympathetic and parasympathetic components of the autonomic nervous system (ESTERHUIZEN et al., 1968). These autonomic neurons are referred to as the extrinsic nerve supply, but nerve cell bodies are sometimes observed within the islets. These latter neurons are called intrinsic neurons and are likely to be postganglionic parasympathetic nerves (SMITH and PORTE, 1976).

Flourescence microscopy has clearly demonstrated that biogenic amines are present not only in islet nerve endings but also within the A and B cells (CEGRELL, 1968). The type and amount of amines found within the islet cells vary according to age, species, and pigmentation of the animal. Dopamine and serotonin have been identified specifically in isolated islets and form part of the evidence that these APUD cells are of neuroectodermal origin. Dopamine may be an intracellular regulator of both insulin and glucagon release (PORTE et al., 1976). Of the two catecholamine-degrading enzymes, MAO and COMT, the former appears to be primarily responsible for the degradation of intracellular amines.

B cells, which produce insulin, have been shown histochemically to synthesize and store dopamine (CEGRELL et al., 1964). However, the function of this catecholamine in the B cell is not understood. When administered exogenously, dopamine or its precursor L-Dopa produce hyperglycemia, which is accompanied by inhibition of insulin release. This effect has been observed in mice (HAKANSON et al., 1967) and in man (VAN WOERT et al., 1973). HAKANSON et al. (1967) suggested that the hyperglycemic activity of dopamine is mediated through a direct inhibitory effect on pancreatic B cells because dopamine did not provoke hyperglycemia in alloxan diabetic mice.

Extracellular catecholamines can also control secretory activity of pancreatic islets. There are three primary sources of extracellular catecholamines: (a) postganglionic sympathetic nerve endings secreting norepinephrine; (b) adrenochromaffin cells within the islets that contain dopamine; and (c) adrenochromaffin cells in the adrenal medulla and in nerve endings outside the islets. Certain other substances (somatostatin and prostaglandins) functionally related to the nervous system can presumably modulate the response of islets to blood-borne catecholamines.

Stimulation of sympathetic nerves either centrally or peripherally affect both A and B cell function. Stimulation of splanchnic nerves (PORTE et al., 1973) or the ventromedial hypothalamus (FROHMAN and BERNADIS, 1971) elicits inhibition of insulin release and concurrently stimulation of glucagon release. The effect of neuronally released catecholamines is complicated further by differing activities of the substances on α- and β-adrenoceptors. Moreover, the individual hormones of the pancreas — insulin, glucagon, and somatostatin—can influence the function of the other pancreatic cells, leading to other complicated interactions. For example, insulin plays a major role in regulating A cell function, glucagon can stimulate the B cell, and somatostatin can influence the function of both the A and B cell.

1. Insulin

COORE and RANDLE (1964) first reported inhibition of glucose-induced insulin secretion by epinephrine from incubating pieces of rabbit pancreas. The inhibitory effect of epinephrine has been confirmed numerous times in vivo and in vitro in a great variety of species including man (KARAM et al., 1966; PORTE et al., 1966), monkey (KRIS et al., 1966), baboon (ELLIS et al., 1975), dog (CAMPBELL and RASTOGI, 1966), pig (HERTELENDY et al., 1966), sheep (HERTELENDY et al., 1969), rabbit (MORATINOS et al., 1977), and rat (MALAISSE et al., 1967).

Moreover, epinephrine not only inhibited glucose-induced insulin release but also abolished insulin released in response to glucagon (PORTE et al., 1966), theophylline (MALAISSE et al., 1970), dibutyryl-cyclic AMP (MALAISSE et al., 1970), tolbutamide (MALAISSE et al., 1967), amino acids (HERTELENDY et al., 1968), and short-chain fatty acids (HERTELENDY et al., 1968).

Although epinephrine stimulates both α- and β-adrenoceptors, the inhibition of insulin release appears to be mediated by α-adrenoceptors. This supposition is supported by the fact that α-adrenoceptor antagonists abolished the inhibitory effect of epinephrine, whereas β-adrenoceptor antagonists failed to do so (MALAISSE et al., 1967; PORTE, 1967; TURTLE et al., 1967). The inhibitory effect of epinephrine and other α-adrenoceptor agonists is apparently mediated ultimately through a decrease in available Ca^{2+} in the B cell (MALAISSE and MALAISSE-LAGAE, 1970).

The physiologic modulation of catecholamine-induced inhibition of insulin secretion under conditions of stress and exercise is mediated by α-adrenoceptors and is related to the increased need for metabolic fuels, i.e., glucose production by the liver and free fatty acids and glycerol release by adipose tissue. Thus, by suppressing insulin secretion, metabolic substrates become more readily available to peripheral tissues, especially muscle and brain. Under pathophysiologic conditions, e.g., in patients with Pheochromocytoma, excessive circulating catecholamines account for the hyperglycemia accompanied by depressed insulin levels and elevated glucagon levels.

Structure-activity relationships for alteration of insulin secretion by adrenergic drugs have been studied using analogs of catecholamines in vitro (FELDMAN et al., 1971) and in vivo (POTTER et al., 1975). These studies have been complicated by species differences and by the fact that some drugs seem to act as partial agonists. Nevertheless, some generalizations can be made regarding adrenergic drugs and insulin secretion. With regard to inhibition of insulin release, deamination of catecholamines results in loss of the inhibitory effect. Aromatic hydroxyls are more essential for the inhibitory effect than the β-hydroxyl group, i.e., dopamine has a moderate inhibitory effect, but tyramine and phenylethylamine are much weaker. In terms of stimulatory effects, isoproterenol is much more active in releasing insulin than drugs that are relatively selective stimulants of β_2-adrenoceptors.

Whereas activation of α-adrenoceptors inhibits glucose-induce insulin release, stimulation of β-adrenoceptors augments insulin release. Isoproterenol, a relatively nonselective β-adrenoceptor stimulant, elevates plasma insulin levels in a variety of

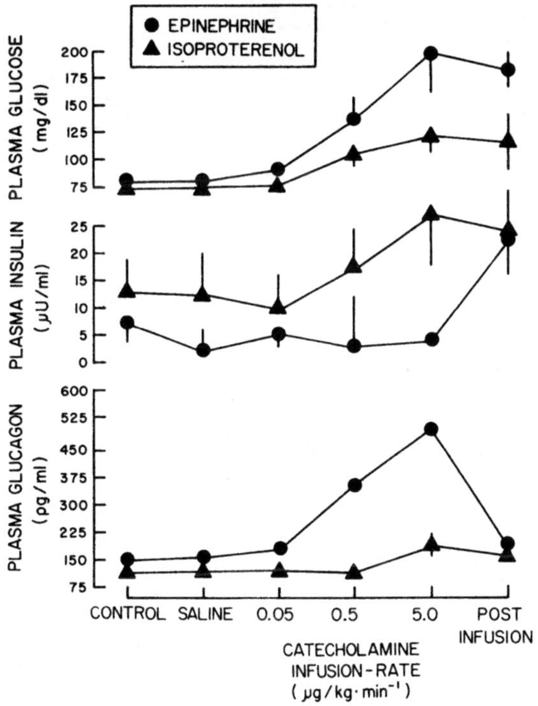

Fig. 3. Changes in plasma glucose, immunoreactive insulin, and glucagon produced by epinephrine and isoproterenol in fasted rabbits. *Symbols* and *vertical lines* represent the mean ±SE. Reproduced, with permission, from POTTER et al. (1978)

species including man (PORTE, 1967), rat (MALAISSE et al., 1967; POTTER and ELLIS, 1975), dog (LOUBATIERES et al., 1971), rabbit (MORATINOS et al., 1977), and baboon (POTTER et al., 1975). A number of relatively selective β_2-adrenoceptor stimulants including metaproterenol, carbuterol, salbutamol and terbutaline also promote insulin release although these agents are generally less active than isoproterenol in baboons (POTTER et al., 1975b) and in man (SANDERS et al., 1977). The β-adrenoceptor mediating insulin release appears to be functionally independent of the glucose receptor in that diabetic patients who had no acute response to glucose responded normally to isoproterenol (ROBERTSON and PORTE, 1973). Stimulation of β-adrenoceptors is thought to influence insulin secretion by activation of adenylyl cyclase, which results in intracellular accumulation of cyclic AMP and the activation of the secretory process.

There is some evidence that the balance of α- and β-adrenoceptors of the pancreatic B cell can differ from species to species and that this balance strongly influences the metabolic effects of catecholamines, particularly the hyperglycemic activity (POTTER and ELLIS, 1975). For example, the hyperglycemic activity of isoproterenol in rats is markedly augmented by chemical destruction of B cells with alloxan (POTTER et al., 1974). Moreover, the responsiveness of adrenoceptor stimulation can also be influenced by environmental factors (TABACHNICK and GULBENKIAN, 1969).

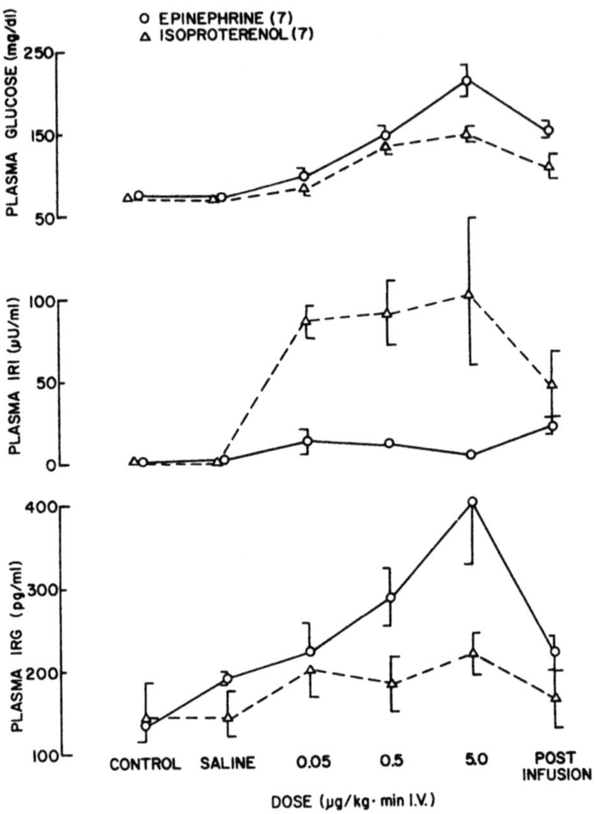

Fig. 4. Catecholamine-induced alterations in plasma glucose, immunoreactive insulin, and glucagon in fasted dogs. *No. in parentheses* represent the No. of dogs for which the mean ±SE were calculated. Reproduced, with permission, from the doctoral dissertation of LEE C. WOODSON (1977)

BURR et al. (1971) have suggested that endogenous catecholamines maintain appropriate concentrations of cyclic AMP in the pancreatic B cell by a β-adrenergic mechanism, while an α-adrenergic mechanism prevents complete expression of this effect as insulin release. PORTE and ROBERTSON (1973) have demonstrated the dualism of epinephrine. They suggested that although α-adrenoceptor stimulation inhibits glucose-stimulated insulin secretion initially, insulin output can be maintained, probably by simultaneous β-adrenoceptor stimulation. Thus, during prolonged infusions of epinephrine, stimulation of insulin release has been observed in dogs. Probably most catecholamines, including isoproterenol, can exhibit dualism depending on, among other things, the dose being used, the species being studied, and the type of experiment being performed (in vivo or in vitro).

BURR et al. (1971) have postulated that adrenergic control may contribute to the postulated regulation of the basal metabolic state of the B cell. Exposure of pancreatic islets to epinephrine prior to a glucose challenge resulted in marked enhancement of glucose-induced biphasic insulin release. The work of BASABE et al. (1977) lends support to this idea. The biphasic pattern of glucose-induced insulin secretion was clearly impaired in reserpine-treated rats, whereas basal levels of insulin secretion was higher.

Norepinephrine perfusion prior to glucose stimulation of the reserpine-treated rat pancreas restored to normal the amount and pattern of both phases of insulin secretion. Administration of 6-hydroxydopamine, an agent that produces selective chemical sympathectomy in vivo, induced glucose intolerance and impaired insulin secretion in rats (BURR et al., 1974). The effects of 6-hydroxydopamine appeared to impair B cell function secondary to adrenergic insufficiency.

Basal or glucose-stimulated levels of circulating insulin tend to increase whenever α-adrenoceptor antagonists, e.g., phentolamine, were administered in vivo (BUSE et al., 1970). This effects is presumed to be due in part to antagonism of the inhibitory effect of endogenously secreted catecholamines (PORTE, 1969). Administration of phentolamine prior to a challenge with epinephrine allowed release of insulin through β-adrenoceptor stimulation (PORTE, 1967). These data do not exclude, however, a possible direct effect of phentolamine on the B cell independent of the α-adrenoceptor. On the other hand, β-adrenoceptor antagonists tended to inhibit not only isoproterenol-induced insulin release (PORTE, 1967) but also basal and glucose-stimulated insulin secretion as well (CERASI et al., 1972; ROBERTSON and PORTE, 1973a; FURMAN and TAYO, 1973). Moreover, CERASI et al. (1972) have also suggested that propranolol directly inhibits the mediation of the glucose signal in the B cell by membrane stabilization or by inhibition of adenyl cyclase activity. Likewise, IMURA et al. (1971) demonstrated that adrenoceptor mechanisms are such that α-receptor blockade and/or β-receptor blockade suppressed insulin secretion. Using selective adrenergic drugs such as practolol (a β_1-adrenoceptor antagonist) and salbutamol (a β_2-adrenoceptor agonist), LOUBATIERES et al. (1971) proposed that catecholamine-induced insulin release is a function of β_2-adrenoceptors and is not dependent upon simultaneous stimulation of β_1-adrenoceptors.

Impaired insulin release during fasting may be mediated partially by changes in endogenous catecholamine activity (FELDMAN et al., 1973). Drugs that interfere with the synthesis, storage, and/or release of catecholamines partially reverse the decreased insulin secretion of fasting in the golden hamster (LEBOVITZ and FELDMAN, 1973). Results with reserpine, α-methyl-p-tyrosine, and p-chlorophenylalanine suggest that endogenous monoamines may contribute to impaired insulin secretion of fasting. Insulin secretion in the fasting state may be altered by circulating catecholamines or by local stores of catecholamines. However, chronic adrenergic insufficiency in man in the form of either bilateral adrenalectomy or cervical sympathectomy was not associated with abnormalities in basal insulin secretion or glucose-induced insulin release (BRODOWS et al., 1974). Although these results seem to indicate that neither central adrenergic tone nor circulating epinephrine plays an important role in modulating basal insulin release in man, one cannot exclude the possibility that extraneuronal sources of catecholamines in the islet may have some role in regulating B cell function.

2. Glucagon

Epinephrine and glucagon are similar in that both agents produce hyperglycemia by an action on hepatic glycogenolysis and gluconeogenesis (EXTON and PARK, 1969). For some time it was thought that both hormones played a physiological role in glucose homeostasis; however, several authors have reported that epinephrine's hyperglycemic activity was less when administered directly into the portal circulation than into the systemic circulation (SHERLOCK, 1949; EZDINLI and SOKAL, 1966). From this latter observation, it was suggested that the hyperglycemic action of epinephrine is mediated in part by the release of glucagon (SOKAL et al., 1964).

This hypothesis was given support indirectly when LECLERQ-MEYER et al. (1971) demonstrated that epinephrine increased glucagon output from pieces of rat pancreas. At about the same time FROHMAN and BERNARDIS (1971) demonstrated that adrenalectomy and administration of antiglucagon serum reduced the hyperglycemic response to stimulation of the ventromedial hypothalamus. Subsequently it was shown that stimulation of sympathetic splanchnic nerves also inhibited insulin release while concurrently eliciting glucagon release (PORTE et al., 1973).

Administration of naturally occurring catecholamines or their precursors to man and laboratory animals also stimulates glucagon release. GERICH et al. (1976) demonstrated initially that epinephrine stimulates glucagon release in man. Intravenously and orally administered L-Dopa also evokes glucagon secretion in monkeys and human subjects, respectively (GEORGE and RAYFIELD, 1974; RAYFIELD et al., 1975). There are several mechanisms by which L-Dopa may produce this effect. One possibility is that L-Dopa or its products stimulates glucagon release through adrenoceptors in the hypothalamus (FROHMAN and BERNARDIS, 1971). Another possibility is that L-Dopa is converted to norepinephrine in the periphery and that norepinephrine promotes the release of glucagon (IVERSEN, 1973). Recent results with carbidopa, a peripheral decarboxylase inhibitor, would suggest that L-Dopa can exert an effect on pancreatic or gastrointestinal A cells without stimulating adrenoceptors in the hypothalamus (GARFINKEL et al., 1977). Plasma glucagon levels in normal subjects declined during treatment with carbidopa, which could be attributed to inhibition of synthesis of L-Dopa to dopamine in the peripheral tissues.

Recent evidence indicates that the stimulation of glucagon release by catecholamines in most mammals is probably due to activation of the β-adrenoceptor as demonstrated in a variety of in vitro and in vivo studies of various mammalian species (EATON et al., 1972; IVERSEN, 1973; LINDSEY and FALOONA, 1973; LUYCKX and LEFEBVRE, 1972). In the duck, stimulation of α-adrenoceptors appears to promote elevation of glucagon levels (TYLER and KAJINUMA, 1972). Interestingly, in Japanese quail the administration of β-adrenoceptor agonists produced hyperglycemia and a profound fall in plasma immunoreactive glucagon levels (POTTER and ROWLAND, 1979). However, there are some reports that α- and not β-adrenoceptor blockade attenuated glucagon secretion by catecholamines in man (GERICH et al., 1972), rats (HARVEY et al., 1972), and ducks (TYLER and KAJINUMA, 1972). Moreover, isoproterenol was found to raise plasma glucagon levels in human subjects while methoxamine, an α-adrenoceptor stimulant, diminished glucagon secretion. Selective β_2-adrenoceptor stimulants were demonstrated to be less active than isoproterenol and epinephrine in elevating glucagon levels in the baboon (POTTER et al., 1975).

The relative inactivity of isoproterenol in releasing glucagon in the rat and other species may be explained in part by the elevation of insulin levels by isoproterenol, which in turn tends to suppress glucagon secretion (TOYOTA et al., 1975; WOODSON et al., 1976). This possibility was substantiated by demonstrating that isoproterenol-induced glucagon release and hyperglycemia are augmented by destruction of B cells with alloxan (WOODSON et al., 1976). Furthermore, the augmented hyperglycemia and

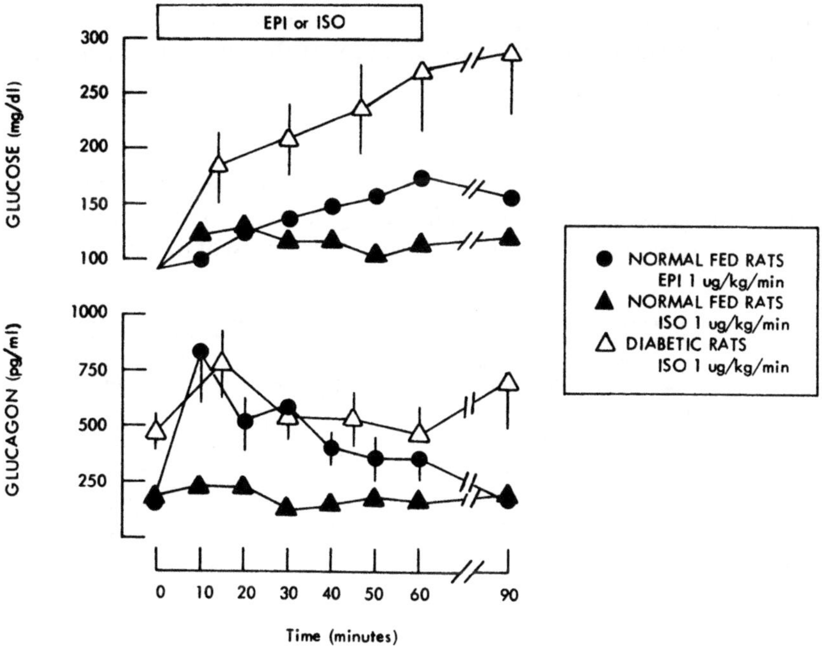

Fig. 5. Hyperglycemic- and glucagon-releasing effects of catecholamines in normal, fed and in alloxan-diabetic, insulin-controlled, fed rats. *Symbols* represent the mean response ±SE except where they cover over SE. *EPI*, epinephrine; *ISO*, isoproterenol. Reproduced, with permission, from the doctoral dissertation of LEE C. WOODSON (1977)

hyperglucagonemia produced by isoproterenol in diabetic rats can be suppressed markedly by coadministration of somatostatin (WOODSON and POTTER, 1979).

GERICH et al. (1976) demonstrated that epinephrine released more glucagon in diabetic subjects than in normal ones. Both somatostatin and propranolol prevented elevation of glucagon in diabetic subjects. These data indicate that, as in normal subjects, epinephrine-induced glucagon secretion in diabetic subjects occurs through a β-adrenergic mechanism. These findings are in general agreement with animal experiments by WOODSON and POTTER (1977).

Similarly, administration of L-propranolol and pindolol suppressed changes in plasma free fatty acids and glucagon that were produced by forced swimming exercise in rats (LUYCKX and LEFEBVRE, 1976). In contrast, HARVEY et al. (1972) reported that propranolol potentiated exercise-induced increases in plasma glucagon in rats. However, propranolol produced hypoglycemia in the experiments of HARVEY et al., and the glucose changes may have accounted for the glucagon response more so than circulating catecholamines. Insulin combined with propranolol produced lower blood glucose levels than those produced by insulin alone (BAIRD and CARTER, 1974). The more intense hypoglycemia produced by propranolol plus insulin may be responsible for the higher glucagon levels measured under these conditions.

Reserpine administration depletes catecholamine stores of adrenergic nerve endings in the brain, sympathetic nerve endings, and to a lesser degree in the adrenal medulla. This depleting agent produced moderate hyperglycemia, hyperglucagonemia, and marked hyperinsulinemia (LUYCKX and LEFEBVRE, 1976). The higher resting blood glucose levels in reserpinized rats has been attributed to the hyperglucagonemia (TAYLOR, 1972).

3. Somatostatin

Somatostatin, a peptide capable of inhibiting release of numerous polypeptide hormones including growth hormone, insulin, and glucagon, was originally isolated from the hypothalamus but is now recognized also as being present in the D cells of the pan-

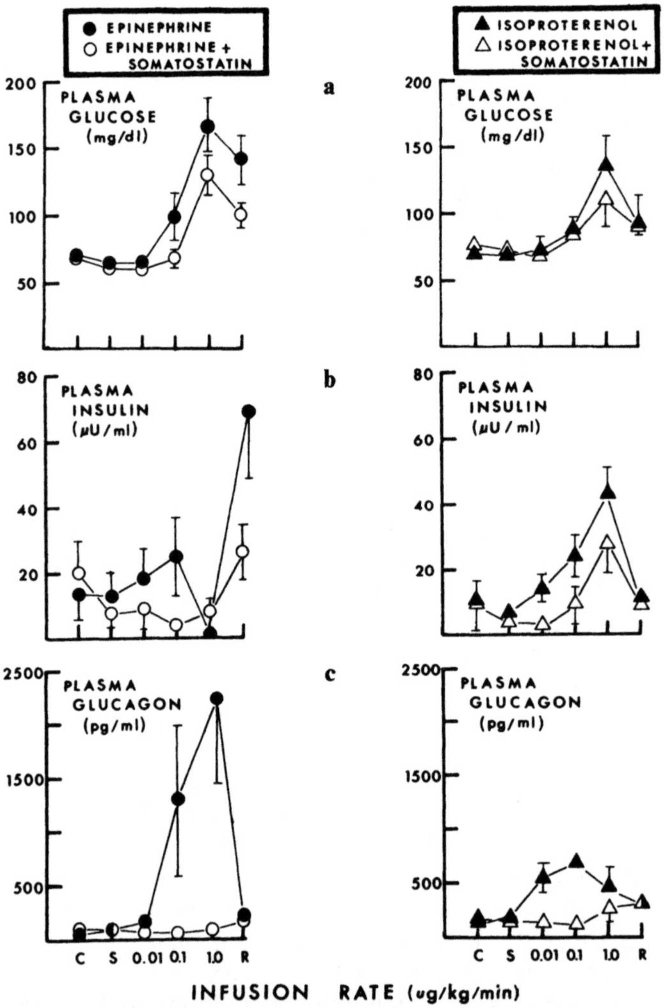

Fig. 6a–c. Inhibition by somatostatin of epinephrine- and isoproterenol-induced changes in plasma (*a*) glucose, (*b*) insulin, and (*c*) glucagon in fasted baboons. Somatostatin infusions were begun 15 min before and continued throughout the period of catecholamine infusion. Recovery samples were drawn 30 min after termination of drug infusions. *C* control; *S* control during saline or somatostin infusion; *R* recovery. *Brackets* show the SE of the mean when it is larger than the symbol. Reproduced, with permission, from the doctoral dissertation of LEE C. WOODSON (1977)

creatic islets. The highest concentrations of somatostatin are found in the nerve endings within the median eminence and arcuate nucleus of the rat hypothalamus (Brownstein et al., 1975); however, the greatest quantities are found in the rat stomach and pancreas (Polak et al., 1975).

Very little is known regarding the effects of adrenergic drugs on somatostatin release. However, agents such as theophylline, which elevate tissue cyclic AMP levels, caused a marked stimulation of somatostatin release, suggesting that catecholamines might also be effective (Barden et al., 1976). Work by Smith et al. (1977) has raised the possibility of a role of α-adrenoceptors in somatostatin-induced inhibition of pancreatic glucagon secretion. An infusion of phentolamine disinhibited somatostatin-induced suppression of glucagon release, suggesting that α-adrenergic mechanisms influence the ability of somatostatin to suppress release of pancreatic glucagon.

Infusion of isoproterenol (2 µg/ml) for 10 min stimulated secretion of somatostatin, glucagon, and insulin from the perfused canine pancreas (Samols et al., 1977). Prior infusion of propranolol blocked the stimulatory effect of isoproterenol on pancreatic hormone secretion. Infusion of epinephrine (2 µg/ml) following prior administration of propranolol inhibited secretion of somatostatin and insulin with variable effects on glucagon. Addition of epinephrine (2 µg/ml) to isolated rat islets inhibited the release of immunoreactive somatostatin (Schauder et al., 1976). Thus, β-adrenoceptor agonism stimulated somatostatin secretion whereas α_1-adrenoceptor agonism inhibited secretion.

Somatostatin has been a very useful tool in elucidating the role of glucagon in catecholamine-induced alterations in glucose homeostasis. The hyperglycemic activity of catecholamines correlated very well with increases in glucagon concentration in rat, rabbit, dog, and baboon (Woodson and Potter, 1977), and in man (Gerich et al., 1976). Somatostatin suppressed catecholamine-induced hyperglucagonemia and concurrently inhibited hyperglycemia as well.

VI. Adrenergic Drugs and the Kidney

Hormonal agents known to be elaborated by the kidney include vitamin D, renin, erythropoietin, prostaglandins, and kallikrein. The sympathetic nervous system can affect the generation and release of most of these hormones by a direct action on the renal tissue and/or by changes in renal blood flow. Likewise, drugs that alter the function of sympathetic neurons and adrenoceptors may also modify the secretion of renal hormones. In turn, the renal hormones may cause secondary reactions within the kidney, either through the nervous system, through other hormonal systems like the adrenal, or directly when the hormonal substances return to the kidney.

It has been clearly demonstrated that the kidney is richly innervated by sympathetic postganglionic nerve fibers. These fibers are particularly numerous along the afferent arterioles and are closely associated with the juxtaglomerular cells (Wagermark et al., 1968; Ayers et al., 1969). Thus, morphological evidence is consistent with the view that juxtaglomerular cells receive sympathetic secretomotor innervation.

1. Renin-Angiotensin

There are three major mechanisms which increase renin release: (1) decrease in sodium load to the distal tubule (macula densa) (2) decrease in stretch of renal afferent arterioles; and (3) stimulation of β-adrenoceptors in the kidney by nerve stimulation or by drugs (DAVIS, 1971).

There is considerable evidence that the sympathetic nervous system can affect renin secretion. Stimulation of the renal nerves, the pressor region of the medulla oblongata, and the midbrain increase renin secretion (LOEFFLER et al., 1972; PASSO et al., 1971; UEDA et al., 1967). Other indirect means of sympathetic activation, such as hypoglycemia, carotid occlusion, changes in posture, and vasodilation by drugs also increase renin secretion (OTSUKA et al., 1970; BUNAG et al., 1966a; GORDON et al., 1966; BUNAG et al., 1966b). Selective denervation of the kidney will block the effect of brainstem stimulation whereas denervation of the adrenal inhibits the response to hypoglycemia, indicating that both stimulation of sympathetic nerves to the kidney and release of catecholamines from the adrenal medulla can play a role in renin release.

Infusions of catecholamines also increase renin secretion (SCORNIK and PALADINI, 1964; VANDER, 1965; PESKAR et al., 1970). Epinephrine and isoproterenol have greater renin-stimulating activity than norepinephrine, suggesting that the adrenoceptor involved is a β-receptor (ASSAYKEEN and GANONG, 1971). Depending on the dose administered, dopamine may increase (high dose) or have no effect on renin secretion in dogs (AYERS et al., 1969; OTSUKA et al., 1970). L-Dopa administered orally to humans has been reported to depress or cause no change in renin secretion (BARBEAU et al., 1969; MICHELAKIS and ROBERTSON, 1970). Methoxamine and metaraminol, synthetic adrenergic drugs that stimulate α-adrenoceptors predominately, have also been reported to have renin stimulating activity (MAEBASHI et al., 1968; WINER et al., 1969). Tyramine, which releases catecholamines from nerve endings, also increases renin output from the kidney (BUNAG et al., 1966a).

Adrenergic agonist drugs can stimulate renin secretion by one or more mechanisms depending upon dose and spectrum of adrenoceptor activation. Agents that stimulate α-adrenoceptors could act by constricting renal afferent arterioles, thus decreasing both GFR and stretch on the juxtaglomerular cells. Alternatively, adrenergic agonists can alter sodium delivery to renin-rich portions of the kidney by redistributing intrarenal blood flow. Another possibility is that catecholamines could act directly on β-adrenoceptors on juxtaglomerular cells, probably by activating formation of cyclic AMP, which in turn promotes renin secretion. There is considerable evidence that the catecholamines, epinephrine, norepinephrine, and isoproterenol stimulate renin secretion by an intrarenal effect that is largely independent of changes in renal perfusion pressure (VANDONGEN and GREENWOOD, 1975). Moreover, there is evidence that β-adrenoceptor stimulation results in increased renin secretion whereas α-adrenoceptor stimulation of juxtaglomerular cells inhibits renin secretion (JOHNSON et al., 1976; PETTINGER et al., 1976).

In vitro and in vivo experiments using D,L- or L-propranolol, a nonselective β-receptor antagonist, have confirmed that renin release is a β-adrenoceptor mediated effect (WEINBERGER et al., 1975; JOHNSON et al., 1976). Whereas propranolol suppressed epinephrine-, norepinephrine-, and isoproterenol-induced renin secretion, α-adrenoceptor blockade with phentolamine or phenoxybenzamine did not. Moreover, methoxamine, which is an α-adrenoceptor agonist with some β-adrenoceptor antagonist activity, also inhibited isoproterenol-induced renin release from rat kidney slices (WEINBERGER et al., 1976). In a clinical situation propranolol will inhibit the sympathetically-mediated increase in renin activity that results from administration of vasodilator drugs (AMER, 1977).

Other types of adrenergic drugs also inhibit renin secretion. Agents such as clonidine and α-methyldopa are antihypertensive agents that lower blood pressure in part by central inhibition of sympathetic tone. These drugs presumably activate α-adrenoceptors within the medulla oblongata, which results in suppression of sympathetic outflow (VAN ZWIETEN, 1973). However, clonidine in particular can also activiate presynaptic α-adrenoceptors that are inhibitory to norepinephrine release (VAN ZWIETEN, 1973). Blockade of α-adrenoceptors with clozapine or phenoxybenzamine reversed the inhibition of serum renin activity by clonidine in rats (PETTINGER, 1976). Moreover, ganglionic blockade enhanced the inhibitory effect of clonidine on renin secretion. The fact that ganglionic blockade did not alter the effect of clonidine would suggest a peripheral effect of clonidine, perhaps at inhibitory intrarenal α-adrenoceptors.

Clonidine also lowers plasma renin and aldosterone activity in human subjects (WEBER et al., 1976; KARLBERG et al., 1977). However, neither the sympathetic nervous system effect nor the effect on intrarenal α-adrenoceptors appear to be involved in the renin response to sodium depletion because under these circumstances clonidine was ineffective (WEBER et al., 1976). Thus, although clonidine suppresses serum or plasma renin activity, this does not appear to be its primary mode of lowering blood pressure.

2. Erythropoietin

Erythropoietin is a humoral substance that stimulates bone marrow to increase the rate of red cell formation, produces a reticulocytosis, increases red cell mass after prolonged injections, and accelerates the rate of iron incorporation into hemoglobin of newly formed red blood cells (FISHER, 1972). A number of pharmacological agents can stimulate erythropoietin production by acting through a renal hypoxic mechanism. Any chemical that decreases renal blood flow, increases renal oxygen utilization, or interferes with renal utilization of oxygen can promote the generation of erythropoietin.

Any drug that will reduce renal blood flow below 1.0 ml/g kidney/min will produce hypoxia sufficient to stimulate erythropoietin production. The reduction in blood flow to the kidney caused by 0.4 μg/kg/min of norepinephrine is sufficient to elevate plasma erythropoietin (FISHER et al., 1968). Norepinephrine infused into dogs was not as active as angiotensin in elevating plasma erythropoietin activity.

3. Prostaglandins

These derivatives of essential fatty acids have been suggested to have a role in the endocrine control of blood pressure at the level of the kidney and also at the peripheral arterioles (LEE and ATTALAH, 1975). The kidney is a major site of production for prostaglandins E_2, $F_{2\alpha}$, and possibly A_2. Since the renal cortex arteries are innervated by adrenergic nerve fibers (MCKENNA and ANGELAKOS, 1968), one might predict that stimulation of these nerves might result in renal vasoconstriction and perhaps increased formation of prostaglandins by the kidney.

Stimulation of the sympathetic nerves and intra-arterial injection of angiotensin or bradykinin promote release of prostaglandins into the renal vein blood (Peart, 1977).

Epinephrine and norepinephrine produced vasoconstriction and prostaglandin release when administered to the isolated perfused rabbit kidney (Needleman et al., 1974). Dopamine was much less active than epinephrine in producing prostaglandin release and isoproterenol was inactive. These data suggest that catecholamine-induced prostaglandin release is an α-adrenergic effect; this was confirmed by demonstrating that prostaglandin production was inhibited by phenoxybenzamine but not propranolol. Prostaglandin release by renal nerve stimulation was also antagonized by phenoxybenzamine; however, α-adrenoceptor blockade did not suppress prostaglandin release induced by angiotensin II or by renal ischemia.

Norepinephrine and epinephrine administration also produced levels of prostaglandin E in the renal venous blood of dogs (Terashima et al., 1974). Since renal blood flow was kept constant, the changes in prostaglandins could not be attributed to changes in total renal blood flow. α-Adrenoceptor blockade with phenoxybenzamine did not prevent the rise in prostaglandin E levels by the catecholamines. There is no apparent reason for the effectiveness of phenoxybenzamine in blocking prostaglandin release from the rabbit kidney but not from the dog kidney.

E. Concluding Remarks

Adrenergic drugs have proven to be important research tools in providing further insight into the interrelationship of the sympathetic nervous system and the endocrine system. Moreover, several adrenergic drugs are being used clinically to treat various endocrine disorders. For example, bromoergocryptine is being used for the treatment of abnormal lactation and amenorrhea in patients with hyperprolactinemia.

Further work is needed to resolve contradictory data gathered from different species, to distinguish effects produced by alteration of the biologic activity of endogenous catecholamines from those produced by administration of exogenous catecholamines, to establish the physiological role of catecholamines in controlling endocrine function, and to develop new adrenergic drugs that can be used to treat endocrinopathy.

References

Abdulla, Y.H., McFarlane, E.: Control of adenylate kinase by prostaglandins E_2 and E_3. Biochem. Pharmacol. *20*, 1726–1730 (1971)

Amer, M.S.: Mechanism of action of β-blockers in hypertension. Biochem. Pharmacol. *26*, 171–175 (1977)

Amer, M.S., Marquis, N.R.: The effect of prostaglandins, epinephrine, and aspirin on cyclic AMP phosphodiesterase activity of human blood platelets and their aggregation. In: Prostaglandins in Cellular Biology (Eds.) Ramwell, P.W., Pharris, B.B. New York: Plenum Press 1972, pp. 93–110

Anden, N.E., Dahlstrom, A., Fuxe, K., Olson, L., Ungerstedt, V.: Ascending monoamine neurons to the telencephalon and diencephalon. Acta Physiol. Scand. *67*, 313–326 (1966)

Aoki, V.S., Wilson, W.R., Theilan, E.O.: Studies of the reputed augmentation of the cardiovascular effects of catecholamines in patients with spontaneous hyperthyroidism. J. Pharmacol. Exp. Ther. *181*, 362–368 (1972)
Assaykeen, T.A., Ganong, W.F.: The sympathetic nervous system and renin secretion. Front. Endocrinol. *2*, 67–102 (1971)
Ayers, C.R., Harris, Jr., R.H., Lefer, L.G.: Control of renin release in experimental hypertension. Circ. Res. *24*, (Suppl. 1) 103–112 (1969)
Axelrod, J.: Relationship between catecholamines and other hormones. Rec. Prog. Horm. Res. *31*, 1–35 (1975)
Axelrod, J., Shein, H., Wurtman, R.: Stimulation of C^{14}-melatonin synthesis from C^{14}-tryptophan by noradrenaline in rat pineal organ culture. Proc. Natl. Acad. Sci. USA *62*, 544–549 (1969)
Backstrom, M.: Selective β-adrenoceptor antagonism of induced formation of ^{14}C-*N*-acetylserotonin in rat pineal glands in organ culture. Life Sci. *20*, 1763–1770 (1977)
Backstrom, M., Wetterberg, L.: Increased *N*-acetylserotonin and melatonin formation induced by D-amphetamine in rat pineal gland organ culture via a β-adrenergic receptor mechanism. Acta Physiol. Scand. *87*, 113–120 (1973)
Baird, J.R.C., Carter, A.J.: Assessment of effects of β-blocking drugs on blood glucose levels and insulin hypoglycemia in rats. Eur. J. Pharmacol. *25*, 275–278 (1974)
Baldwin, D.S., Gombos, E.A., Chasis, H.: Changes in sodium and water excretion induced by epinephrine and L-norepinephrine in normotensive and hypertensive subjects. J. Lab. Clin. Med. *61*, 832–857 (1963)
Barbeau, A., Gillo-Joffroy, L., Boucher, R., Nowaczynski, W., Genest, J.: Renin-aldosterone system in Parkinson's disease. Science *165*, 291–292 (1969)
Barden, N., Avalrado-Urbias, G., Cote, J.-P., Dupont, A. Cyclic AMP-dependent stimulation of somatostatin secretion by isolated rat islets of Langerhans. Biochem. Biophys. Res. Commun. *71*, 840–844 (1976)
Barker, J.L., Crayton, J.W., Nicoll, R.A.: Antidromic and orthodromic responses of paraventricular and supraoptic neurosecretory cells. Brain Res. *33* , 353–366 (1971 a)
Barker, J.L., Crayton, J.W., Nicoll, R.A.: Noradrenaline and acetylcholine responses of supraoptic neurosecretory cells. J. Physiol. (Lond.) *218*, 19–32 (1971 b)
Barraclough, C.A., Sawyer, C.H.: Blockade of the release of pituitary ovulating hormone in the rat by chlorpromazine and reserpine: Possible mechanisms of action. Endocrinology *61*, 341–351 (1957)
Barraclough, C.A., Sawyer, C.H.: Inhibition of the release of pituitary ovulatory hormone in the rat by morphine. Endocrinology *57*, 329–337 (1955)
Basabe, J.C., Farina, J.M.S., Udrisar, D.P., Chieri, R.: Effect of pancreatic adrenergic tone modifications prior to glucose-induced insulin secretion. Horm. Metab. Res. *9*, 108–113 (1977)
Berridge, M.J.: The interaction of cyclic nucleotides and calcium in the control of cellular activity. In: Adv. Cyclic Nucleotide Res. Greengard, P., Robinson, G.A. (Eds.), *6*. New York: Raven Press 1975, 1–80
Betz, D., Ganong, W.F.: Effect of chlorpromazine on pituitary-adrenal function in the dog. Acta Endocrinol. *43*, 264–270 (1963)
Bhattachary, A.N., Marks, B.H.: Effects of pargyline and amphetamine upon acute stress responses in rats. Proc. Soc. Exp. Biol. Med. *130*, 1194–1198 (1969)
Bhattacharya, A.N., Dierschke, D.J., Yamaji, Knobil, E.: The pharmacologic blockade of the circadial mode of LH secretion in the ovarectomized Rhesus monkey. Endocrinology *90*, 778–786 (1972)
Billing, R.J., Barbiroli, B., Smellie, R.M.S.: The mode of action of oestradiol I. The transport of RNA precursors. Biochim. Acta *190*, 52–65 (1969)
Bisset, G.W., Clark, B.J., Errington, M.L.: The hypothalamic neurosecretory pathways for the release of oxytocin and vasopressin in the cat. J. Physiol. (Lond.) *217*, 111–131 (1971)
Bower, A., Hadley, M.E., Hruby, V.J.: Biogenic amines and control of melanophore stimulating hormone release. Science *184*, 70–72 (1974)
Bridges, T.E., Hillhouse, E.W., Jones, M.T.: The effect of dopamine on neurohypophysial hormone release in vivo and from the rat neural lobe and hypothalamus in vitro. J. Physiol. (Lond.) *260*, 647–666 (1976)

Brodows, R.G., Pi-Sunyer, F.X., Campbell, R.G.: Insulin secretion in adrenergic insufficiency in man. J. Clin. Endocrinol. Metab. *38*, 1103–1108 (1974)

Brownstein, M., Arimura, A., Sato, H., Schally, A.V., Kizer, J.S.: The regional distribution of somatostatin in the rat brain. Endocrinology *96*, 1456–1461 (1975)

Bunag, R.D., Page, I.H., McCubbin, J.W.: Neural stimulation of release of renin. Circ. Res. *19*, 851–858 (1966a)

Bunag, R.D., Page, I.H., McCubbin, J.W.: Influence of dietary sodium on stimuli causing renin release. Am. J. Physiol. *211*, 1383–1386 (1966b)

Burr, I.M., Balant, L., Stauffacher, W., Renold, A.E.: Adrenergic modification of glucose-induced biphasic insulin release from perifused rat pancreas. Eur. J. Clin. Invest. *1*, 216–224 (1971)

Burr, I.M., Jackson, A., Culbert, S., Sharp, R., Felts, P., Olson, W.: Glucose tolerance and impaired insulin release following 6-hydroxydopamine administration to intact rats. Endocrinology *94*, 1072–1076 (1974)

Buse, M.G., Johnson, A.H., Kuperming, D., Buse, J.: Effect of alpha-adrenergic blockade on insulin secretion in man. Metabolism *19*, 219–225 (1970)

Camanni, F., Massara, F., Belforte, L., Rosatello, A., Molinatti, G.M.: Effect of dopamine on plasma growth hormone and prolactin levels in normal and acromegalic subjects. J. Clin. Endocrinol. Metab. *44*, 465–473 (1977)

Campbell, J., Rastogi, K.S.: Effects of glucagon and epinephrine on serum insulin and insulin secretion in dogs. Endocrinology *79*, 830–835 (1966)

Canary, J.J., Schaaf, M., Duffy, B.J., Kyle, L.H.: Effects of oral and intramuscular administration of reserpine in thyrotoxicosis. N. Engl. J. Med. *257*, 435–442 (1957)

Care, A.D., Bates, R.F.L., Gitelman, H.J.: Evidence for a role of cyclic AMP in the release of calcitonin. Ann. N.Y. Acad. Sci. *186*, 317–326 (1971)

Cegrell, L.: The occurrence of biogenic monoamines in the mammalian endocrine pancreas. Acta Physiol. Scand. (Suppl.) *314*, 1–60 (1968)

Cegrell, L., Falck, B., Hellman, B.: Monoaminergic mechanisms in the endocrine pancreas. In: The Structure and Function of the Pancreatic Islets. Proc. Third Inter. Symp. Stockholm: Pergamon Press, London 1964

Cerasi, E., Luft, R., Efendic, S.: Effect of adrenergic blocking agents on insulin response to glucose infusion in man. Acta Endocrinol. *69*, 335–346 (1972)

Chambers, J.W., Brown, G.M.: Neurotransmitter regulation of growth hormone and ACTH in the Rhesus monkey: Effects of biogenic amines. Endocrinology *98*, 420–428 (1976)

Christensen, N.J.: Increased levels of plasma noradrenaline in hypothyroidism. J. Clin. Endocrinol. Metab. *35*, 359–363 (1972)

Clemens, J.A.: Neuropharmacological aspects of the neural control of prolactin secretion. In: Current topics in Molecular Endocrinology, Hypothalamus, and Endocrine Function. Labric, F., Meites, J., Pelletier, G. (Eds.). New York: Plenum Press 1976, pp. 283–301

Clemens, J.A., Smalstig, E.B., Sawyer, B.D.: Antipsychotic drugs and prolactin release. Psychopharmacologia *40*, 123–127 (1974a)

Clemens, J.A., Shaar, C.J., Smalstig, E.B., Bach, N.J., Kornfeld, E.C.: Inhibition of prolactin in secretion by ergolines. Endocrinology *94*, 1171–1176 (1974b)

Code, C.F.: The inhibition of gastric secretion: A review. Pharmacol. Rev. *3*, 59–106 (1951)

Coleoni, A.H.: Effects of the administration of catecholamine-depleting drugs on the thyroid function of the rat. Pharmacology *8*, 300–310 (1972)

Collu, R., Franschini, F., Visconti, P., Martini: Adrenergic and serotoninergic control of growth hormone secretion in adult male rats. Endocrinology *90*, 1231–1237 (1972)

Coore, H.G., Randle, P.J.: Regulation of insulin secretion studied with pieces of rabbit pancreas incubated *in vitro*. Biochem. J. *93*, 66–78 (1964)

Coppola, J.A., Leonardi, R.G., Lippman, W., Perrine, J.W., Ringler, I.: Induction of pseudopregnancy in rats by depletors of endogenous catecholamines. Endocrinology *77*, 485–490 (1965)

Dallman, M.F., Yates, F.E.: Anatomical and functional mapping of central neural input and feedback pathways of the adrenocortical system. Mem. Soc. Endocrinol. *17*, 39–72 (1968)

Davis, J.O.: What signals the kidney to release renin? Circ. Res. *28*, 301–306 (1971)

Deguchi, T., Axelrod, J.: Control of circadian change of serotonin *N*-acetyltransferase activity in the pineal organ by the β-adrenergic receptor. Proc. Natl. Acad. Sci. USA *69*, 2547–2550 (1972)

Del Pozo, E., Del Re, R.B., Varga, L., Friesen, H.: The inhibition of prolactin secretion in man by CB-154 (2-Br-α-ergocryptine). J. Clin. Endocrinol. Metab. *35*, 768–771 (1972)

De Wied, D., DeJong, W.: Drug effects and hypothalamic-anterior pituitary function. Ann. Rev. Pharmacol. *14*, 389–412 (1974)

Dickerman, S., Clark, J., Dickerman, E., Meites, J.: Effects of haloperidol on serum and pituitary prolactin and on hypothalamic PIF in rats. Neuroendocrinology *9*, 332–340 (1972)

Dratman, M.B., Crutchfield, F.L., Axelrod, J., Utiger, R.D., Marsh, E.: Triiodothyronine in rat submaxillary salivary gland: Effects of altered adrenergic function. Pharmacology *15*, 193–207 (1977)

Dubois, M.P.: Immunoreactive somatostatin is present in discrete cells of the endocrine pancreas. Proc. Natl. Acad. Sci. USA *72*, 1340–1343 (1975)

Durand, D., Martin, J.B., Brazeau, P.: Evidence for a role of α-adrenergic mechanisms in regulation of episodic growth hormone secretion in the rat. Endocrinology *100*, 722–728 (1977)

Eaton, R., Conway, M., Buckman, M.: Role of alpha-adrenergic blockade on alanine-induced hyperglucagonemia. Metabolism *21*, 371–373 (1972)

Ellis, S., Kempen, R.R., Potter, D.E.: Metabolic responses to catecholamines in baboons and monkeys. Sixth Int. Congr. Pharmacol. (Helsinki), p. 230 (1975)

Eranko, A.: Loss of histochemically demonstrable catecholamines and acetylcholinesterase from sympathetic nerve fibers of the pineal body of the rat after chemical sympathectomy with 6-hydroxydopamine. Histochem. J. *3*, 357–363 (1971)

Ericson, L.E., Melander, A., Owman, Ch., Sundler, F.: Endocytosis of thyroglobulin and release of thyroid hormone in mice by catecholamines and 5-hydroxytryptamine. Endocrinology *87*, 915–923 (1970)

Esterhuizen, A.C., Spriggs, T.L.B., Lever, J.D.: Nature of islet-cell innervation in the cat pancreas. Diabetes *17*, 33–36 (1968)

Ezdinli, E.Z., Sokal, J.E.: Comparison of glucagon and epinephrine effects in the dog. Endocrinology *78*, 47–54 (1966)

Exton, J.H., Park, C.R.: Control of gluconeogenesis in liver. III. Effects of L-lactate, pyruvate, fructose, glucagon, epinephrine, and adenosine 3′,5′-monophosphate on gluconeogenic intermediates in the perfused rat liver. J. Biol. Chem. *244*, 1424–1432 (1969)

Feldman, J.M., Boyd III, A.E., Lebovitz, H.E.: Structural determinants of catecholamine action on *in vitro* insulin release. J. Pharmacol. Exp. Ther. *176*, 611–621 (1971)

Feldman, J.M., Lebovitz, H.E., Bowman, J.: Role of pancreatic monoamines in the impaired insulin secretion of the fasting state. Endocrinology *92*, 1469–1474 (1973)

Fischer, J.A., Blum, J.W., Binswanger, U.: Acute parathyroid hormone response to epinephrine *in vivo*. J. Clin. Invest. *52*, 2434–2440 (1973)

Fisher, D.A.: Norepinephrine inhibition of vasopressin antidiuresis. J. Clin. Invest. *47*, 540–547 (1968)

Fisher, J.W.: Erythropoietin: pharmacology, biogenesis, and control of production. Pharmacol. Rev. *24*, 459–508 (1972)

Fisher, J.W., Samuels, A.I., Langston, J.: Effects of angiotensin, norepinephrine, and renal artery constriction on erythropoietin production. Ann. N.Y. Acad. Sci. *149*, 308–317 (1968)

Fortier, C.: Nervous control of ACTH secretion. In: The Pituitary Gland. Hariss, G.W., Donovan, B.T. (Eds.). London: Butterworth 1966, p. 195

Frantz, A.G.: The regulation of prolactin secretion in humans. In: Frontiers in Neuroendocrinology. Ganong, W.F., Martini, L. (Eds.). New York: Oxford University Press 1973, p. 337

Frantz, A.G., Suh, H.K.: L-Dopa and the control of prolactin secretion. Adv. Neurol. *5*, 447–459 (1974)

Frantz, A.G., Habif, D.V., Hyman, G.A., Suh, H.K.: Remission of metastatic breast cancer after reduction of circulating prolactin in patients treated with L-dopa. Clin. Res. *20*, 864 (1972)

Friesen, H., Guyda, H., Hwang, P., Tyson, J.E., Barbeau, A.: Functional evaluation of prolactin secretion: A guide to therapy. J. Clin. Invest. *51*, 706–709 (1972)

Frohman, L.A., Bernardis, L.L.: Effect of hypothalamic stimulation on plasma glucose, insulin, and glucagon levels. Am. J. Physiol. *221*, 1596–1603 (1971)
Furman, B.L., Tayo, F.M.: Inhibitory effect of propranolol on insulin secretion. Br. J. Pharmacol. *49*, 145P (1973)
Fuxe, K.: Evidence for the existence of monoamine neurons in the central nervous system. III. The monoamine nerve terminal. Z. Zellforsch. *65*, 573–596 (1965)
Fuxe, K., Hokfelt, T.: Catecholamines in the hypothalamus and the pituitary gland. In: Frontiers in Neuroendocrinology. Ganong, W.F., Martini, L. (Eds.). New York, Oxford: University Press 1969, p. 47
Fuxe, K., Hokfelt, T., Nilsson, O.: Activity changes in the tuberoinfundibular dopamine neurons of the rat during various stages of the reproductive cycle. Life Sci. *6*, 2057–2061 (1967)
Fuxe, K., Lofstrom, A., Eneroth, P., Gustafsson, J.-A., Hokfelt, T., Scott, P., Wuttke, W., Fraser, H., Jeffcoate, S.: Interactions between hypothalamic catecholamine nerve terminals and LRF containing neurons. Further evidence for an inhibitory dopaminergic facilitatory noradrenergic influence. In: Basic Applications and Clinical Uses of Hypothalamic Hormones. Charro Salgado, A.L., Fernandez-Durango, R., Lopez del Campo, J.G. (Eds.). New York: Excerpta Medica, American Elsivier Publishing Co., 1976, p. 165
Ganong, W.F.: Evidence for a central noradrenergic system that inhibits ACTH secretion. In: Brain-Endocrine Interaction. Median Eminence: Structure and Function. Knigge, K.M., Scott, D.E., Weindl, A. (eds.), p. 254. Basel: Karger 1972
Ganong, W.F.: Pharmacological aspects of neuroendocrine integration. Prog. Brain Res. *38*, 41–74 (1972)
Ganong, W.F.: Biogenic amines, sympathetic nerves, and renin secretion. Fed. Proc. *32*, 1782–1784 (1973)
Ganong, W.F., Maickel, R.P., Martini, L., Marles, B.H.: Monoamines and control of glucocorticoid secretion. Neurosci. Res. Bull. *9*, 235–242 (1971)
Gautvik, K., Weintraub, B.D., Graeber, C.T., Maloof, F., Zuckerman, J.E., Tashjian, Jr., A.H.: Serum prolactin and TSH: Effects of nursing and pyroglu-His-ProNH_2 administration in postpartum women. J. Clin. Endocrinol. Metab. *37*, 135–139 (1973)
Garfinkel, P.E., Warsh, J.J., Stancer, H.C., Godse, D.D., Brown, G.M., Vranic, M.: The effect of a peripheral decarboxylase inhibitor (carbidopa) on monoamine and neuroendocrine function in man. Neurology *27*, 443–447 (1977)
George, D.T., Rayfield, E.J.: L-Dopa-induced plasma glucagon release. J. Clin. Endocrinol. Metab. *39*, 618–621 (1974)
Gerich, J.E., Karam, J.H., Forsham, P.H.: Reciprocal adrenergic control of pancreatic alpha- and beta-cell function in man. Diabetes *21*, 332 (1972)
Gerich, J.E., Lorenzi, M., Tsalikian, E., Karam, J.H.: Studies on the mechanism of epinephrine-induced hyperglycemia in man. Diabetes *25*, 65–71 (1976)
Ghione, S., Pellegrini, M., Buzzigoli, G., Carpi, A., Valori, C., Donado, L.: Plasma and urinary catecholamine levels and thyroid activity in relation to cardiovascular changes in hyper- and hypothyroids. Horm. Metab. Res. *6*, 93 (1974)
Gordon, R.D., Wolfe, L.K., Island, D.P., Liddle, G.W.: A diurnal rhythm and plasma renin activity in man. J. Clin. Invest. *45*, 1587–1592 (1966)
Grimm, Y., Reichlin, S.: Thyrotropin-releasing hormone (TRH): Neurotransmitter regulation of secretion by mouse hypothalamic tissue *in vitro*. Endocrinology *93*, 626–631 (1973)
Grossman, M.I.: Neural and hormonal stimulation of gastric secretion of acid. In: Handbook of Physiology. Lode, C.F. (Ed.), Washington, D.C.: Physiological Society, 1967, Sect. 6, Vol. 2, pp. 835–863
Grossman, M.I.: The gut as an endocrine organ. J. Endocrinol. *70*, 1P–2P (1976)
Hadden, D.R., Bell, T.K., McDevitt, D.G., Shanks, R.G., Montgomery, D.A.D., Weaver, J.A.: Propranolol and the utilization of radioiodine by the human thyroid gland. Acta Endocrinol. *61*, 393–399 (1969)
Hakanson, R., Lundquist, I., Rerup, C.: On the hyperglycaemic effect of dopa and dopamine. Eur. J. Pharmacol. *1*, 114–119 (1967)
Harrison, T.S.: Adrenal medullary and thyroid relationships. Physiol. Rev. *44*, 161–185 (1964)

Harvey, W., Faloona, G., Unger, R.: Effect of adrenergic blockade on exercise-induced hyperglucagonemia. Clin. Res. *20*, 752 (1972)
Hausmann, W.: Treatment of hyperthyroidism. Hormones *3*, 313–331 (1972)
Hayes, J.R., Ardill, J., Kennedy, T.L., Shanks, R.G., Buchanan, K.D.: Stimulation of gastrin release by catecholamines. Lancet *I*, 819–821 (1972)
Hayward, J.N.: Neural control of the posterior pituitary. Annu. Rev. Physiol. *37*, 191–210 (1975)
Heidingsfelder, S.A., Blackard, W.G.: Adrenergic receptor control mechanism for growth hormone secretion. J. Clin. Invest. *47*, 1407–1414 (1968)
Hertelendy, F., Machlin, L.J., Gordon, R.S., Horino, M., Kipnis, D.M.: Lipolytic activity and inhibition of insulin release by epinephrine in the pig. Proc. Soc. Exp. Biol. Med. *121*, 675–677 (1966)
Hertelendy, F., Machlin, L.J., Takahashi, Y., Kipnis, D.M.: Insulin release from sheep pancreas *in vitro*. J. Endocrinol. *41*, 605–606 (1968)
Hertelendy, F., Machlin, L., Kipnis, D.M.: Further studies on the regulation of insulin and growth hormone secretion in the sheep. Endocrinology *84*, 192–199 (1969)
Hiroshige, T., Abe, K.: Role of brain biogenic amines in the regulation of ACTH secretion. In: Neuroendocrine Control. Yagi, K., Yoshida, S. (Eds.). New York: John Wiley and Sons, 1973, p. 205
Hokfelt, T., Fuxe, K.: On the morphology and the neuroendocrine role of the hypothalamic catecholamine neurons. In: Brain-Endocrine Interaction. Median Eminence: Structure and Function. Knigge, K.M., Scott, D.E., Weindl, A. (Eds.). New York: S. Karger 1972, pp. 181–223
Hokfelt, T., Fuxe, K., Goldstein, M., Johansson, O.: Immunohistochemical evidence for the existence of adrenaline neurons in the rat brain. Brain Res. *66*, 235–251 (1974)
Holz, R., Deguchi, T., Axelrod, J.: Stimulation of serotonin *N*-acetyltransferase in pineal organ culture by drugs. J. Neurochem. *22*, 205–209 (1974)
Hoskins, R.G.: The thryoid-pituitary apparatus as a servo (feedback) mechanism. J. Clin. Endocrinol. *9*, 1429–1431 (1949)
Hsu, W.H., Cooper, C.W.: Hypercalcemic effect of catecholamines and its prevention by thyrocalcitonin. Calcif. Tissue Res. *19*, 125–137 (1975)
Hsu, W.H., Cooper, C.W.: Serum gastrin in the rat: cholinergic and adrenergic effects. Proc. Soc. Exp. Biol. Med. *154*, 401–406 (1977)
Hsu, T.-H., Hsu, C.-K., Gann, D.S.: Potentiation of the ACTH response to metyrapone by L-dopa in the monkey. Endocrinology *99*, 1115–1118 (1976)
Imura, H., Kato, Y., Ikeda, M., Morimoto, M., Yawata, M.: Effect of adrenergic-blocking or -stimulating agents on plasma growth hormone, immunoreactive insulin, and blood free fatty acid levels in man. J. Clin. Invest. *30*, 1069–1078 (1971)
Iturriza, F.C., Kasal-Iturriza, M.: Noradrenalin inhibition of MSH release in incubates of toad pars intermedia. Gen. Comp. Endocrinol. (Suppl.) *3*, 108–113 (1972)
Iversen, J.: Adrenergic receptors and the secretion of glucagon and insulin from the isolated perfused canine pancreas. J. Clin. Invest. *52*, 2102–2116 (1973)
Jacobson, E.D.: The circulation of the stomach. Gastroenterology *48*, 85–109 (1965)
Jaim-Etcheverry, G., Zieher, L.: Ultrastructural cytochemistry and pharmacology of 5-hydroxytryptamine in adrenergic nerve endings. III. Selective increase of norepinephrine in the rat pineal gland consecutive to depletion of neuronal 5-hydroxytryptamine. J. Pharmacol. Exp. Ther. *178*, 42–48 (1971)
Johnson, J.A., Davis, J.O., Gotshall, R.W., Lohmeier, T.E., Davis, J.L., Braverman, B., Tempel, G.E.: Evidence for an intrarenal beta receptor in control of renin release. Am. J. Physiol. *230*, 410–418 (1978)
Johnson, M., Ramwell, P.W.: Prostaglandin modification of membrane-bound enzyme activity: a possible mechanism of action? Prostaglandins *3*, 703–719 (1973)
Kalra, P.S., Kalra, S.P., Krulich, L., Fawcett, C.P., McCann, S.M.: Involvement of norepinephrine in transmission of the stimulatory influence of progesterone on gonadotropin release. Endocrinology *90*, 1168–1176 (1972)
Kalra, S.P., McCann, S.M.: Effects of drugs modifying catecholamine synthesis on plasma LH and ovulation in the rat. Neuroendocrinology *15*, 79–91 (1974)

Kamber, J.H., Schneider, H.P.G., McCann: Action of dopamine to induce release of FSH-releasing factor (FRF) from hypothalamic tissue *in vitro*. Endocrinology *86*, 278–284 (1970)
Kamberi, I.A., Mical, R.S., Porter, J.C.: Luteinizing hormone-releasing activity in hypophysial stalk blood and elevation by dopamine. Science *166*, 388–390 (1969)
Kamberi, I.A., Schneider, H.P.G., McCann, S.M.: Action of dopamine to induce release of FSH-releasing factor (FRF) from hypothalamic tissue in vitro. Endocrinology *86*, 278–284 (1970)
Kamberi, I.A., Mical, R.S., Porter, J.C.: Effects of anterior pituitary perfusion and intraventricular injection of catecholamines on prolactin release. Endocrinology *88*, 1012–1020 (1971)
Karam, J.H., Grasso, S.G., Wegienka, L.C., Grodsky, G.M., Forsham, P.H.: Effect of selected hexoses, of epinephrine and of glucagon on insulin secretion in man. Diabetes *15*, 571–587 (1966)
Karlberg, B.E., Nilsson, O., Tolagen, K.: Clonidine in primary hypertension: Effects on blood pressure, plasma renin activity, plasma and urinary aldosterone. Curr. Ther. Res. *21*, 10–20 (1977)
Kato, Y., Dupre, J., Beck, J.C.: Plasma growth hormone in the anesthetized rat: Effects of dibutyryl cyclic AMP, prostaglandin E, adrenergic agents vasopressin, chlorpromazine, amphetamine, and L-dopa. Endocrinology *93*, 135–146 (1973)
Kato, Y., Chihara, K., Ohgo, S., Imura, H.: Effects of hypothalamic surgery and somatostatin on chlorpromazine-induced growth hormone release in rats. Endocrinology *95*, 1608–1613 (1974)
Kendall, J.W.: Feedback control adrenocorticotropic hormone secretion. In: Frontiers in Neuroendocrinology. Martin, L., Ganong, W.F. (Eds.). New York: Oxford University Press, 1971, p. 177
Kenny, A.D.: Effect of catecholamines on serum calcium and phosphorus levels in intact and parathyroidectomiced rats. Naunyn-Schmiedebergs Arch. exp. Path. Pharmak. *248*, 144–152 (1964)
Kitay, J.I., Holub, D.A., Jailer, M.W.: "Inhibition" of pituitary ACTH release after administration of reserpine or epinephrine. Endocrinology *65*, 548–554 (1959)
Kizer, J.S., Polkovits, M., Zivin, J., Browstein, M., Saavedra, J.M., Kopin, J.J.: The effects of endocrinological manipulation on tyrosine hydroxylase and dopamine-β-hydroxylase activities in the individual hypothalamic nuclei of the adult male rat. Endocrinology *95*, 799–812 (1974)
Klein, D., Rowe, J.: Pineal gland in organ culture. I. Inhibition by harmine of serotonin-^{14}C oxidation, accompanied by stimulation of melatonin-^{14}C production. Mol. Pharmacol. *6*, 164–171 (1970)
Klein, D.C., Berg, G.R., Weller, J.: Melatonin synthesis: adenosine 3′,5′-monophosphate and norepinephrine stimulate *N*-acetyl-transferase. Science *168*, 979–980 (1970a)
Klein, D.C., Weller, J.C.: Indole metabolism in the pineal gland: A circadian rhythm in *N*-acetyltransferase. Science *169*, 1093–1095 (1970b)
Klein, L.A., Liberman, B., Laks, M., Kleeman, C.R.: Interrelated effects of antidiuretic hormone and adrenergic drugs on water metabolism. Am. J. Physiol. *221*, 1657–1665 (1971)
Kotani, M., Onaya, T., Yamada, T.: Acute increase of thyroid hormone secretion in response to cold and its inhibition by drugs which act on the autonomic or central nervous system. Endocrinology *92*, 288–294 (1973)
Krieger, D.T.: Lack of responsiveness to L-dopa in Cushing's disease. J. Clin. Endocrinol. Metab. *36*, 277–284 (1973)
Krieger, H.P., Krieger, D.T.: Chemical stimulation of the brain: effect on adrenal corticoid release. Am. J. Physiol. *213*, 1632–1641 (1970)
Kris, A.O., Miller, R.G., Wherry, F.E., Mason, J.W.: Inhibition of insulin secretion by infused epinephrine in rhesus monkeys. Endocrinology *78*, 87–99 (1966)
Kronborg, O., Pedersen, T., Stadil, F., Rehfeld, J.F.: The effect of beta-adrenergic blockade upon gastric acid secretion and gastrin secretion during hypoglycaemia before and after vagotomy. Scand. J. Gastroent. *9*, 173–176 (1974)
Krulich, L., Illner, P., Fawcett, C.P., Quijada, M., McCann, S.M.: Dual hypothalamic regulation of growth hormone secretion. In: Growth and Growth Hormone. Pecile, A., Muller, E.E. (Eds.). Amsterdam: Excerpta Medica Foundation 1972, p. 306

Krulich, L., Giachetti, A., Marchlewska-Koj, A., Hefco, E., Jameson, H.E.: On the role of the central noradrenergic and dopaminergic systems in the regulation of TSH secretion in the rat. Endocrinology *100*, 496–505 (1977)
Kukreja, S.C., Hargis, G.K., Bower, E.N., Henderson, W.J., Fisherman, E.W., Williams, G.A.: Role of adrenergic stimuli in parathyroid hormone secretion in man. J. Clin. Endocrinol. *40*, 478–481 (1975)
Kukreja, S.C., Hargis, G.K., Rosenthal, I.M., Williams, G.A.: Pheochromocytoma causing excessive parathyroid hormone production and hypercalcemia. Ann. Int. Med. *79*, 838–840 (1973)
Kukreja, S.C., Johnson, P.A., Ayala, G., Banerjee, P., Bowser, E.N., Hargis, G.K., Williams, G.A.: Role of calcium and beta-adrenergic system in control of parathyroid hormone secretion. Proc. Soc. Exp. Biol. Med. *151*, 326–328 (1976)
Lacy, P.E., Greider, M.H.: Ultrastructural organization of mammalian pancreatic islets. In: Endocrine Pancreas. Handbook of Physiology. Steiner, D.F., Freinkel, N. (Eds.), Sect. 7. Baltimore: Williams and Wilkins, 1972, Vol. 1, 77–90
Ladosky, W., Kesikowski, W.M., Gaziri, I.F.: Effects of a single injection of chlorpromazine into infant male rats on subsequent gonadotrophin secretion. J. Endocrinol. *48*, 151–158 (1970)
Lal, S., Martin, J.B., De la Vega, C.E.: Comparison of the effect of apomorphine and L-DOPA on serum growth hormone levels in normal men. Clin. Endocrinol. *4*, 277–285 (1975)
Landsberg, L., Axelrod, J.: Influence of pituitary, thyroid, and adrenal hormones on norepinephrine turnover and metabolism in the rat heart. Circ. Res. *22*, 559–571 (1968)
Leblanc, H., Lachelin, G.C.L., Abu-Fadil, S., Yen, S.S.C.: Effects of dopamine infusion on pituitary hormone secretion in humans. J. Clin. Endocrinol. Metab. *43*, 668–674 (1976)
Lebovitz, H.E., Feldman, J.M.: Pancreatic biogenic amines and insulin secretion in health and disease. Fed. Proc. *32*, 1797–1802 (1973)
Leclercq-Meyer, V., Brisson, G.R., Malaisse, W.J.: Effect of adrenaline and glucose on release of glucagon and insulin *in vitro*. Nature New Bioly. *231*, 2–3 (1971)
Lee, J.B., Attallah, A.A.: Renal prostaglandins. Nephron *15*, 350–368 (1975)
Lindsey, C.A., Faloona, G.: Adrenergic blockade in shock-induced hyperglucagonemia. Diabetes *22*, 301 (1973)
Lippmann, W., Leonardi, R., Ball, J., Coppola, J.A.: Relationship between hypothalamic catecholamines and gonadotrophin secretion in rats. J. Pharmacol. Exp. Ther. *156*, 258–266 (1967)
Liberman, B., Klein, L.A., Kleeman, C.R.: Effect of adrenergic blocking agents on the vasopressin inhibiting action of norepinephrine. Proc. Soc. Exp. Biol. Med. *133*, 131–134 (1970)
Lode, C.F.: The inhibition of gastric secretion: A review. Pharmacol. Rev. *3*, 59–106 (1951)
Loeffler, J.R., Stockigt, J.R., Ganong, W.F.: Effect of alpha- and beta-adrenergic blocking agents on the increase in renin secretion produced by stimulation of the renal nerves. Neuroendocrinology *10*, 129–138 (1972)
Loubatieres, A., Mariani, M.M., Sorel, G., Savi, L.: The action of β-adrenergic blocking and stimulating agents on insulin secretion. Characterization of the type of β-receptor. Diabetalogia *7*, 127–132 (1971)
Lovinger, R., Holland, J., Kaplan, S., Grumbach, M., Boryczka, A.T., Shackelford, R., Salmon, J., Reid, I.A., Ganong, W.F.: Pharmacological evidence for stimulation of growth hormone secretion by a central noradrenergic system in dogs. Neuroscience *1*, 443–450 (1976)
Lu, K.H., Meites, J.: Effects of serotonin precursors and melatonin on serum prolactin release in rats. Endocrinology *93*, 152–155 (1973)
Luyckx, A.S., Lefebvre: Role of catecholamines in exercise-induced glucagon secretion in rats. Diabetes *21*, 334 (1972)
Luyckx, A.S., Lefebvre, P.J.: Mechanisms involved in the exercise-induced increase in glucagon secretion in rats. Diabetes *23*, 81–93 (1974)
Luyckx, A.S., Lefebvre, P.J.: Pharmacological compounds affecting plasma glucagon levels in rats. Biochem. Pharmacol. *25*, 2703–2708 (1976)
Maayan, M.L., Ingbar, S.H.: Effects of epinephrine on iodine and intermediary metabolism in isolated thyroid cells. Endocrinology *87*, 588–595 (1970)

Maayan, M.L.: Epinephrine. Effect on uptake of iodine by dispersed cells of calf thyroid gland. Science *162*, 124–125 (1968)
Macleod, R.M.: Regulation of prolactin secretion. In: Frontiers in Neuroendocrinology. Ganong, W.F., Martini, L. (Eds.). New York: Raven Press, 1975, Vol. 4, p. 169
Maebashi, M., Mivra, Y., Yoshinaga, K.: Plasma renin activity in pheochromocytoma. Jpn. Circ. J. *32*, 1427–1423 (1968)
Maickel, R.P., Westermann, O., Brodie, B.B.: Effects of reserpine and cold-exposure on pituitary-adrenocortical function in rats. J. Pharmacol. Exp. Ther. *134*, 167–175 (1961)
Malaisse, W.J., Malaisse-Lagae, F.: A possible role for calcium in the stimulus-secretion coupling of glucose-induced insulin secretion. Acta Diabet. Lat. 7, (Suppl. 1) 264–275 (1970)
Malaisse, W.J., Brisson, B., Malaisse-Lagae, F.: The stimulus-secretion coupling of glucose-induced release-I. Interaction of epinephrine and alkaline earth cations. J. Lab. Clin. Med. *76*, 895–902 (1970)
Malaisse, W.J., Malaisse-Lagae, F., Wright, P.H., Ashmore, J.: Effects of adrenergic and cholinergic agents upon insulin secretion *in vitro*. Endocrinology *80*, 975–978 (1967)
Malarkey, W.B., Jacobs, L.S., Daughaday, W.H.: Levodopa suppression of prolactin in nonpeurperal galactorrhea. N. Engl. J. Med. *285*, 1160–1163 (1971)
Marks, B.H., Hall, M.M., Bhattacharya, A.N.: Psychopharmacological effects and pituitary-adrenal activity. Prog. Brain Res. *32*, 58–70 (1970)
Massara, F., Strumia, E.: Increase in plasma growth hormone concentration in man after infusion of adrenaline-propranolol. Endocrinology *47*, 95–100 (1970)
Martin, J.B., Reichlin, S., Brown, G.M.: Neural regulation of water and salt metabolism: physiologic function and disease. In: Clinical Neuroendocrinology. Plum, F., McDowell, F.H. (Eds.). Philadelphia: F.A. Davis, 1977
Martin, J.B.: Plasma growth hormone (GH) response to hypothalamic or extra hypothalamic electrical stimulation. Endocrinology *91*, 107–115 (1972)
Martin, J.B.: Neural regulation of growth hormone secretion. Medical progress report. N. Engl. J. Med. *228*, 1384–1393 (1973)
Martin, J.B., Kontor, J., Mead, P.: Plasma GH responses to hypothalamic, hippocampal, and amygdaloid electrical stimulation; effects of variation in stimulus parameters and treatment with α-methyl-p-tyrosine (α-MT). Endocrinology *92*, 1354–1361 (1973)
McCann, S.M.: Regulation of secretion of follicle-stimulation hormone and luteinizing hormone. In: Handbook of Physiology. Greep, R.O., Astwood, E.B. (Eds.), Sect. 7. Endocrinology, Part 1, American Physiological Society. Baltimore: Williams and Wilkins, 1974, Vol. 4, p. 489
McCann, S.M., Kalra, P.S., Donoso, A.O., Bishop, W., Schneider, H.P.G., Fawcett, C.P., Krulich, L.: The role of monoamines in the control of gonadotropin and prolactin secretion. In: Brain-Endocrine Interaction: Median Eminence. Structure and Function. Kinigge, K.M., Scot, D.E., Weindl, A. (Eds.). Basel: S. Karger, 1972, pp. 224–235
McKenna, O.C., Angelakos, E.T.: Adrenergic innervation of the canine kidney. Circ. Res. *22*, 345–354 (1968)
Meites, J., Lu, K.H., Wuttke, W., Welsch, C.W., Nagasawa, H., Quadri, S.K.: Recent studies on functions and control of prolactin secretion in rats. Recent Prog. Horm. Res. *28*, 471–526 (1972)
Meites, J.: Evaluation of research on control of prolactin secretion. Adv. Exp. Med. Biol. *80*, 135–152 (1977)
Melander, A.: Amines and mouse thyroid activity. Release of thyroid hormone by catecholamines and indoleamines and its inhibition by adrenergic blocking drugs. Acta Endocrinol. (Kbh) *65*, 371–384 (1970)
Melander, A.: Thyroid hormone secretion. Its regulation by intrathyroidal amines. Acta Physiol. Scand. (Suppl.) *370*, 7–31 (1971)
Melander, A.: Sympathetic innervation of the thyroid: Variation with species and with age. Endocrinology *96*, 102–106 (1975)
Melander, A., Sundler, F.: Interactions between catecholamines, 5-hydroxytryptamine and TSH on the secretion of thyroid hormone. Endocrinology *90*, 188–193 (1972)
Melander, A., Nilsson, E., Sundler, F.: Sympathetic activation of thyroid hormone secretion in mice. Endocrinology *90*, 194–199 (1972)

Melander, A., Ericson, L., Sundler, F., Westgren, U.: Intrathyroidal amines in the regulation of thyroid activity. Rev. Physiol. Biochem. Pharmacol. *73*, 39–71 (1973)
Melander, A., Ericson, L.E., Sundler, F., Ingbar, S.H.: Sympathetic innervation of the mouse thyroid and its significance in thyroid hormone secretion. Endocrinology *94*, 959–966 (1974)
Melander, A., Ranklev, E., Sundler, F., Westgren, U.: $Beta_2$-adrenergic stimulation of thyroid hormone secretion. Endocrinology *97*, 332–336 (1975)
Melander, A., Bulow, K., Burger, A., Ericson, L.E., Ingemansson, S., Ljunggren, J.-G., Norberg, K.-A., Persson, B., Sundquist, S.-B., Sundler, F., Tibblin, S., Westgren, U.: Influence of the sympathetic nervous system on thyroid activity in man. In: Thyroid Research (Proceedings of 7th International Thyroid Conference, Boston, Mass.). Amsterdam: Excerpta Medica, 1976, p. 100
Myerson, B., Sawyer, C.H.: Monoamines and ovulation in the rat. Endocrinology *83*, 170–176 (1968)
Michelakis, A.M., Robertson, D.: Plasma renin activity and levodopa in Parkinson's disease. J. Am. Med. Assoc. *213*, 83–85 (1970)
Mills, L.C.: Drug treatment in thyroid disease. Sem. Drug Treatment *3*, 377–402 (1974)
Minneman, K.P., Wurtman, R.J.: The pharmacology of the pineal gland. Ann. Rev. Pharmacol. *16*, 33–51 (1976)
Miura, K., Aida, M., Mihara, A., Kato, K., Ojima, M., Demura, R., Demura, H., Okuyama, M.: Treatment of Cushing's disease with reserpine and pituitary irradiation. J. Clin. Endocrinol. Metab. *41*, 511–526 (1975)
Miyai, K., Onishi, T., Hosokawa, M., Ishibashi, K., Kumahara, Y.: Inhibition of thyrotropin and prolactin secretions in primary hypothyroidism by 2-Br-α-ergocyptine. J. Clin. Endocrinol. Metab. *39*, 391–394 (1974)
Moratinos, J., Ellis, S., Potter, D.E.: Catecholamine-induced changes in plasma glucose and insulin levels in the unanesthetized rabbit. Pharmacology *15*, 407–414 (1977)
Moss, R.L., Dyball, R.E.J., Cross, B.A.: Responses of antidromically identified supraoptic and paraventricular units to acetylcholine, noradrenaline, and glutamate applied iontophoretically. Brain Res. *35*, 573–575 (1971)
Müller, E.E.: Catecholamines and control of growth hormone secretion. Neurosci. Res. Prog. Bull. *9*, 232–235 (1971)
Müller, E.E., Cocchi, D., Villa, A., Zambotti, F., Fraschini, F.: Involvement of brain catecholamines in the gonadotropin-releasing mechanism(s) before puberty. Endocrinology *90*, 1267–1276 (1972)
Müller, E.E., Dal Pra, D., Pecile, A.: Influence of brain neurohumors injected into the lateral ventricle of the rat in growth hormone release. Endocrinology *83*, 893–896 (1968)
Müller, E.E., Gil-Ad, I., Paneri, A.E., Secchi, C., Liuzzi, A., Chiodini, P.G., Silvestrini, F.: Involvement of brain monoamines in the control of growth hormone secretion. In: Basic Applications and Clinical Uses of Hypothalamic Hormones. Charro-Salgado, A.L., Fernandez-Durango, R., Lopez de Campo, J.G. (Eds.). New York: Exerpta Medica American Elsevier Publishing Co., Inc., 1976, p. 211
Müller, E.E., Locchi, D., Jalanbo, H., Udeschini, G.: Antagonistic role for norepinephrine (NE) and dopamine (DA) in the control of growth hormone (GH) secretion in the rat. Ineffectiveness of serotonin (5-HT). Endocrinology *92*, A 248 (Abstract) (1973)
Needleman, P., Douglas, Jr., J.R., Jakschik, B., Stoecklein, P.B., Johnson, Jr., E.M.: Release of renal prostaglandin by catecholamines: Relationship to renal endocrine function. J. Pharmacol. Exp. Ther. *188*, 453–460 (1974)
Noel, G.L., Suh, H.K., Frantz, A.G.: L-Dopa suppression of TRH-stimulated prolactin release in man. J. Clin. Endocrinol. Metab. *36*, 1255–1258 (1973)
Noel, G.L., Suh, H.K., Stone, J.G., Frantz, A.G.: Human prolactin and growth hormone release during surgery and other conditions of stress. J. Clin. Endocrinol. Metab. *35*, 840–851 (1972)
Ojeda, J.R., McCann, S.M.: Evidence for participation of a catecholaminergic mechanism in the post-castration rise in plasma gonadotropins. Neuroendocrinology *12*, 295–315 (1973)
Otsuka, K., Assaykeen, T.A., Goldfien, A., Ganong, W.F.: The effect of hypoglycemia on plasma renin activity in dogs. Endocrinology *87*, 1306–1317 (1970)

Passo, S.S., Assaykeen, T.A., Otsuka, K., Wise, B.L., Goldfien, A., Ganong, W.F.: Effect of stimulation of the medulla oblongata on renin secretion in dogs. Neuroendocrinology *7*, 1–10 (1971)

Pearse, A.G.E.: The cytochemistry and ultrastructure of polypeptide hormone-producing cells of the APUD series and the embryologic, physiologic, and pathologic implications of the concept. J. Histochem. Cytochem. *17*, 303–313 (1969)

Pearse, A.G.E.: Evolutionary and development relationships among the cells producing peptide hormones. In: Peptide Hormones. Parsons, J.A. (Ed.). Baltimore: University Park Press, 1976, pp. 33–46

Pearse, A.G.E.: Diffuse neuroendocrine system: Peptides common to brain and intestine and their relationship to the APUD concept. In: Centrally Acting Peptides. Hughes, J. (Ed.). Baltimore: University Park Press, 1978, pp. 49–57

Peart, W.S.: The kidney as an endocrine organ. Lancet *II*, 543–547 (1977)

Peck, W.A., Carpenter, J., Messinger, K.: Cyclic 3′,5′-adenosine monophosphate in isolated bone cells. II. Response to adenosine and parathyroid hormone. Endocrinology *94*, 148–154 (1974)

Pellegrino de Iraldi, A., Suburo, A.: Effect of tyramine on the compartments of the granulated vesicles in rat pineal nerve endings. Eur. J. Pharmacol. *19*, 251–259 (1972)

Peskar, B., Meyer, D.K., Tauchmann, U., Hertting, G.: Influence of isoproterenol, hydralazine, and phentolamine on renin activity of plasma and renal cortex of rats. Eur. J. Pharmacol. *9*, 394–396 (1970)

Pettinger, W.A., Keeton, T.K., Campbell, W.B., Harper, D.C.: Evidence for a renal α-adrenergic receptor inhibiting renin release. Circ. Res. *38*, 338–346 (1976)

Phillipo, M., Bruce, J.B., Lawrence, C.B.: The effect of adrenaline on calcitonin secretion in conscious sheep. J. Endocrinol. *46*, XII (Abstract) (1970)

Polak, J., Grimelius, L., Pearse, A.: Growth hormone release-inhibiting hormone in gastrointestinal and pancreatic D cells. Lancet *1*, 1220–1222 (1975)

Porte, Jr., D.: A receptor mechanism for the inhibition of insulin release by epinephrine in man. J. Clin. Invest. *46*, 86–94 (1967)

Porte, Jr., D.: Sympathetic regulation of insulin secretion. Its relation to diabetes mellitus. Arch. Int. Med. *123*, 252–260 (1969)

Porte, Jr., D., Graber, A.L., Kuzuya, T., Williams, R.H.: The effect of epinephrine on immunoreactive insulin levels in man. J. Clin. Invest. *45*, 228–236 (1966)

Porte, Jr., D., Girardier, L., Seydoux, J., Kanazawa, Y., Posternak, J.: Neural regulation of insulin secretion in the dog. J. Clin. Invest. *52*, 210–214 (1973)

Porte, Jr., D., Robertson, R.P.: Control of insulin secretion by catecholamines, stress, and the sympathetic nervous system. Fed. Proc. *32*, 1792–1796 (1973)

Porte, Jr., D., Smith, P.H., Ensinck, J.W.: Neurohumoral regulation of pancreatic islet A and B cells. Metabolism XXV (Suppl.) *1*, 1453–1456 (1976)

Potter, D.E., Ellis, S.: Isoproterenol- and epinephrine-induced changes in blood glucose and tissue glycogen levels in normal and diabetic rats: The influence of alteration in endogenous insulin levels and state of nourishment. J. Pharmacol. Exp. Ther. *193*, 576–584 (1975)

Potter, D.E., Kempen, R.R., Ellis, S.: Comparative metabolic and cardiovascular responses to isoproterenol (I), metaproterenol (M), salbutamol (S), and carbuterol (C) in baboons. Pharmacologist *17*, 223 (1975)

Potter, D.E., Wilson, L.M., Ellis, S.: Isoproterenol-induced insulin release in normal rats and hyperglycemia in alloxan-diabetic rats: a preliminary report. Res. Commun. Chem. Pathol. Pharmacol. *7*, 787–790 (1974)

Potter, D.E., Barnett, J.W., Woodson, L.C.: Catecholamine-induced changes in plasma glucose, glucagon, and insulin in rabbits: Effects of somatostatin. Horm. Metab. Res. *10*, 373–377 (1978)

Potter, D.E. and Rowland, J.M.: Effect of β-adrenergic drugs on plasma glucose and glucagon in Japanese quail: A preliminary report. Res. Comm. Chem. Pathol. Pharmacol. *26*, 421–424, 1979.

Ramwell, P.W., Shaw, J.E.: Biological significance of prostaglandins. Recent. Prog. Horm. Res. *26*, 139–187 (1970)

Rasmussen, H.: Cell communication, calcium ion, and cyclic adenosine monophosphate. Science *170*, 404–412 (1970)

Rayfield, E.J., George, D.T., Eichner, H.L., Hsu, T.H.: L-Dopa stimulation of glucagon secretion in man. N. Engl. J. Med. *293*, 589–591 (1975)

Robertson, R.P., Porte, Jr., D.: Adrenergic modulation of basal insulin secretion in man. Diabetes *22*, 1–8 (1973a)

Robertson, R.P., Porte, Jr., D.: The glucose receptor: A defective mechanism in diabetes mellitus distinct from the β-adrenergic receptor. J. Clin. Invest. *52*, 870–876 (1973b)

Rodan, S.B., Rodan, G.A.: The effect of parathyroid hormone and thyrocalcitonin on the accumulation of cyclic adenosine 3′:5′-monophosphate in freshly isolated bone cells. J. Biol. Chem. *249*, 3068–3074 (1974)

Rubinstein, L., Sawyer, C.H.: Role of catecholamines in stimulating the release of pituitary ovulating hormone(s) in rats. Endocrinology *86*, 988–995 (1970)

Ruch, W., Mixter, R.C., Russell, R.M., Garcia, J.F., Gale, C.C.: Aminergic and thermoregulatory mechanisms in hypothalamic regulation of growth hormone in cats. Am. J. Physiol. *2*, E61–E69 (1977)

Samols, E., Weir, G.C., Ramseur, R., Day, J.A., Patel, Y.C.: Modulation of pancreatic somatostatin by adrenergic and cholinergic agonism by hyper- and hypoglycemic sulfonamides. Metabolism 27 (Suppl.) 1219–1221 (1978)

Sanders, J.P., Potter, D.E., Ellis, S., Bee, D., Grant, J.A.: Metabolic and cardiovascular effects of carbuterol and metaproterenol. J. Allergy Clin. Immunol. *60*, 174–179 (1977)

Sawyer, C.H., Hilliard, J., Kanetmatsu, S., Scaramuzzi, R., Blake, C.A.: Effects of intraventricular infusions of norepinephrine and dopamine on LH release and ovulation in the rabbit. Neuroendocrinology *15*, 328–337 (1974)

Sawyer, C.R., Markee, J.E., Hollinshead, W.H.: Inhibition of ovulation in the rabbit by the adrenergic-blocking agent, dibenamine. Endocrinology *41*, 395–402 (1947)

Scanlon, M.F., Mora, B., Shale, D.J., Hall, R., Weightman, D.R., Heath, M., Snow, M.H.: Evidence for dopaminergic control of thyrotrophin secretion in man. Lancet *II*, 421–423 (1977)

Scapagnini, U., Preziozi, P.: Receptor involvement in the central noradrenergic inhibition of ACTH secretion in the rat. Neuropharmacology *12*, 57–62 (1973)

Schauder, P., McIntosh, C., Arends, J., Arnold, J., Arnold, R., Fredrichs, H., Creutzfeldt, W.: Somatostatin and insulin release from isolated rat pancreatic islets stimulated by glucose. FEBS Letts. *68*, 225–227 (1976)

Schneider, H.P.G., McCann, S.M.: Possible role of dopamine as transmitter to promote discharge of LH-releasing factor. Endocrinology *85*, 121–132 (1969a)

Schneider, H.P.G., McCann, S.M.: Effect of dopamine on release of LH-releasing factor by stalk median eminence (SME) tissue *in vitro*. Fed. Proc. *28*, 381 (1969b)

Schneider, H.P.G., McCann, S.M.: Mono- and indolamines and control of LH secretion. Endocrinology *86*, 1127–1133 (1970a)

Schneider, H.P.G., McCann, S.M.: Estradiol and the neuroendocrine control of LH release *in vitro*. Endocrinology *87*, 330–338 (1970b)

Schneider, H.P.G., McCann, S.M.: Possible role of dopamine as transmitter to promote discharge of LH-releasing factor. Endocrinology *85*, 121–132 (1969a)

Schrier, R.W., Berl, T.: Mechanism of effect of alpha-adrenergic stimulation with norepinephrine. J. Clin. Invest. *53*, 219–227 (1974)

Scornik, O.A., Paladini, A.C.: Angiotensin blood levels in hemorrhagic hypotension and other related conditions. Am. J. Physiol. *206*, 553–556 (1964)

Sherlock, S.: Comparison of the carbohydrate effect of adrenalin infused into the femoral vein, carotid artery, aorta, and portal vein of rats. Am. J. Physiol. *157*, 52–58 (1949)

Shimamoto, K., Miyahara, M.: Effect of norepinephrine infusion on plasma vasopressin levels in normal human subjects. J. Clin. Endocrinol. Metab. *43*, 201–204 (1976)

Silver, M.J., Smith, J.B.: Prostaglandins as intracellular messengers. Life Sci. *16*, 1635–1648 (1975)

Smith, P.H., Porte, Jr., D.: Neuropharmacology of the pancreatic islets. Ann. Rev. Pharmacol. Toxicol. *16*, 269–285 (1976)

Smith, P.H., Woods, S.C., Ensinck, J.W., Porte, Jr., D.: Phentolamine prevents the somatostatin-mediated inhibition of pancreatic glucagon secretion. Metabolism *26*, 841–845 (1977)
Smythe, C. McC., Nickel, J.F., Bradley, S.E.: The effect of epinephrine (USP), *l*-epinephrine, and *l*-norepinephrine on glomerular filtration rate, renal plasma flow, and the urinary excretion of sodium, potassium, and water in normal man. J. Clin. Invest. *31*, 499–506 (1952)
Soderberg, U.: Temporal characteristics of thyroid activity. Physiol. Rev. *39*, 777–810 (1959)
Sokal, J.E., Sarcione, E.J., Henderson, A.M.: Relative potency of glucagon and epinephrine as hepatic glycogenolytic agents: Studies with the isolated rat liver. Endocrinology *74*, 930–938 (1964)
Speidel, C.C.: Further comparative studies in other fishes of cells that are homologous to the large irregular glandular cells in the spinal cord of the skates. J. Comp. Neurol. *34*, 303 (1922)
Stadil, F.: Effect of vagotomy on gastrin release during insulin hypoglycaemia in ulcer patients. Scand. J. Gastroenterol. *7*, 225–231 (1972)
Stadil, R., Rehfeld, J.F.: Release of gastrin by epinephrine in man. Gastroenterology *65*, 210–215 (1973)
Stewart, J.: Genetic studies on the mechanism of action of aldosterone in mice. Endocrinology *96*, 711–717 (1975)
Stout, B.D., Weiner, L., Cox, J.W.: Combine α and β sympathetic blockade in hyperthyroidism: Clinical and metabolic effects. Ann. Int. Med. *70*, 963–970 (1969)
Szego, C.M.: In: Hormones and Antagonists. Hubinot, P.O., Hendeles, S.M., Preumont, P. (Eds.). New York: S. Karger, 1972, p. 387
Tabachnick, I.I.A., Gulbenkian, A.: Adrenergic changes due to pertussis: Insulin, glucose, and free fatty acids. Eur. J. Pharmacol. *7*, 186–195 (1969)
Takahara, L., Arimura, A., Schally, A.V.: Effects of catecholamines on the TRH-stimulated release of prolactin and growth hormone from sheep pituitaries *in vitro*. Endocrinology *95*, 1490–1494 (1974)
Taylor, A.N., Wilson, R.W.: Electrophysiological evidence for the action of light on the pineal gland in the rat. Experientia *26*, 267–270 (1970)
Taylor, A.W.: Free fatty acid levels in exercised and nonexercised reserpinized rats. Am. J. Physiol. *223*, 319–322 (1972)
Terashima, R., Anderson, F.L., Jubiz, W., Tsagaris, T.J., Kuida, H.: Influence of adrenergic drugs on prostaglandin E release from the dog kidney. Proc. Soc. Exp. Biol. Med. *147*, 449–452 (1974)
Tice, L.W., Creveling, C.R.: Electron microscopic identification of adrenergic nerve endings on thyroid epithelial cells. Endocrinology *97*, 1123–1129 (1975)
Toivola, P.T.K., Gale, G.C.: Stimulation of growth release by microinjection of norepinephrine into hypothalamus of baboons. Endocrinology *90*, 895–902 (1972)
Toyota, T., Sato, S-I., Kido, M., Abe, K., Goto, Y.: Secretory regulation of endocrine pancreas: cyclic AMP and glucagon secretion. J. Clin. Endocrinol. Metab. *41*, 81–89 (1975)
Tuomisto, J., Ranta, T., Mannisto, P., Saarinen, A., Leppaluoto, J.: Neurotransmitter control of thyrotropin secretion in the rat. Eur. J. Pharm. *30*, 221–229 (1975)
Turner, P.: β-Adrenergic receptor blocking drugs in hyperthyroidism. Drugs *7*, 48–54 (1974)
Turtle, J.R., Littleton, G.K., Kipnis, D.M.: Stimulation of insulin secretion by theophylline. Nature (London) *213*, 727–728 (1967)
Tyler, J.M., Kajinuma, H.: Influence of beta-adrenergic and cholinergic agents *in vivo* on pancreatic glucagon and insulin secretion. Diabetes *21*, 332 (1972)
Ueda, H., Yasuda, H., Takabatake, Y., Iizuka, M., Iizuka, T., Jori, M., Yakamoto, M., Sakamoto, Y.: Increased renin release evoked by mesencephalic stimulation in the dog. Japan-Heart, J. *8*, 498–506 (1967)
Uemura, H., Kobayashi, H.: Effects of norepinephrine and dibenamine implanted in the median eminence on the estrous cycle of the rat. Horm. Res. *5*, 89–111 (1974)
Vander, A.J.: Effect of catecholamines and the renal nerves on renin secretion in anesthetized dogs. Am. J. Physiol. *209*, 659–662 (1965)
Vandongen, R., Greenwood, D.M.: The stimulation of renin secretion by non-vasoconstrictor infusions of adrenaline and noradrenaline in the isolated rat kidney. Clin. Sci. Mol. Med. *49*, 609–612 (1975)

Van Loon, G.R.: Brain catecholamines in the regulation of ACTH secretion. In: Recent Studies of Hypothalamic Function. Lederis, K., Cooper, K.E. (Eds.). Basel: S. Karger, 1974, p. 100
Van Woert, M.H., Mueller, P.S., Ambani, L.M.: Abnormal insulin secretion in Parkinson's disease before and during L-dihydroxyphenylalanine (L-dopa) therapy. J. Endocrinology *59*, 523–534 (1973)
Van Zwieten, P.A.: The central action of antihypertensive drugs mediated via central α-receptors. J. Pharm. Pharmacol. *25*, 89–95 (1973)
Veda, H., Yasuda, H., Takabatake, Y., Iizuka, T., Iizuka, M., Iori, M., Yamamoto, M., Inoue, I., Sakamoto, Y.: The mechanism of renin secretion following electrical stimulation of the midbrain. Jpn. Circ. J. *31*, 1931–1932 (1967)
Vernikos-Danellis, J., Marks, B.H.: Epinephrine-induced release of ACTH in normal human subjects: A test of pituitary function. Endocrinology *70*, 525–531 (1962)
Vigas, M., Malatinsky, J., Nemeth, S., Juriovicova, J.: Alpha adrenergic control of growth hormone release during surgical stress in man. Metabolism *26*, 399–402 (1977)
Wagermark, J., Ungerstedt, V., Ljunquist, A.: Sympathetic innervation of the juxtaglomerular cells of the kidney. Circ. Res. *22*, 149–153 (1968)
Weber, M.A., Case, D.B., Baer, L., Sealey, J.E., Drayer, J.I.M., Lopez-Overjero, J.A., Laragh, J.H.: Renin and aldosterone suppression in the antihypertensive action of clonidine. Am. J. Cardiol. *38*, 825–830 (1976)
Weinberger, M.H., Aoi, W., Henry, D.P.: Direct effect of beta-adrenergic stimulation on renin release by the rat kidney slice *in vitro*. Circ. Res. *37*, 318–324 (1975)
Weiss, B.: Similarities and differences in the norepinephrine- and sodium fluoride-sensitive adenylcyclase system. J. Pharmacol. Exp. Ther. *166*, 330–338 (1969)
Wells, H., Lloyd, W.: Inhibition of the hypocalcemic action of thyrocalcitonin by theophylline and isoproterenol. Endocrinology *82*, 468–474 (1968)
Wiersinga, W.M. and Touber, J.L.: The influence of beta-adrenoceptor blocking agents on plasma thyroxine and triiodothyronine. J. Clin. Endocrinol. Metab *45*, 293–298, 1977.
Williams, G.A., Hargis, G.K., Bowser, E.N., Henderson, W.J., Martinez, N.J.: Evidence for a role of adenosine 3′,5′-monophosphate in parathyroid hormone release. Endocrinology *92*, 687–691 (1973)
Winer, N., Choksi, D.S., Yoon, M.S., Freedman, A.D.: Adrenergic receptor mediation of renin secretion. J. Clin. Edocrinol. *29*, 1168–1175 (1969)
Woodson, L.C., Barnett, J.B., Potter, D.E.: Catecholamine-induced glucagon (IRG) release and hyperglycemia in normal and diabetic rats: Effect of somatostatin (SRIF). Pharmacologist *18*, 248 (1976)
Woodson, L.C.: The role of increased glucagon release in the production of hyperglycemia by catecholamines. Doctoral Dissertation, University of Texas, Medical Branch, Galveston, 1977
Woodson, L.C., Potter, D.E.: Catecholamine-induced alterations in glucose homeostasis in baboons, dogs, rabbits, and rats: Comparative effects of somatostatin. Metabolism, *27* (Suppl.): 1441–1444 (1978).
Woodson, L.C., Potter, D.E.: The influence of glucagon release on hyperglycemic responses to catecholamines in normal fed and diabetic rats. J. Pharmacol. Exp. Ther. *210*, 458–464 (1979)
Wurtman, R., Shein, H., Levin, F.: Mediation by β-adrenergic receptors of effect of norepinephrine on pineal synthesis of [^{14}C] serotonin and [^{14}C] melatonin. J. Neurochem. *18*, 1683–1687 (1971)
Wurtman, R.J., Axelrod, J.: The pineal gland. Sci. Am. *213* (1), 50–60 (1965)

CHAPTER 5

Systemic Pharmacology of Adrenergic Activators and Inhibitors: Effects on the Genital System

M. SAS and L. KOVÁCS

A. Introduction

The prime effect of adrenergic activators on the female genital system is on the myometrium; and the effect in influencing the activity of the fallopian tubes is significant only to a smaller extent.

The reduction of myometrium activity and the inhibition of premature labour have posed a problem in obstetrics for a long time, and it has not yet been solved. It was first observed by FEGERL and NARIK (1951), who noted that adrenaline reduces the tone of the uterus and inhibits contraction. On the basis of their data SZENDI (1952) carried out successful treatment with adrenaline in cases of imminent miscarriage and premature labour. Of course, the intensive sympathomimetic effects limited the obstetric treatment. The next step was the clinical administration of isoxsuprine — a catecholamine derivative — in the USA at the beginning of the 1960s. This drug had fewer, although still considerable, side-effects (BISHOP and WOUTERSZ, 1961; HENDRICKS et al., 1961).

Depending on the nature of the substituents in their amino groups, the adrenergic catecholamines have different effects. On the basis of the two main types of these effects AHLQUIST (1948) suggested the terms α- and β-adrenergic receptors. Later LANDS et al. (1967) demonstrated that the β-receptors can be divided into two subgroups — β_1- and β_2-receptors. The activation of the β_1-receptors results in cardiac effects and lipolysis, while that of the β_2-receptors causes dilatation of the bronchi, a decrease in the tone of the myometrium and vasodilatation. As a result of pharmacological research, preparations with selective effects on the β_1- and β_2-receptors have been developed, thus more and more appropriate adrenergic activators for obstetric treatment have been produced. The fact that in the Federal Republic of Germany 1 million ampoules and 6 million pills of a β-sympathomimetic drug, fenoterol (Editorial, 1979), are used annually indicates widespread obstetric administration of such drugs.

The experience gained in the course of this widespread administration has called attention to numerous important side-effects besides the obstetric indispensability of the drug. The observations referring to the effects appearing in the foetus and later in the newborn are also important and, since they are in close connection with obstetric administration, they are also dealt with in this study.

B. Effect of Beta-Sympathomimetics on the Myometrium in Pregnancy

In clinical practice in obstetrics — on the basis of experiences from a period of nearly two decades — β-sympathomimetics have proved to be very effective as uterine muscle-relaxing drugs in the treatment of early or excessive uterine activity. (Data referring to this can be found in Sect. E.)

Clinical administration was preceded by numerous experimental examinations. In experimental circumstances in vitro, the effect of β-sympathomimetics on the uterus of rats, mice, rabbits, and also of humans was examined. The effect of the drugs was measured by triggering spontaneous or oxytocin-induced uterine contractions. LISH et al. (1960) demonstrated the inhibiting effect of isoxsuprine on the motility of animal and human myometrium. The effect of nylidrin was observed on rat uterus and sections of human myometrium by MOSLER and SCHWALM (1965). On the pregnant uterus a relaxing effect was found, while in the non-pregnant uterus nylidrin aggravated the muscle tone.

SEEWALD et al. (1973) demonstrated the contraction-inhibiting effect, depending on the dose, of buphenine, orciprenaline, and fenoterol on human myometrium in vitro.

Although the examinations differed in many details and in vitro results can only be extrapolated to in vivo circumstances with reservations, on the basis of these data clinical examinations could also be carried out.

POSE et al. (1962) and ZUSPAN et al. (1962) examined the result of L-epinephrine treatment and checked uterine activity by measuring the intra-uterine pressure. Uterine activity could be suspended by a dose of 5–20 mcg/min. Twenty minutes after the treatment the contractions returned.

Since the beginning of the 1960 s, examinations have been carried out with isoxsuprine. It was stated that a dosage of 0.5–1 mg/min successfully inhibits uterine activity and that it is also effective orally (HENDRICKS et al., 1961; STANDER et al., 1964). Further examinations with orciprenaline (ESKES et al., 1966) and with ritodrine (BAUMGARTEN, 1970) proved that these agents are sufficient in inhibiting uterine activity. On the basis of these experiences widespread clinical administration started.

I. Connection Between the Structure and Effect of Beta-Sympathomimetics

A considerable amount of research work was carried out to find sympathomimetics which have a possible mild circulatory effect along with a strong uterine relaxing effect. This effort seemed reasonable since, on the basis of various examinations, it could be supposed that the adrenergic β-receptors are not entirely of the same character and that the β-receptors of various organ systems do not have the same degree of sensitivity to a given β-sympathomimetic. It is also possible that with the chemical structure changed, through the changing physical–chemical characteristics of the agent, the tissue distribution and the receptor affinity can be so modified that the desired favourable changes occur.

The myometrium-relaxing effects of various agents were compared in the uterus of pregnant rats in vitro by LORENZ (1972) with special regard to the modification of the effect on the uterus and circulation as a result of changes occurring in the structure of the molecule. Some of the results can be seen in Fig. 1. Together with the extending substitution on the amino group of adrenaline, the stimulating effect of the β-receptor increases. It is mainly the two phenol OH groups in para and meta positions on the

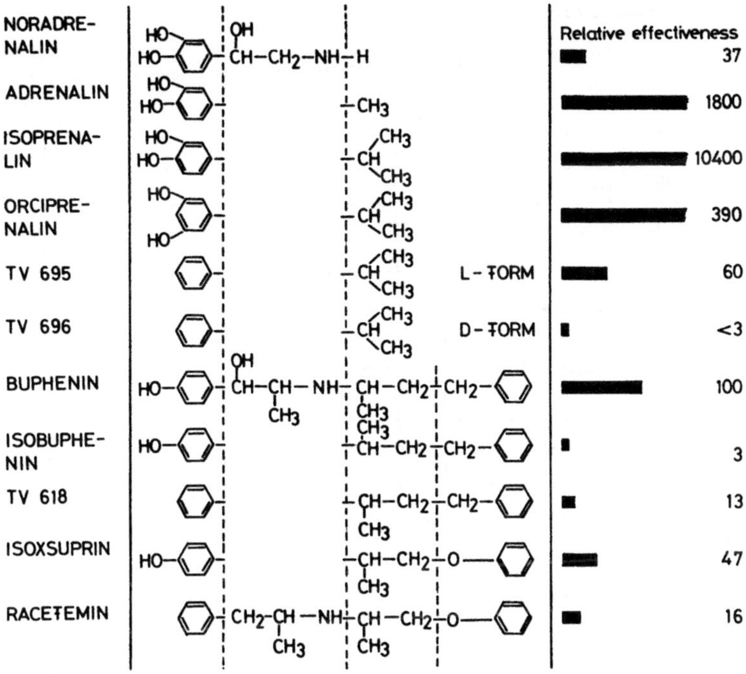

Fig. 1. Relation between chemical structure and effectiveness on the pregnant rat myometrium of different β-sympathicomimetic compounds in vitro (LORENZ, 1972)

benzol ring that are responsible for the circulatory effects. If the two phenol OH groups are in meta position, the uterus-relaxing effect also decreases, but the circulatory effects show such a decrease that the agent becomes suitable for therapeutic administration (e.g. orciprenaline).

For a satisfactory uterus-relaxing effect a single phenol group in para position can be sufficient as in the buphenine and isoxsuprine molecules. If there is no phenol OH group on the benzol ring, either because it is absent or because it was involved in an etheral connection, the uterus-relaxing effect decreases considerably. The secondary alcoholic OH group is also important in the uterus-relaxing effect. Its absence (e.g., racefemine) or its transformation into a keto group causes a considerable decrease in the uterine effect.

The chemical structure is significant in respect of the duration of the effect as well. Two enzymes have an important role in the inactivation of the catecholamine derivatives: the catechol-O-methyltransferase inactivates the hydroxyl groups on the benzol ring, while the mono-aminooxidase inactivates the groups which belong to the nitrogen atom. It is obvious that slower decomposition, i.e., longer duration of effect can be achieved by deviating from the natural catecholamine molecule. As opposed to the 3 and 4 position, the 3 and 5 position of the phenol OH groups results in a considerable deceleration of the inactivation and thus makes it possible for the drug to be also effective per os (PERSSON and PERSSON, 1972).

The line of β-sympathomimetic catecholamine derivatives developed on the basis of the connections realized between the structure and the effect can be seen in Fig. 2.

General structural formula:

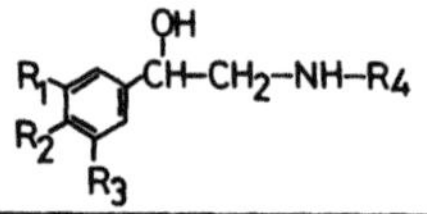

		R_1	R_2	R_3	R_4
1906	Adrenalin	H	OH	OH	CH_3
1941	Isoprenalin	H	OH	OH	$CH(CH_3)_2$
1961	Orciprenalin	OH	H	OH	$CH(CH_3)_2$
1969	Salbutamol	H	OH	CH_2OH	$C(CH_3)_3$
1970	Terbutalin	OH	H	OH	$C(CH_3)_3$
1970	Hexoprenalin	H	OH	OH	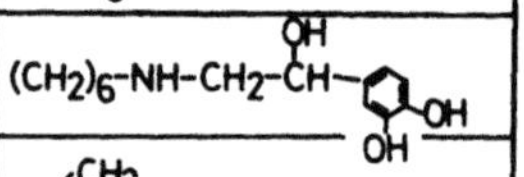
1971	Fenoterol	OH	H	OH	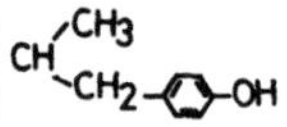
1976	Reproterol	OH	H	OH	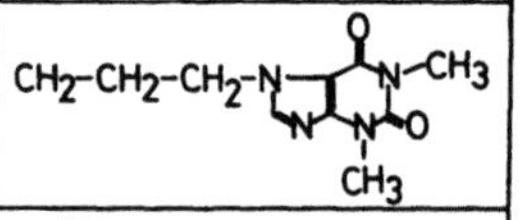
1977	Clenbuterol	Cl	NH_2	Cl	$C(CH_3)_3$

Fig. 2. Development of beta-sympathomimetic drugs

II. Mechanism of Action

The mechanism of the uterus-relaxing effect of β-sympathomimetics is not quite clear. They carry out their effect through the so-called β-receptors in the cell membrane. These β-receptors are considered to be iso-enzymes (DAVIS et al., 1967). The fact that the β-receptors are closely linked with the adenylcyclase enzyme seems certain. According to SUTHERLAND et al. (1965) the β-adrenergic activators, by stimulating the adenylcyclase, raise the cyclic adenosine 3',5'-monophosphate (cAMP) level. Cyclic-AMP acts as second messenger in the intracellular regulation. It has been demonstrated in numerous examinations that the cAMP level rises together with the relaxation induced by the β-sympathomimetic in the uterus of rats (POLACEK and DANIEL, 1971; HARBON and CLAUSER, 1971; DOBBS and ROBISON, 1968). With β-blockers both the rise of the cAMP level and the uterus relaxation can be inhibited. According to certain examinations the exogenic cAMP also inhibits the contraction activity of the uterus and decreases the muscle tone in the uterus of rats (MITZNEGG et al., 1970).

The role of cAMP in this respect seems to be proved by the fact that, as a result of the methyl-xanthin treatment, paralysing phosphodiesterase, the accumulated cAMP level also induces muscle relaxation in the cells of the myometrium.

The nature of the mechanism through which cAMP carries out the relaxation is not known exactly. Calcium must play a major role in the process. As an effect of cAMP the calcium content of the microsomal fraction of the uterus muscle cells increases considerably and, at the same time, the free calcium level of the myoplasm decreases, which leads to relaxation (RASMUSSEN and TENENHOUSE, 1968).

The effect of the sympathomimetics on the uterus is also influenced by the hormonal state. The in vitro examination of human myometrium showed that oestrogens sensibilize the α-receptors and make it possible for the catecholamines to induce muscle contractions. To a limited extent progesteron can also sensibilize the α-receptors; but a considerable progesterone dominance leads to the sensibilization of the β-receptors and helps the muscle-relaxing effect of the β-sympathomimetics (KLÖCK, 1977).

The exclusive role of cAMP in the β-sympathomimetic-induced uterus muscle relaxation is not supported by all the data. In examinations carried out by KORDS (1975c) on the uterus of pregnant rats, fenoterol in an amount under 0.1 mcg/ml did not influence contractions in the oxytocin-stimulated uterus, but it increased the cAMP level in the same way as in the case of relaxation of the uterus. POLACEK and DANIEL (1971), with isoproterenol treatment, caused relaxation and cAMP level rise in the isolated rat uterus. As an effect of propranolol, uterine contractions occurred together with a further increase in the cAMP level. These data support the fact that the increase in the cAMP level cannot be the only explanation for the uterus-relaxing effect of the β-sympathomimetics.

According to examinations carried out by VESIN and HARBON (1974) and HARBON et al. (1976) the prostaglandins also carry out their effect by stimulating the adenylate-cyclase, as do the β-sympathomimetics. By the intracellular accumulation of the cAMP level the myometrial effect is the opposite: it causes contraction. This observation also supports the idea that the adenylate-cyclase-cAMP system cannot be accepted as the single primary intracellular mediator in the β-sympathomimetic myometrial contraction inhibition.

FALKAY et al. (1978) demonstrated in vitro in the microsomal fraction of pregnant myometrium that isoxsuprine in a low concentration (0.1 m*M*) induces biosynthesis of prostaglandins (E_2, $F_{2\alpha}$). According to these examinations, the stimulation of the β-receptors of the human myometrium activates not only the adenylate-cyclase, but also the prostaglandin synthetase system. This interaction could be an explanation for the rebound effect observed occasionally in β-sympathomimetic treatment.

III. Metabolism and Pharmacokinetics

In the course of clinical application the β-sympathomimetics are administered mainly in the form of intravenous infusion and orally, rarely in the form of intramuscular injection or aerosol inhalation. Absorption, tissue distribution and excretion depend on the form of administration.

The kinetics and metabolism of fenoterol were examined in pregnant guinea-pigs by KORDS (1977). Tritium-marked fenoterol was administered intravenously (4.5 mcg/kg body wt.) to the pregnant animals. Radioactivity in the plasma after the administration decreased exponentially, the half-period was 36 min. The metabolism of the fenoterol was very fast, 10 min after administration only 10% of the radioactivity came from non-metabolized fenoterol. Due to the fast metabolism the observable effects of the drug passed quickly; only for the 35 min following administration was it possible to demonstrate the positive chronothropic effect of the drug on the heart of the pregnant animals. If the fenoterol was administered to the pregnant guinea-pigs in infusion form (0.45 mcg/min for 60 min), the non-metabolized material did not exceed 10% of the radioactivity in the plasma during the examination. The inactivation and excretion of the fenoterol took place almost entirely in the form of glucuronide metabolites.

Examinations carried out by BUCHELT and ROMINGER (1972) and ROMINGER and POLLMANN (1972) with tritium-marked fenoterol proved that the drug is also absorbed fast from the gastro-intestinal system of rats, dogs, and humans. The blood level reaches its maximum immediately after intravenous and 2 h after oral administration. The compound is distributed in the tissues quickly and is eliminated mainly through the kidneys and, to a smaller extent, through the gall-bladder. The half-period of renal excretion is 6–7 h and 24 h after administration the excretion is practically completed. The 6–7 h half-period refers to the already conjugated drug, the expected half-period of the biologically active material is about 1 h. From the data on renal excretion gained after oral and intravenous administration the absorption proportions can be calculated. The are as follows: rat, 42%, dog, 85%, human, 60%. Fenoterol is excreted mainly in a conjugated form, in rats in the form of glucuronide, in dogs in the form of glucuronide and sulphate, in man in the form of sulphate conjugate. In the decomposition of fenoterol the catechol-*O*-methyltransferase and the mono-amino-oxidase have no role (BUCHHELT and ROMINGER, 1972).

The examination of the tissue and organ distribution indicated that apart from temporary fenoterol accumulation in the secretory organs (kidney, liver) fenoterol does not accumulate in any other organ. The brain is an exception in one respect, namely that according to autoradiographic examinations and according to chemical examinations of tissue samples neither fenoterol nor its metabolites could be detected in the brain.

Terbutaline, after oral administration, reaches its maximal blood level in 1–3 h, too. Its decomposition and excretion take place in a different way from those of the catecholamines. It is inactivated and excreted mainly in the form of sulphate conjugate. After oral intake 50%, while after intravenous administration 90% will be eliminated in the urine, the rest in the bile and the excrement (NILSSON et al., 1972).

C. Effect of Beta-Sympathomimetics on the Non-Pregnant Uterus

Besides the great practical significance of the relaxing effect of the β-sympathomimetics on the pregnant uterus, little attention was paid to their effect on the non-pregnant uterus. The spontaneous motility of the uterus is under hormonal control and the motility in cycles, which are anovulational, due to hormonal contraceptive therapy differs from the motility characteristic of physiological cycles (FRÖHLICH et al., 1972).

The results of examinations carried out on the human uterus in vivo by means of an intra-uterine open-tip catheter, with α- and β-receptor stimulating and blocking drugs, show that the drugs had their effects independently of the degree of hormonal influence on the uterus: the administration of the β-mimetics [isoprenaline, orciprenaline, fenoterol (Partusisten)] resulted in the relaxation of the uterus and in the suspension of the spontaneous activity in any period of the cycle, either in amenorrhoea or after the menopause, while β-blockers (propranolol, practolol) stimulated the uterus (HEIN, 1975).

The effect of the β-sympathomimetics which influence the non-pregnant uterus is not used in clinical practice. Although it was proposed for the treatment of dysmenorrhoea, it did not become a widely used treatment mainly because of the side-effects.

D. Effect of Beta-Sympathomimetics on the Fallopian Tubes

α- and β-adrenoceptors have always been found in the fallopian tubes in every species which has been studied so far. Stimulation of the β-receptors results in the inhibition of the contractility of the smooth muscles of the fallopian tube.

Isoprenaline inhibits the motility of the fallopian tube in rabbits (HODGSON and PAUERSTEIN, 1974), and this effect could be inhibited with propranolol. In the presence of phenoxybenzamine the stimulating effect of noradrenaline was reversed and became inhibitory (UEDA et al., 1973).

According to examinations carried out by KENDLE and LAM SHAM LEEN (1976) the reaction of the circular and longitudinal tube muscles differs as a result of the effect of β-mimetics. In the presence of practolol the contraction caused by adrenaline was aggravated in the circular muscles of the fallopian tube in rabbits, but not in the longitudinal muscles. A β_2 agonist drug, salbutamol, caused inhibition of the longitudinal muscles but did not affect the circular muscles.

The examination of human fallopian tubes produced contradictory results. With noradrenaline both stimulating and inhibiting effects could be induced and the explanation of the contradictory effects could be the actual hormonal dominance (NAKANISHI and WOOD, 1968; SENIOR and SPENCER-GREGSON, 1969).

The reaction of the fallopian tubes to β-sympathomimetic drugs, i.e., their responsiveness to these drugs, is significant in respect of the control of reproduction, more precisely the control of ovum transport. According to examinations carried out in this field, adrenaline (500 mcg/kg body wt./6 h SC) accelerated ovum transport in rabbits when administered 60 and 72 h after coitus (POLIDORO et al., 1973). Isoprenaline had no effect on ovum transport in rabbits even when the dose was lethal, in the case of 50% of the animals (POLIDORO et al., 1976). Ritodrine did not decrease fertility in rabbits (HODGSON et al., 1975), while in the case of mice it was salbutamol and isoprenaline which had no effect (JOHNS et al., 1975).

On the basis of these results it may be suggested that the β-sympathomimetics also decrease the contractility of human fallopian tubes, but that no practical significance can be attached to this effect.

E. Administration of Beta-Sympathomimetic Drugs in Obstetrics

I. Clinical Studies

Today it is a unanimously accepted fact that the β-sympathomimetic drugs effectively decrease or suspend the activity of the uterine muscles, and that in human clinical practice they are capable of suspending excessively strong or premature uterine contractions. Effective contraction inhibition has been proved by double-blind clinical examination by the administration of buphenine (WOLFF, 1967), ritodrine (WESSELIUS DE CASPARIS et al., 1971), terbutaline (INGEMARSSON, 1976), isoxsuprine (CSAPÓ and HERCZEG, 1977), and by the application of a placebo.

The first clinical reports related the administration of isoxsuprine (BISHOP and WOUTERSZ, 1961; HENDRICKS et al., 1961), then buphenine (WOLFF, 1967; MOSLER and ROSENBOOM, 1972; KOVÁCS et al., 1973), and orciprenaline (BAILLIE et al., 1970). Later, β_2-activator drugs with a more and more selective effect followed and spread and are used today, e.g., ritodrine (BAUMGARTEN et al., 1971; BIENIARZ et al., 1972), fenoterol (BODEN and CRABBEN, 1970; WEIDINGER and WIEST, 1971, 1973a; JUNG et al., 1971), terbutaline (INGEMARSSON, 1976), and salbutamol (LIGGINS and VAUGHAN, 1973).

II. Drugs Applied in Clinical Practice

The names and chemical names of preparations used in obstetrics are as follows:

Name of the preparation	*Chemical name*
Duvadilan, Vasodilan	isoxsuprine
Dilatol	buphenine, nylidrin
Alupent	orciprenaline
Prepar	ritodrine
Partusisten, Berotec	fenoterol, Th 1165a
Bricanyl	terbutaline
Salbutamol	salbutamol.

Comparative clinical examinations have indicated that there are no significant differences in the drugs as fas as the effect on the decrease in uterine activity is concerned: salbutamol and terbutaline were compared by RYDEN (1977), fenoterol and ritodrine by GUMMERUS (1977), fenoterol and orciprenaline by CASTELAZO AYALA and KARCHMER (1977). On the basis of comparing the frequency of side-effects CASTELAZO AYALA and KARCHMER (1977) consider fenoterol more favourable than orciprenaline; on the same basis HÜTER et al. (1972) drew up the following order of preference: fenoterol, ritodrine, buphenine.

III. Indications

The main accepted indications of obstetric treatment are as follows:

1. Long-term treatment for threatened premature birth and spontaneous abortion.

2. Short-term treatment:

a) Irregular uterine activity during labour (hypertonic hyperkinetic contractions).
b) Uterine hypertonus during the administration of oxytocin or prostaglandin.
c) Operations on the pregnant uterus or other operations performed during pregnancy.
d) Emergencies in delivery (prolapse of the umbilical cord, version of the foetus, incarceration of the placenta, etc.).
e) Suspension of contractions in acute foetal distress to improve the utero-placental circulation (intra-uterine reanimation of the foetus).

IV. Contra-Indications

Contra-indications of the treatment are serious cardiac and circulatory disease of the patient, glaucoma, and hyperthyreosis; a relative contra-indication is diabetes mellitus. Contra-indications of prolonged treatment are intra-uterine infection and serious foetal developmental disorders, as well as foetal diseases which can be given extra-uterine treatment more successfully.

V. Methods

As for *the method of treatment,* views are more or less unanimous. The introduction of prolonged treatment starts with intravenous dosage, the first dose being larger to fill the system; further doses, depending on uterine activity, become smaller, serving a mantaining purpose. Usual doses of fenoterol are 1–3 mcg/min (WEIDINGER and WIEST, 1973a; MOSLER and LINKA, 1975), of terbutaline 5–25 mcg/min (INGEMARSSON, 1976), of salbutamol 5–35 mcg/min (RYDEN, 1977), and of isoxsuprine 0.1–1.0 mcg/min (CSAPÓ and HERCZEG, 1977). Infusion treatment can be continued after 12–24 h by per os treatment. The first pill must be administered in the last hour of the infusion to maintain the appropriate β-mimetic blood level, then the administration must be repeated every 4–6 h. Doses of per os treatment with fenoterol are 15–30 mg/die (WEIDINGER and WIEST, 1973 a), with terbutaline 15–20 mg/die (INGEMARSSON, 1976), with salbutamol 10 mg/die (RYDEN, 1977), and with isoxsuprine 80 mg/die (CSAPÓ and HERCZEG, 1977). In acute treatment 50 mcg of fenoterol can be administered in the form of an intravenous injection bolus, and this can be repeated several times (WEIDINGER, 1977). As an acute form of administration, aerosol inhalation seems to be an adequate way. Successful treatment with fenoterol inhalation has been related by ZAHN (1973), LIPSHITZ and BAILLIE (1976), and KOVÁCS and HERCZEG (1978); and with salbutamol by HASTWELL (1975).

A simultaneous administration of calcium antagonistic drugs has been proposed by numerous authors to decrease the side-effects of the β-mimetic treatment (WEIDINGER and WIEST, 1973 b; WEIDINGER, 1977; GUMMERUS, 1977), although others doubt the point of the combination. A proposed dose of verapamil (Isoptin) is 30–150 mcg/min in the form of intravenous infusion, then 240–480 mg/die per os (WEIDINGER and WIEST, 1973a; MOSLER and LINKA, 1975; GUMMERUS, 1977).

VI. Effectiveness

The success of prolonged β-mimetic treatment can be judged only with difficulty, the rate of success being between 25% and 95% (BAUMGARTEN, 1977). The explanation could be that at the beginning of the treatment it is difficult to decide whether tocolysis is needed or whether the pregnancy would continue without it, or the treatment is in vain because it is too late and is therefore going to be unsuccessful. Furthermore, the criteria of the success of the treatment are not uniform.

The premature labour score proposed by BAUMGARTEN (1977) is very helpful in judging the prognosis of the treatment. It takes into account the presence or absence of the three main symptoms of threatened premature birth with regard to the dilatation of the cervix using a 0–4 scoring, the sum being the premature labour score (tocolysis index) Table 1.

Table 1. Premature labour score (BAUMGARTEN, 1977)

	0	1	2	3	4
Contractions		Irregular	Regular	–	–
Membranes	Intact	–	Ruptured high	–	Ruptured low
Bleeding	Nil	Spotting	Bleeding	–	–
Dilatation	Nil	1 cm	2 cm	3 cm	4 cm or more

If the score is 7 or over there is no point in applying tocolysis since it would be hopeless. In the case of the score being between 1 and 4 the initiation of the treatment is supported by the fact that the possibility of successful continuation of the pregnancy is 72%, whereas in the case of scores between 5 and 8 it is only 8% (BAUMGARTEN, 1977).

Criteria of success are given in various ways. Tocolysis is considered successful by most authors if it prolongs the pregnancy by a week after the start of treatment (MOSLER et al., 1974; RYDEN, 1977) while RICHTER (1978) considers cases where birth occurs within 2 weeks unsuccessful. Further criteria of success are the completion of the 37 th week, a birth weight of 2,500 g or more and a 1-week survival after birth. Success is highly influenced by the gestation period in which treatment was started, so this also must be taken into consideration when evaluating.

Treatment with *β*-sympathomimetic drugs is very common in obstetric practice; 5%–40% of hospitalized pregnant women receive such therapy (WARKENTIN, 1978). The value of the treatment is not in doubt but it needs a high degree of technical knowledge and careful attention to patients to bring about and to avoid maternal and foetal side-effects.

F. Maternal Side-Effects of Tocolysis Carried out With Beta-Sympathomimetics

The effects of the *β*-sympathomimetics outside the genital system do not belong to the field of interest of our present study. Only the effects which occurred as side-effects during tocolysis carried out with *β*-sympathomimetics in the course of the treatment of pregnant women will be dealt with since these effects can cause problems in clinical practice.

I. Cardiac Effects

The *β*-receptor stimulating drugs significantly increase the inflow of calcium ions into the cells of the myocardium. Thus the ATPase activity which depends on the calcium ions also increases in the myofibrilla and this leads to elevated ATP consumption. Contractility increases and so does oxygen demand during the period of restitution because of the intensive ATP resynthesis (FLECKENSTEIN et al., 1978). The positive chronothropic and positive dromothropic effects of the β-receptor stimulators are also caused by the increased calcium ion inflow. So the increase of the sinus automatia, the rate of the atrioventricular conduction and that of the contractility of the atrium and the cardiac chamber are accompanying effects of the β-mimetic treatment, so one must be prepared to face these cardiac phenomena during tocolysis.

By increasing the dose the effect of the β-mimetics can cause significant pathological cardiac changes. RONA et al. (1959) observed necrosis in rat myocardium after isoproteronol treatment. Acute sympathetic overstimulation of the myocardium makes it possible for a considerable amount of calcium to get into the myocardiac muscle cells, and the level of ATP and creatin-phosphate decreases because of over consumption and damages occur in the mitochondrium structure and function with a loss of phosphorilating capacity. If the process exceeds a critical point, structural changes similar to those occurring after hypoxia or ischaemia might develop in the myocardium (FLECKENSTEIN et al., 1978).

It is known from SELYE's works (1960) that certain drugs (e.g., corticosteroids, vitamin D) help to develop myocardium necrosis caused by stress. FLECKENSTEIN et al. (1978) demonstrated in rats that β-sympathomimetics and 9-α-fluor-cortisolacetate or dihydrotachysterol have a significant potentiating effect in the increase of the intracellular Ca^{++} level of the myocardium and in the development of necrosis.

The role of the potentiating factors must be referred to for clinical practice since, in order to prevent idiopathic respiratory distress syndrome in the newborn, it is a common practice to apply corticosteroid therapy to pregnant women, as well as the administration of vitamin D, and calcium; and the development of hypokaliaemia is not infrequent. More seldom narcotics and β-mimetics are administered at the same time. In this respect it is important to mention that halothane greatly potentiates the cardiac effects of β-mimetics.

In vitro experiments and experiments with animals have clarified the effects and dangers of β-mimetics on the heart, but during clinical tocolysis serious heart complications are rare. On the basis of clinical reports it is easy to see that generally speaking a mild or serious tachycardia, the decrease of diastolic and, to a smaller extent, systolic blood pressure, the feeling of palpitation and hot flushes are accompanying effects of the treatment. These symptoms occur mainly at the beginning of the treatment, they are generally tolerable and very rarely do they make it necessary to stop the treatment.

The occurrence of myocardium necrosis and hypertrophic cardio-myopathia are not mentioned in the literature describing tocolytic treatment in thousands of cases.

Serious foetal cardiac damage after tocolysis has been mentioned recently in connection with some case reports (TROLP et al., 1978; URBANEK et al., 1978) (see also Sect. E). It was possible to demonstrate in in vitro cell cultures that lesion of the foetal myocardiac muscle cells occurred as an effect of β-mimetics. This effect could be avoided by the administration of verapamil into the incubation medium (WEIDINGER et al., 1978). Despite these important data serious foetal cardiac effects must be considered as exceptionally rare since the pathological examination of infants who died perinatally following tocolytic treatment did not indicate myocardium necrosis – apart from the above-mentioned casuistics (HILLEMANNS, 1978; WEIDINGER and WIEST, 1978).

II. Metabolic Effects

1. Carbohydrate Metabolism

The effect of β-sympathomimetics on the metabolism of carbohydrates is present during tocolytic treatment as well. Maternal and foetal effects and the possibilities of the avoidance of the effects on carbohydrate metabolism have been described in numerous studies. Each drug that has been examined so far has an effect on the metabolism, although the rate of the effect is not the same. For example, the blood sugar level is not raised by isoxsuprine to such an extent as it is by buphenine. In this respect the effect of fenoterol is even weaker (Lippert et al., 1972; Amendt and Gödel, 1975; Weidinger and Mohr, 1973).

During the course of a 4-h fenoterol infusion using a therapeutic dose (3 mcg/min) into healthy pregnant women, a continuous increase in the blood glucose level was found 70.7–101.3 mg-%. The insulin level increased more intensively, reaching a value twice as high as the starting value after 0.5 h; after 1 h it was three times as high as the starting value and thereafter it remained on this level. An hour after the end of the treatment both values decreased considerably. The lactate and pyruvate serum concentration increased significantly and continuously, it was four times as high as the normal starting value and the level decreased minimally during the 1st h after the treatment (Unbehaun et al., 1974). The observed changes can be considered as symptoms of glycogenolysis resulting from β-mimetic effect, the significant and continuous increase of lactate concentration indicating that the decomposition of muscle glycogen takes place. Lipshitz and Vinik (1978) after the intravenous bolus administration of 10 mcg hexoprenaline found a significant increase in the glucose level in pregnant women. It reached its peak after 30 min and returned to the starting value after 60 min. The insulin level trebled in 10 min and the value measured in 1 h was the same as the starting value. The value of the glucagon increased considerably, too, reaching its maximal level 20 min after the treatment and returning to the normal value in an hour. The results of both examinations support the fact that the insulin increase is the immediate effect of β-mimetic treatment and that it is not the result of the increasing glucose level.

Weidinger and Mohr (1973) observed an average 40 mg/100 ml blood glucose level increase and a significant insulin level increase at the same time following treatment with 5 mg fenoterol PO. The whole process lasted for 1.5 h. The examination was repeated 2 days later with an additional administration of 5 mg verapamil i.v. The increase in blood sugar and insulin was half as intensive. A simultaneous administration of 0.08 mg fenoterol together with the intravenous glucose tolerance test of healthy pregnant women showed high-reaching but swiftly decreasing glucose and insulin values.

Similar treatments cause a considerably milder reaction in the case of pregnant women *already undergoing β-mimetic treatment*. The administration of 5 mg fenoterol per os during fenoterol tocolysis causes an insignificant increase in blood sugar. The intravenous glucose tolerance test showed normal values during long-term tocolysis (Weidinger and Mohr, 1973). It seems that in the course of β-mimetic treatment a certain adaptation or habituation develops in connection with carbohydrate metabolism. Data obtained by Unbehaun et al. (1975) indicate this, too. In the course of a week-long fenoterol treatment of pregnant women the blood sugar and insulin values, after increasing during the 1st day, returned to the starting value, while the lactate concentration remained higher during the first 6 days of the treatment.

On the basis of these results, it is understandable that during long-term tocolysis such significant differences cannot be observed in carbohydrate metabolism. Continuous β-mimetic treatment of pregnant women suffering from diabetes is also possible if the carbohydrate metabolism is monitored very carefully, especially at the beginning of the treatment (AMENDT and GÖDEL, 1975; MOHR and WEIDINGER, 1977).

As for the foetal implications of the changes in carbohydrate metabolism during β-mimetic tocolysis, the continuous increase in the lactate level is significant. Because of the diaplancental transport of the lactate in cases of infants born after unsuccessful tocolysis or β-mimetic treatment during labour, metabolic acidosis can be expected more frequently. This observation is supported by examinations carried out by LEHMANN (1977), who, by examining maternal and foetal blood samples taken simultaneously after the administration of 50 mcg fenoterol intravenously, declared that 25 min after the treatment a significantly increased lactate level was observed in the foetus (the lactate level then was the same as in the mother); the value measured 90 min later in the foetus was higher than in the mother.

Maternal hyperglycaemia which occurs during the β-mimetic treatment for reanimation of the distressed foetus during labour, can play a useful role as a source of energy for the foetal metabolism (LIPSHITZ and VINIK, 1978).

2. Lipid Metabolism

After starting the β-mimetic treatment of pregnant women, serum changes linked to lipolysis can be indicated in a short time: free fatty acid concentration, free glycerine level, neutral fat level increase and increase in β-hydroxy-butyric acid and acet-acetic acid indicate that there are certain disturbances in lipid metabolism (UNBEHAUN et al., 1974; LIPSHITZ and VINIK, 1978). After a single drug-administration, the changes take place during a few hours. In the course of a long-term treatment the changes could not be traced after the 1st day (UNBEHAUN et al., 1975). The observed changes have no significance in the case of healthy pregnant women. Similarly to the changes in carbohydrate metabolism the changes in lipid metabolism are significant as long as they contribute to shifting the metabolism in an acidotic direction and they can have a pathological significance mainly in the case of maternal diabetes. They must also be taken into consideration in respect of an aggravated acidosis-affinity of the infant.

3. Blood Gases and Acid-Base Balance

As a result of changes in carbohydrate and lipid metabolism considerable changes occur in the acid-base balance and in the values of blood gases in the course of β-sympathomimetic treatment of pregnant women. The base excess and pH decrease considerably as a sign of a shift in the direction of metabolic acidosis, which is induced mainly by lipolysis and the increasing lactate concentration. The decrease of PCO_2 and the increase of PO_2 are signs of partial respiratory conpensation. The results of examinations carried out by CONRADT et al. (1977) during a 4-h fenoterol infusion

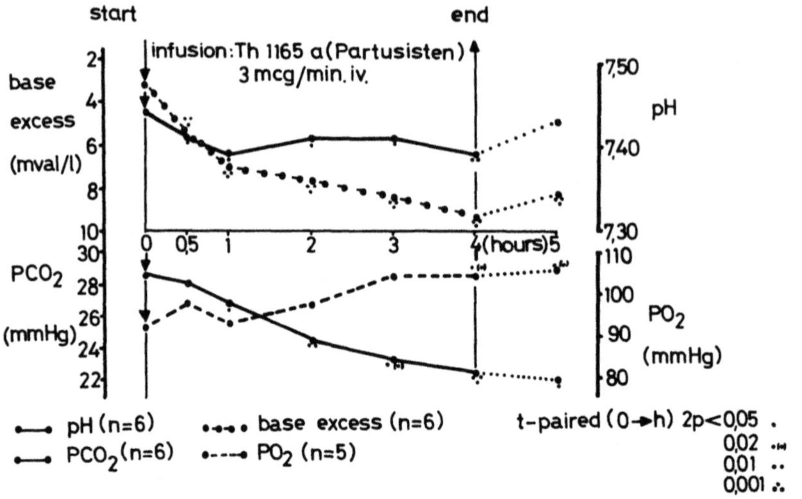

Fig. 3. Acid-base equilibrium during fenoterol (Partusisten) infusion (CONRADT et al., 1977)

treatment demonstrate the changes (Fig. 3). Restitution starts 1 h after the administration of the drug. During long-term tocolytic treatment no blood gas changes can be demonstrated. LEHMANN (1977) in an acute experiment observed the following changes: 25 min after the administration of 50 mcg fenoterol maternal pH decreased from 7.43 to 7.40; the base excess increased from 5.6 to 8.0 mmol/litre and, while foetal pH decreased from 7.33 to 7.30, the base excess increased from 7.6 to 9.9 mmol/litre.

The significance of the changes concerning the acid-base metabolism is that acidosis develops in the foetus and in the mother simultaneously, and in the case of infants who were born following a β-mimetic treatment during labour metabolic acidosis can be expected more frequently.

4. Electrolytes

The examination of serum electrolytes revealed changes first of all in the potassium level. Temporary decrease in the serum potassium level were observed following β-sympathomimetic treatment by a number of authors. The starting 4.3 mval/litre serum level decreased to a level of 2.9 mval/litre in the 60th min after the infusion of 3 mcg/min fenoterol in an examination carried out by UNBEHAUN et al. (1974). During a long-term tocolytic treatment, after an initial decrease, the level of serum potassium becomes normal by the following day and stays normal (UNBEHAUN et al., 1975).

WEIDINGER and WIEST (1973 b) found normal serum potassium levels during continuous tocolysis with fenoterol and verapamil. With the decrease in the serum potassium level, potassium excretion in the urine does not increase; in the 4th h of salbutamol tocolysis the serum potassium level decreased from the starting 3.85 mmol/litre to 2.62 mmol/litre in examinations carried out by SMITH and THOMPSON (1977), potassium excretion in the urine did not change (36.25 mmol/litre). It is suggested that this phenomenon is due to the temporary redistribution of potassium from the extra-cellular to the intra-cellular space. According to in vitro examinations potassium accumulates in the striated and smooth muscles as an effect of β-sympathomimetics and this supports the above theory (WANG and CLAUSEN, 1976: BÜLBRING et al., 1976).

No mention is made of any pathological consequences of the hypokaliaemia which occurs at the beginning of tocolysis. Hypokaliaemia which develops during β-mimetic treatment does not require special treatment and since the patients do not lose potassium the administration of potassium might be harmful. The serum potassium level of patients undergoing β-mimetic treatment must be evaluated in full knowledge of this phenomenon, attention must be paid to clinical symptoms of hypokaliaemia and the administration of potassium should be considered depending on the symptoms.

5. Thrombocyte Function

Since it is well known that the β-sympathomimetics have an effect on thrombocyte metabolism, several examinations deal with the state of the thrombocyte function during tocolysis.

In the first few hours after tocolysis a low-rate thrombocyte aggregation inhibition occurs which, according to some examinations, comes to an end after the first day of treatment (BRIEL et al., 1978), according to others it lasts for several days (STOSIEK and WIEST, 1976). The thrombocyte count does not change essentially; BRIEL et al. (1978) observed an 8% decrease on the 2nd day of the treatment, while the increase was 12% on the 10th–14th days. Thus no clinically significant difference occurs in the thrombocyte function during β-mimetic tocolysis. This is further supported by the observation that in the cases of labour following tocolysis inclination to haemorrhage does not increase (WEIDINGER and WIEST, 1973b). Increased attention should be paid to the tocolytic treatment of patients suffering from thrombocytopathia and to the administration of thrombocyte aggregation inhibiting drugs during tocolysis.

G. Therapy of the Side-Effects of Beta-Sympathomimetic Treatment

A sympathomimetic with a selective effect on the β_2-receptors has not yet been developed, so there is no way of avoiding the side-effects of tocolytic treatment. The effort being made to work out therapeutic procedures to reduce the side-effects is understandable.

I. Beta-Receptor Blockers

One possibility seemed to be the simultaneous administration of β-receptor blockers, since there are more or less selective β_1-blockers. The examinations carried out by MÜLLER-TYL et al. (1974) and REINOLD and MÜLLER-TYL (1977), in which they administered Bunitrolol during fenoterol tocolysis resulted in a successful alleviation of the β-mimetic-induced tachycardia by the β-blocker, but uterine contractions also returned at the same time. So for the time being this is not a suitable way since the avoidance of the side-effects of the β-sympathomimetics results in the suspension of the tocolytic effect.

II. Calcium Antagonists

The examination of the mechanism of action of β-mimetics revealed that a considerable part of the cardiac effects are caused by calcium ions flowing into the cells of the myocardium. This inflow can be blocked by calcium antagonist drugs which have no effect either on the β-receptors of the myometrium or on those of the myocardium.

It has been declared of the calcium antagonist drugs that, besides their contractility inhibiting effect on the mammal heart, they have a similar effect on the myometrium. Depending on the dose they inhibit the transmitting function of the calcium ions between the stimulus and the contraction, and thus they reduce the strength and rate of the myometrium contractions. The observations of FLECKENSTEIN et al. (1972) on the isolated uterus of mice were supported by those of GRÜN et al. (1972) on isolated human myometrium. On the basis of these observations a clinical therapy practice developed in which the administration of β-sympathomimetics is combined with that of calcium antagonists. The different myometrium-relaxing effects on different points might be epitomized in that the drugs are synergic, but, what is more important, they have contradictory cardiac effects so the calcium antagonists — mainly verapamil is used in practice — reduce the uncomfortable cardiovascular side-effects of the β-mimetics. The results of clinical examinations only partially proved the theoretical suggestions. RIPPERT et al. (1971) observed a satisfactory reduction in the cardiac side-effects by administering $5 \times 1-2$ (40 mg) pills verapamil in 24 h as an addition to ritodrine and fenoterol (Berotec) treatment. Several other clinical reports confirm the fact that by additional verapamil treatment, the usual dose of which is fenoterol: verapamil = 1:40, tachycardia and the decrease of blood pressure as well as mainly the subjective side-effects (palpitation, hot flushes, trembling, head-ache, indisposition) can be reduced considerably (MOSLER et al., 1974; WEIDINGER and WIEST, 1971, 1972, 1973a).

WEIDINGER and WIEST (1973a) experienced no essential alteration either in connection with the heart and circulation or with the metabolic parameters during the fenoterol and verapamil treatment of 100 pregnant women and they consider it a favourable combination.

It was also indicated that the simultaneous administration of verapamil reduces the β-sympathomimetic induced glycogenolysis considerably, by nearly 50% (WEIDINGER and MOHR, 1973).

The foetal heart rate was found to be practically unchanged during a combined β-mimetic and verapamil treatment, and it is supposed to be due to the favourable effect of verapamil (WEIDINGER et al., 1973).

The usefulness of the additional verapamil treatment is confirmed by the result of an in vitro examination. According to this, β-mimetic-induced cell damage in the foetal cardiac muscle culture could be avoided by verapamil administration (WEIDINGER et al., 1978).

At the same time, during clinical application it became obvious that in the dose used in human therapy the additional relaxing effect of the calcium antagonist does not exist in the course of tocolysis, contrary to the results of experiments with animals and those of in vitro examinations (WEIDINGER and WIEST, 1978). Verapamil addition did not result in the expected reduction of the tocolytic dose of the β-mimetics. Even the negative chronotropic and negative inotropic effect of verapamil in the dose used in the supplemented treatment of tocolysis was questioned on the basis of examinations carried out by HILTMANN et al. (1976).

The non-desired effects of β-sympathomimetic tocolysis could not be avoided completely by the calcium antagonists. However, since their usefulness is proved, their administration in addition to tocolytic treatment is justified.

H. Foetal Effects of Tocolysis Carried out With Beta-Sympathomimetics

In clinical practice β-sympathomimetics are used in a wide spectrum for the treatment of pregnant women. In the course of treatment foetal effects must be expected, too. The foetal effects can be direct and indirect. Besides the *direct* effects of the drug or its metabolites which penetrate to the foetus from the maternal system, certain *indirect* effects of the drug on the blood circulation of the uterus, on the utero-placental circulation and on the placental transport must also be taken into consideration during the course of the treatment.

I. Diaplacental Penetration

Because of the fast metabolization of β-sympathomimetics, the temporarily high blood level decreases quickly in the blood of pregnant animals after a single treatment and thus considerable placental transport does not take place. MEISSNER and PREIL (1974) after a single venous injection of tritium-marked fenoterol into pregnant rabbits could detect only a minimal amount of marked material in the foetus. In rats KRAMER and KLINGSPOHR (1974) examined the distribution of [^{3}H]fenoterol with autoradiographic methods. They observed that the amount of material which penetrates to the foetus after a single injection is so small that it could not be detected by autoradiography. During a 4-h infusion of tritium-marked fenoterol and afterwards in the examination of the tritium concentration in the maternal and foetal organs lower values were found for the foetus than for the mother as far as the maternal serum and the amniotic fluid were concerned (MEISSNER and KLOSTERMANN, 1976). These data support the theory that the transplacental penetration of β-mimetics from the mother to the foetus is blocked to a certain extent.

The published data always refer to the rate and distribution of radioactivity and do not make it clear whether the agent is the active β-mimetic or one of its ineffective metabolites. It is known on the basis of experiments with animals as well as from human examinations that the radioactive marked β-sympathomimetic metabolizes very fast, and that 86% of the radioactivity which can be detected in the plasma of rabbits 30 min after administration indicates the material already in conjugated form (ROMINGER, 1973, cited by MEISSNER and KLOSTERMANN, 1976). Little information is known about the metabolism of β-sympathomimetics which have penetrated to the foetus. According to examinations carried out by KORDS (1975a) on pregnant guinea-pigs during a 1-h infusion of marked fenoterol only 2%–6% of the radioactivity found in the foetal plasma came from non-conjugated active material and the conjugate concentration was always higher in the plasma of the foetus than in that of the mother animal.

On the basis of these animal experimental data it seems that the foetal β-mimetic level and β-mimetic effect are inhibited by two factors: the rendered penetration of the drug through the placenta and the considerable conjugating capacity of the foetus.

In human examination in the case of women who received tritium-marked fenoterol treatment preceding abortion in the first trimester it was observed that the radioactivity could be detected in the foetus and in the placenta, so fenoterol does pass through the placenta (WIEST et al., 1977).

In later phases of pregnancy the placentary penetration of β-mimetics can be deduced only from foetal cardiac effects, but the possibility that these effects are the result of the changed placental circulation cannot be excluded.

II. Effect on the Utero-Placental Circulation

During β-sympathomimetic treatment two effects, possibly with opposing results on the blood perfusion of the uterus, can be expected. On the one hand the circulation resistance decreases because of the relaxation of the myometrium, which may increase the blood perfusion of the uterus, and, on the other hand, the maternal arterial blood pressure also decreases and this can lead to a decrease in the blood flow.

Detailed examinations were carried out on sheep to decide which was the dominant effect of the two and to see what the joint result of the two effects during treatment is. WERNICKE et al. (1977) carried out examinations, on 14 pregnant sheep near term, into changes of maternal blood pressure, the cardiac frequency, the uterine artery blood flow, the foetal cardiac frequency, arterial blood pressure, umbilical vein blood flow and the PO_2, PCO_2, and pH of the maternal and foetal arterial blood during differing dosages of fenoterol infusions. With low doses the decrease of the circulation resistance and the increase of the cardiac output were balanced; even an increase in the blood flow of the uterus and foetal arterial PO_2 increase occurred. With high doses the increase of the cardiac output did not continue, the circulation resistance decreased and so did the blood flow of the uterus and the foetal PO_2 value (Fig. 4).

The consequences of the results for human clinical practice lead to the conclusion that during a β-mimetic treatment using the usual therapeutic dose the utero-placental circulation does not decrease, instead it improves and so does the oxygen supply to the foetus. However, in the course of increasing the dose the maternal circulation parameters must be monitored carefully because if hypovolaemia develops, a decrease in the blood flow which might be dangerous to the life of the foetus might develop.

WALLENBURG (1975) demonstrated by radioangiographic examinations which he carried out between the 110th and 140th days of pregnancy on rhesus monkeys that the intravenous infusion of metaproterenol (Alupent) increases and accelerates the utero-placental blood flow. The effect could be inhibited by propranolol.

The changes in the blood flow are even more explicit during uterine contractions. KÜNZEL and KASTENDIECK (1977) declared in connection with sheep that in the course of contractions induced by oxytocin infusion, while the intra-amnial pressure increased from 13 mm Hg to 33 mm Hg, the uterine artery blood flow decreased from 400 to 290 ml/min. The decrease could be stopped by the administration of 50 mcg fenoterol during a 30-s period; the blood flow returned to a normal value in 98 s. In respect of the oxygen supply to the foetus these data are very important since it is

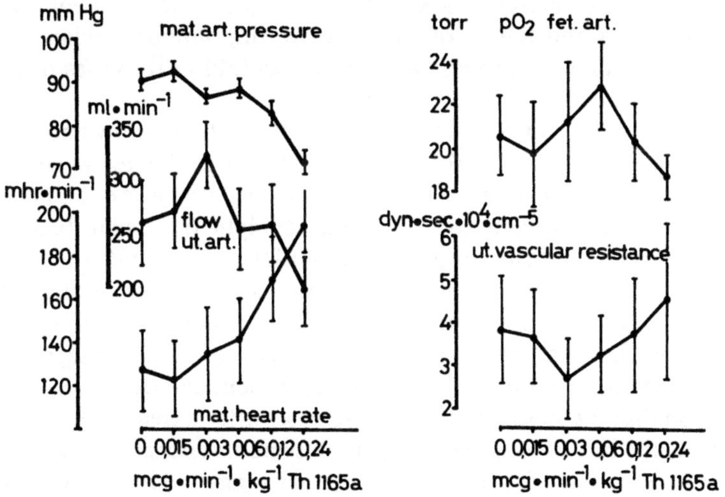

Fig. 4. Uterine blood flow, uterine vascular resistance and fetal arterial PO_2 during increasing dose fenoterol (Partusisten) infusion (WERNICKE et al., 1977)

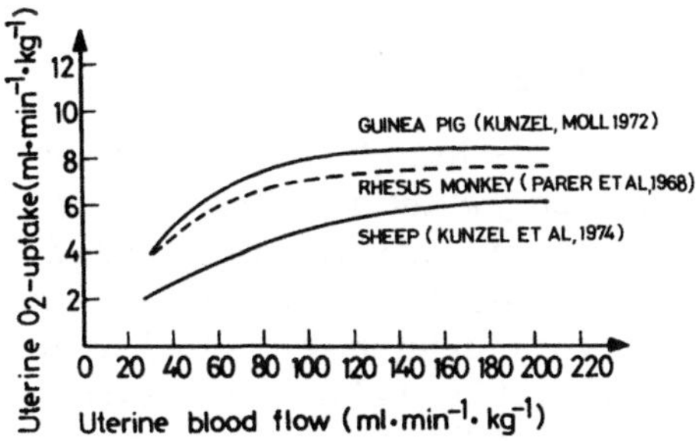

Fig. 5. Uterine O_2-uptake related to uterine blood flow in guinea-pig (KÜNZEL and MOLL, 1972), rhesus monkey (PARER et al., 1968) and sheep (KÜNZEL et al., 1974). Parabolic regression lines are shown which were adapted to the respective data (KÜNZEL and KASTENDIECK, 1977)

known that in various animal species there is a close connection between the blood flow and the oxygen intake of the uterus and it is likely that this connection is the same in man (KÜNZEL et al., 1974; PARER et al., 1968; KÜNZEL, 1974), (Fig. 5).

In the suspension of foetal hypoxia following prolonged uterine contractions it is very important to stop the contractions with β-mimetics and to recover the blood flow of the uterus and the oxygen supply to the foetus in this way (intra-uterine reanimation of the foetus).

The increase in the foetal oxygen level during β-mimetic treatment in the course of human examinations in the non-hypoxic foetus was also observed. LEHMANN (1977) in the course of fenoterol treatment during labour found that in foetal scalp blood samples the PO_2 increased from 20 mm Hg to 22.1 mm Hg. This increase means that it is possible for the foetal blood oxygen saturation to increase by 12%.

The increased *placental transport* due to the aggravated utero-placental blood flow was demonstrated not only in connection with gases. WINDORFER and PRINGSHEIM

(1979), on the basis of maternal and foetal serum concentration values of diazepam following diazepam and fenoterol treatment during labour, declared that the diaplacental penetration of diazepam was nearly twofold in the cases of those who received β-mimetic treatment.

On the basis of the increase in the utero-placental blood flow and the consecutive rise of placental transport it could be suggested that prolonged β-sympathomimetic treatment increases the growth of the foetus as well. RIPPERT et al. (1971) relate the increased rate of foetal weight growth during tocolytic treatment. Examinations carried out later did not confirm this observation. MELCHIOR and BERNARD (1974), LANG et al. (1975), on the basis of results of ultrasonic examinations during pregnancy and on the basis of data referring to the body weight of infants, found the dynamism of foetal growth unchanged under tocolysis. In the course of analysing data referring to 200 cases of prolonged β-sympathomimetic treatment carried out by us, we came to the conclusion that foetal weight growth increases after a treatment lasting more than 2 weeks, while the rate of longitudinal growth remains unchanged. The positive effect of prolonged tocolysis on foetal growth is further suggested in our material by the fact that in cases of twin pregnancy in groups treated by β-mimetics and bed-rest the growth of the biparietal diameter of the skull was greater than in the group which had bed-rest only (KOVÁCS et al., 1978).

III. Effect on the Foetal Heart

The characteristic feature of foetal heart function which can best be examined in clinical circumstances is the frequency of the heart beat. Numerous facts are known about the connection between β-sympathomimetic treatment and the foetal heart rate. The majority of the publications relate the increase of the foetal heart rate: descriptions of foetal heart rate increase are found in works by KARIM (1963), SHENKER (1965), STANDER et al. (1964), KOVÁCS et al. (1976) during isoxsuprine treatment, POSEIRO et al. (1968), ZILIANTI and ALLER (1971) during orciprenaline treatment, SIVASAMBOO (1972), RENAUD et al. (1974) after ritodrine treatment, DAWSON and DAVIES (1977) during salbutamol treatment, KOVÁCS et al. (1976) during fenoterol treatment. There are observations which declare that the foetal heart rate does not change during tocolytic treatment. BAUMGARTEN (1967) during isoxsuprine treatment, LANDESMAN et al. (1971) during ritodrine treatment, WEIDINGER and WIEST (1972) during the administration of fenoterol and verapamil did not observe any change in heart rate.

Foetal tachycardia is generally mild, the changes do not increase as much as the values for the maternal heart rate increase.

The increase of the foetal heart rate is in proportion to the dose of β-sympathomimetic administered to the mother. In our own examinations in the 17th–20th weeks of pregnancy the dose of the intravenously administered fenoterol was increased from 0.1 mcg/min by 0.1 mcg/min every 15 min up to a dose of 0.4 mcg/min. In the meantime the maternal and the foetal heart rates were registered continuously. With 3 and 4 mcg/min doses the foetal heart rates exceeded the starting value significantly: $P < 0.02$ and < 0.01 (KOVÁCS et al., 1976) (Fig. 6).

The in vitro examination of the foetal heart rate also proved that the effects of β-sympathomimetics observed in vivo exist in vitro as well. In animal experiments it was demonstrated by KORDS (1975b) in guinea-pigs that fenoterol had the same chrono-

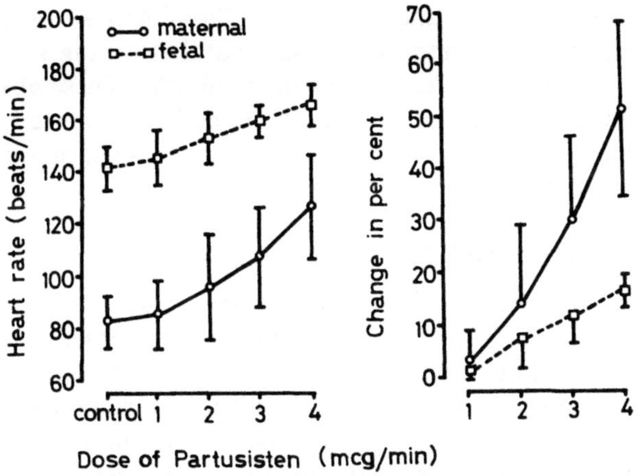

Fig. 6. Changes in maternal and fetal heart rate during increasing dose fenoterol (Partusisten) infusion to the mother (KOVÁCS et al., 1976)

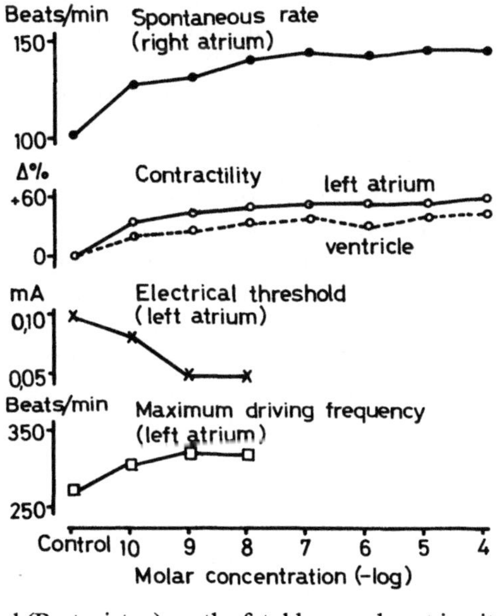

Fig. 7. Effects of fenoterol (Partusisten) on the fetal human heart in vitro (KOVÁCS et al., 1976)

tropic effects in vitro on the maternal and on the foetal heart. In the human foetal heart in vitro RESCH et al. (1978) managed to demonstrate the effect of fenoterol and isoxsuprine on the increase in frequency and the excitability and contractility of the myometrium from the 6th or 7th week of the embryo. In vitro examinations of foetal hearts with therapeutic concentrations of fenoterol and isoxsuprine, previously exposed to a β-mimetic effect in vivo with the same drugs, used, indicated the increase in frequency, atrial and ventricular contractility and the shortening of the atrial and ventricular refractory period (KOVÁCS et al., 1976) (Fig. 7).

These results seem to prove that the β-sympathomimetics have a direct effect on the changes in foetal heart functions in vivo and that these changes are not the indirect consequence of the changes in utero-placental circulation. These observations are indirect evidence of the fact that the β-sympathomimetics penetrate the placenta in an active form. Furthermore, they prove that the β-receptors are present in the myocardium from an early foetal age.

IV. Myocardium Lesion and Tocolysis

After isoproterenol treatment "infarct-like" lesions occurred in rat myocardium according to RONA et al. (1959). In animal experiments it was observed several times that catecholamines in large doses might cause myocardium necrosis for which the calcium ions flowing into the myocardium in great quantities are responsible. Recently some publications have called attention to the fact that in some infants born after tocolysis circulation disturbances were observed which could be derived from myocardium damage (TROLP et al., 1978; URBANEK et al., 1978). What is more, fatal myocardium necrosis was also mentioned (HILLEMANS and TROLP, 1977).

In tissue cultures of the human foetal heart, as an effect of therapeutic concentration of β-mimetics, damage to myocardium cells was detected by light and electron microscopic examinations. With verapamil added to the nutrition medium, the damage could be avoided (WEIDINGER et al., 1978).

These data contradict experiences which have accumulated in the course of thousands of tocolytic treatments and which seem to be supported by the results of pathological examinations of infants who were born and who died after tocolytic treatment, i.e., that neither pathological nor clinical data referred to the development of myocardium lesion. In animal experiments on pregnant rats NOTMAN et al. (1977) with a high-dose fenoterol and isoprenaline treatment could not detect tissue changes in the foetal heart or an increase in the weight of the heart, or increased calcium inflow. Treatment with a dose many times higher than the therapeutic dose caused easily observable changes in the heart of the mother animals, although these changes did not go as far as necrosis. The immunity of the foetal heart is thought to be due to the fact that the β-mimetic could be detected in the foetal heart only in a very low concentration.

On the basis of data gathered so far, no damage to the cardiac muscle can be expected during normal β-sympathomimetic clinical treatment of pregnant women. Any additional treatment, however, which can increase the calcium level and the cellular inflow can thus be a necrosis-inducing factor (catecholamines, corticosteroids, calcium, vitamin D) must be carefully thought over. The foetal heart can be protected by β-mimetic treatment combined with verapamil (WEIDINGER and WIEST, 1978).

V. The Effect of Beta-Sympathomimetics on Foetal Pulmonary Maturation

Among the drugs and hormone-compounds which are supposed to accelerate the maturation of foetal lungs in animal experiments and in clinical practice the special significance of the β-sympathomimetics is attributed to by the fact that they are used mainly in cases of imminent premature labour and therefore besides their main effect — the suspension of the contractions of the uterus — this possible side-effect would be very favourable in respect of the final aim of the treatment, i.e., to save the foetus.

The question is significant since the joint administration of corticosteroids, which are used to improve the maturation of the foetal lung, and the β-mimetics is contraindicated according to some authors, since the foetal myocardium-damaging effect of β-mimetics might be aggravated by the corticosteroid.

The first account of *clinical observations* was published by KERO et al. (1973) who did not observe a single case of respiratory distress syndrome in 38 infants whose mothers had undergone isoxsuprine treatment during labour. BOOG et al. (1975) also stated that ritodrine treatment before labour reduced the incidence of idiopathic respiratory distress syndrome of newborns considerably, although the difference was significant only in the case of premature infants of a body weight less than 2,300 g.

BERGMAN and HEDNER (1978) carried out examinations on the effect of terbutaline on 24 premature newborns whose mothers had been treated with β-sympathomimetics and on 17 premature newborns whose mothers had not been previously treated. Terbutaline treatment — except in eight cases — was prolonged, lasting for several weeks. Significantly fewer cases of respiratory distress syndrome (RDS) occurred among the infants whose mothers had been treated with β-sympathomimetics ($P<0.05$).

HASTWELL (1977) published his observations on salbutamol treatment preceding labour and its effects on the respiration capacity of premature infants. According to his observations the favourable effect is considerable if labour takes place within 4 h after the treatment is stopped. In his prospective study — on a small group of 12 pregnant women — he states that in respect of the RDS-threatened infants no case of RDS occurred if the mother was given 250–500 mcg salbutamol 3 h before labour.

DUDENHAUSEN et al. (1978) examined the maturity of foetal lung during tocolytic treatment by defining the lecithin content of the amniotic fluid and came to different conclusions from those of the above authors. They observed that in the amniotic fluid (157 examinations in 60 pregnant women) of the pregnant women who received prolonged tocolytic treatment with fenoterol (Partusisten) the lecithin values were significantly lower than in the untreated control group (211 examinations in 190 pregnant women). The low values referring to the immaturity of the lung (3 mg lecithin per 100 ml amniotic fluid) were a lot more frequent in the group treated with prolonged tocolysis than in the control group.

In the course of studying the question by means of animal experiments WYSZOGRODSKI et al. (1974) observed that after the intramuscular isoxsuprine treatment of premature rabbits the lung showed better respiratory capacities than those of the nontreated controls. The effect was attributed to the isoxsuprine-induced surfactant release. Later, in a similarly arranged experiment ENHORNING et al. (1977) found that the surface activity of the pulmonary liquid of foetuses which had been treated by isoxsuprine was higher, the lecithin–sphingomyelin (L/S) ratio was higher in the liquid and fewer lamellar bodies were found in the granulated pneumocytes than in the control animals. All this supported the theory of drug-induced surfactant release. ENHORNING et al. (1979) carried out examinations in animal experiments in which the arrangements were closer to human therapy. Rabbits were treated by isoxsuprine infusion on the 28 th day of pregnancy, 2.5 mg/kg body wt. dose was administered in 50 ml 5% glucose (this is about three times as much as the maximum human therapeutic dose). After the infusion a lethal dose of pentobarbital was administered then the dead foetuses were removed by caesarian section. The examination of the pulmonary liquid and the histological process of the lungs both proved the surfactant release as opposed to the 5% glucose treated control group.

GERNER et al. (1977) studied the effect of β-sympathomimetics on the phospholipoid synthesis of the foetal lung by examining the incorporation of [^{14}C]cholin into the lecithin fraction of the pulmonary tissue in rats. Following buphenine (Dilatol) and fenoterol treatment no significant difference was found in either group compared to the untreated control group of animals.

The explanation of the favourable effect suggested by clinical observations and the mechanism of action are not clear. One possible explanation, supported by the results of animal experiments, could be that β-mimetics cause a quick release of the surface-active materials into the alveolae. The results of DUDENHAUSEN et al. (1978) in connection with amniotic fluid do not correspond well with clinical observations. It is suggested that the quick release of the surface-active material as an effect of β-mimetics is followed by a lower surfactant level. This is, however, contrasted by the fact that BERGMAN and HEDNER (1978) experienced more favourable pulmonary maturation in premature infants even after prolonged tocolysis. The possibility that the treatment induces the dilatation of the lower trachea or causes changes in pulmonary circulation and that these changes play a favourable role in post-natal pulmonary maturation cannot be excluded.

Examinations which have been carried out so far have not clarified the effect of β-sympathomimetics on foetal pulmonary maturation, but several data, on the basis of the results of clinical and animal experiments, support the theory that the effect is favourable.

VI. Effect on Newborns of Beta-Sympathomimetic Treatment of Pregnant Women

In summarizing it can be stated that β-sympathomimetic treatment can have a manifold effect on the foetus. Certain effects can be favourable, others unfavourable from the point of view of the foetus and the newborn. However, considerably unfavourable changes were observed very rarely. According to examinations carried out on a large population of infants β-mimetic treatment during pregnancy and labour rather improves the adaptation of the infant to extra-uterine life (CASTRÉN et al., 1972) and metabolism, blood count, ECG, EEG, and neurological examinations carried out on newborns and infants showed normal values (WEIDINGER et al., 1973). The most important effect of the treatment on the foetus is that, by postponing premature labour, intra-uterine life is prolonged and the development, growth and maturation of the foetus can continue without the treatment having significant risks.

References

Ahlquist, R.P.: Study of adrenotropic receptors. Am. J. Physiol. *153*, 586–600 (1948)

Amendt, U., Gödel, E.: Akute und Langzeittokolyse mittels Buphenin (Dilatol) bei insulinpflichtigen diabetischen Schwangeren. Zentralbl. Gynaekol. *97*, 1607–1613 (1975)

Baillie, P., Meehan, F.P., Tyack, A.J.: Treatment of premature labour with orciprenaline. Br. Med. J. *4*, 154–155 (1970)

Baumgarten, K.: Die Beeinflußung der Uterusmotilität. Wien: Hollinek 1967

Baumgarten, K.: Uterusmotilität beim weiblichen Zyklus. Geburtshilfe Frauenheilkd. *30*, 921–933 (1970)
Baumgarten, K.: Criteria in the treatment of threatening premature labour with betamimetics (tokolyse-index), premature labour score. In: Labour inhibition. Betamimetic drugs in obstetrics. Weidinger, H. (ed.), pp. 185–195. Stuttgart, New York: Fischer 1977
Baumgarten, K., Fröhlich, H., Seidl, A., Sokol, K., Lim-Rachmat, F., Hager, R.: A new beta-sympathicomimetic preparation for intravenous and oral inhibition of uterine contractions. Eur. J. Obstet. Gynecol. *2*, 69–73 (1971)
Bergman, B., Hedner, T.: Antepartum administration of terbutaline and the incidence of hyaline membrane disease in preterm infants. Acta Obstet. Gynecol. Scand. *57*, 217–221 (1978)
Bieniarz, J., Motew, M., Scommegna, A.: Uterine and cardiovascular effects of ritodrine in premature labor. Obstet. Gynecol. *40*, 65–73 (1972)
Bishop, E.H., Woutersz, T.B.: Arrest of premature labour. JAMA *178*, 812–814 (1961)
Boden, W., Crabben, H.: Wehenhemmung mit einer neuen beta-adrenergen Substanz. Med. Welt *21*, 1342–1349 (1970)
Boog, G., Ben Brahim, M., Gandar, R.: Betamimetic drugs and possible prevention of respiratory distress syndrome. Br. J. Obstet. Gynaecol. *82*, 285–288 (1975)
Briel, R.C., Kunz, S., Kidess, E.: Die Thrombozytenfunktion bei intravenöser Langzeittokolyse mit Fenoterol-Verapamil. Z. Geburtshilfe Perinatol. *182*, 424–427 (1978)
Buchelt, L., Rominger, K.L.: Pharmacokinetics and metabolism of Th 1165a in man. Int. Z. Klin. Pharmakol. Ther. Toxikol. [Suppl.] *4*, 37–41 (1972)
Bülbring, E., Goodford, P.J., Setekleiv, J.: The action of adrenaline on the ionic content and on sodium and potassium movements in the smooth muscle of the guinea-pig taenia coli. Br. J. Pharmacol. *28*, 296–307 (1966)
Castelazo Ayala, L., Karchmer, S.: Comparative study of utero-inhibiting action of two beta-adrenomimetic drugs. Acta Obstet. Gynecol. Scand. *56*, 287–291 (1977)
Castrén, O., Gummerus, M., Saarikoski, S., Soiva, K.: Zur Wirkung der Beta-Sympathomimetika während der Geburt auf die Adaptation des Neugeborenen. Geburtshilfe Frauenheilkd. *32*, 943–948 (1972)
Conradt, A., Schlotter, C.M., Unbehaun, V.: Lipolysis, ketonaemia, estrogen, and gestagen concentrations during short time infusion therapy with betamimetics. In: Labour inhibition. Betamimetic drugs in obstetrics. Weidinger, H. (ed.), pp. 103–110. Stuttgart, New York: Fischer 1977
Csapó, A.I., Herczeg, J.: Arrest of premature labor by isoxsuprine. Am. J. Obstet. Gynecol. *129*, 482–491 (1977)
Davis, C.H., Schliselfeld, L.H., Wolf, D.P., Laevitt, C.A., Krebs, E.G.: Interrelationships among glycogen phosphorylase isoenzymes. J. Biol. Chem. *242*, 4824–4833 (1967)
Dawson, A.M., Davies, H.J.: The effect of intravenous and oral salbutamol on fetus and mother in premature labour. Br. J. Obstet. Gynaecol. *84*, 348–353 (1977)
Dobbs, J.W., Robison, G.A.: Functional biochemistry of beta receptors in the uterus. Fed. Proc. *27*, 352–352 (1968)
Dudenhausen, J.W., Kynast, G., Lange-Lindberg, A.M., Saling, E.: Influence of long-term beta-mimetic therapy on the lecithin content of amniotic fluid. Gynecol. obstet. invest. *9*, 205–209 (1978)
Editorial: Drugs in threatened preterm labour. Br. Med. J. 1979 *I*, 71–71
Enhorning, G., Chamberlain, D., Contreras, C., Burgoyne, R., Robertson, B.: Isoxsuprine-induced release of pulmonary surfactant in the rabbit fetus. Am. J. Obstet. Gynecol. *129*, 197–202 (1977)
Enhorning, G., Chamberlain, D., Contreras, C., Burgoyne, R., Robertson, B.: Isoxsuprine infusion to the pregnant rabbit and its effect on fetal lung surfactant. Biol. Neonate *35*, 43–51 (1979)
Eskes, T.K.A.B., Seelen, J., van Gent, I.: The effect of betamimetic adrenergic drugs on the activity of the pregnant-human uterus, tested with the intrauterine pressure method. Arzneim. Forsch. *16*, 762–766 (1966)
Falkay, G., Herczeg, J., Kovács, L.: Effect of beta-mimetic isoxsuprine on prostaglandin biosynthesis in pregnant human myometrium in vitro. Life Sci. *23*, 2689–2696 (1978)
Fegerl, H., Narik, G.: Die Beeinflußung der Wehentätigkeit durch das sympathische und parasympathische Nervensystem. Geburtshilfe Frauenheilkd. *11*, 822–834 (1951)

Fleckenstein, A., Grün, G., Byon, K.Y.: Hemmung der Uterus-Kontraktilität durch Ca^{++}-antagonistische Inhibitoren der elektro-mechanischen Koppelung. In: Methoden der pharmakologischen Geburtserleichterung und Uterus Relaxation. Jung, H. (ed)., pp. 107–116. Stuttgart: Thieme 1972
Fleckenstein, A., Janke, J., Fleckenstein-Grün, G.: Kardiotoxische Wirkungen beta-adrenergen Tokolytika – Kardioprotektion durch Ca^{++}-Antagonisten. In: Kardiale Probleme bei der Tokolyse. Hillemanns, H.G., Trolp, R. (eds.), pp. 54–67. Stuttgart: Enke 1978
Fröhlich, H., Baumgarten, K., Seidl, A.: Der Einfluß von Ovulationshemmern auf die Aktivität des Uterus. In: Methoden der pharmakologischen Geburtserleichterung und Uterus-Relaxation. Jung, H. (ed.), pp. 184–192. Stuttgart: Thieme 1972
Gerner, R., Halberstadt, E., Schwartz, H., Stein, W.W.: Zur Wirkung der Tokolytika auf die Phospholipid-Synthese in der fetalen Lunge. Arch. Gynaekol. *224*, 215–216 (1977)
Grün, G., Hillemanns, H.G., Fleckenstein, A.: Hemmung der Kontraktilität des graviden Myometrium durch Ca^{++}-Antagonisten und Sympathikomimetika. In: Methoden der pharmakologischen Geburtserleichterung und Uterus-Relaxation. Jung, H. (ed.), pp. 116– 122. Stuttgart: Thieme 1972
Gummerus, M.: Die Behandlung der vorzeitigen Wehentätigkeit und Antagonisierung der Nebenwirkungen der tokolytischen Therapie mit Verapamil. Z. Geburtshilfe Perinatol. *181*, 334–340 (1977)
Harbon, S., Clauser, H.: Cyclic adenosine 3′,5′-monophosphate levels in rat myometrium under the influence of epinephrine, prostaglandins and oxytocin, correlations with uterus motility. Biochem. Biophys. Res. Commun. *44*, 1496–1503 (1971)
Harbon, S., Do Khac, L., Vesin, M.F.: Cyclic AMP binding to intracellular receptor proteins in rat myometrium. Effect of epinephrine and prostaglandin E_1. Mol. Cell. Endocrinol. *6*, 17–34 (1976)
Hastwell, G.: Salbutamol aerosol in premature labour. Lancet 1975 *II*, 1212–1213
Hastwell, G.: Salbutamol and respiratory distress syndrome. Lancet 1977 *II*, 354–354
Hein, P.R.: Der Einfluß von Th 1165a und Alupent auf die Aktivität des nichtschwangeren Uterus. In: Th 1165a (Partusisten) bei der Behandlung in der Geburtshilfe und Perinatologie. Jung, H., Klöck, F.K. (eds.), pp. 29–35. Stuttgart: Thieme 1975
Hendricks, C.H., Cibils, L.A., Pose, S.V., Eskes, T.K.: The pharmacologic control of excessive uterine activity with isoxsuprine. Am. J. Obstet. Gynecol. *82*, 1064–1078 (1961)
Hillemanns, H.G.: Einführung. In: Kardiale Probleme bei der Tokolyse. Hillemanns, H.G., Trolp, R. (eds.), pp. 1–8. Stuttgart: Enke 1978
Hillemanns, H.G., Trolp, R.: Tokolyse Symposion. Kurzreferat. Geburtshilfe Frauenheilkd. *37*, 191–193 (1977)
Hiltmann, W.D., Weidinger, H., Wiest, W.: Änderung der maternalen cardiovasculären Parameter während der Tokolyse und beim Rückenlagenschocksyndrom. Z. Geburtshilfe Perinatol. *180*, 366–374 (1976)
Hodgson, B.J., Pauerstein, C.J.: The effect of ovulation on the responses of the rabbit oviduct to adrenergic agonists in vitro. Biol. Reprod. *10*, 346–353 (1974)
Hodgson, B.J., Fremming, B.D., Daly, S.: Effects of adrenergic drugs administered during ovum transport and chemical sympathectomy of the oviduct on fertility in rabbits. Biol. Reprod. *13*, 142–146 (1975)
Hüter, J., Rippert, C., Meyer, C.: Wehenhemmung mit welchen Beta-Mimetikum (Berotec, Ritodrine, Dilatol)? Geburtshilfe Frauenheilkd. *32*, 97–103 (1972)
Ingemarsson, I.: Effect of terbutaline on premature labor. A double-blind placebo-controlled study. Am. J. Obstet. Gynecol. *125*, 520–524 (1976)
Johns, A., Chlumecky, J., Cottle, M.K.W., Paton, D.M.: Effect of chemical sympathectomy and adrenergic agonists on the fertility of mice. Contraception *11*, 563–570 (1975)
Jung, H., Abramowski, P., Klöck, F.K., Schwenzel, W.: Zur Wirkung alfa- und beta-adrenergischer Substanzen am menschlichen Uterus und Nebenwirkungen auf Mutter und Kind. Geburtshilfe Frauenheilkd. *31*, 11–27 (1971)
Karim, M.: Isoxsuprine and the human parturient uterus. J. Obstet. Gynaecol. Br. Commonw. *70*, 1335–1337 (1963)
Kendle, K.E., Lam Shan Leen, Y.K.: Further investigation of responses of the mammalian oviduct to catecholamines. J. Reprod. Fertil. *46*, 231–233 (1976)

Kero, P., Hirvonen, T., Välimäki, J.: Prenatal and postnatal isoxsuprine and respiratory distress syndrome. Lancet 1973 *II*, 198–198

Klöck, F.K.: The action of sympathomimetic drugs on uterine muscle. In: Labour inhibition. Betamimetic drugs in obstetrics. Weidinger, H. (ed.), pp. 27–39. Stuttgart, New York: Fischer 1977

Kords, H.: Kreislaufwirkungen, Plazentapassage, Pharmakokinetik und Metabolismus von Fenoterol (Partusisten) beim trächtigen Meerschweinchen. Z. Geburtshilfe Perinatol. *179*, 30–36 (1975a)

Kords, H.: In vitro Wirkungen von Fenoterol (Partusisten) auf die fetale und materne Herzfrequenz. Z. Geburtshilfe Perinatol. *179*, 37–39 (1975b)

Kords, H.: Wirkung von Fenoterol (Partusisten) auf die Motilität und den Gehalt des cyclischen Adenosin 3′,5′-Monophosphat des isolierten Rattenuterus. Z. Geburtshilfe Perinatol. *179*, 40–44 (1975c)

Kords, H.: Pharmacology and pharmacokinetics of Partusisten (Fenoterol). In: Labour inhibition. Betamimetic drugs in obstetrics. Weidinger, H. (ed.), pp. 41–46. Stuttgart, New York: Fischer 1977

Kovács, L., Herczeg, J.: Tokolyse mit Berotec-Aerosol. Zentralbl. Gynaekol. *100*, 106–109 (1978)

Kovács, L., Resch, B., Sztanó, P.: A koraszülés megakadalyozása beta-receptor izgatokkal. Orv. Hetil. *114*, 2537–2538 (1973)

Kovács, L., Resch, B., Herczeg, J., Apro, G., Papp, J.G.: Maternal and fetal cardiac response to beta adrenergic stimulants with tocolytic properties. Proceedings of the I. Intercongress of Asian Federation of Obstetrics and Gynaecology, Vol. II. Chan, L. (ed.), pp. 553–554. Singapore: Eurasia 1976

Kovács, L., Gellén, J., Resch, B., Gyöngyösi, J.: Effect of long-lasting tocolysis on intrauterine development. In: Perinatal medicine, Abstracts of free communications. Thalhammer, O., Pollak, A. (eds.), pp. 178. Vienna: Novographic 1978

Kramer, J., Klingspohr, H.J.: Ganztierautoradiographische Untersuchungen über die Verteilung und die diaplazentare Passage von Fenoterolhydrobromid (Th 1165a) an Ratten. Arzneim. Forsch. *24*, 1210–1213 (1974)

Künzel, W., Kastendieck, E.: Uterine blood flow, fetal oxygenation and betamimetic drugs (Partusisten). In: Labour inhibition. Betamimetic drugs in obstetrics. Weidinger, H. (ed.), pp. 87–97. Stuttgart, New York: Fischer 1977

Künzel, W., Moll, W.: Uterine O_2 consumption and blood flow of the pregnant uterus. Z. Geburtshilfe Perinatol. *176*, 108–117 (1972)

Künzel, W., Klöck, F.K., Junge, H.D., Moll, W.: Uterine blood flow, oxygen uptake, and vascular resistance of pregnant sheep near term. J. Perinat. Med. *2*, 101–105 (1974)

Landesman, R., Wilson, K.H., Coutinho, E.M., Klima, I.M., Marcus, R.S.: The relaxant action of ritodrine, a sympathomimetic amine, on the uterus during term labor. Am. J. Obstet. Gynecol. *110*, 111–114 (1971)

Lands, A.M., Luduena, F.P., Buzzo, H.J.: Differentiation of receptors responsive to isoproterenol. Life Sci. *6*, 2241–2249 (1967)

Lang, N., Hansmann, M., Bellmann, O., Nocke, W., Weitzel, H.: Langzeitbeobachtungen bei Th 1165a-Behandlung unter Einbeziehung von Ultraschall und endokrinologischen Parametern. In: Th 1165a (Partusisten) bei der Behandlung in der Geburtshilfe und Perinatologie. Jung, H., Klöck, F.K. (eds.), pp. 155–161. Stuttgart: Thieme 1975

Lehmann, V.: Einwirkung auf den maternen und fetalen Stoffwechsel, Säure-Basen-Haushalt und die Blutgase bei dem therapeutischen Einsatz von Partusisten unter der Geburt. Z. Geburtshilfe Perinatol. *181*, 20–24 (1977)

Liggins, G.C., Vaughan, G.S.: Intravenous infusion of salbutamol in the management of premature labour. J. Obstet. Gynaecol. Br. Commonw. *80*, 29–32 (1973)

Lippert, T.H., Kubli, F., Rüttgers, H.: Die hyperglykämische Aktivität von Tokolytika. Klin. Wochenschr. *50*, 119–121 (1972)

Lipshitz, J., Baillie, P.: The effect of the fenoterol hydrobromide (Partusisten) aerosol on uterine activity and the cardiovascular system. Br. J. Obstet. Gynaecol. *83*, 864–869 (1976)

Lipshitz, J., Vinik, A.I.: The effects of hexoprenaline, a $beta_2$-sympathomimetic drug, on maternal glucose, insulin, glucagon, and free fatty acid levels. Am. J. Obstet. Gynecol. *130*, 761–764 (1978)

Lish, P.M., Hillyard, J.W., Dungan, K.W.: The uterine relaxant properties of isoxsuprine. J. Pharmacol. Exp. Ther. *129*, 438–444 (1960)
Lorenz, D.: Untersuchungen mit beta-adrenergisch wirksamen Substanzen am wehenbereiten isoierten Uterus der trächtigen Ratte. In: Methoden der pharmakologischen Geburtserleichterung und Uterus-Relaxation. Jung, H. (ed.), pp. 159–169. Stuttgart: Thieme 1972
Meissner, J., Klostermann, H.: Distribution and diaplacental passage of infused ^{3}/H-fenoterol hydrobromide (Partusisten) in the gravid rabbit. Int. J. Clin. Pharmacol. Biopharm. *13*, 27–35 (1976)
Meissner, J., Preil, P.: Untersuchungen über Verteilung und Passage von T-markiertem Fenoterol-Hydrobromid (Th 1165 a) am trächtigen und laktierenden Kaninchen. Arzneim. Forsch. *24*, 1213–1217 (1974)
Melchior, J., Bernard, N.: Present treatment of premature labor. Results and factors which influence success. In: Recent progress in obstetrics and gynaecology. Persianinov, L.S., Chervakova, T.V., Presl, J. (eds.), pp. 75–84. Amsterdam: Excerpta Medica 1974
Mitznegg, P., Heim, F., Meythaler, B.: Influence of endogenous and exogenous cyclic 3′,5′-AMP on contractile responses by oxytocin and calcium in isolated rat uterus. Life Sci. *9*, 121–128 (1970)
Mohr, D., Weidinger, H.: The effect of betamimetics on pregnant diabetics. In: Labour inhibition. Betamimetic drugs in obstetrics. Weidinger, H. (ed.), pp. 125–130. Stuttgart, New York: Fischer 1977
Mosler, K.H., Linka, F.: Klinische Pharmakologie in der Geburtshilfe: Uterusregulation. Med. Klin. *70*, 798–805 (1975)
Mosler, K.H., Rosenboom, H.G.: Neuere Möglichkeiten einer tokolytischen Behandlung in der Geburtshilfe. Z. Geburtshilfe Perinatol. *176*, 85–96 (1972)
Mosler, K.H., Schwalm, H.: Vergleichende Untersuchungen tokolytisch und relaxierend wirkender Substanzen am isolierten Uterus. Zentralbl. Gynaekol. *87*, 603–613 (1965)
Mosler, K.H., Dornhöfer, W., Linka, F.: Hemmung vorzeitiger Wehen. Med. Klin. *69*, 97–101 (1974)
Müller-Tyl, E., Reinold, E., Hernuss, P.: Gleichzeitige Anwendung einer beta-mimetischen und beta-rezeptoren-blockierenden Substanz bei der Wehenhemmung. Z. Geburtshilfe Perinatol. *178*, 128–134 (1974)
Nakanishi, H., Wood, C.: Effects of calcium and magnesium on sympathetic transmission in human fallopian tube. Arch. Int. Pharmacodyn. Ther. *174*, 469–480 (1968)
Nilsson, H.T., Persson, K., Tegner, K.: The metabolism of terbutaline in man. Xenobiotica *2*, 363–373 (1972)
Notman, J., Rominger, K.L., Niggeschulze, A., Arndts, D.: Experimental investigation of possible cardiotoxic effects on the offspring of rats treated with high doses of fenoterol. J. Perinat. Med. *5*, 206–213 (1977)
Parer, J.T., De Lannoy, C.W., Hoversland, A.S., Metcalfe, J.: Effect of decreased uterine blood flow on uterine oxygen consumption in pregnant macaques. Am. J. Obstet. Gynecol. *100*, 813–820 (1968)
Persson, K., Persson, K.: The metabolism of terbutaline in vitro by rat and human liver O-methyltransferases and monoamine oxidases. Xenobiotica *2*, 375–382 (1972)
Polacek, J., Daniel, E.E.: Effect of α- and β-adrenergic stimulation on the uterine motility and adenosine 3′,5′-monophosphate level. Can. J. Physiol. Pharmacol. *49*, 988–998 (1971)
Polidoro, J.P., Howe, G.R., Black, D.L .: The effects of adrenergic drugs on ovum transport through the rabbit oviduct. J. Reprod. Fertil. *35*, 331–337 (1973)
Polidoro, J.P., Heilman, R.D., Culver, R.M., Reo, R.R.: Effects of adrenergic drugs or denervation on ovum transport in rabbits. In: Ovum transport and fertility regulation. Harper, M.J.K., Pauerstein, C.J., Adams, C.E., Coutinho, E.M., Croxatto, H.B., Paton, D.M. (eds.), pp. 331–341. Copenhagen: Scriptor 1976
Pose, S.V., Cibils, L.A., Zuspan, F.P.: Effect of L-epinephrine infusion on uterine contractility and cardiovascular system. Am. J. Obstet. Gynecol. *84*, 297–306 (1962)
Poseiro, J.J., Guevara-Rubio, G., Magan, J.M., Caldeyro-Barcia, R.: Accion de la orciprenalina (Alupent) sobre la contractilidad del utero humano gravido, el sistema cardiovascular materno y la frequencia cardiaca fetal. Arch. Ginecol. Obstet. (Montevideo) *23*, 99–118 (1968)
Rasmussen, H., Tenenhouse, A.: Cyclic adenosine monophosphate CA^{++} and membranes. Proc. Natl. Acad. Sci. USA *59*, 1364–1370 (1968)

Reinold, E., Mueller-Tyl, E.: Tocolysis with betamimetics and beta-blockers. In: Labour inhibition. Betamimetic drugs in obstetrics. Weidinger, H. (ed.), pp. 135–138. Stuttgart, New York: Fischer 1977
Renaud, R., Irrmann, M., Gandar, R., Flynn, M.J.: The use of ritodrine in the treatment of premature labour. J. Obstet. Gynaecol. Br. Commonw . *81*, 182–186 (1974)
Resch, B., Apró, G., Papp, G.: Effect of $beta_2$ mimetic agents on heart function in the human embryo. Acta Physiol. Acad. Sci. Hung. *51*, 176–177 (1978)
Richter, R.: Wirksamkeit der Langzeittokolyse mit Betamimetika zur Behandlung der drohenden Frühgeburt. Z. Geburtshilfe Perinatol. *182*, 417–423 (1978)
Rippert, C., Hüter, J., Bärtschi, R.: Intravenöse Langzeit-Wehenhemmung mit Beta-Mimetika und Antagonisierung der Nebenwirkungen. Geburtshilfe Frauenheilkd. *31*, 710–714 (1971)
Rominger, K.L., Pollmann, W.: Vergleichende Pharmakokinetik von Fenoterol-Hydrobromid bei Ratte, Hund und Mensch. Arzneim. Forsch. *22*, 1190–1196 (1972)
Rona, A., Chappel, C.I., Balázs, T., Gaudry, R.: An infarct like myocardial lesion and other toxic manifestations produced by isoproterenol in the rat. Arch. Pathol. *67*, 443–455 (1959)
Ryden, G.: The effect of salbutamol and terbutaline in the management of premature labour. Acta Obstet. Gynecol. Scand. *56*, 293–296 (1977)
Seewald, H.J., Hauschild, R., Zorn, C.: Pharmakologische Beeinflussung der Aktivität des menschlichen Myometriums im in-vitro-Versuch. Zentralbl. Gynaekol. *95*, 1473–1475 (1973)
Selye, H.: Elektrolyte, Streß und Herznekrose. Basel, Stuttgart: Schwabe 1960
Senior, J.B., Spencer-Gregson, R.N.: The effects of sympathomimetic drugs and bradykinin on the human fallopian tube in vitro using isometric recording methods. J. Obstet. Gynaecol. Br. Commonw. *76*, 652–655 (1969)
Shenker, L.: Effect of isoxsuprine on fetal heart rate and fetal electrocardiogram. Obstet. Gynekol. *26*, 104–108 (1965)
Sivasamboo, R.: Premature labor. In: Proceedings of the International Symposium on the treatment of fetal risks. Baumgarten, K., Wesselius de Casparis, A. (eds.), pp. 16–21. Wien: University of Vienna 1972
Smith, S.K., Thompson, D.: The effect of intravenous salbutamol upon plasma and urinary potassium during premature labour. Br. J. Obstet. Gynaecol. *84*, 344–347 (1977)
Stander, R.W., Barden, T.P., Thompson, J.T., Pugh, W.R., Werts, C.E.: Fetal cardiac effects of maternal isoxsuprine infusion. Am. J. Obstet. Gynecol. *89*, 792–800 (1964)
Stosiek, U., Wiest, W.: Veränderungen der Blutgerinnung und der Thrombocytenaggregation bei Langzeitwehenhemmung. Z. Geburtshilfe Perinatol. *180*, 209–214 (1976)
Sutherland, E.W., Oye, I., Butcher, R.W.: The action of epinephrine and the role of the adenylcyclase system in hormone action. Recent Progr. Hormone Res. *21*, 623–646 (1965)
Szendi, B.: Erhaltung der Schwangerschaft bei drohender (habitueller) Fehl- und Frühgeburt mittels Arzneimittel der viszeralen Nerven, besonders Adrenalin. Zentralbl. Gynaekol. *74*, 1690–1697 (1952)
Trolp, R., Haastert, H.P., Böhm, N., Ullrich, K.: Falldemonstration von drei Fällen mit pathologischen Erscheinungen am Herzen bei Kindern nach Tokolyse. In: Kardiale Probleme bei der Tokolyse. Hillemanns, H.-G., Trolp, R. (eds.), pp. 18–46. Stuttgart: Enke 1978
Ueda, M., DeMattos, C.E.R., Countinho, E.M.: The influence of adrenergic activation and blockade on the motility of the circular and longitudinal muscle layers of the rabbit oviduct in vitro. Fertil. Steril. *24*, 440–447 (1973)
Unbehaun, V., Conradt, A., Schlotter, C.M., Schneider, V.: Stoffwechselveränderungen während Infusion von Th 1165a. Z. Geburtshilfe Perinatol. *178*, 118–127 (1974)
Unbehaun, V., Conradt, A., Schlotter, C.M.: Untersuchungen über das Verhalten von Parametern des Kohlenhydrat- und Fettstoffwechsels sowie von humanem placentaren Lactogen (HPL) und Serum-Kalium während oraler Langzeitmedikation von Th 1165a. In: Th 1165a (Partusisten) bei der Behandlung in der Geburtshilfe und Perinatologie. Jung, H., Klöck, F.K. (eds.), pp. 191–195. Stuttgart: Thieme 1975
Urbanek, R., Schmidt-Redemann, B., Pringsheim, W., Haastert, H.P., Vogt, J.: Myocardveränderung nach Tokolyse. Monatsschr. Kinderheilkd. *126*, 340–341 (1978)
Vesin, M.F., Harbon, S.: The effects of epinephrine, prostaglandins, and their antagonists on adenosine cyclic 3′,5′-monophosphate concentrations and motility of the rat uterus. Mol. Pharmacol. *10*, 457–473 (1974)

Wallenburg, H.C.S.: Effect of metaproterenol (Alupent) on the angiographically visualized uteroplacental circulation in the rhesus monkey. In: Th 1165 a (Partusisten) bei der Behandlung in der Geburtshilfe und Perinatologie. Jung, H., Klöck, F.K. (eds.), pp. 147–154. Stuttgart: Thieme 1975
Wang, P., Clausen, T.: Treatment of attacks in hyperkalaemic familial periodic paralysis by inhalation of salbutamol. Lancet 1976 *I*, 221–223
Warkentin, B.: Die Tokolyse an der Universitäts-Frauenklinik Freiburg. In: Kardiale Probleme bei der Tokolyse. Hillemanns, H.G., Trolp, R. (eds.), pp. 17–18. Stuttgart: Enke 1978
Weidinger, H.: Current status of tocolysis. Labour inhibition. In: Labour inhibition. Betamimetic drugs in obstetrics. Weidinger, H. (ed.), pp. 243–261. Stuttgart, New York: Fischer 1977
Weidinger, H., Mohr, D.: Blutglukose und immunoreaktives Insulin unter dem Einfluß vom Th 1165 a und Isoptin bei Schwangeren mit und ohne tokolytische Therapie. Z. Geburtshilfe Perinatol. *177*, 244–251 (1973)
Weidinger, H., Wiest, W.: Behandlung der vorzeitigen Wehentätigkeit mit einem neuen Tokolytikum und Isoptin. Fortschr. Med. *89*, 1380–1381 (1971)
Weidinger, H., Wiest, W.: Die Behandlung der drohenden Frühgeburt mit Th 1165 a und Verapamil und deren Wirkung auf die Mutter, den Föten und das Neugeborene. In: Proceedings of the International Symposium on the treatment of fetal risks. Baumgarten, K., Wesselius de Casparis, A. (eds.), pp. 39–44. Wien: University of Vienna 1972
Weidinger, H., Wiest, W.: Die Behandlung des Spätabortes und der drohenden Frühgeburt mit Th 1165 a in Kombination mit Isoptin. Z. Geburtshilfe Perinatol. *177*, 233–237 (1973 a)
Weidinger, H., Wiest, W.: Die Auswirkungen lang dauernder Wehenhemmung mit Th 1165 a und Isoptin auf Herz-, Kreislauf-, Organ- und Stoffwechselparameter der Mutter. Z. Geburtshilfe Perinatol. *177*, 238–244 (1973 b)
Weidinger, H., Wiest, W.: Tokolyse. Fortschritt mit möglichen Gefahren. In: Kardiale Probleme bei der Tokolyse. Hillemanns, H.G., Trolp, R. (eds.), pp. 9–16. Stuttgart: Enke 1978
Weidinger, H., Wiest, W., Dietze, S., Witzel, K.: Wirkungen der Wehenhemmung mit Th 1165 a und Isoptin auf den Fetus, das Neugeborene und den Säugling. Z. Geburtshilfe Perinatol. *177*, 366–372 (1973)
Weidinger, H., Hofmann, W.-D., Wiest, W., Schleich, H., Shröter, D.: Histologische Befunde nach Inkubation von fötalen menschlichen Herzen mit Partusisten. In: Kardiale Probleme bei der Tokolyse. Hillemanns, H.G., Trolp, R. (eds.), pp. 74–77. Stuttgart: Enke 1978
Wernicke, K., Schulz, J., Berg, D.: The effect of the labour inhibitor Partusisten on cardiovascular parameters: blood gases and pH values of dam and fetus in sheep. In: Betamimetic drugs in obstetrics. Weidinger, H. (ed.), pp. 81–86. Stuttgart, New York: Fischer 1977
Wesselius de Casparis, A., Thiery, M., Yo Le Sian, A., Baumgarten, K., Brosens, I., Gammissans, O., Stolk, J.G., Vivier, W.: Results of double-blind, multicentre study with ritodrine in premature labour. Br. Med. J. *3*, 144–147 (1971)
Wiest, W., Weidinger, H., Zsolnai, B., Somogyi, J., Rominger, K.L.: Diaplacental transfer of Partusisten in humans. In: Labour inhibition. Betamimetic drugs in obstetrics. Weidinger, H. (ed.), pp. 47–51. Stuttgart, New York: Fischer 1977
Windorfer, A., Pringsheim, W.: Untersuchungen über den Einfluß einer tokolytischen Behandlung schwangerer Frauen mit Diazepam und Fenoterol auf die Bilirubin-Konzentration und Apgarwerte von Neugeborenen. Klin. Paediatr. *191*, 51–60 (1979)
Wolff, C.H.: Die medikamentöse Behandlung der vorzeitigen Wehentätigkeit. Z. Geburtshilfe Gynaekol. *167*, 68–76 (1967)
Wyszogrodski, I., Taeusch, H.W., Avery, M.E.: Isoxsuprine-induced alterations of pulmonary pressure-volume relationships in premature rabbits. Am. J. Obstet. Gynecol. *119*, 1107–1111 (1974)
Zahn, V.: Tokolyse mit einem Th 1165 a Dosier-Aerosol. Geburtshilfe Frauenheilkd. *33*, 818–821 (1973)
Zilianti, M., Aller, J.: Action of orciprenaline on uterine contractility during labor, maternal cardiovascular system, fetal heart rate and acid-base balance. Am. J. Obstet. Gynecol. *109*, 1073–1079 (1971)
Zuspan, F.P., Cibils, L.A., Pose, S.V.: Myometrial and cardiovascular responses to alterations in plasma epinephrine and norepinephrine. Am. J. Obstet. Gynecol. *84*, 841–851 (1962)

CHAPTER 6

Effects of Adrenergic Activators and Inhibitors on Kidney Function

H. OSSWALD and J. GREVEN

A. Introduction

For a long time the role of renal nerves in the regulation of renal function was considered to be of low importance. SMITH stated in 1951: "Renal denervation in unanaesthetized normal dogs and men does not produce renal hyperemia, the vasoconstrictor pathways being quiescent under basal conditions; nor does renal denervation have any significant effect upon the normal urine flow, upon water diuresis, or pituitary antidiuresis." The demonstration of rich sympathetic innervation of the juxtaglomerular apparatus and tubular epithelium (for review see BARAJAS, 1978) is the basis for the action of the nervous system and catecholamines on the kidney. Electrical stimulation of the renal nerves was found by VANDER (1965) to increase renal venous renin activity. It was only recently that a direct effect of renal nerve stimulation on tubular electrolyte reabsorption was clearly demonstrated by DIBONA (1977). Thus, there is morphological and functional evidence that renal sympathetic nerves are intimately involved in the regulation of the secretory and excretory function of the kidney.

B. Renal Hemodynamics

Renal blood flow constitutes 15%–25% of the cardiac output, which gives an average flow per gram of renal tissue of 3–5 ml/min. This average reflects mainly cortical flow, whereas the medulla and papilla are perfused by about 10% of the cortical flow. Despite the large amount of blood perfusing the renal cortex, renal blood flow and glomerular filtration rate remain remarkably constant over wide variations in arterial pressure. Our knowledge about regulation of renal blood flow is still incomplete and hence the contribution of catecholamines to renal blood flow regulation is poorly understood. Since the physiologic principles of the circulatory processes in the kidney are the basis for understanding the effect of drug action of renal blood flow, the reader may refer to some comprehensive reviews of renal hemodynamics written by THURAU (1964), BARGER and HERD (1973), and AUKLAND (1976).

I. Effects of Alpha-Adrenergic Activators

1. Adrenaline and Noradrenaline

a) Total Renal Blood Flow

The first observation of a catecholamine-induced renal vasoconstriction in the isolated perfused rabbit kidney using adrenaline was by RICHARDS and PLANT (1922). Despite renal vasoconstriction a simultaneous swelling of the kidney was observed.

This phenomenon has been confirmed by other data (for review see SMITH, 1951). It was suggested that adrenaline induced constriction mainly of the efferent glomerular arterioles leaving glomerular filtration rate unchanged while renal blood flow was reduced. In man, doses of 1 mg adrenaline s.c. or 10–40 μg/min i.v. reduced renal blood flow by 20%–40% whereas glomerular filtration rate was unaffected (SMITH, 1943; RANGES and BRADLEY, 1943). The effects of adrenaline and noradrenaline were almost indistinguishable (WESSON, 1969). More detailed analysis of the catecholamine effects on renal hemodynamics was done on laboratory animals. BALINT and CHATEL (1967) studied in anesthetized dogs the renal effects of intravenous infusion of adrenaline and noradrenaline in doses of 0.5–8.0 μg/kg/min. In lower doses renal blood flow was reduced only slightly while glomerular filtration rate was increased which suggests constriction of the efferent glomerular arterioles. Marked vasoconstriction (50% and more) and a fall in glomerular filtration rate were noted in doses of 5–8 μg/kg/min of either catecholamine.

In two recent studies the effect of noradrenaline on renal hemodynamics was investigated in Munich Wistar rats using micropuncture techniques. MYERS et al. (1975) reported an equal increase in afferent and efferent glomerular arteriolar resistance following intravenous infusion of 2.0–4.0 μg/kg/min of noradrenaline. When the increase in systemic blood pressure was not allowed to be transmitted to the kidney by partial aortic constriction above the renal arteries, noradrenaline increased only the resistance of the efferent glomerular arterioles. The authors concluded that the noradrenaline action is confined primarily to the efferent arterioles, thereby confirming the first suggestion of RICHARDS and PLANT (1922). However, ANDREUCCI et al. (1976) using the same rat strain and similar techniques, with the only difference being in the anesthetic employed (pentobarbital 60 mg/kg, in comparison to thiobutabarbital in the study of MYERS et al., 1975), reported a decrease in the hydrostatic pressure of the glomerular capillaries following noradrenaline intravenous infusion (2–4 μg/kg/min) and concluded that the afferent arterioles were constricted by noradrenaline, whereas no resistance changes occurred at the efferent arterioles. In this study no attempt was made to prevent the increase of blood pressure perfusing the kidneys. It was found that adrenaline, in contrast to noradrenaline, elevated the hydrostatic pressure in the glomerular capillaries. But again the conclusion was a predominant afferent arteriolar constriction with no change in efferent vascular resistance (ANDREUCCI et al., 1976).

The majority of the reports suggests that adrenaline and noradrenaline are able to constrict the efferent glomerular arterioles as indicated by an increase of filtration fraction. However, no definite conclusion can be reached (from both micropuncture studies cited above) as to why opposite effects of noradrenaline on the hydrostatic pressure in the glomerular capillaries were seen.

In toads *(Bufo arenarum)* noradrenaline (1.6 μg/min for 10 min intravenous infusion) increased glomerular capillary pressure when systemic blood pressure was also increased (URANGA, 1973).

In conscious rats intravenous infusion of 0.5 and 5.0 μg/kg/min of adrenaline and noradrenaline were compared in their effect on total renal blood flow and its fraction of cardiac output (GOLDMAN, 1966). The low dose of adrenaline increased renal blood flow and its fraction of cardiac output while noradrenaline in both dosages lowered renal blood flow and did not alter cardiac output. The high dose of adrenaline (5 μg/kg/min) did not change absolute renal blood flow but its fraction of cardiac output was still higher than in controls. Similar results were reported for the anesthetized rat. The fraction of cardiac output perfusing the kidney was significantly increased by 10 μg/kg adrenaline infused for 1–2 min. Absolute renal blood flow was also enhanced (LORENZETTI, 1970).

b) Intrarenal Blood Flow Distribution

Several studies were done to analyze the effect of adrenaline and noradrenaline on intrarenal blood flow distribution. The different techniques used to measure intrarenal blood flow include dye dilution, washout of inert gases like ^{85}Kr or ^{133}Xe, ^{32}P labeled erythrocytes, regional hydrogen clearances by means of implanted platinum electrodes, heated thermocouples, radioactive labeled microspheres, and the use of extractable substances such as p-aminohippurate and diodrast. A description of the different methods and a discussion of their validity are given by BARGER and HERD (1973) by CARRIÈRE (1975) and recently by AUKLAND (1980). Using implanted thermoelements in dog kidneys, GEBER (1966) concluded that 1 μg adrenaline or noradrenaline injected into the renal artery produced a marked decrease of outer cortical blood flow whereas flow to the juxtamedullary region had increased. However, changes in local heat production may not reflect absolute flow through an anatomically defined area.

POMERANZ et al. (1968), CARRIÈRE (1969), KILCOYNE and CANNON (1971), and BOMZON et al. (1975) estimated intrarenal blood flow distribution by means of the inert gas washout technique and concluded similarly that adrenaline and noradrenaline shifted blood flow from the outer to the inner cortex.

However, AUKLAND (1968) using hydrogen clearance measured by implanted platinum electrodes in dog kidneys demonstrated uniform reduction of cortical blood flow following intra-arterial or intravenous infusion of adrenaline or noradrenaline. This finding was confirmed by TYSSEBOTN and KIRKEBØ (1975) using the same technique (Fig. 1).

In this study renal perfusion pressure was kept constant by aortic constriction. As PROSNITZ et al. (1977) pointed out intrarenal blood flow distribution can be affected merely by changes in renal perfusion pressure. In agreement with AUKLAND's (1968) finding a uniform vascular sensitivity of the renal cortex of man to adrenaline was reported by EPSTEIN et al. (1970).

Studies using radioactively labeled microspheres to analyze intrarenal blood flow distribution in dogs in vivo (RECTOR et al., 1972; STEIN et al., 1973) clearly demonstrated a parallel decrease of renal blood flow in all layers of the cortex following adrenaline or noradrenaline administration.

JOSE et al. (1972) suggested that high renal resistance in young puppies, which is associated with a redistribution of renal blood flow toward the inner cortex, might be due to a heightened sensitivity to circulating catecholamines. They indeed demonstrated an increased sensitivity of the renal vasculature of the young puppy to adrenaline, particularly in the outer cortex in comparison with the inner cortex (JOSE et al., 1974).

GOTTSHALL and ITSKOVITZ (1977) studied in blood perfused dog kidney the effect on renal blood flow distribution of renal nerve stimulation and noradrenaline infusion (250–500 ng/min) into the renal artery; they reported that the inner zone of the cortex was more constricted. These results, which conflict with the data of RECTOR et al.

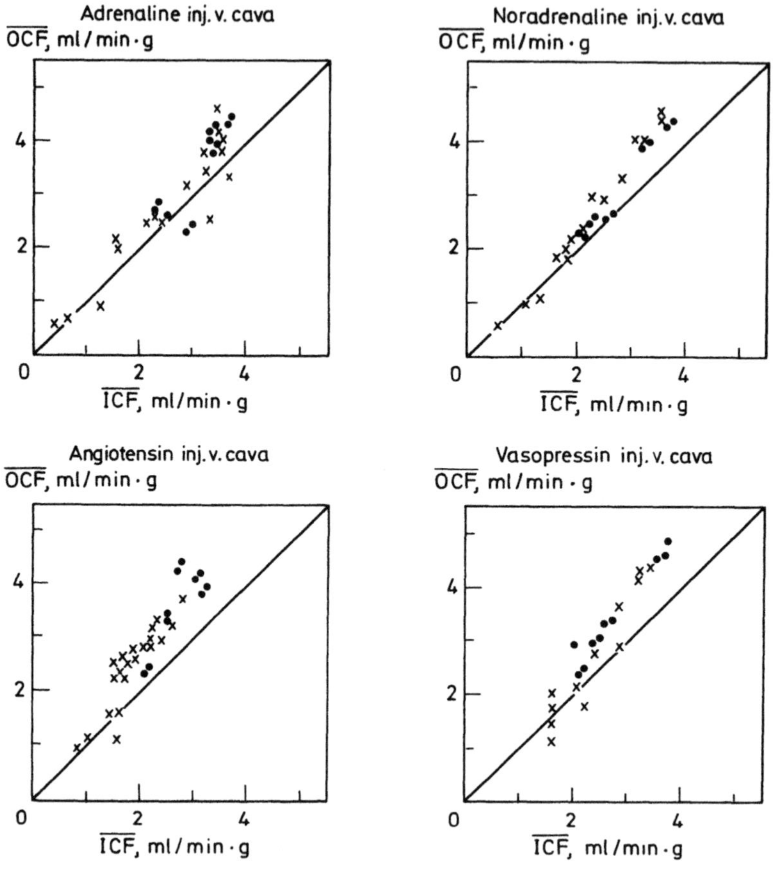

Fig. 1. Mean blood flow in outer cortex (OCF) related to mean flow in inner cortex (ICF) during intravenous infusion of vasoactive agents to dogs. Closed circles, control period; crosses, test period (TYSSEBOTN and KIRKEBØ, 1975)

(1972) and STEIN et al. (1973), have to be related to the different preparation of the kidneys and the artifacts due to isolated kidney perfusion.

In cats it is possible to collect separately venous blood from the superficial and deep cortex. Adrenaline preferentially reduced the deep cortical blood flow (NISSEN and GALSKOV, 1972).

GRÄNGSJÖ and PERSSON (1971) measured cortical and medullary blood flow in dog kidney by means of implanted heated thermocouples. They found that adrenaline administered intravenously or intrarenally reduced cortical and medullary flow; this effect was dose dependent. Noradrenaline had similar effects when injected into the renal artery. However, continuous infusion of noradrenaline (0.6 µg/kg/min) increased blood pressure slightly, reduced cortical flow, but increased medullary flow. Further increase of the dose of noradrenaline reduced blood flow in all the regions of the kidney. Methoxamine (0.17–0.6 mg/kg), metaraminol (0.6–1.3 µg/kg) and *N*-ethyl-normetaoxedrin (10–20 µg/kg) injected into the renal artery had identical effects as high doses of noradrenaline; as long as the hypertensive effect was seen, cortical and medullary blood flow were reduced to an equal extent.

Dietary induced hypercholesterolemia in baboons increased vascular sensitivity to noradrenaline mainly in the outer cortex. However, these effects could be attributed to the higher increase of systemic blood pressure compared to normocholesterolemic baboons (BOMZON et al., 1978). Redistribution of renal blood flow from the outer cortex to the juxtamedullary region accompanied by enhanced renal vascular sensitivity to noradrenaline in baboons with experimental obstructive jaundice was reported by BLOOM et al. (1974, 1976).

2. Other Alpha-Adrenergic Activators

The effects of α-adrenergic activators on renal hemodynamics reported in the older literature are reviewed by SMITH (1951) and WESSON (1969). The effects are qualitatively and in higher doses quantitatively very similar to those of noradrenaline (GRÄNGSJÖ and PERSSON, 1971; SWAIN et al., 1975; HEYNDRICKX et al., 1976). N-n-Dimethyldopamine was found to be an α-adrenergic agonist in the renal vascular bed. Phentolamine did inhibit the renal vasoconstriction (KITZEN et al., 1976). CHRYSANT and LAVENDER (1975) reported a decrease in effective renal plasma flow following intrarenal infusion of 1.2 μg/min clonidine; glomerular filtration rate was unchanged. The effects of clonidine on renal function in man have been reviewed recently by SCHMITT (1977).

3. Factors that Influence Renal Hemodynamic Response to Vasoconstrictive Catecholamines

In *neonates* renal blood flow is much lower than in adults. A recent review on perinatal renal pharmacology has been written by HOOK and BAILIE (1979). Adrenaline when infused intravenously at a rate of 21–31 ng/g kidney weight/min decreased cortical blood flow by 92% in puppies but only by 27% in the adult (JOSE et al., 1974). Cortical blood flow was redistributed to the inner cortex. Noradrenaline, 22–120 μg/kg injected into the umbilical circulation of sheep fetus (3 kg), increased markedly renal vascular resistance of the fetal kidney whereas maternal renal blood flow was unchanged (RANKIN and PHERNETTON, 1976).

Cold exposure of 3-day-old lambs increased the potency of noradrenaline (10 μg/kg/min) to constrict the renal vasculature whereas the adrenaline effects were not changed by cold exposure (ALEXANDER et al., 1972). In isolated perfused adult rabbit kidneys, noradrenaline had a higher constrictive potency when perfusion fluid was kept at 25 °C than at 37 °C (FONTELES and KAROW, 1976). In an additional study these authors reported that slow cooling to 15 °C at a rate of 0.6 °C/min did enhance whereas rapid cooling (at 6 °C/min) did not enhance vascular sensitivity to noradrenaline in the isolated perfused rabbit kidney (FONTELES and KAROW, 1978).

In *isolated saline perfused kidneys* of the rat the vasoconstrictive potency of adrenaline was found to be lost with time and to be attenuated by omitting calcium from the perfusion fluid (HYSELL and BOHR, 1970). In another study on vascular sensitivity of isolated saline perfused rat kidney, COLLIS and VANHOUTTE (1976) reported an increased vasoconstriction following noradrenaline infusion in the kidney of spontaneously hypertensive rats when compared to their controls. The renal vascular response to noradrenaline is also dependent on renal perfusion pressure (MYERS et al.,

1975; PROSNITZ et al., 1977) in that increased perfusion pressure enhances noradrenaline-induced vasoconstriction (MCNAY and KISHIMOTO, 1969a; KENDRICK and MATSON, 1973).

Salt diet is another factor influencing renal vascular response to noradrenaline. HOLLENBERG et al. (1971) found in normal men that a low sodium diet enhanced renal vascular sensitivity to noradrenaline by a factor of 10, whereas vascular sensitivity to angiotensin II was markedly reduced when compared to men with normal sodium intake. However, OLIVER and CANNON (1978) did not observe any correlation between sodium intake or plasma renin activity and renal vasoconstrictor response to noradrenaline in anesthetized dogs. Inhibition of conversion of angiotensin I to angiotensin II by SQ 20,881 in sodium-depleted dogs did not affect the noradrenaline-induced renal vasoconstriction (OLIVER and CANNON, 1978). In contrast to this finding, BOMZON and ROSENDORFF (1975) found a significant attenuation of noradrenaline renal vasoconstriction by SQ 20,881 or by saralasin, an angiotensin II antagonist, in anesthetized baboons.

In trained dogs BURGER et al. (1976) evaluated the effect of barbiturate anesthesia on renal vascular response to noradrenaline (0.3–3.0 µg/min intrarenal). In this study it was demonstrated that anesthesia enhanced the renal vascular response to noradrenaline and blunted responsiveness to angiotensin II. High salt diet and agents interfering with the renin-angiotensin system partially reversed the effect of anesthesia. They concluded that in barbiturate anesthesia the increased sensitivity of the renal vasculature to noradrenaline is angiotensin mediated. However, higher doses of noradrenaline 2 µg/kg (single injection i.v.) elicited a more pronounced vasoconstriction in the conscious dog (LONGO and SANTA, 1968). The difference in salt diet, anesthesia, dose, and route of administration of noradrenaline may explain the observed discrepancies.

When tubular sodium reabsorption was inhibited by ethacrynic acid in dogs vascular responsiveness to noradrenaline and angiotensin II was reduced. Infusion of 0.5 µg/min angiotensin into the renal artery during ethacrynic acid diuresis restored renal vascular sensitivity to noradrenaline. The vasculature of the hind limb did not show such an effect (MCNAY and KISHIMOTO, 1969b). MCGIFF and FASY (1965) reported that acute denervation did not affect vascular response of the dog kidney to noradrenaline and adrenaline but blunted the response to angiotensin II. These results could not be reproduced by GELLER and KENDRICK (1967). These authors reported reduced renal vascular responses to noradrenaline and angiotensin II at high carotid sinus pressure. This effect was independent of kidney innervation. Chronic denervation of the kidney is known to enhance renal vascular response to constrictive catecholamines (KORNER et al., 1967; NOVELLI et al., 1969; WESSON, 1969; MILLARD et al., 1972).

Prostaglandins seem to be involved in the response of renal vasculature to noradrenaline. In the anesthetized cat, inhibitors of prostaglandin synthesis such as indomethacin or meclofenamate increased renal vascular resistance. The vasoconstrictor response to noradrenaline was enhanced, that to renal nerve stimulation or angiotensin II was unaffected (CHAPNICK et al., 1977). However, in conscious dogs indomethacin and meclofenamate did not increase vascular resistance per se but renal response to vasoconstrictors (methoxamine and angiotensin) was enhanced by indomethacin (SWAIN et al., 1975).

Adenosine, which is constrictive in the renal vasculature, potentiates the vasoconstrictor response of the kidney to noradrenaline (HASHIMOTO and KOKUBUN, 1971). Dipyridamol, an inhibitor of adenosine uptake by the cells, also potentiated noradrenaline-induced renal vasoconstriction (HASHIMOTO et al., 1970).

HEDQVIST et al. (1978) could demonstrate that adenosine inhibited noradrenaline release from the kidney following renal nerve stimulation but enhanced vasoconstrictor response to nerve stimulation and noradrenaline. The renal adenosine effects can be antagonized by theophylline (OSSWALD, 1975) but not by phosphodiesterase inhibitors like R020–174 or ZK 62.711 (HEDQVIST et al., 1978).

Cadmium inhibited dose-dependent and reversible adrenaline and noradrenaline induced vasoconstriction in the dog kidney (BIERY et al., 1972).

II. Effects of Alpha-Adrenergic Inhibitors

As in other vascular beds α-adrenergic inhibitors antagonize catecholamine induced renal vasoconstriction. Simultaneous administration of 1–2 μg/kg/min of noradrenaline and 1–2.7 μg/kg/min phentolamine intravenously over a period of 3 h resulted in a fall of renal blood flow by 17%–22% in dogs. Noradrenaline alone reduced renal blood flow by 28%–58% (CIMMINO et al., 1976). In baboons the rise in renal vascular resistance by intrarenally infused noradrenaline (5.0 μg/min) was nearly completely antagonized by infusion of 100 μg/min phenoxybenzamine (ROSENDORFF et al., 1973). NC 7,197, a nitrogen-substituted tetrahydroisoquinilon derivative, in doses of 1–1,000 mg was found to antagonize noradrenaline induced renal vasoconstriction in dogs (LOHMOELLER et al., 1973).

In most of the other studies on renal hemodynamics α-adrenergic inhibitors were used to evaluate the contribution of vasoconstrictive catecholamines to the renal vascular resistance under various experimental and clinical conditions.

MCGIFF and FASY (1965) studied the influence of substances interfering with adrenergic transmission on the angiotensin II (A II) induced renal vasoconstriction in dogs. Renal blood flow was decreased by 0.1 μg/kg of AII i.v. Acute denervation of the kidney abolished the renal vasoconstrictive effect of intravenous AII, whereas intrarenally infused AII (0.01–0.05 μg/kg/min) was still constrictive. Spinal cord transection (C1) had the same effect as denervation. Tyramine could partially restore renal vascular sensitivity to intravenous AII. Guanethidine also inhibited renal vascular response to intravenous AII, while tyramine reversed the guanethidine effects. Phentolamine and hexamethonium were without effect on intravenous AII-induced renal vasoconstriction. Bretylium (5 mg/kg) and hydralazine (2 mg/kg) attenuated the AII-induced renal vasoconstriction whereas the noradrenaline effect on renal blood flow was unchanged. The authors concluded that the autonomic nervous system can modify the renal vascular response to AII.

In rats, FINK and BRODY (1978) also observed no effect of bretylium (100 μg/min intrarenal) on noradrenaline-induced renal vasoconstriction, whereas the increase in renal vascular resistance following nerve stimulation could be diminished by bretylium.

In several studies on renal hemodynamic response to hemorrhage α-adrenergic inhibitors like phentolamine of phenoxybenzamine were used. It is beyond the scope of this chapter to discuss the neural and humoral mechanisms involved in renal response to hemorrhagic shock. An extensive review on renal circulation in hemorrhage has been written by SELKURT (1974a, b). The increase of renal vascular resistance following hemorrhage in unanesthetized rabbit could be prevented in "de-efferented animals" (adrenalectomy, guanethidine, atropine). However, chronic denervation of one kidney resulted in a more severe renal vasoconstriction compared to the innervated kidney. It was concluded that the chronic denervated kidney responded with an increase of sensitivity to enhanced levels of circulating vasoconstrictors such as catecholamines, angiotensin II and vasopressin during hemorrhage (KORNER et al., 1967). In comparison, exercise in dogs with experimental heart failure was accompanied with increased renal vascular resistance sensitive to denervation and α-adrenergic blockade (MILLARD et al., 1972). In contrast, TRUNINGER et al. (1971) could not find a difference between innervated and chronic denervated dog kidneys in their response to hemorrhagic hypotension. Using phenoxybenzamine these authors (GRANDCHAMP et al., 1971 b) concluded that circulating catecholamines are mainly responsible for the renal response to hemorrhagic hypotension.

The fraction of cardiac output perfusing the kidney was similar whether hemorrhage (25 ml/kg) was induced or adrenaline and noradrenaline (1.0–1.5 μg/kg/min) were infused into dogs (BUCKLEY et al., 1967), emphasizing the importance of catecholamines in hemorrhagic shock. In moderate hemorrhage (10 ml/kg) in dogs, ganglionic blockade by trimetaphan and blockade of α- and β-adrenoceptors by phenoxybenzamine and propranolol did not alter renal hemodynamics when compared to saline infused controls (ZEIG et al., 1968). Similar results were obtained by VATNER (1974) in conscious dogs and baboons. In severe hypotensive hemorrhage in dogs, which reduced blood pressure to 50 mm Hg, CARRIÈRE and DAIGNEAULT (1970) observed that phentolamine only partly antagonized the marked decrease in cortical RBF. GRANDCHAMP et al. (1971 a) reducing blood pressure to 70 mm Hg by hemorrhage could bring cortical blood flow to control levels by administration of phenoxybenzamine, while renin release stimulation due to hemorrhage was three times higher in phenoxybenzamine treated dogs. STEIN et al. (1973) compared renal nerve stimulation and hypotensive hemorrhage on intrarenal blood flow distribution. Nerve stimulation reduced renal blood flow by 40% without redistribution to the inner zone. Hypotensive hemorrhage, however, caused redistribution which was unaffected by phenoxybenzamine, phentolamine, propranolol, or atropine. A second transfusion after bleeding to restore blood pressure to normal values did not increase cortical blood flow to the levels prior to hemorrhage; however, phentolamine or phenoxybenzamine brought cortical blood flow nearly to normal (BELL and LISTER, 1970; CARRIÈRE and DAIGNEAULT, 1970).

In conclusion, α-adrenoceptor blocking agents can only partially antagonize renal cortical ischemia seen in hypotensive hemorrhage, which suggests that catecholamines are not the only factor responsible for increased renal vascular resistance during acute hemorrhage.

In the renal response to endotoxin shock "blunted sympathetic nervous system" (DIETZMANN et al., 1973) or administration of phenoxybenzamine (SHANBOUR et al., 1971) were found to improve renal function.

Increased renal vascular resistance due to anesthesia (BURGER et al., 1976) in dogs could not be antagonized by phentolamine or phenoxybenzamine, but by propranolol and an angiotensin II antagonist. Similarly, phentolamine (3 mg/min) infused into the renal artery of normal man kept on a low sodium died dit not increase net renal perfusion or alter its intrarenal pattern (HOLLENBERG et al., 1971).

Increased renal vascular resistance seen in hypoxia could only partly be inhibited by phentolamine infusion (BURSAUX et al., 1976). In severe respiratory acidosis phenoxybenzamine attenuated the increase of renal vascular resistance, while denervation of the kidney was without effect (BERSENTES and SIMMONS, 1967). Renal vasoconstriction due to intrarenally injected mercury chloride could be reduced by phenoxybenzamine (SOLOMON and HOLLENBERG, 1975). Phentolamine or propranolol did not affect oxytocin-induced renal vasoconstriction (BARNES, 1970). Also angiotensin II-induced renal vasoconstriction could not be antagonized by phentolamine (HORNYCH et al., 1972).

α-Adrenoceptor blocking agents were found to be useful in preventing vasospasm in kidneys of patients in agony, in kidney preservation, and to improve renal function post transplantation (MANDELBAUM et al., 1967; CORTESINI and NOVELLI, 1968; NOVELLI et al., 1969; PRYOR et al., 1971; PRYOR, 1972; MILLER and ALEXANDER, 1972; BELL et al., 1974; KAPUR and KHARSIING, 1974; MILLER et al., 1974; TOLEDO-PEREYRA et al., 1974; WEBER et al., 1976).

Ganglionic stimulants such as nicotine, 1,1-dimethyl-4-phenylpiperazinium (DMPP), and acetylcholine (in high doses or together with atropine) when injected into the renal artery increase renal vascular resistance (McGIFF and FASY, 1965; McGIFF et al., 1967; UEDA et al., 1968; CONCHA and NORRIS, 1968; DISALVO and FELL, 1971). The effect of DMPP and acetylcholine could only be demonstrated in innervated kidneys (DISALVO and FELL, 1971), while hexamethonium and atropine attenuated DMPP induced vasodilatation in denervated kidneys. The constrictor response in innervated kidneys could be blocked by phentolamine, guanethidine, reserpine, and hexamethonium (McGIFF et al., 1967; CONCHA and NORRIS, 1968; UEDA et al., 1968; DISALVO and FELL, 1971). The authors conclude that the ganglionic stimulants enhance intrarenal noradrenaline release and thereby elicit renal vascoconstriction.

III. Effects of Dopamine

Dopamine causes vasodilatation when injected into the renal artery of dogs (McDONALD et al., 1964; McNAY et al., 1965; DRESSLER et al., 1974; ROBIE et al., 1974a, b; BELL and MYA, 1977). This vasodilatation in the presence of phenoxybenzamine and propranolol appeared to be different from that commonly associated with sympathomimetic amines since it cannot be demonstrated when dopamine is injected into the femoral artery and cannot be antagonized by administration of β-adrenoceptor inhibitors. Among 44 phenylethylamines, epinine, a *N*-methyl analog of dopamine, was found to possess dopaminelike activity (GOLDBERG et al., 1968). Recently, conformational requirements for action on dopaminergic and β_2-adrenergic vascular receptors were investigated (VOLKMAN et al., 1978). 2-Amino-6,7-dihydroxy-1,2, 34,-tetrahydronaphthalene (A-6,7 DTN) and its *N*-methyl derivative exhibited pronounced dopamine agonist activity and minimal β_2-adrenergic activity. In contrast A-5,6-DTN and its *N*-methyl derivative exerted pronounced β_2-adrenergic activity but were inactive as dopamine agonists. It was concluded that the molecular structural requirements for dopamine-like renal vasodilatation are more specific than those for the α- and β-adrenergic effects of sympathomimetic amines on renal vasculature (GOLDBERG et al., 1968; VOLKMAN et al., 1978). In rats dopamine (6–20 μg injected into the renal artery) caused vasoconstriction (AIHARA et al., 1972; AUGUSTIN et al., 1977). This constrictive effect of dopamine in the rat kidney may have been the result of the preparation (isolated perfused kidney) and of the dose, which is high compared to dog experiments. In fact, BROTZU (1970) could show that doses of 20 μg injected into the renal artery of dogs reduced renal blood flow. This constriction was reversed by phentolamine. Chlorpromazine (3 mg/kg) prevented dopamine but not isoproterenol-induced renal vasodilatation (BROTZU, 1970). Haloperidol shifted the dose-response curve of dopamine-induced renal vasodilatation to the right while morphine (2–6 mg/kg) antagonized the renal vascular dopamine effect in a noncompetitive manner (DRESSLER et al., 1974). As measured with intrarenal microsphere distribution the dopamine-induced increase in renal blood flow was greater in the deep than in the superficial layers of the cortex (HARDAKER and WECHSLER, 1973). However, using a hydrogen washout technique TYSSEBOTN and KIRKEBØ (1979) could not find a redistribution of renal blood flow in dogs either at vasodilating or vasoconstricting doses of dopamine.

ANDREUCCI et al. (1976) measured in Munich Wistar rats a marked increase of glomerular capillary pressure following intravenous dopamine infusion (15–25 μg/min) and suggested afferent arteriolar dilatation. Dobutamine is a weak renal vasodilatator (ROBIE et al., 1974b; LEIGHTON and BRUCE, 1976).

Reviews on cardiovascular and renal actions of dopamine and its clinical applications were written by GOLDBERG (1972) and by LOUIS and SAMPSON (1974).

IV. Effects of Beta-Adrenergic Activators

SPENCER (1956) reported renal vasodilatation following intrarenal injection of isoproterenol. This observation has been confirmed by numerous experimentators (AVIADO et al., 1958; MURPHY et al., 1965; MCNAY and GOLDBERG, 1966; CHATEL et al., 1968; MANDELBAUM and SHUMACKER, 1968; CARRIÈRE, 1969; NEELY and WINDHAM, 1970; HARDT et al., 1971). In man intravenous injection of 0.5 mg orciprenaline did not change renal hemodynamics (SCHIRMEISTER et al., 1966).

Higher doses of isoproterenol similar to dopamine can cause renal vasoconstriction (SPENCER, 1956), which can be antagonized by phentolamine or phenoxybenzamine (MARK et al., 1969). Propranolol reverses isoproterenol-induced renal vasodilatation and uncovers the vasoconstrictive component of the renal vascular response to isoproterenol (Fig. 2) (MARK et al., 1969; DISALVO and FELL, 1970). Practolol was not as efficient as propranolol in preventing renal vasodilatation following isoproterenol in rats (DEBRECZENI and FENYVESI, 1971).

Comparing the effect of isoproterenol and salbutamol on renal vascular resistance, TAIRA et al. (1977) found that salbutamol on the weight basis was only 1/240 as potent as isoproterenol and that the slope of the dose-response curve for salbutamol was less steep than that for isoproterenol. The dose-response curve for isoproterenol below constrictive concentrations was shifted to the right more markedly by intravenous administration of pindolol than by intravenous or intrarenal practolol. It was suggested that the renal vascular bed consists of both β_1- and β_2-adrenoceptors (TAIRA et al., 1977).

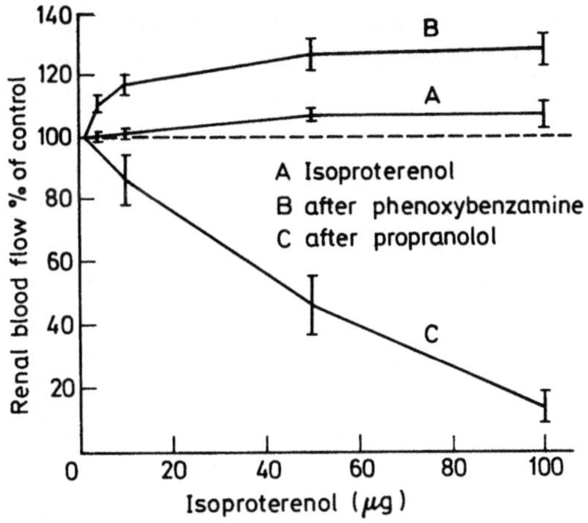

Fig. 2. Effects of isoproterenol on renal blood flow: dotted line, control blood flow. Mean responses to intra-arterial bolus injections of 1, 5, 10, 50, and 100 μg of isoproterenol are shown. Small vertical bars represent ±1 SE. (*A*) Responses to isoproterenol alone in nine dogs. (*B*) Responses after intra-arterial infusion of phenoxybenzamine (5 mg/kg) in four dogs. (*C*) Responses after intra-arterial bolus injection of propranolol (5 mg) in three dogs (DiSalvo and Fell, 1971)

Evidence was presented for intrarenal redistribution of glomerular filtration rate from the outer to the inner cortex following intravenous isoproterenol infusion in rats (Greven, 1974a). Propranolol had the opposite effect. No change of renal blood flow or glomerular filtration rate was seen following isoproterenol in isolated perfused dog kidneys (Hwang et al., 1970). Kovach et al. (1970) reported an increase (30%) of cortical renal blood flow following injection of 15 mg/kg of a β-adrenergic substance, 1-(4-oxy-phenyl)-2n-butyl-aminoethanol hydrochloride, in dogs.

V. Effects of Beta-Adrenergic Inhibitors

Since it was found that exogenous administered β-sympathomimetic drugs can cause renal vasodilatation, specific β-adrenoceptor inhibitors were used to define whether there is a β-adrenergic controlled basal nervous tone of the renal vasculature. In man intravenous injection of propranolol (0.02–0.2 mg/kg) reduced glomerular filtration rate and PAH clearance by an average of 10%. However, orciprenaline did not alter renal hemodynamics (Schirmeister et al., 1966). In rats nethalide (1 mg) did not affect glomerular filtration rate or renal blood flow (Lees and Lockett, 1963). In dogs, however, propranolol (0.5 mg/kg i.v.) reduced renal blood flow by about 30% whereas glomerular filtration rate was unchanged (Laubie and Drouillat, 1968). In the unanesthetized dogs 1 mg/kg of propranolol i.v. increased renal vascular resistance while 1 μg/kg of isoproterenol i.v. was without an effect (Granata et al., 1970). Nakamura et al. (1974) found no change of renal blood flow or redistribution in the dog kidney after bunitrolol (0.5 mg/kg) administration. Absence of significant changes in renal blood flow and glomerular filtration rate following propranolol in isolated perfused dog kidneys was reported by McCombs and Berkowitz (1976). The redistribution of renal blood flow to the inner cortex seen following a low sodium diet could be inhibited by propranolol in conscious rabbits (WARREN and LEDINGHAM, 1975). In agreement with the other studies these authors did not see an effect of propranolol on renal blood flow in rabbits kept on normal sodium diet. Thus, since the majority of the studies did not see altered total renal blood flow or glomerular filtration rate following β-adrenoceptor inhibitors, it appears that β-adrenergic controlled vascular tone in the kidney is questionable. However, changes in the distribution of intrarenal glomerular filtration rate due to β-adrenoceptor activators or inhibitors as reported by GREVEN (1974a) may point to a β-adrenergic control of intrarenal circulation.

Autoregulation of renal blood flow and glomerular filtration rate was not affected by propranolol (ANDERSON et al., 1975). Reduction of renal blood flow by propranolol, oxprenolol, and pindolol in dogs was interpreted as the result of the concomitant fall in cardiac output (ABDEL-RAZZAK, 1978). Pindolol and practolol were used to differentiate between β_1- and β_2-adrenoceptors in the renal vascular bed (TAIRA et al., 1977); with the result suggesting that the renal vessels have both receptor types.

VI. Use of Catecholamines in Renal Angiography

The renal vascular action of adrenaline, noradrenaline, metaraminol, and phenylephrine were evaluated by angiography. When blood pressure was increased by 30–50 mm Hg following administration of the drugs, renal blood flow was markedly reduced in dogs (CAREY et al., 1969). Phenoxybenzamine enlarged the width of the intrarenal arteries, prevented outer cortical vasoconstriction following hypotensive hemorrhage, and reversed adrenaline-induced renal vasoconstriction in dogs (ELKIN et al., 1973). The use of vasodilating and vasoconstrictive drugs to improve the value of a renal angiography in various kidney abnormalities was recommended by BOOKSTEIN and ERNEST (1972), EKELUND et al. (1972), APITZSCH (1975), and VESIN et al. (1976). EKELUND et al. (1978) reexamined in man the hazard of intrarenally injected vasoconstrictive drugs and suggested the use of 2–5 μg adrenaline for intrarenal injection instead of 10–25 μg as practiced in the past.

VII. Conclusion

Similar to other vascular beds α-adrenoceptor agonists constrict the resistance vessels in the kidney. The α-adrenergic receptors in the renal vascular bed seem to greatly outnumber the β-receptors. The physiologic significance of isoproterenol or dopamine-induced renal vasodilatation is still unclear. Depending upon experimental or clinical conditions the renal vascular response to catecholamines is modified by a number of factors such as the renin-angiotensin system, state of salt and water balance, tubular electrolyte transport capacity (diuretics), the prostaglandin system, renal perfusion pressure and preexisting vascular tone, temperature, and surely also by unknown factors. Since in the kidney hemodynamics are closely related to tubular transport and since the vascular pole of the glomerulus is intimately connected with the juxtaglomerular apparatus (including the macula densa), a satisfactory understanding of the catecholamine effects on renal hemodynamics is not possible unless the elements that control renal vascular resistance and filtration dynamics are better defined.

C. Renin Release

The physiologic mechanisms of renin release are being actively investigated and have been reviewed recently by LARAGH and SEALEY (1973), DAVIS (1976), DAVIS and FREEMAN (1976), R.H. MCDONALD et al., (1977), and ZANCHETTI et al. (1977). The biochemistry of the renin-angiotensin system and its mechanisms of action in controlling electrolyte and water balance are reviewed extensively by BLAIR-WEST (1976), PEACH (1977), and GANTEN and GROSS (1977). Therefore, we shall not repeat a review of the older literature in this chapter, but restrict ourselves to describing conclusive experiments on catecholamine mediated renin release reported in the last 5 years. Due to the limited space, we will not review experimental work which is directed to elucidate the influence of calcium ions, prostaglandins, cyclic nucleotides, and diuretics on renal renin release, although adrenergic activators and inhibitors were also included in these studies.

I. Evidence for Neural Control of Renin Release

As reviewed by GANONG and REID (1976), ZEHR (1976), and ZANCHETTI and STELLA (1976), electrical stimulation of areas in the brain which are part of the vasomotor center induces marked renin release from innervated kidneys despite an increase in blood pressure. Renin release from the contralateral denervated kidney was unchanged. Prevention of the stimulus-induced renal vasoconstriction in the innervated kidney by intrarenally infused phenoxybenzamine, or prevention of increase of renal artery pressure by aortic constriction, increased renin release due to brain stem stimulation even further. The mechanism responsible for this increase in renin release following vasomotor stimulation is sensitive to β-adrenoceptor blockade because after propranolol renin release was unchanged (ZANCHETTI and STELLA, 1976).

Renin release is also controlled by adrenergic reflex activation. Denervation of the kidney abolished tilting-induced increase in renin release (ZANCHETTI and STELLA, 1976). Besides the reflex-induced increase of renin release elicited by carotid sinus hypotension, cardiopulmonary receptors with vagal afferents exhibit a tonic restraining influence on renin release, as demonstrated in cats by MANCIA et al. (1975), ZEHR (1976), YUN et al. (1976), THAMES (1977); STELLA et al. (1978), in *dogs* by JARECKI et al. (1978), THAMES et al. (1978), THAMES (1979), and in *man* by KIOWSKI and JULIUS (1978). Atrial hypotension did not increase renin release in patients with denervated renal transplants or propranolol treated normal volunteers (KIOWSKI and JULIUS, 1978). Renal nerves when stimulated at very low frequency (0.25 Hz) augmented the nonneural stimulated renin release by furosemide or suprarenal aortic constriction (THAMES and DIBONA, 1979).

The data on neuronal influences on renin release clearly demonstrate that the sympathetic nervous system plays a key role in regulation of renin release. The identification of the stimulatory effect of the vasomotor center, the reflex mediated inhibition (cardiopulmonary receptors), and potentiation (carotid sinus) of the central sympathetic activity responsible for renin release, and the potentiation of nonneural stimuli for renin release by low level stimulation of renal nerves allows a better interpretation of the discrepancies between the results obtained by various groups under different experimental conditions.

II. Effects of Beta-Adrenergic Activators and Inhibitors

Since DAVIS and FREEMAN (1976) could review convincing evidence that β-adrenergic activators stimulate renin release and that β-adrenergic inhibitors prevent this stimulation, a large number of papers have confirmed this concept in several species including man. It seems to be nearly impossible, and does not improve understanding of the topic, to cite every published paper which deals in some way with plasma renin activity, β-adrenergic blockade, and the clinical implication of drugs that interfere with the renin-angiotensin system in hypertension. The reader may refer to the extensive review articles cited above. Here we shall only consider papers that appeared later than 1974.

Adrenaline, noradrenaline, and isoproterenol increased renin release which was prevented by administration of β-adrenergic inhibitors in denervated autotransplanted *dog* kidneys (ALMGARD and LJUNDQVIST, 1975), in isolated perfused kidneys of *rats* (QUESADA et al., 1975; VANDONGEN and GREENWOOD, 1975; HOFBAUER et al., 1976; SINAIKO and MIRKIN, 1978), isolated perfused kidneys of *cats* (LESTER and RUBIN, 1977; HARADA and RUBIN, 1978), of *rabbits* (VISKOPER et al., 1976), in renal cortical *slices* of rats (DESAULLES et al., 1975; WEINBERGER et al., 1975; AOI et al., 1976; CAPPONI et al., 1977; HENRY et al., 1977; DESAULLES et al., 1978) and in suspensions of isolated *glomeruli* (B.J. MORRIS et al., 1976), and in renal *cortical cells* (JOHNS et al., 1975). Thus, β-adrenergic stimulation of renin release can be shown to occur in the absence of systemic, intrarenal, and tubular factors.

Similar conclusions were reported from experiments in dogs (TAHER et al., 1976). Stimulation of renal nerves which did not alter renal or systemic hemodynamics or urinary electrolyte excretion resulted in a marked increase in renal renin release. Intrarenally infused D-propranolol was ineffective whereas L-propranolol abolished nerve stimulation induced renin secretion (TAHER et al., 1976). Renin release from sodium depleted dogs was decreased by intrarenal infusion of 50 μg/kg/h propranolol. The same dose infused intravenously failed to alter renin release (JOHNSON J.A. et al., 1976). Denervated "nonfiltering" kidneys also responded with a decreased renin release rate following intrarenal propranolol infusion (JOHNSON J.A. et al., 1976). OSBORN et al. (1977) presented evidence that the effect of D-propranolol (1 mg/kg plus 1 mg/kg per hour) on the nonfiltering and denervated kidney, to inhibit furosemide stimulated renin release, can be explained on the basis of its local anesthetic action since lidocaine was equally effective.

β-Adrenergic inhibitors were successfully used as tools to demonstrate the β-adrenergic nature of sympathetic nerve reflex mediated increases in renin release in laboratory animals and man: ATTMANN et al. (1975), CAMPBELL et al. (1975), MELADA et al. (1975), O'MALLEY et al. (1975), PETTINGER and KEETON (1975), PETTINGER et al. (1975), WEBER et al. (1975a), WERNZE et al. (1975), DAVIES and SLATER (1976), GRAHAM et al. (1976), HÖFGEN et al. (1976), KEETON et al. (1976), VIOL et al. (1976), ZEHNER et al. (1975, 1976), BONELLI et al. (1977), DAVIES et al. (1977), GIUDICELLI et al. (1977), GUTKIN et al. (1977), LIEBAU et al. (1977), PLANCHETTA et al. (1977), YUN et al. (1977), WIGGINS et al. (1978).

Attempts were made to differentiate the β-adrenergic stimulation of renin release by means of "β_1"- and "β_2"-adrenoceptor inhibitors. AMERY et al. (1974) and WEBER et al. (1974) proposed that renin release may be mediated by β_2-agonists. Using metoprolol ATTMANN et al. (1975) suggested that β_1-adrenoceptors may be involved in renin release in man. In comparison, it was suggested by LAMMINTAUSTA et al. (1977) that basal unstimulated levels of plasma renin activity in man may be reduced by β_2-adrenergic inhibitors while exercise-induced increase in plasma renin activity could be inhibited by β_1-antagonists. JOHNSON B.F. et al. (1976) could block salbutamol-induced increases in plasma renin activity in healthy volunteers by practolol and concluded that a β_1 type of adrenoceptor might be responsible for changes in plasma renin activity. MEURER et al. (1976) could not support the clear discrimination of the two receptor types responsible for renin release in man.

β-Adrenergic inhibitors were used to evaluate to what extent the sympathetic nervous system might contribute to the stimulation of renin release by sodium depletion. There is clear evidence that reduction of plasma sodium chloride concentration is a stimulus for renin secretion (for review see LARAGH and SEALEY, 1973; BLAIR-WEST, 1976; DAVIS and FREEMAN, 1976). However, sodium depletion leads to a decrease in the extracellular fluid volume (including intravascular volume), decrease of glomerular filtration rate, increase of tubular electrolyte reabsorption (including changes of transepithelial sodium gradients across the ascending limb of Henle's loop and macula densa) and to an increase in renal vascular resistance. Several of these factors could modify the balance of activating and inhibiting influences of the sympathetic nervous system on the renin releasing cells.

A number of observations could demonstrate a decrease of renin secretion initially stimulated by sodium depletion after application of β-adrenergic inhibitors. SULLIVAN et al. (1976) found that propranolol intravenously injected at a low dose (9–18 μg/kg) lowered the renal renin secretion rate only in patients kept on a low sodium diet (10 mmol/day) whereas patients with a daily sodium intake of 200 mmol did not respond to propranolol.

LOWENSTEIN and STEELE (1977) could prevent the increase of plasma renin activity following a low sodium diet with propranolol in man. Similar findings of inhibition of renin release by propranolol in sodium-depleted hypoparathyroid patients were reported by WEBER et al. (1975b). These findings are in agreement with earlier reports (see for ref. LARAGH and SEALEY, 1973; DAVIS and FREEMAN, 1976). However, OMVIK et al. (1976) studied 33 healthy normotensive volunteers in their response to low, normal, and high sodium intake. The known hyperbolic relationship between plasma renin activity and daily sodium intake was confirmed. This correlation was unaffected by 60 mg propranolol per day.

In sodium depleted *dogs* propranolol (1–5 mg/kg followed by 0.6–1.8 mg/kg/h) did markedly depress high plasma renin activity suggesting the importance of β-adrenergic activation of renin secreting cells in the low sodium state (YUN et al., 1977). In contrast, SPARKS and SUSIC (1977) did not prevent in rats the marked increase in plasma renin activity following low sodium diet by propranolol.

Keeping in mind the dynamic balance of central and reflex mediated sympathetic nervous activity regulating renin release it may be very difficult to have identical experimental conditions in studies on humans and animals. Therefore, it can be concluded that the contribution of the sympathetic nervous system to the renin release stimulated by low sodium diet can vary. The different results obtained with β-adrenergic inhibitors on plasma renin activity do not alter the fact that sodium chloride or chloride by itself is an important, well established factor in the control of renin release (KIRCHNER et al., 1978; CHURCHILL et al., 1978; ABBOUD et al., 1979).

III. Effects of Dopamine

CUCHE et al. (1972) have shown in man that the increase in plasma renin activity with upright posture is associated with a decrease in urinary dopamine and increase in noradrenaline and adrenaline excretion. ALEXANDER et al. (1974) have reported that sodium-depleted subjects respond to dietary or intravenous sodium loading with an increase in urinary dopamine and a decrease in urinary noradrenaline. Thus, maneuvers which alter plasma renin activity seem to be inversely related to urinary dopamine excretion. WILCOX et al. (1974) could show an increase of plasma renin activity in man following intravenous infusion of dopamine (10 μg/min/kg). IMBS et al. (1975) infused 6 μg/kg/min dopamine into the denervated kidney of dogs and observed a threefold increase in renin secretion rate which was prevented by intrarenal haloperidol but not by propranolol infusion. The dopamine dose did not alter blood pressure, diuresis, or potassium in the plasma, but renal blood flow was increased. In another study in dogs the same authors (IMBS et al., 1976) reported that apomorphine induced an increase in renin release which was prevented by haloperidol infusion. Dopamine stimulated renin release was not affected by the neuroleptic drug pimozide. The authors assume that specific dopamine receptors are present in the kidney. Stimulation of renin release by dopamine in the isolated perfused rat kidney could be antagonized by propranolol but not by haloperidol (QUESADA et al., 1979).

In two recent studies using rat kidney cortical slices (HENRY et al., 1977; LOPEZ et al., 1979) dopamine was able to increase renin release. In the study of HENRY et al. (1977) phentolamine, haloperidol, or cocaine did not antagonize dopamine-induced renin release, whereas in both studies propranolol antagonized the dopamine effect.

Infusion of ergometrine into the renal artery of dogs diminished the increase of angiotensin II concentration in the arterial blood associated with moderate hemorrhage and suprarenal aortic constriction (BELL and LANG, 1978). The increase in angiotensin II concentration in central venous blood was not affected by ergometrine. Thus, there is some evidence for a dopamine action on renin release. However, the underlying mechanism(s) of this dopamine effect remains to be clarified.

An interesting observation was reported by CAREY et al. (1979) in healthy volunteers. Following administration of metoclopramide (10 mg), a specific dopaminergic antagonist, plasma aldosterone levels rose (together with prolactin) twofold above control levels. The stimulatory effect of angiotensin II infusion (2–6 pmol/kg/min) on plasma aldosterone was potentiated. Plasma renin activity was not altered by metoclopramide. Bromocriptin, a dopamine receptor agonist did not change basal or angiotensin II stimulated plasma aldosterone levels. The authors conclude that the adrenal aldosterone production is under maximum tonic inhibition by dopamine in man. It appears to be premature at the present time to define the role of dopamine in the mechanisms of renin release.

IV. Effects of Alpha-Adrenergic Activators and Inhibitors

It was reported by PETTINGER et al. (1972) using the unanesthetized rat that low doses of noradrenaline caused a dose-related decrease in plasma renin activity, whereas adrenaline and isoproterenol stimulated renin release. An α-adrenoceptor mediated inhibition of renin secretion was suggested. This hypothesis was tested further by using different experimental protocols.

MEYER et al. (1975a, b) could inhibit the isoproterenol stimulated renin release by phenylephrine. LAUTERWEIN et al. (1975) observed that phenylephrine abolished the furosemide-induced stimulation of renin release. In additional studies MEYER et al. (1977) could present evidence that there is an α-adrenergic mediated inhibition of renin release. Denervation of the kidney, pretreatment with a ganglionic blocker (trimethidinium), with guanethidine or with reserpine, all potentiated the isoproterenol-induced stimulation of renin release. In addition, phenoxybenzamine enhanced the isoproterenol effect. In support of this observation MEYER and HERRMANN (1978) reduced the isoproterenol-stimulated renin release by tyramine in conscious rats. This effect was again abolished by phenoxybenzamine, reserpine, and denervation.

PETTINGER et al. (1976) also presented evidence for α-adrenergic mediated inhibition of renin release in conscious rats. In addition, cortical slices from rat kidneys showed inhibition of renin release by noradrenaline (10 μM) an effect which could be reversed to stimulation of renin release by the addition of phenoxybenzamine (10 μM) into the medium (CAPPONI and VALLOTTON, 1976; LOPEZ et al., 1978). However, in isolated perfused rat kidneys, phenylephrine failed to depress renin secretion rate (STRANG et al., 1977).

In normal volunteers methoxamine (1.6 and 5.9 µg/kg/min) and isoproterenol (0.015 and 0.026 µg/kg/min) caused dose dependent equal elevations of plasma renin activity which were prevented by 0.125 mg/kg of propranolol. The concept of α-adrenergic agonist mediated inhibition of renin release was therefore questioned (LEENEN et al., 1975). Similar conclusions were made by VETTER et al. (1976) based on observations obtained in patients with pheochromocytoma. However, in two studies on healthy subjects HSU et al. (1977) and LEVY et al. (1977) provided clear evidence for an α-adrenergic agonist mediated renin release inhibition. Amylnitrite inhalation and cold pressure testing failed to alter plasma renin activity. Applying both stimuli after α-adrenergic receptor inhibition, plasma renin activity was increased. Phenylephrine lowered phentolamine-elevated basal plasma renin levels (HSU et al., 1977). Recently, VANDONGEN et al. (1979) found suppression of isoproterenol stimulated renin release by phenylephrine in isolated perfused rat kidneys. This phenylephrine effect was abolished by phenoxybenzamine but not by dihydralazine. Thus, it appears that the controversial point of an α-adrenergic control of renin release seems to be clarified in that α-adrenergic activators lower and α-adrenergic inhibitors enhance renin release.

The actions of clonidine on the cardiovascular and sympathetic system including renin release are extensively reviewed by SCHMITT (1977).

V. Conclusion

The experimental data reported in the last 5 years have added substantial evidence for the assumption that the efferent renal sympathetic nerves control renal renin release via a β-adrenergic mechanism. There is a dynamic balance between the reflex-mediated and central nervous activity influencing renin release which appears to be as complex as other neurohumoral systems. As shown in a simplified model (Fig. 3) other factors besides the nervous system affect renin release. Among these factors the renal perfusion pressure is a powerful stimulus (when it is decreased) for renin release inde-

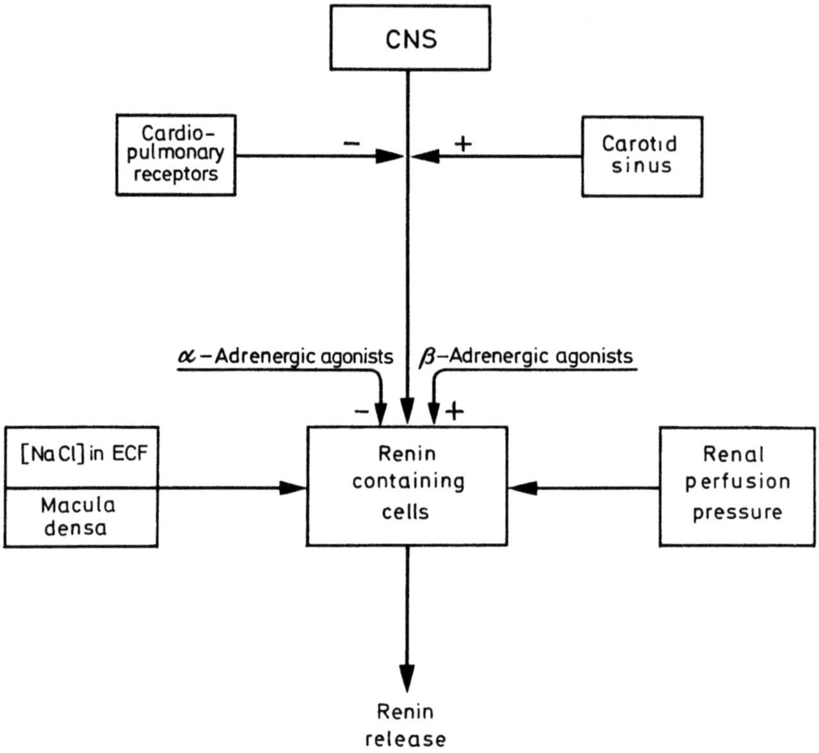

Fig. 3. Simplified schematic model of the factors controlling renal renin release. CNS, central nervous system; [NaCl] in ECF, sodium chloride concentration in the extracellular fluid; cross, stimulation; minus, inhibition. For explanation see Sect. C, renin release I–V

pendent from renal nerves. Evidence was presented to suggest that prostaglandins are involved in the "baroreceptor" controlled renin release (ROMERO et al., 1976; DATA et al., 1978; BERL et al., 1979; CAMPBELL et al., 1979; FRÖLICH et al., 1979; HEURICH et al., 1979). Although it is desirable to separate functionally the different control systems of renin release, the observation of THAMES and DIBONA (1979) that very low level stimulation of renal nerves changes the gain of the nonneural factors to release renin emphasizes again the close interaction of the neural and nonneural elements that control renin release. It seems also to be established that α-adrenoceptor activation is inhibitory in renin release, at least under certain circumstances.

The response of the renin secreting cells to low sodium or to low chloride diet seems to involve at least in parts the sympathetic nervous system, since β-adrenergic antagonists can attenuate the stimulation of renin release due to sodium chloride depletion. To what extent the intrarenal sodium chloride concentrations and transtubular chloride gradients affect the renin secreting cells via the macula densa segment cannot be said clearly at present. However, a suggestion might be presented. Adenosine depresses markedly renal renin release (TAGAWA and VANDER, 1970; OSSWALD et al., 1978). Intrarenal load with sodium chloride leads to an increase in renal tissue content of adenosine (OSSWALD and NABAKOWSKI, 1979) and to a decrease of renin release (SPIELMAN, 1979) which can be prevented by the adenosine antagonist theophylline. Adenosine inhibits renal release of noradrenaline following nerve stimulation (HEDQ-

VIST et al., 1978). Evidence was presented which assumed that adenosine is the mediator in the vascular response to increased sodium chloride load to the ascending limb of Henle's loop, i.e., tubuloglomerular feedback (OSSWALD and NABAKOWSKI, 1979; OSSWALD and HERMES, 1980). According to that hypothesis the ascending limb of Henle's loop transforms the signal of luminal sodium chloride concentration by generating adenosine which then acts on the juxtaglomerular apparatus. It is beyond the aim of this chapter to discuss in detail the mechanisms controlling renin release besides the effects of catecholamines. Since in the kidney renal blood flow, tubular electrolyte reabsorption, and renin release are functionally coupled, consideration of one aspect (renin release) without taking into account the other elements of renal function may lead to misinterpretation.

D. Tubular Electrolyte and Water Transport

I. Effects of Beta-Adrenergic Activators

There is considerable evidence that indicates that β-adrenoceptor stimulation affects the tubular handling of fluid and electrolytes. Thus, it has been established by a lot of investigators that systemic application of β-adrenoceptor agonists is associated with an antidiuretic response (Fig. 4) in the *rat* (BOTTING et al., 1961; BOTTING and LOCKETT, 1961; FARMER and LOCKETT, 1961; LEES and LOCKETT, 1963; LEHR et al., 1967; HEINTZE, 1968; HEINTZE and HEIDENREICH, 1968; LEES, 1968; FÜLGRAFF et al., 1968, 1969; PESKAR et al., 1969; LEVI et al., 1971; GREVEN, 1974a, b; KLEIN, 1975a; MCDONALD et al., 1977; SHIBOUTA et al., 1978), in the *dog* (BLAKE, 1955; AVIADO et al., 1958; HEIDENREICH, 1967; PEARSON and WILLIAMS, 1968; HEIDENREICH et al., 1966, 1969; KLEIN et al., 1971; BERL et al., 1974c; SCHRIER, 1974; SCHRIER et al., 1972, 1975) and in *man* (LEVI and KLEEMAN, 1973; NADJMABADI et al., 1975; KORDS et al., 1976; LEVI et al., 1976; SCHEITZA et al., 1976, with the exception of SCHIRMEISTER et al., 1966). Only in the *ckicken* did isoproterenol, the most frequently chosen β-adrenoceptor agonist, have no effect on water or sodium excretion (MAY and CARTER, 1970) whereas in *turkeys* isoproterenol induced a diuresis (FREGLY et al., 1976; PALMORE et al., 1977).

As a consequence of their marked cardiovascular effects, it is sometimes difficult to distinguish direct renal effects of β-adrenoceptor stimulating drugs from those due to changes in renal hemodynamics, secondary to alterations in systemic hemodynamics. However, since antidiuresis has also been observed with constant or even increased glomerular filtration rate (FARMER and LOCKETT, 1961; HEIDENREICH, 1967; HEIDENREICH et al., 1966, 1969; SCHRIER et al., 1972; GREVEN, 1974a, b; KORDS et al., 1976; SHIBOUTA et al., 1978; GREVEN and PANTEL, 1979, unpublished observations) renal hemodynamics do not seem to play a main role in the diminished kidney excretory function observed after β-adrenoceptor stimulation.

There exists, however, controversy concerning whether antidiuresis results from direct tubular effects or from interaction with antidiuretic hormone. There is evidence for each of these mechanisms.

1. Evidence for Direct Tubular Effects

Antidiuresis and increased tubular sodium reabsorption have been observed in isolated kidneys of the cat (LEES and LOCKETT, 1965), the rat (BESARBAB et al., 1977), and

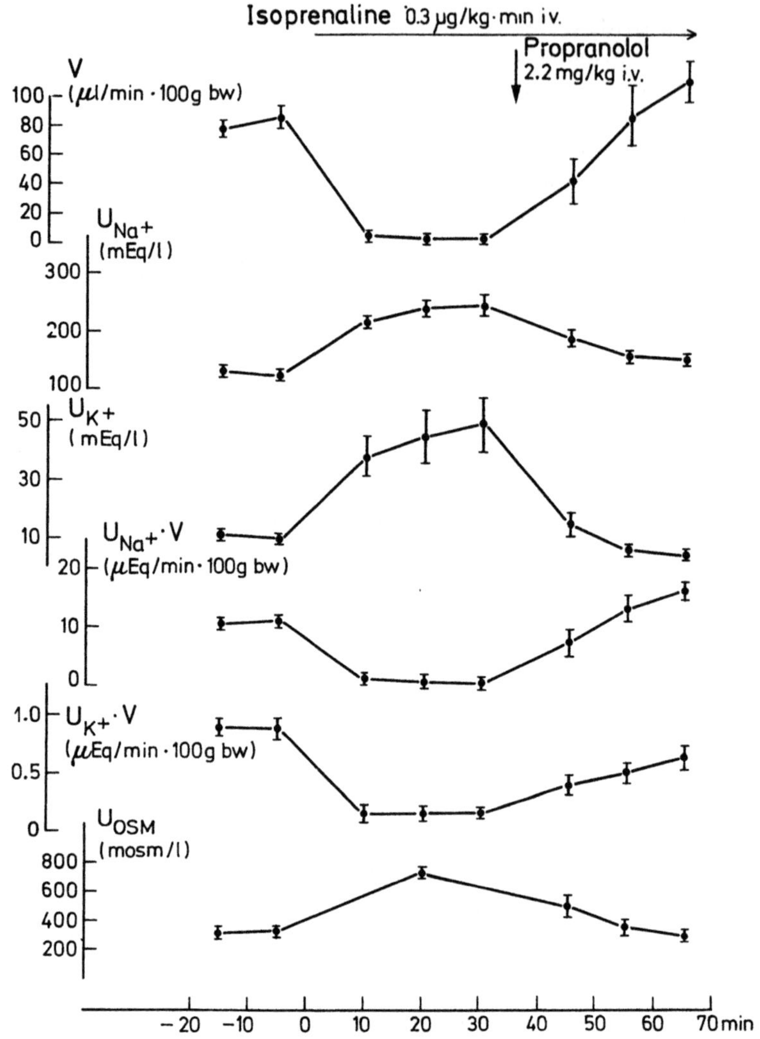

Fig. 4. Urine volume (V), sodium and potassium concentration in urine (U_{Na^+}, U_{K^+}), sodium and potassium excretion ($U_{Na^+} \cdot V$, $U_{K^+} \cdot V$) and urine osmolarity (U_{osm}) after isoprenaline with subsequent blocking of the renal β-receptors by propranolol (GREVEN, 1974a)

the dog (WILLIAMS et al., 1972). Thus, β-adrenergic activators may affect kidney function in the absence of antidiuretic hormone.

Evidence for direct tubular effects of β-adrenoceptor stimulating drugs is indicated by micropuncture studies in the rat. Orciprenaline (10^{-5} *M*) and dopamine (10^{-4} *M*) injected directly into the lumen of the proximal and isoproterenol (10^{-4} *M*) injected into the distal convoluted tubules (Fig. 5) stimulated tubular fluid reabsorption (FÜLGRAFF et al., 1968, 1969; GREVEN and HEIDENREICH, 1975; GREVEN and KLEIN, 1977) as measured by the split oil droplet method of GERTZ which is independent of changes in renal hemodynamics. Since these effects were abolished by propranolol they were thought to be due to stimulation of β-adrenoceptors.

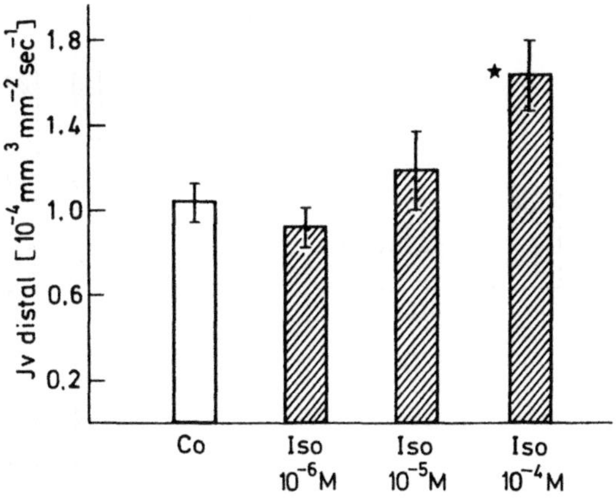

Fig. 5. Effect of isoprenaline on the distal transtubular volume fluxes (Jv). Isoprenaline was injected into the distal tubular lumen. Co, control; Iso, isoprenaline; *$P < 0.01$ (GREVEN and HEIDENREICH, 1975)

It has been postulated that antidiuresis after β-adrenergic stimulation mainly results from enhanced fluid and sodium reabsorption in the distal parts of the nephron, since the increase in proximal reabsorption was entirely compensated for by decreased reabsorption from the loops of Henle (GREVEN and HEIDENREICH, 1975).

With respect to dopamine, which in contrast to isoproterenol or orciprenaline increases renal sodium and fluid excretion (for review see GOLDBERG, 1972; KUCHEL et al., 1978), the exact site of natriuretic action within the nephron has not been defined yet. Free flow micropuncture studies demonstrated that intravenously infused dopamine did not influence fractional reabsorption of fluid in the proximal tubules in dogs; the increase in urine flow and sodium excretion has been assumed, but not proven, to be the result of a depressive action of the drug on the distal tubules (DAVIS et al., 1968).

Clearance studies in dogs (HEIDENREICH, 1967; HEIDENREICH et al., 1966, 1969) revealed that the maximal rate of tubular glucose reabsorption was significantly increased by intravenous orciprenaline. Since tubular glucose reabsorption is linked to proximal tubular sodium reabsorption (for review see KINNE and SCHWARTZ, 1978) this finding also points to a direct influence of β-adrenoceptor stimulating drugs on tubular sodium reabsorption. In these experiments free water clearance remained positive despite a decrease in urine flow and therefore antidiuretic hormone secretion did not seem to be an important factor in diminishing urine flow. It has also been observed that antidiuretic hormone exerted an antidiuretic effect in rats only undergoing water diuresis but not saline diuresis, whereas isoproterenol induced antidiuresis in both conditions (GREVEN, 1974b).

Other authors (BLENDIS et al., 1972; STEIN et al., 1972) using free flow micropuncture in the dog, failed to detect a significant effect on proximal tubular sodium reabsorption of β-adrenoceptor stimulation. However, the isoproterenol dose (0.036 and 0.018 μg/kg/min, respectively) these authors used was too small to induce changes in overall kidney sodium and urine excretion and therefore no effect on tubular function could be expected.

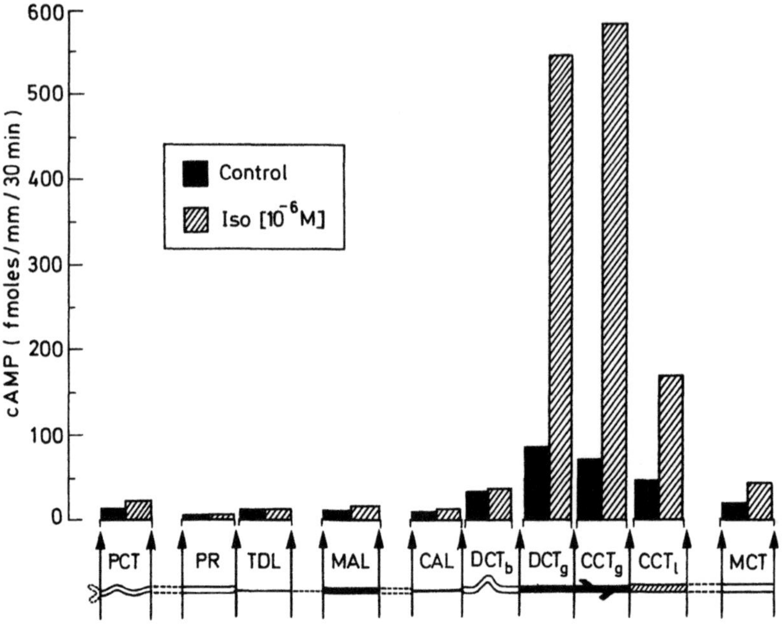

Fig. 6. Distribution of isoproterenol sensitive adenylate cyclase activity along the rabbit nephron. The ten different segments tested are schematically represented in the abscissa. In ordinate, the size of each bar corresponds to the mean value of six to eight samples from two experiments. PCT, proximal convoluted tubule; PR, pars recta of the proximal tubule; TDL, thin descending limb of the loop of Henle; MAL, portion of the thick ascending limb located in the outer medulla; CAL, portion of the thick ascending limb located in the cortex; DCT, distal convoluted tubule; CCT, cortical collecting tubule; MCT, portion of the collecting tubule located on the outer medulla. Subscripts b, g, l, refer to the microscopic appearance being "bright", "granular", and "light", respectively (CHABARDÈS et al., 1975)

It has been claimed from studies with an isolated kidney papilla preparation of rats that isoproterenol does not alter water handling by a direct action on the water permeability of the kidney (RAYSON et al., 1978). These authors demonstrated that isoproterenol exerted no effect on its own on diffusing water permeability of collecting ducts within the papilla. However, by perfusing isolated rabbit cortical tubules in vitro, it could recently be established that isoproterenol (10^{-6} *M*) added to the bath stimulated chloride transport and caused the negative potential difference of cortical collecting ducts to become more positive (IINO and BRENNER, 1979).

In well defined segments of the rabbit nephron, isolated by microdissection, CHARBADÈS et al. (1975) demonstrated that isoproterenol (10^{-6} *M*) stimulated adenylate cyclase activity in the second (granular) portion of the distal convoluted tubule, in the granular, and in the light portions of the cortical collecting tubule (Fig. 6). In the medullary portions of the collecting duct, a main target site for vasopressin (IMBERT et al., 1975), the adenylate cyclase response to isoproterenol was rather poor. The isoproterenol effects were completely suppressed by propranolol, indicating that these effects are mediated by β-receptors. Whether these actions of isoproterenol are causally related to the observed changes in electrolyte transport of these tubule segments needs further clarification.

Direct actions of β-adrenergic activators on other electrolyte transporting epithelia have also been demonstrated. β-Adrenergic stimulation has been found to be associated with activation of water and salt movements across frog skin (McAfee, 1970; Ambalavanar et al., 1973; Tomlinson and Wood, 1976, 1978), toad bladder (Handler et al., 1968), frog cornea (Montoreano et al., 1976), and excretory duct of submandibular gland of rats and rabbits (Martin and Young, 1971; Schneyler and Thavornthon, 1973; Denniss et al., 1978).

Additional evidence of direct influence of catecholamines on tubular function may be derived from electron-microscopic, histochemical, and nerve stimulating studies. Müller and Barajas (1972) and Barajas and Müller (1973) for the first time demonstrated adrenergic nerve terminals in direct contact with proximal and distal tubular epithelium of monkey and rat kidneys, whereas previous studies failed to demonstrate adrenergic tubular nerves. In the dog kidney DiBona (1977) recently demonstrated similar adrenergic innervation.

An increase in tubular sodium reabsorption was found in dogs after stimulation of renal sympathetic nerves at low frequencies which did not influence glomerular filtration rate, total renal blood flow or its intrarenal distribution (DiBona, 1977), and micropuncture studies in the rat revealed, with unchanged nephron filtration rate, a decrease in water and sodium reabsorption by the proximal tubule after renal denervation (Bello-Reuss et al., 1975). These studies indicate sympathetic involvement in renal tubular water and sodium reabsorption. This issue has been covered recently by three comprehensive reviews (DiBona, 1977; Gottschalk et al., 1978; Gottschalk, 1979) and will not be further discussed here in detail.

2. Evidence for Renal Effects Mediated Through Changes in Release of Antidiuretic Hormone

Thus, while there is considerable evidence that indicates that β-adrenoceptor stimulation exerts a direct intrarenal effect on the tubular handling of water and electrolytes, there are also studies which favor the view that the decrease in urine flow may be mediated, at least in part, through changes in endogenous release of antidiuretic hormone.

Since some authors have found (in contrast to Heidenreich et al., 1969; Aviado et al., 1958) that isoproterenol caused diuresis rather than antidiuresis after intrarenal infusion to dogs in amounts which were too small to exert systemic effects (Pearson and Williams, 1968; Gill and Casper, 1971; Schrier, 1974; Schrier et al., 1972, 1975), an extrarenal mechanism of the antidiuretic effect of intravenous isoproterenol has been claimed. Several papers have been published which suggest that the antidiuretic effect observed after systemic β-adrenergic activation involves the integrity of the hypothalamic-neurohypophysic system and the release of antidiuretic hormone.

Thus, patients with untreated diabetes insipidus did not respond with antidiuresis after isoproterenol application whereas normal subjects, undergoing a water diuresis did (Berl et al., 1974a). Similar results were obtained in the dog (Schrier et al., 1972) and the rat (McDonald et al., 1977, with the exception of Levi et al., 1971).

Although in the dog (Klein et al., 1971) no increase in systemic ADH levels could be observed after β-adrenoceptor stimulation, the same group (Levi and Kleeman,

1973) demonstrated in man that the isoproterenol antidiuresis was associated with increased peripheral ADH plasma concentration.

In dogs, intracarotic infusion of isoproterenol, which was estimated to produce drug concentrations comparable to those achieved during intravenous infusion, induced no change in renal water excretion (BERL et al., 1974c). It was therefore suggested that isoproterenol regulates antidiuretic hormone release by way of its effects on vascular baroreceptors. In agreement with this assumption are experiments in dogs which show that when carotid baroreceptors were denervated isoproterenol induced no antidiuresis (BERL et al., 1974c).

In summary, systemic application of β-adrenoceptor agonists is usually associated with decreased urine flow, free water clearance, and urinary electrolyte excretion. Changes in renal hemodynamics seem not to be a prerequisite for this antidiuretic effect. There is evidence to indicate that β-adrenoceptor stimulation exerts direct intrarenal effects on tubular electrolyte transport and water excretion as well as an effect mediated by the release of antidiuretic hormone.

II. Effects of Beta-Adrenergic Inhibitors

It has been well established that β-adrenoceptor blocking agents induce an increase in urine and electrolyte excretion in the rat (HEINTZE, 1968; HEINTZE and HEIDENREICH, 1968; LEES, 1968; FÜLGRAFF et al., 1968, 1969; GREVEN, 1974a, b; CARRARA and BAINES, 1976; SHIBOUTA et al., 1979). These effects frequently occurred without changes in glomerular filtration rate. This points to a direct effect of β-adrenoceptor blockers on renal tubules of the rat. By micropuncture, GREVEN (1974c) could demonstrate that propranolol inhibited sodium reabsorption in the loops of Henle of rats.

In contrast to the rat, the effect of β-adrenoceptor blockade on tubular function in the dog has revealed conflicting results. Infusion of propranolol directly into the renal artery of dog kidneys induced no change in urinary fluid and electrolyte excretion (HEIDENREICH et al., 1969; NIES et al., 1971). Also in an isolated dog kidney preparation propranolol exerted no tubular effects (ADER et al., 1977).

Systemic application of propranolol or pronethalol to dogs, however, decreased renal sodium excretion (WAUGH, 1970; NIES et al., 1971). This effect probably was caused by changes in renal hemodynamics secondary to alteration in systemic hemodynamics, but a direct tubular action of systemic propranolol in the dog (URBAITES and WAUGH, 1969; CACCIAGUIDA et al., 1973) has also been suggested.

Propranolol was able to reverse the antinatriuresis of chronic bile duct ligation in the dog. This was thought to be mediated by an extrarenal effect of the β-adrenergic blockade (WINAVER et al., 1978).

In man, no effect (EPSTEIN and BRAUNWALD, 1966; SCHIRMEISTER et al., 1966; GIBSON, 1972; SABBAH, 1976; SALVETTI et al., 1977), an antidiuretic effect (RAHN et al., 1968; MROCZEK et al, 1970; HEIERLI et al., 1977), and a diuretic effect (IMBS et al., 1976, 1977) have all been observed after β-adrenergic inhibition.

In summary, the observed effects of β-adrenoceptor blocking agents on renal function are highly variable and may be the net results of direct renal actions and indirect systemic responses which are highly dependent upon doses, routes of administration, and species used.

III. Effects of Alpha-Adrenergic Activators

In contrast to β-adrenoceptor stimulation systemic application of noradrenaline is usually associated with an increase in urine formation. This has been demonstrated in the *dog* (HANDLEY and MOYER, 1954; BLAKE, 1955; PEARSON and WILLIAMS, 1968; EARLEY and FRIEDLER, 1966; LAUBIE et al., 1967; KLEIN et al., 1971; LIANG and YANG, 1972; SCHRIER and BERL, 1973), the *rat* (DEXTER and STONER, 1952; EVERSOLE et al., 1952; HORRES et al., 1960; BOTTING and LOCKETT, 1961, GREEN and SIM, 1961; HEINTZE, 1968; HEINTZE and HEIDENREICH, 1968; FÜLGRAFF et al., 1969; KLEIN, 1975b), the *aligator* (HERNANDEZ and COULSON, 1956) and in *man* (SMYTHE et al., 1952; BALDWIN et al., 1963; FISHER, 1968; WILSON et al., 1969). A natriuretic effect was also observed in *isolated perfused rat kidneys* (STEELE and UNDERWOOD, 1978).

In contrast to systemic application, infusion of noradrenaline directly into the renal artery of dogs induced an antidiuresis (BARGER et al., 1959; PEARSON and WILLIAMS, 1968; GILL and CASPER, 1972). Injection of noradrenaline into the third ventricle of rats (M. MORRIS et al., 1976) and sheep (BEAL and BLIGH, 1976) also decreased urinary excretion of fluid.

The effect of systemic application of adrenaline seems to be dose-dependent (BOTTING and LOCKETT, 1961) in that low doses (5–30 μg/kg s.c.) exerted an antidiuretic, high doses (50–200 μg/kg s.c.) a diuretic effect in rats. Thus, it is not surprising that variable effects of systemic adrenaline on urine excretion have been claimed. An increase (RYDIN and VERNEY, 1938; GREEN and SIM, 1961; BANK et al., 1970; FORSTER et al., 1972) as well a decrease (DEXTER and STONER, 1952; BERNE et al., 1953; NICKEL et al., 1954; OGLE, 1968), or no effects (HORRES et al., 1960) have been reported. Antidiuretic and diuretic effects in the same animals have also been observed (LAUBIE et al., 1967; LIANG and YOUNG, 1972).

GILL and CASPER (1972) suggested from clearance studies in dogs that noradrenaline infused directly into the renal artery increases proximal but not distal tubular reabsorption of sodium by a direct action on renal tubules. In these experiments, hypophysectomized animals were used, and β-adrenergic blockade was achieved by infusion of propranolol into the renal artery.

However, micropuncture studies designed to demonstrate direct tubular effects of noradrenaline or adrenaline were without success. FÜLGRAFF et al. (1969) did not find an effect of noradrenaline or adrenaline on tubular reabsorption in the proximal convolution. These authors injected the catecholamines directly into the tubular lumen and measured the reabsorptive capacity of the proximal tubular epithelium photographically by the split oil droplet method of GERTZ (1963). Free flow micropuncture studies in rats (MYERS et al., 1975) and dogs (BLENDIS et al., 1972) were also unable to demonstrate direct tubular effects of noradrenaline.

However, an interaction of α-receptor stimulating agents with the cellular action and with the release of antidiuretic hormone seems to be well established. Noradrenaline interferes with antidiuretic hormone antidiuresis in man and animals (NICKEL et al., 1954; FISHER, 1968; LIBERMAN et al., 1970; KLEIN et al., 1971) and inhibits the antidiuretic hormone induced cAMP generation in rat (KUROKAWA and MASSRY,

1973a) and dog renal medulla (BECK et al., 1972), as it does in the toad bladder (OMACHI et al., 1974). Noradrenaline may also antagonize the antidiuretic hormone induced increase of water permeability in the toad bladder (HANDLER et al., 1968; STRAUCH and LANGDON, 1969).

In hypophysectomized dogs intravenous or intrarenal applicated noradrenaline was not associated with changes in either urinary osmolarity or free water clearance (SCHRIER and BERL, 1973), which indicates that the water diuresis induced by intravenous noradrenaline may be mediated by suppression of antidiuretic hormone release. Further studies of the same group suggested that noradrenaline suppresses antidiuretic hormone release by altering autonomic baroreceptor tone rather than by a central effect of the catecholamine (BERL et al., 1974b).

In addition clonidine has been found to increase urine flow and urinary sodium, potassium, and chloride excretion in rats and dogs and again inhibition of antidiuretic hormone release has been claimed to be, at least partly, the underlying mechanism. The effects of clonidine on the kidneys have recently been reviewed extensively (SCHMITT, 1977) and will not be discussed here further.

In summary there is conclusive evidence that water diuresis associated with systemic α-adrenergic stimulation results from interaction with cellular action and release of antidiuretic hormone. It is not established if α-adrenoceptor stimulating agents exert a direct tubular effect.

IV. Effects of Alpha-Adrenergic Inhibitors

Only a few papers are available with respect to α-adrenoceptor blockade and renal excretory function. Subcutaneous injection of phentolamine to awake rats induced no changes in the pattern of renal fluid and electrolyte excretion (HEINTZE, 1968; HEINTZE and HEIDENREICH, 1968; FÜLGRAFF et al., 1969).

Infusion of phentolamine or phenoxybenzamine directly into the renal artery of dogs was associated with an increase in urine flow, free water (GILL and CASPER, 1971), and sodium excretion (STRANDHOY et al., 1974). In these experiments the doses (0.09 μg/kg/min) of the α-blockers used induced no changes in renal hemodynamics. Also in isolated perfused rabbit kidneys an increase in urine flow was observed after adding phenoxybenzamine to the perfusing medium (ERCAN et al., 1977). If the doses (10–35 μg/kg/min), however, were high enough to induce a fall in mean arterial pressure phentolamine reduced urine flow and sodium excretion (LOCKETT and WADLEY, 1969).

In dogs with normovolemic hemorrhagic shock phenoxybenzamine caused significant increases in the excretion rates for sodium and potassium but also an increase in renal blood flow. The observed changes in the renal excretion rates, when phenoxybenzamine was given, were thought to reflect drug-induced changed in renal hemodynamics (FEIGEN et al., 1977).

Whereas GILL and CASPER (1971) concluded from their clearance studies in dogs that α-adrenoceptor blockade affects proximal tubular sodium reabsorption, direct micropuncture studies in dogs (STRANDHOY et al., 1974) detected no change in proximal sodium reabsorption although natriuresis occurred in these experiments. The authors concluded that the phenoxybenzamine-induced natriuresis indicates decreased sodium reabsorption in more distal segments of the nephron.

E. Kidney Intermediary Metabolism

I. Effects of Adrenergic Activators and Inhibitors on Kidney cAMP Content and Its Relation to Renal Gluconeogenesis

Studies concerning the effect of catecholamines on renal metabolism have been mainly addressed to renal gluconeogenesis. Most experiments were performed using rat kidneys, since it was found that in this species the gluconeogenetic capacity of the kidneys may be even higher than that of the liver (KREBS and YOSHIDA, 1963).

It has been well established that catecholamines may increase renal gluconeogenesis. Increased renal glucose production has been demonstrated in vitro in rat renal cortical slices (KLAHR et al., 1973; ROOBOL and ALLEYNE, 1973) or isolated rat kidney cortex tubules (MARX et al., 1972; FRIEDRICHS and SCHONER, 1973; KUROKAWA and MASSRY, 1973c; GUDER and RUPPRECHT, 1974, 1975a; MCDONALD and SAGGERSON, 1977). In vivo studies in rats suggested enhanced renal gluconeogenesis after adrenergic activation (GREVEN, 1974b; GREVEN et al., 1974, 1975). Renal uptake of lactate and free fatty acids was unchanged by isoprenaline in these in vivo experiments, but noradrenaline enhanced uptake of free fatty acids coinciding with a depression of lactate uptake in dogs (DIES et al., 1970). In dogs noradrenaline and adrenaline did not increase the oxygen consumption of the kidneys (BALINT and CHATEL, 1967), whereas dopamine did (JOHANNESEN et al., 1976).

Since catecholamines may enhance the cellular content of cAMP in isolated tubules or renal cortical slices of animals (MELSON et al., 1970; BECK et al., 1972; MARX et al., 1972; KLAHR et al., 1973; KUROKAWA and MASSRY, 1973a, b, c; BELL, 1974; KUROKAWA et al., 1977; CHRISTENSEN, 1978) and since studies in man also suggested a stimulating effect of catecholamines on renal adenylate cyclase (BALL et al., 1972; MULVEHILL et al., 1976) it was assumed that enhanced renal gluconeogenesis is mediated through the adenylate cyclase-cAMP system (KLAHR et al., 1973; KUROKAWA and MASSRY, 1973c; KUROKAWA et al., 1977). This assumption is strengthened by the finding that cAMP on its own may stimulate gluconeogenesis in isolated perfused kidneys (BOWMAN, 1970), renal cortical slices (PAGLIARA and GOODMAN, 1969; NAGATA and RASMUSSEN, 1970; KLAHR et al., 1973; ROOBOL and ALLEYNE, 1973), and in isolated tubules (RASMUSSEN and NAGATA, 1970; GUDER and WIELAND, 1972).

The increase in renal gluconeogenesis and cAMP production was observed not only after noradrenaline and adrenaline but also after isoproterenol application. Since in some experiments these effects could be abolished by propranolol, it was suggested that catecholamines enhance gluconeogenesis in renal cortical tubules by the stimulation of β-adrenoceptors (MARX et al., 1972; KUROKAWA and MASSRY, 1973c; GREVEN, 1974b; GREVEN et al., 1974, 1975; KUROKAWA et al., 1977). In support of this assumption it was found by KUROKAWA et al. (1977) that phentolamine had no effect on noradrenaline-induced rises in cAMP concentration of isolated renal tubules and it was postulated that the renal cortex where gluconeogenesis takes place lacks significant α-adrenoceptor activity.

It is noteworthy that dopamine, which is known to stimulate the renal adenylate cyclase system in man (VLACHOYANNIS et al., 1974, 1976) and animals (AUGUSTIN et al., 1975; NAKAJIAMA et al., 1977; NAKAJIAMA and NAITOH, 1977) increased renal glucose release when infused intravenously to anesthetized rats at a dose of 4.7 $\times 10^{-6}$ mol/kg/h (GREVEN and CHARL, 1977). Renal glucose release was estimated from the difference in glucose concentration in the arterial and renal venous plasma and from renal plasma flow. The glycogen content of the kidneys was found to be too small to account for the observed renal glucose release by glycogenolysis and the increase of renal glucose release was assumed to reflect enhanced renal gluconeogenesis. The effect of dopamine on renal glucose release could be abolished by propranolol, suggesting again β-adrenoceptor mediated stimulation of renal gluconeogenesis.

However, studies by GUDER and co-workers (GUDER and RUPPRECHT, 1974, 1975a) led to completely opposite conclusions. These authors observed that the different catecholamines stimulated gluconeogenesis of isolated kidney cortex tubules of starved rats in parallel to their α-adrenergic potency. They also claimed that this α-receptor mediated effect is independent from stimulation of renal adenylate cyclase, since phenylephrine was the best stimulator of gluconeogenesis but had no effect on cAMP. Whereas isoproterenol was by far the most effective drug in raising cAMP, it was without effect on glucose formation. Phentolamine prevented the stimulatory effect of noradrenaline on gluconeogenesis, whereas the β-blocker propranolol did not abolish the hormone effect below a concentration of 5×10^{-4} M. At higher concentrations both blockers inhibited stimulated gluconeogenesis but this was thought to be due to unspecific effects.

Similar results to the group of GUDER were obtained by MCDONALD and SAGGERSON (1977). In their studies with tubule fragments from the renal cortex of fed rats, gluconeogenesis from pyruvate was stimulated by adrenaline and the selective α-adrenoceptor agonists oxymetazoline and amidephrine. Isoproterenol and salbutamol were ineffective. The adrenaline effect was blocked by phentolamine but was unaffected by propranolol. Although oxymetazoline increased gluconeogenesis it had no effect on cAMP or cGMP tissue content.

Thus, according to these authors, renal gluconeogenesis may be increased by α- but not by β-adrenoceptor stimulation, independent of changes in cAMP or cGMP tissue levels. However, interpretation of the changes in renal tissue content of cyclic nucleotides has to take into account the extreme heterogeneity of nephron segments in response to hormonal stimulation (for review see OSSWALD and NORTHRUP, 1978).

In summary, most authors agree that catecholamines increase renal gluconeogenesis by a direct tubular effect. However, it remains a matter of controversy whether these effects are mediated by α- or β-adrenoceptors and whether cyclic nucleotides are involved in these effects of catecholamines.

II. Miscellaneous Effects

An interaction between noradrenaline and parathyroid hormone has been described by GUDER and RUPPRECHT (1975b) and GUDER (1976). Using isolated rat kidney cortex tubules, the authors could show that adrenaline in a concentration of 5×10^{-7} M, which itself had no effect on cAMP levels, inhibited by 50% the ability of parathyroid hormone to increase cAMP tissue content. This effect of the catecholamine could be completely abolished by the addition of phentolamine. Whether the antagonism between noradrenaline and parathyroid hormone may be related to renal transport processes is not established. Noradrenaline should then counteract the inhibiting effect of parathyroid hormone on proximal tubular sodium reabsorption, but experimental evidence to support this hypothesis is still lacking.

L-Adrenaline (1 m*M*) was found to enhance prostaglandin biosynthesis in rabbit kidneys by way of stimulating synthesis of endoperoxide (TAI, 1976). It has also been observed that noradrenaline at doses which decreased renal blood flow stimulated erythropoietin release from dog kidneys (FISHER et al., 1971). The mechanism of these effects and the functional implications remain to be established.

F. Summary of Effects of Catecholamines on Kidney Function

Catecholamines when circulating or being intrarenally released from the terminal nerves affect kidney function mainly in four ways:
1) Tubular electrolyte and water reabsorption
2) Renin release
3) Renal hemodynamics
4) Renal gluconeogenesis.

The effects of catecholamines on each of these processes have clearly been shown and can occur independently from each other.

Under normal resting conditions the effect of circulating and intrarenally released catecholamines on total renal blood flow seems to be rather small. However, low frequency stimulation of the efferent renal nerves results in an increase in tubular electrolyte reabsorption, decreased urine flow, and sodium excretion. Increased sodium chloride reabsorption in the proximal tubule results in a decrease of sodium chloride delivery to the macula densa region and changes thereby one signal to be integrated by the juxtaglomerular apparatus. Minute changes in intrarenal flow and filtrate distribution might occur although this has not been demonstrated yet.

Renal nerve stimulation also results in an increase of release of renin into the renal vein. Renin may increase via angiotensin II formation the secretion rate of aldosterone from the adrenals. The result of increased aldosterone levels is an increased rate of sodium reabsorption in the kidney.

As an overall effect elevated sympathetic tone tends to increase water and electrolyte conservation by the kidney whereas low renal sympathetic nerve activity favors excretion of salt and water

Acknowledgments. Research from the authors' laboratories mentioned in this article was supported by the Deutsche Forschungsgemeinschaft (Grants OSSWALD 42/1–5 and GREVEN 532/1–5). Secreterial assistance of E. ABRAHAMS is gratefully acknowledged.

References

Abboud, H.E., Luke, R.G., Galla, J.H., Kotchen, T.A.: Stimulation of renin by acute selective chloride depletion in the rat. Circ. Res. *44*, 815–821 (1979)
Abdel-Razzak, M.: Effect of some β-adrenergic blocking drugs on the renal blood flow in dogs. Arch. Int. Pharmacodyn. Ther. *229*, 227–234 (1978)
Ader, J.L., Serres, P., Moatti, J.P., Haas, S., Mousteou, F., van Tran, T.: Etude des effects du blocage de récepteurs β-adrénergiques sur les fonctions de reins isolés et perfusés. J. Physiol. (Paris) *73*, 131–153 (1977)
Aihara, H., Kasai, A., Sakai, T.: The effect of dopamine on peripheral vasculature of the rat. Jpn. J. Pharmacol. *22*, 617–627 (1972)

Alexander, G., Bell, A.W., Setchell, B.P.: Regional distribution of cardiac output in young lambs: Effect of cold exposure and treatment with catecholamines. J. Physiol. (Lond.) *220*, 511–528 (1972)

Alexander, R.W., Gill, J.R., Jr., Yamabe, H., Lovenberg, W., Keiser, H.R.: Effects of dietary sodium and of acute saline infusion on the relationship between dopamine excretion and adrenergic activity in man. J. Clin. Invest. *54*, 194–200 (1974)

Almgard, L.E., Ljundqvist, A.: Effect of circulating norepinephrine on the renin release from the denervated kidney. Scand. J. Urol. Nephrol. (Paris) *9*, 125–128 (1975)

Ambalavanar, S., Foster, R.W., Schnieden, H.: The adrenoceptors mediating catecholamine effects in frog isolated skin. J. Pharm. Pharmacol. *25*, 55–59 (1973)

Amery, A., Billiet, L., Fagard, R.: Letter: Beta receptors and renin release. N. Engl. J. Med. *290*, 284/31 (1974)

Anderson, R.J., Taher, M.S., Cronin, R.E., McDonald, K.M., Schier, R.W.: Effect of beta-adrenergic blockade and inhibitors of angiotensin II and prostaglandins on renal autoregulation. Am. J. Physiol. *229*, 731–736 (1975)

Andreucci, V.E., Dal Canton, A., Corradi, A., Stanziale, R., Migone, L.: Role of the efferent arteriole in glomerular hemodynamics of superficial nephrons. Kidney Int. *9*, 475–480 (1976)

Aoi, W., Henry, D.P., Weinberger, M.H.: Evidence for a physiological role of renal sympathetic nerves in adrenergic stimulation of renin release in the rat. Circ. Res. *38*, 123–126 (1976)

Apitzsch, D.E.: Angiographic technique in assessment of renal mass lesions. ROEFO *122*, 74–77 (1975)

Attmann, P.O., Aurell, M., Johnsson, G.: Effects of metoprolol and propranolol on furosemide-stimulated renin release in healthy subjects. Eur. J. Clin. Pharmacol. *8*, 201–204 (1975)

Augustin, H.J., Huland, H., Kaukel, E.: Der Einfluß von Dopamin auf den intrarenalen cAMP-Gehalt der Niere. Verh. Dtsch. Ges. Inn. Med. *81*, 1029–1032 (1975)

Augustin, H.J., Baumgarten, H.G., Huland, H., Leichtweiss, H.P.: The vasoconstrictive effect of dopamine in the isolated, perfused rat kidney after catecholamine depletion. Res. Exp. Med. (Berl.) *169*, 1–5 (1977)

Aukland, K.: Effect of adrenaline, noradrenaline, angiotensin and renal nerve stimulation on intrarenal distribution of blood flow in dogs. Acta Physiol. Scand. *72*, 498–509 (1968)

Aukland, K.: Renal blood flow. Int. Rev. Physiol. Volume 11, Kidney and Urinary Tract Physiology II, University Park Press, Baltimore, London, Tokyo 25–79 (1976)

Aukland, K.: Methods for measuring renal blood flow: Total flow and regional distribution. Ann. Rev. Physiol. *42*, 543–555 (1980)

Aviado, D.M., Jr., Wnuck, A.L., DeBeer, E.J.: The effects of sympathomimetic drugs on renal vessels. J. Pharmacol. Exp. Ther. *124*, 238–244 (1958)

Baldwin, D.S., Gombos, E.A., Chasis, H.: Changes in sodium and water excretion induced by epinephrine and l-norepinephrine in normotensive and hypertensive subjects. J. Lab. Clin. Med. *61*, 832–857 (1963)

Balint, P., Chatel, R.: Die Wirkung von Adrenalin und von Noradrenalin auf die Nierenhaemodynamik beim Hund. Naunyn Schmiedebergs Arch. Pharmacol. *258*, 24–36 (1967)

Ball, I.H., Kaminsky, N.I., Hardman, I.G., Broadus, A.E., Sutherland, E.W., Liddle, G.W.: Effects of catecholamines and adrenergic blocking agents on plasma and urinary cyclic nucleotides in man. J. Clin. Invest. *51*, 2124–2129 (1972)

Bank, N., Aynedjian, H.S., Bansal, V.K., Goldman, D.M.: Effect of acute hypertension on sodium transport by the distal nephron. Am. J. Physiol. *219*, 275–280 (1970)

Barajas, L.: Innervation of the renal cortex. Fed. Proc. *37*, 1192–1201 (1978)

Barajas, L., Müller, I.: The innervation of the juxtaglomerular apparatus and surrounding tubules: A quantitative analysis by serial section electron microscopy. J. Ultrastruct. Res. *43*, 107–132 (1973)

Barger, A.C., Herd, J.A.: Renal vascular anatomy and distribution of blood flow. In: Handbook of physiology, Sect. 8: Renal Physiology. Orloff, J., Berliner, R.W. (eds.), pp. 249–314. Washington, D.C.: American Physiological Society 1973

Barger, A.C., Muldowney, F.P., Liebowitz, M.R.: Role of the kidney in the pathogenesis of congestive heart failure. Circulation *20*, 273–285 (1959)

Barnes, A.B.: The effect of oxytocin on total renal blood flow and its distribution in the dog. Surg. Forum *21*, 414–416 (1970)
Beal, A.M., Bligh, J.: Renal electrolyte excretion following injection of carbachol, noradrenaline and 5-hydroxytryptamine into the lateral cerebral ventricle of conscious sheep. J. Physiol. (Lond.) *263*, 188P–189P (1976)
Beck, N.P., Reed, S.W., Murdaugh, H.V., Davis, B.B.: Effects of catecholamines and their interaction with other hormones on cyclic 3′,5′-adenosine monophosphate of the kidney. J. Clin. Invest. *51*, 939–944 (1972)
Bell, C., Lang, W.J.: Effect of renal dopamine receptor and beta-adrenoceptor blockade on rises in blood angiotensin after haemorrhage, renal ischaemia and furosemide diuresis in the dog. Clin. Sci. Mol. Med. *54*, 17–23 (1978)
Bell, C., Mya, M.K.: Is the renal vasodilatation induced by beta-adrenoceptor stimulants in the dog mediated through dopamine receptor? Experientia *33*, 638–639 (1977)
Bell, G., Lister, G.D.: The effect of noradrenaline and phenoxybenzamine on the renal response to hemorrhage. Surg. Gynecol. Obstet. *130*, 813–821 (1970)
Bell, N.H.: Evidence for a separate adenylate cyclase system responsive to β-adrenergic stimulation in the renal cortex of the rat. Acta Endocrinol. (Kbh.) *77*, 604–611 (1974)
Bell, P.R., Quin, R.O., Calman, K.C.: Donor pretreatment and organ preservation. Transplant. Proc. *6*, 245–248 (1974)
Bello-Reuss, E., Colindres, R.E., Pastoriza-Munoz, E., Müller, R.A., Gottschalk, C.W.: Effects of acute unilateral renal denervation in the rat. J. Clin. Invest. *56*, 208–217 (1975)
Berl, T., Harbottle, J.A., Schrier, R.W.: Effect of α- and β-adrenergic stimulation on renal water excretion in normal subjects and patients with diabetes insipidus. Kidney Int. *6*, 247–253 (1974a)
Berl, T., Cadnapaphornchai, P., Harbottle, J.A., Schrier, R.W.: Mechanism of supression of vasopressin during α-adrenergic stimulation with norepinephrine. J. Clin. Invest. *53*, 219–227 (1974b)
Berl, T., Cadnapaphornchai, P., Harbottle, J.A., Schrier, R.W.: Mechanism of stimulation of vasopressin release during β-adrenergic stimulation with isoproterenol. J. Clin. Invest. *53*, 857–867 (1974c)
Berl, T., Heurich, W.L., Erickson, A.L., Schrier, R.W.: Prostaglandins in the beta-adrenergic and baroreceptor-mediated secretion of renin. Am. J. Physiol. *236*, F472–477 (1979)
Berne, R.M., Kagan, W.K., Levy, M.N.: Response of the normal and denervated kidney to l-epinephrine and l-norepinephrine. Am. J. Physiol. *171*, 564–571 (1953)
Bersentes, T.J., Simmons, D.H.: Effects of acute acidosis on renal hemodynamics. Am. J. Physiol. *212*, 633–640 (1967)
Besarbab, A., Silva, P., Landsberg, L., Epstein, F.H.: Effect of catecholamines on tubular function in the isolated perfused rat kidney. Am. J. Physiol. *233*, F39–45 (1977)
Biery, D.N., Thind, G.S., Baum, S.: The effect of cadmium on catecholamines and angiotensin responses in the dog kidney. Acta. Radiol. [Suppl.] (Stockh.) *319*, 245–249 (1972)
Blair-West, J.R.: Renin-angiotensin system and sodium metabolism. Int. Rev. Physiol. Volume 11, Kidney and Urinary Tract Physiology II, University Park Press, Baltimore, London, Tokyo 95–143 (1976)
Blake, W.D.: Pathways of adrenaline action on renal function with observations on a blood pressure reflex regulating water and electrolyte excretion. Am. J. Physiol. *181*, 399–416 (1955)
Blendis, L.M., Auld, R.B., Alexander, E.A., Levinsky, N.: Effect of renal β- and α-adrenergic stimulation on proximal sodium reabsorption in dogs. Clin. Sci. Mol. Med. *43*, 569–576 (1972)
Bloom, D., McCalden, T.A., Rosendorff, C.: Proceedings: The effects of jaundiced plasma on vascular sensitivity to noradrenaline. J. Physiol. (Lond.) *241*, 109P–110P (1974)
Bloom, D.S., Bomzon, L., Rosendorff, C., Kew, M.C.: Renal blood flow in obstructive jaundice: An experimental study in baboons. Clin. Exp. Pharmacol. Physiol. *3*, 461–472 (1976)
Bomzon, L., Rosendorff, C.: Renovascular resistance and noradrenaline. Am. J. Physiol. *229*, 1649–1653 (1975)
Bomzon, L., Rosendorff, C., Scriven, D.R., Farr, J.: The effect of noradrenaline, adrenergic blocking agents, and tyramine on the intrarenal distribution of blood flow in the baboon. Cardiovasc. Res. *9*, 314–322 (1975)

Bomzon, L., Kew, M.C., Rosendorff, C.: Renovascular hypersensitivity to noradrenaline in dietary-induced hypercholesterolaemia in baboons. Clin. Exp. Pharmacol. Physiol. *5*, 181–185 (1978)
Bonelli, J., Waldhaesel, W., Magometschnigg, D., Schwarzmeier, J., Korn, A.: Effect of exercise and of prolonged oral administration of propranolol on haemodynamic variables, plasma renin concentration, plasma aldosterone and c-AMP. Eur. J. Clin. Invest. *7*, 337–343 (1977)
Bookstein, J.J., Ernest, C.B.: Pharmacoangiographic manipulation of renal collateral flow. An important adjunct in evaluating hemodynamic significance of renal artery stenosis. Radiology *102*, 433–434 (1972)
Botting, R.M., Lockett, M.F.: Threshold effect of subcutaneous adrenaline, noradrenaline and isoprenaline on water diuresis in rats. Arch. Int. Physiol. Biochim. *69*, 36–45 (1961)
Botting, R.M., Farmer, J.B., Lockett, M.F.: The effect of subcutaneous adrenaline and isoprenaline on the excretion of electrolytes by rats. Arch. Int. Physiol. Biochim. *69*, 203–212 (1961)
Bowman, R.H.: Gluconeogenesis in the isolated perfused rat kidney. J. Biol. Chem. *245*, 1604–1612 (1970)
Brotzu, G.: Inhibition by chlorpromazine of the effects of dopamine on the dog kidney. J. Pharm. Pharmac. *22*, 664–667 (1970)
Buckley, N.M., Frank, M.H., Zeig, N.J., Bass, B.G., Macy, Jr. J.: Effects of acute hemorrhage during catecholamine infusion in splenectomized dogs. Am. J. Physiol. *212*, 579–588 (1967)
Burger, B.M., Hopkins, T., Tulloch, A., Hollenberg, N.K.: The role of angiotensin in the canine renal vascular response to barbiturate anesthesia. Circ. Res. *38*, 196–202 (1976)
Bursaux, E., Poyart, C., Bohn, B.: Renal hemodynamics and renal O_2 uptake during hypoxia in the anesthetized rabbit. Pfluegers Arch. *365*, 213–220 (1976)
Cacciaguida, R.J., Pablo, N.C., Basilio, R.D., Porush, J.: Antinatriuresis associated with propranolol administration in the dog. Nephron *11*, 58–64 (1973)
Campbell, W.B., Pettinger, W.A., Keeton, K., Brooks, S.N.: Vasodilating antihypertensive drug-induced aldesterone release – a study of endogenous angiotensin-mediated aldosterone release in the rat. J. Pharmacol. Exp. Ther. *193*, 166–175 (1975)
Campbell, W.B., Graham, R.M., Jackson, E.K.: Role of renal prostaglandins in sympathetically mediated renin release in the rat. J. Clin. Invest. *64*, 448–456 (1979)
Capponi, A.M., Vallotton, M.B.: Renin release by kidney slices incubated in vitro. Role of sodium and of alpha- and beta-adrenergic receptors, and effect of vincristine. Circ. Res. *39*, 200–203 (1976)
Capponi, A.M., Gourjon, M., Valloton, M.B.: Effect of beta-blocking agents and angiotensin II on isoproterenol – stimulated renin release from rat kidney slices. Circ. Res. *40*, I-89–I-93 (1977)
Carey, J.P., Stemmer, E.A., List, J.W., Chin, S.C., Heber, R., Connolly, J.E.: The hazards of using vasoactive drugs to augment peripheral and cerebral blood flow. Am. Surg. *35*, 12–22 (1969)
Carey, R.M., Thorner, M.O., Ortt, E.M.: Effects of metoclopramide and bromocriptine on the renin-angiotensin-aldosterone system in man. J. Clin. Invest. *63*, 727–735 (1979)
Carrara, M.C., Baines, A.D.: Propranolol induces acute natriuresis by β-blockade and dopaminergic stimulation. Can. J. Physiol. Pharmacol. *54*, 683–691 (1976)
Carrière, S.: Effect of norepinephrine, isoproterenol and adrenergic blockers upon the intrarenal distribution of blood flow. Can. J. Physiol. Pharmacol. *47*, 199–208 (1969)
Carrière, S.: Factors affecting renal cortical blood flow. A review. Can. J. Physiol. Pharmacol. *53*, 1–20 (1975)
Carrière, S., Daigneault, B.: Effect of retransfusion after hemorrhagic hypotension on intrarenal distribution of blood flow in dogs. J. Clin. Invest. *49*, 2205–2215 (1970)
Chapnick, B.M., Paustian, P.W., Feigen, L.P., Joiner, P.D., Hyman, A.L., Kadowitz, P.J.: Influence of inhibitors of prostaglandin synthesis on renal vascular resistance and on renal vascular responses to vasopressure and vasodilator agents in the cat. Circ. Res. *40*, 348–354 (1977)
Charbadès, D., Imbert-Teboul, M., Montegut, M., Clique, A., Morel, F.: Catecholamine sensitive adenylate cyclase activity in different segments of the rabbit nephron. Pfluegers Arch. *361*, 9–15 (1975)

Chatel, R., Forgacs, I., Visy, M.: The effect of isopropylnoradrenaline on renal haemodynamics. Acta Physiol. Acad. Sci. Hung. *34*, 77–83 (1968)
Christensen, S.: Dissociation between antidiuretic response and renal medullary cyclic AMP levels in the rat. Pfluegers Arch. *374*, 229–234 (1978)
Chrysant, S.G., Lavender, A.R.: Direct renal hemodynamic effects of clonidine. Arch. Int. Pharmacodyn. Ther. *218*, 202–211 (1975)
Churchill, P.C., Churchill, M.C., McDonald, F.D.: Renin secretion and distal tubule Na^+ in rats. Am. J. Physiol. *235*, F611–616 (1978)
Cimmino, V.M., Bove, E.L., Argenta, L.C., Brown, J.W.: The effect of simultaneous administration of levaterenol and phentolamine on renal blood flow. Ann. Thorac. Surg. *21*, 158–163 (1976)
Collis, M.G., Vanhoutte, P.M.: Vascular reactivity in the isolated perfused kidney of the spontaneously hypertensive rat. Arch. Int. Pharmacodyn. Ther. *223*, 164–165 (1976)
Concha, J., Norris, B.: Studies on renal vasomotion. Br. J. Pharmacol. *34*, 277–290 (1968)
Cortesini, C., Novelli, G.P.: On renal transplantation. Renal vasomotor changes in rejection and alpha-receptor blocking. Boll. Soc. Ital. Biol. Sper. *44*, 2091–2092 (1968)
Cuche, J.L., Kuchel, O., Bartean, A., Baucher, R., Genest, I.: Relationship between the adrenergic nervous system and renin during adaption to upright posture; a possible role for 3,4-dihydroxy-phenyl-ethylamine (dopamine). Clin. Sci. Mol. Med. *43*, 481–491 (1972)
Data, J.L., Gerber, J.G., Crump, W.J., Frölich, J.C., Hollifield, J.W., Nies, A.S.: The prostaglandin system. Circ. Res. *42*, 454–458 (1978)
Davies, R., Slater, J.D.: Is the adrenergic control of renin release dominant in man? Lancet II, 594–596 (1976)
Davies, R., Slater, J.D., Rudolf, M., Geddes, D.M.: The effect of isoprenaline on plasma renin activity in man: A dose-response curve. Clin. Endocrinol. (Oxf.) *6*, 395–399 (1977)
Davis, B.B., Walter, M.J., Murdaugh, H.V.: The mechanism of the increase in sodium excretion following dopamine infusion. Proc. Soc. Exp. Biol. Med. *129*, 210–213 (1968)
Davis, J.O.: The control of renin release. Am. J. Med. *55*, 333–350 (1976)
Davis, J.O., Freeman, R.H.: Mechanisms regulating renin release. Physiol. Rev. *56*, 1–56 (1976)
Debreczeni, L., Fenyvesi, T.: Effect of beta-adrenoceptor blocking compounds (propranolol, practolol and LB46) on isoprenaline induced changes in regional blood flow in the rat. Br. J. Pharmacol. *41*, 171–176 (1971)
Denniss, A.R., Schneyer, L.H.; Sucanthapree, C., Youngh, J.: Actions of adrenergic agonists on isolated excretory ducts of submandibular glands. Am. J. Physiol. *235*, 548–557 (1978)
Desaulles, E., Forler, C., Velly, J., Schwartz, J.: Effect of catecholamines on renin release in vitro. Biomedicine *22*, 433–439 (1975)
Desaulles, E., Miesch, F., Schwartz, J.: Evidence for the participation of beta 1-adrenoceptors in isoprenaline – induced renin release from rat kidney slices in vitro. Br. J. Pharmacol. *65*, 421–425 (1978)
Dexter, D., Stoner, H.B.: The role of the adrenal medulla in water diuresis in rats. J. Physiol. (Lond.) *118*, 486–499 (1952)
DiBona, G.F.: Neurogenic regulation of renal tubular sodium reabsorption. Am. J. Physiol. *233*, F73–81 (1977)
Dies, F., Herrera, J., Matos, M., Avelar, E., Ramos, G.: Substrate uptake by the dog kidney in vivo. Am. J. Physiol. *218*, 405–410 (1970)
Dietzmann, R.H., Beckman, C.B., Romero, L.H., Schultz, L.S., Lillehei, R.C.: Effects of blunted sympathetic nervous system response on regional tissue perfusion in experimental endotoxic shock. J. Surg. Res. *14*, 412–419 (1973)
DiSalvo, J., Fell, C.: Drug-evoked neural responses in the canine renal vascular bed. Am. J. Physiol. *220*, 1586–1592 (1971)
DiSalvo, J., Fell, C.: Stimulation of renal "alpha receptors" with isoproterenol. Proc. Soc. Exp. Biol. Med. *133*, 1435–1438 (1970)
Dressler, W.E., D'Alonzo, G., Rossi, G.V., Orzechowski, R.F.: Modification of certain vascular responses to dopamine by morphine. Eur. J. Pharmacol. *28*, 108–113 (1974)
Earley, L.E., Friedler, R.M.: The effects of combined renal vasodilatation and pressor agents on renal hemodynamics and the tubular reabsorption of sodium. J. Clin. Invest. *45*, 542–551 (1966)

Ekelund, L., Goethlin, J., Olin, T.: Arteriovenous fistulae in rabbit kidney studied by dye-dilution technique and by angiography. Scand. J. Urol. Nephrol. *6*, 84–90 (1972)

Ekelund, L., Gerlock. J., Jr., Goncharenko, V.: The epinephrine effect in renal angiography revisited. Clin. Radiol. *29*, 387–392 (1978)

Elkin, M., Meng, C.H., Mendez, L.: Renal vascularity in the dog:alpha-adrenergic blockade and acute hemorrhage. AJR *119*, 748–756 (1973)

Epstein, M., Hollenberg, N.K., Merrill, J.P.: The pattern of the renal vascular response to epinephrine in man. Proc. Soc. Exp. Biol. Med. *134*, 720–724 (1970)

Epstein, S.E., Braunwald, E.: The effect of β-adrenergic blockade on patterns of urinary sodium excretion. Ann. Intern. Med. *65*, 20–27 (1966)

Ercan, Z.S., Tuerker, R.K., Bor, N., Torunoglu, M.: Interaction of phenoxybenzamine with angiotensin II in the isolated perfused rabbit kidney. Arzneim. Forsch. *27*, 1996–1997 (1977)

Eversole, W.J., Giere, F.A., Rock, M.H.: Effects of adrenal medullary hormones on renal excretion of water and electrolytes. Am. J. Physiol. *170*, 24–30 (1952)

Farmer, J.B., Lockett, M.F.: The effect of small subcutaneous doses of adrenaline and isoprenaline on the excretion of water and isotonic solutions of sodium and potassium chloride by rats. Arch. Int. Physiol. Biochim. *69*, 277–283 (1961)

Feigen, L.P., Coleman, B., Glaviano, V.V.: Effects of α-adrenergic blockade on renal function in hemorrhagic shock. Am. J. Physiol. *232*, F409–415 (1977)

Fink, G.D., Brody, M.J.: Continuous measurement of renal blood flow changes to renal nerve stimulation and intraarterial drug administration in the rat. Am. J. Physiol. *234*, H219–H222 (1978)

Fisher, D.A.: Norepinephrine inhibition of vasopressin antidiuresis. J. Clin. Invest. *47*, 540–547 (1968)

Fisher, J.W., Roh, B.L., Malgor, L.A., Noveck, R.J.: Effects of vasoactive agents on erythropoietin production. Isr. J. Med. Sci. *7*, 977–985 (1971)

Fonteles, M.C., Karow, A.M.: An alpha-adrenotypic study of the isolated rabbit kidney at normo- and hypothermia. Arch. Int. Pharmacodyn. Ther. *223*, 196–214 (1976)

Fonteles, M.C., Karow, A.M.: Vascular alpha adrenotropic responses of the isolated rabbit kidney at 15 degrees C. Arch. Int. Pharmacodyn. Ther. *227*, 195–205 (1978)

Forster, R.P., Goldstein, L., Rosen, J.K.: Intrarenal control of urea reabsorption by renal tubules of the marine elasmobranch, squalus acanthias. Comp. Biochem. Physiol. *42*, 3–12 (1972)

Fregly, M.I., Simpson, C.F., Palmore, W.P.: Some β-adrenergic responses to administration of d,l-isoproterenol to turkeys. Proc. Soc. Exp. Biol. Med. *152*, 348–353 (1976)

Friedrichs, D., Schoner, W.: Stimulation of renal gluconeogenesis by inhibition of the sodium pump. Biochim. Biophys. Acta *304*, 142–160 (1973)

Frölich, J.C., Hollifiels, J.W., Michelakis, A.M., Vesper, B.S., Wilson, J.P., Shand, D.G., Seyberth, H.J., Frölich, W.H., Oates, J.A.: Reduction of plasma renin activity by inhibition of the fatty acid cyclooxygenase in human subjects. Circ. Res. *44*, 781–787 (1979)

Fülgraff, G., Meiforth, A., Osswald, H., Heidenreich, O.: Die Wirkung von α- und β-Sympathomimetica auf die lokale Transportkapazität im proximalen Konvolut von Rattennieren. Naunyn Schmiedebergs Arch. Pharmacol. *260*, 116 (1968)

Fülgraff, G., Heidenreich, O., Heintze, K., Osswald, H.: Die Wirkung von α- und β-Sympathomimetica und Sympatholytica auf die renale Exkretion und Resorption von Flüssigkeit und Elektrolyten in Ausscheidungs- und Mikropunktionsversuchen an Ratten. Naunyn Schmiedebergs Arch. Pharmacol. *262*, 295–308 (1969)

Ganong, W.F., Reid, I.A.: Role of the sympathetic nervous system and central α- and β-adrenergic receptors in regulation of renin secretion. In: Regulation of blood pressure by central nervous system. Onesti, G. et al. (ed.), pp. 261–273. New York: Grune & Stratton 1976

Ganten, D., Gross, F.: Interference with the renin-angiotensin system and their effects on high blood pressure. In: Handbook of experimental pharmacology. Vol. 39: Antihypertensive agents. Gross, F. (ed.), pp. 518–546. Berlin, Heidelberg, New York: Springer 1977

Geber, W.F.: Pharmacologic study of the relationship between the total and intrarenal blood flows. Arch. Int. Pharmacodyn. Ther. *160*, 55–65 (1966)

Geller, R.G., Kendrick, J.E.: Reduction in renal vascular responses to angiotensin and norepinephrine during carotid sinus stimulation. Circ. Res. *20*, 321–327 (1967)
Gertz, K.H.: Transtubuläre Natriumchloridflüsse und Permeabilität für Nichtelektrolyte im proximalen und distalen Konvolut der Rattenniere. Pflügers Arch. *276*, 336–356 (1963)
Gibson, D.G.: Effects of practolol administration on cardiac and renal function in patients with chronic atrial fibrillation. Acta Cardiol. (Brux.) *25*, 279–280 (1972)
Gill, J.R., Jr., Casper, A.G.T.: Depression of proximal tubular sodium reabsorption in the dog in response to renal β-adrenergic stimulation by isoproterenol. J. Clin. Invest. *50*, 112–118 (1971)
Gill, J.R., Jr., Casper, A.G.T.: Effect of renal α-adrenergic stimulation on proximal tubular sodium reabsorption. Am. J. Physiol. *223*, 1201–1205 (1972)
Giudicelli, J.F., Richer, C., Chauvin, M., Idrissi, N., Berdeaux, A.: Comparative beta-adrenoceptor blocking effects and pharmacokinetics of penbutolol and propranolol in man. Br. J. Clin. Pharmacol. *4*, 135–140 (1977)
Goldberg, L.I.: Cardiovascular and renal actions of dopamine: Potential clinical applications. Pharmacol. Rev. *24*, 1–29 (1972)
Goldberg, L.I., Sonneville, F., McNay, J.L.: An investigation of the structural requirements for dopamine-like renal vasodilation: phenylethylamines and apomorphine. J. Pharmacol. Exp. Ther. *163*, 188–197 (1968)
Goldman, H.: Catecholamine-induced redistribution of blood flow in the unanesthetized rat. Am. J. Physiol. *210*, 1419–1423 (1966)
Gottshall, R.W., Itskovitz, H.D.: Redistribution of renal cortical blood flow by renal nerve stimulation and norepinephrine infusion. Proc. Soc. Exp. Biol. Med. *154*, 60–64 (1977)
Gottschalk, C.W.: Renal nerves and sodium excretion. Annu. Rev. Physiol. *41*, 229–240 (1979)
Gottschalk, C.W., Colindres, R.E., Spielman, W.S.: Neural involvement in renal function. In: Proceedings VIIth Int. Congress of Nephrology, Montreal 1978, pp. 545–552, S. Karger, London, New York, Sydney
Grängsjö, G., Persson, E.: Influence of some vaso-active substances on regional blood flow in the dog kidney. A study on normovolaemic and hypovolaemic dogs. Acta Anaesthesiol. Scand. *15*, 71–95 (1971)
Graham, R.M., Oates, H.F., Weber, M.A., Stockes, G.S.: Suppression of renin release by timolol. Arch. Int. Pharmacodyn. Ther. *219*, 205–210 (1976)
Granata, L., Braga, E.C., Cevese, A., Data, P.G.: Beta adrenergic receptor activity in peripheral vascular beds of the unanesthetized dog. Pfluegers Arch. *320*, 64–78 (1970)
Grandchamp, A., Ayer, G., Truniger, B.: Pathogenesis of redistribution of intrarenal blood flow in haemorrhagic hypotension. Eur. J. Clin. Invest. *1*, 271–276 (1971a)
Grandchamp, A., Veyrat, R., Rosset, E., Scherrer, J.R., Truniger, B.: Relationship between renin and intrarenal hemodynamics in hemorrhagic hypotension. J. Clin. Invest. *50*, 970–978 (1971b)
Green, A.F., Sim, M.F.: Diuresis in rats: Effects of sympathomimetic and sympathetic blocking agents. Br. J. Pharmacol. Chemother. *17*, 464–472 (1961)
Greven, J.: Evidence for redistribution of filtrate among nephrons after β-adrenergic stimulation and blockade. Naunyn Schmiedebergs Arch. Pharmacol. *282*, 171–180 (1974a)
Greven, J.: Clearance-, Mikropunktions- und Stoffwechselversuche zur renalen Wirkung von Sympathomimetica und Sympatholytica. Habilitationsschrift, Aachen, 1974b
Greven, J.: Fluid reabsorption in the loops of Henle and the distal convoluted tubules of the rat kidney after β-adrenergic stimulation and blockade. Naunyn Schmiedebergs Arch. Pharmacol. *285*, R23 (1974c)
Greven, J., Charl, F.J.: Effect of dopamine on the glucose release of the rat kidney in vivo (abstr.). Joint Meeting of German and Italian Pharmacologists 1977, p. 315
Greven, J., Heidenreich, O.: A micropuncture study of the effect of isoprenaline on renal tubular fluid and electrolyte transport in the rat. Naunyn Schmiedebergs Arch. Pharmacol. *287*, 117–128 (1975)
Greven, J., Klein, H.: Effects of dopamine on whole kidney function and proximal transtubular volume fluxes in the rat. Naunyn Schmiedebergs Arch. Pharmacol. *296*, 289–292 (1977)
Greven, J., Jacobs, W., van Eys, B.: Glucose release of the rat kidney in vivo after β-adrenergic stimulation and blockade. Naunyn Schmiedebergs Arch. Pharmacol. *282*, R27 (1974)

Greven, J., van Eys, B., Jacobs, W.: Stimulation of glucose release of the rat kidney in vivo by epinephrine and isoprenaline. Pharmacology *13*, 265–271 (1975)
Guder, W.G.: Hormonal regulation of renal gluconeogenesis in isolated tubule fragments. Curr. Probl. Clin. Biochem. *6*, 202–213 (1976)
Guder, W.G., Rupprecht, A.: α-adrenergic stimulation of renal gluconeogenesis in isolated kidney tubules. Hoppe Seylers Z. Physiol. Chem. *355*, 1200 (1974)
Guder, G., Rupprecht, A.: Metabolism of isolated kidney tubules. Independent actions of catecholamines on renal cyclic adenosine 3′,5′monophosphate levels and gluconeogenesis. Eur. J. Biochem. *52*, 283–290 (1975a)
Guder, W.G., Rupprecht, A.: Antagonism between parathyroid hormone and norepinephrine on cyclic adenosine-3′:5′-monophosphate (cAMP) levels in isolated tubules from rat kidney cortex. Pfluegers Arch. *354*, 177–186 (1975b)
Guder, W.G., Wieland, O.H.: Metabolism of isolated kidney tubules. Additive effects of parathyroid hormone and free-fatty acids on renal gluconeogenesis. Eur. J. Biochem. *31*, 69–79 (1972)
Gutkin, M., Das, B., Chin, B.K., Mezey, K., Modlinger, R.S.: Synergistic effects of hydralazine and alpha- or beta-adrenergic blockers: The role of plasma renin activity. J. Clin. Pharmacol. *17*, 509–518 (1977)
Handler, J.S., Bensinger, R., Orloff, J.: Effect of adrenergic agents on toad bladder response to ADH, 3′- 5′AMP, and theophylline. Am. J. Physiol. *215*, 1024–1031 (1968)
Handley, C.A., Moyer, J.H.: Unilateral adrenergic blockade and the renal response to vasopressor agents and to hemorrhage. J. Pharmacol. Exp. Ther. *112*, 1–7 (1954)
Harada, E., Rubin, R.P.: Stimulation of renin secretion and calcium efflux from the isolated perfused cat kidney by noradrenaline after prolonged calcium deprivation. J. Physiol. (Lond.) *274*, 367–379 (1978)
Hardaker, W.T., Wechsler, A.S.: Redistribution of cortical blood flow during renal vasodilation in dogs. Circ. Res. *33*, 437–444 (1973)
Hardt, D., Gross, R., Kirchheim, H.: Demonstration of a beta adrenergic dilatation of renal vessels in the awake dog. Pfluegers Arch. *327*, 152–166 (1971)
Hashimoto, K., Kokubun, H.: Adenosine-catecholamine interaction in the renal vascular response. Proc. Soc. Exp. Biol. Med. *136*, 1125–1128 (1971)
Hashimoto, K., Yasuda, K., Sato, S.: Renal vascular effect of dipyridamole: Potentiation of norepinephrine and adenosine. Eur. J. Pharmacol. *10*, 385–388 (1970)
Hedqvist, P., Fredholm, B.B., Ölundh, S.: Antagonistic effects of theophylline and adenosine on adrenergic neuroeffector transmission in the rabbit kidney. Circ. Res. *43*, 592–598 (1978)
Heidenreich, O.: Die Wirkung von Sympathomimetica auf die Nierenfunktion und ihre Beeinflussung durch alpha- und beta-Rezeptorenblocker. In: Beta-Rezeptorenblockade in Klinik und Experiment. Internationales Symposion in Wien am 17. und 18. 3. 1967. Moser, K., Lujf, A. (Hrsg.). Wien: Hollinek 1967
Heidenreich, O., Laaff, H., Fülgraff, G., Balshüsemann, E.: Die Wirkung von Orciprenalin, Isoprenalin und Propranolol auf die Nierenfunktion des Hundes. Naunyn Schmiedebergs Arch. Pharmacol. *255*, 23–24 (1966)
Heidenreich, O., Fülgraff, G., Laaff, H., Balshuesemann, E.: Die Wirkung von β-Sympathomimetica und Sympatholytica auf die Nierenfunktion von Hunden. Naunyn Schmiedebergs Arch. Pharmacol. *263*, 439–449 (1969)
Heierli, D., Thoelen, H., Radielovic, P.: Renal function following a single dose of pindolol in hypertensive patients with varying degrees of impairment of renal function. Int. J. Clin. Pharmacol. Biopharm. *15*, 65–71 (1977)
Heintze, K.: Die Wirkung von Sympathomimetica und Sympatholytica auf die renale Elektrolyt- und Wasserausscheidung bei Ratten. Inauguraldissertation, Freiburg 1968
Heintze, K., Heidenreich, O.: Die Wirkung von Sympathicomimetica und α- und β-Receptorenblockern auf die Nierenfunktion von Ratten. Naunyn Schmiedebergs Arch. Pharmacol. *260*, 137–138 (1968)
Henry, D.P., Aoi, W., Weinberger, M.H.: The effects of dopamine on renin release in vitro. Endocrinology *101*, 279–283 (1977)
Hernandez, T., Coulson, R.A.: Sympathomimetic action of xanthine diuretics in the alligator. Am. J. Physiol. *185*, 201–204 (1956)

Heurich, W.L., Schrier, R.W., Berl, T.: Mechanism of renin secretion during hemorrhage in the dog. J. Clin. Invest. *64*, 1–7 (1979)
Heyndrickx, G.R., Boettcher, D.H., Vatner, S.F.: Effects of angiotensin, vasopressin, and methoxamine on cardiac function and blood flow distribution in conscious dogs. Am. J. Physiol. *231*, 1579–1587 (1976)
Höfgen, K.U., Laudage, G., Von Lilienfeld-Toal, H., Gugler, R., Bodem, G.: Relationship between the blood level and the inhibitory effect of renin activation under beta-receptor blockade using pindolol. Verh. Dtsch. Ges. Inn. Med. *82*, 1337–1339 (1976)
Hofbauer, K.G., Zschiedrich, H., Gross, F.: Regulation of renin release and intrarenal formation of angiotensin. Studies in the isolated perfused rat kidney. Clin. Exp. Pharmacol. Physiol. *3*, 73–93 (1976)
Hollenberg, N.K., Adams, D.F., Rashid, A., Epstein, M., Abrams, H.L., Merrill, J.P.: Renal vascular response to salt restriction in normal man. Evidence against adrenergic mediation. Circulation *43*, 845–851 (1971)
Hook, J.B., Bailie, M.D.: Perinatal renal pharmacology. Annu. Rev. Pharmacol. Toxicol. *19*, 491–509 (1979)
Hornych, H., Beaufils, M., Richet, G.: The effect of exogenous angiotensin on superficial and deep glomeruli in the rat kidney. Kidney Int. *2*, 336–372 (1972)
Horres, A.D., Eversole, W.J., Rock, M.: Adrenal hormones in water diuresis. Proc. Soc. Exp. Biol. Med. *75*, 58–61 (1960)
Hsu, L., Lilley, J.J., Stone, R.A.: Endogenous adrenergic regulation of renin release in normotensive man. Clin. Endocrinol. (Oxf.) *7*, 233–243 (1977)
Hwang, C.T., Tsutsumi, E., Suzuki, H., Takano, K., Matoba, N.: Experimental study of the isolated canine kidney perfusion with special reference to effects of various vasodilator agents. Tohoku J. Exp. Med. *101*, 161–173 (1970)
Hysell, J.W., Bohr, D.F.: Renal vascular response to plasma and to known vasoactive substances. Proc. Soc. Exp. Biol. Med. *135*, 930–933 (1970)
Iino, Y., Brenner, B.M.: Stimulation of chloride transport by isoproterenol in isolated rabbit cortical collecting tubule. Kidney Int. *16*, 821 (1979)
Imbert, M., Charbadès, D., Montegut, M., Clique, A., Morel, F.: Vasopressin dependent adenylate cyclase in single segments of rabbit kidney tubule. Pfluegers Arch. *357*, 173–187 (1975)
Imbs, J.L., Schmidt, M., Schwartz, J.: Effect of dopamine on renin secretion in the anesthetized dog. Eur. J. Pharmacol. *33*, 151–157 (1975)
Imbs, J.L., Schmidy, M., Spach, M.O., Schwartz, J.: Effet de propranolol sur la concentration des urines. Nouv. Presse Med. *5*, 211 (1976)
Imbs, J.L., Spach, M.O., Smidy, M., Schwartz, J.: Effet du propranolol sur la concentration des urines. Therapie *32*, 329–335 (1977)
Jarecki, M., Thoren, P.N., Donald, D.E.: Release of renin by the carotid baroreflex in anesthetized dogs. Circ. Rec. *42*, 614–619 (1978)
Johannesen, J., Lie, M., Mathisen, O., Kiil, F.: Dopamine-induced dissociation between renal metabolic rate and sodium reabsorption. Am. J. Physiol. *230*, 1126–1131 (1976)
Johns, E.J., Richards, H.K., Singer, B.: Effects of adrenaline, noradrenaline, isoprenaline and salbutamol on the production and release of renin by isolated renal cortical cells of the cat. Br. J. Pharmacol. *53*, 67–73 (1975)
Johnson, B.F., Smith, I.K., Labrooy, J., Bye, C.: The nature of the beta-adrenoceptor controlling plasma renin activity in man. Clin. Sci. Mol. Med. *51*, 113 s–115 s (1976)
Johnson, J.A., Davis, J.O., Gotshall, R.W., Lohmeier, T.E., Davis, J.l., Braverman, B., Tempel, G.E.: Evidence for an intrarenal beta receptor in control of renin release. Am. J. Physiol. *230*, 410–418 (1976)
Jose, P.A., Logan, A., Slotkoff, L.M., Lilienfield, L., Calcagno, P.L., Eisner, G.: Block: Intrarenal flow distribution in canine puppies. In: Intrarenal blood flow distribution in the maturing kidney. Blaufox, M.D., Funck-Brentano, J.L. (eds.), pp. 87–91. New York: Grune & Stratton 1972
Jose, P.A., Slotkoff, L.M., Lillienfield, L.S., Calcagno, P.L., Eisner, G.M.: Sensitivity of neonatal renal vasculature to epinephrine. Am. J. Physiol. *226*, 796–799 (1974)
Kapur, B.M., Kharsiing, W.: Evaluation of regional adrenergic blockade of donor kidney in canine renal allotransplantation. Indian J. Med. Res. *62*, 1247–1250 (1974)

Keeton, T.K., Pettinger, W.A., Campbell, W.B.: The effects of altered sodium balance and adrenergic blockade on renin release induced in rats by angiotensin antagonism. Circ. Res. *38*, 531–539 (1976)
Kendrick, J.E., Matson, G.L.: Effects of carotid occlusion on the renal and iliac vascular resistance during constant flow and constant pressure perfusion. Proc. Soc. Exp. Biol. Med. *142*, 1306–1309 (1973)
Kilcoyne, M.M., Cannon, P.J.: Neural and humoral influences on intrarenal blood flow distribution during thoracic caval occlusion. Am. J. Physiol. *220*, 1231–1237 (1971)
Kinne, R., Schwartz, I.L.: Isolated membrane vesicles in the evaluation of the nature, localisation and regulation of renal transport processes. Kidney Int. *14*, 547–556 (1978)
Kiowski, W., Julius, S.: Renin response to stimulation of cardiopulmonary mechanoreceptors in man. J. Clin. Invest. *62*, 656–663 (1978)
Kirchner, K.A., Kotchen, T.A., Galla, J.H., Luke, R.B.: Importance of chloride for acute inhibition of renin by sodium chloride. Am. J. Physiol. *235*, F444–450 (1978)
Kitzen, J.M., Ilhan, M., Cannon, J.G., Long, J.P.: α-Adrenergic activity of N, N-dimethyldopamine (DMDA). Eur. J. Pharmacol. *38*, 365–372 (1976)
Klahr, S., Nawar, T., Schoolwerth, A.: Effects of catecholamines on ammoniagenesis and glucogenesis by renal cortex in vivo. Biochim. Biophys. Acta *304*, 161–168 (1973)
Klein, L., Liberman, B., Laks, M., Kleeman, C.: Interrelated effects of antidiuretic hormone and adrenergic drugs on water metabolism. Am. J. Physiol. *221*, 1657–1665 (1971)
Klein, L.A.: β-adrenergic (isoproterenol) regulation of antidiuretic hormone. Invest. Urol. *12*, 285–290 (1975a)
Klein, L.A.: α-adrenergic (norepinephrine) effect on antidiuretic hormone activity. Invest. Urol. *13*, 159–164 (1975b)
Kords, H., Scheitza, E., Rodt, C.H.: Nierenfunktion und renaler Wasser- und Elektrolyttransport bei intravenöser Behandlung mit dem Tokolytikum Fenoterol (Partusisten). Geburtshilfe Perinatol. *180*, 266–270 (1976)
Korner, P.I., Stokes, G.S., White, S.W., Chalmers, J.P.: Role of the autonomic nervous system in the renal vasoconstriction response to hemorrhage in the rabbit. Circ. Res. *20*, 676–685 (1967)
Kovach, A.G., Szentagothai, K., Hamar, J., D'Ora, E., Nyary, I.: Effect of 1-(4-oxyphenyl)-2n-butylamino-ethanone hydrochloride on blood circulation. 2. Blood supply of hypothalamus, liver, renal cortex, myocardium and hindlimb. Arzneim. Forsch. *20*, 1659–1662 (1970)
Krebs, H.A., Yoshida, T.: Renal gluconeogenesis. II. The gluconeogenetic capacity of the kidney cortex of various species. Biochem. J. *89*, 398–400 (1963)
Kuchel, O., Buu, N.T., Unger, T.: Dopamine-sodium relationship. – Is dopamine a part of the endogenous natriuretic system? Contrib. Nephrol. *13*, 27–36 (1978)
Kurokawa, K., Massry, S.G.: Interaction between catecholamines and vasopressin on renal medullary cyclic AMP of rat. Am. J. Physiol. *225*, 825–829 (1973a)
Kurokawa, K., Massry, S.G.: Evidence for two seperate adenyl cyclase systems responding independently to parathyroid hormone and β-adrenergic agents in the renal cortex of the rat. Proc. Soc. Exp. Biol. Med. *143*, 123–126 (1973b)
Kurokawa, K., Massry, S.G.: Evidence for stimulation of renal gluconeogenesis by catecholamines. J. Clin. Invest. *52*, 961–964 (1973c)
Kurokawa, K., Lenchner, G., Massry, S.G.: Interaction between parathyroid hormone and catecholamines on renal cortical cyclic AMP. Nephron *18*, 60–67 (1977)
Lammintausta, R., Sylvaelahti, E., Iisalo, E., Kanto, J., Maentylae, R.: Selective and non-selective beta-blockade in renin release. Acta Pharmacol. Toxicol. (Kbh.) *41*, 489–496 (1977)
Laragh, J.H., Sealey, J.E.: The renin-angiotensin-aldosteron humoral system and regulation of sodium, potassium, and blood pressure homeostasis. In: Handbook of Physiology. Sect. 8: Renal Physiology. Orloff, J., Berliner, R.W. (eds.), pp. 831–908. Washington, D.C.: American Physiological Society 1973
Laubie, M., Drouillat, M.: Effects hémodynamique du propranolol chez le chien. Arch. Int. Pharmacodyn. Ther. *175*, 470–481 (1968)
Laubie, M., Drouillat, M., Rémy, C., Roblin, M.: Action de la noradrénaline sur la fonction rénale du chien (Hémodynamie-métabolisme-excrétion de l'eau et des électrolytes). Arch. Int. Pharmacodyn. Ther. *165*, 227–240 (1967)

Lauterwein, B., Boll, H., Meyer, D.K., Hertting, G.: Inhibition of furosemide-induced renin release by vasoconstrictors. Naunyn Schmiedebergs Arch. Pharmacol. *290*, 307–314 (1975)
Leenen, F.H.H., Redmond, D.P., McDonald, R.H., Jr.: Alpha and beta adrenergic-induced renin release in man. Clin. Pharmacol. Ther. *18*, 31–38 (1975)
Lees, P.: The influence of β-adrenoceptive receptor blocking agents on urinary function in the rat. Br. J. Pharmacol. *34*, 429–444 (1968)
Lees, P., Lockett, M.F.: A study of the β-adrenoceptors in rat kidneys. Br. J. Pharmacol. *20*, 135–138 (1963)
Lees, P., Lockett, M.F.: Some actions of isoprenaline and orciprenaline on perfused cat kidneys. Br. J. Pharmacol. *25*, 152–157 (1965)
Lehr, D., Mallow, J., Krukowski, M.: Copious drinking and simultaneous inhibition of urine flow elicited by β-adrenergic stimulation and α-adrenergic stimulation. J. Pharmacol. Exp. Ther. *158*, 150–163 (1967)
Leighton, K.M., Bruce, C.: Dobutamine and general anaesthesia: A study of the response of arterial pressure, heart rate and renal blood flow. Can. Anaesth. Soc. J. *23*, 176–184 (1976)
Lester, G.E., Rubin, R.P.: The role of calcium in renin secretion from the isolated perfused cat kidney. J. Physiol. (Lond.) *269*, 93–108 (1977)
Levi, J., Kleeman, C.R.: Effect of isoproterenol on water diuresis. Proc. Eur. Dial. Transplant. Assoc. *10*, 422–426 (1973)
Levi, J., Grinblat, J., Kleeman, C.R.: Effect of isoproterenol on water diuresis in rats with congenital diabetes insipidus. Am. J. Physiol. *221*, 1728–1732 (1971)
Levi, J., Coburn, J., Kleeman, C.R.: Mechanism of the antidiuretic effect of β-adrenergic stimulation in man. Arch. Intern. Med. *136*, 25–29 (1976)
Levy, S.B., Holle, R., Hsu, L., Lilley, J.J., Stone, R.A.: Physiologic and pharmacologic influences on adrenergic regulation of renin release. Clin. Pharmacol. Ther. *22*, 511–518 (1977)
Liang, C.C., Yang, M.M.: Re-investigation of the effect of adrenaline and noradrenaline on renal function in situ. J. Physiol. *220*, 19–32 (1972)
Liberman, B.L., Klein, A., Kleeman, C.R.: Effect of adrenergic blocking agents on the vasopressin inhibiting action of norepinephrine. Proc. Soc. Exp. Biol. Med. *133*, 131–134 (1970)
Liebau, G., Beyer, J., Larbig, D., Schick, K., Sekania, G., Hayduk, K.: Hemodynamic changes after angiotensin II blockade by saralasin. Klin. Wochenschr. *55*, 647–649 (1977)
Lockett, M.F., Wadley, R.: Renal actions of dihydroergocristine and of phentolamine in anaesthetized cats. Br. J. Pharmacol. *37*, 595–608 (1969)
Lohmoeller, R.M., Lohmoeller, G.J., Frohlich, E.D.: Systemic and renal hemodynamic effects of a new alpha-adrenergic blocking agent: NC 7197. Arch. Int. Pharmacodyn. Ther. *204*, 170–180 (1973)
Longo, T., Santa, A.: The effects of catecholamines on renal artery flow before and after alpha receptor blockade. Comparative experimental research on the conscious and anesthetized dog. J. Cardiovasc. Surg. (Torino) *9*, 195–200 (1968)
Lopez, G.A., Reid, I.A., Rose, J.C., Ganong, W.F.: Effect of norepinephrine on renin release and cyclic AMP content of rat kidney slices: Modification by sodium deficiency and α-adrenergic blockade. Neuroendocrinology *27*, 63–73 (1978)
Lorenzetti, O.J.: Influence of epinephrine infusion on the blood flow rate in the rat. Arch. Int. Pharmacodyn. Ther. *187*, 5–12 (1970)
Louis, W.J., Sampson, R.: Renal and vascular of dopamine and their clinical significance. Prog. Biochem. Pharmacol. *9*, 22–28 (1974)
Lowenstein, J., Steele, J.M., Jr.: Aldosterone production during dietary sodium restriction and beta-adrenergic blockade. Kidney Int. *11*, 128–135 (1977)
Mancia, G., Romero, J.C., Snepherd, J.T.: Continous inhibition of renin release in dogs by vagally innervated receptors in the cardiopulmonary region. Circ. Res. *36*, 529–535 (1975)
Mandelbaum, I., Shumacker, H.B., Jr.: The effect of mannitol and low molecular weight dextran upon renal vascular resistance during controled renal blood flow. Ann. Surg. *167*, 533–538 (1968)
Mandelbaum, I., Silbert, M., Berry, J.: Phenoxybenzamine (dibenzyline) and renal blood flow during extracorporeal circulation. J. Cardiovasc. Surg. (Torino) *8*, 73–76 (1967)
Mark, A.L., Eckstein, J.W., Abboud, F.M., Wendling, M.G.: Renal vascular responses to isoproterenol. Am. J. Physiol. *217*, 764–767 (1969)

Martin, C.J., Young, J.A.: A microperfusion investigation of the effects of a sympathomimetic and a parasympathomimetic drug on water and electrolyte fluxes in the main duct of the rat submaxillary gland. Pfluegers Arch. *327*, 303–323 (1971)
Marx, S.J., Fedak, S.A., Aurbach, G.D.: Preparation and characterization of a hormone-responsive renal plasma membrane fraction. J. Biol. Chem. *247*, 6913–6918 (1972)
May, D.G., Carter, M.K.: Effect of vasoactive agents on urine and electrolyte excretion in the chicken. Am. J. Physiol. *218*, 417–422 (1970)
McAfee, R.D.: The action of β-adrenergic site stimulating catecholamines on isolated frog skin. Biochim. Biophys. Acta *203*, 104–110 (1970)
McCombs, P.R., Berkowitz, H.D.: Adrenergic blockade and renal hemodynamics. Surgery *80*, 246–251 (1976)
McDonald, D.W., Saggerson, E.D.: Hormonal control of gluconeogenesis in tubule fragments from renal cortex of fed rats. Effects of α-adrenergic stimuli, glucagon, theophylline and papaverine. Biochem. J. *168*, 33–42 (1977)
McDonald, K.M., Kuruvila, K.C., Aisenbrey, G.A., Schrier, R.W.: Effect of α- and β-adrenergic stimulation on renal water excretion and medullary tissue cyclic AMP in intact and diabetes insipidus rats. Kidney Int. *12*, 96–103 (1977)
McDonald, R.H., Goldberg, L.I., McNay, J.L., Tuttle, E.P.: Effect of dopamine in man: Augmentation of sodium excretion, glomerular filtration rate and renal plasma flow. J. Clin. Invest. *43*, 1116–1124 (1964)
McDonald, R.H., Jr., Corder, C.N., Leenen, F.H.: Alpha and beta blockers: Effects on renin release. Prog. Brain. Res. *47*, 409–416 (1977)
McGiff, J.C., Fasy, T.M.: The relationship of the renal vascular activity of angiotensin II to the autonomic nervous system. J. Clin. Invest. *44*, 1911–1923 (1965)
McGiff, J.C., Burns, R.B., Blumenthal, M.R.: Role of acetylcholine in the renal vasoconstrictor response to sympathetic nerve stimulation in the dog. Circ. Res. *20*, 616–629 (1967)
McNay, J.L., Goldberg, L.I.: Comparison of the effects of dopamine isoproterenol, norepinephrine and bradykinine on canine renal and femoral blood flow. J. Pharmacol. Exp. Ther. *151*, 23–31 (1966)
McNay, J.L., Kishimoto, T.: Association between autoregulation and pressure dependency of renal vascular responsiveness in dogs. Circ. Res. *24*, 599–605 (1969a)
McNay, J.L., Kishimoto, T.: Selective renal vascular effects of ethacrynic acid. J. Pharmacol. Exp. Ther. *174*, 159–168 (1969b)
McNay, J.L., McDonald, R.H., Jr., Goldberg, L.I.: Direct renal vasodilation produced by dopamine in the dog. Circ. Res. *16*, 510–517 (1965)
Melada, G.A., Goldman, R.H., Luetscher, J.A., Zager, P.G.: Hemodynamics, renal function, plasma renin, and aldosterone in man after 5–14 days of bedrest. Aviat. Space Environ. Med. *46*, 1049–1055 (1975)
Melson, G.L., Chase, L.R., Aurbach, G.D.: Parathyroid hormone sensitive adenyl cyclase in isolated renal tubules. Endocrinology *86*, 511–518 (1970)
Meurer, K.A., Maxrath, L., Helber, A., Kaufman, W.: Participation of beta 1- and beta 2-adrenergic receptors on the renin-liberation. Verh. Dtsch. Ges. Inn. Med. *82*, 1296–1299 (1976)
Meyer, D.K., Herrmann, M.: Inhibitory effect of tyramine-induced release of catecholamines on renin secretion. Naunyn Schmiedebergs Arch. Pharmacol. *303*, 139–144 (1978)
Meyer, D.K., Hertting, G., Mittermayer, C.: Suppression of isoprenaline-induced increase in plasma renin concentration by vasoconstrictors in rats with nonfunctioning macula densa. Naunyn Schmiedebergs Arch. Pharmacol. *290*, 315–321 (1975a)
Meyer, D.K., Boll, H., Lauterwein, B., Hertting, G.: Inhibition of isoprenaline-induced increase in plasma renin concentration by vasoconstrictors. Experientia *31*, 1071–1072 (1975b)
Meyer, D.K., Kempter, A., Boll, H., Eisenreich, M., Hertting, G.: Alpha-adrenoceptor-mediated inhibitory effect of the sympathetic nervous system on the isoprenaline-induced increase in plasma renin concentration. Naunyn Schmiedebergs Arch. Pharmacol. *299*, 77–82 (1977)
Millard, R.W., Higgins, C.B., Franklin, D., Vatner, S.F.: Regulation of the renal circulation during serve exercise in normal dogs and dogs with experimental heart failure. Circ. Res. *31*, 881–888 (1972)

Miller, H.C., Alexander, J.W.: Use of phentolamine (regitine) to prevent and dissipate vasospasm in donor kidneys. Surg. Forum *23*, 273–275 (1972)

Miller, H.C., Alexander, J.W., Smith, E.J., Fidler, J.P.: Salutary effect of Phentolamine (regitine) on renal vasoconstriction in donor kidneys. Experimental and clinical studies. Transplantation *17*, 201–210 (1974)

Montoreano, R., Candia, O.A., Cook, P.: α- and β-adrenergic receptors in regulation of ionic transport in frog cornea. Am. J. Physiol. *230*, 1487–1493 (1976)

Morris, B.J., Nixon, R.L., Johnston, C.I.: Release of renin from glomeruli isolated from rat kidney. Clin. Exp. Pharmacol. Physiol. *3*, 37–47 (1976)

Morris, M., McCann, S.M., Orias, R.: Evidence for hormonal participation in the natriuretic and kaliuretic responses to intraventricular hypertonic saline and norepinephrine. Proc. Soc. Exp. Biol. Med. *152*, 95–98 (1976)

Mroczek, W.I., Davidov, M., Gavilovich, L., Finnerty, F.A., Jr.: The response of hypertensive patients to a hypertonic saline load after β-adrenergic blockade. Clin. Res. *18*, 511 (1970)

Müller, I., Barajas, L.: Electron microscopic and histochemical evidence for a tubular innervation in the renal cortex of the monkey. J. Ultrastruct. Res. *41*, 533–549 (1972)

Mulvehill, J.B., Hui, Y.S., Barnes, L., Palumbo, P.J., Dousa, T.P.: Glucagon-sensitive adenylate-cyclase in human renal medulla. J. Clin. Endocrinol. Metab. *42*, 380–384 (1976)

Murphy, G.P., Homsy, E.G., Scott, W.W.: Evaluation of pharmacologically induced renal vasodilatation. J. Surg. Res. *5*, 525–37 (1965)

Myers, B.D., Deen, W.M., Brenner, B.M.: Effects of norepinephrine and angiotensin II on the determinants of glomerular ultrafiltration and proximal tubule fluid reabsorption in the rat. Circ. Res. *37*, 101–110 (1975)

Nadjmabadi, M.H., Purschke, R., Tarbiat, S., Lennartz, H., Bircks, W.: Vergleichende Untersuchungen über den Einfluß von Dopamin bzw. Orciprenalin auf Herz- und Nierenfunktion nach kardiochirurgischen Eingriffen. Thoraxchir. Vask. Chir. *23*, 552–559 (1975)

Nagata, N., Rasmussen, H.: Parathyroid hormone, 3′,5′AMP, Ca^{++}, and renal gluconeogenesis. Proc. Natl. Acad. Sci. USA *65*, 368 (1970)

Nakajiama, T., Naitoh, F.: Elevation of adenosine 3′,5′-monophosphate in the perfusate of rat kidney after addition of dopamine. Eur. J. Pharmacol. *45*, 195–198 (1977)

Nakajiama, T., Naitoh, F., Kuruma, I.: Dopamine-sensitive adenylate cyclase in the rat kidney particulate preparation. Eur. J. Pharmacol. *41*, 163–169 (1977)

Nakamura, M., Nose, Y., Tomoike, H., Shirai, T., Kuroiwa, A.: Effects of koe 1366 on the distribution of intrarenal blood flow in normal canine kidneys. Arzneim. Forsch. *24*, 1325–1328 (1974)

Neely, W.A., Windham, T.L.: Cardiac and renal blood flow. Comparison of the effects of isoproterenol, phenoxybenzamine and levarterol. Arch. Surg. *100*, 249–252 (1970)

Nickel, J.F., Smythe, C.McC., Papper, E.M., Bradley, S.E.: A study of the mode of action of the adrenal medullary hormones on sodium, potassium and water excretion in man. J. Clin. Invest. *33*, 1687–1699 (1954)

Nies, A.S., McNeil, J.S., Schrier, R.W.: Mechanism of increased sodium reabsorption during propranolol administration. Circulation *44*, 596–604 (1971)

Nissen, O.I., Galskov, A.: Direct measurements of superficial and deep venous flow in the cat kidney. Effects of epinephrine, angiotensin, microspheres, and renal nerve stimulation. Circ. Res. *30*, 82–96 (1972)

Novelli, G.P., Cortessini, C., Pagliai, P., Francini, R.: Interpretation of adrenergic vasoconstriction as an aspecific rejection factor of renal homotransplants. Minerva Anestesiol. *35*, 1280–1285 (1969)

Ogle, C.W.: Urinary output of rats in response to subcutaneous injections of adrenaline. Experienta *24*, 496–497 (1968)

Oliver, J.A., Cannon, P.J.: The effect of altered sodium balance upon renal vascular reactivity to angiotensin II and norepinephrine in the dog. Mechanism of variation in angiotensin responses. J. Clin. Invest. *61*, 610–623 (1978)

Omachi, R.S., Roblie, D.E., Handler, J.S., Orloff, I.: Effects of ADH and other agents on cyclic AMP accumulation in toad bladder epithelium. Am. J. Physiol. *226*, 1152–1157 (1974)

O'Malley, K., Velasco, M., Wells, J., McNay, J.L.: Control plasma renin activity and changes in sympathetic tone as determinants of minoxidil-induced increase in plasma renin activity. J. Clin. Invest. *55*, 230–235 (1975)

Omvik, P., Enger, E., Eide, I.: Effect of sodium depletion on plasma renin concentration before and during adrenergic beta-receptor blockade with propranolol in normotensive man. Am. J. Med. *61*, 608–614 (1976)
Osborn, J.L., Hook, J.B., Bailie, M.D.: Control of renin release. Effects of d-propranolol and renal denervation on furosemide-induced renin release in the dog. Circ. Res. *41*, 481–486 (1977)
Osswald, H.: Renal effects of adenosine and their inhibition by theophylline. Naunyn Schmiedebergs Arch. Pharmacol. *288*, 79–86 (1975)
Osswald, H., Hermes, H.: Potentiation and inhibition of tubuloglomerular feedback by adenosin synergistic and antagonistic substances (abstr.). Fed. Proc. *39*, 1084 (1980)
Osswald, H., Nabakowski, G.: Correlation between renal sodium transport and kidney tissue levels of ATP and adenosine. Pfluegers Arch. [Suppl.] *382*, R 15 (1979)
Osswald, H., Northrup, T.E.: Renal adenylate cyclase systems. Contrib. Nephrol. *14*, 74–86 (1978)
Osswald, H., Schmitz, H.J., Kemper, R.: Renal action of adenosine: Effect on renin secretion in the rat. Naunyn Schmiedebergs Arch. Pharmacol. *303*, 95–99 (1978)
Pagliara, A., Goodman, A.D.: Effect of adenosine 3′,5′monophosphate on production of glucose and ammonia by renal cortex. J. Clin. Invest. *48*, 1408–1413 (1969)
Palmore, W.P., Fregly, M.J., Simpson, C.F.: Isoproterenol-induced diuresis in turkeys. Proc. Soc. Exp. Biol. Med. *154*, 602–605 (1977)
Peach, M.: Renin-angiotensin system: Biochemistry and mechanisms of action. Physiol. Rev. *57*, 313–370 (1977)
Pearson, I.E., Williams, R.L.: Analysis of direct renal actions of α- and β-adrenergic stimulation upon sodium excretion compared to acetylcholine. Br. J. Pharmacol. *33*, 223–241 (1968)
Peskar, B., Leodolter, S., Hertting, G.: Die Wirkung von Hydralazin und Dihydralazin sowie anderer blutdrucksenkender Pharmaka auf Wasseraufnahme und -abgabe bei Ratten. Naunyn Schmiedebergs Arch. Pharmacol. *264*, 292–293 (1969)
Pettinger, W.A., Keeton, K.: Altered renin release and propranolol potentiation of vasodilatory drug hypotension. J. Clin. Invest. *55*, 236–243 (1975)
Pettinger, W.A., Augusto, L., Leon, A.S.: Alteration of renin release by stress and adrenergic receptor drugs in unanesthetized rats. In: Comparative pathophysiology of circulatory disturbances. Bloor, C.M. (ed.), pp. 105–117. New York: 1972
Pettinger, W.A., Tanaka, K., Keeton, K., Campbell, W.B., Brooks, S.N.: Renin release, an artifact of anesthesia and its implications in rats. Proc. Soc. Exp. Biol. Med. *148*, 625–630 (1975)
Pettinger, W.A., Keeton, T.K., Campbell, W.B., Harper, D.C.: Evidence for a renal alpha-adrenergic receptor inhibiting renin release. Circ. Res. *38*, 338–346 (1976)
Plancheta, P., Singer, E., Kraupp, O.: Untersuchungen über die Beeinflussung der Plasmareninaktivität normotoner Ratten durch den Beta-Rezeptorenblocker Bupanolol. Arzneim. Forsch. *27*, 2063–2066 (1977)
Pomeranz, B.H., Birtch, A.G., Barger, A.C.: Neural control of intrarenal blood flow. Am. J. Physiol. *215*, 1067–1081 (1968)
Prosnitz, E.H., Zambraski, E.J., DiBona, G.F.: Mechanism of intrarenal blood flow redistribution after carotid artery occlusion. Am. J. Physiol. *232*, F167–F172 (1977)
Pryor, J.P.: Some methods of improving the immediate function of cadaver kidneys after transplantation. Ann. R. Coll. Surg. Engl. *50*, 256–267 (1972)
Pryor, J.P., Keaveny, T.V., Reed, T.W., Belzer, F.O.: Improved immediate function of experimental cadaver renal allografts by elimination of agonal vasospasm. Br. J. Surg. *58*, 184–187 (1971)
Quesada, T., Del Rio, C.G., Alba, F., De la Torre, M., Osorio, J.: Effect of somatostatin on renin secretion of isolated perfused rat kidney. Rev. Esp. Fisiol. *32*, 107–110 (1975)
Quesada, T., Garcia-Torres, L., Alba, F., Garcia del Rio, C.: The effects of dopamine on renin release in the isolated perfused rat kidney. Experientia *35*, 1205 (1979)
Rahn, K.H., Johnson, L.E., McNay, I.L.: A comparison of the β-adrenergic blocking effects and the influence on sodium excretion of propranolol and M.I. 1999. Circulation *6*, 159 (1968)

Ranges, H.A., Bradley, S.A.: Systemic and renal circulatory changes following the administration of adrenine, ephedrine and paredrinol to normal man. J. Clin. Invest. *22*, 687 (1943)
Rankin, J.H., Phernetton, T.M.: Effect of norepinephrine on the ovine umbilical circulation. Proc. Soc. Exp. Biol. Med. *152*, 312–317 (1976)
Rasmussen, H., Nagata, N.: Renal gluconeogenesis: Effects of parathyroid hormone and dibutyryl 3′5′AMP. Biochim. Biophys. Acta *215*, 17–28 (1970)
Rayson, B.M., Ray, C., Morgan, T.: A study of the interaction of catecholamines and antidiuretic hormone on water permeability and the cyclic AMP system in isolated papillae of the rat. Pfluegers Arch. *373*, 99–103 (1978)
Rector, J.B., Stein, J.H., Bay, W.H., Osgood, R.W., Ferris, T.F.: Effect of hemorrhage and vasopressor agents on distribution of renal blood flow. Am. J. Physiol. *222*, 1125–1131 (1972)
Richards, A.N., Plant, H.O.: Urine formation in the perfused kidney. The influence of adrenaline on the volume of the perfused kidney. Am. J. Physiol *59*, 184–190 (1922)
Robie, N.W., Goetter, W.E., Goldberg, L.I.: Systemic and renal hemodynamic effects of dopamine and prostaglandine A alone and in combination. Blood Vessels *11*, 86–95 (1974a)
Robie, N.W., Nutter, D.O., Mody, C., McNay, J.L.: In vivo analysis of adrenergic receptor activity of dobutamine. Circ. Res. *34*, 663–671 (1974b)
Romero, J.C., Dunlap, C.L., Strong, C.G.: The effect of indomethacin and other anti-inflammatory drugs on the renin-angiotensin system. J. Clin. Invest. *58*, 282–288 (1976)
Roobol, A., Alleyne, G.O.: Regulation of renal gluconeogenesis by calcium ions, hormones and adenosine 3′5′ cyclic monophosphate. Biochem. J. *134*, 157–165 (1973)
Rosendorff, C., Bomzon, L., Farr, J., Scriven, D.: Intrarenal distribution of blood flow in the baboon: Effect of noradrenaline and adrenergic blocking agents. Clin. Sci. Mol. Med. *45*, 7p (1973)
Rydin, H., Verney, E.B.: The inhibition of water diuresis by emotional stress and by muscular exercise. Q. J. Exp. Physiol. *27*, 343–374 (1938)
Sabbah, A.: Action des β-bloquants dans les cirrhoses décompensées. Nouv. Presse Med. *5*, 91 (1976)
Salvetti, A., Sassano, P., Poli, L., Pedrinelli, R., Arzilli, F.: The effect of the β-adrenergic blockade on patterns of urinary sodium excretion, blood pressure and plasma renin activity in patients with essential and renovascular hypertension. Eur. J. Clin. Invest. *7*, 331–336 (1977)
Scheitza, E., Rodt, C., Kords, H., Müller, G., Wernze, H.: Der Einfluß des Betamimetikums Fenoterol auf den renalen Transport von Wasser und Elektrolyten sowie auf Plasmarenin und Plasma-Aldosteron bei Normalpersonen, Schwangeren und Urämiepatienten. Verh. Dtsch. Ges. Inn. Med. *82*, 1529–1532 (1976)
Schirmeister, J., Decot, M., Hallauer, W., Willmann, H.: β-Receptoren und renale Hämodynamik des Menschen. Arzneim. Forsch. *16*, 847–849 (1966)
Schmitt, H.: The pharmacology of clonidine and related products. In: Handbook of experimental pharmacology. Vol. 39: Antihypertensive agents. Gross, F. (ed.), pp. 354–356. Berlin, Heidelberg, New York: Springer 1977
Schneyler, L.H., Thavornthon, T.: Isoproterenol-induced stimulation of sodium absorption in perfused salivary duct. Am. J. Physiol. *224*, 136–139 (1973)
Schrier, R.W.: Effects of adrenergic nervous system and catecholamines on systemic and renal hemodynamics, sodium and water excretion and renin secretion. Kidney Int. *6*, 291–306 (1974)
Schrier, R.W., Berl, T.: Mechanism of effect of α-adrenergic stimulation with norepinephrine on renal water excretion. J. Clin. Invest. *52*, 502–511 (1973)
Schrier, R.W., Lieberman, R., Ufferman, R.: Mechanism of antidiuretic effect of β-adrenergic stimulation. J. Clin. Invest. *51*, 97–111 (1972)
Schrier, R.W., Berl, T., Harbottle, J.A., McDonald, K.M.: Catecholamines and renal water excretion. Nephron *15*, 186–196 (1975)
Selkurt, E.E.: Current status of renal circulation and related nephron function in hemorrhage and experimental shock. I. Vascular mechanisms. Circ. Shock *1*, 3–15 (1974a)
Selkurt, E.E.: Current status of renal circulation and related nephron function in hemorrhage and experimental hemorrhagic shock. II. Neurohumoral and tubular mechanisms. Circ. Shock *1*, 89–97 (1974b)

Shanbour, L.L., Lindeman, R.D., Archer, L.T., Tung, S.H., Hinshaw, L.B.: Improvement of renal hemodynamics in endotoxin shock with dopamine, phenoxybenzamine and dextran. J. Pharmacol. Exp. Ther. *176*, 383–388 (1971)

Shibouta, Y., Inada, Y., Terashita, Z.-I., Nishikawa, K., Kikuchi, S.: Antidiuresis induced by β_1- and β_2-adrenergic agonists in ethanol-anesthetized rats. Eur. J. Pharmacol. *47*, 149–159 (1978)

Shibouta, Y., Nishikawa, K., Kikucki, S., Shimamoto, K.: Renal effects of propranolol, practolol and butoxamine in pentobarbital-anesthetized rats. Eur. J. Pharmacol. *53*, 201–208 (1979)

Sinaiko, A.R., Mirkin, B.L.: Isoproterenol-evoked renin release from the in situ perfused kidney. Dose response characteristics in spontaneously hypertensive and normotensive wistar rats. Circ. Res. *42*, 381–385 (1978)

Smith, H.W.: Lectures on the kidney. Lawrence, Kansas: University Extension Division, University of Kansas 1943

Smith, H.W.: The kidney. Structure and function in health and disease. New York: Oxford University Press 1951

Smythe, C.M., Nickel, J.F., Bradley, S.E.: The effect of epinephrine (USP), l-epinephrine, and l-norepinephrine on glomerular filtration rate, renal plasma flow, and the urinary excretion of sodium, potassium, and water in normal man. J. Clin. Invest. *31*, 499–506 (1952)

Solomon, H.S., Hollenberg, N.K.: Catecholamine release: Mechanism of mercury-induced vascular smooth muscle contraction. Am. J. Physiol. *229*, 8–12 (1975)

Sparks, J.C., Susic, D.: The effects of propranolol on plasma renin concentration in rats on normal and sodium deficient diets. Pharmacol. Res. Commun. *9*, 479–487 (1977)

Spencer, M.P.: The renal vascular response to vasodepressor sympathomimetics. J. Pharmacol. Exp. Ther. *116*, 237–244 (1956)

Spielman, W.S.: Blockade of the hypertonic saline induced decrease in renin release by theophylline. Kidney Int. *16*, 838 (1979)

Steele, T.H., Underwood, J.L.: Blunted norepinephrine natriuresis in the isolated spontaneously hypertensive rat kidney. Am. J. Physiol. *235*, F425–430 (1978)

Stein, J.H., Osgood, R.W., Ferris, T.F.: The effect of β-adrenergic stimulation on proximal tubular sodium reabsorption. Proc. Soc. Exp. Biol. Med. *141*, 901–905 (1972)

Stein, J.H., Boonjarern, S., Mauk, R.C., Ferris, T.F.: Mechanism of the redistribution of renal cortical blood flow during hemorrhagic hypotension in the dog. J. Clin. Invest. *52*, 39–47 (1973)

Stella, A., Dampney, R.A.L., Golin, R., Zanchetti, A.: Afferent vagal control of renin release in the anesthetized cat. Circ. Res. *43*, 107–111 (1978)

Strandhoy, I. W., Schneider, E.G., Willis, L.R., Knox, F.: Intrarenal effects of phenoxybenzamine on sodium reabsorption. J. Lab. Clin. Med. *83*, 263–269 (1974)

Strang, K.D., Vandongen, R., Poesse, M.H., Birkenhäger, W.H.: Failure of alpha-adrenergic stimulation by phenylephrine to enhance renin secretion in the isolated rat kidney. Eur. J. Pharmacol. *45*, 141–144 (1977)

Strauch, B.S., Langdon, R.G.: Tyramine, catecholamines and the action of vasopressin stimulation of water flux in toad bladders. Arch. Biochem. Biophys. *129*, 277–283 (1969)

Sullivan, J.M., Adams, D.F., Hollenberg, N.K.: Beta-adrenergic blockade in essential hypertension: Reduced release despite renal vasoconstriction. Circ. Res. *39*, 532–536 (1976)

Swain, J.A., Hyndrickx, G.R., Boettcher, D.H., Vatner, S.F.: Prostaglandin control of renal circulation in the unanesthetized dog and baboon. Am. J. Physiol. *229*, 826–830 (1975)

Tagawa, H., Vander, A.J.: Effects of adenosine compounds on renal function and renin secretion in dogs. Circ. Res. *26*, 327–338 (1970)

Taher, M.S., McLain, L.G., McDonald, K.M., Schrier, R.R.W., Gilbert, L.K., Aisenbrey, G.A., McCool, A.L.: Effect of beta-adrenergic blockade on renin response to renal nerve stimulation. J. Clin. Invest. *57*, 459–465 (1976)

Tai, H.H.: Mechanism of prostaglandin biosynthesis in rabbit kidney medulla. A rate-limiting step and the differential stimulatory actions of l-adrenaline and glutathione. Biochem. J. *160*, 577–581 (1976)

Taira, N., Yabuuchi, Y., Yamashita, S.: Profile of beta-adrenoceptors in femoral, superior mesenteric and renal vascular beds of dogs. Br. J. Pharmacol. *59*, 577–583 (1977)

Thames, M.D.: Reflex suppression of renin release by ventricular receptors with vagal afferents. Am. J. Physiol. *233*, H181–H184 (1977)
Thames, M.D.: Acetylstrophanthidin-induced reflex inhibition of canine renal sympathetic nerve activity mediated by cardiac receptors with vagal afferents. Circ. Res. *44*, 9–15 (1979)
Thames, M.D., DiBona, G.F.: Renal nerves modulate the secretion of renin mediated by non-neural mechanisms. Circ. Res. *44*, 645–652 (1979)
Thames, M.D., Jarecki, M., Donald, D.E.: Neural control of renin secretion in anesthetized dogs. Circ. Res. *42*, 237–245 (1978)
Thurau, K.: Renal hemodynamics. Am. J. Med. *36*, 698–719 (1964)
Toledo-Pereyra, L.H., Moberg, A.W., Najarian, J.S.: Optimal management of warm ischemic kidneys prior to hypothermic preservation. Transplant. Proc. *6*, 279–282 (1974)
Tomlinson, W.S., Wood, A.W.: Catecholamine-induced changes in ion transport in short-circuited frog skin and the effect of β-blockade. J. Physiol. *257*, 515–530 (1976)
Tomlinson, R.W.S., Wood, A.W.: Effect of amiloride on catecholamine-induced changes in ion transport in short-circuited frog skin. J. Membr. Biol. *40*, 135–150 (1978)
Truninger, R., Rosen, S.M., Grandchamp, A., Strebel, H., Kriek, H.R.: Redistribution of renal blood flow in haemorrhagic hypotension, role of renal nerves and circulating catecholamines. Eur. J. Clin. Invest. *1*, 277–280 (1971)
Tyssebotn, I., Kirkebø, A.: Effect of vasoactive agents on the distribution of renal cortical blood flow in dogs. Acta Physiol. Scand. *95*, 318–328 (1975)
Tyssebotn, I., Kirkebø, A.: Renal cortical blood flow distribution measured by hydrogen clearance during dopamine and acetylcholine infusion. Effect of electrode thickness and position in the cortex. Acta Physiol. Scand. *106*, 385–393 (1979)
Ueda, J., Kishimoto, T., Shimizu, H., Yamamoto, K.: Renal vascular response to ganglionic stimulants in the dog. Jap. Circulation J. *32*, 705–714 (1968)
Uranga, J.: Effect of glomerulopressin, oxytocin, and norepinephrine on glomerular pressure in the toad. Gen. Comp. Endocrinol. *20*, 515–521 (1973)
Urbaites, B.K., Waugh, W.H.: Renal effect of a lipokinetic arylomine in saline diuresis. Fed. Proc. *28*, 831 (1969)
Vander, A.J.: Effect of catecholamines and the renal nerves on renin secretion in anesthetized dogs. Am. J. Physiol. *209*, 659–662 (1965)
Vandongen, R., Greenwood, D.M.: The stimulation of renin secretion by non-vasoconstrictor infusions of adrenaline and noradrenaline in the isolated rat kidney. Clin. Sci. Mol. Med. *49*, 609–612 (1975)
Vandongen, R., Stranf, K.D., Poesse, M.H., Birkenhäger, W.H.: Suppression of renin secretion in the rat kidney by a nonvascular α-adrenergic mechanism. Circ. Res. *45*, 435–439 (1979)
Vatner, S.V.: Effects of hemorrhage on regional blood flow distribution in dogs and primates. J. Clin. Invest. *54*, 225–235 (1974)
Vesin, S., Lerlova, L., Serfova, O.: The effectiveness of vasopressors and vasodilators for pharmaco-dynamic renal angiography. ROEFO *124*, 216–225 (1976)
Vetter, H., Vetter, W., Warnholz, C., Bayer, J.M., Kaester, H., Vielhaber, K., Krueck, F.: Renin and aldosterone secretion in pheochromocytoma. Effect of chronic alpha-adrenergic receptor blockade. Am. J. Med. *60*, 866–871 (1976)
Viol, G.W., Smith, E.K., Fitzegerald, J.D.: Comparison of metoprolol and propranolol in modification of haemodynamic and renin-aldosterone responses to tilting in humans. Clin. Sci. Mol. Med. *51*, 533s–535s (1976)
Viskoper, R.J., Rosenfeeld, S., Maxwell, M.H., De Lima, J., Lupu, A.M., Rosenfeeld, J.B.: Effect of Ca 2+ binding by egta on renin release in the isolated perfused rabbit kidney. Proc. Soc. Exp. Biol. Med. *152*, 415–418 (1976)
Vlachoyannis, J., Weismueller, G., Brecht, H.M., Schoeppe, W.: Das Verhalten von Nierenfunktion und Adenyl-Cyclasensystem unter Einwirkung von Dopamin bei Kranken mit eingeschränkter Nierenleistung. Verh. Dtsch. Ges. Inn. Med. *80*, 659–665 (1974)
Vlachoyannis, J., Weismueller, G., Schoeppe, W.: Effects of dopamine on kidney function and on the adenyl-cyclase phosphodiesterase system in man. Eur. J. Clin. Invest. *6*, 131–137 (1976)
Volkman, P.H., Kohli, J.D., Goldberg, L.I., Cannon, J.G., Lee, T.: Conformational requirements for dopamine-induced vasodilation. Proc. Natl. Acad. Sci. USA *74*, 3602–3606 (1978)

Warren, D.J., Ledingham, J.G.: Effects of beta-adrenergic receptor blockade on the renal vascular response to a low sodium diet in the rabbit. Clin. Sci. Mol. Med. *48*, 533–535 (1975)
Waugh, W.H.: Evidence that renal sympathetic tone modulates the degree of natriuresis upon volume expansion. Fed. Proc. *29*, 459 (1970)
Weber, M.A., Stockes, G.S., Gain, J.M.: Comparison of the effects on renin release of beta-adrenergic antagonists with differing properties. J. Clin. Invest. *54*, 1413–1419 (1974)
Weber, M.A., Thronell, I.R., Graham, R.M., Stokes, G.S.: Beta-adrenoceptor blockade in the conscious rabbit: Effects on plasma renin activity and blood pressure. Life Sci. *17*, 959–967 (1975a)
Weber, M.A., Kleerekoper, M., Thornell, I.R., Stokes, G.S.: Effects of sodium depletion on plasma renin activity and on the urinary excretion of cyclic AMP and aldosterone in hypoparathyroid patients. J. Clin. Endocrinol. Metab. *40*, 982–987 (1975b)
Weber, T.R., Freier, D.T., Salles, C.A., Ramsburgh, S.R., Lindenauer, S.M.: Effect of phentolamine on perfusate flow characteristics during renal preservation. J. Surg. Res. *21*, 21–25 (1976)
Weinberger, M.H., Aoi, W., Henry, D.P.: Direct effect of beta-adrenergic stimulation on renin release by the rat kidney slice in vitro. Circ. Res. *37*, 318–324 (1975)
Wernze, H., Hilfenhaus, M., Rietbrock, I., Schuettke, R., Kuehn, K.: Plasma renin activity and plasma aldosterone during anaesthesia and operative stress and beta-adrenergic blockade. Anesthesiology *24*, 471–476 (1975)
Wesson, L.G.: Physiology of the human kidney, pp. 109–113. New York, London: Grune & Stratton 1969
Wiggins, R., Davies, R., Basar, I., Slater, J.D.: The inhibition of adrenergically provoked renin release by salbutamol in man. Br. J. Clin. Pharmacol. *5*, 213–215 (1978)
Wilcox, C.S., Aminoff, M.J., Kurtz, A.B., Slater, J.D.: Comparison of the renin response to dopamine and noradrenaline in normal subjects and patients with autonomic insufficiency. Clin. Sci. Mol. *46*, 481–488 (1974)
Williams, R.L., Maines, J.E., Pearson, J.E.: Comparison of cholinergic and adrenergic stimulation in the autoperfused kidney. Arch. Int. Pharmacodyn. Ther. *196*, 393–403 (1972)
Wilson, R.J., Mills, I.H., de Bono, E.: Cardiovascular reflexes and the control of aldosterone production and sodium excretion. Proc. R. Soc. Med. *62*, 1257–1258 (1969)
Winaver, J., Chaimovitz, C., Better, O.S.: Natriuretic effect of propranolol on dogs with chronic bile-duct ligation. Clin. Sci. Mol. Med. *54*, 603–607 (1978)
Yun, J.C., Delea, C.S., Bartter, F.C., Kelly, G.: Increase in renin release after sionaortic denervation and cervical vagotomy. Am. J. Physiol. *230*, 777–783 (1976)
Yun, J.C., Kelly, G., Bartter, F.C.: Suppression of renin secretion by propranolol in salt-depleted dogs. Life Sci. *21*, 237–244 (1977)
Zanchetti, A., Stella, A.: Renin release by central and reflex regulation. In: Regulation of blood pressure by central nervous system. Onesti, G. et al. (Eds.) pp. 235–250. New York: Grune & Stratton 1976
Zanchetti, A., Stella, A., Leonetti, G.: Regulation of renin secretion. Contrib. Nephrol. *8*, 44–56 (1977)
Zehner, J., Klaus, D., Klumpp, F., Lemke, R.: The influence of propranolol, practolol and theophylline on the plasma renin activity. Res. Exp. Med. (Berl.) *166*, 275–282 (1975)
Zehner, J., Klaus, D., Klumpp, F., Lemke, R.: Cyclic AMP and plasma renin activity in renal vein blood after amitryptiline, theophylline, furosemide, and beta-adrenergic blocking substances. Klin. Wochenschr. *54*, 1085–1093 (1976)
Zehr, J.E.: Neurally mediated inhibition of renin release. In: Regulation of blood pressure by central nervous system. Onesti, G. et al. (eds.) pp. 221–234. New York: Grune & Stratton 1976
Zeig, N.J., Buckley, N.M., Macy, J., Jr.: Effects of acute hemorrhage after adrenergic blockade in splenectomized dogs. Am. J. Physiol. *214*, 33–40 (1968)

CHAPTER 7

Effects of Adrenergic Activators and Inhibitors on the Urinary Tract

J. HANNAPPEL

A. The Upper Urinary Tract

I. Morphology of the Upper Urinary Tract

1. Anatomy

In the adult man the ureter is a thick-walled tube, about 25 to 30 cm in length, which arises within the renal sinus as a funnel-shaped renal pelvis into which open the calyces and renal pyramids and ends in the bladder (NOTLEY, 1978). A multicalyceal kidney is found in man and pig whereas in the rat, guinea pig, rabbit, dog, and sheep it is unicalyceal. The ureter is blood-supplied by a variable number of long arteries arising from the aorta or its branches. These arteries give off secondary branches which form a plexus on the surface of the ureter and this plexus sends small twigs into the substance of the ureter (DANIEL and SHACKMAN, 1952). The ureter receives sympathetic innervation from the spinal cord segments thoracic 6 to lumbar 2, and parasympathetic innervation in the upper two-thirds from the vagus nerve. The lower ureteral third is parasympathetically innervated from the spinal cord segments sacral 2 and 3 (SCHREYER, 1974). As early as 1869, ENGELMANN described how a number of nerves enter the ureter at two points: at the hilus renalis are a few branches from the plexus renalis; and, at the bladder end, a few somewhat larger branches arise from the sympathetic plexus. These nerve trunks build a plexus with large and long meshes in the outer fibrous coat along the whole length of the ureter. SATANI (1919) found that the outer fibrous coat of the ureter is an important seat of nerves and blood vessels. Nerve trunks which enter this coat at several points – starting from the plexus renalis, vesicalis, and spermaticus, as well as from the inferior mesenteric and other ganglia – make numerous divisions successfully connecting each other to make a plexus with long and rhomboidlike meshes.

2. Histology

In early publications, the ureter was thought to have a muscle coat of three definite layers: a circular coat which is especially strong in the middle part of the ureter, and an outer and inner longitudinal layer which increase in thickness towards the bladder (SATANI, 1919). Later, the arrangement of ureteral muscle fibers was described as a single layer which consists of bundles forming an interlacing series of spirals, each beginning as longitudinal strands in the outer region of the musculature, forming a middle circular layer as they describe their spiral turn before terminating as longitudinal fibers adjacent to the lamina propria (SCHNEIDER, 1939). The outer surface of the muscle layer is covered by the adventitia, a loose connective tissue sheath in which lie the small blood vessels, lymphatic vessels, and the bundles of unmyelinated nerves running to and from the ureter. Deep in the muscular layer lies the lamina propria, which is followed by the transitional epithelium. In transverse section, the epithelium and lamina propria tend to fall into an irregular zigzag pattern as the outer elastic layers of the ureter pull the epithelium into longitudinal folds so that the ureteric lumen is normally closed (NOTLEY, 1978).

BERGMANN (1958) described intercellular bridges in the smooth muscle layer of the ureter and suggested that they may provide a pathway for the conduction of excitation between the muscle cells. At these points, the basement membranes of the contiguous cells become fused with each other so that the plasma membrane of the two cells lie in close apposition to each other without an intervening basement membrane (NOTLEY, 1978). As to the nerve supply of ureteral musculature, there have been long discussions in the literature: SATANI (1919) described that the nerve elements in the muscle layer are usually very scanty. WEIN et al. (1972b) made histochemical observations in dogs and detected adrenergic innervation to the ureter predominantly around the blood vessels. The smooth muscle of the ureter did not appear to be innervated by adrenergic nerves. HOYES et al. (1976) stated that the low density of both adrenergic and cholinergic terminals in the intramuscular nerves implies that the autonomic nervous system plays only a secondary part in controlling the muscle activity. DEANE (1967) found a rich nerve fiber system in the adventitia of the ureter, but no nerve cells or nerve fibers in the muscle coat or in the transitional epithelium. ENGELMANN (1869) saw ganglion cells in the lowermost 3 or 4 cm of the outer fibrous coat of the ureter. At the hilus renalis and in the renal pelvis, he occasionally found a few small ganglia, whereas the ganglia in the lower ureter contained a large number of cells. The ganglia gave off numerous small branches inside the muscle coat, some of them ending as very fine fibrils between the muscle fibers, others terminating in the transitional epithelium. In the electron microscopic studies of NOTLEY (1968) it was noted that the ureter had neither ganglia nor plexus, but showed an abundant distribution of sympathetic nerve fibers in the blood vessels. NOTLEY states that some axons displaying the characteristics of terminal areas are seen in close proximity to smooth muscle cells of the ureter and, by analogy with neuromuscular junctions in other organs, they can be thought to represent efferent nerve endings. By fluorometric assay, significant concentrations of catecholamines in the ureter have been demonstrated as well as radioactive noradrenalin uptake by reserpine pretreatment. This suggests that there is significant sympathetic innervation of the ureter. However, these catecholamine data do not demonstrate whether the sympathetics innervate the blood vessels or the ureteral musculature itself (BOYARSKY et al., 1966a). DUARTE-ESCALANTE et al. (1969) made different histochemical studies and concluded that both cholinergic and adrenergic components innervate the ureter. The cholinergic innervation is better developed than the adrenergic at the ureterovesical and ureteropelvic junction. They stated that these findings are consistent with the observed actions of catecholamines on the ureter. Whichever of the two commonly postulated mechanisms proves to be correct for the ureteral smooth muscle, e.g., directly discharged on the smooth muscle or indirectly through the changes in the blood flow, there is no doubt that the innervation is rich. They observed that adrenergic and cholinergic fibers synapse at multiple points around and along the muscle fibers. These contacts include axonal varicosities containing the catecholamines or acetylcholine in granular or soluble form. Ganglion cells are consistently found in clusters in the lower ureteral segment and in a scattered distribution along the middle and the upper segments. The authors conclude that the ganglion cells might act as modulating units and even as independent units to elicit and regulate rhythmic activity. SCHULMAN (1976) in his histochemical study of fluorescent catecholamines and acetylcholinesterase has demonstrated a dual adrenergic and cholinergic innervation of human and rabbit ureter. The ureteric innervation is characterized by terminal nerve fibers and ganglia located in the terminal portion of the ureter. These ganglia are composed of cholinergic and adrenergic elements. Terminal nerve fibers do not innervate each muscle cell, and chemical transmitters liberated from *en passage* varicosities may influence at distance several muscle cells in a muscle bundle. These influences on some of the ureteric smooth muscle cells can be transmitted myogenically to the other cells via the abovementioned intercellular bridges with low electrical resistance.

II. Functional Studies in the Upper Urinary Tract

1. Pharmacologic Studies in Isolated Calyx and Renal Pelvis Preparations

In most cases, autonomic drugs do not act on nerve endings but directly on effector cells. Therefore, it might be argued that the effect of adrenergic activators and inhibitors on ureteral activity does not indicate the presence of autonomic innervation. Nevertheless pharmacologic studies are of value, presumably due to a cellular "receptive substance" which responds to nervous stimuli as well as to autonomic drugs, while such a physico-chemical differentiation does not exist in cells which do not receive nervous stimuli (KIIL, 1957). Isolated preparations of rabbit renal calyx and pelvis undergo spontaneous rhythmic changes in tension. Adrenalin and noradrenalin in-

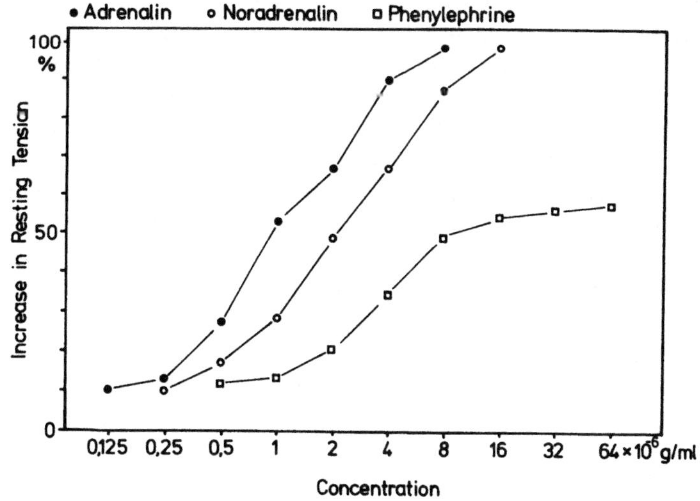

Fig. 1. Dose response curves for the effects of adrenalin, noradrenalin, and phenylephrine on isolated smooth muscle strips from pig renal calyx. The increase in resting tension is mediated via α-adrenoceptors. (LONGRIGG, 1974)

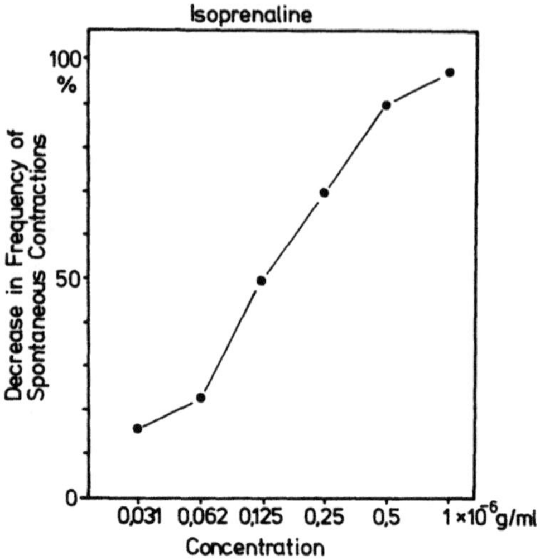

Fig. 2. Dose response curve for the effect of isoprenaline on the spontaneous activity of porcine calyx preparations. This effect can be inhibited by the application of β-receptor blocking substances. A 100% decrease in frequency means complete cessation of spontaneous activity. (LONGRIGG, 1974)

crease both the rate of contractions and the resting tone of the preparations (GOSLING and WAAS, 1971). Also in preparations of human minor calyces, adrenalin, and noradrenalin did effectively increase resting tension and frequency of spontaneous contractions. Phenylephrine (a predominantly α-stimulating agent) caused similar effects. The actions were antagonized by phentolamine, and it was noted that an EC_{50} dose of noradrenalin could be prevented by prior incubation with a dose of phentolamine as low as 1.6×10^{-7} g/ml. This high degree of specificity of the antagonism is suggestive of the observed responses to adrenalin, noradrenalin, and phenylephrine having been mediated via α-adrenoceptors. Isoprenaline, a synthetic catecholamine with predominantly β-stimulatory actions, was completely devoid of inhibitory effects upon the frequency and resting tension of the spontaneously contracting human minor calyx when used in a dosage similar to that used effectively in pig tissue. However, when the dose of isoprenaline was increased, there appeared an excitatory response resembling α-adrenoceptor stimulation, and this response could be abolished by phentolamine but not by propranolol. Thus, no evidence could be produced to support the presence of β-adrenoceptors in the smooth muscle of human minor calyces (DEL TACCA et al., 1974; LONGRIGG, 1975b). Other experiments were made to ascertain the effect of thyramine on isolated minor calyces from pigs. Thyramine is a sympathomimetic amine and predominantly acting by the release of noradrenalin from sympathetic postganglionic nerve endings. Its addition to the organ bath fluid in high concentrations caused a response similar to α-adrenoceptor stimulation. However, pretreatment of the tissue with cocaine (thus preventing the neuronal uptake of thyramine) did not alter this response, and it was concluded that the effect upon the calyx was direct upon smooth muscle cells and unrelated to noradrenalin release. After liberation of noradrenalin from adrenergic nerves, the major route of inactivation is an

Table 1. Effects of adrenergic activators and inhibitors on the renal calyx and pelvis

Author	Species	Method	α-Receptors	β-Receptors
Björk (1976)	Human	In vivo cineradiography	Adrenalin: phasic and tonic activation	
Del Tacca et al. (1974)	Human, rabbit	In vitro muscle strips	Phenylephrine, adrenalin, and noradrenalin: phasic and tonic activation; blocked by phentolamine	Isoprenaline: no response
Finberg and Peart (1970)	Rat	In vitro muscle strips	Adrenalin and noradrenalin: phasic and tonic activation	Isoprenaline: phasic inhibition
Golenhofen and Hannappel (1978)	Pig, rabbit	In vitro muscle strips	Adrenalin: phasic and tonic activation (in rabbits only phasic)	
Gosling and Waas (1971)	Rabbit	In vitro muscle strips	Adrenalin and noradrenalin: phasic and tonic activation; blocked by phentolamine, not changed by propranolol	
Hannappel and Golenhofen (1974)	Rat, guinea pig, dog	In vitro muscle strips, in vivo electromyogram	In the most intrarenal areas α-receptors predominant	In the pyeloureteral junction β-receptors predominant
Longrigg (1974)	Pig	In vitro muscle strips	Phenylephrine, adrenalin, and noradrenalin: phasic and tonic activation, blocked by phentolamine	Adrenalin after pretreatment with phentolamine and isoprenaline: phasic and tonic inhibition; blocked by propranolol
Longrigg (1975b)	Human	In vitro muscle strips from calyx	Phenylephrine, adrenalin, and noradrenalin: phasic and tonic activation; blocked by phentolamine	Isoprenaline: no response
Longrigg (1975c)	Human	In vitro muscle strips from renal pelvis	Phenylephrine, adrenalin, and noradrenalin: phasic and tonic activation; blocked by phentolamine	Isoprenaline: no response
Vereecken et al. (1972)	Dog	In vivo electromyogram and pressure	α-Receptors predominant in renal calyx and pelvis	

active reuptake by the nerve terminals. This uptake process does not only apply to the intact animal, but also to exogenously administered noradrenalin on an isolated tissue preparation. Abolition of neuronal uptake can be obtained by treating the tissue with cocaine which prevents active transport of noradrenalin from the extracellular fluid to the intra-axonal storage areas, and thereby potentiates the effect of this drug. However, no quantitative difference in response of the calyx to noradrenalin could be determined before and after treatment with cocaine. The results from experiments with cocaine and thyramine suggest that the innervation is relatively sparse (LONGRIGG, 1974). These findings are consistent with anatomical studies of the region (DIXON and GOSLING, 1971). It was demonstrated that the renal pelvis of rats and dogs has a much higher sensibility to α-adrenergic drugs than the same tissue from guinea pigs. In renal pelvis strips from guinea pigs, also no β-adrenergic response could be found (GOLENHOFEN and HANNAPPEL, 1972). In pigs, EC_{50} values calculated for the α-adrenergic effects of adrenalin and noradrenalin, revealed a far greater sensibility to these drugs of calyceal compared with pelvic muscle, the latter in turn being more sensitive than preparations of the ureter (LONGRIGG, 1976).

2. Pharmacologic Studies in Isolated Ureter Preparations

Myogenic pacemaker areas are localized for unicalyceal kidneys in the utmost renal ends of the pelvis and for multicalyceal systems in the calyces. Here ureteral peristalsis takes its origin and is conducted myogenically towards the bladder (GOLENHOFEN and HANNAPPEL, 1973a). In isolated ureter preparations, the effects of various drugs on the ureteric musculature can be studied excluding the influences on pacemaker activity. DEANE and GARRY (1966) using isolated porcine ureters found that adrenalin (10^{-7} g/ml) and noradrenalin (10^{-7} g/ml) both caused an increase in tone and frequency of concentration. In the presence of phenoxybenzamine (10^{-7}–10^{-5} g/ml),

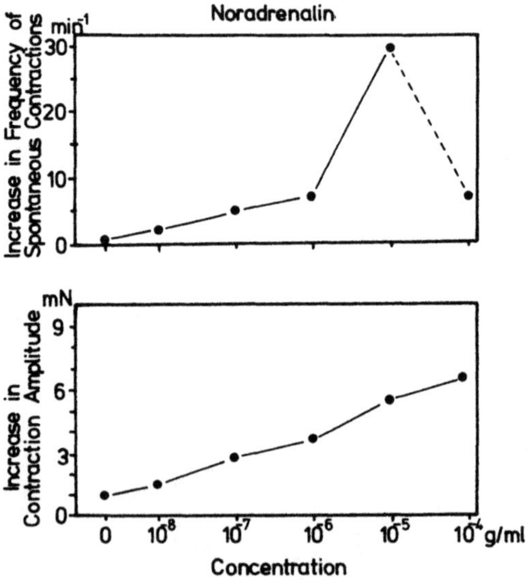

Fig. 3. In vitro dose response curves for the α-excitatory effects on ureteral musculature from dogs. (MALIN et al., 1968)

adrenalin and noradrenalin decreased tone and abolished contractions. Isoprenaline (10^{-7} g/ml) decreased tone and activity, and this action was abolished by pronethalol at concentrations from 10^{-7}–10^{-5} g/ml. There is thus evidence for the existence of both α- and β-adrenergic receptors in the smooth muscle of the ureter. The α-receptors are "dominant" and motor in effect. When these are blocked, "recessive" β-receptors are revealed which are inhibitory (DEANE, 1967). Also in isolated ureters of dogs, the whole muscle becomes more excitable after application of adrenalin as is shown by the conduction velocity, the increase of contraction frequency, and the occurrence of antiperistaltic contractions. Here, too, the activation produced by adrenalin runs along the α-receptors since α-blockers abolish the effects. The inhibition of the ureter activity produced by adrenalin after phenoxybenzamine administration may be an effect on the recessive β-adrenergic receptors (VEREECKEN et al., 1972). These results are also valid for human specimens (MALIN et al., 1970). Isolated guinea pig and rat ureters are not spontaneously active under normal conditions. Activity can easily be induced by adrenalin and noradrenalin in rat ureter, but not in guinea pig ureter (HANNAPPEL and GOLENHOFEN, 1974). The isolated rabbit ureter also fails to contract spontaneously and remains unresponsive to a variety of drugs, inclusive adrenergic substances (GOSLING and WAAS, 1971; HANNAPPEL and LUTZEYER, 1978).

The neonatal rabbit ureter undergoes a greater degree of diametral change in response to an applied intraluminal pressure than does the adult ureteral segment. After application of noradrenalin (10^{-5} mol/l), the degree of deformation of the neonatal ureter approximates the magnitude of deformation of the adult ureter in response to a given pressure load. This concentration of noradrenalin has no significant effects on adult ureteral segments. The reasons for the differences in the sensitivity of the isolated neonatal and isolated adult ureters to catecholamines is unknown (AKIMOTO et al., 1977). Perhaps this result relates to the incomplete development of sympathetic innervation of young ureters, as described by SCHULMAN (1974).

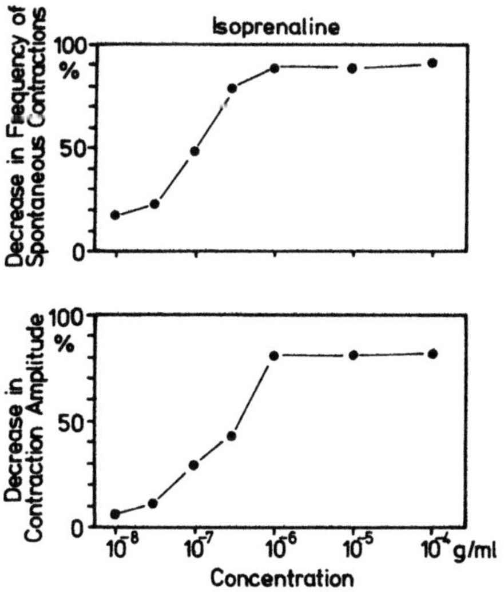

Fig. 4. In vitro dose response curves for the β-inhibitory effects on ureteral musculature from dogs. (MALIN et al., 1968)

Table 2. Effects of adrenergic activators and inhibitors on the ureter

Author	Species	Method	α-Receptors	β-Receptors
ANCILL et al. (1971)	Rat	In vivo electromyogram		Adrenalin, noradrenalin, and isoprenaline: inhibition of phasic activity; blocked by propranolol
ANCILL et al. (1972)	Rat	In vivo electromyogram renal vessels ligated ureter perfused		Adrenalin, noradrenalin, and isoprenaline: inhibition of phasic activity; blocked by propranolol
BOATMAN et al. (1967)	Dog	In vivo pressure recordings	Adrenalin and noradrenalin: increase in perfusion pressure; blocked by phentolamine	Adrenalin after pretreatment with phentolamine and isoprenaline: no change in perfusion pressure
BOYARSKY et al. (1966b)	Dog	In vivo pressure recordings	Adrenal compression: bilateral phasic activation; blocked by phentolamine	
CASTEELS et al. (1971)	Guinea pig	In vitro intracellular recordings	Adrenalin and noradrenalin: phasic and tonic activation, prolongation of action potential; activating effects of phenoxybenzamine and phentolamine	Isoprenaline: inhibition of tonic activity, no influence on action potential
DEANE and GARRY (1966)	Pig	In vitro pressure recordings	Adrenalin and noradrenalin: phasic and tonic activation	Adrenalin and noradrenalin after pretreatment with phenoxybenzamine: inhibition of phasic and tonic activity, blocked by pronethalol
DEANE (1967)	Pig	In vitro pressure recordings	Adrenalin and noradrenalin: phasic and tonic activation	Isoprenaline: inhibition of phasic and tonic avtivity
GOLENHOFEN and HANNAPPEL (1972)	Rat, guinea pig, dog	In vitro muscle strips	Activation predominant in proximal regions	Inhibition predominant in distal regions
GONZALES (1973)	Rat	In vitro sucrose gap	Noradrenalin: increase in spike activity	
GOSLING and WAAS (1971)	Rabbit	In vitro muscle strips	No spontaneous activity, no activity after α-receptor stimulation	

HANNAPPEL and GOLENHOFEN (1974)	Rat, guinea pig, dog	In vitro muscle strips, in vivo electromyogram	Adrenalin and noradrenalin after pretreatment with propranolol: increase in phasic activity	Noradrenalin and orciprenaline after pretreatment with phentolamine: decrease in phasic activity
HANNAPPEL and LUTZEYER (1978)	Rabbit	In vitro muscle strips	No spontaneous activity, no activity after α-receptor stimulation	
HAUBENSACK and MÜLLER (1973)	Human	In vitro electromyogram and pressure recordings	Adrenalin and noradrenalin: phasic and tonic activation; blocked by phentolamine	Adrenalin after pretreatment with phentolamine and orciprenaline: inhibition of phasic activity
JACKSON et al. (1970)	Rat	In vivo electromyogram		Adrenalin, noradrenalin, and isoprenaline: inhibition of phasic activity; blocked by propranolol
KAPLAN et al. (1968)	Dog	In vivo cineradiography pressure recordings flow studies	Adrenalin and noradrenalin: phasic and tonic activation; blocked by phenoxybenzamine	Adrenalin after pretreatment with phenoxybenzamine: sometimes slight activation
KIIL and KJEKSHUS (1967)	Dog	In vivo cineradiography pressure recordings flow studies	Adrenalin and noradrenalin: phasic and tonic activation; phenoxybenzamine is not able to block this effect completely	Isoprenaline: inhibition of phasic activity
LONGRIGG (1975a)	Human	In vivo pressure recordings	Blockade of α-receptors with phentolamine: inhibition of phasic and tonic activity	Isoprenaline: inhibition of phasic activity
MALATINSKY and HAUBENSACK (1971)	Dog	In vivo electromyogram	Adrenalin: phasic activation	
MALIN et al. (1968)	Human, dog	In vitro muscle strips	Noradrenalin: phasic activation	Isoprenaline: inhibition of phasic activity
MALIN et al. (1970)	Human	In vitro length recordings	Adrenalin and noradrenalin: phasic and tonic activation	Isoprenaline: inhibition of phasic activity (only in the lower third of the ureter)
MELCHIOR et al. (1971a)	Dog	In vivo pressure recordings flow studies	Adrenalin and noradrenalin: phasic activation; blocked by phentolamine and phenoxybenzamine	Isoprenaline: inhibition of phasic activity
MELCHIOR et al. (1971a)	Human, dog	In vivo pressure recordings flow studies		Isoprenaline: inhibition of phasic activity
RAZ et al. (1972b)	Rat	In vitro muscle strips	α-Receptors predominant after estrogen pretreatment	β-Receptors predominant after progesterone pretreatment

Table 2 (continued)

Author	Species	Method	α-Receptors	β-Receptors
Reid et al. (1974)	Dog	In vivo pressure recordings		Isoprenaline: inhibition of phasic activity
Struthers (1973)	Dog	In vivo pressure recordings	Phenylephrine: phasic activation; blocked by phentolamine	Isoprenaline: inhibition of phasic activity
Tindall (1972)	Rat	In vivo electromyogram	Activation, predominant in proximal regions	Inhibition, predominant in distal regions
Tsuchida and Sakamoto (1974)	Dog	In vivo electromyogram	Adrenalin and noradrenalin: phasic activation; blocked by phentolamine	Isoprenaline: inhibition of phasic activity; blocked by propranolol
Tsuchida et al. (1873)	Dog	In vivo electromyogram	Phenylephrine, adrenalin, and noradrenalin: phasic activation	Adrenalin after pretreatment with phentolamine: inhibition of phasic activity
Vereecken et al. (1971)	Guinea pig	In vitro intracellular recordings	Adrenalin and noradrenalin: slight depolarization of resting potential and prolongation of action potential	
Vereecken et al. (1972)	Dog	In vivo electromyogram and pressure recordings, in vitro pressure recordings	Adrenalin and noradrenalin: phasic and tonic activation; blocked by phenoxybenzamine	Isoprenaline: inhibition of phasic activity (only in the lower part of the ureter)
Washizu (1968)	Guinea pig	In vitro intracellular recordings	Adrenalin: slight depolarization of resting potential and prolongation of action potential	

3. Pharmacologic Studies in Isolated Pyeloureter Preparations

An isolated pyeloureter of the guinea pig will contract in the organ bath at 37 °C at its normal in situ rate only if the preparation includes the utmost renal ends of the pelvis. This spontaneous activity was not affected under the influence of tetrodotoxin up to a concentration of 3×10^{-6} g/ml. Therefore, the contribution of nervous elements can be excluded, and thus the spontaneous generation of excitation in the pyeloureter is myogenic (GOLENHOFEN and HANNAPPEL, 1973b). In such a completely isolated pyeloureter of a guinea pig containing the primary pacemaker, adrenalin, and noradrenalin have weak effects in a normal concentration range (up to 10^{-6} g/ml). However, pronounced reactions to adrenalin and noradrenalin can be found in completely isolated pyeloureter preparations of dog and rat. MALIN et al. (1970) demonstrated α-adrenergic receptors in the human ureter; β-adrenergic receptors could be found only in the distal regions. In isolated pyeloureter preparations of the rat could be observed (after blockade of the α-component with phenoxybenzamine) that the activity in the renal pelvis continued at the normal rate during administration of adrenalin, while the activity in the distal ureter was completely suppressed due to a conduction block. Thus, adrenergic activation is strongest in the proximal regions and declines towards distal parts, whereas β-adrenergic inhibition increases towards distal regions of the pyeloureter (GOLENHOFEN and HANNAPPEL, 1973b).

In isolated rat pyeloureter, adrenalin, and noradrenalin have very similar effects; in dog pyeloureter, adrenalin exerts pure α-stimulation, and noradrenalin stimulates both α- and β-receptors. This observation indicates that species differences exist in the affinity of adrenergic receptors to adrenalin and noradrenalin. This could be additionally demonstrated in the differences of the effect of phentolamine, which is generally, in comparison with phenoxybenzamine, the less specific α-blocker. Phentolamine (10^{-6} g/ml) acts as a specific blocking agent in the dog, both in situ and in the isolated pyeloureter. In the pyeloureter of the rat, however, in addition to the α-blockade, phentolamine produces a direct α-excitatory effect, already measurable at a concentration of 10^{-6} and very strong at 10^{-5} g/ml. This indicates that the α-adrenergic receptors of the pyeloureteral system are less differentiated in rats than in dogs (HANNAPPEL and GOLENHOFEN, 1974).

Recently, the differentiation between phasic and tonic contractions in the smooth muscle system was improved by the findings that some substances of the so-called calcium antagonistic drugs are able to suppress phasic or tonic activations selectively. This led to the concept that in smooth muscle, two chemically different calcium activation systems exist which have been called the p-system (mainly responsible for phasic activity) and the t-system (mainly responsible for tonic activity). Application of adrenalin on spontaneously active renal pelvis preparations leads to an increase in contraction frequency and to an increase in tension which appears similar to the development of a tetanic contraction in skeletal muscle. The calcium antagonist nifedipine (3×10^{-7} mol/l) completely inhibits the spontaneous rhythmic activity and, under these conditions, adrenalin induces a purely tonic contraction. This shows that the adrenalin reaction cannot be interpreted as a tetanic summation of phasic contractions: it is rather a summation of phasic contractions (p-component) and a tonic activation in the strict sense (t-component). Isolated strips of ureteral smooth muscle exhibit very low spontaneous phasic activity and respond to an increasing concentration of adrenalin with a progressive increase of contraction frequency, sometimes with a fusion of the single contractions. In contrast to the pelvis preparations, the adrenalin reaction of the ureter was virtually completely inhibited by nifedipine. This indicates that in contrast to the renal pelvis, the ureter is only capable of producing phasic contractions (p-component) which sometimes may give the appearance of an incomplete tetanic contraction. These results, first obtained with porcine preparations, are also valid for the human pyeloureter (GOLENHOFEN and HANNAPPEL, 1978).

4. In Vivo Studies in the Pyeloureteral System

There are numerous publications with the results of in vivo studies in the pyeloureteral system after application of various drugs. It is often difficult to distinguish whether the alterations in ureteral peristalsis have been caused directly by the effect of drugs on the smooth muscle cell itself, or indirectly through nerve excitation. Other possibilities are changes in the blood flow to the ureter or the kidney, the latter causing changes in urine production and thus influencing the activity of the pyeloureteral system.

Some investigators failed to demonstrate α- or β-receptors in the upper urinary tract. BOATMAN et al. (1967) were unable to produce ureteral dilatation in dogs with isoproterenol. Moreover, absence of relaxation was noted with adrenalin following pretreatment with phentolamine. So they concluded lack of β-receptors in ureteral muscle. Similar to these results, STRUTHERS (1973) found a marked increase in the frequency of ureteric contractions, and a slight rise in pelvis pressure after stimulation with phenylephrine 2×10^{-5} g/min to a total dose of 1.4×10^{-4} g. When phentolamine was given to block the α-receptors, and the ureter again challenged with phenylephrine, no change in ureteric contraction was observed. Isoproterenol was given to stimulate the β-receptors, and was infused in a rate of 5×10^{-6} g/min to a total dose of 2.5×10^{-5} g, but no clear effects were observed. He had done his experiments in dogs with pelvicostomy at one side and nephrostomy at the other side. Contrary results were presented by ANCILL et al. (1972). They tried to exclude indirect ureteric responses to catecholamine application and, therefore, perfused in situ the ureter from a reservoir. Thereafter, the effect of isoprenaline, noradrenalin, and adrenalin was always a reduction in the frequency of peristalsis. Since the inhibitory response of all three amines was prevented by propanolol, they concluded that these drugs probably act on β-adrenoceptors, and that there might be no α-receptors in the rat ureter.

However, in most of the in situ studies on ureteral activity, α- as well as β-receptors have been demonstrated. The effect of adrenalin was investigated in various animals using different in vivo methods like electromyogram, ureteral pressure recordings, and transureteral flow studies. Many investigators found activation concerning contraction frequency and pressure amplitude.

α-Blocking substances like phentolamine or phenoxybenzamine suppressed these effects, and even caused β-receptor mediated inhibition following the application of adrenalin (BOATMAN et al., 1967; TSUCHIDA et al., 1973; HANNAPPEL and GOLENHOFEN, 1974; TSUCHIDA and SAKAMOTO, 1974). Even after adrenal compression, ureteral peristalsis was stimulated in dogs, probably by the release of endogenous catecholamines (BOYARSKY et al., 1966b). The threshold concentration for the α-excitatory effect of adrenalin on ureteral activity was found at 0.5×10^{-7}–10^{-6} g/kg × min (HANNAP-

PEL and GOLENHOFEN, 1974). TINDALL (1972) recorded electrical and mechanical activity from the rat ureter in situ and demonstrated with a close arterial injection technique that the proximal ureter behaves as if it possessed α-receptors, and the distal end as if it had β-receptors. These findings are consistent with the above-mentioned results in isolated pyeloureters. During angiography of the kidneys it was observed that intra-arterial adrenalin injections produce not only arterial constriction, but also considerable contraction changes in the renal pelvis (BJÖRK, 1976). Isoproterenol inhibits ureteral peristalsis in the same way as noradrenalin during α-blockade, the threshold being found at 2.5×10^{-7}–5×10^{-7} g/kg × min. Orciprenaline also had similar effects (HANNAPPEL and GOLENHOFEN, 1974; TSUCHIDA and SAKAMOTO, 1974). The same results were obtained by LONGRIGG (1975a) in female patients by the use of open-ended indwelling catheters. The effect of noradrenalin infusions alone is less uniform, but uniform reactions can be obtained after application of adrenergic blocking agents: an increase of peristaltic rate during β-blockade (propranolol 1 mg/kg) or a decrease of the frequency after α-blockade (phentolamine 1 mg/kg). This explains the variability under normal conditions: α-excitatory as well as β-inhibitory effects are produced by noradrenalin (HANNAPPEL and GOLENHOFEN, 1974). Although α- and β-adrenergic responses are clearly demonstrated in ureteral peristalsis, the fact that adrenergic blockers alone have little influence signifies that under normal conditions catecholamines and sympathetic nerve terminals might not intervene in ureteral peristalsis; they probably only have regulating function in particular conditions (KIIL and KJEKSHUS, 1967; VEREECKEN et al., 1972; WEIN et al., 1972a; TSUCHIDA et al., 1973; TSUCHIDA and SAKAMOTO, 1974).

B. The Lower Urinary Tract

I. Morphology of the Lower Urinary Tract

1. Anatomy

In the human bladder, only the upper portion is covered by peritoneum. The prevesical area is filled with loose fatty tissue, and the bladder itself is supported by the pelvic floor. The posterior vesical wall is in close contact with the rectum in males and with the uterus and vagina in females. The inner side of the bladder is covered with transitional epithelium. Topographically, the organ can be divided into detrusor dome and body, vesical neck with trigone, and urethra. The ureters describe an oblique passage through the bladder wall, emptying in the region of the bladder neck close to the internal urethral orifice, and forming with the latter the trigone. Embryologically, the bladder is endodermal in origin except for the trigone which finds its origin, with the ureters, in the mesoderm (DOWNIE et al., 1975). The muscular coat of the bladder is meshwork; it consists of fascicles running in many directions, and changing planes and orientation. In the region of the bladder neck, muscle bundles reach the internal urethral orifice in radial direction. As they contract, the urethral aperture is pulled upon radially (WOODBURNE, 1968). Several components are responsible for tight closure of bladder neck and urethra: elastic tissue, vascular sinuses, an inner longitudinal and an outer circular smooth muscle layer (the so-called sphincter internus), and the striated muscle portion of the urethra known as sphincter externus (WOODBURNE, 1960; LAPIDES, 1958; RÁZ et al., 1972a).

The arterial blood supply of the bladder is derived from the superior and inferior vesical arteries which are branches of the anterior division of the hypogastric arteries. The veins of the bladder drain into large plexuses which empty into the hypogastric vein (LICH et al., 1978). In earlier papers, the term "sympathetic" was used to denote that part of the autonomic system which leaves the spinal cord in the thoracicolumbar region, whereas the term "parasympathetic" was used for the part of the autonomic system leaving the sacral region of the cord. The so-called sympathetic nerves pass through the hypogastric plexus, and about the level of the first part of the sacrum they are divided into the two *hypogastric nerves*. Each hypogastric nerve ends in a corresponding hypogastric ganglion. The parasympathetic nerves of the bladder are derived from the anterior primary division of the second and the third sacral nerves on both sides. They join the hypogastric ganglia via the *pelvic nerves*. From the anterior borders of the hypogastric ganglia emerge several branches of distribution, the *vesical nerves*, containing both sympathetic and parasympathetic fibers for the bladder. The striated external sphincter receives somatic fibers by way of the *pudic nerves* which spring from the anterior primary divisions of the third and fourth sacral nerves (LEARMONTH and GLAS, 1931). More recent studies exhibited that there are in no way pure sympathetic or parasympathetic nerves. Experiments in anesthetized cats provided evidence for the existence of an adrenergic inhibitory mechanism in vesical parasympathetic ganglia mediated via α-receptors (SAUM and DE GROAT, 1972). In vivo electrical stimulation of the hypogastric nerves of the guinea pig induced contraction of the urinary bladder. The antiadrenergic (bretylium and guanethidine) and adrenergic blocking agents (phenoxybenzamine and dihydroergotamine) at lower doses were not able to impair the responses of the urinary bladder. On the other hand, contractions of the urinary bladder were greatly potentiated by prostigmine and physostigmine. Thus, the guinea pig hypogastric nerves contain motor fibers innervating the urinary bladder which are certainly not adrenergic, but may be cholinergic in nature (MANTEGAZZA and NAIMZADA, 1967). ALM and ELMER (1975) made histochemical investigations in nondenervated bladders and in bladders denervated 10–14 days earlier. They concluded that the urinary bladder of the rat is supplied by postganglionic adrenergic fibers mainly via the pelvic nerves but also via the hypogastric nerves, having their cell bodies outside the bladder wall.

2. Histology

The smooth muscle bundles of the bladder consist of 12–15 muscle cells enclosed in a collagen capsule. Postganglionic axons develop varicosities at points of close contact with one or more of these fibers. Postganglionic motor neurons, when activated, cause the release of a transmitter agent from the synaptic vesicles of axon varicosities. Since many cells do not have close contact to axon varicosities, excitation in these cells can be produced by diffusion of a transmitter agent from axon bundles. This may be the principal mode of neuromuscular transmission in bladder muscles (BRADLEY and SCOTT, 1978). The catecholamines in the urinary bladder of the toad were localized using histochemical techniques: only a few of these smooth muscle bundles were innervated by fine, varicose, fluorescent nerve fibers running in parallel with the axis of the bundle. In general, the intensity of the fluorescence in the nerves supplying these muscle bundles was low compared with those innervating blood vessels (MCLEAN and

BURNSTOCK, 1966). Also in the bladder dome and body of dogs, only scant cholinergic and adrenergic innervation was found (RAEZER et al., 1973). But the muscle of the trigone and the underlying detrusor muscle contain an abundant number of cholinergic nerves, intensely stained cholinergic ganglion cell bodies, and an abundant number of adrenergic nerve fibers (RAEZER et al., 1976).

II. Functional Studies in the Lower Urinary Tract

1. Pharmacologic Studies in Isolated Bladder Dome and Body Preparations

In strip preparations of human detrusor muscle (dome), phenylephrine (10^{-5} g/ml) consistently caused contraction of the preparation while the other adrenergic substances, such as adrenalin, noradrenalin, and isoprenaline, had an inhibitory action (TODD and MACK, 1969). The experiments of MALIN and BOYARSKY (1970) established the presence of both cholinergic and adrenergic receptors in canine detrusor muscle. The threshold response (10^{-8} g/ml) was well within the range attributed to receptor stimulation. Reversal of noradrenalin response following blockade with phentolamine was further evidence of receptor site stimulation.

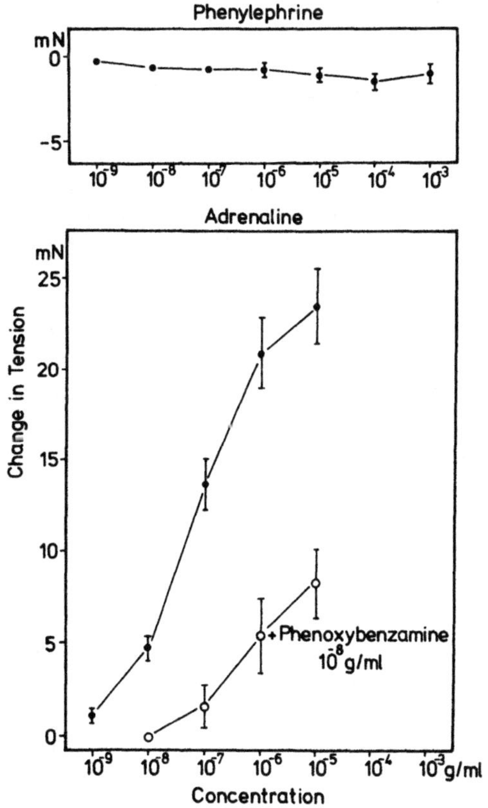

Fig. 5. Effects of α-adrenergic substances on muscle strips from human bladder dome (*above*) and bladder neck (*below*). In bladder dome musculature no α-excitatory response. In the bladder neck after application of adrenalin strong increase in tension, which is antagonized by the α-blocker phenoxybenzamine. (AWAD et al., 1974)

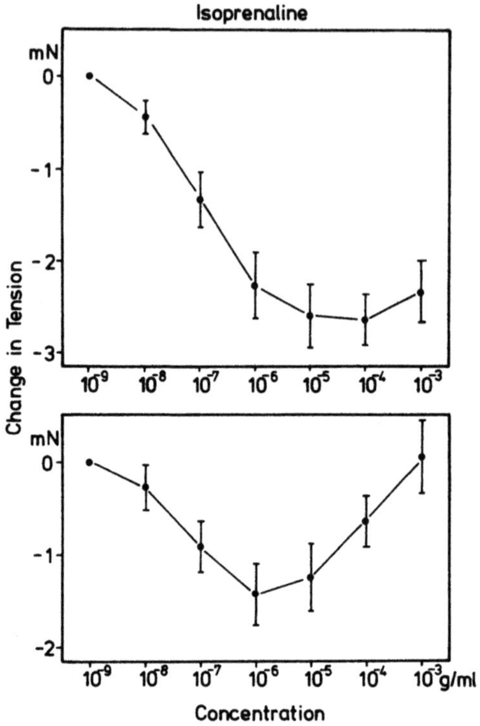

Fig. 6. Effects of β-adrenergic substances on muscle strips from human bladder dome (*above*) and bladder neck (*below*). The dose response curves reveal higher sensibility to β-receptor mediated inhibition in bladder dome than in bladder neck musculature. (AWAD et al., 1974)

Cholinergic receptor stimulation readily produced an increase in muscle tension. Adrenergic receptor stimulation produced a less uniform response. The presence of both adrenergic receptors (α and β) and the stimulation of these receptors by sympathomimetic pharmacologic agents may produce contraction and inhibition of contraction under varying circumstances. The use of blocking agents demonstrated this dual possibility.

AWAD et al. (1974) verified in the bladder dome of man a predominance of inhibitory β-adrenoceptors, though it was possible to demonstrate also the presence of excitatory α-adrenoceptors. In detrusor strips from rabbits, administration of noradrenalin caused a relaxation of muscle specimen. Frequency and amplitude were the first to be affected, then followed by a fall of muscle tonus. Isoprenaline equally inhibited muscle contraction in a concentration of 10^{-9} g/ml. This inhibitory action was prevented by the β-blocking drug propranolol. Blockade of the α-receptors with phenoxybenzamine slightly facilitated the action of isoprenaline. Nerve bladder preparations obtained from adult guinea pigs were stimulated. Here, too, the results indicated the presence of an inhibitory β-adrenoceptor and suggested the possibility of an excitatory α-adrenoceptor (DAVE and DHATTIWALA, 1976).

Contradictory are other results in guinea pig bladder strips: noradrenalin and isoprenaline depressed the reactions of the bladder strips to an imposed external stimulus. The action of isoprenaline could be completely blocked by propranolol, whereas the relaxing effect of noradrenalin could be abolished only by blocking α- as well as β-receptors. Thus, it is concluded that at the level of the guinea pig bladder, both α- and β-adrenergic receptors are present, whereby activation of both types of receptors induces a reaction in the same direction, relaxation (DE SY, 1971). The results of other investigators provide evidence only for the presence of inhibitory β-receptors (ROHNER et al., 1971; LEONI et al., 1973; GANGULY and VEDASIROMONI, 1976). SUNDIN et al. (1977) even denied the existence of α-receptors in the normal human detrusor muscle. SALIMI et al. (1969) stated that the response of the urinary bladder to drugs which act both on adrenergic α- and β-receptors depends on the magnitude of the given dose. The inhibitory response is most sensitive, and small doses of adrenalin produce an inhibition only, while higher doses are necessary to stimulate the excitatory receptors. Not consistent are the results of ANDERSON et al. (1971) who found in strips of rabbit detrusor muscle that higher concentrations of isoprenaline markedly depressed all parameters of activity, whereas at very low concentrations a stimulation of the contraction force was observed. By means of α- and β-blocking substances it was shown that the inhibition at high concentrations was a β-adrenergic response, and that the stimulation at low concentration was mediated via α-receptors. BENSON et al. (1975) studied the response of bladder dome strips from dogs to adrenergic stimulation. At length, near the resting length, noradrenalin (10^{-6}–10^{-5} g/ml) invariably caused a reduction in spontaneous activity and a decrease in base line tension (β-response). This effect was unaltered by pretreatment with phentolamine or atropine, but was blocked by propranolol. As the length was increased, however, noradrenalin, at the same concentration, caused an increase in base line tension and amplitude in 28 of 40 strips tested. This change from β- to α-response occurred at an average of 180% of the resting length. In no instance was a β-response converted to an α-response by increasing noradrenalin concentration.

By means of histochemistry and muscle strip studies it was found in the normal feline detrusor that, although α-receptors might exist, β-receptors dominate strongly. However, after parasympathetic denervation there appears to be a change in the relation between α- and β-receptors in favor of β-receptors (NORLÉN et al., 1976). Consistent are the results from human bladder strips, indicating the existence of an α-adrenergic receptor function only in the parasympathetically denervated detrusor from patients with lower motor neuron lesion (SUNDIN et al., 1977). Also after chronic bladder outlet obstruction in dogs, a change in the usual response of detrusor muscle to noradrenalin was observed. Bladder dome and body muscle strips demonstrated α-adrenergic contractile responses instead of β-adrenergic relaxing responses, probably caused by decrease in β-receptor function or increase in α-receptor sensitivity (ROHNER et al., 1978). CREED (1971) studied the membrane potential in muscle cells from the guinea pig bladder. In the presence of tetrodotoxin (2×10^{-7} g/ml), no change was observed in the spontaneous action potentials. This suggests that the electrical changes were not initiated by neural activity. In the absence of spontaneous activity, adrenalin (5×10^{-5} g/ml) produced no hyperpolarization. In preparations with spontaneous activity, adrenalin sometimes had no effect. In many preparations, however, adrenalin decreased the frequency of spike activity or abolished it. Even when marked depolarization had occurred, adrenalin did not produce hyperpolarization of the membrane. The action of noradrenalin was identical to that of adrenalin in all cases.

Table 3. Effects of adrenergic activators and inhibitors on the bladder dome and body

Author	Species	Method	α-Receptors	β-Receptors
ANDERSON et al. (1971)	Rabbit	In vitro muscle strips	Isoprenaline at very low concentrations, blocked by phenoxybenzamine and phentolamine	Isoprenaline at higher concentrations: inhibition
AWAD et al. (1974)	Human	In vitro muscle strips	Phenylephrine after pretreatment with propranolol: activation	Isoprenaline and phenylephrine: inhibition; blocked by propranolol
BENSON et al. (1975)	Dog	In vitro muscle strips	In stretched muscles α-excitation predominant	In non-stretched muscles β-inhibition predominant
BENSON et al. (1976b)	Dog	In vitro muscle strips	Dopamine: activation; blocked by phentolamine	Noradrenaline: inhibition; blocked by propranolol
CARPENTER (1970)	Rat	In vitro muscle strips	Phenylephrine: no response	Noradrenalin and isoprenaline: inhibition; blocked by propranolol
DAVE and DHATTIWALA (1976)	Guinea pig	In vitro, nerve-bladder preparations	Adrenalin after pretreatment with propranolol: slight activation	Adrenalin, noradrenalin, and isoprenaline: inhibition; blocked by propranolol
DE SY (1971)	Guinea pig	In vitro muscle strip	Noradrenalin: inhibition! blocked by phentolamine	Noradrenalin and isoprenaline: inhibition; blocked by propranolol
DHASMANA et al. (1970)	Dog	In vivo intravesical pressure		Adrenalin, noradrenalin, and isoprenaline: inhibition
DOWNIE et al. (1975)	Rabbit	In vitro muscle strips	Phenylephrine and noradrenalin after pretreatment with propranolol: activation	
EDVARDSEN (1968a)	Cat	In vivo intravesical pressure	Phenoxybenzamine: no response	Propranolol: decrease of bladder capacity
ELMÉR (1974)	Rat	In vivo intravesical pressure	Phenylephrine, adrenalin, and noradrenalin: contraction; blocked by dihydroergotamine	Isoprenaline: relaxation; blocked by propranolol
GANGULY and VEDASIROMONI (1976)	Guinea pig, rat	In vitro muscle strip	Adrenalin and isoprenaline after pretreatment with propranolol: activation	Adrenalin and isoprenaline after pretreatment with phenoxybenzamine: inhibition
GREGG et al. (1970)	Dog, cat	In vivo intravesical pressure	Phenylephrine increases voiding pressure, lowers bladder capacity	Isoprenaline lowers voiding pressure, increases bladder capacity

Homsy (1967)	Dog	In vivo intravesical pressure	Adrenalin: activation	
Kondo (1976)	Rabbit	In vitro muscle strips		Noradrenalin and isoprenaline: inhibition; blocked by propranolol
Leoni et al. (1973)	Dog	In vitro muscle strips		Noradrenalin after pretreatment with phentolamine, isoprenaline and soterenol: inhibition
Malin and Boyarsky (1970)	Dog	In vitro muscle strips	Noradrenalin after pretreatment with propranolol: activation	Noradrenalin and isoprenaline: inhibition; augmented by phentolamine, blocked by propranolol
Nergardh and Boréus (1972)	Human, cat	In vitro muscle strips	Phenylephrine and metoxamine: no response	Isoprenaline: inhibition; not augmented by phentolamine, blocked by propranolol
Norlén (1977)	Cat	In vivo intravesical pressure	Noradrenalin after pretreatment with propranolol: activation	Noradrenalin: inhibition
Raezer et al. (1973)	Dog	In vitro muscle strips	Adrenalin and noradrenalin after pretreatment with β-blocker: activation	Adrenalin, noradrenalin, and isoprenaline after pretreatment with α-blocker: inhibition
Rohner et al. (1978)	Dog	In vitro muscle strips	Noradrenalin after chronic bladder outlet obstruction: activation; blocked by phentolamine	Noradrenalin in normal bladder strips: inhibition; blocked by sotalol
Rohner et al. (1971)	Dog	In vitro muscle strips		Noradrenalin: inhibition; blocked by propranolol
Salimi et al. (1969)	Rabbit	In vitro muscle strips	Adrenalin and noradrenalin after pretreatment with propranolol: activation	Adrenalin, noradrenalin, and isoprenaline: inhibition; blocked by propranolol
Sjöstrand et al. (1972)	Rabbit, cat	In vivo intravesical pressure	Adrenalin and noradrenalin after pretreatment with propranolol: increase in pressure; blocked by phentolamine	Adrenalin and isoprenaline: decrease in pressure
Sundin et al. (1977)	Human	In vitro muscle strips	α-Receptors only in parasympathetically denervated bladders, not in normal ones	Isoprenaline: inhibition
		In vivo intravesical pressure	Bladder volume increase after α-adrenergic blockade	
Todd and Mack (1969)	Human	In vitro muscle strips	Phenylephrine: activation; blocked by hydergine	Adrenalin, noradrenalin, and isoprenaline: inhibition; blocked by propranolol

2. Pharmacologic Studies in Isolated Bladder Neck and Urethra Preparations

AWAD et al. (1974) were able to verify that the human bladder shows a predominance of α-adrenoceptors in the bladder neck. It was also possible to demonstrate the presence of recessive β-adrenoceptors in the same region. NERGARDH and BORÉUS (1972) studied autonomic receptor function in smooth muscle strips from the lower urinary tract of children and cats. In the bladder base, as well as in the proximal urethra, cholinergic and both α- and β-adrenergic receptors were found. Noradrenalin and adrenalin in concentrations of 2.5×10^{-6} and 10^{-6} mol/l produced contractile responses in all strips taken from the dog bladder neck and trigone areas. This α-adrenergic response was completely blocked by phentolamine (10^{-4} mol/l), but was not altered by the β-adrenergic blocking agent propranolol (10^{-4} mol/l) (ROHNER et al., 1971).

Similar results are reported from BENSON et al. (1976a) and KONDO (1976) who found no appreciable β-adrenergic activity in this region. SALIMI et al. (1969) described that in tissues from rabbit bladder base, inhibition is elicited by small doses of adrenalin. But the inhibition usually is overcome by the excitatory response when higher doses of adrenalin and noradrenalin are used. NERGARDH (1974a, b) made in vitro studies in bladder base and urethra from cats. Isometric contractions in the longitudinal musculature and changes in resistance to transurethral flow were registrated. α-adrenergic stimulation with phenylephrine increased while β-adrenergic stimulation with isoprenaline decreased flow resistance. The β-adrenergic reaction was far more sensitive than the α-adrenergic reaction, and was of longer duration. So he suggests that the β-adrenoceptor induced relaxation might be a physiologic mechanism which opens the internal sphincter at micturition. This is in contrast with the normally accepted theory that during the filling phase, the bladder dome is relaxed via β-receptors, and the bladder neck is closed via α-adrenoceptors, whereas at micturition detrusor muscle contraction is mediated by cholinergic transmitter substances.

3. In Vivo Studies in Bladder Dome and Body

In cystometric recordings, in cats propranolol had a rising effect on intravesical pressure which may reasonably be attributed to a blockade of β-adrenergic inhibitory receptors. On the other hand, the unchanged micturition contraction after the administration of this drug suggests that adrenergic inhibitory receptors do not operate during the expulsion of urine. Phenoxybenzamine did not affect the bladder pressure significantly, which indicated that adrenergic excitatory receptors are not brought into play by the collection of urine (EDVARDSEN, 1968). Partly not consistent are the results of GREGG et al. (1969), which have shown in dogs that isoprenaline lowers the maximum voiding pressure, raises the bladder capacity, and impairs the emptying of the bladder. This effect was reversed by sotalol, a specific blocker of β-receptors. But also this study confirms the presence of sympathetic β-adrenergic receptors in the bladder. Phenylephrine (10 mg/kg × min i.a.), an α-adrenergic agonist, raised voiding pressure and decreased bladder capacity, thus giving evidence for the presence of α-adrenoceptors (GREGG et al., 1970). The experiments of SJÖSTRAND et al. (1972) in anesthetized rabbits and cats showed, too, that there are excitatory α-receptors and inhibitory β-receptors, the latter being predominant.

By in vivo studies in cats it was found that the bladder relaxation following hypogastric nerve stimulation appears to be β-adrenergic. After pretreatment with atropine to abolish the parasympathetically mediated bladder contraction, a relaxation of the detrusor muscle was found when the pelvic or the hypogastric nerves were stimulated. This relaxation of the bladder was totally abolished by the nonselective β-adrenoceptor blocking agent propranolol, or a β_2-blocking agent indicating that the inhibitory effect of adrenergic nerve stimulation is exerted by action on β_2-receptors (NORLÉN, 1977). Terbutaline, a selective β_2-receptor stimulating agent, and isoprenaline, a general β-receptor stimulating agent, were tested: after terbutaline, the maximum increase in the bladder volume was 10% and on an average around 5%; after isoprenaline, the maximum increase in the bladder volume was 15% and on an average around 5% (NORLÉN et al., 1978). These results obtained in rat and man are opposite to the observations of NERGARDH (1977) who found in smooth muscle strips from the feline bladder only β_1-adrenoceptors. In the human bladder he found that the β-receptors are neither of the β_1 nor of the β_2-group. He suggested that they are of a third type (NERGARDH et al., 1977).

Stimulation of vesical afferents in cats activates a spinal sympathetic reflex which results in closing of the internal sphincter and a depression of bladder activity. The latter occurs by a direct depression of detrusor smooth muscle as well as a block of the neural input to the bladder. This vesico-sympathetic reflex represents a negative feed-back mechanism which may have an important role in the maintenance of urinary continence. The data provide evidence for the existence in the bladder of two distinct sympathetic inhibitory mechanisms: (1) ganglionic inhibition mediated by α-adrenergic receptors, and (2) inhibition of vesical smooth muscle mediated by β-adrenergic receptors (DE GROAT and SAUM, 1971; DE GROAT and THEOBALD, 1976). NORLÉN (1977) found in parasympathetically denervated bladders that noradrenalin caused a bladder contraction without previous β-adrenergic blockade in most of the denervated cats which was never the case in normal cats. Thus it is concluded that parasympathetic denervation induces α-receptor activity in the detrusor. In good agreement are the findings of ELMÉR (1974) who observed that the rat bladder developed supersensitivity to parasympathetic agents, and in the case of α-receptors mediated effects also to sympathomimetic agents after parasympathetic and sympathetic denervation. Regarding the adrenergic β-receptor effects, however, no supersensitivity developed after the denervation procedures.

4. In Vivo Studies in Bladder Neck and Urethra

Phenoxybenzamine, a potent long-acting α-adrenergic blocker, has clearly demonstrable effects on urethral function in dogs. In a dose of 0.5 mg/kg it caused a significant lowering of the resting urethral pressure (KHANNA and GONICK, 1975). The sympathetic activity in the proximal urethra was investigated by recording the fall of internal sphincter pressure produced by a dose of phentolamine which completely blocked all α-adrenergic sympathetic activity. It was found in dogs with empty bladders that the mean fall of internal sphincter pressure was 7.1 cm H_2O; but when the bladder was partially filled, the mean fall was 17.6 cm H_2O. After use of reserpine which creates a "pharmacologic sympathectomy", no sympathetic activity was demonstrated (TULLOCH, 1975).

Table 4. Effects of adrenergic activators and inhibitors on the bladder neck and urethra

Author	Species	Method	α-Receptors	β-Receptors
Awad et al. (1974)	Human	In vitro muscle strips	Isoprenaline in high concentrations and adrenalin: activation; blocked by phenoxybenzamine	Isoprenaline in low concentrations: inhibition; blocked by propranolol
Benson et al. (1976a)	Human	In vitro muscle strips	Noradrenalin: activation; blocked by phentolamine	Isoprenaline: slight inhibition
Benson et al. (1976b)	Dog	In vitro muscle strips	Noradrenalin and dopamine: activation; blocked by phentolamine	
	Human	In vivo, urethral closure pressure	Levodopa: increase in closure pressure	
Dhasmana et al. (1970)	Dog	In vivo, urethral closure pressure	Adrenalin and noradrenalin: increase in closure pressure; blocked by phenoxybenzamine	Isoprenaline: decrease in closure pressure
Domer et al. (1978)	Cat	In vivo, urethral closure pressure	Ephedrine, metoxamine, and noradrenalin: increase in closure pressure; blocked by phentolamine	
Downie et al. (1975)	Rabbit	In vitro muscle strips	Metoxamine, phenylephrine, and noradrenalin after pretreatment with propranolol: strong activation	
Khanna et al. (1975)	Dog	In vivo, urethral closure pressure	Imipramine: increase in closure pressure; blocked by phenoxybenzamine	
Khanna and Gonick (1975)	Dog	In vivo, urethral closure pressure	Blockade of α-Receptors with phenoxybenzamine: decrease in closure pressure	
Kondo (1976)	Rabbit	In vitro muscle strips	Noradrenalin and isoprenaline: activation; blocked by phenoxybenzamine	
McGuire and Herlihy (1977)	Cat	In vivo, urethral closure pressure	Blockade of α-receptors with phentolamine: decrease in closure pressure	
Nergardh and Boréus (1972)	Cat	In vitro muscle strips	Phenylephrine and metoxamine: activation; blocked by phentolamine	Isoprenaline: inhibition; blocked by propranolol

NERGARDH (1974a)	Cat	In vitro and in vivo, urethral closure pressure	Phenylephrine: increase in closure pressure	Isoprenaline: decrease in closure pressure (β-adrenergic reaction far more sensitive than the α-adrenergic one)
NERGARDH (1974b)	Cat	In vitro, urethral closure pressure	Adrenalin and noradrenalin in higher concentrations: increase in closure pressure	Adrenalin and noradrenalin in lower concentrations: decrease in closure pressure
NERGARDH and GIERUP (1974)	Human	In vivo, urethral closure pressure	Phenylephrine: increase in closure pressure	Isoprenaline: decrease in closure pressure
NORLÉN (1977)	Cat	In vivo, urethral closure pressure	Noradrenalin: increase in closure pressure; augmented by propranolol, blocked by phenoxybenzamine or phentolamine	Noradrenalin after pretreatment with phentolamine: decrease in closure pressure
RAEZER et al. (1976)	Dog	In vitro muscle strips	Noradrenalin: activation; augmented by propranolol, blocked by phentolamine	
RAZ et al. (1973)	Cat	In vitro muscle strips	Noradrenalin: activation; blocked by methergin	
ROHNER et al. (1971)	Dog	In vitro muscle strips	Noradrenalin: activation; not augmented by propranolol, blocked by phentolamine	
SALIMI et al. (1969)	Rabbit	In vitro muscle strips	Adrenalin and noradrenalin: activation	
SUNDIN et al. (1977)	Human	In vivo, urethral closure pressure	Blockade of α-receptors with phenoxybenzamine or phentolamine: decrease in closure pressure	
TULLOCH (1975)	Dog	In vivo, urethral closure pressure	Blockade of α-receptors with phentolamine: decrease in closure pressure	
WHITEFIELD et al. (1976)	Human	In vivo, urethral closure pressure	Blockade of α-receptors with phentolamine: decrease in closure pressure	Blockade of β-receptors with propranolol: no change in closure pressure

In 25 patients, α-blockade with 0.1 mg/kg phentolamine intravenously caused a mean percentage fall in the urethral pressure profile of 31.9% (WHITFIELD et al., 1976). Thus, it is concluded that the predominant mechanism of urethral resistance is α-adrenergic activity in smooth muscle. But besides the predominant α-receptors, also inhibitory β-receptors could be demonstrated in the bladder neck and urethra in situ (NORLÉN, 1977; LAVAL et al., 1978). Consistent with these results are the observations of MCGUIRE and HERLIHY (1977) who found that in cats urethral resistance to urine flow was not influenced by curare administration, but was markedly decreased by phentolamine administration. By pelvic nerve stimulation in anesthetized cats, it was demonstrated that urethral relaxation occurs prior to and during detrusor activity. Urethral smooth muscular pressure loss can be blocked with propranolol, suggesting that β-receptors are involved in this response (MCGUIRE, 1978). Even in children with myelomeningocele and, thus, lacking sympathetic bladder innervation from spinal centers, vital adrenergic muscle receptors have been demonstrated. The increase in outflow resistance in response to α-adrenergic stimulation, and the reduction in this resistance in response to β-adrenergic muscle relaxation, are in agreement with abovementioned findings (NERGARDH and GIERUP, 1974). In dogs, imipramine caused a sharp rise in the resting urethral pressure. Phenoxybenzamine completely blocked this effect. It is thus concluded that the basic mode of imipramine action is the stimulation of α-adrenergic receptors in the bladder neck and the urethra (KHANNA et al., 1975). TANAGHO et al. (1969) described, in disagreement with the results of others, that the sympathetic nerves apparently have their effect solely on the vascular bed of the urethra rather than on the urethral intrinsic musculature. In dogs, they observed only sometimes an increase in the intraurethral pressure after the application of sympathomimetic drugs (adrenalin 2.5 µg/kg), which they attributed to the known effects on the blood vessels in the same segment (TANAGHO and MEYERS, 1969). Also EDVARDSEN (1968) doubts the importance of α-adrenergic bladder closure. He observed urinary continence in cats after complete blockade of α-adrenoceptors and suggests that the elastic forces of the bladder outlet are capable of keeping the latter closed without muscular support induced by adrenergic excitatory receptors.

References

Akimoto, M., Biancani, P., Weiss, R.M.: Comparative pressure-length-diameter relationships of neonatal and adult rabbit ureters. Invest. Urol. *14*, 297–300 (1977)

Alm, P., Elmer, M.: Adrenergic and cholinergic innervation of the rat urinary bladder. Acta Physiol. Scand. *94*, 36–45 (1975)

Ancill, R.J., Jackson, D.M., Redfern, P.H.: The effect of sympathomimetic drugs and sympathetic nerve stimulation on the activity of the rat ureter in vivo. J. Physiol. (Lond.) *213*, 67P–68P (1971)

Ancill, R.J., Jackson, D.M ., Redfern, P.H.: The pharmacology of the rat ureter in vivo. Br. J. Pharmacol. *44*, 628–633 (1972)

Anderson, G.F., Pierce, J.M., Fredericks, C.M., Atkinson, G.M., Goellner, P.: A pharmacologic evaluation of the adrenergic receptors of the rabbit detrusor muscle. Arch. Int. Pharmacodyn. Ther. *191*, 220–230 (1971)

Awad, S.A., Bruce, A.W., Carro-Ciampi, G., Downie, J.W., Lin, M., Marks, G.S.: Distribution of alpha- and beta-adrenoceptors in human urinary bladder. Br. J. Pharmacol. *50*, 525–529 (1974)

Benson, G.S., Raezer, D.M., Wein, A.J., Corrière, J.N. Jr.: Effect of muscle length on adrenergic stimulation of canine detrusor. Urology *5*, 769–772 (1975)

Benson, G.S., Wein, A.J., Raezer, D.M., Corrière, J.N. Jr.: Adrenergic and cholinergic stimulation and blockade of the human bladder base. J. Urol. *116*, 174–175 (1976a)
Benson, G.S., Raezer, D.M., Anderson, J.R., Saunders, C.D., Corrière, J.N. Jr.: Effect of levodopa on urinary bladder. Urology *7*, 24–28 (1976b)
Bergmann, R.A.: Intercellular bridges in ureteral smooth muscle. Bull. John Hopkins Hosp. *102*, 195–202 (1958)
Björk, L.: Effect of epinephrine on the contractions in the normal renal pelvis in man. A cineradiographic investigation. Acta Radiol. [Diagn.] (Stockh.) *1*, 93–96 (1976)
Boatman, D.L., Lewin, M.L., Culp, D.A., Flocks, R.H.: Pharmacologic evaluation of ureteral smooth muscle. A technique for monitoring ureteral peristalsis. Invest. Urol. *4*, 509–520 (1967)
Boyarsky, S., Kirshner, N., Labay, P.: Catecholamine content of the normal dog ureter. Invest. Urol. *4*, 97–102 (1966a)
Boyarsky, S., Labay, P., Kirshner, N.: Acceleration of ureteral peristalsis by adrenal compression. Science *154*, 669 (1966b)
Bradley, E.W., Scott, F.B.: Physiology of the urinary bladder. In: Campbell's urology. Harrison, J.H., Gittes, R.F., Perlmutter, A.D., Stamey, T.A., Walsh, P.C. (eds.), Vol. 1. Philadelphia: Saunders 1978, pp. 87–124
Carpenter, F.G.: Antagonism of smooth muscle contractility by catecholamines. Am. J. Physiol. *219*, 1539–1543 (1970)
Casteels, R., Hendrickx, H., Vereecken, R., Bülbring, E.: Effects of catecholamines on the electrical and mechanical activity of the guinea-pig ureter. Br. J. Pharmacol. *43*, 429 (1971)
Creed, K.E.: Effects of ions and drugs on the smooth muscle cell membrane of the guinea-pig urinary bladder. Pflügers Arch. *326*, 127–141 (1971)
Daniel, O., Shackman, R.: Blood supply of the human ureter in relation to ureterocolic anastomosis. Br. J. Urol. *24*, 334–343 (1952)
Dave, K.C., Dhattiwala, A.S.: Adrenoreceptors of the guinea-pig urinary bladder. Br. J. Pharmacol. *58*, 37–41 (1976)
Deane, R.F.: Functional studies of the ureter: Its behaviour in the domestic pig (sus scrofa domestica) as recorded by the technique of Trendelenburg. Br. J. Urol. *39*, 31–37 (1967)
Deane, R.F., Garry, R.C.: The behaviour of the ureter of the pig recorded by the Trendelenburg technique. J. Physiol. (Lond.) *183*, 36P–37P (1966)
De Groat, W.C., Saum, W.R.: Adrenergic inhibition in mammalian parasympathetic ganglia. Nature *231*, 188–189 (1971)
De Groat, W.C., Theobald, R.J.: Reflex activation of sympathetic pathways to vesical smooth muscle and parasympathetic ganglia by electrical stimulation of vesical afferents. J. Physiol. (Lond.) *259*, 223–237 (1976)
Del Tacca, M., Lecchini, S., Stacchini, B., Tonini, M., Frigo, G.M., Mazzanti, L., Crema, A.: Pharmacological studies of the rabbit and human renal pelvis. Naunyn Schmiedebergs Arch. Pharmacol. *285*, 209–222 (1974)
De Sy, W.: The reactivity of isolated urinary bladder strips of the guinea-pig towards electric stimulation. Arch. Int. Physiol. Biochim. *79*, 459–468 (1971)
Dhasmana, K.M., Gupta, G.P., Bhargava, K.P.: Analysis of the adrenergic receptors in the urinary tract of dog. Jpn. J. Pharmacol. *20*, 461–466 (1970)
Dixon, J.S., Gosling, J.A.: Histochemical and electron microscopic observations on the innervation of the upper segment of the mammalian ureter. J. Anat. *110*, 57–66 (1971)
Domer, F.R., Wessler, G., Brown, R.L., Charles, H.C.: Involvement of the sympathetic nervous system in the urinary bladder internal sphincter and in penile erection in the anesthetized cat. Invest. Urol. *15*, 404–407 (1978)
Downie, J.W., Dean, D.M., Carro-Ciampi, G., Awad, S.A.: A difference in sensitivity to alpha-adrenergic agonists exhibited by detrusor and bladder neck of rabbit. Can. J. Physiol. Pharmacol. *53*, 525–530 (1975)
Duarte-Escalante, O., Labay, P., Boyarsky, S.: The neurohistochemistry of mammalian ureter: A new combination of histochemical procedures to demonstrate adrenergic, cholinergic, and chromaffin structures in ureter. J. Urol. *101*, 803–811 (1969)
Edvardsen, P.: Nervous control of urinary bladder in cats. 3. Effects of autonomic blocking agents in the intact animal. Acta Physiol. Scand. *72*, 183–193 (1968)

Elmèr, M.: Action of drugs on the innervated and denervated urinary bladder of the rat. Acta Physiol. Scand. *91*, 289–297 (1974)

Engelmann, T.W.: Zur Physiologie des Ureters. Pflügers Arch. *2*, 243–293 (1869)

Finberg, J.P., Peart, W.S.: Function of smooth muscle of the rat renal pelvis – response of the isolated pelvis muscle to angiotensin and some other substances. Br. J. Pharmacol. *39*, 273–281 (1970)

Ganguly, D.K., Vedasiromoni, J.R.: β-adrenoceptors in urinary bladder. Arch. Int. Pharmacodyn. Ther. *222*, 193–199 (1976)

Golenhofen, K., Hannappel, J.: Vergleichende Untersuchungen zur Ureterdynamik von Ratte, Meerschweinchen und Hund. Pflügers Arch. [Suppl.] *332*, R 77 (1972)

Golenhofen, K., Hannappel, J.: Normal spontaneous activity of the pyeloureteral system in the guinea pig. Pflügers Arch. *341*, 257–270 (1973 a)

Golenhofen, K., Hannappel, J.: Spontaneous generation of excitation in the pyeloureteral system and the effect of adrenergic substances. In: Urodynamics, upper and lower urinary tract. Lutzeyer, W., Melchior, H. (eds.), pp. 46–56. Berlin, Heidelberg, New York: Springer 1973 b

Golenhofen, K., Hannappel, J.: A tonic component in the motility of the upper urinary tract (renal pelvis – ureter). Experientia *34*, 64–65 (1978)

Gonzales, E.T. Jr.: The sucrose gap technique. Autonomic drugs and electrical characteristics of the ureter. Invest. Urol. *11*, 75–79 (1973)

Gosling, J.A., Waas, A.N.: The behaviour of the isolated rabbit calix and pelvis compared with that of the ureter. Eur. J. Pharmacol. *16*, 100–104 (1971)

Gregg, R.A., Boyarsky, S., Labay, P.: Blocking of β-adrenergic receptors in the urinary bladder using sotalol. South. Med. J. *62*, 1366–1373 (1969)

Gregg, R.A., Boyarsky, S., Labay, P., Levie, B.B.: Presence of β-adrenergic receptors in urinary bladder of dog and cat: response to isoproterenol. Arch. Phys. Med. Rehabil. *51*, 88–94 (1970)

Hannappel, J., Golenhofen, K.: The effect of catecholamines on ureteral peristalsis in different species (dog, guinea-pig, and rat). Pflügers Arch. *350*, 55–68 (1974)

Hannappel, J., Lutzeyer, W.: Pacemaker localization in the renal pelvis of the unicalyceal kidney. In vitro study in the rabbit. Eur. Urol. *4*, 192–194 (1978)

Haubensack, K., Müller, K.D.: Die Abhängigkeit der Motilität des menschlichen Harnleiters in vitro von Druck und Pharmaka. Urol. Int. *28*, 274–281 (1973)

Homsy, G.E.: The dynamics of the ureterovesical and vesicourethral junctions. II. Effect of autonomic and somatic excitation on the resistance to flow of the distal ureter and lower urinary tract. Invest. Urol. *4*, 408–418 (1967)

Hoyes, A.D., Bourne, R., Martin, B.G.H.: Ureteric vascular and muscle coat innervation in the rat. Invest. Urol. *14*, 38–43 (1976)

Jackson, D.M., Redfern, P.H., Ancill, R.J.: Pharmacology of the ureter. Lancet *1970 I*, 575

Kaplan, N., Elkin, M., Sharkey, J.: Ureteral peristalsis and the autonomic nervous system. Invest. Urol. *5*, 468–482 (1968)

Khanna, O.P., Gonick, P.: Effects of phenoxybenzamine hydrochloride on canine lower urinary tract: Clinical implications. Urology *6*, 323– 330 (1975)

Khanna, O.P., Elkouss, G., Heber, D., Gonick, P.: Imipramine hydrochloride: Pharmacodynamic effects on lower urinary tract of female dogs. Urology *6*, 49–51 (1975)

Kiil, F.: The function of the ureter and renal pelvis. Oslo: University Press 1957

Kiil, F., Kjekshus, J.: The physiology of the ureter and renal pelvis. Proc. 3rd Int. Congr. Nephrol. Washington, Vol. 2, pp. 321–335. Basel, New York: Karger 1967

Kondo, A.: Response of urinary bladder to cholinergic and adrenergic agents. Nagoya J. Med. Sci. *39*, 37–42 (1976)

Lapides, J.: Structure and function of the internal vesical sphincter. J. Urol. *80*, 341–353 (1958)

Laval, K.U., Hannappel, J., Lutzeyer, W.: Effects of β-adrenergic stimulating and blocking agents on the dynamics of the human bladder outlet. Urol. Int. *33*, 366–369 (1978)

Learmonth, J.R., Glas, C.M.: A contribution to the neurophysiology of the urinary bladder in man. Brain *54*, 147–176 (1931)

Leoni, J.V., Wein, A.J., Raezer, D.M., Schoenberg, H.W.: The effect of β-adrenergic stimulation on the contractile response of canine detrusor muscle. Invest. Urol. *10*, 419–425 (1973)

Lich, R., Howerton, L.W., Amin, M.: Anatomy and surgical approach to the urogenital tract in the male. In: Campbell's urology. Harrison, J.H., Gittes, R.F., Perlmutter, A.D., Stamey, T.A., Walsh, P.C. (eds.), Vol. 1. Philadelphia: Saunders 1978, pp. 3–33
Longrigg, N.: Autonomic innervation of the renal calyx. Br. J. Urol. *46*, 357–370 (1974)
Longrigg, N.: The effect of some autonomic receptor agonists and antagonists on motor activity of the human ureter. Br. J. Surg. *62*, 160–161 (1975a)
Longrigg, N.: In vitro studies on the human renal calices. J. Urol. *114*, 325–331 (1975b)
Longrigg, N.: In vitro studies on smooth muscle of the human renal pelvis. Eur. J. Pharmacol. *34*, 293–298 (1975c)
Longrigg, N.: The relationship of extrinsic nerves to motor activity of the upper urinary tract. Invest. Urol. *13*, 313–317 (1976)
Malatinsky, E., Haubensack, K.: Die pharmakologische Beeinflussung der Harnleitertätigkeit mit Sympathomimetika. Urologe *10*, 181–183 (1971)
Malin, J.M. Jr., Boyarsky, S., Labay, P., Gerber, C.: In vitro isometric studies of ureteral smooth muscle. J. Urol. *99*, 396–398 (1968)
Malin, J.M. Jr., Boyarsky, S.: The effects of cholinergic and adrenergic drug stimulation of detrusor muscle. Invest. Urol. *8*, 286–291 (1970)
Malin, J.M. Jr., Deane, R.F., Boyarsky, S.: Characterisation of adrenergic receptors in human ureter. Br. J. Urol. *42*, 171–174 (1970)
Mantegazza, P., Naimzada, K.M.: Responses of the guinea-pig vas deferens and urinary bladder to hypogastric nerve stimulation in vivo. Eur. J. Pharmacol. *1*, 402–406 (1967)
McGuire, E.J.: Experimental observations on the integration of bladder and urethral function. Invest. Urol. *15*, 303–307 (1978)
McGuire, E.J., Herlihy, E.: The influence of urethral position in urinary continence. Invest. Urol. *15*, 205–207 (1977)
McLean, J.R., Burnstock, G.: Histochemical localization of catecholamines in the urinary bladder of the toad (bufo marinus). J. Histochem. Cytochem. *14*, 538–548 (1966)
Melchior, H., Diemer, K.F., Simhan, K., Lutzeyer, K., Lutzeyer, W.: Ureterdynamik. II. Der Einfluß des autonomen Nervensystems auf die Ureterdynamik. Ein Beitrag zur Physiologie des Ureters. Z. Urol. Nephrol. *64*, 93–101 (1971a)
Melchior, H., Lymberopoulos, S., Lutzeyer, W.: Spasmolyse durch β-adrenergica. Ein Beitrag zur konservativen Behandlung der Urolithiasis. Urologe *10*, 183–188 (1971b)
Nergårdh, A.: The functional role of adrenergic receptors in the outlet region of the urinary bladder. An in vitro and in vivo study in the cat. Scand. J. Urol. Nephrol. *8*, 100–107 (1974a)
Nergårdh, A.: The interaction between cholinergic and adrenergic receptor functions in the outlet region of the urinary bladder. An in vitro study in the cat. Scand. J. Urol. Nephrol. *8*, 108–113 (1974b)
Nergårdh, A.: Characterization of the beta-adrenergic receptors in the lower urinary tract of the cat. Scand. J. Urol. Nephrol. *11*, 211–217 (1977)
Nergårdh, A., Borèus, L.O.: Autonomic receptor function in the lower urinary tract of man and cat. Scand. J. Urol. Nephrol. *6*, 32–36 (1972)
Nergårdh, A., Gierup, J.: Adrenergic receptor function in the urinary bladder. Observations in five children with myelomeningocele. Scand. J. Urol. Nephrol. *8*, 114–119 (1974)
Nergårdh, A., Borèus, L.O., Naglo, A.S.: Characterization of the adrenergic beta-receptor in the urinary bladder of man and cat. Acta Pharmacol. Toxicol. (Kbh.) *40*, 14–21 (1977)
Norlén, L.: Effects on the urinary bladder and urethra of different pharmacological treatments. An in-vivo study in normal and parasympathetically denervated cats. Scand. J. Urol. Nephrol. *11*, 7–16 (1977)
Norlén, L., Dahlstroem, A., Sundin, T., Svedmyr, N.: The adrenergic innervation and adrenergic receptor activity of the feline urinary bladder and urethra in the normal state and after hypogastric and/or parasympathetic denervation. Scand. J. Urol. Nephrol. *10*, 177–184 (1976)
Norlén, L., Sundin, T., Waagstein, F.: Effect of beta-adrenoceptor stimulation on the human bladder in vivo. Urol. Int. *33*, 355–358 (1978)
Notley, R.G.: Electron microscopy of the upper ureter and the pelviureteric junction. Br. J. Urol. *40*, 37–52 (1968)

Notley, R.G.: Ureteral morphology. Anatomic and clinical considerations. Urology *12*, 8–14 (1978)
Raezer, D.M., Wein, A.J., Jacobowitz, D., Corrière, J.N. Jr.: Autonomic innervation of canine urinary bladder. Cholinergic and adrenergic contributions and interaction of sympathetic and parasympathetic nervous systems in bladder function. Urology *2*, 211–221 (1973)
Raezer, D.M., Benson, G.S., Greenberg, S.H., Corrière, J.N. Jr., Jacobowitz, D.M., Wein, A.J.: Innervation of trigonal area of canine urinary bladder. Urology *7*, 369–375 (1976)
Raz, S., Caine, M., Zeigler, M.: The vascular component in the production of intraurethral pressure. J. Urol. *108*, 93–96 (1972a)
Raz, S., Zeigler, M., Caine, M.: Hormonal influence on the adrenergic receptors of the ureter. Br. J. Urol. *44*, 405–410 (1972b)
Raz, S., Zeigler, M., Caine, M.: The effect of methergin on the lower urinary tract. Urol. Res. *1*, 79–82 (1973)
Reid, R.E., Herman, R., Teng, C.S.: Attempts at altering ureteral activity in the unanesthetized, conditioned dog with commonly employed drugs. Invest. Urol. *12*, 74–78 (1974)
Rohner, T.J., Raezer, D.M., Wein, A.J., Schoenberg, H.W.: Contractile responses of dog bladder neck muscle to adrenergic drugs. J. Urol. *105*, 657–661 (1971)
Rohner, T.J., Hannigan, J.D., Sanford, E.J.: Altered in vitro adrenergic responses of dog detrusor muscle after chronic bladder outlet obstruction. Urology *11*, 357–361 (1978)
Salimi, M., Setekleiv, J., Skobba, T.J.: The sensitivity of adrenergic excitatory and inhibitory receptors in the smooth muscle of the rabbit urinary bladder. Acta Pharmacol. Toxicol. (Kbh.) *27*, 213–224 (1969)
Satani, Y.: Histologic study of the ureter. J. Urol. *3*, 247–267 (1919)
Saum, W.R., De Groat, W.C.: Parasympathetic ganglia: Activation of an adrenergic inhibitory mechanism by cholinomimetic agents. Science *175*, 659–661 (1972)
Schneider, W.: Die Muskulatur der oberen harnableitenden Wege. Anat. Entwicklungsgesch. *109*, 187–196 (1939)
Schreyer, H.: Röntgenphysiologie und -pathophysiologie. In: Radiologische Diagnostik der Harnorgane. Vogler, E. (ed.), pp. 188–234. Stuttgart: Thieme 1974
Schulman, C.C.: Development of adrenergic innervation in the ureter and vas deferens in rabbits. Experientia *30*, 790–792 (1974)
Schulman, C.C.: Etude histochimique et ultrastructurale de l'innervation de l'uretère. Ann. Histochim. *21*, 163–178 (1976)
Sjöstrand, S.E., Sjögren, C., Schmiterlöw, C.G.: Responses of the rabbit and cat urinary bladders in situ to drugs and to nerve stimulation. Acta Pharmacol. Toxicol. (Kbh.) *31*, 241–254 (1972)
Struthers, N.W.: An experimental model for evaluating drug effects on the ureter. Br. J. Urol. *45*, 23–27 (1973)
Sundin, T., Dahlström, A., Norlén, L., Svedmyr, N.: The sympathetic innervation and adrenoceptor function of the human lower urinary tract in the normal state and after parasympathetic denervation. Invest. Urol. *14*, 322–328 (1977)
Tanagho, E.A., Meyers, F.H.: The internal sphincter: Is it under sympathetic control? Invest. Urol. *7*, 79–89 (1969)
Tanagho, E.A., Meyers, F.H., Smith, D.R.: Urethral resistance: Its components and implications. I. Smooth muscle component. Invest. Urol. *7*, 136–149 (1969)
Tindall, A.R.: Preliminary observations on the mechanical and electrical activity of the rat ureter. J. Physiol. (Lond.) *223*, 633–647 (1972)
Todd, J.K., Mack, A.J.: A study of human bladder detrusor muscle. Br. J. Urol. *41*, 448–454 (1969)
Tsuchida, S., Sakamoto, K.: An electroureterographic study of the effects of autonomic drugs on ureteral peristalsis. Urol. Int. *29*, 280–290 (1974)
Tsuchida, S., Sugawara, H., Matsumura, S., Shibuya, Y., Nishiyama, A.: The effect of autonomic drugs on the canine electroureterogram. Tohoku J. Exp. Med. *110*, 235–245 (1973)
Tulloch, A.G.S.: Sympathetic activity of internal urethral sphincter. Urology *5*, 353–355 (1975)
Vereecken, R., Hendrickx, H., Casteels, R.: Modification of the action potential of the guineapigs ureter by catecholamines. Arch. Int. Pharmacodyn. Ther. *192*, 208 (1971)

Vereecken, R., Houben, F., Verduyn, H.: Effects of catecholamines and their antagonists on the dog ureter. Acta Urol. Belg. *40*, 18–27 (1972)
Washizu, Y.: Epinephrine on potential, tension, and ionic content of guinea-pig ureter. Eur. J. Pharmacol. *4*, 411–415 (1968)
Wein, A.J., Leoni, J.V., Gregory, J.G., Schoenberg, H.W., Jacobowitz, D.: The effect of 6-hydroxydopamine on canine ureteral contractility: Further evidence in favor of a non-neurogenic theory of ureteral function. J. Urol. *108*, 402–405 (1972a)
Wein, A.J., Leoni, J.V., Schoenberg, H.W., Jacobowitz, D.: A study of the adrenergic nerves in the dog ureter. J. Urol. *108*, 232–233 (1972b)
Whitfield, H.N., Doyle, P.T., Mayo, M.E., Poopalasingham, N.: The effect of adrenergic blocking drugs on outflow resistance. Br. J. Urol. *47*, 823–827 (1976)
Woodburne, R.T.: Structure and function of the urinary bladder. J. Urol. *84*, 79–85 (1960)
Woodburne, R.T.: Anatomy of the bladder and bladder outlet. J. Urol. *100*, 474–487 (1968)

CHAPTER 8

Miscellaneous Effects: Effects of Adrenergic Activators and Inhibitors on the Eye

Á. Kahán

A. Introduction

The ever valid advice "first anatomy, then physiology" cannot be disregarded when attempting to survey the effects of adrenergic activators and inhibitors on the eye. The eyes are multilayered organs, harboring in close proximity to each other quite different strata, in terms of their ontogeny, anatomy, and biochemistry, which – as regards pharmacology – behave as quite different, sometimes antagonistic targets of adrenergic drugs.

Another peculiarity of the eyes may be characterized by the concept splendid isolation. Some structures of the eye, for example, the lens, have no direct contact with systemic circulation, others (e.g. the uvea) constitute the most dense vascular bed of the organism, the retina – in spite of its very high oxygen demands – is between the two. Vascular supply, on the other hand, does not warrant free access of circulating adrenergic agents to the receptors of ocular structures (blood-retina barrier, blood-aqueous barrier). This splendid isolation is a misnomer, however. Adrenergic control of ocular functions is highly realized via adrenergic innervation, and light inputs acting on the retina control the circadian rhythm of the whole organism, and inter alia the functions of the eyes themselves.

Before discussing the effects of adrenergic agents on the eye it is necessary to summarize:

1) the targets of adrenergic agents in the eye and its adnexa, and
2) the adrenergic interactions between the eye and the organism

I. Targets of Adrenergic Agents in the Eye and Its Adnexa

The aim of this section is to provide a map of ocular targets on which adrenergic activators and inhibitors may act (Fig. 1). This map should include, besides the limited number of preganglionic fibers (Macri, 1971), the adrenergic neurons, its terminals, and in particular the α- and β-receptors. At first sight it would be intriguing to mark α- and the different β-receptors with different signs or colors. Natural and even synthetic catecholamines may bind, however, to different receptors at the same time. Blocking agents are much more receptor-specific (Radius and Langham, 1973), and form the tool by which site and number of different receptors can be determined.

The radio-labeled α- or β-antagonists, [^{3}H]dihydroergocryptine or [^{3}H]dihydroalprenolol were used to mark the α- or β-receptors, respectively, of prepared membranes, or in vivo; and the radioactivity was measured or made visible by autoradiography (Neufeld and Page, 1977; Neufeld et al., 1978). 9-Amino-acridin-pro-

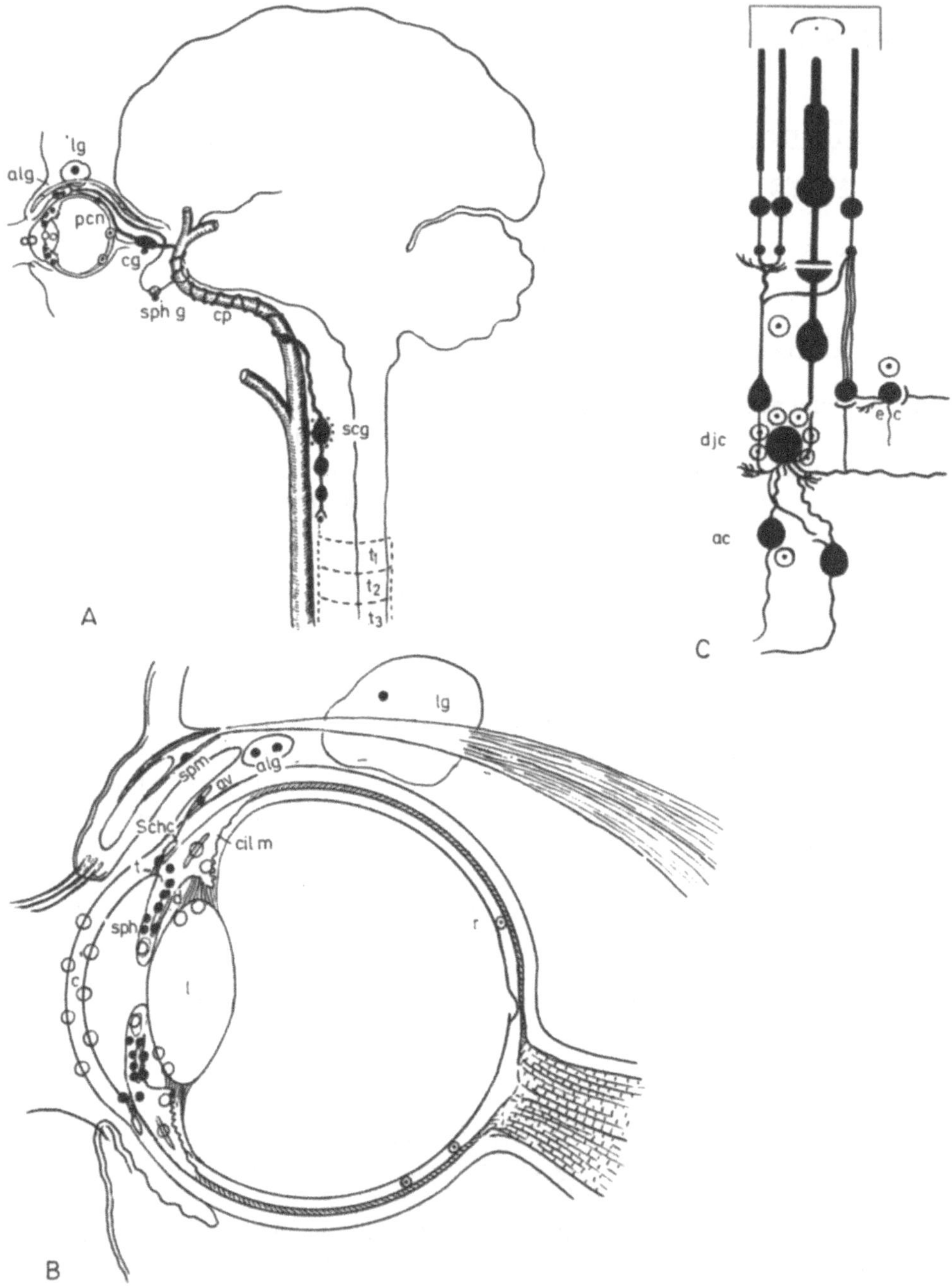

Fig. 1. A–C. Adrenergic structures of the eye and of its adnexa. **A** Origin and pathways of adrenergic innervation of the eye and of its adnexa. **B** Adrenergic structures of the eye and of its adnexa. **C** Adrenergic structures of the retina. Abbreviations: *ac* alloganglionic cell; *alg* accessory lacrimal gland; *av* aqueous vein; *c* cornea; *cg* ciliary ganglion; *cil m* ciliary muscle; *cp* carotid plexus; *d* dilator muscle, pupil; *djc* dopaminergic junctional cell; *e* eremite cell; *l* lens; *lg* lacrimal gland; *pcn* posterior ciliary nerve; *r* retina; *scg* superior cervical ganglion, sympathetic; *Schc* SCHLEMM's canal; *sph* sphincter muscle, pupil; *sph g* spheno-palatine ganglion; *spm* superior palpebral (smooth) muscle; *t* trabeculae of ant. chamber; t_1, t_2, t_3 thoracic 1st, 2nd and 3d segment of the cord, site of the cilio-spinal center; ● α-adrenergic, ○ β-adrenergic, ⊙ dopaminergic structures

pranolol treatment made visible even the β-receptors by fluorescence (LAHAV et al., 1978). Retinal [^{3}H]dopamine was identified by chromatography and its retinal site detected by radioautography (KRAMER, 1971; KRAMER et al., 1971). This latter method was applied to demonstrate the site of retinal serotonin (EHINGER and FLORÉN, 1978). Before the advent of these modern methods, the site and the quality of intracellular catecholamines was determined by the FALCK and HILLARP method, preceded by different pharmacologic treatments, e.g., releasing agents, followed by l-Dopa and Mao inhibitors, to demonstrate dopamine only (EHINGER and FALCK, 1969; KNYIHÁR et al., 1969).

In plotting the map of ocular adrenergic targets, it is fortunate that the sites of most intense adrenergic activities coincide with those which are almost completely explored. Most publications deal and most effects are concerned with aqueous humor dynamics. Modern experimental (perfusion) studies, and clinical (fluorimetric and tonographic) investigations made it possible to discern between (decreased or increased) outflow and (increased or decreased) aqueous humor production, manifesting in the elevation or drop of intraocular pressure, respectively.

1. Adrenergic Effects on Outflow of Aqueous Humor

The development of pathology and clinical investigation permitted the distinction between angle closure and primary open angle glaucoma, respectively. This distinction changed the pharmacology of aqueous humor outflow. Before this change it was believed that outflow only occurs under acetylcholinergic control (CHIOU and ZIMMERMAN, 1975). All systemic medicaments having the slightest adrenergic stimulating side effect were declared contraindicated in glaucoma before the era of distinction between angle closure and open angle glaucoma. At present, we are aware of the fact that angle closure can be stopped by cholinergic drugs, however, pulling backwards of the irisplane can be augmented by α-receptor blocking agents inducing relaxation of the dilator (HALASA and RUTKOWSKI, 1973), and even β-receptor blocking agents can reduce the β-receptor stimulation-induced inhibition of the sphincter (LAHAV et al., 1978). On the other hand, in eyes without angle closure (i.e., normals, or those suffering from primary open angle glaucoma), it is mainly stimulation of α-receptors that increase outflow. This effect is due to, and simulated by, the increased cAMP concentration of the aqueous humor. As in man, the activity of adenylate cyclase is increased at a higher rate by epinephrine than by norepinephrine, both activators increase outflow without denying the outflow-increasing effects of acetylcholinergic drugs (SEARS, 1978).

2. Adrenergic Effects on Aqueous Humor Secretion

In the ciliary processes movement of Na^+ and H_2O towards the posterior chamber is accomplished by the same forces which reabsorb Na^+ and H_2O from glomerular filtrate in the renal proximal tubuli [Na(K)ATPase pump]. Stimulation of β-receptors inhibits this pump and decreases aqueous humor production (SEARS, 1978). Prevalance of β-receptors has been demonstrated in the epithelium and the core of the ciliary processes by the [^{3}H]dihydroalprenolol and the 9-amino-acridin-propranolol methods, respectively (NEUFELD et al., 1978; LAHAV et al., 1978).

3. Intraocular Smooth Muscles as Targets of Adrenergic Agents

The dilator of the iris contracts on α-receptor stimulation. Mixed α- and β-receptor stimulators and even high concentrations of β-receptor stimulators may evoke mydriasis, which is only inhibited by α-receptor blocking agents (e.g., phenoxybenzamine).

The sphincter of the iris is inhibited by β-receptor stimulating agents. The longitudinal muscles of the ciliary body respond to β-stimulation (inhibitory effect of epinephrine on accomodation) (v. ALPHEN, 1976).

Norepinephrine increases the synthesis of phosphatidic acid, phosphatidylserine and phosphatidyl-inositol in the iris dilator (ABDEL-LATIF and SMITH, 1976). The ground plexus of the iris is the most abundant source of intraocular norepinephrine.

4. Retinal Targets of Adrenergic Drugs

The transformation of light into visual excitations and their conveyance across the retina and into the optic pathways is a rapidly developing field.

Catecholamines were only demonstrated, by the method of FALCK and HILLARP, in the layers already conveying evoked visual excitations, and not in the photoreceptors. Their main localization is in the inner plexiform layer corresponding to the amacrine cells ("adrenergic junctional cells"). Moreover, catecholamine-containing cells were found at the inner border of the inner nuclear layer ("eremite cells"), some catecholamine-containing fibers reaching the outer plexiform layer. Some catecholamine fluorescence was found in the ganglion cell layer as well ("alloganglionic cells"). By prior treatment with releasing agents, then administering l-Dopa and MAO inhibitors, it was concluded that the catecholamine demonstrated was dopamine only (EHINGER and FALCK, 1969). Later studies (KRAMER, 1971; KRAMER et al., 1971) confirmed this view, and revolutionized the concepts of transretinal transfer of visual excitations.

a) It was proven by chromatography of extracted retinal catecholamines, after in vivo administered different catecholamines, that only dopamine was retained in the retina.

b) The site of the retained dopamine coincided with the amacrines ("dopaminergic junctional cells").

c) The main discovery consisted in the measurement of the frequency-proportional release of this labeled dopamine on intermittent light-stimulation of the eye-cup preparations.

KRAMER'S well-founded claim was that dopamine is a retinal neurotransmitter acting by inhibition. The question arises whether dopamine is the only catecholamine playing a role in visual excitation. It was demonstrated, that the retina only takes up [^{3}H]dopamine, and never [^{3}H]norepinephrine from the vitreous body, and that dopamine β-hydroxylase activity is absent from the retina (RENTZHOG, 1975); that retinal homogenates release cAMP on stimulation by dopamine. Intact retinas responded at a higher rate to apomorphine (BUCHER and SCHORDERET, 1974; BROWN and MAKMAN, 1973). EHINGER and FLORÉN (1978) were the first to challenge the autocracy of dopamine in the transmission of visual excitations; they found that the amacrines could take up alternately labeled dopamine or [^{3}H]serotonin; the latter was inhibited by chlorimipramine. The transport of labeled leucine along the visual pathways is accelerated by both dopamine and serotonin (GUY et al., 1978).

However, as regards the transformation of light inputs into visual excitation only occurring in the photoreceptors, the role of inhibition of cGMP (and cAMP) formation is proven, inducing hyperpolarization (MILLER et al., 1971). This inhibitory phenomenon is induced by bleached photoproducts of visual pigments and by an increased phosphodiesterase activity (BROWN and MAKMAN, 1972; PANNBACKER et al., 1972; BITENSKY et al., 1973). Till now, no *direct* effects of catecholamines have been disclosed at this level.

5. Targets of Adrenergic Agents in the Cornea

The corneal epithelium is densely packed with β-receptors accepting the specific radiolabel [^{3}H]dihydroalprenolol. Its acceptance is abolished by both epinephrine and practolol (NEUFELD et al., 1978). Stimulation of this receptor has four effects: inhibition of cell-sliding to replace surface defects; inhibition of mitosis; loosening of epithelial adhesion to the stroma; decreased production of collagenase in the cornea. Stimulator of corneal β adrenergic receptors may be epinephrine leaking out from the blood vessels (KREJCI and HARRISON, 1957; NEUFELD et al., 1978). All four effects delay healing of corneal wounds and of corneal ulcers. Practolol may cause dry eyes with corneal ulceration. In frogs Cl^- is moving outwards through the corneal epithelium, in man Na^+ is pumped inwards. On the stimulation of the corneal β-receptors, even in man Cl^- is moving outwards (KLYCE et al., 1972; ZADUNAISKY et al., 1973). Of course, the decreased concentration of tears in Cl^- on epinephrine is not due to the above described change of corneal ion pump. Topical epinephrine therapy is decreasing the number of endothelial cells, without increasing corneal thickness (WALTMAN et al., 1977).

6. Targets of Adrenergic Agents of the Lens

The lens is suspended in the aqueous humor containing more or less norepinephrine, according to its changing release from its most ample intraocular store, the iris. Moreover, minute amounts of epinephrine may leak from the circulation into the aqueous humor. Almost every catecholamine may enter the aqueous humor if administered topically. The lens responds to every catecholamine, however, in producing cAMP the most effective is epinephrine. The former's main role in the lens is to increase protein-kinase activity, as the scanty energy yield of lenticular anaerobic glycolysis is spent mostly on its lifelong protein synthesis. The potential role of false transmitters, decreasing the storage, and release of norepinephrine in cataractogenesis is obvious, and this side effect of α-methyl-Dopa therapy was observed by the author (unpublished).

Another interesting role of catecholamines in the growth of the lens is their synergism with chalones, proteins with the specific activity of inhibiting mitosis of the lens epithelium. In the neighborhood of the iris, in the epithelium of the anterior lens surface there is almost no mitosis. Mitosis is restricted to the equatorial area of the lens, which is remote from the iris, the source of norepinephrine and some leaking epinephrine. Of course, epinephrine would be more active in the presence of chalones than norepinephrine (FROOMBERG and VOADEN, 1966; VOADEN and FROOMBERG, 1967; VOADEN, 1968).

7. Targets of Adrenergic Agents in the Orbita

The striped muscles in the orbit consist of an external red muscle layer securing tonic contractions, and an internal white muscle layer responsible for the rapid eye movements (SCOTT and COLLINS, 1973). The levator of the superior lid corresponds to the external red muscle layer. Moreover, the superior lid is kept in an elevated position by the tonic contraction of the superior tarsal smooth muscle having only adrenergic innervation. It responds mainly to epinephrine, and to the dominance of adrenergic hyphothalamic centers induced by hyperthyroidism (Graefe's sign). The same central effects of thyroxine inhibit, via adrenergic innervation, the accomodation, and the absence of accomodation leads to a decrease of convergence (Moebius sign): the outer red muscle layer of the lateral rectus muscle being in tonic contraction simultaneously. In experimental animals the epinephrine induced contraction of the orbital muscle of MÜLLER causes exophthalmos.

In this context, the easily measurable retraction of the nictitating membrane of cats should be mentioned. This retraction is due to the contraction of a smooth muscle responding mainly to epinephrine. This phenomenon proved to be a very useful tool in the pharmacology of adrenergic activators and inhibitors.

It should be emphasized that the somewhat frightening aspect of extremely open-kept, shining eyes looking at the distance, characteristic of stressed or hyperthyreotic individuals, is mediated by adrenergic innervation. Retraction of the nictitating membrane is an analog to the Graefe's sign.

The lachrymal glands have double innervation. The accessory lachrymal glands providing the basic supply of tears are governed by the sympathetic (in addition to cholinergic control), and excessive lacrimation is elicited by the cholinergic innervation of the main lachrymal glands (DUKE-ELDER, 1968).

II. Adrenergic Interactions Between the Eye and the Organism

These interactions were the first to point to an indirect influence of adrenergic mediation of light responses at the level of photoreceptors.

These interactions are two directional (Fig. 2).

1. Retinal Light Stimulation and the Circadian Rhythm

From the light stimulated retinas of mammals, the inferior accessory optic tracts and the medial forebrain bundles conduct inhibitory stimuli to the superior ganglion of the cervical sympathetic nerve (AXELROD, 1971). From this ganglion, postganglionic fibers carry serotoninergic impulses into the pineal gland, suppressing its melatonin synthesis and release. This result is attained by the decreased activity of the enzyme serotonin-*N*-acetylase, the rate limiting factor of melatonin synthesis; the enzyme 5-hydroxyindol-*O*-methyltransferase is present in excess. On the other hand, stimulation of the superior cervical ganglion melatonin synthesis in the pineal gland increases. This may be attained inter alia by disjoining the inhibitory pathways by blinding, by section of the inferior accessory optic tract, superior cervical sympathetic ganglionectomy, or by depleting norepinephrine by reserpine. The same occurs in the dark phase of the normal circadian rhythm.

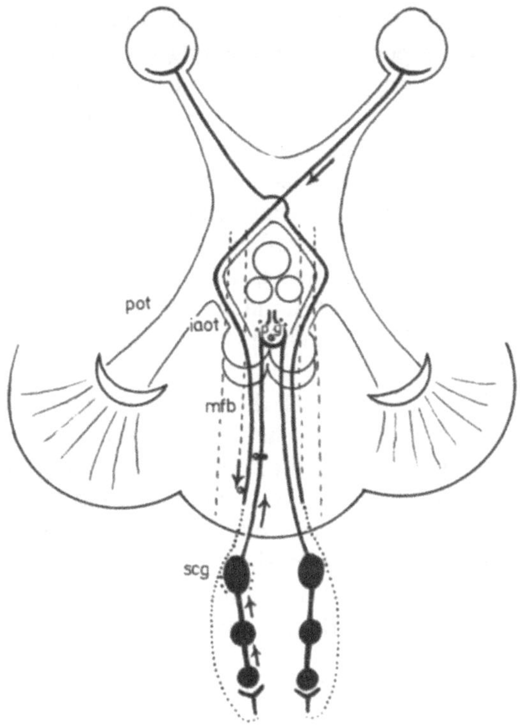

Fig. 2. Interconnections of the eyes and of the pineal gland; *iaot* inferior accessory optic tract; *mfb* medial forebrain bundle; *pg* pineal gland; *pot* primary optic tract; *scg* superior cervical ganglion (sympathetic). ●: α-adrenergic. ◑: serotoninergic structures. ↓: Pathway of serotoninergic impulses inhibiting melatonin-synthesis in the pineal gland. ↑ Common pathway of α-adrenergic (exitatory) and serotoninergic (inhibitory) impulses from cervical sympathetic ganglia towards the pineal gland

Melatonin is a hormone counteracting the activity of most stimulating hormones of the pituitary (ANTON-TAY, 1971; MOSZKOWSKA et al., 1971): it is active as antiadrenocorticotrophine (decreasing aldosteron effects and cortisol secretion), antigonadotrophine (abolishing estrus and retarding puberty), antimelanocyte stimulating hormone (contracting the melanocytes). This latter effect led to the discovery, purification, synthesis, and former measurement of melatonin (LERNER and CASE, 1959; LERNER et al., 1959; LERNER et al., 1960).

The pineal gland is responsible for the light-induced, adrenergic control of the circadian rhythm of the endocrine system. In blind persons the cortisol rhythm of the serum, peaking normally in the morning, is missing or reversed. By administering the peripheral hormones, the extent of secretion of melatonin can be decreased (JOÓ and KAHÁN, 1975).

2. Ocular Targets of Melatonin and of Its Antagonist MSH

There is no wonder that melatonin has been demonstrated in the photoreceptors of the mammalian retina (BUBENIK et al., 1978). In the pineal organ of fish, reptiles, and amphibia, there are photoreceptors fulfilling the same biologic clock role as the pineal gland of mammals, without the need of any retinal input. Even during the fetal ontogeny of mammals, there is a period when the *anlage* of the pineal gland does contain photoreceptors. As regards phylogenesis and ontogeny, retinal photoreceptors and the pineal gland are related structures (KAHÁN, 1971). Melatonin seems to have its role in the shedding of rod's discs in the morning hours, while the discs of cones are prone to phagocytosis in the evening hours, governed by the adrenergically controlled increase or decrease, respectively, of retinal melatonin. In the evening, melatonocyte stimulating hormone (MSH) may prevail (BUBENIK et al., 1978).

These authors described an accumulation of melatonin in the harderian glands of rats in the dark phase. This extraorbital lachrymal gland is highly fluorescent from its porphyrin content, which is an indicator of melatonin secretion of the pineal gland (JOÓ and KAHÁN, 1975).

Disregarding the porphyrin contents, the salivary glands of rats are in the proximity of, and more or less resemble, the harderian glands. From one of the salivary glands, the submaxillary glands of adult male mice a protein promoting the growth and hypertrophy of noradrenergic neurons, nerve growth factor (NGF), can be extracted and purified (LEVI-MONTALCINI and ANGELETTI, 1968). The complete protein of molecular weight 140,000 (VARON et al., 1967) is most active, however, one of its subunits (VARON et al., 1968) is still active (COHEN, 1960):

1) in promoting the growth of the cervical sympathetic ganglia, even that of the noradrenergic ground plexus of the iris,

2) in increasing the activity of the enzyme tyrosine-hydroxylase (IVERSEN et al., 1974),

3) as antigen, injected into rabbits with FREUND'S adjuvant is active in yielding an antiserum against NGF. This anti-NGF serum , injected into newborn animals, is producing immunosympathectomy.

B. Adrenergic Alpha- and Beta-Receptor Activators

I. Adrenergic Receptors

In the eye or its adnexa, there are (at least) four kinds of receptors for binding adrenergic receptor stimulators:

1) α-Receptors, the stimulation of which manifests in vascular constriction of the conjunctiva (pale eyes), mydriasis consequent to contraction of the iris dilator, slow decrease of intracular pressure consequent to increased facility of outflow;

2) β_1-Receptors, the stimulation of which results, especially if the stimuli are repeated, in an increase of intraocular pressure (consequent to a decreased facility of outflow), without conjunctival pallor or mydriasis. If the β_1-stimulators are applied in very high concentrations, mydriasis and conjunctival pallor may appear, however, due to α-receptor stimulation. These signs may be inhibited by the α-receptor blocking agent phenoxybenzamine, however, not by the β-receptor blocking agent propranolol. As side effects, ventricular contractions of the heart may occur.

3) β_2-Receptors. Their stimulation manifests in an early decrease of intraocular pressure, due to an early release of cAMP increasing facility of outflow. A later effect is the decreased rate of aqueous production, consequent to a decrease of the $Na^+(K^+)$ ATPase pump activity in the ciliary processes. Side effect of β_2-receptor stimulation

may be bronchospasms (LAMBLE, 1973; SEARS and NEUFELD, 1975; WETTRELL and PANDOLFI, 1975; SEARS, 1978).

β-Receptors (without any distinction made between β_1 or β_2) are present in the lachrymal glands, cornea, lens, sphincter of the iris (with inhibitory activity), longitudinal smooth muscles of the ciliary body (inhibiting accomodation), and in the retina.

4) Dopaminergic receptors are characteristic of the retina. Their specific inhibitor is chlorimipramine (EHINGER and FLORÉN, 1978), however, the most effective (specific) dopaminergic receptor blocking agent is haloperidol (BROWN and MAKMAN, 1973). Without paying respect to the different localization and to the difference of their blocking agents, dopaminergic receptors have much in common with α-receptors. Of course retinal dopaminergic receptors are inhibitory; α-receptors have an augmentative effect, a fact justifying their separate description.

II. Adrenergic Receptor Stimulators

As regards the stimulators, distinction should be made between the agonist(s) physiologically present, and between the pharmacologic stimulators that may be administered.

It has been proven that within the eye there is no phenylaethanolamine-*N*-methyltransferase: even after glycocorticosteroid pretreatment [^{3}H]epinephrine was never formed from [^{3}H]l-Dopa injected into different sites of the eye (RENTZHOG, 1975). Hence it must be concluded that as physiologic adrenergic stimulators mainly primary catecholamines – norepinephrine and dopamine – may act on the receptors of the eye. From the circulating blood only small quantities of epinephrine may diffuse into ocular tissues and media. In the retina, the above cited experiments of RENTZHOG demonstrated the absence of dopamine-β-hydroxylase activity, hence in the retina dopamine is the main active adrenergic physiologic stimulator. In spite of the minor amounts of norepinephrine having been measured in the retina (KAHÁN and OLÁH, 1975), it is questionable whether it can stimulate the dopaminergic receptors of the retina. Preliminary experiments (KAHÁN and OLÁH, 1972) suggest the role of retinal norepinephrine in the mediation of antidromic impulses reaching the covered eye from the fellow eye, which is receiving intermittent light stimuli.

Here it should be pointed out the fact that certain structures (lachrymal glands, cornea, lens, certain intraocular smooth muscles, and mainly the ciliary processes) are provided with the β-type of adrenergic receptors (in addition to cholinergic ones), and the released physiologic adrenergic agonist in norepinephrine. Of course, norepinephrine may bind to, and stimulate, β-receptors, however, to a lower degree than pharmacologically administered $\beta(+\alpha)$- or β-receptor activators.

The pharmacologically administrable adrenergic activators are the following:

l-norepinephrine: $\alpha(+\beta)$-receptor activator,

l-epinephrine, dipivalylepinephrine: $\beta(+\alpha)$-receptor activators,

l-isoproterenol: β_1-receptor activator,

l-salbutamol, l-soterenol: β_2-receptor activators (probably d-isoproterenol conforms more to β_2-receptors, than l-isoproterenol does),

dopamine: dopamine-receptor activator, with some α-receptor activator effects (mydriasis, decrease of intraocular pressure).

As evident from the above list of adrenergic receptor activators, they are not completely specific activators of a single kind of receptors. Receptor blocking agents are much more specific for certain receptors than are activators (RADIUS and LANGHAM, 1973). The effects of activators depend on the dose or concentration of the activator, on the route of administration, and on the availability of the responding receptors in a species or an individual.

Nevertheless, it may be stated that epinephrine is the most potent activator of all, increasing the adenylate-cyclase activity at the highest rate when compared to other adrenergic activators (NEUFELD et al., 1978).

1. Norepinephrine

Topical administration of 50 μl of 0.1 *M* norepinephrine (chloride or bitartrate) into the cul-de-sac of rabbits yields the typical signs of α-receptor stimulation: pallor of the conjunctiva, mydriasis, and decrease of intraocular pressure with slow onset, due to increased facility of outflow. It is striking to compare the huge concentration of instilled norepinephrine (0.1 *M*) with that of perfused norepinephrine flowing through the anterior chamber and outflow channels of cannulated rabbits (10^{-5} *M*), yielding the same results (SEARS and NEUFELD, 1975). All depends on the availability of α-receptors: if the perfusion is performed after surgical sympathectomy, the empty receptors respond equally to 10^{-7} *M* norepinephrine.

2. Epinephrine

Primates (monkey, man) are less responsive to norepinephrine, however they exhibit a typical triple response to the mixed $\beta(+\alpha)$-receptor activator epinephrine. In the early phase there are, applying 1%–2% epinephrine (borate or borate-phosphate) topically, signs of α-receptor stimulation: pallor of the conjunctiva, mydriasis, and a decrease of intraocular pressure with early onset. This is followed by a sustained decrease of intraocular pressure, when pallor and mydriasis are already over (β-receptor response, releasing cAMP into the outflow channels causing increased outflow). β-Receptor response may also cause decreased aqueous humor production. This intermediate (β) response is followed by long lasting decrease of intraocular pressure, due to the depolymerization of glicans coating the aqueous humor outflow channels (SEARS and NEUFELD, 1975; SEARS, 1978).

Even in the case of epinephrine it is striking that to obtain the same effect, huge concentrations (10^{-1} *M*) of epinephrine are required if instilled onto the conjunctiva, and very high dilutions (10^{-5}) of it, if perfused. Obviously corneal epithelium is the major obstacle of the penetration of the hydrophilic epinephrine salts. Corneal epithelium can be loosened, and the penetration of epinephrine increased if the solutions contains 5% polyoxyethylene sorbitan monolaurate (Tween 20, Atlas Chem. Ind. Inc.). The dipivalyl ester of epinephrine is 100-fold more lipid soluble, and 10-fold more efficient if instilled onto the conjunctiva (CHAU-PO WEI et al., 1978).

3. Beta-Receptor Stimulators

β-Receptor stimulators applied topically exert an immediate effect on intraocular pressure.

l-Isoproterenol in lower concentrations does not dilate the pupil, its higher concentrations induce mydriasis which may be prevented by prior administration of phenoxybenzamine (α-receptor blocking agent). Four percent l-isoproterenol may decrease intraocular pressure, however, this effect is reversed, if applied repeatedly, by decreasing outflow. This fact, and the induction of cardiac venticular contractions, preclude the clinical application of this β_1-agonist.

The β_2-agonists salbutamol (2%) and soterenol do not dilate the pupil and immediately decrease intraocular pressure by lowering production of aqueous humor. They do not cause cardiac side effects.

Both the aqueous humor outflow-inhibiting and the ventricular contractions-inducing effects seem to be bound to the l-enantiomer of isoproterenol. d-l-Isoproterenol (3%), and d-isoproterenol (4.4%) proved to be safe in reducing intraocular pressure without cardiac effects. d-salbutamol has also been tried with success (SEIDEHAMEL et al., 1975).

4. Systemic Administration of Adrenergic Receptor Stimulators

When applied systemically, α-receptor stimulators decreased intraocular pressure, β-receptor stimulators caused an increase (NEETENS and BERNARD, 1973). The effects of systemic β-receptor stimulators are probably realized in cerebral areas governing intraocular pressure (GLOSTER and GREAVES, 1957). If [^{3}H]dopamine or [^{3}H]norepinephrine were injected via the carotid artery, the former was transformed to, and the latter retained as [^{3}H]norepinephrine in the iris, or ciliary processes (KRAMER and POTTS, 1971; KRAMER et al., 1972). The effect of systemic α-receptor stimulators may be explained by vasoconstriction: both norepinephrine and epinephrine when injected into the long ciliary arteries caused decreased flow in the choroid and the ciliary body (CHANDRA and FRIEDMAN, 1972). Stimulation of the cervical sympathetic nerve increased the circulation of the iris, that of the ciliary processes to a lesser degree, that of the retina remained unaltered. This was measured by trapping microspheres carrying a radiolabel, injected into the left ventricle of the heart (ALM, 1977).

5. Administration of Catecholamine Precursors

Systemic l-Dopa administration may increase the catecholamine contents within the eye. This result may be extreme if care is taken by previous administration of MAO inhibitors to save the catecholamines from breakdown.

The blood-brain barrier precludes the entrance of systemically administered catecholamines (and of serotonin) into the brain. This difficulty can be avoided by filling up dopaminergic or noradrenergic cerebral areas by administering a MAO inhibitor plus l-Dopa (or l-HTP for serotonin-enrichment) (SCHÜMANN, 1960; UDENFRIEND et al., 1957). The same holds true for the retina: its dopamine contents can be raised maximally by MAO inhibitors plus l-Dopa. From the latter, only minor quantities of norepinephrine are formed. On the other hand, the norepinephrine contents of the iris and ciliary body increase tremendously (5.5 µg/g) with this treatment. The increase of norepinephrine is not in the aqueous humor, but in the tissue itself, in contrast to topical administration of the ready adrenergic receptor-activators. The same high-values of norepinephrine were found in surgically removed human iris samples, to put an end to attacks of angle closure glaucoma. Local administration of acetylcholine- and cholinesterase-inhibitors increased at almost the same rate the norepinephrine contents of rabbit iris (KAHÁN and OLÁH, 1975).

6. Factors Determining the Different Effects of Adrenergic Receptor Stimulators in the Eye

As has been described previously, the effects of different adrenergic receptor-stimulators are quite dissimilar as regards quality and quantity in different structures of the eye, in different species, and in different individuals; as will be demonstrated, even pretreatment with inhibitors of prostaglandin-synthetase activity can basically change the answers. The development of these factors is the most modern achievement in the study of adrenergic receptor-stimulation in the eye.

a) Density of Alpha- or Beta-Receptors at Different Sites of the Eye

One of determining factors is the different density of α- or β-receptors at different sites in the eye, in different species or individuals, and the avidity of binding of different stimulators to the receptors. As already mentioned, the tritiated α-receptor blocking agent [^{3}H]dihydroergocryptine is the most specific marker of the α-receptors, the tritiated β-receptor blocking agent [^{3}H]dihydroalprenolol is an even more specific marker of the β-receptors. In the rabbit, the iris is densely packed with α radiolabel accepting receptors. The radiolabel is displaced almost equally by epinephrine and norepinephrine, almost not by isoproterenol. The cornea and the ciliary body are densely packed with the β radiolabel accepting receptors. The radiolabel is displaced by isoproterenol and epinephrine, less by norepinephrine. Epinephrine treatment decreases the acceptance of the β-radiolabel both in the cornea and the ciliary-body. 6-*OH*-dopamine increases the β radiolabel acceptance in the ciliary body (NEUFELD and PAGE, 1977; NEUFELD et al., 1978). The β-receptors were made visible under the fluorescence microscope, applying the acridine-coupled β-antagonist propranolol (LAHAV et al., 1978).

b) Dosage, Concentration of Adrenergic Receptor Stimulators

The most important factor determining whether an adrenergic receptor stimulator applied topically is active in reducing intraocular pressure depends on its ability to increase cAMP concentration of the aqueous. Cyclic-AMP injected into the anterior chamber decreased intraocular pressure by opening the outflow channels. For example, rabbits respond at a higher rate to norepinephrine, primates more efficiently to β-receptor stimulation as regards both cAMP production and decrease of intraocular pressure (NEUFELD et al., 1972b). d-Isoproterenol was inactive as regards cAMP production: it binds to the β-receptor, but acts rather as a β-receptor blocking agent, not unlike timolol (NEUFELD and PAGE, 1977).

c) Genetic Factors Determining Epinephrine Responsivity in Man

Populations were tested as regards their dexamethason sensitivity. There were individuals responding to local dexamethason treatment of the eye with primary open angle glaucoma (POAG); in others no changes of intraocular pressure occurred. To each group belonged 25% of the population. The remaining 50% responded with transitory elevations of intraocular pressure to dexamethason treatment. From the study of family-trees, it became evident that people reacting with POAG to dexamethason were homozygotes for the dexamethason sensitivity gene (gg), the nonresponders were homozygotes as regards the nonsensitivity gene (nn); the remaining 50% were heterozygotes (ng). It was found that almost every patient suffering from POAG belonged to the gg group. Their intraocular pressure was much more responsive to topical epinephrine, it was their remedy of choice, without applying the latter they developed severe field defects, not characteristic of the ng or nn group. Their epinephrine sensitivity was not confined to their aqueous humor dynamics. It was these patients who, when aphakic, developed macular edema on epinephrine treatment, which disappeared on cessation of this therapy.

This epinephrine responsiveness is even not confined to the eyes. The side effect of conjunctival epinephrine instillations in the gg group is pointing already to the systemic epinephrine responsiveness: premature ventricular contractions of the heart, extrasystoles. The T-lymphocytes may be transformed into lymphoblasts by the presence of phytohemagglutinine (PHA), which phenomenon can be measured by the increased uptake of [^{3}H]thymidine. The T-lymphocytes of the gg group, or POAG patients show 50% decrease of PHA-induced transformation if they are in contact with $3 \cdot 10^{-5}$ *M* epinephrine (or theophylline or dibutyryl-cAMP), in contrast to T-lymphocytes of the nn or ng group. Prednisolone phosphate seems to have a permissive effect on cAMP effects upon the cells of the gg group; dexamethason elicites cortisol release suppression in this group (BECKER and SHIN, 1976; PALMBERG et al., 1977a, b; BECKER et al., 1977). Members of the gg group and patients suffering from POAG belong to the HLA-B_{12} and HLA-B_7 groups. POAG is more prevalent between the maternal ancestors.

d) Modulation of Adrenergic Receptor Stimulators

Local application of high concentrations of norepinephrine (10^{-1} *M*) may dilate conjunctival vessels and increase intraocular pressure. This is due to an increased activity of prostaglandin synthetase occurring in the receptors consequent to α-receptor stimulation. Prostaglandin E_1 and E_2 is in feed-back relation to norepinephrine release; consequent to this feed-back effect, the release of norepinephrine decreases. Dilation of vessels and increased intraocular pressure is the effect of prostaglandins, which may manifest on cervical sympathetic ganglionectomy as well, and which may be abolished by the simultaneous administration of indomethacine (COLASANTI and BÁRÁNY, 1978; WAITZMAN et al., 1979). One of the effects of prostaglandins is to dilate intrascleral venous channels, inhibiting the outflow of aqueous humor (LANGHAM and KRIEGLSTEIN, 1975). On the administration of prostaglandin E_1 and E_2 major increases of intraocular pressure occur in experimental animals, prostaglandin $F_{2\alpha}$ is less active as regards intraocular pressure. On administration of prostaglandin $F_{2\alpha}$ and prostaglandin E_2 mainly the vessels of the ciliary body and of the iris-root dilate. Prostaglandin E_1 dilates the vessels of the entire iris. The increase of vascular permeability on the administration of every prostaglandin is tremendous (WHITELOCKE and EAKINS, 1973; LATIES et al., 1976; NEUFELD et al., 1972a).

C. Adrenergic Transmitter Releasing Agents

As the blood-brain barrier hinders the entrance of systemically administered adrenergic receptor stimulators into the brain, their releasing agents are of utmost importance giving rise to a new discipline: psychopharmacology. In the eye, only the retina is relatively less accessible to its neurotransmitter dopamine and more effects may be attained by the administration of its precursor l-Dopa together with that of MAO inhibitors and releasing agents.

On the other hand, the anterior segment of the eye is readily accessible to the adrenergic transmitters themselves, and their releasing agents have some significance, however, less than in the case of the brain and the retina.

This is the reason why the releasing agents are handled in this section in their broadest sense:

1) all the agents which can increase the stores of transmitters disposable to release (MAO inhibitors and the inhibitors of catecholamine-*O*-methyltransferase),

2) the agents inhibiting re-uptake into the storing vesicles of the adrenergic neurons (dibenzoazepines and dibenzosuberons),

3) the agents chemically related to the catecholamines, being simple or hydroxylated phenylalkylamines, expelling thereby the transmitters from the storing vesicles. Even cocaine belonges to this group as regards to its effects.

4) The drug clonidine (Catapresane) was first described as an adrenergic α-receptor blocking agent. It proved to be five times more active than epinephrine in displacing the radioligand [^{3}H]dihydroergocryptine from the α-receptors (NEUFELD and PAGE, 1977). However, in the eye its effects on the α-receptors were those of an agonist rather than of an antagonist. Its effects will be described in this section.

I. Agents Increasing the Stores of Transmitters

The retina may be maximally enriched as regards its transmitter dopamine by administering its precursor l-Dopa, after prior treatment with MAO antagonists (iproniazid, nialamide) and the re-uptake inhibiting desipramine, allowing spreading of the transmitter (EHINGER and FALCK, 1969). The physiologic releasers are light-inputs reaching the retina, which bleach the visual pigments of the photoreceptor. These bleached products increase the phosphodiesterase activity and decrease the cAMP contents of photoreceptors. Dopamine too is an inhibitory transmitter. Due to its release, reserpine causes photophobia. In the retina almost devoid of extracellular space, MAO is mainly responsible for the breakdown of the transmitter. In the elderly and in patients suffering from primary angle closure glaucoma, the adrenergic nerve-ends degenerate, not unlike their state after surgical cervical sympathetic ganglionectomy. In these states, the released norepinephrine is prone to be inactivated by catecholamine-*O*-methyltransferase. The activity of this enzyme may be inhibited by 3′4′-dihydroxy-2-methylpropiophenone, resulting in mydriasis and reduction of intraocular pressure (BAUSHER and SEARS, 1976).

II. Agents Inhibiting Re-Uptake into the Storing Vesicles

Topically applied protryptiline (a tricyclic methylaminopropyl derivative) plus norepinephrine caused submaximal mydriasis, decrease of intraocular pressure, and a fourfold increase of cAMP concentration in the aqueous humor. Neither norepinephrine, nor the potentiator alone evoked these effects. The same is attained after surgical cervical sympathetic ganglionectomy. Electric stimulation of the cervical sympathetic nerve reduces intraocular pressure, because of the decrease of circulation in the ciliary processes (Radius and Langham, 1973; Langham and Rosenthal, 1966). Scurvy also induces decreased storage and release of norepinephrine (Sears, 1973).

III. Simple or Hydroxylated Phenylalkylamines

From the group of the simple and hydroxylated phenylalkylamines, ephedrine is sometimes used locally or systemically as conjunctival vasoconstrictor or against hypersensitivity states, respectively. As vasoconstrictor naphazoline (privine) is preferred. It is noteworthy that 4-hydroxyphenyl-methylamino-(β)ethanol is, as a secondary amine, an adrenergic β-transmitter releasing agent. Its isomer, m-(3-)hydroxyphenyl-methylaminoethanol (phenylephrine, Neo-Synephrine) is an α-transmitter releasing agent, inducing, in 10% solution, in a very short time maximal mydriasis, without weakening accomodation. Its use is sometimes indispensable in ophthalmologic therapy and surgery.

Cocaine also releases norepinephrine from the adrenergic terminals, besides inducing surface anesthesia. More cocaine is bound to the pigmented iris, and hence less may serve to release norepinephrine (Patil, 1972). In the elderly less epinephrine is stored in the vesicles, and consequently the mydriatic effect of cocaine is of a lower degree.

The central effect of cocaine is due to norepinephrine liberation from the posterolateral (adrenergic) nuclei of the hypothalamus. One of the targets of thyroxine is the same, inducing adrenergic dominance in the hypothalamus. The ocular signs of hyperthyreosis are partly due to its central effect, and partly to peripheral norepinephrine release in the smooth muscles in the orbita. Amplitudes of all ERG waves are increased (Wirth and Stirpe, 1965). The same has been observed as side effect of l-Dopa therapy in Parkinson's disease.

IV. Clonidine

Clonidine, 0.5%–1.5% solutions have been found useful in the therapy of primary open angle glaucoma. The intraocular pressure decreases, pallor of conjunctiva and mydriasis are prominent. Concomitantly, blood pressure decreases as well (Bill and Heilman, 1975). The effect is due partly to adrenergic α-receptor stimulation, and partly to the decreased pressure of intrascleral venous channels. Moreover, its administration into the vertebral artery proved to be the most efficient. It seems to act upon the α-receptors of cerebral areas supplied by the vertebral arteries. This seems to support the views of Gloster and Greaves (1957) on the important role of cerebral centers governing intraocular pressure (Junemee and Zwieten, 1979).

D. Adrenergic Alpha- and Beta-Receptor Blocking Agents

I. General Considerations

An ideal adrenergic blocking agent should correspond to the following criteria:

1) It should be liable to bind to one kind of adrenergic receptors only (to α, to β_1, or to β_2, or to dopamine adrenergic receptors only). This binding is measurable by the

displacement of the α-radioligand [^{3}H]dihydroergocryptine or of the β_1-radioligand [^{3}H]dihydroalprenolol (NEUFELD and PAGE, 1977).

2) This binding should be strongly specific to one kind of adrenergic receptors.

3) This binding should not be accompanied by stimulation of the respective adrenergic receptor.

4) This binding should conceal the respective adrenergic receptor from any contact with the respective adrenergic receptor stimulator, however, it should not stabilize the membranes of the sensitive nerve-ends.

These are pharmacologic criteria, which are more, or less, or almost not fulfilled by the agents at our disposal.

As regards the effects exerted upon the eye, these considerations require further amplification.

5) Stimulation of adrenergic α-receptors increases facility of outflow of aqueous humor, and causes mydriasis. Hence adrenergic α-receptor blocking agents (a) decrease the facility of outflow, unfavorable in primary open angle glaucoma; (b) cause miosis, favorable in attacks of angle closure glaucoma, and (c) create adrenergic β-receptor dominance, decreasing the production of aqueous humor.

6) Stimulation of β_1-receptors decreases facility of outflow. Consequently, adrenergic β_1-receptor blocking agents (a) increase facility of outflow, (b) this effect is potentiated by creating α-receptor dominance, increasing facility of outflow, (c) unchanged or increased stimulated state of β_2-receptors decrease the production of aqueous humor.

Together, a, b, and c promise an increasing usage of β_1-receptor blocking agents in the treatment of primary open angle glaucoma, alone or in combination with epinephrine.

7) Stimulation of β_2-receptors does not decrease the facility of outflow. Hence the adrenergic β_2-receptor blocking agents do not increase facility of outflow, and probably increase aqueous humor production. They are less useful in the treatment of open angle glaucoma.

8) Fortunately there are adrenergic β-receptor blocking agents that are not specific for either of the two receptors: $(\beta_1+\beta_2)$ blocking agents. Among them is the most active adrenergic β blocking agent, timolol, which proved the most useful in the treatment of open angle glaucoma.

II. Effects of Alpha-Receptor Blocking Agents

1) After surgical cervical sympathetic ganglionectomy in rabbits, norepinephrine is released from the degenerating adrenergic terminals, inducing mydriasis and decreased intraocular pressure, because of the increased cAMP contents of the aqueous humor, opening the outflow channels. The appearance of both the above-described developments may be prevented by prior administration of the adrenergic α-receptor blocking agents dibenamine, penoxybenzamine (long lasting effects), or by phentolamine (SEARS and NEUFELD, 1975; LANGHAM and DIGGS, 1974). Even the mydriasis following the administration of high concentration of the adrenergic β-$_1$-stimulator isoproterenol is due to α-stimulation. It may be prevented by administration of the

Table 1. Different effects, side effects, and dosages (against open angle glaucoma) of adrenergic β-receptor blocking agents

Blocking agent	β_1 blocking effect	β_2 blocking effect	Surface anesthetic effect	Intrinsic sympatho-mimetic activity	Dosage systemic (g)	Dosage eye-drops (%)	Systemic side effects
Propranolol	+	+	+	–	2×0.040	–	–
Timolol	+	+	–	–	2×0.040	0.5–1.5	–
Practolol[a]	+	–	–	+	2×0.100	4	Heart failure
Atenolol	+	–	–	–	2×0.050	1–4	Heart failure
Alprenolol	+	–	–	–	2×0.040	–	Heart failure
Pindolol	–	+	–	+	–	1	–

[a] evoking in some individuals oculomucocutaneous syndrome

adrenergic α-receptor blocking agents phenoxybenzamine, phentolamine (LANGHAM and DIGGS, 1974; v. ALPHEN, 1976). The sequence of stimulators used to increase the facility of outflow and the concentration of cAMP is in general: epinephrine > norepinephrine > isoproterenol. These effects were prevented by phenoxybenzamine (NEUFELD et al., 1972b)

2) Clonidine does not correspond to the demand 3 described in the general considerations: it *does* stimulate the adrenergic α-receptors, and not only shield them. Hence it stimulates the adrenergic α-receptors of the pontomedullary area. This stimulation may be inhibited by the simultaneous administration of the α-receptor blocking agent piperoxan (JUNEMEE and ZWIETEN, 1979).

3) Against attacks of angle closure glaucoma, 0.5% solution of thymoxymine was instilled frequently (every minute for a quarter of an hour), inducing maximal miosis (HALASA and RUTKOWSKI, 1973).

4) Ergotamine salts reduce pulsation of intracranial arteries, relieving migraine. Hydergin was found useful in the treatment of occlusions of the central retinal vessels.

III. Effects of Beta-Receptor Blocking Agents

1. Synopsis of Their Different Effects

Administration of all adrenergic β-receptor blocking agents induce α-receptor dominance. This may be proven, as in the case of norepinephrine effect, by the increased synthesis of phosphatidic acid, phosphatidyl-serine, and phosphatidyl-inositol in the muscles of the iris (ABDEL-LATIF and SMITH, 1976). α-Receptor dominance is characterized, even in man and more so in rabbits, by increased aqueous humor-cAMP inducing increased outflow facility (NEUFELD et al., 1972b) (see Table 1).

2. $Beta_1$- and $Beta_2$-Receptor Blocking Agents

Of all the stimulators and blocking agents the most effective in displacing the adrenergic β-receptor radioligand [^{3}H]dihydroalprenolol in iris-ciliary body membrane preparations were the β_1- and β_2-receptor blocking agents propranolol and timolol (NEUFELD and PAGE, 1977). Timolol was the most effective in this respect, 100-fold more active than epinephrine.

In clinical therapy (primary open angle glaucoma), timolol has been found to be the β-receptor blocking agent of choice (ZIMMERMAN and KAUFMAN, 1977a, b). The pupil remained unchanged (JOHNSON et al., 1978), the decrease of intraocular pressure to normal values was due to reduction of aqueous humor production (SONNTAG et al., 1978). The effects of propranolol were slight in inhibiting epinephrine activity, maximal in antagonizing that of isoproterenol. The receptors of corneal epithelium are β-receptors, stimulated by the almost only available physiologic transmitter norepinephrine, stimulated, however, (and destroyed) by instilled epinephrine. These effects could be blocked totally by propranolol (RADIUS and LANGHAM, 1973).

Practolol, atenolol (ELLIOT et al., 1975; WETTRELL and PANDOLFI, 1977), and alprenolol are both chemically and pharmacologically related substances. Chemically all three are phenoxyalkanolamine derivatives, with somewhat different side-chains. Pharmacologically they are blocking agents of the adrenergic β_1-receptor. In the eye, this manifests in the increase of aqueous humor outflow facility (WETTRELL and PANDOLFI, 1975). One danger of practolol therapy consists in the possibility of inducing oculomucocutaneous syndrome (FELIX et al., 1974; RAHI et al., 1976). Its appearance may be predicted from the decrease of tears' lysozyme-activity, and by the appearance of antinuclear and antiintercellular-cement antibodies, leading to Sjögren's syndrome. Even drug-induced pemphigus may appear.

Pindolol reduces intraocular pressure by decreasing the rate of aqueous humor production. This effect is slight, however (BONOMI and STEINDLER, 1975).

IV. Dopaminergic Receptor Blocking Agents

They act upon the dopaminergic receptors of the retina. Chlorimipramine is the specific blocking agent of retinal dopaminergic receptors; the most effective (specific) dopaminergic receptor blocking agent is haloperidol (BROWN and MAKMAN, 1973).

E. Adrenergic Nerve-End Inhibitors, Neural Transmitter Depleting Agents and False Transmitters

I. General Considerations

The main effect of all these agents is to decrease, at least at a certain limited phase of their activity, the release of the adrenergic receptor stimulator norepinephrine from the adrenergic nerve-ends.

1) In the case of adrenergic true nerve-end inhibitors (TM_{10} = cholin-2,6-xylyl-etherbromide, bretylium tosylate), the adrenergic neurons reveal their stimulated

state by giving rise to electric peaks, however, the nerve-ends fail to release norepinephrine. The responsiveness of the receptors remain undisturbed by norepinephrine, if delivered artificially to the latter, in contrast to their shielded state after administration of blocking agents.

2) In the case of transmitter depleting agents (e.g., reserpine, tetrabenazine), storing of the transmitters is disturbed. The first phase of their activity results in an increased release of the transmitters, followed by the second phase when little or no epinephrine remains to be released. In the first phase they resemble adrenergic transmitter releasing agents; in the second phase they differ from them.

3) Increased release, followed by absence of stored true transmitters, and the supersensitivity of the empty receptors may be attained by the administration of "false" transmitters, which like cuckoos extrude the true transmitters from their nests, the storing vesicles. In this context it should be remembered that both amphetamine and sympaethamine, the typical adrenergic transmitter releasing agents, are α-methylated phenylaethylamine derivatives, much the same as the false transmitter α-methyldopa is, however the latter is stored more avidly by the vesicles, being more resemblant to the true transmitter; both α-methyl-norepinephrine and norepinephrine are catecholamines.

Consequently, in describing the effects on the eye of all the three groups of agents, due attention will be paid to the normal sensitivity or supersensitivity of the receptors, and to the initially decreased or increased release of the adrenergic transmitter from the adrenergic nerve-end.

II. Effects of Adrenergic Nerve-End Inhibitors on the Eye

1) TM_{10} and bretylium (Darenthin) inhibit the release of norepinephrine from the adrenergic nerve-ends. This manifests in the eye in an extreme miosis, as TM_{10} has muscarine-like side effects too.

2) Guanethidine (Ismeline) also inhibits the release of norepinephrine from the adrenergic terminals. This results in a decreased aqueous production and in miosis. Moreover, guanethidine initially increases the release of norepinephrine stores, acting rather in the beginning as an adrenergic depleting agent. This initial phase of activity manifests in an increased outflow of aqueous. On continuation of this therapy, the stores of adrenergic transmitters evacuate and the receptors devoid of the transmitters for long, become more and more sensitive to the latter, as if they had been denervated. This epinephrine hypersensitivity created by guanethidine suggested the combined local use of 2.5% guanethidine plus 0.5% epinephrine in a borate-phosphate buffer, pH 7.4 with preservatives, in the therapy of primary open angle glaucoma. They act by increasing outflow and decreasing inflow of aqueous, and by a further increase of the responsiveness of primary open angle glaucoma to epinephrine (Roth, 1973; Jones et al., 1975; Editorial, 1975).

The increased norepinephrine response probably increases the prostaglandin-synthetase activity in the anterior segment of the eye, which becomes evident in vascular dilatation and pain, sometimes precluding continuation of this therapy.

Another side effect of guanethidine that becomes apparent after 5–6 days of instillation, when the initially increased release of norepinephrine is already changing towards a decreased release, is ptosis. This may be of value in abolishing Graefe's sign of hyperthyreotic patients.

Systemic administration of guanethidihe may inhibit the release of, or deplete, dopamine from retinal dopaminergic junctional cells, the absence of this photopic inhibitory transmitter manifesting in photophobia.

III. Effects of Adrenergic Transmitter Depleting Procedures and Agents on the Eye

Depletion of adrenergic transmitters may be attained by cervical sympathetic superior ganglionectomy. After having performed this procedure the storing vesicles of the adrenergic terminals initially degenerate, this process may be followed ultrastructurally (FLACH and WOOD, 1978). The release of norepinephrine increases the outflow of aqueous humor, leading to a decreased intraocular pressure. Later the adrenergic nerve terminals become depleted, and less adrenergic activator is delivered to the receptors, hence their increased norepinephrine responsiveness. Administration of reserpine prior to denervation was found to abolish the initial response to denervation, i.e., the increased norepinephrine concentration of the aqueous humor, the increased facility of outflow, reserpine having had already depleted the transmitter from the adrenergic nerve-ends that should be released by denervation. Simultaneous administration of reserpine with denervation, on the other hand, increased the release of norepinephrine and its ocular signs. Of course, not only prior administration of reserpine, but all pharmacologic pretreatments that may either inhibit the biosynthesis of norepinephrine (e.g., α-methyl-p-tyrosine, decreasing tyrosine hydroxylase activity), or decrease storage of the transmitter (e.g., α-methyl-m-tyrosine, transformed into metaraminol in the storing vesicles) may decrease denervation effects (SEARS and NEUFELD, 1975). Denervation may be performed by injecting very young animals with antinerve-growth factor containing sera, or pharmacologically. Without paying respect to the method of denervation, prior administration of reserpine decreases, while simultaneous reserpinization increases the early signs of denervation.

Reserpine depletes dopamine from the retinal junctional cells, causing photophobia (KRAMER, 1971).

IV. False Transmitters

1) The most frequently used false transmitter is α-methyl-Dopa being transformed in the anterior segment of the eye to α-methyl-noradrenaline (Cobefrin). Continuous administration of this agent causes, after initial rise of the concentration of norepinephrine in the aqueous humor, a decrease of the latter. As protein synthesis of the lens is protein-kinase (cAMP- and consequently norepinephrine-) dependent, α-methyl-Dopa therapy may be presumed, and has been found to be cataractogenous.

2) α-Methyl-m-tyrosine is used mostly in pharmacologic experiments to deplete adrenergic transmitters, as it is formed to metaraminol(3-hydroxyphenyl-α methyl-β hydroxy-aethanolamine). Its administration stops melatonin synthesis in the pineal gland.

3) Both pharmacologically and in the therapy of primary open angle glaucoma, the false transmitter 6-hydroxy-dopamine is of utmost importance.

a) Its pharmacologic effects on the eye, after having been injected subconjunctivally, may be divided into three periods:

initial release of norepinephrine, followed by

perfect depletion of norepinephrine from the adrenergic nerve-ends, and dominance of acetylcholinergic innervation,

days later, a hypersensitivity of receptors to epinephrine develops, as it appears after denervation ("pharmacologic denervation").

These stages are shown by:

pupil diameter: mydriasis, followed by miosis, and later mydriasis after instillation of very low concentrations of epinephrine;

intraocular pressure: decrease, followed by increase, later by epinephrine-induced decreases (HOLLAND and MIMS, 1971). The corresponding ultrastructural changes were followed by EM studies (FLACH and WOOD, 1978).

According to radioligand-displacement studies, 6-*OH*-dopamine decreases the density of free β-receptors in iris-ciliary body preparations (NEUFELD et al., 1978).

b) Clinical effects. Solutions of 0.2 ml of 2% 6-hydroxy-dopamine were injected subconjunctivally in patients suffering from primary open angle glaucoma.

Pupil changes: mydriasis, followed by miosis, and later hypersensitivity to epinephrine occurred.

Intraocular pressure decreased by 20 Hgmm, due to 70% increase of outflow facility.

These effects of one single treatment lasted for 86 days (longer, than those of some surgical interventions) (DIAMON, 1976).

F. Summary

The four types of agents, and their subtypes acting on adrenergic structures of the eye and of its adnexa were dealt with in different sections and subsections of this chapter as if their effects were not interconnected with each other. Of course, they are interconnected, which is shown by synergism or antagonism. To get a bird's eye view of ocular autonomic interactions, two aspects of autonomic regulation should be kept in mind.

1) In the autonomic regulations, both adrenergic and acetylcholinergic neurons and their receptors are involved. In the hypothalamic centers adrenergic dominance is always stressed by the simultaneous decrease of its antagonist-transmitter serotonin, and vice versa. In contrast to the centers in the peripheral organs, e.g., the eye, trends toward homeostasis sometimes prevail: administration of cholinergic agents increase the concentration of norepinephrine in the iris. In other respects an antagonism between all the adrenergic stimulators and the acetylcholinergic agents becomes apparent, for example, in the intraocular smooth muscles.

2) There is a second antagonism between adrenergic α- and β-receptors. For example, adrenergic α-receptor blocking agents induce β-receptor dominance, blocking

of β-receptors create α-dominance. Timolol seems to be the most effective β_1- and β_2-receptor blocking agent in the treatment of primary open angle glaucoma. Other instances suggest a veritable synergism of adrenergic α- and β-receptors, e.g., as regards facility of outflow, or a synergism as regards the end result (decrease of intraocular pressure: α-receptors increasing facility of outflow of, β-receptors decreasing inflow of aqueous humor). It sounds like a joke, but it is reality that even cholinergic stimulators, e.g., pilocarpine, yield the same end effect: the decrease of intraocular pressure by increasing facility of outflow. This end result is counteracted to some extent, however, not abolished by the simultaneous increase of aqueous humor production. There are basic differences, however, in the responsiveness of different glaucomas: *primary open angle glaucoma is genetically determined to be epinephrine responsive, primary angle closure glaucoma is anatomically determined to respond mainly to cholinergic stimuli.*

3) As regards effects the most intricate are the interconnections of nerve-end inhibitors and false transmitters with other adrenergic agents: in the beginning, the release of norepinephrine prevails, later the absence of it, concomitantly with the hypersensitivity towards epinephrine. Consequently, the effects of guanethidine or 6-*OH*-dopamine may be potentiated by the simultaneously administered epinephrine.

4) Interconnections of adrenergic receptor stimulators and prostaglandins.

High concentrations of norepinephrine or epinephrine increase the signs of prostaglandin dominance. Prostaglandin E_1 and E_2 decrease the release of norepinephrine. The disturbing signs of prostaglandin dominance may be abolished by indomethacine.

Increasing knowledge of interactions between agents of autonomic regulations both verify old observations and create new possibilities for their combined administration.

References

Abdel-Latif, H.A., Smith, J.P.: Effects of D,L-propranolol on the synthesis of glycerolipids by rabbit iris muscle. Biochem. Pharmacol. *25*, 1697–1704 (1976)

Alm, A.: The effect of sympathetic stimulation on blood flow through the uvea, retina and optic nerve in monkeys (Macaca irus). Exp. Eye Res. *25*, 19–24 (1977)

van Alphen, G.W.H.M.: The adrenergic receptor of the intraocular muscles of the human eye. Invest. Ophthalmol. *15*, 502–505 (1976)

Anton-Tay, F.: Pineal-brain relationships. The pineal gland, a Ciba Foundation symposium, Wolstenholme, G.E.W., Knight, J. (eds.), pp. 213–220. Edinburgh, London: Churchill Livingstone 1971

Axelrod, J.: Neural control of indoleamine metabolism in the pineal. The pineal gland, a Ciba Foundation symposium, Wolstenholme, G.E.W., Knight, J. (eds.), pp. 35–47. Edinburgh, London: Churchill Livingstone 1971

Bausher, L.P., Sears, M.L.: Potentiation of the effects of topical epinephrine on the pupil and intraocular pressere in the sympathetically denervated rabbit eye by a catechol-0-methyl transferase inhibitor. Invest. Ophthalmol. *15*, 854–857 (1976)

Becker, B., Shin, D.H.: Response to topical epinephrine, a practical prognostic test in patients with ocular hypertension. Arch. Ophthalmol. *94*, 2057–2058 (1976)

Becker, B., Montgomery, S.W., Kass, M.A., Shin, D.H.: Increased ocular and systemic responsiveness to epinephrine in primary open angle glaucoma. Arch. Ophthalmol. *95*, 789–790 (1977)

Bill, A., Heilman, K.: Ocular effects of clonidin in cats and monkeys. Exp. Eye Res. *21*, 481–488 (1975)
Bitensky, M.W., Miki, N., Marcus, F.R., Kleirns, J.J.: The role of cyclic nucleotids in visual excitation. Life Sci. *13*, 145–147 (1973)
Bonomi, L., Steindler, P.: Effect of Pindolol on intraocular pressure. Br. J. Ophthalmol. *59*, 301–303 (1975)
Brown, J.H., Makman, M.H.: Stimulation by dopamine of adenylate cyclase in retinal homogenates and of adenosine 3'-5'-cyclic monophosphate formation in intact retina. Proc. Natl. Acad. Sci. USA *69*, 539–543 (1972)
Brown, J.H., Makman, M.H.: Influence of neuroleptic drugs and apomorphine on dopamine-sensitive adenylate cyclase of retina. J. Neurochem. *21*, 477–479 (1973)
Bubenik, G.A., Purtill, R.A., Brown, G.M., Grota, L.J.: Melatonin in the retina and the Harderian gland. Exp. Eye Res. *27*, 323–333 (1978)
Bucher, M.B., Schorderet, M.: Apomorphine-induced accumulation of cyclic AMP in isolated retinas of the rabbit. Biochem. Pharmacol. *23*, 3079–3082 (1974)
Chandra, S.R., Friedmann, E.: Choroidal blood flow. II. The effects of autonomic agents. Arch. Ophthalmol. *87*, 67–69 (1972)
Chau-Po Wei, Anderson, J.A., Leopold, I.: Ocular absorption and metabolism of topically applied epinephrine, and a dipivalyl ester of epinephrine. Invest. Ophthalmol. *17*, 315–321 (1978)
Chiou, C.Y., Zimmerman, T.J.: Ocular hypotensive effects of autonomic drugs. Invest. Ophthalmol. *14*, 416–417 (1975)
Cohen, S.: Purification of a nerve growth promoting protein from the mouse salivary gland and its neurocytotoxic antiserum. Proc. Natl. Acad. Sci. USA *46*, 302–311 (1960)
Colasanti, B.K., Bárány, E.H.: Reduction by indomethacin of the degeneration increase in outflow facility after superior cervical ganglionectomy in the rabbit. Invest. Ophthalmol. *17*, 802–805 (1978)
Diamon, J.G.: 6-hydroxydopamine in treatment of open angle glaucoma. Arch. Ophthalmol. *94*, 41–47 (1976)
Duke-Elder, S., Gloster, J.: The physiology of the eye and of vision. System of ophthalmol. Duke-Elder, S. (Ed.), Vol. IV, pp. 426–427. London: Kimpton 1968
Editorial: A sympathetic approach to open-angle glaucoma. Br. J. Ophthalmol. *59*, 295 (1975)
Ehinger, B., Falck, B.: Morphological and pharmacohistological characteristics of adrenergic retinal neurons of some mammals. Graefes Arch. Ophthalmol. *178*, 295–305 (1969)
Ehinger, B., Florén, I.: Quantitation fo the uptake of indolamines and dopamine in the rabbit retina. Exp. Eye Res. *26*, 1–11 (1978)
Elliot, M.J., Cullen, P.M., Phillips, C.I.: Ocular hypotensive effect of atenolol. Br. J. Ophthalmol. *59*, 296–300 (1975)
Felix, R.H., Ive, F.A., Dahl, M.G.C.: Cutaneous and ocular reactions to practolol. Br. Med. J. *4*, 321–324 (1974)
Flach, A., Wood, I.: An electron microscopic study of degeneration of nerve terminals after administration of epinephrine. Exp. Eye Res. *27*, 377–385 (1978)
Froomberg, D., Voaden, M.J.: An investigation of mitotic control in the rabbit lens epithelium. Exp. Eye Res. *5*, 1–9 (1966)
Gloster, J., Greaves, D.P.: Effect of diencephalic stimulation upon intraocular pressure. Br. J. Ophthalmol. *41*, 513–532 (1957)
Guy, J., Quigley, H.A., Andersen, D.R.: The effect of biogenic monoamines on rapid axonal transport in the rabbit optic nerve. Invest. Ophthalmol. *17*, 296–300 (1978)
Halasa, A.H., Rutkowski, P.C.: Thymoxamine therapy for angle closure glaucoma. Arch. Ophthalmol. *90*, 177–179 (1973)
Holland, M.G., Mims, J.L.: Anterior segment chemical sympathectomy by 6-hydroxy-dopamine. Invest. Ophthalmol. *10*, 120–143 (1971)
Iversen, L.L., Hendry, I.A., Mackay, A.V.P.: Assay of nerve growth factor (NGF) in mouse tissue and the role of NGF and depolarizing stimuli in the long-term regulation of tyrosine-hydroxylase activity in adrenergic neurons. Dynamics of degeneration and growth in neurons. Fuxe, K., Olson, L., Zotterman, Y. (eds.), pp. 329–345. Oxford: Pergamon 1974

Johnson, S.J., Brubaker, R.F., Trautman, J.C.: Absence of an effect of timolol on the pupil. Invest. Ophthalmol. *17*, 924–926 (1978)
Jones, D.E.P., Norton, D.A., Harvey, J., Davies, D.J.G.: Effect of adrenaline and guanethidine in reducing intraocular pressure in rabbits' eyes. Br. J. Ophthalmol. *59*, 304–307 (1975)
Joó, I., Kahán, Á.: The porphyrin content of Harderian glands is rats and the melatonine-melanocyte stimulating hormone-system. Endokrinologie *65*, 308–312 (1975)
Junemee, H.C., Zwieten, P.A.: The central ocular hypotensive effect of clonidine. Graefes Arch. Ophthalmol. *210*, 93–102 (1979)
Kahán, Á.: The role of blood in the pathogeny and therapy of retinal disorders. Thesis, Acad. Sci. Hung. 1971
Kahán, Á., Oláh, M.: Catecholamine-contents of the retina and uvea and their significance. Szemészet *112*, 182–185 (1975)
Klyce, S.D., Neufeld, A.H., Zadunaisky, J.A.: Actions of epinephrine and other cAMP mediator agents on the chloride transport of the frog cornea. Invest. Ophthalmol. *11*, 644–650 (1972)
Knyihár, K., Ristovky, G., Csillik, B.: Chemical sympathectomy: Histochemical and submicroscopical consequences of 6-hydroxy-dopamine treatment in the rat iris. Experientia *25*, 518–520 (1969)
Kramer, S.G.: Dopamine: a retinal neurotransmitter. I. Retinal uptake, storage, and light-stimulated release of H 3-dopamine in vivo. Invest. Ophthal. *10*, 438–452 (1971)
Kramer, S.G., Potts, A.M.: Catecholamine metabolite formation in the iris and ciliary body in vivo. Am. J. Ophthalmol. *72*, 939–946 (1971)
Kramer, S.G., Potts, A.M., Mangnall, Y.: Dopamine: A retinal neurotransmitter. II. Autoradiographic localization of H 3-dopamine in the retina. Invest. Ophthalmol. *10*, 617–624 (1971)
Kramer, S.G., Potts, A.M., Mangnall, Y.: Autoradiographic localization ofcateholamines in the uveal tract. I. Light-microscopic study. Am. J. Ophthalmol. *74*, 129–134 (1972)
Krejci, L., Harrison, R.: Epinephrine effects on corneal cells in tissue culture. Arch. Ophthalmol. *83*, 451–454 (1957)
Lahav, M., Melamed, E., Dafna, Z., Alas, D.: Localization of beta-receptors in the anterior segment of the rat eye by a fluorescent analogue of propranolol. Invest. Ophthalmol. *17*, 645–651 (1978)
Lamble, J.W.: Some factors affecting the intraocular hypotensive and mydriasis responses of the rabbit to topically administered L-adrenaline bitartrate. Exp. Eye Res. *17*, 473–482 (1973)
Langham, M.E., Diggs, E.: Beta-adrenergic responses in the eyes of rabbits, primates, and man. Exp. Eye Res. *19*, 281–295 (1974)
Langham, M.E., Krieglstein, G.K.: Die Wirkung wiederholter Adrenalin-Applikation auf intraokularen Druck und Pupille beim Kaninchen. Graefes Arch. Ophthalmol. *196*, 267–277 (1975)
Langham, M.E., Rosenthal, R.: Role of cervical sympathetic nerve in regulating intraocular pressure and circulation. Am. J. Physiol. *210*, 786–794 (1966)
Laties, A.L., Neufeld, A.H., Veggs, T., Sears, L.: Differential reactivity of rabbit iris and ciliary process to topically applied prostaglandin E_2 (Dinoprostone). Arch. Ophthalmol. *94*, 1966–1971 (1976)
Lerner, A.B., Case, J.D.: Pigment cell regulatory factors. J. Invest. Dermatol. *32*, 211–221 (1959)
Lerner, A.B., Case, J.D., Heinzelman, R.V.: Structure of melatonin. J. Am. Chem. Soc. *81*, 6084–6085 (1959)
Lerner, A.B., Case, J.D., Takayaski, Y.: Isolation of melatonin and 5-methoxyindol-3-acetic acid from bovine pineal glands. J. Biol. Chem. *235*, 1992–1997 (1960)
Levi-Montalcini, R., Angeletti, P.U.: Nerve growth factor. Physiol. Rev. *48*, 534–569 (1968)
Macri, F.J.: Vasoconstriction produced in the iris-ciliary body of the cat by stimulation of local ganglion-like receptors. Invest. Ophthalmol. *10*, 581–588 (1971)
Miller, W.H., Gorman, R.E., Bitensky, M.W.: Cyclic adenosine monophosphate function in photoreceptors. Science *174*, 295–297 (1971)

Moszkovska, A., Kordon, C., Ebels, I.: Biochemical fractions and mechanisms involved in the pineal modulation of pituitary gonadotropin release. The pineal gland, a Ciba Foundation symposium, Wolstenholme, G.E.W., Knight, J. (eds.), pp. 241–256. Edinburgh, London: Churchill Livingstone 1971
Neetens, A., Bernard, P.J.: The influence of adrenergic drugs on intra-ocular pressure in the anaesthetized dog. Exp. Eye Res. *17*, 427–433 (1973)
Neufeld, A.H., Page, E.D.: In vitro determination of the ability of drugs to bind to adrenergic receptors. Invest. Ophthalmol. *16*, 1118–1124 (1977)
Neufeld, A.H., Jampol, L.M., Sears, M.L.: Aspirin prevents the disruption of the blood-aqueous barrier in the rabbit eye. Nature *238*, 158–159 (1972a)
Neufeld, A.H., Jampol, L.M., Sears, M.L.: Cyclic-AMP in the aqueous humor. The effects of adrenergic agents. Exp. Eye Res. *14*, 242–250 (1972b)
Neufeld, A.H., Zawistowski, K.A., Page, E.D., Bromberg, B.B.: Influences on the density of beta adrenergic receptors in the cornea and iris-ciliary body of the rabbit. Invest. Ophthalmol. *17*, 1069–1075 (1978)
Palmberg, P.F., Hajek, S., Cooper, D., Becker, B.: Increased ocular and systemic responsiveness to epinephrine in primary open angle glaucoma. Arch. Ophthalmol. *95*, 789–790 (1977a)
Palmberg, P.F., Hajek, S., Cooper, D., Becker, B.: Increased cellular responsiveness to epinephrine in primary open angle glaucoma. Arch. Ophthalmol. *95*, 855–856 (1977b)
Pannbacker, R.G., Fleischman, D.E., Reed, D.W.: Cyclic nucleotide diesterase: high activity in mammalian photoreceptors. Science *175*, 757–758 (1972)
Patil, P.N.: Cocaine-binding by the pigmented and the nonpigmented iris and its relevance to the mydriatic effect. Invest. Ophthalmol. *11*, 739–746 (1972)
Radius, R., Langham, M.E.: Cyclic AMP and the ocular response to norepinephrine. Exp. Eye Res. *17*, 219–229 (1973)
Rahi, A.H.S., Chapman, C.M., Garner, A., Wright, P.: Pathology of practolol-induced ocular toxicity. Br. J. Ophthalmol. *60*, 312–323 (1976)
Rentzhog, L.: Synthesis of catecholamines in the eye after local injection of ^{3}H-precursors. Acta Physiol. Scand. *94*, 459–466 (1975)
Roth, J.A.: Guanethidine and adrenaline used in combination in chronic simple glaucoma. Br. J. Ophthalmol. *57*, 507–510 (1973)
Schümann, H.J.: Formation of adrenergic transmitters. Adrenergic mechanisms. Ciba Foundation symposium. Vane, J.J., Wolstenholme, G.E.W., O'Connor, M. (eds.), pp. 6–16. London: Churchill Livingstone 1960
Scott, A.B., Collins, C.C.: Division of labor in human extraocular muscle. Arch. Ophthalmol. *90*, 319–327 (1973)
Sears, M.L.: Adrenergic supersensitivity of the scorbutic iris. Trans. Am. Ophthalmol. Soc. *71*, 536–557 (1973)
Sears, M.L.: Perspectives in glaucoma research. Invest. Ophthalmol. *17*, 6–20 (1978)
Sears, M.L., Neufeld, A.H.: Adrenergic modulation of the outflow of aqueous humor. Invest. Ophthalmol. *14*, 83–86 (1975)
Seidehamel, R.J., Dungan, K.W., Hickey, T.E.: Specific hypotensive and antihypertensive ocular effects of D-isoproterenol in rabbits. Am. J. Ophthalmol. *79*, 1018–1025 (1975)
Sonntag, R., Brindley, G.O., Shields, M.B.: Effect of timolol therapy on outflow facilities. Invest. Ophthalmol. *17*, 293–296 (1978)
Udenfriend, S., Weissbach, H., Bogdanski, P.F.: Increase in tissue serotonin following administration of its precursor 5-hydroxy-tryptophan. J. Biol. Chem. *224*, 803–810 (1957)
Varon, S., Nomura, J., Shooter, E.M.: The isolation of the mouse nerve growth factor protein in a high molecular weight form. Biochemistry *6*, 2202–2209 (1967)
Varon, S., Nomura, J., Shooter, E.M.: Reversible dissociation of the mouse nerve growth factor protein into different subunits. Biochemistry *7*, 1296–1303 (1968)
Voaden, M.J.: A chalone in the rabbit lens. Exp. Eye Res. *7*, 326–331 (1968)
Voaden, M.J., Froomberg, D.: Topography of a mitotic inhibitor in the rabbit lens. Exp. Eye Res. *6*, 213–218 (1967)

Waitzmann, M.B., Woods, W.D., Cheek, W.V.: Effects of prostaglandins and norepinephrine on ocular pressure and pupil size in rabbits following bilateral cervical ganglionectomy. Invest. Ophthalmol. *18*, 52–60 (1979)
Waltman, S.R., Yarian, D., Hart, W., Becker, B.: Corneal endothelial changes with long term topical epinephrine therapy. Arch. Ophthalmol. *95*, 1357–1358 (1977)
Wettrell, K., Pandolfi, M.: Effect of oral administration of various beta-blocking agents on the intraocular pressure in healthy volunteers. Exp. Eye Res. *21*, 451–456 (1975)
Wettrell, K., Pandolfi, M.: Effect of topical atenolol on intraocular pressure. Br. J. Ophthalmol. *61*, 334–338 (1977)
Whitelocke, R.A.F., Eakins, K.E.: Vascular changes in the anterior uvea of the rabbit produced by prostaglandins. Arch. Ophthalmol. *89*, 495–499 (1973)
Wirth, A., Stirpe, M.: The electroretinogram in thyroid dysfunction. Current topics in thyroid research. New York: Academic Press 1965
Zadunaisky, J.A., Lande, M.A., Chalfie, M., Neufeld, A.H.: Ion pumps in the cornea and its stimulation by epinephrine and cAMP. Exp. Eye Res. *15*, 577–584 (1973)
Zimmerman, T., Kaufman, H.E.: Timolol. A beta-adrenergic blocking agent for the treatment of glaucoma. Arch. Ophthalmol. *95*, 601–605 (1977a)
Zimmerman, T., Kaufman, H.E.: Timolol. Dose, response and duration of action. Arch. Ophthalmol. *95*, 605–607 (1977b)

CHAPTER 9

Effects of Adrenergic Activators and Inhibitors on the Sweat Glands

D. ROBERTSHAW

A. Classification of Sweat Glands

Sweat glands have been defined as all those cutaneous glands other than sebaceous glands that produce a secretion onto the surface of the skin. This loose definition encompasses a wide variety of structures with a broad range of functions. Some, such as the dermal glands of the hippopotamus or the nasal disc of the pig, have never been identified as sweat glands, whereas other glands are so specialized that it is difficult to decide how they might be classified. On a purely anatomical and embryological basis BLIGH (1967) coined the terms epitrichial to refer to glands associated with hair follicles, and atrichial for those that open onto the epidermal surface independent of hair follicle units. SCHIEFFERDECKER (1917, 1922) classified glands associated with hair follicles as apocrine and those that have a duct which spirals through the epidermis and are independent of hair follicles or sebaceous glands as eccrine. This is the more conventional terminology although it is based on a suggested mode of secretion that is probably erroneous (JENKINSON, 1967). There does, however, appear to be a physiologic distinction between the two types of glands since eccrine glands are innervated largely by cholinergic nerves and apocrine glands by adrenergic nerves. Thus it is possible to examine sudomotor transmission alone without having to classify them on the basis of structure or function of the gland. In fact, there is considerable functional overlap. For example, in man and many primates, eccrine glands are concerned with thermoregulation, whereas in cattle and horses apocrine glands serve this function. Likewise, the sweat glands on the foot pad of the cat and dog aid frictional resistance and are eccrine, whereas those on the feet of the koala bear are apocrine. In many species, including man, the apocrine glands are odoriferous, which may have been the original function of phylogenetically primitive glands. The function of the primitive eccrine gland was probably to assist in prehension, and its distribution was therefore localized to glabrous friction areas of skin, e.g. foot pads of animals and palms and soles of man. In the case of man and some primates, eccrine glands have extended in the course of evolution to the general body surface where they have assumed a thermoregulatory function. As a result, the palmar glands of man respond to two different types of stimuli: emotion and heat exposure; the former being related to prehensile function and the latter to heat dissipation. Thus, the palmar glands may posses a double innervation with two separate central connections within the central nervous system.

Three cell types are involved in sweating. The cells of the secretory coil elaborate the primal secretion whose composition and volume may be changed by the cells that line the excretory duct. In addition the secretory cells are surrounded by myoepithelial cells that are assumed to be contractile although this has never been observed directly or recorded. Fluctuations in sweat output observed from continuous records of cutaneous moisture loss are usually attributed to myoepithelial activity although they may be due to changes in rate of secretion. Theoretically, therefore, the control of the rate and composition of sweat can be influenced at each of these sites although this aspect of sweat secretion has not been fully investigated.

Students of physiology are usually taught that transmission from postganglionic sympathetic nerve endings is effected by the release of noradrenaline and that sudomotor eccrine transmission by acetylcholine represents an exception to this rule. This finding is based in part on the experiments of DALE and FELDBERG (1934) who detected acetylcholine in the blood that drains the paw of the cat during plantar nerve stimulation. However, ICHIBASHI (1936) demonstrated that iontophoretic administration of adrenaline would also stimulate eccrine sweat glands, an observation that has been confirmed many times and resulted in much speculation on its physiologic significance.

Apocrine sweat glands have been shown to be adrenergic, but in some species, e.g. the horse, they can also be stimulated by the local application of acetylcholine (EVANS and SMITH, 1956). Thus, the division of eccrine and apocrine glands on the basis of neural transmission is seen to be less specific than was suggested by the original observations. The whole issue has been reactivated recently by the work of UNO (1977) who has demonstrated that both apocrine and eccrine glands of man and macaque monkeys have a cholinergic and adrenergic nerve supply. The presence of adrenergic nerves was detected by light microscopy using the formaldehyde fluorescence method (FALCK, 1962) and by electron microscopy using 6-hydroxydopamine, a substance that causes selective degeneration of adrenergic nerve terminals. Although UNO (1977) found that the innervation of eccrine glands is predominantly cholinergic and that of apocrine glands adrenergic, the physiologic significance of the secondary innervation remains to be elucidated.

B. Apocrine Glands

In many species, especially those of the orders Perissodactyla and Artiodactyla, apocrine glands on the general body surface can be stimulated by heat exposure and are concerned to varying degrees with temperature regulation. Sudomotor transmission, therefore, can be readily studied since the natural stimulus is known.

I. Perissodactyla

1. Equidae

Two species of horse have been studied, *Equus equus* and *Equus asinus*. The glands can be stimulated by the intradermal administration of adrenaline and isoprenaline at much lower concentrations than noradrenaline. Intravenous adrenaline and isoprenaline, but not noradrenaline are potent sudorific agents (EVANS and SMITH, 1956; ALLEN and BLIGH, 1969; ROBERTSHAW and TAYLOR, 1969b). Isolated perfused skin responds in a similar manner (JOHNSON, 1975). The glands can also be stimulated by cholomimetic agents but only at high concentrations relative to adrenergic compounds; the volume of sweat produced by acetylcholine is small and sweating is of

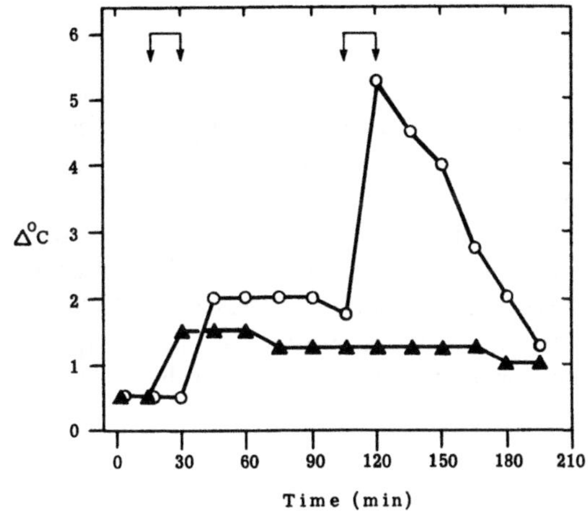

Fig. 1. Record of cutaneous moisture loss from the midside of a donkey exposed to an air temperature of 40 °C. Δ °C is the difference of wet bulb temperatures of ambient air and that of a stream of air passing through a capsule placed on the skin. Control experiment (○); the effect of propranolol (▲) infused between the *arrows* at 15–30 min. Adrenaline was infused (0.25 μg/kg · min) in both experiments at 105–120 min as shown by the arrows. (After ROBERTSHAW, 1974, with permission)

short duration when compared to that produced by adrenaline or isoprenaline (EVANS and SMITH, 1956). These findings are taken as evidence that not only is sweating under adrenergic control but also that β-receptors are involved. The presence of β-receptors has been confirmed using the β-receptor blocking drug propranolol, which blocks both heat- and adrenaline-induced sweating (ROBERTSHAW, 1974; Fig. 1). LANDS et al. (1967) subdivided β-receptors into β_1 and β_2 types. The β_1-receptors are located in the heart, whereas most receptors elsewhere are β_2-receptors. SNOW (1977) concluded that since sweating is not suppressed by the β_1-receptor blocking drug metroprolol, the receptors at the sweat glands are the β_2-variety. BELL and EVANS (1956) were unable to produce sweating by sympathetic nerve stimulation and proposed that sweating in the horse is caused by blood-borne adrenaline and that no sudomotor nerves exist. However, sweating in response to heat exposure does not occur from sympathetically denervated skin although exercise and i.v. adrenaline infusion have a sudorific effect (ROBERTSHAW and TAYLOR, 1969b). Furthermore, bethanidine, an adrenergic-neurone blocking agent that does not influence adrenomedullary secretion (BOURA and GREEN, 1963) effectively inhibits heat-induced sweating (ROBERTSHAW and TAYLOR, 1969b). The conclusion from these observations is that exercise-induced sweating combines both neural and humoral components whereas thermal sweating is under neural control only. The presence of a nerve supply has been confirmed anatomically by both light and electron microscopy (JENKINSON and BLACKBURN, 1968; BELL and MONTAGNA, 1972; JENKINSON et al., 1978).

2. Rhinocerotidae

A few studies on the black rhinocerus *(Diceros bicornis)* suggest that the sweat gland system may be similar to that of the horse (ROBERTSHAW, 1975).

II. Artiodactyla

1. Camelidae

Both the South American llama *(Lama peruana)* and the single-humped camel *(Camelus dromedarius)* sweat on heat exposure and following i.v. adrenaline administration (ALLEN and BLIGH, 1969; SCHMIDT-NIELSEN et al., 1957). In addition, i. v. isoprenaline administration will stimulate the glands, an effect that can be blocked by propranolol, whereas atropine has no effect on the sweating of heat exposure (ROBERTSHAW and TAYLOR, unpublished observations). Although these results indicate that sweating of the Camelidae is similar to that of Equidae, ROLLINSON et al. (1972) were unable to demonstrate a nerve supply to the sweat glands by light microscopy.

2. Bovidae

The most intensively studied members of this family are cattle, sheep, goats, and some feral species. In all species the glands can be activated by heat exposure although the importance of sweating as an evaporative heat loss mechanism varies, being greater in larger species (ROBERTSHAW and TAYLOR, 1969a). For example, at 40 °C the cutaneous moisture loss of cattle represents approximately 80% of the total evaporative heat loss whereas in sheep only 20% of the total evaporative heat loss is derived from the skin, the remainder being from the respiratory tract.

Table 1 shows the effect of the ID injection of various drugs on the activity of the sweat glands of cattle. Threshold concentrations, i.e., the smallest concentration evoking sweat gland activity, are also given and provide a rough assessment of the relative sensitivity of the gland to various agents. Similar results are obtained with the sheep and goat, and all species show a positive sudomotor response to i.v. adrenaline and in some instances to noradrenaline (FERGUSON and DOWLING, 1955; WAITES and VOGLMAYR, 1963; FINDLAY and ROBERTSHAW, 1965; ROBERTSHAW, 1968; HOFMEYR et al., 1969; ALLEN and Bligh, 1969; Johnson, 1971; Jenkinson and ROBERTSHAW, 1971).

Table 1. The threshold dosage of various drugs (in 0.1 ml) required to stimulate the sweat glands of cattle

Drug	Dosage
Adrenaline	1–10 ng
Noradrenaline	10–100 ng to 10–100 µg
Isoprenaline	0.1–1 µg
Nicotine	100 µg
Acetylcholine	Negative
Methacholine	Negative
Carbachol	Negative
Pilocarpine	Negative
Neostigmine	Negative
Physostigmine	Negative
Oxytocin	Negative

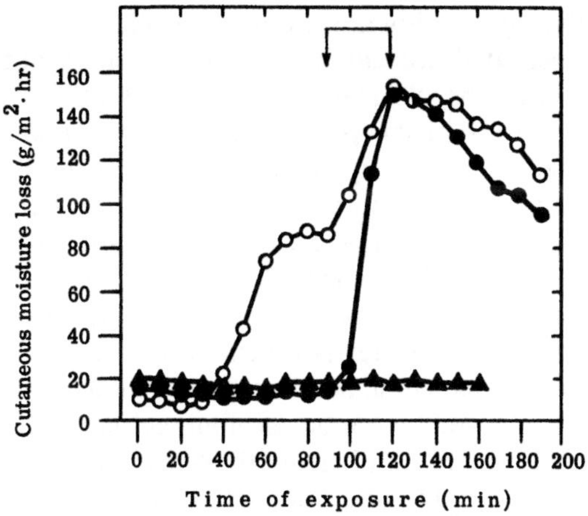

Fig. 2. Cutaneous moisture loss measured from the skin of the thorax of a cow exposed to an air temperature of 30 °C. Control experiment (○); after bethanidine (1 mg/kg) given 1 h before heat exposure (●); after phenoxybenzamine (3 mg/kg) given 30 min before heat exposure (▲). *Arrows* indicate adrenaline infusion (0.25 μg/kg · min). (After FINDLAY and ROBERTSHAW, 1965, with permission)

Surgical denervation prevents sweat gland discharges (WAITES and VOGLMAYR, 1963; FINDLAY and ROBERTSHAW, 1965), but histological studies indicate that nerves do not extend to the sweat glands (JENKINSON et al., 1966; JENKINSON and BLACKBURN, 1967), although electron microscopy has revealed small unmyelinated bundles of fibers in close proximity to blood vessels rather than the sweat glands. In no case have nerves been seen to penetrate the fibrocytic sheath of the glands (JENKINSON et al., 1978). The nature of the final pathway from nerve terminal to receptor is therefore unknown, but a clue may be obtained from the studies of INGRAM et al. (1963) who reported that arterial occlusion of a limb prevented sweating in that limb when the hypothalamus was heated, although sweating occurred elsewhere. This suggested that an intact circulation is required for effective sudomotor transmission and the close association of nerve terminals with blood vessels may thus reflect a neurohumoral type of transmission.

Specific autonomic blocking drugs verify the conclusions made concerning the adrenergic nature of the sweat gland system of Bovidae. The adrenergic-neurone blocking drug bethanidine, which in effect produces a pharmacological sympathectomy inhibits heat-induced but not adrenaline-induced sweating (FINDLAY and ROBERTSHAW, 1965; ROBERTSHAW, 1968). β-Receptor antagonists do not affect sweating, but the α-receptor blocking drug phenoxybenzamine will effectively block both heat- and adrenaline-induced sweating (Fig. 2) (FINDLAY and ROBERTSHAW, 1965). Denervation supersensitivity was not observed in cattle (FINDLAY and ROBERTSHAW, 1965) and sheep (HAYASHI, 1968) although KIMURA and AOKI (1962) claimed that two out of three of their animals demonstrated the phenomenon. Recent experiments on goats indigenous to Sinai failed to confirm the presence of denervation supersensitivity (CHOSHNIAK, DMI'EL, and ROBERTSHAW, unpublished observations). Species or individuals that fail to show denervation supersensitivity are particularly useful to elucidate the role of circulating catecholamines on sweat gland function since any sweat gland activity from denervated skin can be assumed to represent humoral stimulation under physiological conditions. WAITES and VOGLMAYR (1963) and HAYASHI (1968) have concluded that sweating in sheep includes a humoral component. They denervated the skin of the abdomen and thigh by removal of the lumbar sympathetic chain and were able to detect sweating from the denervated area. Adrenomedullary denervation (splanchnicotomy) either completely or partially abolished the sweating of the denervated area, and they therefore concluded that they had removed the humoral component. Such a conclusion is only valid if surgical denervation of the skin is complete; it is possible that the skin of the abdomen receives fibers from both the lumbar sympathetic chain and the splanchnic nerve so that splanchnicotomy might complete the partial denervation achieved by lumbar sympathectomy. The skin of the head receives its total sympathetic nerve supply from the cervical sympathetic nerve. Sectioning this nerve produces a reliable and complete denervation. Using this approach CHOSHNIAK, DMI'EL and ROBERTSHAW (unpublished observations) could detect no sweating from denervated skin. Furthermore, denervated skin remained anhidrotic during exercise and they therefore concluded that the elevation of catecholamines during exercise is insufficient to stimulate sweating, which therefore must be entirely under neural control.

Thus there are four major differences between the sudomotor system of equines and bovines.

1. The receptor types are different: β-receptors are found in Equidae and Camelidae and α-receptors in Bovidae.
2. No definitive nerve supply has been demonstrated in the Bovidae and Camelidae whereas a dense network of nerves exist around the glands of Equidae.
3. Denervated glands of Equidae exhibit denervation supersensitivity whereas those of the Bovidae do not.
4. Circulating catecholamines may supplement the neural control of sweating in Equidae particularly during exercise, but no humoral component of sweating has been described for the Bovidae.

Since adrenaline is a more effective stimulus to sweating than noradrenaline, adrenaline could be considered as the transmitter at sudomotor nerve terminals. On the other hand, the greater sensitivity to adrenaline may be related to the fact that noradrenaline uptake mechanisms remove adrenaline less rapidly than noradrenaline and thereby allow a more prolonged effect of adrenaline (IVERSEN, 1967). The presence of α-receptors would suggest that in the Bovidae noradrenaline rather than adrenaline is the transmitter. The β-receptors of Equidae and Camelidae would be consistent with their responsiveness to circulating catecholamines, particularly adrenaline. Attempts have been made to identify the transmitter at bovine sudomotor nerve endings by the chemical analysis of sweat. MABON (1970) isolated two catecholamine metabolites from bovine sweat, 3 methoxy-4-hydroxymandelic acid (VMA) and 3,4-dihydroxymandelic acid, but this did not provide definite proof that they were metabolites of a sudomotor transmitter substance since the VMA in sweat could be increased when the blood levels of VMA were elevated. The VMA therefore may not have originated at sudomotor nerve terminals but be derived from the circulation. The sweat of horses contains a catecholamine-like substance that has not been positively identified as being either adrenaline or noradrenaline (BRUNAUD and PITRE, 1945).

3. Suidae

The apocrine glands on the general body surface of the pig cannot be stimulated by heat or cholinergic compounds, but i.v. adrenaline and noradrenaline have a sudorific action, adrenaline being about three times more potent than noradrenaline. Since tolazoline will inhibit this response, an α-receptor effect is suggested (INGRAM, 1967).

III. Carnivora

The domestic cat *(Felis catus)* and dog *(Canis familiaris)* possess apocrine glands on the general body surface and eccrine glands on the food pads. There have been no studies on the apocrine glands of the cat whereas those of the dog have been fairly well investigated.

1. Canidae

The apocrine glands respond to both local and i.v. administration of adrenaline and noradrenaline, adrenaline being more potent than noradrenaline (AOKI, 1955; AOKI and WADA, 1951; IWABUCHI, 1967). In addition, they can be stimulated by cholinergic compounds whose effect can be blocked by atropine. The adrenergic effect is mediated by α-receptors since dihydroergotamine inhibits sweating (AOKI, 1955; IWABUCHI, 1967).

There seems little doubt that a functional nerve supply to the glands exists although their terminals have not been detected histologically (JENKINSON and BLACKBURN, 1968; BELL and MONTAGNA, 1972). The nature of neural transmission, however, seems to be in doubt. IWABUCHI (1967) concluded that the glands are innervated by adrenergic sympathetic nerves since sweating, stimulated by asphyxiation, was blocked by sympathetic denervation and more effectively inhibited by dihydroergotamine than atropine. He also demonstrated a lack of denervation supersensitivity and provided evidence for an adrenomedullary component of asphyxiation-induced sweating. In contrast, COTTON and VAN HASSELT (1972) showed by continuously recording moisture loss from the skin, that adrenaline produces only a transient sweat gland response whereas acetylcholine-induced sweating is of much longer duration. Furthermore, an increase in cutaneous moisture loss produced by radiant heating sufficient to produce burning can be reduced by the local administration of atropine. In these experiments they make the assumption that the increase in cutaneous moisture loss is the result of sweat secretion rather than any disintegration of the epidermal layer. They concluded, therefore, that the sudomotor nerve terminals of the dog are cholinergic although they did not perform what might be considered the crucial experiment: namely, inhibition of sweating produced by nervous stimulation using pharmacological blockade with atropine.

IV. Marsupialia

Since the metatherian and eutherian mammals evolved independently it might be expected that they would use different strategies of temperature regulation. This is so; macropod marsupials sweat only in response to exercise and not to heat exposure. Although i.v. adrenaline will stimulate the sweat glands, denervated glands do not secrete during exercise, suggesting that sweat secretion is entirely under neural control (DAWSON et al., 1974). Intradermal injections of adrenaline are a more effective stimulus to the sweat glands than noradrenaline, whereas isoprenaline, acetylcholine, or carbachol have only slight or negative effects (GUBBINS and JOHNSON, 1972). Although specific adrenergic blocking drugs have not been used, the lack of sensitivity of the glands to isoprenaline would suggest that the sweat glands possess α-receptors.

V. Primates

The order primates can be subdivided into two suborders, the Prosimii and the Anthropoidea. The Anthropoidea, which includes man, possess a varying number of apocrine glands on the general body surface. Man probably has the lowest density of apocrine glands that are confined to localized regions, e.g., axilla, anus, and nipple.

1. Prosimii

The Prosimii only have apocrine glands on the general body surface, which in some of the Lorisidae are densely aggregated in certain areas such as the flexor aspect of the arm (ELLIS and MONTAGNA, 1963). The glands of the slow loris *(Nycticebus cougang)* and the potto *(Perodicticus potto)* can be stimulated by the local injection of adrenaline and noradrenaline, the former being the more potent and the specialized brachial glands of the slow loris being particularly sensitive. Isoprenaline is without effect and since the response can be annulled by dihydroergotamine, an α-receptor mediated effect is indicated (AOKI, 1962a).

2. Anthropoidae

The apocrine glands of man only become functional at puberty and respond to emotive stimuli. They have a sporadic adrenergic nerve supply with cholinergic terminals around the ducts (UNO, 1977). They can be stimulated by both local and systemic administration of adrenaline and noradrenaline (SHELLEY, 1951; BELL, 1974), although AOKI (1962b) claims that cholinergic stimulation is effective. It is difficult to explain this difference unless the glands receive a dual motor innervation. Denervation does not abolish the response to emotive sweating (SHELLEY and HURLEY, 1952) which suggests that the glands can react to humoral stimulation presumably by either circulating adrenaline or noradrenaline. There have been no experiments with adrenergic blocking drugs that might give some indication as to the type of adrenergic receptor involved.

C. Eccrine Glands

I. Felidae

The sweat glands on the foot pad of the cat have been used as the model for the study of eccrine sweating. Although DALE and FELDBERG (1934) clearly demonstrated the release of acetylcholine from sudomotor nerve endings, LLOYD (1959) claimed that i.v. noradrenaline and adrenaline will also stimulate sweating. LLOYD used changes in cutaneous impedance as an index of sweating that may detect an increase in secretion sufficient to fill the ducts but not to produce secretion at the skin surface. FOSTER (1968) using a ventilated capsule with an infrared analyzer for moisture detection was able to verify LLOYD's findings in only one animal in five. LLOYD (1963, 1964, 1968) subsequently demonstrated blockade of the sudomotor response to nerve stimulation with large doses of adrenergic blocking agents such as phenoxybenzamine, guanethidine, and bretylium, but FOSTER and WEINER (1970) maintained that these effects were due to a cholinergic blocking action of these drugs. NAKAMURA and HATANAKA (1958) showed that dihydroergotamine will block the stimulatory effect of i.d. adrenaline. They were also able to detect some degree of denervation supersensitivity to both adrenergic and cholinergic agents.

II. Muridae

The sweat glands on the foot pad of the rat appear to be primarily cholinergic in that atropine will block spontaneous sweating. They can be stimulated, however, by the ID administration of adrenaline whose effect can be inhibited by local administration of dihydroergotamine (HAYASHI and NAKAGAWA, 1963).

III. Primates

1. Anthropoidae

The physiologic significance of the responsiveness of human eccrine sweat glands to the local application of adrenergic agents, as originally demonstrated by ICHIBASHI in 1963 is still not understood. Sweating in man can be elicited by two stimuli: heat exposure and emotion. The sweating of exercise may not be due entirely to an increased heat production as there is evidence that a nonthermal stimulus exists, particularly at the onset of exercise (VAN BEAUMONT and BULLARD, 1966). All glands respond to both stimuli but those of the palms and soles are particularly sensitive to emotive stimuli. Atropine will block all types of sweating and the glands then fail to respond to any kind of physiologic stimulation. The observation by HAIMOVICI (1950) that spontaneous sweating can be blocked by the α-receptor antagonist n-dibenzyl-2-chloroethylamine (Dibenamine) is usually interpreted as being due to a central depression of sweating rather than a direct action on the sweat glands. The doses used were large (5 mg/kg) and produced marked central effects, e.g., vomiting. It must be concluded from the studies with atropine that adrenergic stimulation, whether it be neural or humoral, can only modify the magnitude of the response of the secretory cell to stimulation by acetylcholine and does not, in its own right, have any sudomotor activity. It is in this context that one has to try and assess the physiologic significance, if any, of adrenergic stimulation to sweating.

It is convenient to separate the effects of adrenergic agents on primate sweating into local and systemic responses as their mechanism of action appears to be distinct. Local administration is likely to mimic effects produced by neural adrenergic stimulation whereas systemic administration will demonstrate changes in sweat gland activity induced by elevation of plasma catecholamine levels.

a) Local Administration of Adrenergic Agents

The sensitivity of human sweat glands to either i.d. or s.c. injection of catecholamines appears to be approximately equal for adrenaline and noradrenaline although the number of active sweat glands and the volume secreted is less for nordrenaline than for adrenaline (CHALMERS and KEELE, 1951; HAIMOVICI, 1950; KISIN, 1948; SONNENSCHEIN et al., 1951; TANAKA and NAKAMURA, 1955; WADA, 1950). Isoprenaline is usually less effective in producing a response (HAIMOVICI, 1950; TANAKA and NAKAMURA, 1955) although SONNENSCHEIN et al. (1951) report on one subject who manifested a weak response to adrenaline and noradrenaline but was sensitive to isoprenaline. There seems to be no difference in the sensitivity of the glands of the palms and those of the general body surface (CHALMERS and KEELE, 1952). Sensitivity of the glands to catecholamines is not affected by environmental temperature (WADA, 1950) or racial type (SONNENSCHEIN et al., 1951) but is reduced in age groups 1–12 years and 62–84 years (SILVER et al., 1964; WADA, 1950). Although newborn children show the same sensitivity as their mothers, there is a decline after the first week of life (SILVER et al., 1964), which would suggest that the hormonal environment of the fetus and early neonate influence the responsiveness of the sweat glands to catecholamines. There seems to be some divergence of opinion as to the effects of exercise on the catecholamine sensitivity of sweat glands. WADA (1955) noted that after exercise there was a decrease in the threshold concentration of adrenaline for the induction of local sweating whereas OGAWA (1976b) who blocked cholinergic sweating with atropine could find no difference in threshold concentration before and after exercise.

Numerous studies have confirmed the fact that the adrenergic and cholinergic receptors are distinct, pharmacological blockade of one receptor does not interfere with the action of agonists for the other receptor. Receptor antagonists known to block adrenergic sweating are Dibenamine (CHALMERS and KEELE, 1951; SONNENSCHEIN et al., 1951), dihydroergotamine (CHALMERS and KEELE, 1952; SONNENSCHEIN et al., 1951; OGAWA, 1976a), ergotamine (SONNENSCHEIN et al., 1951), dihydroergocristine (CHALMERS and KEELE, 1951), and tolazoline (CHALMERS and KEELE, 1951; COLLINS et al., 1959; KERNEN and BRUN, 1953; OGAWA, 1976a). In contrast WOLF and MAIBACH (1974) were unable to block the sudorific action of adrenaline by i.v. doses of phentolamine, phenoxybenzamine, or propranolol. It is possible that i.v. administration does not produce a concentration at the receptor site that is adequate for receptor blockade.

Adrenaline has variable effects on the sweating produced by acetylcholine administration. HAIMOVICI (1950) reported that the response to cholinergic stimulation "appeared more intense" when adrenaline was given simultaneously. KUNO (1965) confirmed these findings. SONNENSCHEIN et al. (1951) gave subthreshold doses of adrenaline and acetylcholine simultaneously which produced a positive sudomotor response suggesting a potentiating action. However, FOSTER et al. (1970) made quantitative measurements of sweat loss and concluded that the total output of sweat produced by a combination of cholinergic and adrenergic agents is usually less than that resulting from the sum of separate sudorific effects of the two drugs. Inhibition of sweating by adrenaline is thought to be due to its vasoconstrictor effect; vasoconstriction occurs at concentrations that are subthreshold for sweat stimulation, and therefore are always predominant. Vasoconstriction not only reduces the peak sweat response but also prolongs the action of cholinergic compounds particularly when adrenaline is given before cholinergic stimulation (OGAWA, 1976). The in vitro experiments of SATO (1973) would support this conclusion since isolated glands that have no intact blood supply respond equally to cholinergic and adrenergic agents.

OGAWA (1976 b) reported an inhibition of thermal sweating by adrenaline, but if adrenaline was given after local administration of dihydroergotamine or tolazoline, sweating was stimulated. Since this could be blocked by atropine, the author interprets his results as showing a direct action of adrenaline on cholinergic sudomotor nerve endings and not on the secretory cell.

Although COLLINS et al. (1959) found that only half the sweat glands respond to adrenaline, SILVER et al. (1964) maintained that all glands were affected. MELLINKOFF and SONNENSCHEIN (1954) reported that the same gland can be stimulated by adrenaline, acetylcholine, and heat. The mechanism of action of catecholamines is thought to be due to a direct action on the secretory cells. This has been proven by injecting methylene blue i.d. before adrenaline. The appearance of dye in the sweat was taken as evidence of the transfer of extracellular fluid through the cells of the secretory coil although an action on the myoepithelial cells is not ruled out. In this respect there is no difference between the effect of adrenaline, acetylcholine, and heat exposure (HURLEY and WITKOWSKI, 1961). Working with isolated glands SATO (1973) has shown that adrenaline will induce sweat secretion at a rate, and with an electrolyte composition, that is comparable to that produced by acetylcholine. Examination of secretory cells by electron microscopy reveals identical intracellular changes for both modes of stimulation (SATO et al., 1974). On the other hand IKAI and HASEGAWA (1972) found that in vivo, the sodium and potassium concentration of adrenaline-induced sweat is higher than that produced by cholinergic drugs; he concluded that cutaneous vasoconstriction inhibits electrolyte transport mechanisms in the cells lining the duct.

b) Systemic Administration of Adrenergic Agents

The sudorific action of circulating catecholamines has been the subject of investigation largely because several pathological conditions associated with elevated plasma catecholamine levels present generalized and profuse sweating as a symptom.

CHALMERS and KEELE (1951) and BARCROFT and SWAN (1953) were unable to induce sweating by the i.v. injection of adrenaline, and FOSTER et al. (1970) confirmed that i.v. adrenaline does not induce sweating or affect thermal sweating but that intra-arterial adrenaline infusion could cause sweating localized to the area supplied by the artery. Isoprenaline was without effect and the response to adrenaline could be blocked by the α-receptor antagonist phentolamine. Intra-arterial infusion of adrenaline during thermal sweating caused sweating to decrease.

HARRISON and MACKINNON (1963) reported that palmar sweating is inhibited by i.v. adrenaline administration, an effect that still persists after arterial occlusion or pretreatment with phenoxybenzamine; they concluded that the suppression is due to actions of adrenaline on the central nervous system. GORDON and MAIBACH (1965) have confirmed these observations but noted that the effect is variable and that 90% of their subjects who responded were classified as hyperhidrotic. ALLEN et al. (1974) studied one subject with palmar hyperhidrosis who showed an increase in palmar sweating with adrenaline infusion. However, since the magnitude of the response was not directly related to the dose and declined in successive experiments, they concluded

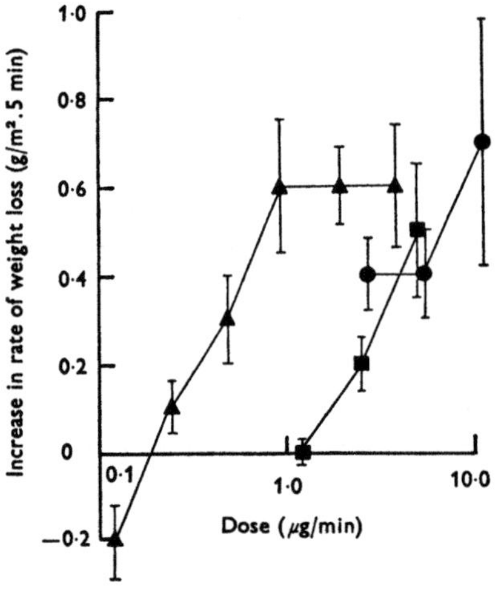

Fig. 3

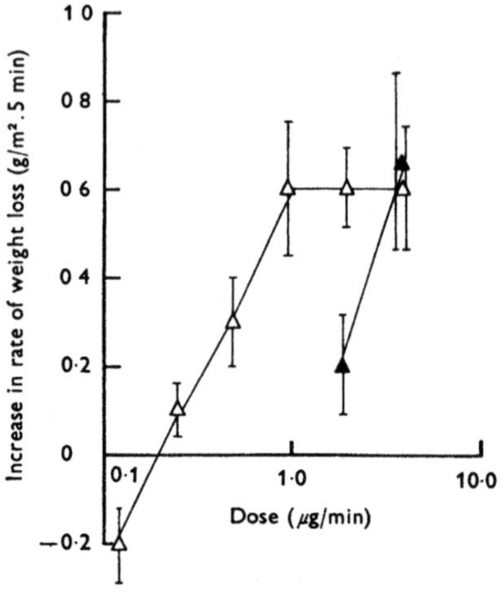

Fig. 4

Fig. 3. Dose-response curves for the weight loss response to i.v. infusion of adrenaline (●), noradrenaline (▲) and isoprenaline (△). (After ALLEN and RODDIE, 1972, with permission)

Fig. 4. Dose-response curves for the weight loss response to IV infusion of isoprenaline before (△) and after (▲) propranolol. (After ALLEN and RODDIE, 1972, with premission)

that the increase in sweating was due to the subjective effects of adrenaline infusion, rather than to a direct action of adrenaline itself on the sweat glands.

By recording total body weight loss with a sensitive balance and correcting for respiratory weight loss, ALLEN and RODDIE (1972) developed a gravimetric system for the measurement of total cutaneous evaporative loss. They noted that adrenaline and noradrenaline infusion increased the rate of weight loss but that isoprenaline was effective at a lower dosage and β-receptor blockade with propranolol reduced the response (Figs. 3 and 4). Cholinergic blockade with atropine had no effect. In a subsequent paper, ALLEN et al. (1974) demonstrated that propranolol did not affect increases in weight loss due to heat exposure or emotive stimulation, suggesting that under these conditions circulating catecholamines do not contribute to sweat gland function. The changes in evaporative loss resulting from catecholamine infusion are small and the source of moisture is not known; it may be from either apocrine or eccrine sweat glands or simply due to an increase in the transepidermal diffusion of water, a phenomenon controlled by the vapor pressure gradient across the skin. If ambient humidity is constant, the vapor pressure gradient is a function of skin temperature. An examination of the records of ALLEN and RODDIE (1972) clearly show no fluctuation in skin temperature that would eliminate such an explanation. The true nature of the phenomenon they describe therefore awaits elucidation.

It would seem that there are two types of adrenergic receptors on human sweat glands: α-receptors are only stimulated when catecholamines are given by close intra-arterial infusion or i.d. injection, whereas the β-receptors are more readily accessible from the circulation but yield such a small increment in sweat rate that it can only be detected by very sensitive methods of measurement. One might speculate that the α-receptor-mediated effect represents stimulation of receptors located at the postsynaptic site of adrenergic sudomotor nerves, and that the β-receptors would be involved if circulating catecholamines have any direct stimulatory action on sweat secretion. KUNO (1965) proposed that elevation of plasma catecholamine levels during exercise might enhance sweating evoked by neural means. ROBERTSHAW et al. (1973) using the stump-tailed macaque *(Macaca speciosa)* showed that the maximum sweat rate at rest in a hot environment could be elevated by as much as 50% with exercise (running on a treadmill). This enhancement of sweating could be abolished by surgical denervation of the adrenal medulla and restored by the i.v. infusion of adrenaline. These findings were interpreted as demonstrating that the increased adrenomedullary secretion of exercise assists in the dissipation of the heat of exercise, a finding that would support KUNO's hypothesis. No studies were performed to determine the type of receptor involved.

D. Pathological Considerations

Sweating is a marked feature of the crisis in phaeochromocytoma, a tumor of the adrenal medulla that intermittently releases large quantities of catecholamines into the circulation. The circulating catecholamines also cause cutaneous vasoconstriction so that sweating occurs onto a cold skin and evaporates slowly. For this reason sweating is often described as profuse because it accumulates on the skin and does not evaporate. In fact, it may not be excessive when compared with thermal sweating, where both skin blood flow and evaporation are high.

The doses of adrenaline and noradrenaline used by various authors (up to 20 μg/min) are considered to elevate plasma catecholamines to levels as high as those found during a phaeochromocytoma crisis (FOSTER et al., 1970). If therefore sweating is due to direct stimulation of the glands by circulating catecholamines, it might be expected that the hyperhidrosis would be suppressed by adrenergic blocking drugs. If on the other hand sweating results from cholinergic neural stimulation, then anticholinergic drugs would be effective. PROUT and WARDELL (1969) showed that the iontophoretic application of the anticholinergic compound hyoscine to the skin of two patients with phaeochromocytoma abolished sweating in the treated area although the glands could still be stimulated by i.d. injections of noradrenaline. Thus, sweating appears to be of central origin. Profound cutaneous vasoconstriction combined with the calorigenic effects of catecholamines are probably sufficient to stimulate heat loss mechanisms, and thus the sweating attacks may simply represent the chief method of dealing with an elevated heat load combined with a decreased convective heat loss. Alternatively, sweating may be the result of the action of circulating catecholamines on the central nervous system. Administration of adrenaline into the hypothalamus of monkeys causes the body temperature to fall, presumably by stimulation of heat loss mechanisms, including sweating (MYERS and YAKSH, 1969). If small amounts of catecholamines therefore can pass the blood brain barrier in the region of the hypothalamus when blood levels are considerably in excess of those that occur in physiologic as opposed to pathological situations, central stimulation of sweating could theoretically occur. VOGT (1975) calculates that the maximal concentration found during physiologic stimulation would be 10 μg/liter plasma, although this would be a rare occurrence. During phaeochromocytoma, levels as high as 87 μg/liter have been recorded (PROUT and WARDELL, 1969). It is possible therefore that these high concentrations might penetrate the barrier although the threshold plasma concentration for this to happen is not known.

It is unlikely that adrenomedullary stimulation produced by insulin hypoglycemia would raise the concentration of plasma catecholamines to a level sufficient to stimulate the sweat glands either directly or via the central nervous system. Thus the sweating of insulin hypoglycemia must be independent of the adrenal medulla, a conclusion that is verified by the fact that adrenalectomized subjects are capable of hypoglycemic sweating (GINSBURG and PATON, 1956).

Many of the symptoms of hyperthyroidism are similar to those associated with elevated plasma catecholamine levels, and excessive sweating is often a feature of thyrotoxicosis. Adrenergic receptor blockade, particularly using β-receptor antagonists such as propranolol, reduces not only the autonomic symptoms but also the hyperhidrosis (SHANKS et al., 1969). There are two possible explanations for these findings: propranolol either reduces heat production or directly reduces a β-receptor-mediated sudorific action of circulating catecholamines. Neither of these possibilities has been fully tested. ALLEN et al. (1972) concluded that since β-receptor blockade had no effect no either thermal or emotive sweating in normal people, the anhidrotic effect of propranolol in hyperthyroidism is related to some other action of the drug. This, however, does not entirely rule out a possible direct effect of propranolol on the sweat glands since hyperthyroidism may stimulate or magnify some latent β-receptor activity. The similarity between the symptoms of hyperthyroidism and generalized sympathetic stimulation are due not so much to elevated plasma catecholamine levels as to an increased sensitivity of adrenergic receptors brought about by elevated plasma levels of thyroid hormones. Thus the effects of normal sympathetic activity become greatly exaggerated and likewise the presence of any β-receptors at the sweat glands would become more readily apparent and thereby be suppressed by the specific blocking drug.

E. Conclusion

There is no doubt that apocrine sweat glands are controlled predominantly by adrenergic nerves, but the type of receptor involved shows species variation. Since there appears to be major cellular differences between the two types of receptors, one has to speculate on whether or not the glands are in any way comparable and should be classified together. It is more likely that they are phylogenetically distinct although they may subserve the same function. On the other hand, eccrine glands are largely under cholinergic control but their function can be modified by adrenergic agents that act through specific adrenergic receptors, there being evidence for the presene of both types of receptor. The physiologic significance of the adrenergic component of eccrine sweating is still in doubt although some evidence has been produced that suggests that catecholamine release during exercise may assist in the dissipation of the heat of exercise.

References

Allen, J.A., Roddie, I.C.: The role of circulating catecholamines in sweat production in man. J. Physiol. (Lond.) *227*, 801–814 (1972)

Allen, J.A., Jenkinson, D.J., Roddie, I.C.: The effect of β-adrenoceptor blockade on human sweating. Br. J. Pharmacol. *47*, 487–497 (1972)

Allen, T.E., Bligh, J.: A comparative study of the temporal patterns of cutaneous water vapour loss from some domesticated mammals with epitrichial sweat glands. Comp. Biochem. Physiol. *31*, 347–363 (1969)

Aoki, T.: Stimulation of the sweat glands in the hairy skin of the dog by adrenaline, noradrenaline, mecholyl and pilocarpine. J. Invest. Dermatol. *24*, 545–556 (1955)

Aoki, T.: The skin of primates. IX. Observations on the functional activity of the sweat glands in *Nycticebus coucang* and *Perodicticus potto*. J. Invest. Dermatol. *39*, 115–122 (1962a)

Aoki, T.: Stimulation of human axillary apocrine sweat glands by cholinergic agents. J. Invest. Dermatol. *38*, 41–44 (1962b)

Aoki, T., Wada, M.: Functional activity of the sweat glands in the hairy skin of the dog. Science *114*, 123–124 (1951)

Barcroft, H., Swan, H.J.C.: Sympathetic control of human blood vessels. In: Monograph of Physiological Society, No. 1. L.E. Bayliss, W. Feldberg, A.L. Hodgkin (eds.). London: Arnold 1953

Bell, F.R., Evans, C.L.: Sweating responses in the horse. J. Physiol. (Lond.) *134*, 421–426 (1956)

Bell, M.: The ultrastructure of human axillary apocrine glands after epinephrine injection. J. Invest. Dermatol. *63*, 147–159 (1974)

Bell, M., Montagna, W.: Innervation of sweat glands in horses and dogs. Br. J. Dermatol. *86*, 160–163 (1972)

Bligh, J.: A thesis concerning the processes of secretion and discharge of sweat. Environ. Res. *1*, 28–45 (1967)

Boura, A.L.A., Green, A.F.: Adrenergic neurone blockade and other acute effects caused by *N*-benzyl-*N′N″*-dimethylguanidine and its ortho chloro derivative. Br. J. Pharmacol. *20*, 36–55 (1963)

Brunaud, M., Pitre, J.: Existe-t-il de l'adrénaline dans la sueur du cheval? Bull. Acad. Vet. France *18*, 339–347 (1945)

Chalmers, T.M., Keele, C.A.: Physiological significance of the sweat response to adrenaline in man. J. Physiol. (Lond.) *114*, 510–514 (1951)

Chalmers, T.M., Keele, C.A.: The nervous and chemical control of sweating. Br. J. Dermatol. *64*, 43–54 (1952)

Collins, K.J., Sargent, F., Weiner, J.S.: Excitation and depression of eccrine sweat glands by acetylcholine, acetyl-β-methylcholine and adrenaline. J. Physiol. (Lond.) *148*, 592–614 (1959)

Cotton, D.W.K., Van Hasselt, P.: Sweating on the hairy surface of the beagle. J. Invest. Dermatol. *59*, 313–316 (1972)

Dale, H.H., Feldberg, W.: The chemical transmission of secretory impulses to the sweat glands of the cat. J. Physiol. (Lond.) *82*, 121–128 (1934)

Dawson, T.J., Robertshaw, D., Taylor, C.R.: Sweating in the red kangaroo: stimulation during exercise but not in the heat. Am. J. Physiol. *224*, 494–498 (1974)

Ellis, R.A., Montagna, W.: The sweat glands of the Lorisidae. In: Evolutionary and Genetic Biology of Primates. J. Buettner-Janusch (ed.). Vol. I. New York: Academic Press 1963

Evans, C.L., Smith, D.F.G.: Sweating responses in the horse. Proc. R. Soc. Lond. [Biol.] *145*, 61–83 (1956)

Falck, B.: Observations on the possibilities of the cellular localization of monoamines by a fluorescence method. Acta Physiol. Scand. *56*, Suppl. 197 (1962)

Ferguson, K.A., Dowling, D.F.: The function of cattle sweat glands. Aust. J. Agr. Res. *6*, 641–644 (1955)

Findlay, J.D., Robertshaw, D.: The role of the sympathoadrenal system in the control of sweating in the ox *(Bos taurus)*. J. Physiol. (Lond.) *179*, 285–297 (1965)

Foster, K.G.: Response of the cats' pad eccrine sweat glands to intravascular injections of catecholamines. J. Physiol. (Lond.) *195*, 331–337 (1968)

Foster, K.G., Weiner, J.S.: Effects of cholinergic and adrenergic blocking agents on the activity of the eccrine sweat glands. J. Physiol. (Lond.) *210*, 883–895 (1970)
Foster, K.G., Ginsburg, J., Weiner, J.S.: Role of circulating catecholamines in human eccrine sweat gland control. Clin. Sci. *39*, 823–832 (1970)
Ginsburg, J., Paton, A.: Effects in man of insulin hypoglycaemia after adrenalectomy. J. Physiol. (Lond.) *133*, 59–60P (1956)
Gordon, B.I., Maibach, H.I.: Effect of systemically administered epinephrine on palmar sweating. Arch. Dermatol. *92*, 192–194 (1965)
Gubbins, S., Johnson, K.G.: Evaporative water loss in the wallaby *(Protemnodon rufogrisea)*. J. Physiol. (Lond.) *226*, 110–111P (1972)
Haimovici, H.: Evidence for adrenergic sweating in man. J. Appl. Physiol. *2*, 512–521 (1950)
Harrison, J., Mackinnon, P.C.B.: Central effect of epinephrine and norepinephrine on the palmar sweat index. Am. J. Physiol. *204*, 785–788 (1963)
Hayashi, H.: Functional activity of the sweat glands in the hairy skin of the sheep. Tohoku J. Exp. Med. *94*, 361–375 (1968)
Hayashi, H., Nakagawa, T.: Functional activity of the sweat glands of the albino rat. J. Invest. Dermatol. *41*, 365–367 (1963)
Hofmeyr, H.S., Guidry, A.J., Waltz, F.A.: Effects of temperature and wool length on surface and respiratory evaporative losses of sheep. J. Appl. Physiol. *26*, 517–523 (1969)
Hurley, H.J., Witkowski, J.A.: Mechanism of epinephrine-induced eccrine sweating in human skin. J. Appl. Physiol. *16*, 652–654 (1961)
Ichibashi, T.: Effect of drugs on the sweat glands by cataphoresis and effective method for suppression of local sweating. J. Orient. Med. *25*, 1401 (1936)
Ikai, K., Hasegawa, Y.: Adrenaline sweating. In: Advances in Climatic Physiology. S. Itoh, K. Ogata, H. Yoshimura (eds.) Tokyo: Igaku Shoin 1972
Ingram, D.L.: Stimulation of cutaneous glands in the pig. J. Comp. Pathol. *77*, 93–98 (1967)
Ingram, D.L., McLean, J.A., Whittow, G.C.: The effect of heating the hypothalamus and the skin on the rate of moisture vaporization from the skin of the ox *(Bos taurus)*. J. Physiol. (Lond.) *169*, 394–403 (1963)
Iversen, L.L.: The uptake and storage of noradrenaline in sympathetic nerves. Cambridge: Cambridge University Press 1967
Iwabuchi, T.: General sweating on the hairy skin of the dog and its mechanisms. J. Invest. Dermatol. *49*, 61–70 (1967)
Jenkinson, D.McE.: On the classification of sweat glands and the question of the existence of an apocrine secretory process. Br. Vet. J. *123*, 311–316 (1967)
Jenkinson, D.McE., Blackburn, P.S.: The distribution of nerves, monoamine oxidase and cholinesterase in the skin of the sheep and goat. J. Anat. *101*, 333–341 (1967)
Jenkinson, D.McE., Blackburn, P.S.: The distribution of nerves, monoamine oxidase and cholinesterase in the skin of the horse. Res. Vet. Sci. *9*, 165–169 (1968)
Jenkinson, D.McE., Robertshaw, D.: Studies on the nature of sweat gland "fatigue" in the goat. J. Physiol. (Lond.) *212*, 455–465 (1971)
Jenkinson, D.McE., Montgomery, I., Elder, H.Y.: Studies on the nature of the peripheral sudomotor control mechanism. J. Anat. *125*, 625–639 (1978)
Jenkinson, D.McE., Sengupta, B.P., Blackburn, P.S.: The ditribution of nerves, monoamine oxidase and cholinesterase in the skin of cattle. J. Anat. *100*, 593–613 (1966)
Johnson, K.G.: The discharge of sweat in Welsh Mountain sheep. J. Physiol. (Lond.) *215*, 743–753 (1971)
Johnson, K.G.: Sweat gland function in isolated perfused skin. J. Physiol. (Lond.) *250*, 633–649 (1975)
Kernen, R., Brun, R.: Expériences sur la transpiration. V. Examens pharmacodynamiques au niveau de la gland sudoripare de l'homme. Dermatologica *106*, 1–13 (1953)
Kimura, S., Aoki, T.: Functional activity of the apocrine sweat gland in the goat. Tohoku J. Exp. Med. *76*, 8–22 (1962)
Kisin, E.E.: A method of pharmacological study of the sweating function of the skin in situ. Vestn. Venerol. i Dermatol. *5*, 27–31 (1948)
Kuno, Y.: The mechanism of human sweat secretion. Proc. Int. Union Physiol. Sci. *4*, 3–16 (1965)

Lands, A.M., Arnold, A., Mc Auliff, J.P., Luduena, F.P., Brown, T.G., Jr.: Differentiation of receptor systems activated by sympathomimetic amines. Nature *214*, 597–598 (1967)

Lloyd, D.P.C.: Response of cholinergically innervated sweat glands to adrenaline and noradrenaline. Nature *184*, 277–278 (1959)

Lloyd, D.P.C.: Action of phenoxybenzamine on neural and humoral activation of sweat glands. J. Physiol. (Lond.) *169*, 116–117P (1963)

Lloyd, D.P.C.: Actions of guanethidine and bretylium on transmission to sweat glands in the cat. J. Physiol. (Lond.) *175*, 74P (1964)

Lloyd, D.P.C.: Effect of phenoxybenzamine on neural and humoral control of sweat glands. Proc. Natl. Acad. Sci. USA *59*, 816–820 (1968)

Mabon, R.M.: Two possible catecholamine metabolites in the secretion from ox skin. Res. Vet. Sci. *11*, 287–288 (1970)

Mellinkoff, S.M., Sonnenschein, R.R.: Identity of sweat glands stimulated by heat, epinephrine and acetylcholine. Science *120*, 997–998 (1954)

Myers, R.D., Yaksh, T.L.: Control of body temperature in the unanaesthetised monkey by cholinergic and aminergic systems in the hypothalamus. J. Physiol. (Lond.) *202*, 483–500 (1969)

Nakamura, Y., Hatanaka, K.: The effect of denervation of the cat's sweat glands on their responsiveness to adrenaline, nicotine and mecholyl. Tohoku J. Exp. Med. *68*, 225–237 (1958)

Ogawa, T.: Effects of subcutaneously administered adrenaline on human eccrine sweating, with special reference to the physiological significance of the adrenergic sweating mechanism. Jap. J. Physiol. *26*, 517–528 (1976a).

Ogawa, T.: Effects of intradermal adrenaline on human eccrine sweating, with special reference to its possible interaction with the cholinergic mechanism. J. Aichi Med. Univ. Ass. *4*, 163–172 (1976b)

Prout, B.J., Wardell, W.M.: Sweating and peripheral blood flow in patients with phaeochromocytoma. Clin. Sci. *36*, 109–117 (1969)

Robertshaw, D.: The pattern and control of sweating in the sheep and the goat. J. Physiol. (Lond.) 198, 531–539 (1968)

Robertshaw, D.: Neural and humoral control of apocrine glands. J. Invest. Dermatol. *63*, 160–167 (1974)

Robertshaw, D.: Catecholamines and control of sweat glands. In: Handbook of Physiology, Endocrinology VI. H. Blaschko, G. Sayers, A.D. Smith (eds.) Washington, D.C.: American Physiological Society 1975

Robertshaw, D., Taylor, C.R.: A comparison of sweat gland activity in eight species of East African bovids. J. Physiol. (Lond.) *203*, 135–143 (1969a)

Robertshaw, D., Taylor, C.R.: Sweat gland function of the donkey *(Equus asinus)*. J. Physiol. (Lond.) *205*, 79–89 (1969b)

Robertshaw, D., Taylor, C.R., Mazzia, L.M.: Sweating in primates: secretion by adrenal medulla during exercise. Am. J. Physiol. *224*, 678–681 (1973)

Rollinson, D.H.L., Injidi, M.H., Jenkinson, D.McE.: The distribution of nerves, monoamine oxidase and cholinesterase in the skin of the camel. Res. Vet. Sci. *13*, 304–305 (1972)

Sato, F., Burgers, M., Sato, K.: Some characteristics of adrenergic human eccrine sweating. Experientia *30*, 40–41 (1974)

Sato, K.: Sweat induction from an isolated eccrine sweat gland. Am. J. Physiol. *225*, 1147–1152 (1973)

Schiefferdecker, P.: Die Hautdrüsen des Menschen und der Säugetiere, ihre biologische und rassenatomische Bedeutung, sowie die Muscularis sexualis. Biol. Zentr. *37*, 534–562 (1917)

Schiefferdecker, P.: Die Hautdrüsen des Menschen und der Säugetiere, ihre biologische und rassenatomische Bedeutung, sowie die Muscularis sexualis. Zoologica *72*, 1–154 (1922)

Schmidt-Nielsen, K., Schmidt-Nielsen, B., Jarnum, S.A., Houpt, T.R.: Body temperature of the camel and its relation to water economy. Am. J. Physiol. *188*, 103–112 (1957)

Shanks, R.G., Hadden, D.R., Lowe, D.C., Mc Devitt, D.G., Montgomery, D.A.D.: Controlled trial of propranolol in thyrotoxicosis. Lancet *i*, 993–994 (1969)

Shelley, W.B.: Apocrine sweat. J. Invest. Dermatol. *17*, 255 (1951)

Shelley, W.B., Hurley, H.J.: Methods of exploring human apocrine gland physiology. Arch. Dermatol. Syphilol. *66*, 165–161, 172–179 (1952)

Silver, A., Montagna, W., Karacan, I.: Age and sex differences in spontaneous, adrenergic and cholinergic human sweating. J. Invest. Dermatol. *43*, 255–266 (1964)
Snow, D.H.: Identification of the receptor involved in adrenaline mediated sweating in the horse. Res. Vet. Sci. *23*, 246–247 (1977)
Sonnenschein, R.R., Kobrin, H., Janowitz, H.D., Grossman, M.I.: Stimulation and inhibition of human sweat glands by intradermal sympathomimetic agents. J. Appl. Physiol. *3*, 573–581 (1951)
Tanaka, I., Nakamura, T.: Action of adrenaline, noradrenaline, and isopropylnoradrenaline on the sweat glands in young healthy men. Kumamoto Med. J. *8*, 26–28 (1955)
Uno, H.: Sympathetic innervation of the sweat glands and piloarrector muscles of macaques and human beings. J. Invest. Dermatol. *69*, 112–120 (1977)
Van Beaumont, W., Bullard, R.W.: Sweating: exercise stimulation during circulatory arrest. Science *152*, 1521–1523 (1966)
Vogt, M.: Influence of circulating catecholamines on the central nervous system. In: Handbook of Physiology, Vol. VI, Endocrinology. H. Blaschko, G. Sayers, A.D. Smith (eds.). Washington, D.C.: American Physiological Society 1975
Wada, F.: Effects of exercise on excitability of local sweat glands. Japan J. Physical Fitness. *5*, 246–247 (1955)
Wada, M.: Sudorific action of adrenaline on the human sweat glands and determination of their excitability. Science *111*, 376–377 (1950)
Waites, G.M.H., Voglmayr, J.K.: The functional activity and control of the apocrine sweat glands of the scrotum of the ram. Aust. J. Agr. Res. *14*, 839–851 (1963)
Wolf, J.E., Maibach, H.I.: Palmar eccrine sweating–the role of adrenergic and cholinergic mediators. Br. J. Dermatol. *91*, 439–446 (1974)

Section V: Kinetics, Biotransformation, Toxic Effects and Clinical Implications

CHAPTER 1

Kinetics and Biotransformation of Adrenergic Activators and Inhibitors: Adrenergic Alpha- and Beta-Receptor Activators

K.H. Rahn

A. Alpha-Receptor Activators*

I. Etilephrine

Etilephrine (Fig. 1) is a sympathomimetic used almost exclusively by oral administration for the treatment of hypotension. Its distribution in the rat and its disposition in humans have been studied by Hengstmann et al. (1975).

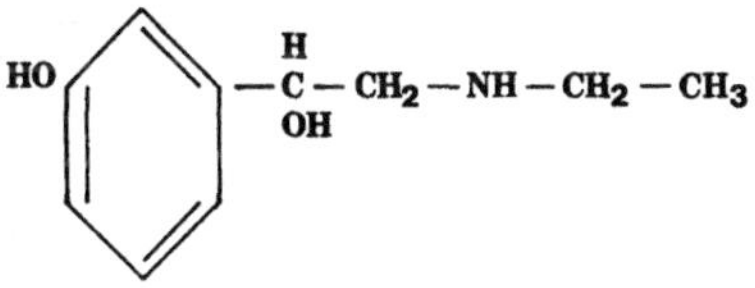

Fig. 1. The structure of etilephrine

1. Metabolism

After oral or intravenous application of ^{3}H-etilefrine to man most of the radioactivity is excreted in urine in the form of conjugates, as revealed by treatment of the urine with glucuronidase-arylsulfatase. It is not clear which of the conjugates prevails, since no studies were done using glucuronidase separately. Independent of the route of administration, very little etilefrine, i.e., about 3% of a dose, is metabolized to form hydroxymandelic acid.

The extent of conjugation largely depends upon the route of administration. Thus, after intravenous application 28% of the dose is excreted in urine as unchanged etilefrine and 44% as conjugates. Of an oral dose, only 7% is eliminated in urine as free etilefrine, however, 73% as conjugates. Therefore, conjugation probably takes place within the intestinal wall and/or in the liver. Based upon these findings, one would expect a first-pass metabolism.

2. Kinetics

In man, etilefrine is rapidly absorbed from the gastrointestinal tract, peak plasma levels being achieved about 30 min after an oral dose. After both oral and intravenous

* The metabolism (Kopin, 1972) and the distribution (Holzbauer and Sharman, 1972) of noradrenaline and adrenaline have been extensively reviewed. The same is true for dopamine (Holzbauer and Sharman, 1972; Sandler, 1972). Therefore, these amines will not further be mentioned in the present review

application of ^{3}H-etilefrine, about 80% of the radioactivity appears in urine, indicating good intestinal absorption. However, after oral application the area under the plasma curve of etilefrine is only about 50% of the area obtained after an intravenous injection. Thus, one must assume a significant first-pass effect.

The binding of etilefrine to human serum albumin is 8.5% as compared with 23% binding to human plasma. Obviously, part of etilefrine is bound to plasma proteins other than albumin. In rats injected intravenously with ^{3}H-etilefrine, higher concentrations of radioactivity were found in the liver, kidneys, and gut wall than in plasma.

In patients, serum levels of etilefrine ranging from 5–20 ng/ml were measured 10–360 min after an oral dose of 7 mg of the drug. After an intravenous dose of 0.75 mg, serum concentrations of 0.4–25 ng/ml were obtained. Elimination half-life was about 150 min. In man, etilefrine and its metabolites are almost exclusively eliminated via the kidneys, since of an oral or intravenous dose of the tritium labeled drug about 80% are excreted in urine within 24 h.

II. Phenylephrine

Phenylephrine (Fig. 2), a vasoconstrictor sympathomimetic agent is mainly used locally as a decongestant.

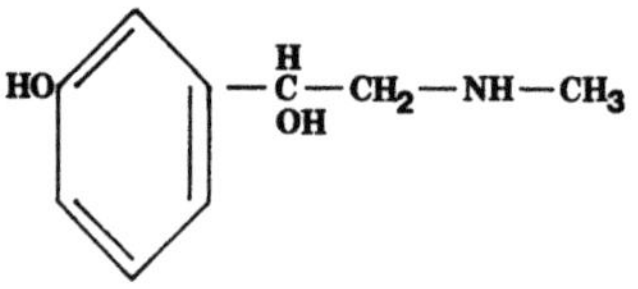

Fig. 2. The structure of phenylephrine

1. Metabolism

The metabolism of phenylephrine has been studied in man after oral application of 10 mg of the drug (BRUCE and PITTS, 1968). Only conjugates of phenylephrine could be detected in urine, most of them being sulfates. A small fraction was excreted as the glucuronide.

2. Kinetics

After oral application of ^{3}H-phenylephrine as hydrochloride, peak plasma levels are obtained after 1 h in human volunteers (BOGNER and WALSH, 1964). A more gradual rise and decline of plasma radioactivity was observed after ^{3}H-phenylephrine given orally in a sustained release form (CAVALITTO et al., 1963; BOGNER and WALSH, 1964). Within 24 h of an oral dose of 10 mg phenylephrine, about 80% of the dose could be recovered from urine in the form of phenylephrine conjugates (BRUCE and PITTS, 1968). From these data, one may conclude that phenylephrine is rapidly and almost completely absorbed from the gastrointestinal tract. However, since there are no data on plasma levels of the unchanged drug, the bioavailability of phenylephrine given orally remains unknown. In view of the results obtained with etilefrine, it seems most probable that there is a significant first-pass metabolism for phenylephrine as well.

After oral doses of 9 mg ^{3}H-phenylephrine hydrochloride, peak plasma levels of total radioactivity corresponding to 207 ng/ml phenylephrine base were measured (BOGNER and WALSH, 1964).

When ^{3}H-phenylephrine was given orally to normal volunteers in a sustained release form, about 15% of the dose was excreted in urine within 24 h. Considerably more radioactivity, i.e., about 45% of the dose, was eliminated in urine within 1 day when the ^{3}H-phenylephrine was given as tablets containing the hydrochloride of the drug (CAVALITTO et al., 1963; BOGNER and WALSH, 1964). These differences obviously are due to the slow intestinal absorption and hence delayed elimination of phenylephrine contained in a slow release preparation. As has already been mentioned, a much higher percentage – namely about 80% – of an oral dose was eliminated in urine within 24 h in the study by BRUCE and PITTS (1968). These authors, however, had maintained by the administration of ammonium chloride an urine pH of 5.6 or below in the subjects studied. As BRUCE and PITTS (1968) exclusively measured phenylephrine conjugates, the data suggest that the renal elimination of these metabolites is strongly dependent upon the pH of the urine.

B. Beta-Receptor Activators

I. Isoprenaline

The β-receptor stimulating agent isoprenaline (Fig. 3) is used in the treatment of asthma, it is mostly given as an aerosol. Furthermore, the drug is infused intravenously in the treatment of shock and of atrioventricular conduction disturbances. Several studies on its biotransformation and its kinetics have been performed using different routes of application.

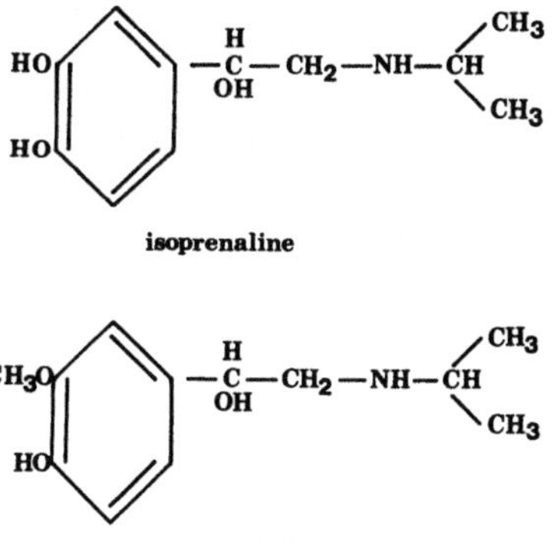

Fig. 3. The structure of isoprenaline and of 3-o-methylisoprenaline

1. Biotransformation

The metabolism of D,L-isoprenaline has been investigated in the rat (HERTTING, 1964), in the cat (KADAR et al., 1978), in the dog (CONWAY et al., 1968; MORGAN et al., 1969 b), and in man (MORGAN et al., 1969 a, b; CONOLLY et al., 1972). As could be expected from the fact that isoprenaline has an isopropyl group attached to the N-atom,

Table 1. Excretion of ^{3}H-isoprenaline and its metabolites in urine[a]

Species	Application	Unchanged isoprenaline	3-o-Methyl-isoprenaline	Conjugated isoprenaline	Conjugated 3-o-methyl-isoprenaline	Reference
Rat	Intravenous	10	14	18	36	HERTTING (1964)
Man	Intravenous	40	4	0	32	PATERSON and
	Oral	4	2	65	10	CONOLLY (1971)
	Aerosol	1–2	1–2	81–95	4–6	

[a] The data for isoprenaline and its metabolites are given in % of the dose. Urine was collected for 24 h after application of the drug

the drug does not undergo deamination. Isoprenaline is metabolized by catechol-o-methyltransferase to form the 3-o-methylisoprenaline (Fig. 3). Both, the parent drug and its 3-o-methyl metabolite are conjugated. MORGAN et al. (1969 b), using a sulfatase-β-glucuronidase separately, demonstrated that predominantly the sulfate conjugates are formed. The same findings were obtained in man (CONOLLY et al., 1972).

The metabolic pattern of isoprenaline injected intravenously into rats has been studied by HERTTING (1964). Within 24 h of the injection, more than 75% of the dose is recovered from urine, however, only 10% in the form of the unchanged drug (Table 1). Conjugated 3-o-methylisoprenaline represents the main metabolite.

In man, the metabolic pattern of isoprenaline greatly depends on the route of administration (BLACKWELL et al., 1970; DOLLERY et al., 1971; PATERSON and CONOLLY, 1971; CONOLLY et al., 1972). Within 24 h of intravenous injection of ^{3}H-isoprenaline, 40% of the dose is recovered from urine in the form of the parent drug (Table 1). The main metabolite is conjugated 3-o-methylisoprenaline. In contrast, very little unchanged isoprenaline is excreted in urine when the substance is given orally or as an aerosol (Table 1). After both forms of application, conjugated isoprenaline represents the main metabolite. The similarities in metabolic pattern after oral ingestion and inhalation suggest that a considerable part of the isoprenaline given as aerosol is swallowed and absorbed in the intestine.

The metabolism of isoprenaline in man gained much interest when SPEIZER et al. (1968 a, b) found an association of the increased death-rate from asthma with the use of pressurized aerosols containing beta-receptor stimulating drugs. Furthermore, resistance towards the positive chronotropic effect of inhaled and ingested isoprenaline could be demonstrated in patients with asthma who had been using aerosol preparations of the drug (PATERSON et al., 1968). Surprisingly, 3-o-methylisoprenaline was found to exert beta-receptor blocking activity (PHILIPPOT et al., 1965; PATERSON et al., 1968; REICHL et al., 1971). It seemed possible that the diminished efficacy of isoprenaline in patients with asthma was due to the formation of 3-o-methylisoprenaline which could block the effects of the parent compound. However, REICHL et al. (1971) clearly demonstrated that 3-o-methylisoprenaline is at least 100 times weaker than propranolol as a beta-receptor blocking agent. Considering this and the relatively small percentage of isoprenaline which is converted to 3-o-methyl-isoprenaline, one must conclude that the formation of this metabolite can not be the underlying cause of the decreased efficacy of isoprenaline in asthmatic patients.

2. Kinetics

Studies in dogs, where the increase in heart rate was used as an indirect measure of absorption, showed that isoprenaline is readily absorbed in the gastrointestinal tract except for the empty stomach (MINATOYA et al., 1965a). Comparison of the areas under the curve demonstrated that the effect increased with the doses given (MINATOYA et al., 1965b). The rapid intestinal absorption of the drug was confirmed in dogs by CONOLLY et al. (1972) using tritiated isoprenaline. Asthmatic patients who were given oral doses of 0.044–0.21 mg/kg ^{3}H-isoprenaline excreted 59%–107% of the radioactivity in urine within 30–48 h after injection. From feces, 12%–27% of the radioactivity was recovered (CONOLLY et al., 1972). In spite of the good intestinal absorption, intravenous isoprenaline is about 1000 times more potent in increasing heart rate than oral doses of the substance (DOLLERY et al., 1971). These findings are explained by the earlier mentioned fact that after oral application almost all the drug is excreted in the form of metabolites, whereas after intravenous doses a considerable portion is excreted in urine as unchanged isoprenaline. Apparently, almost all of the drug absorbed in the intestine is metabolized prior to reaching the systemic circulation resulting in an extremely low bioavailability. Investigations, where intraduodenal administration and intraportal infusion of isoprenaline were compared in dogs, make it likely that the metabolism of the drug occurs largely in the intestinal wall and to a lesser extent in the liver (CONOLLY et al., 1972).

One may assume that this gut wall first-pass metabolism mainly results in the formation of a sulfate conjugate, since, as has been mentioned earlier, a conjugate is the major metabolite of oral isoprenaline. Furthermore, only very litte, if any, isoprenaline is metabolized to glucuronides. If the assumption mentioned above is true, drugs such as salicylamide, which themselves are conjugated with sulfate, could inhibit the metabolic degradation of isoprenaline in the gut wall and thereby enhance its effects. In fact, BENNETT et al. (1975) have shown that in dogs the bioavailability of oral isoprenaline is increased by salicylamide. At present, the significance of these findings for therapeutics is not yet clear.

Ten min after intravenous injection of ^{3}H-isoprenaline in rats, the highest concentrations of radioactivity were found in kidneys, adrenals, lungs, liver, and heart (HERTTING, 1964); less radioactivity was recovered from blood; with more of the radioactivity in the form of 3-o-methylisoprenaline than in the form of the parent drug. Similar results were obtained in cats (KADAR et al., 1978). In rats, 2 h after the injection, there was a sharp decrease of radioactivity in all organs except for kidneys and liver. Most probably, the relatively high concentrations of radioactivity in kidneys and liver are due to accumulation of isoprenaline and its metabolites in urine and bile, respectively, with little radioactive material being present in the organ cells themselves.

Plasma levels of isoprenaline were followed in dogs after intravenous injection of 0.27–0.64 μg/kg of the tritiated substance (CONOLLY et al., 1972). Concentrations of the unchanged drug were in the order of 0.2–6.0 ng/ml. Levels of 3-o-methylisoprenaline were considerably lower. No significant amounts of conjugates were found. Plasma levels of isoprenaline declined biphasically after the injection, the half-life of the rapid phase being 1–2 min. This half-life appeared to be related to the decline of the positive chronotropic effects of isoprenaline on the heart.

In one normal subject in whom 0.063 µg/kg ^{3}H-isoprenaline was injected intravenously within 1 min, plasma levels of the unchanged drug fell in a biexponential way from 0.39 to 0.046 ng/ml in the following 210 min (CONOLLY et al., 1972). Half-life was about 5 min during the rapid and approximately 2.5 h during the slow phase. Concentrations of 3-o-methylisoprenaline were considerably lower than the levels the parent compound. As in dogs, no conjugates of isoprenaline or 3-o-methylisoprenaline were found in plasma.

No unchanged isoprenaline could be detected in the plasma of a patient who was given 0.2 mg/kg ^{3}H-labeled drug orally (CONOLLY et al., 1972). However, high concentrations of conjugated isoprenaline were measured. Not surprisingly, there was a clear cut dissociation in the time course of total plasma radioactivity and of the rise in heart rate.

In rats which were given ^{3}H-isoprenaline intravenously, 60%–70% of the radioactivity was excreted in urine, 34%–42% in the bile (HERTTING, 1964). The latter fraction contained a conjugate of 3-o-methylisoprenaline. When bile of rats who had received labeled isoprenaline was injected into the duodenum of other rats, very little radioactivity was excreted in urine and bile of the latter animals (HERTTING, 1964). Therefore, one must conclude that most of the radioactivity present in the bile of rats which were given ^{3}H-isoprenaline is eliminated via the feces. In dogs, apparently very little radioactivity is excreted via the bile after intravenous injection of ^{3}H-isoprenaline (CONOLLY et al., 1972).

As has already been mentioned, asthmatic patients who were given an oral dose of ^{3}H-isoprenaline excreted 59%–107% of the radioactivity in urine and 12%–27% in feces within 30–48 h (CONOLLY et al., 1972). It seems possible that the radioactivity contained in feces does not represent the portion of drug not absorbed in the intestine but rather metabolites of isoprenaline excreted via the bile. However, data on the radioactivity in feces after intravenous injection of ^{3}H-isoprenaline are lacking in man. Another possibility could be that 3-o-methylisoprenaline, a basic compound, diffuses from plasma into the acidic medium of the stomach being not absorbed during passage through the gut.

II. Orciprenaline

Orciprenaline, the 1-(3,5-dihydroxyphenyl)-*N*-isopropyl-ethanolamine (Fig. 4), has preferably β-receptor stimulating effects. As isoprenaline, the drug is used as aerosol in patients with asthma and intravenously in patients with cardiogenic shock. Furthermore, the substance is given intravenously and orally to patients with atrioventricular conduction disturbances.

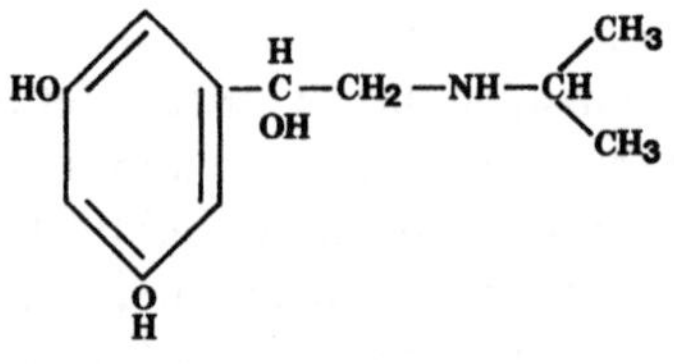

Fig. 4. The structure of orciprenaline

1. Biotransformation

As in the case of isoprenaline, one would expect that due to the isopropyl group attached to the *N*-atom, orciprenaline does not undergo deamination. Furthermore, because of the position of the phenolic hydroxy groups orciprenaline, in contrast to isoprenaline, is no substrate for catechol-o-methyltransferase. In fact, studies in the rat, rabbit, and man suggest that the main metabolic pathway of orciprenaline is conjugate forming with the phenolic hydroxy groups (DENGLER and HENGSTMANN, 1976). In contrast to the other species, the cat metabolized the drug only to a minor degree. Experiments with β-glucuronidase revealed that, in rat and rabbit, most of the orciprenaline conjugates are glucuronides. There is evidence that orciprenaline may undergo ester or ether linkaes of the β-hydroxy group with methanol or ethanol at acidic pH in vitro (DENGLER and HENGSTMANN, 1976). This should be considered in studies of the metabolism of the drug in order to avoid misinterpretations.

2. Kinetics

Orciprenaline seems to be rather poorly absorbed from the gastrointestinal tract of rabbits, rats, and mice as only 35%–45% of the radioactivity given orally to these animals in the form of ^{14}C-orciprenaline could be recovered from urine within 72–120 h (TATSUMI et al., 1970, 1971). In man, too, the intestinal absorption is incomplete (DENGLER and HENGSTMANN, 1976). Thus, only 36% of the radioactivity given as an oral dose of ^{3}H-orciprenaline to patients was eliminated in urine within 72 h compared with 82% in the same period after intravenous application. From these data, an intestinal absorption of 44% may be calculated. Peak plasma levels of orciprenaline were obtained 2–4 h after an oral dose (DENGLER and HENGSTMANN, 1976). This is in good agreement with pharmacodynamic studies where the maximum effect on bronchiolar resistance was observed 2–6 h after oral orciprenaline (BAVING and ULMER, 1970). After an oral dose of ^{3}H-orciprenaline given to patients, 1.2% of the radioactivity was excreted in urine as unchanged drug compared with 12% after intravenous application (DENGLER and HENGSTMANN, 1976). Provided that the urinary excretion of unchanged drug reflects its area under the plasma curve, one may conclude that the bioavailability of orciprenaline is about 10%, a figure coming close to the 5% obtained in pharmacodynamic studies (BAVING and ULMER, 1970). The difference between a bioavailability of 10% and an intestinal absorption of 44% is apparently due to first-pass metabolism of orciprenaline. Studies in patients with portocaval shunt suggest that this occurs in the gut wall (HENGSTMANN and DENGLER, 1975).

Thirty min after intravenous injection of ^{3}H-orciprenaline into rats, high concentrations of radioactivity were found in kidneys, plasma, and liver (DENGLER and HENGSTMANN, 1976). Radioactivity rose rapidly in all organs studied. In plasma, always less than 20% of the radioactivity was represented by the unchanged amine. In contrast, 50%–80% of the radioactivity in heart, lungs, kidneys, and skeletal muscle was in the form of the parent drug even 4 h after the intravenous injection. There could, therefore, be a storage mechanism for orciprenaline in these organs. Other than in rat and rabbit, most of the plasma radioactivity in cats was unchanged orciprenaline up to 180 min after an intravenous injection of the labeled drug (DENGLER and HENGSTMANN, 1976).

In the study by DENGLER and HENGSTMANN (1976), one patient received an infusion with 1.6 mg ^{3}H-orciprenaline (500 μCi) within 12 h. The plasma level curve of the unchanged drug obtained after ending the infusion could be analyzed by means of an open two-compartment model. Elimination half-life was about 6 h.

Little is known about the relation of orciprenaline plasma levels and pharmacodynamic effects. Comparing the concentrations measured by DENGLER and HENGSTMANN (1976) after oral administration of ^{3}H-orciprenaline and the effect on bronchiolar resistance determined by ULMER et al. (1968) and BAVING and ULMER (1970), one can assume that the therapeutic plasma levels of the β-receptor stimulating agent are in the order of 0.5–5 ng/ml.

In the rat, 95% of the radioactivity injected intravenously as ^{3}H-orciprenaline was excreted in the urine within 24 h (DENGLER and HENGSTMANN, 1976). Almost all of the radioactivity in urine was in the form of conjugates of the drug. As has already been mentioned, patients excreted in urine 82% of the radioactivity injected intravenously as 0.8 mg ^{3}H-orciprenaline, 12% of the dose being in the form of the unchanged amine (DENGLER and HENGSTMANN, 1976). In one patient, who was given an infusion with 1.6 mg ^{3}H-orciprenaline, the total clearance of the drug was 1000 ml/min. The renal clearance contributed approximately 10% only (DENGLER and HENGSTMANN, 1976). One may, thus, assume that in man orciprenaline and its metabolites are almost exclusively eliminated via the kidneys. About 90% of a dose of the drug are excreted in the form of metabolites.

III. Salbutamol

Salbutamol (Fig. 5) is a noncatechol β-receptor stimulating agent. It exerts selective effects on β-2-receptors and does not cause tachycardia when bronchodilator doses are taken as aerosol or orally (CHOO-KANG et al., 1969; KENNEDY and SIMPSON, 1969; WARRELL et al., 1970). The drug is widely used in the treatment of asthma.

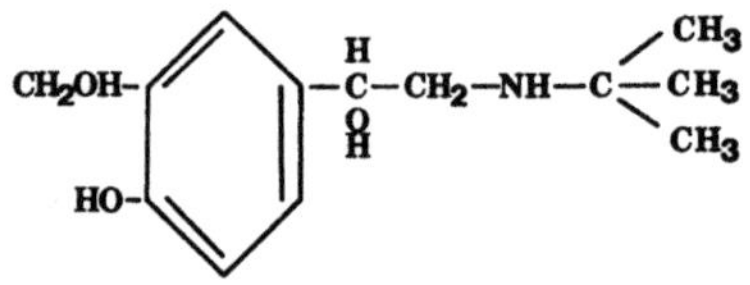

Fig. 5. The structure of salbutamol

1. Biotransformation

In the rat and in the rabbit, salbutamol is metabolized to form a glucuronide (MARTIN et al., 1971). NMR and UV spectra revealed that the phenolic group is substituted. The extend of metabolization varies greatly with the species studied (Table 2). Thus, in the rat, 60% of the radioactivity excreted in urine after an oral dose of ^{3}H-salbutamol was in the form of unchanged drug. The rest was salbutamol glucuronide. In the dog, more than 70% of the radioactivity was salbutamol as compared with only about 10% in the rabbit (MARTIN et al., 1971).

Table 2. Excretion of ^{3}H-salbutamol and its metabolites in urine

Species	Dose	Application	% of dose recovered from urine	% of radioactivity present in urine as unchanged salbutamol	% of dose recovered from feces	Reference
Man	10 mg	Orally	90 within 24 h[a]			MARTIN et al. (1971)
Man	0.1 mg	Aerosol	60–70 within 17 h			MARTIN et al. (1971)
Man	8 mg	Orally	65–84 within 72 h	37–41	1– 7	WALKER et al. (1972)
Man	0.08 mg	Aerosol	78–97 within 72 h	41–54	10–12	WALKER et al. (1972)
Man	0.2–0.22 mg	Topically on bronchi	89 within 24 h	63		SHENFIELD et al. (1976)
Dog	12.5 mg/kg	Orally	72 within 24 h	79		MARTIN et al. (1971)
Rabbit	10–100 mg/kg	Orally	63 within 48 h	10		MARTIN et al. (1971)
Rat	25 mg/kg	Orally	56 within 48 h	60	25–40	MARTIN et al. (1971)

[a] h = hours

In man, unchanged salbutamol and a metabolite were excreted in urine after oral and aerosol dosing of the drug (WALKER et al., 1972). Acid hydrolysis of the metabolite yielded free salbutamol. However, the metabolite was not effected by glucuronidase and by arylsulfatase (WALKER et al., 1972). Nevertheless, LIN et al. (1977) clearly demonstrated that in man the main metabolite of salbutamol is its 4′-o-sulfate ester. The failure of WALKER et al. (1972) to identify this metabolite is explained by the fact that salbutamol sulfate ester is a very poor substrate for arylsulfatase. Large amounts of the enzyme and a long incubation time (17 h) were required for its partial hydrolysis (LIN et al., 1977). Besides salbutamol sulfate ester, a minor metabolite not yet identified is present in urine of patients treated with ^{3}H-salbutamol (LIN et al., 1977). Of the radioactivity excreted in urine of patients given ^{3}H-salbutamol orally or as aerosol, about 40% is in the form of unchanged drug. The rest are metabolites (Table 2). A different pattern was found after topical application of ^{3}H-salbutamol during bronchoscopy. Within 24 h, 87%–91% of the radioactivity applied was recovered from urine, 58%–67% of urinary radioactivity being in the form of unchanged drug (SHENFIELD et al., 1976).

2. Kinetics

About 60% of the radioactivity given orally to rats in the form of ^{3}H-salbutamol is excreted in urine within 96 h, 25%–40% is eliminated with the feces (Table 2). Probably, most of the latter fraction also has been absorbed in the intestine since in rats 20% of an oral dose of ^{3}H-salbutamol were excreted in the bile (MARTIN et al., 1971). Apparently, salbutamol is also well absorbed from the intestine of dogs and rabbits (MARTIN et al., 1971).

In man, 65%–90% of an oral dose of salbutamol is excreted in urine demonstrating good intestinal absorption. Only a small percentage of the dose is recovered from feces (Table 2). The drug is also absorbed from the bronchi when applied locally during bronchoscopy (SHENFIELD et al., 1976). An intravenous injection of 4 µg/kg salbutamol and 200 µg salbutamol given as aerosol produced equal bronchodilation, but differed significantly in hemodynamic and metabolic effects. Thus intravenous salbutamol increased heart rate and plasma insulin whereas salbutamol given as aerosol did not (NEVILLE et al., 1977). One may conclude from these experiments that the dose of salbutamol given as aerosol mainly acted topically on the bronchi. Nevertheless, 60%–97% of the radioactivity given as ^{3}H-salbutamol aerosol to patients is excreted in urine within 17–72 h (Table 2). Most probably, the majority of the aerosol administered dose is swallowed and only a small portion reaches the bronchi directly.

The distribution of salbutamol has been studied in rats and dogs (MARTIN et al., 1971). In rats given ^{3}H-salbutamol orally, the highest concentrations of total radioactivity were measured in liver, fat, muscle, and kidneys. In dogs given an oral dose of 12.5 mg/kg ^{3}H-salbutamol, liver and kidneys were the only organs where radioactivity could be detected after 24 h. ^{3}H-salbutamol given by aerosol was well distributed throughout the lungs of this species.

In dogs given 12.5 mg/kg ^{3}H-salbutamol orally, plasma levels of total radioactivity were about 4 µg/ml expressed as salbutamol 2–4 h after dosing (MARTIN et al., 1971). Concentrations of total radioactivity ranging 1–39 ng/mg salbutamol equivalents were obtained 5 min to 24 h after 1000 µg ^{3}H-salbutamol given as aerosol. In the rabbit, half-life of total radioactivity in plasma was approximately 90 min after oral application of ^{3}H-salbutamol (MARTIN et al., 1971).

In volunteers given 10 mg ^{3}H-salbutamol per os, plasma concentrations of radioactivity ranged between 70 and 120 ng/ml expressed as salbutamol (MARTIN et al., 1971). Comparable concentrations were measured in another study, where further a ratio salbutamol/metabolites of 1:4 was found at the time of peak plasma levels (WALKER et al., 1972). Half-life of total radioactivity in plasma was about 1.5–2 h in the study by MARTIN et al. (1971) and 2.7–5 h in the one by WALKER et al. (1972). WALKER et al. (1972) also found the plasma half-life of unchanged salbutamol to be similar to that of the metabolites. However, one must consider that all these data represent only rough estimates of half-life.

Total radioactivity corresponding to 3.8–6.7 ng/ml salbutamol was found in plasma of one of two subjects given 100 µg ^{3}H-salbutamol as aerosol. In the plasma of the other, no radioactivity was detected at all (MARTIN et al., 1971). In the study by WALKER et al. (1972), peak plasma concentrations of total radioactivity corresponding to 0.6–1.4 ng/ml were seen at 3–5 h after application of 0.04–0.1 mg ^{3}H-salbutamol as aerosol. The ratio of salbutamol/metabolites was 1:4 and the total plasma radioactivity declined with a half-life of 1.7–7.1 h. When 200–220 µg ^{3}H-salbutamol were applied topically to the bronchi during bronchoscopy, peak plasma levels of unchanged drug ranging from 5.7 to 11.4 ng/ml were measured within 10 min of the application (SHENFIELD et al., 1976). At this time, less than 15% of the total radioactivity in plasma was in the form of metabolites of the drug.

After oral doses of ^{3}H-salbutamol, the time course of total radioactivity in plasma was related to the effect of the drug on forced expiratory volume. No such relation could be detected when ^{3}H-salbutamol was given as aerosol. Rather, maximum increase of forced expiratory volume was observed within 15 min of inhalation of salbutamol, whereas peak plasma levels of total radioactivity were measured 3–5 h after the aerosol was given (WALKER et al., 1972).

Salbutamol and its metabolites are mainly excreted in urine (Table 2). In man, only a minor percentage of a dose of ^{3}H-salbutamol is eliminated with the feces. However, in the rat about a third of an oral dose of ^{3}H-salbutamol can be recovered from feces. As has already been mentioned, this portion probably represents radioactivity excreted in the bile.

IV. Terbutaline

Terbutaline (Fig. 6) is a noncatechol which has been shown to act selectively on β-2-adrenoceptors (BERGMANN et al., 1969). The drug is used in the treatment of asthma.

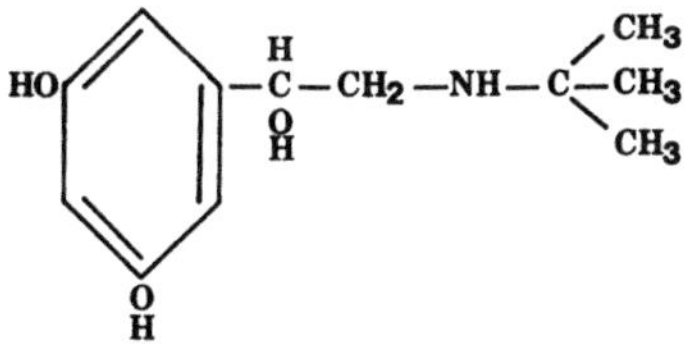

Fig. 6. The structure of terbutaline

Table 3. Excretion of ^{3}H-terbutaline and its conjugates in urine and feces from man[a]

Administration	Urine						Feces
	Dose (mg)	Collection period (h)	Free terbutaline	Conjugated terbutaline	Unidentified	Total radioactivity	Total radioactivity
Oral	5–10	70–185	6	17	—	23	47
Intravenous	0.1	91–120	56	12	15	83	3

[a] The data for terbutaline and its metabolites are given in % of the dose. Feces contained almost exclusively free terbutaline (DAVIES et al., 1974)

1. Biotransformation

Terbutaline is a resorcinol and therefore not a substrate for catechol-o-methyltransferase (PERSSON and PERSSON, 1972). In the rat, terbutaline is extensively metabolized to form a glucuronide (CONWAY et al., 1973). Studies with intraportal and intraperitoneal administration of the drug revealed that the conjugation takes place in the liver. However, there is evidence that part of the terbutaline glucuronide is also formed in the intestinal wall (CONWAY et al., 1973). In the rat and in the guinea pig, terbutaline is not metabolized in the lung (RYRFELDT and NILSSON, 1978).

In dogs, very little if any conjugates of terbutaline are formed after intravenous, intragastric, and intraduodenal administration of the drug (DAVIES et al., 1974).

In man, terbutaline is metabolized to a conjugate (NILSSON et al., 1972; DAVIES et al., 1974). Comparative enzymatic hydrolysis with arylsulfatase/beta-glucuronidase and beta-glucuronidase separately demonstrated that a sulfate conjugate is formed. Furthermore, an unidentified metabolite of terbutaline is excreted in urine after intravenous administration of the drug (DAVIES et al., 1974). The metabolic pattern of terbutaline is greatly dependent upon the route of administration (Table 3). After intravenous injection of ^{3}H-terbutaline, considerable more radioactivity is excreted in the form of the unchanged drug than after oral administration (DAVIES et al., 1974). Similar results were obtained in rats (CONWAY et al., 1973).

2. Kinetics

Terbutaline is absorbed from the intestine when given orally to rats. Urinary excretion of free drug is considerably lower after oral than after intraportal administration suggesting a gut wall first-pass metabolism in this species (CONWAY et al., 1973).

Oral therapy with terbutaline has been shown to be effective in man (FORMGREN, 1970; FREEDMAN, 1971; LEGGE et al., 1971). Of oral doses ranging from 5–10 mg, an average of 23% can be recovered from urine within 70–185 h, 47% from feces (Table 3). Feces contain almost exclusively free terbutaline. Furthermore, very little radioactivity is eliminated via the feces when ^{3}H-terbutaline is injected intravenously (Table 3). One may therefore assume, that terbutaline recovered from feces after an oral dose represents the portion of the drug being not absorbed. Terbutaline as well as isoprenaline is absorbed from the respiratory tract after endotracheal instillation (RYRFELDT and BODIN, 1975). Isolated perfused rat and guinea pig lungs very slowly take terbutaline up from the perfusate (RYRFELDT and NILSSON, 1978).

After intraduodenal administration of 2 μg/kg labeled terbutaline to dogs, peak plasma levels of total radioactivity ranging from 300–653 ng/ml were obtained at 45–57 min (CONOLLY et al., 1971; DAVIES et al., 1974). Since very little, if any, terbutaline is metabolized in this species (DAVIES et al., 1974), the concentrations of total radioactivity mainly represent the parent drug. Plasma radioactivity in the dog declined with a half-life of approximately 3 h (CONOLLY et al., 1971). After intravenous injection of terbutaline in doses of 2.5–18.65 μg/kg to dogs, peak plasma concentrations of total radioactivity ranged from 15.6–341 ng/ml terbutaline equivalents (DAVIES et al., 1974). The increase in heart rate caused by terbutaline given intravenously to dogs did not correspond well with the plasma levels of total radioactivity (DAVIES et al., 1974).

In man, intravenous injection of 100 μg ^{3}H-terbutaline produced plasma concentrations of the unchanged drug ranging from 3–8 ng/ml. In one subject, total radioactivity declined biphasically with a half-life of the slow phase exceeding 3 h (DAVIES et al., 1974). After oral administration of 5–10 mg ^{3}H-terbutaline, plasma levels of total radioactivity ranging from 29–37 ng/ml terbutaline equivalents were measured. In one subject who had received more radioactivity than the others (10 mg terbutaline, 250 μCi^{3}H) a peak of 4.9 ng/ml unchanged drug in plasma was reached after 4 h (DAVIES et al., 1974). Clinical studies have shown that the bronchodilating effect of terbutaline aerosols lasts 4–5 h (TRAUTLEIN et al., 1976; CAPECCHI et al., 1978; CHESTER et al., 1978) and that this drug has a more prolonged action than salbutamol (FREEDMAN, 1972; CHOO-KANG et al., 1973; BROGDEN et al., 1974). In the rat, terbutaline given by oral, subcutaneous, intraperitoneal, and intraportal routes is almost completely excreted in urine and feces within 72 h. Thus, during this time about 40% of an oral, subcutaneous, intraperitoneal, and intraportal dose of ^{3}H-terbutaline was eliminated in urine, approximately 50% in feces (CONWAY et al., 1973). In dogs, 59% of an intragastric dose of ^{3}H-terbutaline was excreted in urine within 24 h. In the same species, 17%–46% of an intravenous dose of the labeled drug was eliminated in urine within 2–4 h, less than 0.2% being excreted via the bile (DAVIES et al., 1974).

In man, practically all the radioactivity given intravenously in the form of ^{3}H-terbutaline appears in urine within 91–120 h (Table 3). From this, one may conclude that terbutaline which has reached the systemic circulation in man is almost exclusively, as unchanged drug and as metabolites, eliminated via the kidneys.

V. Fenoterol

Fenoterol (Fig. 7) acts selectively on adrenergic β-2-receptors. The drug is used in the treatment of asthma. Furthermore, fenoterol as well as some other β-2-receptor stimulating agents is increasingly given in pregnancy in order to decrease contractions

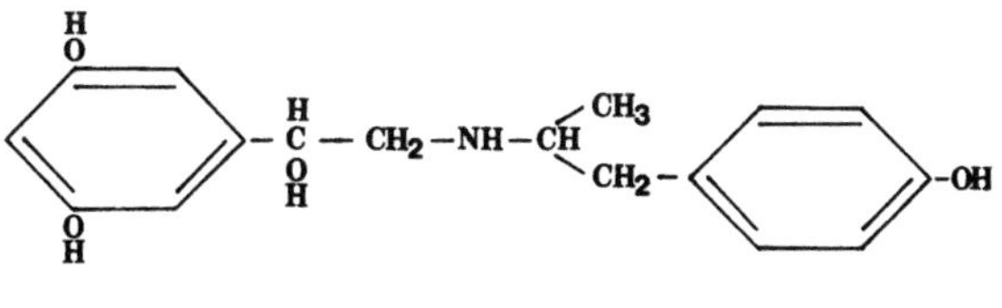

Fig. 7. The structure of fenoterol

of the uterus (MOSLER, 1969; JUNG et al., 1971; STOCKHAUSEN et al., 1972; KÜNZEL and REINECKE, 1973). Therefore, the diaplacental passage of fenoterol deserves special interest.

1. Biotransformation

The metabolism of fenoterol has been studied in rats (ROMINGER and POLLMANN, 1972). In the urine of animals treated with oral and intravenous doses of ^{3}H-fenoterol, two radioactive fractions could be separated. One fraction was basic and, when subjected to thin layer chromatography using five different solvent systems, had the same R_f value as authentic fenoterol. Thus, this fraction is most probably identical with the unchanged drug. The second fraction was acidic as shown by ion exchange chromatography. When treated with a mixture of glucuronidase and arylsulfatase, this fraction was quantitatively split to form fenoterol. The above mentioned second fraction, thus, obviously represents conjugates of the parent compound.

Also in the urine of dogs, acidic conjugates of fenoterol were found (ROMINGER and POLLMANN, 1972). Conjugates are formed rapidly and extensively in this species, since they represent more than 90% of the radioactivity excreted in urine collected in the time period 4–5 h after an oral or intravenous dose of ^{3}H-fenoterol. Similar results were obtained in pregnant guinea pigs (KORDS, 1975).

In man, more than 98% of the radioactivity excreted in urine after an oral dose of labeled fenoterol consists of acid conjugates (ROMINGER and POLLMANN, 1972). After an intravenous dose of ^{3}H-fenoterol given to man, 63% of the radioactivity excreted in urine in the first hour was conjugates as compared with 94% in the second hour (ROMINGER and POLLMANN, 1972). More than 99% of the radioactivity excreted in urine within 3 days after ^{3}H-fenoterol given as aerosol to man (Table 4) was in the form of conjugates of the drug (SEYBERTH and RAHN, 1973). These data clearly demonstrate, that in man, too, fenoterol is extensively metabolized independent of the route of application.

2. Kinetics

In the rat, fenoterol is rapidly absorbed from the gastrointestinal tract, peak blood levels of total radioactivity being obtained 1–2 h after an oral dose of tritium-labeled drug. On the bais of the radioactivity excreted via urine and bile, an intestinal absorp-

Table 4. Elimination of radioactivity in man after a dose of 200 μg ^{3}H-fenoterol given as aerosol [a]

Radioactivity excreted in	% of the dose
Urine	19.2 ± 1.1
Feces	62.7 ± 8.9
Urine + feces	81.9 ± 9.2

[a] Urine and feces were collected for at least 3 days. Data represent mean ± standard error of the mean of 5 subjects (SEYBERTH and RAHN, 1973)

tion of 23% was calculated in this study (ROMINGER and POLLMANN, 1972). However, levels of the unchanged compound were neither determined in blood nor in the excreta. Thus, there are no data on bioavailability. In the dog, 78% of the radioactivity given intravenously in the form of ^{3}H-fenoterol was recovered from urine. After oral application to fasting animals, 69% of the radioactivity was excreted in urine, suggesting almost complete intestinal absorption. Less radioactivity was found in urine from animals which had free access to food (ROMINGER and POLLMANN, 1972). In man, about 60% of the radioactivity given intravenously as ^{3}H-fenoterol was recovered from urine, compared with approximately 35% after an oral dose. Maximum plasma levels of total radioactivity were determined 1–3 h after oral application of the drug (ROMINGER and POLLMANN, 1972).

The distribution of fenoterol has been studied in rats and rabbits. After intravenous injection of ^{3}H-fenoterol into rats, radioactivity was found predominantly in the kidneys, less in liver, lungs, and heart (ROMINGER and POLLMANN, 1972; KRAMER and KLINGSPOHR, 1974). In these studies, where counting of the radioactivity (ROMINGER and POLLMANN, 1972) as well as autoradiography (ROMINGER and POLLMANN, 1972; KRAMER and KLINGSPOHR, 1974) were used, little, if any, radioactivity could be detected in the brain indicating a blood-brain barrier for fenoterol. Plasma protein binding of the drug, as measured by means of equilibrium dialysis, was 37% (ROMINGER and POLLMANN, 1972). In gravid rabbits which were given intravenous doses of ^{3}H-fenoterol, the highest concentrations of radioactivity were detected in kidneys, liver, lungs, heart, and uterus (MEISSNER and PREIL, 1974; MEISSNER and KLOSTERMANN, 1976). Again, little, if any, radioactivity was found in the brain. However, in lactating rabbits, higher concentrations of tritium were measured in the mammary glands and in the milk than in serum (MEISSNER and PREIL, 1974).

Studies on the diaplacental passage of ^{3}H-fenoterol in the gravid rabbit revealed that placenta, blood, urine, amniotic fluid, stomach content, and kidney of the fetuses contained radioactivity. However, tritium concentration in alle fetal tissues and fluids was less than one-fifth of the levels measured in the respective maternal material (MEISSNER and KLOSTERMANN, 1976). Similarly, little radioactivity was found in fetal plasma when pregnant guinea pigs were injected or infused intravenously with labeled fenoterol. In this study, 2%–6% of the radioactivity in fetal plasma was identified as unchanged fenoterol (KORDS, 1975). KRAMER and KLINGSPOHR (1974) using autoradiography could barely detect radioactivity in fetuses of pregnant rats injected intravenously with ^{3}H-fenoterol.

Taken together, these studies on the diaplacental passage of fenoterol demonstrate that only small amounts of the drug pass the placenta. These findings are supported by experiments where the effects of fenoterol on maternal and fetal heart rate were compared. Thus, in pregnant guinea pigs injected or infused intravenously with fenoterol, maternal heart rate increased significantly, whereas fetal heart rate did not (KORDS, 1975). In man, intravenous infusion of 0.06 μg/kg/min fenoterol increased maternal heart rate by 35% whereas fetal heart rate remained unchanged (KÜNZEL and REINECKE, 1973). In another study in man, infusion of 1.5–3.0 μg/min fenoterol enhanced maternal heart rate by 25%, fetal heart rate by only 3%–5% (HÜTER et al., 1972).

After intravenous injection of the high dose of 1 mg/kg ^{3}H-fenoterol into rats, blood levels of total radioactivity ranged between 1 and 2 ng/ml. The time course of radioactivity in blood was biphasic with a half-life of the slow phase of about 2 h (ROMINGER and POLLMANN, 1972). In dogs, blood levels of total radioactivity ranging between 0.1 and 6.0 ng/ml fenoterol equivalents were measured after intravenous administration of 2 μg/kg and after an oral dose of 50 μg/kg ^{3}H-fenoterol (ROMINGER and POLLMANN, 1972).

In man, plasma levels of total radioactivity corresponded to 0.5–1.5 ng/ml fenoterol after intravenous injection of 0.9 μg/kg and to 5–50 ng/ml fenoterol after an oral dose of 90 μg/kg of the drug. Elimination half-life after an oral dose was 7 h (ROMINGER and POLLMANN, 1972). After application of 200 μg ^{3}H-fenoterol as an aerosol, total radioactivity in plasma ranged from 0.2 to 0.7 ng/ml fenoterol equivalent 1–12 h after dosage with an elimination half-life of about 6 h (SEYBERTH and RAHN, 1973).

In a body plethysmographic study, maximum effect on airway resistance was measured 10 min after fenoterol given as aerosol. This effect was significantly decreased 1 h after dosage (NOLTE, 1970). In contrast, radioactivity in plasma could be detected not earlier than 1 h after application of ^{3}H-fenoterol as aerosol, maximum concentrations being obtained 3 h after the dose (SEYBERTH and RAHN, 1973). This dissociation in time course between pharmacodynamic effect and plasma levels is compatible with the idea that fenoterol aerosols act locally on the bronchi. The radioactivity measured in plasma after an aerosol dose of ^{3}H-fenoterol most probably stems from substance that has been swallowed and absorbed from the intestine.

After application of ^{3}H-fenoterol to rats (ROMINGER and POLLMANN, 1972) and rabbits (MEISSNER and PREIL, 1974), radioactivity was excreted in urine and bile. In dogs given ^{3}H-fenoterol intravenously, 78% of the radioactivity injected was excreted in urine, 12% in feces within 46 h (ROMINGER and POLLMANN, 1972). The latter fraction apparently represents radioactivity excreted via the bile or by the gut wall. As already has been mentioned, the radioactivity excreted in urine from dogs given oral doses of ^{3}H-fenoterol is depending from whether or not the animals had access to food.

In man, about 60% of the radioactivity injected intravenously in the form of ^{3}H-fenoterol was excreted in urine, 15% in feces. After oral application of ^{3}H-fenoterol, about 35% of the radioactivity given to the volunteers was recovered from urine, 40% from feces (ROMINGER and POLLMANN, 1972). After an aerosol dose of ^{3}H-fenoterol, by far most of the radioactivity was eliminated with the feces (SEYBERTH and RAHN, 1973; Table 4).

References

Baving, G., Ulmer, W.T.: Die Dosis-Wirkungs-Relation von peroral verabreichtem Orciprenalin bei obstruktiven Atemwegserkrankungen. Arzneim. Forsch. *20*, 1083–1088 (1970)

Bennett, P., Blackwell, E., Davies, D.S.: Metabolism of drugs by intestinal mucosa – effect of salicylamide on bio-availability of oral isoprenaline in dogs. Abstracts VI. International Congress of Pharmacology, Helsinki, 1975, p. 583

Bergman, J., Persson, H., Wetterlin, K.: Two new groups of selective stimulants of adrenergic beta-receptors. Experientia *25*, 899–901 (1969)

Blackwell, E.W., Conolly, M.E., Davies, D.S., Dollery, C.T.: The fate of isoprenaline administered by pressurized aerosols. Br. J. Pharmacol. *39*, 194P–195P (1970)

Bogner, R.L., Walsh, J.M.: Sustained-release principle in human subjects utilizing radioactive techniques. J. Pharmac. Sci. *53*, 617–620 (1964)

Brogden, R.N., Speight, T.M., Avery, G.S.: Terbutaline aerosol (bricanyl): an independent report. Med. Progr. Technol. *1*, 19–21 (1974)

Bruce, R.B., Pitts, J.E.: The determination and excretion of phenylephrine in urine. Biochem. Pharmacol. *17*, 335–337 (1968)

Capecchi, V., Cavalli, F., Falcoone, F., Fasano, E.: Comparison of terbutaline and salbutamol aerosols in patients with bronchial asthma. Int. J. Clin. Pharmacol. Biopharm. *16*, 310–312 (1978)

Cavalitto, C.J., Chafetz, L., Miller, L.D.: Some studies of a sustained release principle. J. Pharmac. Sci. *52*, 259–263 (1963)

Chester, E.H., Doggett, W.E., Montenegro, H.D., Schwartz, H.J., Jones, P.K.: Bronchodilating effect of terbutaline aerosol. Clin. Pharmacol. Ther. *23*, 630–634 (1978)

Choo-Kang, Y.F.J., Simpson, W.T., Grant, I.W.B.: Controlled comparison of the bronchodilator effects of three beta-adrenergic stimulant drugs administered by inhalation to patients with asthma. Br. Med. J. *2*, 287–289 (1969)

Choo-Kang, Y.F.J., McDonald, H.C., Harne, N.W.: A comparison of salbutamol and terbutaline aerosols in bronchial asthma. Pactitioner *211*, 801–804 (1973)

Conolly, M.E., Davies, D.S., Dollery, C.T., George, C.F.: Resistance to β-adrenoceptor stimulants (a possible explanation for the rise in asthma deaths). Br. J. Pharmacol. *43*, 389–402 (1971)

Conolly, M.E., Davies, D.S., Dollery, C.T., Morgan, C.D., Paterson, J.W., Sandler, M.: Metabolism of isoprenaline in dog and man. Br. J. Pharmacol. *46*, 458–472 (1972)

Conway, W.D., Minatoya, H., Lands, A.M., Shekosky, J.M.: Absorption and elimination profile of isoprenaline. III. J. Pharmac. Sci. *57*, 1135–1141 (1968)

Conway, W.D., Singhvi, S.M., Gibaldi, M., Boyes, R.N.: The effect of route of administration on the metabolic fate of terbutaline in the rat. Xenobiotica *3*, 813–821 (1973)

Davies, D.S., George, C.F., Blackwell, E., Conolly, M.E., Dollery, C.T.: Metabolism of terbutaline in man and dog. Br. J. Clin. Pharmacol. *1*, 129–136 (1974)

Dengler, H.J., Hengstmann, J.H.: Metabolism and pharmacokinetics of orciprenaline in various animal species and man. Arch. Int. Pharmacodyn. Ther. *223*, 71–87 (1976)

Dollery, C.T., Davies, D.S., Conolly, M.E.: Differences in the metabolism of drugs depending upon their route of administration. Arch. Int. Pharmacodyn. Ther. *192*, Suppl., 214–219 (1971)

Formgren, H.: A clinical comparison of the effects of oral terbutaline and orciprenaline. Scand. J. Respir. Dis. *51*, 195–202 (1970)

Freedman, B.J.: Trial of a new bronchodilator, terbutaline, in asthma. Br. Med. J. *1*, 633–636 (1971)

Freedman, B.J.: Trial of terbutaline aerosol in the treatment of asthma and comparison of its effects with those of a salbutamol aerosol. Br. J. Dis. Chest. *66*, 222–229 (1972)

Hengstmann, J.H., Dengler, H.J.: Pharmacokinetic properties and metabolism of phenolic sympathomimetic amines in man. Abstracts VI. International Congress of Pharmacology, Helsinki 1975, p. 451

Hengstmann, J.H., Weyand, U., Dengler, H.J.: The physiological disposition of etilefrine in man. Eur. J. Clin. Pharmacol. *9*, 179–187 (1975)

Hertting, G.: The fate of ^{3}H-iso-proterenol in the rat. Biochem. Pharmacol. *13*, 1119–1128 (1964)

Holzbauer, M., Sharman, D.F.: The distribution of catecholamines in vertebrates. In: Catecholamines. Blaschko, H., Muscholl, E. (eds.), pp. 110–185. Berlin, Heidelberg, New York: Springer 1972

Hüter, J., Rippert, C., Meyer, C.: Wehenhemmung mit welchem Beta-Mimetikum (Berotec®, Ritodrine®, Dilatol®)? Geburtshilfe Frauenheilkd. *32*, 97–103 (1972)

Jung, H., Abramowski, P., Klöck, F.K., Schwenzel, W.: Zur Wirkung alpha- und beta-adrenergischer Substanzen am menschlichen Uterus und Nebenwirkungen auf Mutter und Kind. Geburtshilfe Frauenheilkd. *31*, 11–27 (1971)

Kadar, D., Lovrics, A.J., Endrenyi, L.: The fate of (7-^{3}H)isoproterenol in cats after intravenous administration. Drug. Metab. Dispos. *6*, 476–480 (1978)

Kennedy, M.C.S.: Simpson, W.T.: Human pharmacological and clinical studies on salbutamol: A specific beta-adrenergic bronchodilator. Br. J. Dis. Chest. *63*, 165–174 (1969)

Kopin, I.J.: Metabolic degradation of catecholamines. The relative importance of different pathways under physiological conditions and after administration of drugs. In: Catecholamines. Blaschko, H., Muscholl, E. (eds.), pp. 270–282. Berlin, Heidelberg, New York: Springer 1972
Kords, H.: Kreislaufwirkungen, Placentapassage, Pharmakokinetik und Metabolismus von Fenoterol (Partusisten) beim trächtigen Meerschweinchen. Z. Geburtshilfe Perinatol. *179*, 30–36 (1975)
Kramer, I., Klingspohr, H.J.: Ganztierautoradiographische Untersuchungen über die Verteilung und die diaplazentare Passage von Fenoterol-hydrobromid (Th 1165a) an Ratten. Arzneim. Forsch. *24*, 1210–1213 (1974)
Künzel, W., Reinecke, J.: Der Einfluß von Th 1165a auf die Gaspartialdrucke und auf kardiovaskuläre Parameter von Mutter und Fetus. Zugleich eine quantitative Analyse der Wehentätigkeit. Z. Geburtshilfe Perinatol. *177*, 81–90 (1973)
Legge, J.S., Gaddie, J., Palmer, K.N.V.: Comparison of two oral selective beta-adrenergic stimulant drugs in bronchial asthma. Br. Med. J. *1*, 637–639 (1971)
Lin, C., Li, Y., McGlotten, J., Morton, J.B., Symchowicz, S.: Isolation and identification of the major metabolite of albuterol in human urine. Drug Metab. Dispos. *5*, 234–238 (1977)
Martin, L.E., Hobson, J.C., Page, J.A., Harrison, C.: Metabolic studies of salbutamol-^{3}H: A new bronchodilator, in rat, rabbit, dog, and man. Eur. J. Pharmacol. *14*, 183–199 (1971)
Meissner, J., Klostermann, H.: Distribution and diaplacental passage of infused ^{3}H-fenoterol hydrobromide (Partusisten®) in the gravid rabbit. Int. J. Clin. Pharmacol. *13*, 27–35 (1976)
Meissner, J., Preil, P.: Untersuchungen über Verteilung und Passage von T-markiertem Fenoterol-hydrobromid (Th 1165a) am trächtigen und laktierenden Kaninchen. Arzneim. Forsch. *24*, 1213–1217 (1974)
Minatoya, H., Lands, A.M., Portmann, G.A.: Absorption and elimination profile of isoproterenol. I. Anesthetized Dogs. J. Pharmac. Sci. *54*, 968–972 (1965a)
Minatoya, H., Lands, A.M., Portmann, G.A.: Absorption and elimination profile of isoproterenol. II. Parenteral, oral, and rectal administration to unanaesthetized dogs. J. Pharmac. Sci. *54*, 973–978 (1965b)
Morgan, C.D., Ruthven, C.R.J., Sandler, M.: The quantitative assessment of isoprenaline metabolism in man. Clin. Chim. Acta *26*, 381–386 (1969a)
Morgan, C.D., Sandler, M., Davies, D.S., Conolly, M., Paterson, J.W., Dollery, C.T.: The metabolic fate of DL-(7-^{3}H)isoprenaline in man and dog. Clin. Chim. Acta *26*, 381–386 (1969b)
Mosler, K.H.: Probleme der Wehenhemmung durch Pharmaka. Med. Klin. *64*, 133–139 (1969)
Neville, A., Palmer, J.B.D., Gaddie, J., May, C.S., Palmer, K.N.V., Murchison, L.E.: Metabolic effects of salbutamol: comparison of aerosol and intravenous administration. Br. Med. J. *1*, 413–414 (1977)
Nilsson, H.T., Persson, K., Tegner, K.: The metabolism of terbutaline in man. Xenobiotica *2*, 363–373 (1972)
Nolte, D.: Das Verhalten von Atemwegs-Resistance und intrathorakalem Gasvolumen nach Inhalation eines Hydroxyphenyl-Derivates des Orciprenalin (Th 1165a). Respiration *27*, 396–405 (1970)
Paterson, J.W., Conolly, M.E.: The clinical pharmacology of inhaled isoprenaline. Proc. Int. Soc. Drug Toxicol. *12*, 138–141 (1971)
Paterson, J.W., Conolly, M.E., Davies, D.S., Dollery, C.T.: Isoprenaline resistance and the use of pressurized aerosols in asthma. Lancet *2*, 426–429 (1968)
Persson, K., Persson, K.: The metabolism of terbutaline in vitro by rat and human liver O-methyltransferases and monoamine oxidases. Xenobiotica *2*, 375–382 (1972)
Philippot, E., Bacq, Z.M., Sulman, E.G.: Actions du 1(3-méthoxy-4-oxyphényl)-1-hydroxy-2-isopropylamino-éthane(3-méthoxy-isoprotérénol). Arch. Int. Pharmacodyn. Ther. *156*, 234–237 (1965)
Reichl, R., Traunecker, W., Engelhardt, A.: Quantitative pharmacological investigations with 3-methoxy-isoprenaline, the primary metabolite of isoprenaline. Proc. Eur. Soc. Drug Tox. *12*, 142–146 (1971)
Rominger, K.L., Pollmann, W.: Vergleichende Pharmakokinetik von Fenoterol-Hydrobromid bei Ratte, Hund und Mensch. Arzneim. Forsch. *22*, 1190–1196 (1972)

Ryrfeldt, A., Bodin, N.O.: The physiological disposition of ibuterol, terbutaline and isoproterenol after endotracheal instillation to rats. Xenobiotica *5*, 521–529 (1975)

Ryrfeldt, A., Nilsson, E.: Uptake and biotransformation of ibuterol and terbutaline in isolated perfused rat and guinea pig lungs. Biochem. Pharmacol. *27*, 301–305 (1978)

Sandler, M.: Catecholamine synthesis and metabolism in man: clinical implications (with special reference to Parkinsonism). In: Catecholamines. Blaschko, H., Muscholl, E. (eds.), pp. 845–899. Berlin, Heidelberg, New York: Springer 1972

Seyberth, H.W., Rahn, K.H.: Pharmakokinetische Untersuchungen am Menschen mit einem als Dosier-Aerosol verwendeten Beta-Sympathomimetikum. Verh. Dtsch. Ges. Inn. Med. *79*, 888–891 (1973)

Shenfield, G.M., Evans, M.E., Paterson, J.W.: Absorption of drugs by the lung. Br. J. Clin. Pharmacol. *3*, 583 (1976)

Speizer, E.E., Doll, R., Heaf, P.: Observations on recent increase in mortality from asthma. Br. Med. J. *1*, 335–339 (1968a)

Speizer, E.E., Doll, R., Heaf, P., Strang, L.B.: Investigation into use of drugs preceding death from asthma. Br. Med. J. *1*, 339–343 (1968b)

Stockhausen, H., Schnell, J., Rüther, K.: Die Tokolyse unter der Geburt – eine tokographische Vergleichsuntersuchung bei Anwendung verschiedener tokolytischer Substanzen. Geburtshilfe Frauenheilkd. *1*, 51–56 (1972)

Tatsumi, K., Yamato, C., Arima, N., Yoshimura, H., Tsukamoto, H.: Metabolism of drugs. LXVIII. Metabolic fate of metaproterenol. Yakugaku Zasshi *90*, 639–643 (1970)

Tatsumi, K., Arima, N., Yoshimura, H.: Metabolism of drugs. LXXIV. Metabolic fate of metaproterenol. Yakugaku Zasshi *91*, 680–683 (1971)

Trautlein, J., Allegra, J., Gillin, M.: A long term study of low dose aerosolized terbutaline sulfate. J. Clin. Pharmacol. *16*, 361–366 (1976)

Ulmer, W.T., Podlesch, I., Heede, C.: Objektivierung von Therapieerfolgen bei chronisch obstruktivem Emphysem. Verh. Dtsch. Ges. Inn. Med. *71*, 964–969 (1968)

Walker, S.R., Evans, M.E., Richards, A.J., Paterson, J.W.: The clinical pharmacology of oral and inhaled salbutamol. Clin. Pharmacol. Ther. *13*, 861–867 (1972)

Warrell, D.A., Robertson, D.G., Newton Howes, J., Conolly, M.E., Paterson, J.W., Beilin, L.J., Dollery, C.T.: Comparison of cardiorespiratory effecs of isoprenaline and salbutamol in patients with bronchial asthma. Br. Med. J. *1*, 65–70 (1970)

CHAPTER 2

Kinetics and Biotransformation of Adrenergic Activators and Inhibitors: Adrenergic Transmitter Releasing Agents

H.A.J. STRUYKER-BOUDIER

A. Tyramine

I. Introduction

Tyramine occurs endogenously in the mammalian body. Studies into the distribution of this agent have been hampered by the lack of sufficiently specific and sensitive methods for its determination (OATES, 1961). Recently, sensitive methods have been developed based on a mass spectrometrical–gas chromatographic technique (PHILIPS et al., 1974, 1975), radio-immunoassay (FARAJ et al., 1975a) or radio-enzymatic assay (TALLMAN et al., 1976a). With these methods, amounts as low as 1 ng can be determined. The mass spectrometric method, moreover, allows separate determination of m- and p-tyramine (PHILIPS et al., 1974, 1975). These sensitive methods have allowed the study of the endogenous distribution as well as the metabolism and kinetics of exogenously applied tyramine in plasma, brain, and other tissues in a number of species. The endogenous distribution of tyramine was recently reviewed by BOULTON (1978).

II. Endogenous Tissue Distribution

The distribution of endogenous tyramine in several species is given in Table 1. These data indicate that tyramine rich organs include heart (especially the atria), kidney, spleen, adrenals, and salivary glands. In the central nervous system regions of relatively high concentration are hypothalamus and striatum. Mass spectrometric studies by PHILIPS et al. (1974, 1975, 1978) indicate that the p-isomer is the major isomer occurring endogenously in mammalian tissues. m-Tyramine only contributes 5%–20% to total tyramine concentration. From the data summarized in Table 1 it can be concluded that there is relatively good agreement between the distribution data in rats obtained with the mass spectrometric technique (PHILIPS et al., 1974, 1975) and the radio-enzymatic technique (TALLMAN et al., 1976a), although the levels reported in the latter study are generally somewhat higher. Apart from differences in the analytical techniques this may reflect strain differences, since Wistar and Sprague-Dawley rats, respectively, were used by these authors. The brain tyramine levels reported for humans (PHILIPS et al., 1978) are somewhat lower, but this could be caused by the fact that these data were obtained 4–10 h postmortem.

Levels in the tissue of rabbits and dogs, measured with the radio-immunoassay technique, are much higher than those in the rat (FARAJ et al., 1975a, b, 1977). Similarly, the earlier fluorometric methods (SPECTOR et al., 1963) gave tyramine levels of approximately 200 ng up to 1 μg/g wet weight of tissue for various brain regions of the rat, rabbit, and dog. An exception in this respect is the study by GUNNE and JONS-

Table 1. Concentration (ng/g wet tissue) of endogenous tyramine in a number of tissues in several species

Tissue	Rabbit (FARAJ et al., 1975)	Dog (FARAJ et al., 1977b)	Rat (PHILIPS et al., 1975)[a]	Rat (TALLMAN et al., 1976a)	Man (PHILIPS et al., 1978)[a]
Plasma	2.5	1.2	1.5 (BOULTON, 1978)[a]		
Heart total	110	132	3.4		
Atria				104	
Ventricles				< 10	
Adrenal	656	1,728			
Spleen	513	691	3.4	5.4	
Lung	183	524	3.0	< 5	
Kidney	163	361	32.7	27.0	
Liver	158	567	1.5	< 5	
Brain total	186	141	2.0	12.9	
Brainstem			2.2	9.6	
Cerebellum			2.3	9.7	0.6
Hypothalamus			11.3	25.7	0.2
Striatum			19.2	39.9	1.3
Cortex			1.6	< 5	0.2

[a] Only the p-isomer is indicated

SON (1965), who did not find levels higher than 30 ng/g in the rabbit brain. It is clear that not only species differences cause these ten- to hundredfold differences in tyramine levels in mammalian tissues. The large amount of closely related chemical structures in body tissues potentially interfering with the tyramine determination forces the use of rigorous analytical techniques of which the radio-enzymatic and mass-spectrometric methods seem, so far, to be the most reliable ones.

The specific pattern of distribution of tyramine in the central nervous system and its presence in a number of peripheral organs such as heart and kidney poses the question of its possible localization in nerve terminals. BOULTON and BAKER (1975) studied the subcellular distribution of p-tyramine in rat brain and found a synaptosomal localization for tyramine with a particulate/soluble ratio close to that of dopamine (LAVERTY et al., 1963). As regards peripheral organs TALLMAN et al. (1976b) performed a superior cervical ganglionectomy in rats. This procedure caused an approximate 50% reduction of salivary gland tyramine content. Also, after chemical sympathectomy with intravenous 6-hydroxydopamine significant reductions in tyramine level in heart atria and salivary gland were found, suggesting that tyramine is localized in nerve terminals (TALLMAN et al., 1976b).

III. Pharmacokinetics

After intravenous administration tyramine plasma levels decline rapidly. In dogs the plasma concentration declines biphasically with half-lifes of 4–5 min for the α-phase and 205 min for the β-phase (FARAJ et al., 1977). Tyramine is rapidly metabolized to p-hydroxyphenylacetic acid and concentrations of this metabolite, tenfold greater than tyramine, are reached in plasma within 5 min. Tyramine is taken immediately into the heart and red blood cells, after an intravenous injection, in rats and dogs (COMMARATO et al., 1969; FARAJ et al., 1977). It is eliminated from erythrocytes biphasically with half-lifes of 3 and 102 min respectively (FARAJ et al., 1977). These half-lifes are similar to those found during the α- and β-phase in plasma. Elimination from the heart follows similar kinetics (COMMARATO et al., 1969). Pargyline increases plasma half-life of tyramine during the α-phase to 13.4 min, indicating the importance of monoamine oxidation in its biotransformation (FARAJ et al., 1977).

When injected into brain ventricles in rats, tyramine is rapidly taken up into different brain areas. It is eliminated from those areas with a half-life of approximately 10–30 min. Again, pargyline pretreatment leads to a substantial increase in half-life, indicating that metabolism is the major route of tyramine elimination (WU and BOULTON, 1974).

Studies in isolated atria indicate that at the level of adrenergic neurons tyramine is retained as two pools: a pool with a rapid turnover (half-life of 3–4 min) in which tyramine is converted quantitatively to p-hydroxyphenylacetic acid and a pool of more firmly bound tyramine (STEINBERG and SMITH, 1971). Once retained in the adrenergic neuron octopamine is synthesized from tyramine through the action of the enzyme dopamine β-hydroxylase (DBH). This metabolite is firmly bound within the adrenergic neurons of the right atria (STEINBERG and SMITH, 1971). Therefore, even though plasma or total organ kinetics would suggest rapid elimination of tyramine, small amounts of this agent can be retained in adrenergic neurons for relatively long periods of time.

A change in endogenous tyramine excretion, neuronal uptake or metabolism has been implicated in various disease states. Abnormal urinary excretion has been reported in patients suffering from Parkinson's disease (BOULTON et al., 1967; SMITH and KELLOW, 1969; BOULTON and MARJERRISON, 1972), schizophrenia (BOULTON, 1971), migraine (YOUDIM et al., 1971; SMITH et al., 1971) or encephalopathic cirrhosis (FISCHER, 1974). These data do not yet allow firm conclusions on a possible role for tyraminergic mechanism in these disease states. However, the recently developed sensitive assays for tyramine in plasma or other tissues can be of great help in further delineating such a role.

IV. Biotransformation

1. Introduction

p-Tyramine is synthesized endogenously by the decarboxylation of tyrosine (DAVID et al., 1974) and dehydroxylation of dopamine (BRANDAU and AXELROD, 1973; BOULTON and WU, 1973). Hydroxylation of phenylethylamine has been suggested as a minor route of synthesis (BOULTON et al., 1974). m-Tyramine can be formed by the same enzymatic processes, although there is a preference for the synthesis of the p-isomer (LOVENBERG et al., 1962; BOULTON and DYCK, 1974; Fig. 1). TALLMAN et al. (1976b) recently found that neither the administration of tyrosine nor that of phenylalanine alone leads to an increase in tyramine levels in rat brains. However, when combined with monoamine oxidase (MAO) inhibition these two amino acids produce a significant rise in tyramine levels. Therefore these authors suggested that in the brain tyramine might be formed by decarboxylation of phenylalanine and hydroxylation of phenylethylamine (TALLMAN et al., 1976b, Fig. 1).

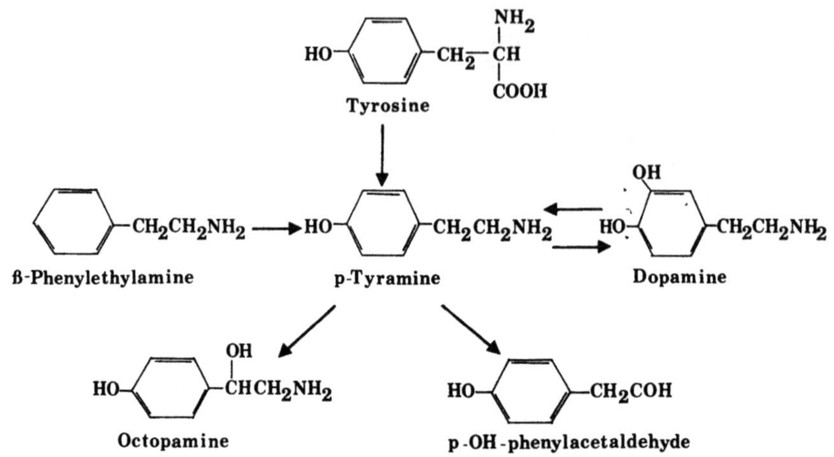

Fig. 1. Major pathways of p-tyramine metabolism

The development of specific and sensitive assays for tyramine has enabled the study of tyramine breakdown in several tissues. p-Tyramine is excreted normally in human urine (PERRY, 1962; DEQUATTRO and SJOERDSMA, 1967). When given exogenously a small (1%–6%) proportion of the total dose is excreted in the urine as unchanged tyramine (HOROWITZ et al., 1964; TACKER et al., 1972). Conjugation with glucuronide, glycine or glutamate does not play a role in tyramine excretion in man (TACKER et al., 1972). Glycine conjugation contributes significantly to tyramine excretion in the rat (TACKER et al., 1970). Sulphate conjugation to tyramine-O-sulphate accounts for 10%–20% of the total dose of tyramine recovered in urine in man after ingesting tyramine orally (MULLEN and SMITH, 1971; SMITH and MITCHELL, 1974). Simultaneous oral ingestion of inorganic sulphate can even increase tyramine-*O*-sulphate excretion by 30%–50% (SMITH and MITCHELL, 1974).

Tyramine can be metabolized in the mammalian body along three major routes: β-hydroxylation, deamination, and ring-hydroxylation (Fig. 1).

2. Beta-C-Hydroxylation

β-Hydroxylation of tyramine produces octopamine, a mechanism that has been demonstrated in a number of animal tissues, including the brain (CARLSSON and WALDECK, 1963; BRANDAU and AXELROD, 1972; BOULTON and WU, 1973; WU and BOULTON, 1974). Inhibition of DBH with FLA-63 (bis (4-methyl-1-homopiperarinyl-thiocarbonyl disulfide)) results in a two- to threefold increase in tyramine level in rat brains, suggesting the importance of β-hydroxylation of tyramine (TALLMAN et al., 1976b). In man, β-hydroxylation of tyramine has been suggested on the basis of the increased urinary concentrations of p-hydroxymandelic acid – a major metabolite of octopamine – after intravenous injection of tyramine (KAKIMOTO and ARMSTRONG, 1962; JONES and POLLITT, 1976). These data were not confirmed in a study by TACKER et al. (1972) who found that p-hydroxyphenylacetic acid accounts, almost exclusively, for tyramine metabolites found in urine. In that study, however, lower doses of tyramine were injected and therefore not enough tyramine might have been taken up into nerve terminals where the β-hydroxylation takes place (JONES and POLLITT, 1976).

3. Deamination

Deamination by MAO is the second major route for tyramine metabolism. The principle product p-hydroxyphenylacetaldehyde is further metabolized to p-hydroxyphenylacetic acid or p-hydroxyphenylethanol (Fig. 1). The formation of the carboxylic acid is by far the most important route for tyramine metabolism in man, as evidenced by the observation that p-hydroxyphenylacetic acid accounts for 60%–90% of the recovery of the total dose of tyramine given to human volunteers (KAKIMOTO and ARMSTRONG, 1962; TACKER et al., 1972; SMITH and MARCH, 1972; JONES and POLLITT, 1976). Also, in rabbits and rats p-hydroxyphenylacetic acid is the major product found in the urine of tyramine-treated animals (LEMBERGER et al., 1966; TACKER et al., 1970).

If p-tyramine is injected into the brain ventricles of rats p-hydroxyphenylacetaldehyde rather than the acid is formed in brain homogenates (WU and BOULTON, 1974). After pretreatment with the MAO inhibitor pargyline, tyramine metabolism via deamination is drastically reduced, especially in the caudate nucleus (WU and BOULTON, 1974). The recent observation by TALLMAN et al. (1976b) that pargyline causes a twofold increase in tyramine levels in the striatum agrees with this primary role for MAO in the brain metabolism of tyramine.

4. Ring-Hydroxylation

The third route for tyramine metabolism involves ring-hydroxylation to form catecholamines (CREVELING et al., 1962; AXELROD et al., 1965; Fig. 1). In vivo studies in rats show that radioactivity of injected labelled tyramine can be found in urinary normetanephrine (CREVELING et al., 1962). Moreover, in vivo studies indicate a ring-hydroxylation of tyramine to form dopamine (AXELROD et al., 1965), probably via the action of a relatively non-specific liver microsomal enzyme. However, in the overall metabolism of tyramine ring-hydroxylation is of minor importance when compared with β-hydroxylation or deamination.

B. Amphetamine and Related Compounds

I. Introduction

The amphetamines form a group of compounds with widely diversifying chemical structures and consequent physicochemical properties. The basic structure of these compounds is that of a phenylethylamine (Fig. 2). This structure is essential for most of the biochemical and pharmacological properties of these agents and is discussed in several other chapters in this volume and elsewhere (BIEL, 1970; VAN ROSSUM, 1970). The kinetics of distribution and metabolism of the amphetamines is determined largely by the physicochemical properties of the chain and ring substitution (HANSCH et al., 1968; BECKETT and BROOKES, 1970; VREE, 1973; Table 2).

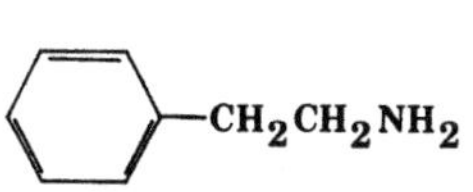

Fig. 2. Basic β-phenylethylamine structure of amphetamines

Table 2. Chemical structures and relevant physicochemical parameters of several amphetamines, ephedrines and phentermines

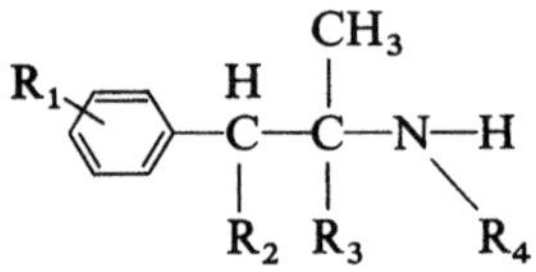

	R_1	R_2	R_3	R_4	pK_a (VREE et al., 1969)	RLS[a]
Amphetamines						
Amphetamine	H	H	H	H	9.90	1
N-Methylamphetamine	H	H	H	CH_3	10.11	2.3
N-Ethylamphetamine	H	H	H	C2H5	10.23	5.6
N-Propylamphetamine	H	H	H	Propyl	9.98	44.2
N-Isopropylamphetamine	H	H	H	Isopr.	10.14	16.9
N-Butylamphetamine	H	H	H	Butyl	—	—
N-Benzylamphetamine	H	H	H	Benzyl	7.50	2,000
p-Hydroxyamphetamine	p-OH	H	H	H	—	—
p-Chloroamphetamine	p-Cl	H	H	H	9.80	1.7
Fenfluramine	m-CF_3	H	H	C2H5	9.10	67.3
Norfenfluramine	m-CF_3	H	H	H	—	—
Ephedrines						
Norephedrine	H	OH	H	H	9.55	0.002
Ephedrine	H	OH	H	CH_3	9.60	0.03
N-Methylephedrine	H	OH	H	di-CH_3	9.30	2.1
p-Hydroxynorephedrine	p-OH	OH	H	H	—	—
Phentermines						
Phentermine	H	H	CH_3	H	10.11	2.1
N-Methylphentermine	H	H	CH_3	CH_3	10.25	2.5
p-Chlorophentermine	p-Cl	H	CH_3	H	9.60	8.3

[a] RLS: Relative lipid solubility calculated from the apparent partition coefficients (chloroform/water) at pH 7.4 with amphetamine taken as 1

The amphetamines can be divided into several major groups of chemical compounds:

1) the amphetamines proper with an H or alkyl substituent on the N;
2) ring-substituted derivatives, such as fenfluramine and norfenfluramine;
3) phentermines, which have a methyl group on the α-C;
4) β-C substituted derivatives, which include the ephedrines with a hydroxy substituent and the aminopropiophenones with a ketone substitution;
5) the cyclohexylisopropylamines: saturated amphetamine derivatives;
6) miscellaneous compounds in which the terminal *N*, α-C and β-C forms part of a cyclic substituent, such as phenmetrazine, fencamfamine, pemoline, and methylphenidate.

In this review only the amphetamines proper, the ephedrines, the phentermines and fenfluramine will be considered, since it is only for these groups that systematic studies on kinetics and biotransformation have been performed. The amphetamines proper will be discussed in this paragraph and the ephedrines, phentermines, and fenfluramine in the following.

Several aspects of the biotransformation and pharmacokinetics have been reviewed previously. The symposium proceedings *Amphetamines and Related Compounds* (Costa and Garattini, 1970) contain pertinent reviews of the older literature. More recently Caldwell (1976) has reviewed a number of in vivo data on the biotransformation and pharmacokinetics of amphetamines. Caldwell's paper (1976) moreover extensively discusses species variations in the metabolism of the amphetamines. Finally, Cho and Wright (1978) recently reviewed in vitro metabolism of amphetamines.

II. Pharmacokinetics

The analysis of the kinetic behaviour of amphetamines in man is based almost exclusively upon renal excretion data of the amphetamines and their metabolites. The blood concentration of these agents, in the doses in which they can be given to man, are extremely low. The strong central stimulating effects do not allow intake of large doses of amphetamines and their relatively large volume of distribution (2–4 litre/kg body weight) also contributes to the low blood levels. The introduction of sensitive detection methods has allowed measurement of amphetamines in blood in the picogram–nanogram range. In particular, gas–liquid chromatography with electron capture detection (Rowland, 1969; Noonan et al., 1969; Bruce and Maynard, 1969; Änggård et al., 1970; Vree, 1973), nitrogen detection (Campbell, 1969; Vree, 1973) or mass spectrometric identification (Cho et al., 1973; Vree, 1973) have led to studies in which blood levels of amphetamines were determined. However, even with these methods only part of the plasma elimination phase can be followed in time, since concentrations reach levels below the minimum detection level within a few hours.

1. Absorption and Distribution

After oral dosing in man amphetamine and its *N*-alkyl derivatives are rapidly absorbed and maximal blood levels are reached within 2 to 3 h (Änggård et al., 1973; Beckett and Shenoy, 1973; Vree, 1973; Hinsvark et al., 1973; Wan et al., 1978). After oral administration of 10 mg (±) amphetamine or one of its isomers, maximal plasma concentrations in man are 10–30 ng/ml (Wan et al., 1978). After a 60 mg dose of (−) amphetamine a maximal plasma concentration of 200–300 ng/ml has been reported (Vree, 1973). Hinsvark et al. (1973) compared the absorption characteristics of resin-bound amphetamine and soluble salt, after oral administration. The absorption rate constant was larger for the soluble salt, thus leading to higher plasma levels. Moreover, the resinate yielded a later and flatter peak than did the soluble salt (Hinsvark et al., 1973).

The volume of distribution of both amphetamine isomers in man is 2–4 litre/kg body weight (Rowland, 1969; Beckett et al., 1969; Änggård et al., 1970; Vree, 1973; Hinsvark et al., 1973; Wan et al., 1978). The distribution volume of *N*-alkyl derivatives of amphetamine is smaller than that of their parent compound (Vree, 1973). The smaller distribution volume is not related to lower lipid solubility or increased protein binding, but rather to the more extensive metabolism of these deriv-

Table 3. Ratio of tissue to plasma amphetamine concentration in several species 1 h after an injection of amphetamine

Tissue	Dog[a] (AXELROD, 1954)	Cat[b] (LATINI et al., 1977)	Rat (LINDENBAUM et al., 1974[c], DANIELSON and BOULTON, 1976[d])
Plasma	1	1	1
Liver	10	10	12–16
Spleen	9	7	10–14
Lung	14	13	13–28
Heart	4	3	3– 4
Muscle	2	2	3.4
Kidney	18	7	30–64
Adipose tissue	0.4	0.4	—
Brain	8	8	6–10
Cerebrospinal fluid	1	0.8	1.1

[a] i.p. injection of 10 mg/kg (+) amphetamine sulphate
[b] i.v. injection of 4 mg/kg (±) amphetamine sulphate
[c] i.v. injection of 0.5–7 mg/kg (+) amphetamine sulphate
[d] i.p. injection of 0.5–7 mg/kg (+) amphetamine sulphate

atives as will be discussed later. The kinetics of organ distribution of several amphetamine derivatives has been studied in experimental animals, e.g., amphetamine, *N*-methyl-amphetamine, and p-hydroxy-amphetamine. In his original studies on the disposition of sympathomimetic amines in the dog AXELROD (1954) found that (+) amphetamine was localized in most tissues rapidly after an intraperitoneal injection of 10 mg/kg (+) amphetamine sulphate. Relatively high concentrations were found in liver, brain, spleen, lung, and kidney. This pattern of distribution agrees with the relative blood flows through these tissues. In later studies similar distribution data for amphetamine were found in the cat (ELLISON et al., 1971; LATINI et al., 1977), rat (YOUNG and GORDON, 1962; MAICKEL et al., 1969; JORI and CACCIA, 1974; LINDENBAUM et al., 1974; DANIELSON and BOULTON, 1976; FULLER et al., 1977; LOKIEC et al., 1978) and mouse (BENAKIS and THOMASSET, 1970; PLACIDI et al., 1972; DEFEUDIS and MARKS, 1973; RIFFEE et al., 1978). In Table 3 some of these distribution studies are summarized.

After a rapid uptake of amphetamine into different organs the ratios of tissue to plasma concentrations remain relatively constant between 0.5 and 2 h after injection (LINDENBAUM et al., 1974; LATINI et al., 1977; RIFFEE et al., 1978). Moreover, DANIELSON and BOULTON (1976) showed that these ratios do not depend on the dose injected in the range they studied in rats (0.5–7 mg/kg). The concentration of amphetamine in plasma and cerebrospinal fluid (CSF) are similar, indicating free passage through the blood–brain barrier (Table 3). This agrees with the observation that the extent of protein binding is less than 40% in a number of species, including man, dog, cat, rat, and mouse (BAGGOT et al., 1972). In man, racemic, (+) and (−) amphetamine are bound to plasma proteins for 16% at concentrations of 10–100 ng/ml (WAN et al., 1978).

Within the central nervous system amphetamine does not distribute homogeneously, although concentrations in several regions do not differ more than a factor of 3 (YOUNG and GORDON, 1962; ELLISON et al., 1971; PLACIDI et al., 1972; LINDENBAUM et al., 1974; HONECKER and COPER, 1975; LATINI et al., 1977). Highest concentrations are found in the grey matter of the cerebral cortex, the hippocampus, the caudate nucleus, the thalamus, the hypothalamus and the hypophysis (PLACIDI et al., 1972; LINDENBAUM et al., 1974; LATINI et al., 1977). In cats, this distribution seems closely related to the pattern of vascularity of the brain (LATINI et al., 1977). However, this parallelism does not hold for the rodents since in these animals the cerebellar cortex and the colliculi are among the most highly vascularized areas (NAIR et al., 1960), whereas relatively low amounts of amphetamine are deposited in these areas.

Although high relative concentrations of a drug in a brain nucleus do not necessarily indicate sites of action, it is of interest that two of the areas taking up high amounts of amphetamine are associated with its major behavioural effects: the caudate nucleus is the primary site for amphetamine-induced stereotyped behaviour (COOLS and VAN ROSSUM, 1970) and the hypothalamus appears to be closely involved in the effects of amphetamine on food intake (LEIBOWITZ, 1975).

In a recent study BAREGGI et al. (1978) studied the correlation of amphetamine and p-hydroxyamphetamine levels in plasma and CSF in dogs with the changes in behaviour and body temperature. The relationship between the CSF amphetamine kinetics and the time-dependent degree of stereotyped behaviour was not linear: maximal amphetamine levels in CSF were found within 3 h, with a rapid decline thereafter, whereas stereotyped behaviour remained constant for at least 6 h after the injection of amphetamine. The effects on body temperature had a time course similar to amphetamine kinetics in CSF and plasma (BAREGGI et al., 1978). Although such studies provide interesting data for the analysis of the pharmacokinetics of a drug in relation to its pharmacodynamic effects, it is a simplification to expect a linear relationship between the concentration of a drug in the biophase and high-order pharmacological effects such as changes in body temperature or stereotyped behaviour (cf. VAN ROSSUM, 1977; STRUYKER-BOUDIER, 1979).

The rate of disappearance of amphetamine from organs closely follows the plasma pattern (LINDENBAUM et al., 1974; HONECKER and COPER, 1975; LATINI et al., 1977). In experimental animals plasma elimination half-lifes have been reported of 7 h in the dog (AXELROD, 1954), 8 h in the cat (LATINI et al., 1977), and 60 min in the rat (MAICKEL et al., 1969; HONECKER and COPER, 1975). In man amphetamine plasma half-life is approximately 6–8 h, but this value may vary greatly at different urine pH, as will be discussed later.

Recently LOKIEC et al. (1978) studied the disappearance curves of (+) and (−) amphetamine from the brain of isolated and aggregated rats. It was known from previous studies (MAICKEL et al., 1969) that the behavioural effects of (+) amphetamine are markedly enhanced in aggregated rats. LOKIEC al. (1978) were able to show that (+) amphetamine is eliminated from the brain of aggregated rats biphasically with half-lifes of 0.9 and 2.3 h, whereas in isolated rats elimination occurs monophasically with a half-life of 1.2 h. The relevance of these data in the explanation of the behavioural effects of (+) amphetamine remains to be further investigated on synaptic level rather than crude brain homogenates.

The distribution of *N*-methyl-amphetamine after intravenous injection has been studied qualitatively in mice with total body autoradiography (VREE and VAN ROSSUM, 1970). Within 1 min after injection large amounts of radioactivity occur in brain, salivary glands, kidney, stomach, and intestines. After 30 min high labelling can be found in brain, liver, and stomach; after 2 h most of the radioactivity has disappeared (VREE and VAN ROSSUM, 1970).

2. Excretion

Amphetamines are excreted almost exclusively in the urine; faecal excretion does not play a significant role in any species. As was discussed before, blood levels of amphetamine are too low to measure with conventional analytical techniques. Therefore, much of the analysis of elimination mechanisms of amphetamines is based upon urinary excretion data. There is a relatively good agreement between kinetics of blood elimination and urinary excretion of amphetamines and their metabolites in man if pH values in urine are controlled (BECKETT et al., 1969; ROWLAND, 1969; VREE, 1973). The relevance of controlling urine pH for reproducible urinary excretion of amphetamines was stressed by Beckett and co-workers (BECKETT et al., 1963). Amphetamines in their unionized form are subject to tubular reabsorption in the kidney. The degree of tubular reabsorption of weak basic drugs like amphetamines is determined by the relative amount of unionized drug in the tubuli. This amount depends on the difference in pH of blood and urine. Since the pH of blood is constant, urine pH is the major factor determining the degree of ionization. Under acidic conditions (pH equals 5.0 ± 0.5) tubular reabsorption plays an insignificant role and urinary excretion of the unchanged drug is maximal. However, under uncontrolled conditions urinary excretion may fluctuate since the pH of urine can vary 4.7–7.5 (BECKETT and BROOKES, 1970). Under such conditions the ratio of metabolites to unchanged drug in the urine varies greatly (BECKETT and BROOKES, 1970).

Relevant elimination parameters of several amphetamines in man are summarized in Table 4. The plasma half-life of 4–8 h for (+) amphetamine under acidic urinary conditions is almost equal to that of (−) amphetamine (VREE, 1973; WAN et al., 1978). Under basic urine conditions plasma half-life is increased to 16 h for (+) amphetamine and 25 h for (−) amphetamine (WAN et al., 1978). The reason for this difference is that with basic urine metabolism is the major route of amphetamine elimination. (+) Isomers of amphetamine derivatives are more extensively deaminated than (−) isomers (DRING et al., 1970).

The half-life of amphetamine calculated from urinary excretion data corresponds well with that in plasma if urine pH is controlled (Table 4). *N*-Alkyl derivatives have a shorter half-life than amphetamine. This is related to the more extensive degree of metabolism of these agents especially of their (+) isomers (Table 4; BECKETT and BROOKES, 1970; VREE et al., 1972; BECKETT and SHENOY, 1973; VREE, 1973; WAN et al., 1978).

The elimination of amphetamine has also been studied in several animal species (ELLISON et al., 1971; BAGGOT and DAVIS, 1972; LINDENBAUM et al., 1974; HONECKER and COPER, 1975; DANIELSON and BOULTON, 1976). The results of a number of these studies are summarized in Table 5. In rats and swine the half-life of amphetamine is short (BAGGOT and DAVIS, 1972; LINDENBAUM et al., 1974; HONECKER and COPER, 1975; DANIELSON and BOULTON, 1976). These two species metabolize amphetamine extensively in contrast to the cat (ELLISON et al., 1971). In the latter species elimination half-life of amphetamine may be as high as 8–10 h (ELLISON et al., 1971; LATINI et al., 1977).

Table 4. Biological half-life ($t^1/_2$), volume of distribution (*Vf*) and relative contribution of excretion of unchanged drug to total elimination ($K_{c\ ren.\ excr.}/K_{c\ el.}$) of several amphetamines in man

Drug	$t^1/_2$ (h)	*Vf* (litres/kg body weight)	$K_{c\ ren.\ excr.}/K_{c\ el.}$ (%)
(+) amphetamine	4–8	2–4	60– 75
(−) amphetamine	5–7	2–4	80
(+) *N*-methylamphetamine	5–7	2–3	50– 80
(−) *N*-methylamphetamine	5–8	2–3	65– 90
(+) *N*-ethylamphetamine	2–5	1–2	20– 50
(−) *N*-ethylamphetamine	5–7	1–2	80–100
(+) *N*-propylamphetamine	2–4	1–2	10– 20
(−) *N*-propylamphetamine	4–7	–	40– 60
(+) *N*-Isopropylamphetamine	2–5	–	10– 50
(−) *N*-Isopropylamphetamine	6–7	–	60– 90
(+) *N*-butylamphetamine	–	–	0
(−) *N*-butylamphetamine	–	–	0
(+) *N*-benzylamphetamine	–	–	0
(−) *N*-benzylamphetamine	–	–	0
(+) *N,N*-dimethylamphetamine	3–5	1	30– 45
(−) *N,N*-dimethylamphetamine	5–7	1	55– 85

Source: Adapted from BECKETT and BROOKES (1970), BECKETT and SHENOY (1973), and VREE (1973)
Urine pH was controlled at 5.0 ± 0.5

Table 5. Biological half-life ($t\ ^1/_2$), plasma protein binding and relative contribution of excretion of unchanged drug to total elimination of amphetamine in several animal species

Species	$t\ ^1/_2$ (h)	Plasma protein binding (%) (BAGGOT et al., 1972)	% Drug excreted unchanged
Rat	1 (HONECKER and COPER, 1975; DANIELSON and BOULTON, 1976)	40	10 (DRING et al., 1970)
Cat	8.5 (ELLISON et al., 1971; LATINI et al., 1977)	26	30 (ELLISON et al., 1971; LATINI et al., 1977)
Dog	4.5 (BAGGOT and DAVIS, 1972)	27	30 (DRING et al., 1970)
Swine	1 (BAGGOT and DAVIS, 1972)	40	—
Mouse	0.5 (RIFFEE et al., 1978)	17	—

III. Biotransformation

1. Introduction

The general pathways involved in the metabolism of amphetamines are given in Fig. 3. The principle routes are:

a) aromatic p-hydroxylation;
b) β-C-hydroxylation;
c) *N*-dealkylation and deamination via
 c′. α-C-oxidation, c″. N-oxidation.

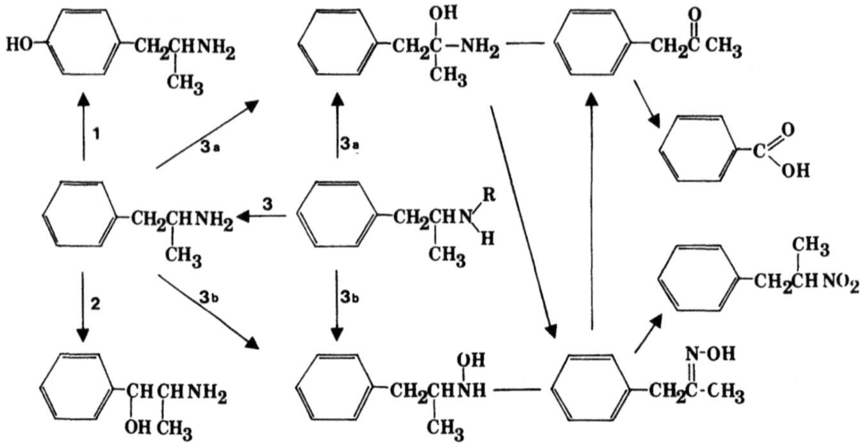

Fig. 3. Major pathways of metabolism of the amphetamines. *1*:*p*-Ring-hydroxylation; *2*: β-C-hydroxylation; *3*: dealkylation; *3a*: α-C-oxidation; *3b*: N-oxidation

Table 6. Relative contribution (%) of different routes of metabolism in the overall elimination of several amphetamines in man on the basis of urinary recovery of unchanged drug or metabolites, including their conjugates

Compound	Unchanged drug	*p*-Ring-hydroxylated metabolites	β-C-Hydroxylated metabolites	*N*-Dealkylated metabolites	Deaminated metabolites
(±) Amphetamine[a, b, c, d]	40–70	3– 7	3–4	—	20–50
(±) *N*-Methylamphetamine[b, c, e]	50–80	15–20	3–4	5–10	10–20
(±) p-Hydroxyamphetamine[f]	80–90	3–10	—	—	—

[a] Data from DRING et al. (1970)
[b] Data from VREE (1973)
[c] Data from BECKETT and SHENOY (1973)
[d] Data from CALDWELL et al. (1972b)
[e] Data from CALDWELL et al. (1972a)
[f] Data from SEVER et al. (1976)

These multiple possibilities for metabolism imply the occurrence of a variety of metabolites. Moreover, these metabolites can be conjugated, thereby further complicating in vivo analysis of metabolism of amphetamines. The extent to which amphetamines are metabolized via either of the above mentioned routes is strongly species-dependent (CALDWELL, 1976). In rats, for instance, aromatic hydroxylation accounts for some 70%–80% of (+) amphetamine metabolism, whereas deamination does not play a significant role. In contrast, up to 30% of a dose of (+) amphetamine given to man may be excreted as deaminated metabolites, whereas aromatic hydroxylation only contributes insignificantly to amphetamine metabolism. Another factor influenc-

Table 7. Relative contribution (%) of different routes of metabolism in the overall elimination of amphetamine in several species on the basis of urinary recovery of unchanged drug or metabolites, including their conjugates

Species	Unchanged drug	*p*-Ring hydroxylated metabolites	*β*-C-Hydroxylated metabolites	Deaminated metabolites
Rat (DRING et al., 1970)	10–20	70–80	1	5
Guinea-pig (DRING et al., 1970)	20	0	—	80
Rabbit (DRING et al., 1970)	5	6–10	—	70–90
Dog (DRING et al., 1970)	30–40	20–30	—	25–35
Man (DRING et al., 1970; CALDWELL et al., 1972b)	40–70	3– 7	3–4	20–50

ing in vivo analysis of amphetamine biotransformation on the basis of urinary excretion data is the strong urinary pH dependence of the relative excretion of amphetamines or their metabolites (BECKETT et al., 1963; see Sect. B.II.2). Table 6 summarizes the contribution of different routes of metabolism of several amphetamines in man, whereas Table 7 contains data pertaining to the species dependency of amphetamine metabolism.

The introduction of isolated liver preparations as well as the recent improvements in chemical analytical techniques has greatly helped the study of the mechanisms underlying the biotransformation of the amphetamines. In the following paragraphs these mechanisms will be discussed individually.

2. Aromatic Para-Hydroxylation

Hydroxylation of the aromatic ring of amphetamine derivatives in vivo is limited to the p-position (DRING et al., 1970). p-Hydroxylation of amphetamine derivatives occurs extensively in the rat, and to a lesser degree in the dog (WILLIAMS et al., 1973; CALDWELL, 1976). In man, p-hydroxylated metabolites represent less than 5% of the total dose excreted (CALDWELL et al., 1972a; BECKETT and SHENOY, 1973; CALDWELL, 1976). The p-hydroxy metabolites are conjugated to sulphates and glucuronides. The relative amount of O-sulphate or O-glucuronide conjugate found in the urine is species-dependent (DRING et al., 1970; CALDWELL et al., 1972a; SEVER et al., 1973, 1976).

The mechanisms involved in p-hydroxylation of amphetamine derivatives are not completely settled. A major problem in this respect has been the difficulty in finding a suitable liver microsomal preparation that is able to form p-hydroxylated metabolites of amphetamine. Even rat liver microsome preparations produce very little or no p-hydroxylated metabolites (DALY et al., 1967; DINGELL and BASS, 1969), although DINGELL and BASS (1969) showed by perfusion of the isolated rat liver that this organ p-hydroxylates amphetamine. JONSSON (1974, 1977) and CHO et al. (1975a) recently showed that rat liver microsomes isolated by special gel filtration techniques can form p-hydroxylated amphetamine metabolites at low substrate concentrations. Rat liver microsome preparations capable of p-hydroxylation of amphetamine can also be obtained by differential centrifugation at 88,000 g (ROMMELSPRACHER et al., 1974; CHO et al., 1975a).

The hydroxylation of amphetamine has a low apparent Km value of approximately 10 μM. Excess substrate concentration (>0.5 mM) inhibits the enzyme system which might explain the lack of effects found in vitro by authors using substrate concentrations in the millimolar range (CHO et al., 1975a). The hydroxylation is NADP-dependent and has an optimum pH of 6.9–7.0 (ROMMELSPRACHER et al., 1974; JONSSON, 1974, 1977). The V max for (+) amphetamine is similar to that for (−) amphetamine, but the Km for the (−) isomer is 22 145es lower than that for (+) amphetamine (JONSSON, 1974). The chemical mechanism of p-hydroxylation probably involves the formation of epoxide intermediates (DALY et al., 1967; UDENFRIEND, 1971; BRODIE et al., 1971).

Amphetamine p-hydroxylation differs from that of other drugs, since phenobarbital or 3-methylcholanthrene cannot induce this enzymatic process (CREAVEN et al., 1970; CHO et al., 1975b). Another difference is the inhibition of the hydroxylation pathway by drugs like the antidepressants desimipramine or iprindole (DINGELL and BASS, 1969; CHO et al., 1975b), MAO inhibitors (LEW et al., 1971), and ethanol (CREAVEN and BARBEE, 1969), although concentrations needed for the latter compound are very high (JONSSON, 1977). p-Hydroxylation of amphetamine in rat liver microsomes is strongly inhibited by carbon monoxide and SKF 525-A (2-diethylaminoethyl-2,2-diphenylvalerate), indicating the involvement of cytochrome P-450 (JONSSON, 1977). Chronic pretreatment of rats with amphetamine reduces microsomal p-hydroxylation without changing cytochrome P-450 levels and without influencing p-hydroxylation of other aromatic compounds (JONSSON, 1977). These data may indicate an altered hepatic metabolism of amphetamine during chronic use of this agent (MAGOUR et al., 1974; ANGGÅRD et al., 1973; JONSSON, 1977). In contrast to the reduced metabolism of amphetamine in isolated liver microsomes of chronically treated rats, such animals excrete significantly more p-hydroxy-amphetamine and its conjugates in the perfusate in liver perfusion experiments (JONSSON, 1977). This increased amount of metabolites in liver perfusate was paralleled by a reduction of excretion in the bile (JONSSON, 1977).

The major site of overall amphetamine metabolism is the liver. However, extrahepatic metabolism may contribute to the pharmacodynamic effects of amphetamine via its metabolites. Nerve tissue of rats can form p-hydroxy-amphetamine both in vivo and in vitro (FREEMAN and SULSER, 1974; KUHN et al., 1978). The nervous system p-hydroxylation of amphetamine can be inhibited by iprindole, suggesting similarities to the liver cytochrome P-450 mixed-function oxidase system route of metabolism (KUHN et al., 1978). However, cytochrome P-450 is barely detectable in brain (GARFINKEL, 1963) and therefore other enzymatic mechanisms must be considered. Central 6-hydroxydopamine pretreatment does not influence the formation of p-hydroxy-amphetamine which indicates an extraneuronal mechanism different from that involved in phenylethylamine hydroxylation to tyramine (BOULTON et al., 1974; KUHN et al., 1978).

3. Beta-C-Hydroxylation

The second route of metabolism of amphetamines is hydroxylation of the carbon in the β-position to the nitrogen. β-Hydroxylation primarily occurs in the catecholaminergic nerve terminals by the activity of the enzyme DBH (GOLDSTEIN et al., 1964).

Amphetamine has to be taken up by catecholaminergic nerve terminals to allow β-hydroxylation. It can then be metabolized to norephedrine or – in case of further p-hydroxylation of the aromatic ring – to p-hydroxynorephedrine (Fig. 3). In the overall metabolism of amphetamine β-hydroxylation plays a minor role in all species investigated (CALDWELL, 1976). In normal humans β-hydroxylation only accounts for 3%, but this value increases in amphetamine tolerant humans (CALDWELL et al., 1972b; SEVER et al., 1973). It was suggested earlier that the development of tolerance to amphetamines is related to the formation of norephedrine and p-hydroxynorephedrine, substances that are regarded to act as false neurotransmitters (THOENEN et al., 1966; BRODIE et al., 1970; LEWANDER, 1971). The relevance of these substances in the behavioural effects of amphetamine has been doubted on the basis of their low concentrations in tissues. However, recent evidence suggests that β-hydroxylated derivatives are accumulated in noradrenergic nerve terminals in contrast to amphetamine, which has a more homogenous distribution inside and outside neurones (WONG et al., 1972; CATTABENI et al., 1973; CHO et al., 1975b; KUHN et al., 1978). The involvement of intraneuronal DBH in the metabolism of amphetamines was further substantiated by KUHN et al. (1978) in a study in which they showed that the DBH inhibitors U 14-624 (2-thiazolyl-2-thiourea) and FLA-63, or the noradrenergic nerve terminal destroying agent 6-hydroxydopamine, inhibit the formation of norephedrine and p-hydroxynorephedrine. DBH exhibits substrate selectivity, since only (+) amphetamine and (+) p-hydroxy-amphetamine are metabolized to form norephedrine and p-hydroxynorephedrine (GOLDSTEIN et al., 1964; CALDWELL et al., 1972b). Moreover, only primary amines seem to be β-hydroxylated by DBH. *N*-substituted derivatives are first metabolized to amphetamine, before β-hydroxylation takes place (CALDWELL et al., 1972a).

4. N-Dealkylation and Deamination

The major route of metabolism of amphetamine itself is deamination. Metabolism of *N*-alkyl derivatives of amphetamines involves both dealkylation and deamination (Fig. 3). An important experimental problem in the study of chemical pathways involved in this route of metabolism has been the instability of the intermediates and the consequent difficulty in detecting these intermediates in blood and urine of humans or animals (AXELROD, 1955; ASATOOR et al., 1965; ELLISON et al., 1966; DRING et al., 1970). It has therefore been impossible, so far, to quantify metabolism via this pathway in vivo in terms of the different metabolites formed along this pathway. Benzoic acid is the major deamination end product excreted in the urine of most species (CALDWELL, 1976). In man, this metabolite is present primarily as its glycine conjugate (DRING et al., 1970; CALDWELL et al., 1972a). In man, benzoic acid and its conjugates contribute approximately 25% of the total amount of the original dose of amphetamine excreted (Table 6; DRING et al., 1970; CALDWELL et al., 1972a). The quantitative contribution of deamination in the metabolism of amphetamine differs per species (Tables 6 and 7; CALDWELL, 1976). In the rat it contributes less than 5% to overall elimination, whereas in the mouse, rabbit, dog, monkey, and man it amounts to 20%–40% (DRING et al., 1970; CALDWELL, 1976). In the guinea pig and horse deamination is even the predominant route of amphetamine elimination contributing some 70% (DRING et al., 1970). The reader is referred to the review of CALDWELL (1976) for a detailed discussion of these species variations.

If amphetamine contains *N*-alkyl substituents deamination involves a complex combination of hydroxylation of the *N* followed by dealkylation and α-*C*-oxidation (Fig. 3). The dealkylation itself therefore proceeds both via *N*- and *C*-oxidation. In vivo studies in man indicate that the importance of dealkylation in the overall elimination of *N*-alkyl substituted amphetamines increases with larger alkyl substituents (VREE et al., 1971, 1972; BECKETT and SHENOY, 1973). Approximately 10% of a dose of methylamphetamine is excreted as amphetamine, whereas this amounts to 20% for ethylamphetamine and 45% for isopropylamphetamine (VREE, 1973; BECKETT and SHENOY, 1973). Moreover, the degree of dealkylation is larger for the (+) isomers of the *N*-alkyl substituted amphetamines than for the (−) isomers (VREE et al., 1971, 1972; VREE, 1973; BECKETT and SHENOY, 1973; HENDERSON et al., 1974). This preference may be related to a lower activation energy of the overall dealkylation of (+) isomers (HENDERSON et al., 1974). In the rat a similar preferential dealkylation of the (+) isomer was shown for methylamphetamine (JENNER and TESTA, 1973) and propylamphetamine (COUTTS et al., 1976b). Finally, *N*-dealkylation of tertiary amphetamines proceeds more rapidly for the first alkyl substituent than for the second group (VREE, 1973; HENDERSON et al., 1974).

It was mentioned earlier that the in vivo study of the mechanisms of *N*-dealkylation and deamination have been hampered by the instability of the intermediates. More recently the use of in vitro liver preparations, the use of stable isotopes (PARLI et al., 1971a; VREE et al., 1971; KAMMERER et al., 1978) and the introduction of mass spectrometry have enabled more sophisticated studies of the N-dealkylation and deamination mechanisms (HUCKER et al., 1971; PARLI et al., 1971a; BECKETT and AL-SARRAJ, 1972b; CHO et al., 1974a; HENDERSON et al., 1974; COUTTS et al., 1976a, b, 1978; BECKETT and HAYA, 1977; WRIGHT et al., 1977a, b; COUTTS and KOVACH, 1977; LINDEKE et al., 1978). Such studies have shown the importance of both *N*- and α-*C*-oxidation in the *N*-dealkylation and deamination. N-Oxidation occurs via the formation of unstable hydroxylamines, whereas unstable carbinolamines are involved in the α-*C*-oxidation. The detailed mechanisms involved in these two pathways will now be discussed.

a) Alpha-C-Oxidation

The oxidation of the α-C of amphetamine derivatives was first proposed as an explanation for the production of phenylacetone from amphetamine by rabbit liver microsomes (AXELROD, 1955). The intermediate in this reaction would be an α-carbinolamine (PARLI et al., 1971a; Fig. 3). According to PARLI et al. (1971a) the α-carbinolamine is either oxidized directly to form the ketone or dehydrated to the imine, which is then further oxidized and hydrolyzed to give the ketone. From a series of experiments in which they used 18–O labelled O_2 in the incubation mixture, PARLI et al. (1971a) concluded that direct hydroxylation accounts for some 30% of the ketone formed on the basis of the amount of 18–O incorporation. Another study indicating the relevance of α-C-oxidation in the metabolism of amphetamines has come from VREE et al. (1971). These authors concluded that insertion of the O in the α-*C*–*H* bond is the rate-limiting step of metabolism of (+) amphetamines on the basis of experiments in which they showed that replacement of the H at the α-*C* by a deuterium isotope significantly slowed deamination of (+) amphetamines. This deuterium effect was not observed for (−) isomers (VREE et al., 1971; VREE, 1973), indicating possible differences in metabolic pathways for these stereoisomers (HENDERSON et al., 1974). An alternative mechanism for the production of the ketone was suggested by BECKETT et al. (1971) and involves oxidation of the terminal N. This mechanism will be discussed later.

Whatever the route by which phenylacetone is formed, the mechanisms of further breakdown are relatively undisputed: (a) phenylacetone may be excreted as a conjugate, (b) it can be reduced to the corresponding alcohol, or (c) it may be degraded to benzoic acid. The contribution of each of these mechanisms is species-dependent (CALDWELL, 1976; COUTTS et al., 1978). Conjugation of the ketone plays a minor role in most species (CALDWELL, 1976). Only in the rabbit is the sulphate conjugate a major excretion product (DRING et al., 1968, 1970). Reduction of phenylacetone produces phenyl-2-propanol. The enzyme responsible for this reaction has been described to be a NADPH-dependent liver enzyme (MCMAHON, 1971). In vivo, phenyl-2-propanol was shown to be a minor excretion product in several species (DRING et al., 1970). Therefore, the major route of phenylacetone degradation is the third mechanism via formation of benzoic acid and its conjugates (AXELROD, 1955; ASATOOR et al., 1965; DRING et al., 1970). Glycine and glucuronic acid conjugates have been described, depending upon the species involved (BRIDGES et al., 1970).

b) N-Oxidation

The role of *N*-oxidation in the deamination of amphetamines was first proposed by HUCKER et al. (1971) and BECKETT et al. (1971). This pathway was not shown earlier because of the instability of the *N*-oxidation intermediates in vivo (BECKETT et al., 1971). HUCKER et al. (1971) used the isolated microsomal fraction of rabbit liver and found that phenyl-2-propanone oxime is the major in vitro metabolite of amphetamine in this preparation. Since this original report numerous other authors have shown the formation of oximes from amphetamines both in vivo (BECKETT and AL-SARRAJ, 1972a; MIDHA et al., 1974) and in vitro (PARLI et al., 1971b; BECKETT and AL-SARRAJ, 1972b; HUCKER, 1973; PARLI and MCMAHON, 1973; BECKETT and MIDHA, 1974; COUTTS and KOVACH, 1977). BECKETT et al. (1971) suggested that the oxime originates from chemical oxidation of hydroxylamine, the primary *N*-hydroxylation product. There has been extensive discussion in the literature whether oximes are formed metabolically (HUCKER et al., 1971; PARLI et al., 1971a, b; PARLI and MCMAHON, 1973) or non-enzymatically from chemical breakdown of the hydroxylamines during extraction and analysis procedures (BECKETT et al., 1971; BECKETT and AL-SARRAJ, 1972a, b; LINDEKE et al., 1973; MIDHA et al., 1974). In a recent study in rabbit liver preparation WRIGHT et al. (1977a) provided new evidence in favour of an enzymatic process on the basis of quantitative differences in conversion between the optical isomers of amphetamines, including *N*-hydroxy-amphetamine. Chemical dehydrogenation of *N*-hydroxy-amphetamine would not be expected to demonstrate stereoselectivity. In the same study WRIGHT et al. (1977a) showed that the formation of the oxime depends strongly on the duration of the incubation. The role of *N*-hydroxy-amphetamine as an intermediate in the oxime production was further substantiated by GAL et al. (1975), who found that although the hydroxylamine is unstable in aqueous solution, it is more stable when protein is present. Strongest evidence for the significance of *N*-hydroxylation comes from studies in which phentermines were used as substrates. These compounds lack the H at the α-C and are therefore not oxidized at this position. However, stable *N*-hydroxylation products of these compounds are found extensively both in vivo (BECKETT and BELANGER, 1974b) and in vitro (CHO et al., 1974b; BECKETT and BELANGER, 1976). These studies have shown that *N*-oxidation is mediated by a NADPH dependent oxidase which is sensitive to carbon monoxide and SKF 525-A (CHO et al., 1974a).

The oxime that is formed by the N-oxidation of amphetamines is metabolized by rabbit liver microsomes to 2-nitrophenylpropane (PARLI and MCMAHON, 1973; COUTTS et al., 1976c). Apparently microsomal metabolism is species-dependent since phenylacetone and phenyl-2-propanol are the major oxime metabolites in rat liver microsomes (HUCKER, 1973). This author proposed that phenylacetone is formed largely via N-hydroxylation of amphetamine derivatives. Recently, however, WRIGHT et al. (1977b) suggested that the ketone is formed independently from *N*-hydroxyl-derivatives on the basis of a study in which the combined incubation of *N*-hydroxy-amphetamine with deuterium labelled amphetamine in rabbit liver homogenates did not lead to isotopic mixing in the deamination product. This implies the existence of a route of ketone formation distinct from pure *N*-hydroxylation. CHO and WRIGHT (1978) speculated that this route involves simultaneous α-*C* and *N*-hydroxylation of amphetamine derivatives and the subsequent formation of the oxime from which the ketone is formed by hydrolysis.

C. Ephedrine and Related Compounds

I. Introduction

The ephedrines differ from the amphetamines by the hydroxyl substituent at the β-C (Table 2). This substituent markedly affects pharmacological activity of these agents as well as their pharmacokinetics and biotransformation. In this respect the much lower lipid solubility of these agents is of great importance.

II. Pharmacokinetics

Similar to the amphetamines, information on the pharmacokinetics of ephedrines is based almost exclusively on urinary excretion data. Also analogous to the previously discussed amphetamines the excretion of unchanged drug and metabolites is greatly influenced by urinary pH (WILKINSON and BECKETT, 1968a). The difference in recovery of unchanged drug between acidic and alkaline urine may be 10–30 fold for methylephedrine and 2–5 fold for ephedrine and norephedrine (WILKINSON and BECKETT, 1968a). Therefore, conclusions on the pharmacokinetics of ephedrines on the basis of urinary excretion data should always be carefully considered in the light of urine pH.

1. Absorption and Tissue Distribution

After oral intake in man ephedrines are rapidly absorbed (WILKINSON and BECKETT, 1968b). Absorption can be described with a single first-order process following a lag period of 0–18 min for ephedrine, 8–67 min for norephedrine and 6–36 min for methylephedrine (WILKINSON and BECKETT, 1968b). In a recent study FROSCH (1977) followed the kinetics of norpseudoephedrine – a stereoisomer of norephedrine. After oral intake of 60 mg of this drug in volunteers, a maximum plasma concentration of approximately 200 ng/ml was reached in 2–3 h. The distribution volume is 1–2 litre/kg body weight (FROSCH, 1977). This volume of distribution is lower than that of amphetamine, which agrees with the lower lipid solubility of norephedrine.

The tissue distribution of norephedrine and ephedrine has been studied in several species by JACQUOT and co-workers (JACQUOT et al., 1974; THIERCELIN et al., 1976). In rats and mice norephedrine is taken up rapidly by the lungs, adrenals, and spleen, and to a slightly lesser degree by the heart (THIERCELIN et al., 1976). The drug is taken up more slowly by the brain. Elimination from these organs and plasma is very rapid with half-lifes of less than 1 h and without specific retention in a certain tissue. The ratio of tissue to plasma concentration is relatively constant between 30 and 120 min with highest ratios for the lungs (16), adrenals (8), and brain (7). A similar pattern of distribution was reported for ephedrine in the rat (BRALET et al., 1968) and guinea pig (JACQOUT et al., 1974). Tissue to plasma ratios are somewhat higher for ephedrine than norephedrine which agrees with the lower lipid solubility of the latter compound (Table 2).

In vitro studies on the uptake of ephedrine and norephedrine by cardiac or nerve tissue indicate that organ uptake of these agents is a passive process (ROSS et al., 1968; JACQUOT et al., 1969a). This process is sensitive to the pH of the extracellular fluid, but does not depend upon the concentration of the amine (JACQUOT et al., 1969a, b). The mechanisms involved in the uptake of these agents differ therefore markedly from those of catecholamines (IVERSEN, 1967).

2. Excretion

Ephedrine, norephedrine, and *N*-methylephedrine are only metabolized to a limited degree in man (RICHTER, 1938; HEIMLICH et al., 1961; WILKINSON and BECKETT, 1968a, b; SINSHEIMER et al., 1973; SEVER et al., 1975; Table 8). Urinary recovery of unchanged ephedrines is much greater in acidic than in alkaline urine due to the lack of tubular reabsorption of the unchanged drugs in acidic urine (WILKINSON and BECKETT, 1968a). Under controlled acidic urinary conditions overall elimination half-life in man is 3 h for ephedrine and norephedrine and 4.5 h for *N*-methylephedrine (WILKINSON and BECKETT, 1968b). These half-lifes agree with the plasma elimination half-life of 3 h for norpseudoephedrine reported by FROSCH (1977).

Table 8. Biological half-life ($t\ ^1/_2$) and relative contribution (%) of different routes of metabolism in the overall metabolism of ephedrines in man on the basis of urinary recovery of unchanged drug or metabolites, including their conjugates

Compound	$t\ ^1/_2$ (h)	Unchanged drug	*N*-Dealkylated metabolites	Deaminated metabolites
(−) Norephedrine	3	95	0	5
(−) Ephedrine	3	70	5–20	10–20
(−) N-Methylephedrine	4.5	70	15	15

Source: WILKINSON and BECKETT, 1968a; SINSHEIMER et al., 1973; SEVER et al., 1975.

III. Biotransformation

The presence of a β-C -hydroxy substituent limits the pathways of biotransformation of ephedrines to p-hydroxylation, *N*-dealkylation, and deamination.

In vivo studies in man indicate that ephedrine and norephedrine are excreted largely unchanged (WILKINSON and BECKETT, 1968a; SINSHEIMER et al., 1973; SEVER et al., 1975). Only 3%–4% of a dose of norephedrine is metabolized in man (SINSHEIMER et al., 1973), whereas the more lipid soluble ephedrine is metabolized some 30% (WILKINSON and BECKETT, 1968a; SEVER et al., 1975). p-Hydroxylated metabolites of ephedrines have not been detected in man (WILKINSON and BECKETT, 1968a; SINSHEIMER et al., 1973; SEVER et al., 1975) or rabbits (AXELROD, 1953; MATSUDA et al., 1971; FELLER and MALSPEIS, 1977) and only minor amounts (less than 3% of the total dose) were found in guinea pigs (JACQUOT et al., 1974). In vitro studies with isolated rabbit liver preparations also do not indicate the formation of significant amounts of p-hydroxylated metabolites by hepatic metabolism (FELLER and MALSPEIS, 1977). In contrast, rats metabolize norephedrine in vivo for some 18% to its p-hydroxylated derivative α-methyloctopamine (THIERCELIN et al., 1976). The low amount of p-hydroxylated metabolites found in the urine of most species does not exclude the possibility that these false transmitters are found in special organs, such as the brain (KUHN et al., 1978). This remains to be further elucidated.

Dealkylation and subsequent deamination is the major route of metabolism of ephedrines in most species, excluding the rat (WILLIAMS et al., 1973). In man ephedrine is demethylated to norephedrine for 5%–20%, whereas methylephedrine is dealkylated to ephedrine and norephedrine for some 15% (WILKINSON and BECKETT, 1968a; SEVER et al., 1975). However, conclusions on the extent of dealkylation cannot be firm, since the dealkylated metabolites are subject to further in vivo metabolism to deaminated products. The major in vivo deaminated metabolites are free and conjugated benzoic acid and 1,2-dihydroxy-1-phenylpropane (SINSHEIMER et al., 1973; SEVER et al., 1975; FELLER and MALSPEIS, 1977). There is a marked difference in the extent of deamination of ephedrines in man and rabbit. Whereas man excretes norephedrine unchanged for 85% or more (WILKINSON and BECKETT, 1968a; SINSHEIMER et al., 1973), rabbits deaminate this drug up to 75% (SINSHEIMER et al., 1973). Similarly unchanged ephedrine is the major urinary excretion product of ephedrine in man (50%–75%; WILKINSON and BECKETT, 1968a; SEVER et al., 1973), whereas rabbits excrete less than 4% as unchanged drug (FELLER and MALSPEIS, 1977). The detailed mechanisms of these metabolic pathways were discussed in the paragraph on the biotransformation of amphetamines (see Sect. B.III).

D. Phentermine and Related Compounds

I. Introduction

The phentermines differ from the amphetamines by the methyl substituent at the α-C (Table 2). Similarly to the ephedrines such substitution greatly influences pharmacodynamic actions, pharmacokinetics and biotransformation. The phentermines are slightly more lipid soluble than the amphetamines (Table 2). This review is limited to a discussion of pharmacokinetics and biotransformation of phentermine, *N*-methylphentermine and p-chlorophentermine, since it is only for these agents that pharmacokinetics and biotransformation have been investigated in detail.

II. Pharmacokinetics

Human pharmacokinetic studies of phentermines are almost exclusively based upon urinary excretion data for reasons similar to those for amphetamines and ephedrines. The kinetics of urinary excretion of phentermines is strongly influenced by urinary pH (BECKETT and BROOKES, 1970, 1971; BECKETT and BÉLANGER, 1977a). This is especially the case for chlorphentermine: after oral administration 75% of the total dose of chlorphentermine is excreted as *N*-oxidized metabolites when urine pH is around 6.5, whereas this amount is only 25% if urine is maintained acidic (pH ≦ 5; BECKETT and BÉLANGER, 1977a).

1. Absorption and Distribution

After oral administration to man phentermine is rapidly absorbed and maximal levels in blood are reached within 2–3 h (HINSVARK et al., 1973; VREE, 1973). After an oral dose of 30–40 mg maximal blood levels of 100–250 ng/ml are reached (HINSVARK et al., 1973; VREE, 1973). HINSVARK et al. (1973) compared the pharmacokinetic profile of phentermine in blood after oral administration of a resin-bound form and the soluble salt. The resinate yielded a lower, later, and flatter peak than the soluble salt (HINSVARK et al., 1973).

The volume of distribution of phentermine in man is approximately 2–3 litre/kg body weight (HINSVARK et al., 1973). A similar relative distribution volume was reported for phentermine in rats (CHO et al., 1973). The tissue distribution of phentermine and chlorphentermine has been studied in several species (DUBNICK et al., 1963, 1968; LÜLLMANN et al., 1973; SEILER and WASSERMANN, 1974). After a single injection in rats or mice phentermine and chlorphentermine are rapidly taken up by a number of organs. Uptake is highest in lung, liver, kidney, adrenals, spleen, and brain and is stronger for chlorphentermine than for phentermine (DUBNICK et al., 1963; LÜLLMANN et al., 1973). The tissue blood concentration ratios for phentermine in rats remain constant during chronic treatment, whereas these ratios increase for a number of organs after repeated chlorphentermine injections (LÜLLMANN et al., 1973). The tissue blood concentration ratio for the lungs increases from 30 on the first day to 170 after 8 weeks (LÜLLMANN et al., 1973). A similar increase was observed for the adrenals. The increased binding of chlorphentermine by these tissues has been related to chlorphentermine-induced accumulation of phospholipids in the adrenal cells and pulmonary free intra-alveolar cells (LÜLLMANN et al., 1973; KARABELNIK et al., 1974; LÜLLMANN-RAUSCH, 1975). The pulmonary accumulation of chlorphentermine is of interest in view of the pulmonary hypertension that has been reported as a complication of chronic anorexigenic use of this compound (cf. LÜLLMANN et al., 1973).

2. Excretion

Under acidic urinary conditions phentermine is excreted almost completely unchanged in man with an elimination half-life of approximately 10 h (BECKETT and BROOKES, 1970, 1971; VREE, 1973, cf. Table 9). Plasma elimination half-life for phentermine from blood is similar (VREE, 1973; HINSVARK et al., 1973). *N*-Methylphentermine is also excreted largely unchanged in man under acid urinary conditions. Its elimination half-life is also approximately 10 h (BECKETT and BROOKES, 1970, 1971; VREE, 1973; cf. Table 9). If urine pH is 6 or more, up to 25% of the original dose of

Table 9. Biological half-life ($t\ ^1/_2$) and relative contribution (%) of different routes of metabolism in the overall metabolism of phentermines in man on the basis of urinary recovery of unchanged drug or metabolites, including their conjugates

Compound	$t\ ^1/_2$ (h)	Unchanged drug	*N*-Dealkylated metabolites	*N*-Oxidized metabolites
Phentermine	9–10	95–100	0	0– 5
N-Methylphentermine	6–20	50– 85	15–20	—
p-Chlorphentermine	12–38	30– 70	0	20–50

Source: Data from Vree, 1973; CALDWELL et al., 1975; BECKETT and BÉLANGER, 1977a

N-methylphentermine may be excreted as the dealkylated product phentermine (BECKETT and BROOKES, 1970, 1971; VREE, 1973).

The urinary excretion of chlorphentermine and its metabolites in man was recently studied in detail by BECKETT and BÉLANGER (1977a). With acidic urine more than 70% of a dose of chlorphentermine is excreted unchanged, whereas without urine pH control the majority (approximately 75% of the total recovered amount) of the original dose was recovered as *N*-oxidized metabolites (BECKETT and BÉLANGER, 1977a). The urine excretion half-life of p-chlorphentermine is much higher than that of phentermine. VREE (1973) reported half-lifes ranging 12–38 h, which agrees with the elimination half-life of ca. 40 h reported by JUN and TRIGGS (1970) on the basis of blood level determinations. The long half-life of chlorphentermine may be related to the high uptake of this compound by a number of tissues and its slow release from these tissues (DUBNICK et al., 1963; LÜLLMANN et al., 1973). Chlorphentermine has a more prolonged anorexigenic effect than amphetamine or phentermine.

III. Biotransformation

Phentermine derivatives are substituted at the *α-C*. This substitution limits pathways for metabolism, specially the α-C-oxidation and possibly also *β-C*-hydroxylation. Other routes of metabolism – ring hydroxylation and *N*-oxidation – have been described for several species both in vivo and in vitro (WEISCHER and OPITZ, 1967; CHO et al., 1974b, 1975a; CHO, 1974; BECKETT and BÉLANGER, 1974a, b, 1976, 1977a, b; CALDWELL et al., 1975).

p-Hydroxylation of phentermines is a minor route of metabolism: only small amounts of p-hydroxyphentermine can be detected in the urine of rats and man after administration of phentermine (WEISCHER and OPITZ, 1967; CHO, 1974). Recently, CHO et al. (1975a) showed p-hydroxylation of phentermine in rat liver microsomes with reaction characteristics similar to those of amphetamine p-hydroxylation.

β-C-Hydroxylated metabolites of phentermines have not yet been described, possibly because of the hindrance exerted by the α-methyl substituent (CHO and WRIGHT, 1978).

The main metabolic route for phentermines is *N*-oxidation. *N*-Hydroxyphentermine has been found as in vivo metabolite of phentermine in contrast to *N*-hydroxyamphetamine (BECKETT and BÉLANGER, 1974b). Similarly, N-hydroxychlorphentermine and its conjugates have been detected in vivo in urine of various species, including man (CALDWELL et al., 1975; BECKETT and BÉLANGER, 1977a). The in vivo presence of *N*-hydroxyphentermines indicates the relative stability of these metabolites when compared with their amphetamine analogues. *N*-Hydroxyphentermines are synthesized in vitro by liver preparations from rabbit, rat, and guinea-pig (CHO et al., 1974b; BECKETT and BÉLANGER, 1974a, 1976). This reaction is NADPH-dependent and has been suggested to proceed via the formation of oxygen radical flavoprotein anion complex with a nitrogen radical cation (BECKETT and BÉLANGER, 1974b). Cytochrome P-450 does not seem to be involved since well-known cytochrome P-450 inhibitors like cyanide or iodine do not decrease the in vitro *N*-oxidation of phentermine (BECKETT and BÉLANGER, 1976).

N-Methylphentermine is both dealkylated and *N*-hydroxylated by rabbit liver microsomes (BECKETT and BÉLANGER, 1977b). The dealkylation proceeds via hydroxylation of the methyl substituent of the *N* (BECKETT and BÉLANGER, 1977b).

N-Hydroxyphentermines are further metabolized in vivo and in vitro to nitroso and nitro compounds (BECKETT and BÉLANGER, 1974a, b, 1976, 1977a, b; CALDWELL et al., 1975). The hydroxyphentermines are also reduced in vivo and in vitro to their parent amines (CHO et al., 1974; BECKETT and BÉLANGER, 1976; SUM and CHO, 1976). This reductase activity can be induced by phenobarbital and is sensitive to SKF 525-A and carbon monoxide, suggesting the involvement of cytochrome P-450 (SUM and CHO, 1976).

E. Fenfluramine

I. Introduction

Fenfluramine differs from amphetamine by its *N*-ethyl and m-benzyl-CF_3 substitutions (Table 2). These substitutions lead to a much greater lipid solubility, which affects its pharmacokinetics and biotransformation. The pharmacology of fenfluramine – including its pharmacokinetics – have been reviewed recently by PINDER et al. (1976).

II. Pharmacokinetics

Similar to other amphetamine derivatives, the pharmacokinetic behaviour of fenfluramine is influenced by the urine pH (BECKETT and BROOKES, 1967). In man, under acid urine conditions, approximately 20% of an original dose of fenfluramine is excreted unchanged and 20% as its de-ethylated metabolite norfenfluramine (BECKETT and BROOKES, 1967). These figures may fall below 10% if urinary pH is not controlled. WESLEY-HADZIJA (1973) reported similar data in subjects on different diets whose urine pH varied widely.

1. Absorption and Distribution

Fenfluramine is rapidly absorbed after oral administration in man. After oral intake of 60 mg maximum plasma concentrations of 25–75 ng/ml are reached within 2–4 h (BRUCE and MAYNARD, 1968; CAMPBELL, 1971). Absorption half-life varies 1–1.4 h (CAMPBELL, 1971). The distribution volume of fenfluramine in man is approximately 10–20 litre/kg body weight (AVERY, 1976). Fenfluramine is rapidly taken up by a number of tissues. An injection of fenfluramine in rats leads to high concentrations of fenfluramine in lung, brain, spleen, and adrenals (EICHELBAUM and SIPES, 1972). Chronic dosage of fenfluramine in dogs leads to relatively high concentrations in the same tissues, as well as in fatty tissues (DUHAULT and FENARD, 1965). The occurrence of relatively high amounts of the fenfluramine metabolite norfenfluramine in a number of tissues has led to the suggestion that this metabolite may cause (part of) the anorectic effect of fenfluramine. Indeed, on the basis of direct stereotaxic application of these agents in the appetite controlling nuclei of the brain, BROEKKAMP et al. (1975) were able to show that norfenfluramine may be the active metabolite.

2. Excretion

Since the rate of urinary excretion of fenfluramine depends upon urine pH, wide variations in elimination half-life have been reported for fenfluramine. Elimination half-lifes in urine of 13–30 h have been reported (BECKETT and BROOKES, 1970; BECKETT and SALMON, 1972), whereas CAMPBELL (1971) calculated a half-life of approximately 20 h on the basis of plasma level measurements.

BECKETT and BROOKES (1967) found less unchanged drug in urine after oral than i.v. administration of fenfluramine. This observation suggests that some of the drug is metabolized in the intestine or on a first-pass through the liver (BECKETT and SALMON, 1972). Indeed, BROOKES (1968, cited in BECKETT and SALMON, 1972) detected the dealkylated metabolite norfenfluramine in the gut after administration of fenfluramine. The long elimination half-life of fenfluramine agrees with the large degree of uptake of this drug by a number of tissues. In a computer simulation of the kinetics of absorption, distribution and elimination of fenfluramine in man, BECKETT and SALMON (1972) needed a three compartment open model to explain the kinetic behaviour of this drug. In this model the overall elimination characteristics of fenfluramine were governed by the rate of release of fenfluramine from a deep compartment including brain, deposits of fat and some tissues with limited blood supplies. Probably the slow elimination from this compartment also explains the long duration of action of fenfluramine (LE DOUAREC and NEVEU, 1970; cf. PINDER et al., 1976).

III. Biotransformation

The presence of the m-CF_3 substituent in fenfluramine hampers metabolism of this drug via ring hydroxylation. In fact, the primary in vivo route of metabolism of fenfluramine is dealkylation to norfenfluramine (BECKETT and BROOKES, 1967; BRUCE and MAYNARD, 1968; BELVEDERE et al., 1972). BRUCE and MAYNARD (1968) reported that norfenfluramine can be further metabolized to 3-trifluoro-methylbenzoic acid and its glycine conjugate. The presence of *N*-oxidation metabolites in vivo was not demonstrated in man. However, BECKETT et al. (1973) showed that approximately 25% of a dose of fenfluramine can be converted to a nitrone in vitro by guinea-pig liver homogenates. The mechanisms whereby dealkylation and N-oxidation occur were discussed extensively in the paragraph on the amphetamines.

Acknowledgements. The author is indebted to T.B. VREE and H. THIJSSEN for reading the manuscript and suggesting improvements and to Mrs. A. LIPPINKHOF for secretarial assistance.

References

Anggård, E., Gunne, L.-M., Niklasson, F.: Gaschromatographic determination of amphetamine in blood, tissue, and urine. Scand. J. Clin. Lab. Invest. *26*, 137–142 (1970)
Anggård, E., Jönsson, L.E., Hogmark, A.L., Gunne, L.-M.: Amphetamine metabolism in amphetamine psychosis. Clin. Pharmacol. Ther. *14*, 870–880 (1973)
Asatoor, A.M., Galman, B.R., Johnson, M.T., Milne, M.D.: The excretion of dexamphetamine and its derivatives. Br. J. Pharmacol. *24*, 293–297 (1965)
Avery, G.S.: Drug treatment. Sydney: ADIS Press 1976
Axelrod, J.: Studies on sympathomimetic amines. I. The biotransformation and physiological disposition of l-ephedrine and l-norephedrine. J. Pharmacol. Exp. Ther. *109*, 62–73 (1953)
Axelrod, J.: Studies on sympathomimetic amines. II. The biotransformation and physiological disposition of d-amphetamine, d-para-hydroxyamphetamine and d-methamphetamine. J. Pharmacol. Exp. Ther. *110*, 315–326 (1954)
Axelrod, J.: The enzymatic deamination of amphetamine. J. Biol. Chem. *214*, 753–763 (1955)
Axelrod, J., Inscoe, J.K., Daly, J.: Enzymatic formation of O-methylated dihydroxy derivatives from phenolic amines and indoles. J. Pharmacol. Exp. Ther. *149*, 16–22 (1965)
Baggot, J.D., Davis, L.E.: Pharmacokinetic study of amphetamine elimination in dogs and swine. Biochem. Pharmacol. *21*, 1967–1976 (1972)
Baggot, J.D., Davis, L.E., Nef, C.A.: Extent of plasma protein binding of amphetamine in different species. Biochem. Pharmacol. *21*, 1813–1816 (1972)
Bareggi, S.R., Gomeni, R., Becker, R.E.: Stereotyped behavior and hyperthermia in dogs: correlation with the levels of amphetamine and p-hydroxyamphetamine in plasma and CSF. Psychopharmacology *58*, 89–94 (1978)
Beckett, A.H., Al-Sarraj, S.M.: The metabolism of (+) and (−) amphetamine and (+) and (−) dimethylamphetamine in rabbits *in vivo*. Biochem. J. *130*, 14P (1972a)
Beckett, A.H., Al-Sarraj, S.M.: The mechanism of oxidation of amphetamine enantiomorphs by liver microsomal preparations from different species. J. Pharm. Pharmacol. *24*, 174–176 (1972b)
Beckett, A.R., Bélanger, P.M.: The identification of three new metabolic products of phentermine after liver microsomal incubation. Xenobiotica *4*, 509–519 (1974a)
Beckett, A.H. Bélanger, P.M.: The mechanism of metabolic N-oxidation of phentermine and chlorphentermine to their hydroxyl-, amino-, and nitrosocompounds. J. Pharm. Pharmacol. *26*, 558–560 (1974b)
Beckett, A.H., Bélanger, P.M.: The microsomal N-oxidation of phentermine. J. Pharm. Pharmacol. *28*, 692–699 (1976)
Beckett, A.H., Bélanger, P.M.: The metabolism, distribution and elimination of chlorphentermine in man. Br. J. Clin. Pharmacol. *4*, 193–200 (1977a)
Beckett, A.H., Bélanger, P.M.: The *in vitro* metabolism of mephentermine. Biochem. Pharmacol. *26*, 1455–1462 (1977b)
Beckett , A.H., Brookes, L.G.: The absorption and urinary excretion in man of fenfluramine and its main metabolite. J. Pharm. Pharmacol. *19*, 42S–49S (1967)
Beckett, A.H., Brookes, L.G.: The effect of chain and ring substitution on the metabolism, distribution, and biological action of amphetamines. In: Amphetamines and related compounds. Costa, E., Garattini, S. (eds.), pp. 109–121. New York: Raven Press 1970
Beckett, A.H., Brookes, L.G.: The metabolism and urinary excretion in man of phentermine, and the influence of N-methyl and p-chlorosubstitution. J. Pharm. Pharmacol. *23*, 288–294 (1971)
Beckett, A.H., Coutts, R.T., Ogunbona, F.A.: N-ethyl-alpha-methyl-alpha (m-trifluoromethylbenzyl) nitrone – the major in vitro metabolic product of fenfluramine in guinea-pig liver microsomal fractions. J. Pharm. Pharmacol. *25*, 190–192 (1973)
Beckett, A.H., Haya, K.: The identification and quantitation of the major metabolites of ethylamphetamine, produced by rabbit liver microsomal preparations. J. Pharm. Pharmacol. *29*, 89–95 (1977)
Beckett, A.H., Midha, K.K.: The identification of four metabolic products after incubation of p-methoxyamphetamine with liver preparations of various species. Xenobiotica *4*, 297–311 (1974)

Beckett, A.H., Salmon, J.A.: Pharmacokinetics of absorption, distribution, and elimination of fenfluramine and its main metabolite in man. J. Pharm. Pharmacol. *24*, 108–114 (1972)
Beckett, A.H., Shenoy, E.V.B.: The effect of N-alkyl chain length and stereochemistry on the absorption, metabolism, and urinary excretion of N-alkylamphetamines in man. J. Pharm. Pharmacol. *25*, 792–799 (1973)
Beckett, A.H., Rowland, M., Turner, P.: Influence of urine pH on excretion of amphetamine. Lancet *1*, 303 (1963)
Beckett, A.H., Salmon, J.A., Mitchard, M.: The relation between blood levels and urinary excretion of amphetamine under controlled acidic and under fluctuating urinary pH values using 14-C-amphetamine. J. Pharm. Pharmacol. *21*, 251–258 (1969)
Beckett, A.H., Van Dijk, J.M., Chissick, H.H., Gorrod, J.W.: Metabolism of amphetamines to oximes as a route of deamination. J. Pharm. Pharmacol. *23*, 560 (1971)
Belvedere, G., Tognoni, S., Morsell, P.: A new sensitive gas-chromatographic method for the determination of fenfluramine in biological specimens. Eur. J. Clin. Pharmacol. *5*, 62–66 (1972)
Benakis, A., Thomasset, M.: Metabolism of amphetamines and their interaction with barbiturates and SKF-525A. In: Amphetamines and related compounds. Costa, E., Garattini, S. (eds.), pp. 153–165. New York: Raven Press 1970
Biel, J.H.: Structure-activity relationships of amphetamines and derivatives. In: Amphetamine and related compounds. Costa, E., Garattini, S. (eds.), pp. 3–21. New York: Raven Press 1970
Boulton, A.A.: Biochemical research in schizophrenia. Nature *231*, 22–28 (1971)
Boulton, A.A.: The tyramines: Functionally significant biogenic amines or metabolic accidents? Life Sci *23*, 659–672 (1978)
Boulton, A.A., Baker, G.B.: The subcellular distribution of beta-phenylethylamine, p-tyramine, and tryptamine in rat brain. J. Neurochem. *25*, 477–481 (1975)
Boulton, A.A., Dyck, L.E.: Biosynthesis and excretion of meta- and para-tyramine in the rat. Life Sci. *14*, 2497–2506 (1974)
Boulton, A.A., Marjerrison, G.L.: Effect of L-dopa therapy on urinary p-tyramine excretion and EEG changes in Parkinson's disease. Nature *236*, 76–78 (1972)
Boulton, A.A., Wu, P.W.: Biosynthesis of cerebral phenolic amines. II. *In vivo* regional formation of p-tyramine and octopamine from tyrosine and dopamine. Can. J. Biochem. *51*, 428–435 (1973)
Boulton, A.A., Pollitt, R.J., Majer, J.R.: Identity of a urinary "pink spot" in schizophrenia and Parkinson's disease. Nature *215*, 132–134 (1967)
Boulton, A.A., Dyck, L.E., Durden, D.A.: Hydroxylation of beta-phenylethylamine in the rat. Life Sci. *15*, 1673–1683 (1974)
Bralet, J., Cohen, Y., Valette, G.: Metabolisme et distribution tissulaire de la dl-ephedrine – 14C. Biochem. Pharmacol. *17*, 2319–2331 (1968)
Brandau, K., Axelrod, J.: The biosynthesis of octopamine. Naunyn. Schmiedebergs Arch. Pharmacol. *273*, 123–133 (1972)
Brandau, K., Axelrod, J.: Ring hydroxylation of N-methylation of noradrenaline and dopamine in the intact rat brain. In: Frontiers in catecholamine research. Usdin, E., Snyder, S. (eds.), pp. 129–133. New York: Pergamon Press 1973
Bridges, J.W., French, M.R., Smith, R.L., Williams, R.T.: The fate of benzoic acid in various species. Biochem. J. *118*, 47–51 (1970)
Brodie, B.B., Cho, A.K., Gessa, G.L.: Possible role of p-hydroxynorephedrine in the depletion of norepinephrine induced by d-amphetamine and in tolerance to this drug. In: Amphetamines and related compounds. Costa, E., Garattini, S. (eds.), pp. 217–231. New York: Raven Press 1970
Brodie, B.B., Cho, A.K., Krishna, G., Reid, W.D.: Drug metabolism in man, past, present, and future. Ann. N.Y. Acad. Sci. *179*, 11–19 (1971)
Broekkamp, C.L.E., Weemaes, A.J.M., Rossum, J.M. van: Does fenfluramine act via norfenfluramine? J. Pharm. Pharmacol. *27*, 129–130 (1975)
Bruce, R.B., Maynard, W.R.: Fenfluramine metabolism. J. Pharm. Sci. *57*, 1173–1179 (1968)
Bruce, R.B., Maynard, W.R.: Determination of amphetamine and related amines in blood by gas chromatography. Anal. Chem. *41*, 977–982 (1969)

Caldwell, J.: The metabolism of amphetamines in mammals. Drug. Metab. Rev. *5*, 219–280 (1976)
Caldwell, J., Dring, L.G., Williams, R.T.: Metabolism of 14-C-methamphetamine in man, the guinea pig and the rat. Biochem. J. *129*, 11–22 (1972a)
Caldwell, J., Dring, L.G., Williams, R.T.: Norephedrines as metabolites of 14-C-amphetamine in urine of man. Biochem. J. *129*, 23–24 (1972b)
Caldwell, J., Koster, U., Smith, R.L., Williams, R.T.: Species variation in the N-oxidation of chlorphentermine. Biochem. Pharmacol. *24*, 2225–2232 (1975)
Campbell, D.B.: A method for the measurement of therapeutic levels of (+) amphetamine in human plasma. J. Pharm. Pharmacol. *21*, 129–131 (1969)
Campbell, D.B.: Plasma concentration of fenfluramine and its metabolite, norfenfluramine, following single and repeated oral administration. Br. J. Pharmacol. *43*, 465–470 (1971)
Carlsson, A., Waldeck, B.: Beta-hydroxylation of tyramine *in vivo*. Acta Pharmacol. Toxicol. (Kbh.) *20*, 371–374 (1963)
Cattabeni, F., Racagni, G., Gropetti, A.: Use of mass fragmentography to detect subcellular localization of drug metabolites acting as false transmitters. Adv. Biochem. Psychopharmacol. *7*, 45–55 (1973)
Cho, A.K.: The identification of p-hydroxyphentermine as a urinary metabolite of phentermine. Res. Commun. Chem. Pathol. Pharmacol. *7*, 67–78 (1974)
Cho, A.K., Wright, J.: Pathways of metabolism of amphetamine and related compounds. Life Sci. *22*, 363–372 (1978)
Cho, A.K., Hodshon, B.J., Lindeke, B., Johnsson, J.: The p-hydroxylation of amphetamine and phentermine by rat liver microsomes. Xenobiotica *5*, 531–538 (1975a)
Cho, A.K., Hodshon, B.J., Lindeke, B., Miwa, G.T.: Application of quantitative GC-mass spectrometry to study of pharmacokinetics of amphetamine and phentermine. J. Pharm. Sci. *62*, 1491–1494 (1973)
Cho, A.K., Lindeke, B., Jenden, D.J.: Gas-chromatography – mass spectrometry in the distribution and metabolism of phentermine. In: Mass spectrometry in biochemistry and medicine. Frigerio, A., Castagnoli, N. (eds.), pp. 83–90. New York: Raven Press 1974a
Cho, A.K., Lindeke, B., Sum, C.Y.: The N-hydroxylation of phentermine-2-methyl-2-amino-1-phenyl propane: Properties of the enzyme system. Drug. Metab. Dispos. *2*, 1–8 (1974b)
Cho, A.K., Schaeffer, J.C., Fischer, J.F.: Accumulation of 4-hydroxy-amphetamine by rat striatal homogenates. Biochem. Pharmacol. *24*, 1540–1542 (1975b)
Commarato, M.A., Brody, T.M., McNeill, J.H.: The effect of various drugs on the uptake and metabolism of tyramine-H^3 in the rat heart. J. Pharmacol. Exp. Ther. *167*, 151–158 (1969)
Cools, A.R., Rossum, J.M. van: Caudate dopamine and stereotyped behavior of cats. Arch. Int. Pharmacodyn. Ther. *187*, 163–173 (1970)
Costa, E., Garattini, S.: Amphetamines and related compounds. New York: Raven Press 1970
Coutts, R.T., Kovach, S.H.: Metabolism in vitro of N-methylamphetamine with rat liver homogenates. Biochem. Pharmacol. *26*, 1043–1049 (1977)
Coutts, R.T., Dawe, R., Dawson, G.W., Kovach, S.H.: In vitro metabolism of 1-phenyl-2-propanone oxime in rat liver homogenates. Drug. Metab. Dispos. *4*, 35–39 (1976a)
Coutts, R.T., Dawson, G.W., Beckett, A.H.: In vitro metabolism of 1-phenyl-2-(n-propylamino)propane (N-propylamphetamine) by rat liver homogenates. J. Pharm. Pharmacol. *28*, 815–821 (1976b)
Coutts, R.T., Dawson, G.W., Kazakoff, C.W., Wong, J.Y.: In vivo phenolic metabolites of N-alkylamphetamines in the rat. Drug. Metab. Dispos. *4*, 256–261 (1976c)
Coutts, R.T., Jones, G.R., Townsend, R.E.: Species differences in the in vitro metabolic reduction of the amphetamine metabolite, 1-phenyl-2-propanone. J. Pharm. Pharmacol. *30*, 415–418 (1978)
Creaven, P.J., Barbee, T.: The effect of ethanol on the metabolism of amphetamine by the rat. J. Pharm. Pharmacol. *21*, 859–860 (1969)
Creaven, P.J., Barbee, T., Roach, M.K.: The interaction of ethanol and amphetamine metabolism. J. Pharm. Pharmacol. *22*, 828–831 (1970)
Creveling, C.R., Levitt, M., Udenfriend, S.: An alternate route for biosynthesis of norepinephrine. Life Sci. *1*, 523–526 (1962)

Daly, J.W., Guroff, G., Udenfriend, S., Witkop, B.: Hydroxylation-induced migrations of tritium in several substrates of liver aryl hydroxylases. Arch. Biochem. Biophys. *122*, 218–223 (1967)

Danielson, I.J., Boulton, A.A.: Distribution and occurrence of amphetamine and p-hydroxyamphetamine in tissues of the rat after injection of d-amphetamine sulphate. Eur. J. Pharmacol. *37*, 257–264 (1976)

David, J.C., Dairman, W., Udenfriend, S.: Decarboxylation to tyramine: A major route of tyrosine metabolism in mammals. Proc. Natl. Acad. Sci. USA *71*, 1771–1775 (1974)

De Feudis, F.V., Marks, J.H.: Studies on the time-course of entry and subcellular distribution of radioactivity of 3H-d-amphetamine in the brains of differentially-housed mice. Experientia *29*, 1518–1520 (1973)

De Quattro, V.L., Sjoerdsma, A.: Origin of urinary tyramine and tryptamine. Clin. Chim. Acta *16*, 227–233 (1967)

Dingell, J.V., Bass, A.D.: Inhibition of the hepatic metabolism of amphetamine by desipramine. Biochem. Pharmacol. *18*, 1535–1538 (1969)

Dring, L.G., Smith, R.L., Williams, R.T.: A precursor of benzyl methyl ketone in amphetamine urine. Biochem. J. *109*, 10P–11P (1968)

Dring, L.G., Smith, R.L., Williams, R.T.: The metabolic fate of amphetamine in man and other species. Biochem. J. *116*, 425–435 (1970)

Dubnick, B., Leeson, G.A., Leverett, R., Morgan, D.F., Phillips, G.E.: Sympathomimetic properties of chlorphentermine: metabolism, metabolic effects, interaction with reserpine and biogenic amines. J. Pharmacol. Exp. Ther. *140*, 85–92 (1963)

Dubnick, B., Towne, C.A., Hartignan, J.M., Phillips, G.E.: Distribution and metabolism of chlorphentermine-C-14 in rats and mice. Biochem. Pharmacol. *17*, 1243–1251 (1968)

Duhault, J., Fénard, S.: Étude sur l'excrétion, la localisation, et le métabolisme d'une nouvelle substance anorexigène: le fenfluramine. Arch. Int. Pharmacodyn. Ther. *158*, 251–264 (1965)

Eichelbaum, M., Sipes, I.C.: The physiological disposition of fenfluramine in the rat. Naunyn. Schmiedebergs Arch. Pharmacol. *274*, Suppl., R31 (1972)

Ellison, T., Gutzait, L., Loon, E.J. van: The comparative metabolism of d-amphetamine C-14 in the rat, dog, and monkey. J. Pharmacol. Exp. Ther. *152*, 383–387 (1966)

Ellison, T., Okun, R., Silverman, A., Siegel, M.: Metabolic fate of amphetamine in the cat during development of tolerance. Arch. Int. Pharmacodyn. Ther. *190*, 135–149 (1971)

Faraj, B.A., Mu, J.Y., Lewis, M.S., Wilson, J.P., Israili, Z.H., Dayton, P.G.: Determination of plasma and tissue levels of tyramine by radioimmunoassay. Proc. Soc. Exp. Biol. Med. *149*, 664–669 (1975a)

Faraj, B.A., Wilson, J.P., Lewis, M.S., Dayton, P.G.: Tissue distribution of tyramine in rabbits and dogs by radioimmunoassay. Fed. Proc. *34*, 712 (1975b)

Faraj, B.A., Dayton, P.G., Camp, V.M., Wilson, J.P., Malveaux, E.J., Schlant, R.C.: Studies on the fate of tyramine in dogs: the effect of monoamine oxidase inhibition, portafemoral shunt and coronary artery ligation on the kinetics of tyramine. J. Pharmacol. Exp. Ther. *200*, 384–393 (1977)

Feller, D.R., Malspeis, L.: Biotransformation of d(−) ephedrine and l(+) ephedrine in the rabbit, in vivo and in vitro. Drug. Metab. Dispos. *5*, 37–47 (1977)

Fischer, J.E.: False neurotransmitters and hepatic coma. Res. Publ. Assoc. Res. Nerv. Ment. Dis. *53*, 53–74 (1974)

Freeman, J., Sulser, F.S.: Formation of p-hydroxynorephedrine in brain following intraventricular administration of p-hydroxyamphetamine. Neuropharmacology *13*, 1187–1190 (1974)

Frosch, F.: Biopharmazeutische Untersuchungen am D-Norpseudo-ephedrin. Arzneim. Forsch. *27*, 665–668 (1977)

Fuller, R.W., Baker, J.C., Molloy, B.B.: Biological disposition of rigid analogs of amphetamine. J. Pharm. Sci. *66*, 271–273 (1977)

Gal, J., Gruenke, L.D., Castagnoli, N.: N-hydroxylation of 1-(2,5-dimethoxy-4-methylphenyl)-2-aminopropane by rabbit liver microsomes. J. Med. Chem. *18* , 683–688 (1975)

Garfinkel, D.: A comparative study of electron transport in microsomes. Comp. Biochem. Physiol. *8*, 367–379 (1963)

Goldstein, M., McKereghan, M.R., Lauber, E.: The stereospecificity of the enzymatic amphetamine-beta-hydroxylase. Biochem. Biophys. Acta *89*, 191–198 (1964)

Gunne, L.M., Jonsson, J.: On the ocurrence of tyramine in the rabbit brain. Acta Physiol. Scand. *64*, 434–438 (1965)
Hansch, C., Lien, E.J., Helmer, F.: Structure-activity correlations in the metabolism of drugs. Arch. Biochem. Biophys. *128*, 319–330 (1968)
Heimlich, K.R., Mcdonnel, D.R., Flanagan, T.L., O'Brien, P.D.: Evaluation of a sustained release form of phenylpropanolamine hydrochloride by urinary excretion studies. J. Pharm. Sci. *50*, 232–237 (1961)
Henderson, P.Th., Vree, T.B., Ginneken, C.A.M. van, Rossum, J.M. van: Activation energies of alpha-C-oxidation and N-oxidation of N-alkyl-substituted amphetamines by rat liver microsomes. Xenobiotica *4*, 121–130 (1974)
Hinsvark, O.N., Truant, A.P., Jenden, D.J., Steinborn, J.A.: The oral bioavailability and pharmacokinetics of soluble and resin-bound forms of amphetamine and phentermine in man. J. Pharmacokinet. Biopharm. *1*, 319–328 (1973)
Honecker, H., Coper, H.: Kinetics and metabolism of amphetamine in the brain of rats of different ages. Naunyn. Schmiedebergs Arch. Pharmacol. *291*, 111–121 (1975)
Horowitz, D., Lovenberg, W., Engelman, K., Sjoerdsma, A.: Monoamine oxidase inhibitions, tyramine and cheese. J. Am. Med. Assoc. *188*, 1108–1110 (1964)
Hucker, H.B.: Phenylacetone oxime an intermediate in amphetamine deamination. Drug. Metab. Dispos. *1*, 332–336 (1973)
Hucker, H.B., Michoriewics, B.M., Rhodes, R.E.: Phenylacetoneoxime. An intermediate in the oxidative deamination of amphetamine. Biochem. Pharmacol. *20*, 2123–2128 (1971)
Iversen, L.L.: Uptake and storage of noradrenaline by sympathetic nerves. Cambridge: Cambridge University Press 1967
Jacquot, C., Bralet, J., Cohen, Y., Valette, G.: Fixation de la dl ephédrine 14-C par le coeur isolé perfusé de rat. Biochem. Pharmacol. *18*, 903–914 (1969a)
Jacquot, C., Bratlet, J., Cohen, Y., Valette, G.: Influence du pH sur la fixation tissulaire de l'amphetamine 3H et de l'ephédrine 14C. Biochem. Pharmacol. *18*, 2415–2424 (1969b)
Jacquot, C., Rapin, J.R., Wepierre, J., Cohen, Y.: Métabolisme et distribution tissulaire de l'ephédrine 14-C chez le cobaye. Arch. Int. Pharmacodyn. Ther. *207*, 298–309 (1974)
Jenner, P., Testa, B.: The influence of stereochemical factors on drug disposition. Drug. Metab. Rev. *2*, 117–184 (1973)
Jones, R.A.D., Pollitt, R.J.: The hydroxylation of p-tyramine in man. J. Pharm. Pharmacol. *28*, 461–462 (1976)
Jonsson, J.A.: Hydroxylation of amphetamine to parahydroxyamphetamine by rat liver microsomes. Biochem. Pharmacol. *23*, 3101–3107 (1974)
Jonsson, J.A.: On the aromatic hydroxylation of amphetamine in rat liver microsomes and perfused liver preparations: effects of long-term administration. Acta Pharmacol. Toxicol. (Kbh.) *40*, 517–528 (1977)
Jori, A., Caccia, S.: Distribution of amphetamine and its hydroxylated metabolites in various areas of the rat brain. J. Pharm. Pharmacol. *26*, 746–748 (1974)
Jun, H.W., Triggs, E.J.: Blood levels of chlorphentermine in man. J. Pharm. Sci. *59*, 306–309 (1970)
Kakimoto, Y., Armstrong, M.D.: On the indentification of octopamine in mammals. J. Biol. Chem. *237*, 422–427 (1962)
Kammerer, R.C., Jonsson, J., Gal, J., Cho, A.K.: Use of stable isotopes in studies on metabolism of amphetamine. Life Sci. *23*, 283–290 (1978)
Karabelnick, D., Zbinden, G., Baumgartner, E.: Drug-induced foam cell reaction in rats. I. Histopathologic and cytochemical observations after treatment with chlorphentermine, RMI 10.391 and Ro 4-4318. Toxicol. Appl. Pharmacol. *27*, 395–407 (1974)
Kuhn, C.M., Schanberg, S.M., Breese, G.R.: Metabolism of amphetamine by rat brain tissue. Biochem. Pharmacol. *27*, 343–351 (1978)
Latini, R., Placidi, G.F., Riva, E., Fornaro, P., Guarneri, M., Morselli, P.L.: Kinetics of distribution of amphetamine in cats. Psychopharmacology *54*, 209–215 (1977)
Laverty, R., Michaelson, I.A., Sharman, D.F., Whittaker, V.P.: The subcellular localization of dopamine and acetylcholine in the dog caudate nucleus. Br. J. Pharmacol. *21*, 482–490 (1963)
Le Douarec, J.C., Neveu, C.: Pharmacology and biochemistry of fenfluramine. In: Amphetamines and related compounds. Costa, E., Garattini, S. (eds.), pp. 75–109. New York: Raven Press 1970

Leibowitz, S.: Amphetamine: Possible site and mode of action for producing anorexia in the rat. Brain Res. *84*, 160–165 (1975)
Lemberger, L., Klutch, A., Kuntzman, R.: The metabolism of tyramine in rabbits. J. Pharmacol. Exp. Ther. *153*, 183–190 (1966)
Lew, C., Iversen, S.D., Iversen, L.L.: Effects of imipramine, desipramine, and monoamine oxidase inhibitors on the metabolism and psychomotor stimulant actions of d-amphetamine in mice. Eur. J. Pharmacol. *14*, 351–359 (1971)
Lewander, T.: On the presence of p-hydroxynorephedrine in the rat brain and heart in relation to changes in catecholamine levels after administration of amphetamine. Acta Pharmacol. Toxicol. (Kbh) *29*, 33–48 (1971)
Lindeke, B., Cho, A.K., Thomas, T.L., Michelson, L.: Microsomal N-Hydroxylation of phenylalkyl amines: identification of N-hydroxylated phenylalkyl amines as their tri-methyl silyl derivatives by gas chromatography/mass spectrometry. Acta Pharm. Suec. *10*, 493–506 (1973)
Lindeke, B., Cho, A.K., Jonsson, U., Paulsen, W.: Chemical stability of beta-hydroxyphenylalkylhydroxylamines and its relevance to metabolism of amphetamines and ephedrines. Life Sci. *23*, 921–926 (1978)
Lindenbaum, A., Marcher, K., Wepierre, J., Cohen, Y.: Barrière hématoencéphalique: I. Cinétique de distribution de l'amphetamine 3H dans les structures du cerveau de rat après administration intraveineuse. Arch. Int. Pharmacodyn. Ther. *212*, 337–347 (1974)
Lokiec, F., Rapin, J.R., Jacquot, C., Cohen, Y.: A comparison of the kinetics of d- and l-amphetamine in the brain of isolated and aggregated rats. Psychopharmacology *58*, 73–77 (1978)
Lovenberg, W., Weissbach, H., Udenfriend, S.: Aromatic L-amino acid decarboxylase. J. Biol. Chem. *237*, 89–93 (1962)
Lüllmann, H., Rossen, E., Seiler, K.U.: The pharmacokinetics of phentermine and chlorphentermine in chronically treated rats. J. Pharm. Pharmacol. *25*, 239–243 (1973)
Lüllmann-Rausch, R.: Chlorphentermine-induced cytoplasmic inclusions in peripheral blood cells of rats and guinea-pigs. Toxicol. Appl. Pharmacol. *32*, 32–39 (1975)
Magour, S., Coper, H., Fälmdrich, Ch.: Effect of chronic intoxication with (+) amphetamine on its concentration in liver and brain and on 14C-leucine incorporation into microsomal and cytoplasmic proteins of rat liver. J. Pharm. Pharmacol. *26*, 105–108 (1974)
Maickel, R.P., Cox, R.H., Miller, F.P., Segal, D.S., Russel, R.W.: Correlation of brain levels of drugs with behavioral effects. J. Pharmacol. Exp. Ther. *165*, 216–224 (1969)
Matsuda, A., Baba, S., Nagasi, Y.: Studies on the analysis of drugs by use of isotopes. VII. Identification of metabolites of ephedrine in rabbit. J. Pharm. Soc. Jap. *91*, 542–545 (1971)
McMahon, R.E.: Microsomal dealkylation of drugs. Substrate specificity and mechanism. J. Pharm. Sci. *55*, 457–466 (1966)
McMahon, R.E.: Enzymatic oxidation and reduction of alcohols, aldehydes, and ketones. In: Handbuch der Experimentellen Pharmakologie. Brodie, B.B., Gillette, J.R. (eds.), Vol. 2, pp. 500–517. Berlin, Heidelberg, New York: Springer 1971
Midha, K.K., Beckett, A.H., Saunders, A.: Identification of the major metabolites of propylhexedrine in vivo (in man) and in vitro (in guinea pig and rabbit). Xenobiotica *4*, 627–635 (1974)
Mullen, P.E., Smith, I.: Tyramine metabolism and migraine: a metabolic effect. Br. J. Pharmacol. *41*, 413P–414P (1971)
Nair, V., Palm, D., Roth, J.L.: Relative vascularity of certain anatomical areas of the brain and other organs of the rat. Nature *188*, 497–498 (1960)
Noonan, J.S., Murdick, P.W., Ray, R.S.: A method for detecting amphetamine using gaschromatography of a halogenated derivative. J. Pharmacol. Exp. Ther. *168*, 205–210 (1969)
Oates, J.A.: Measurement of urinary tryptamine, tyramine, and serotonin. Methods Med. Res. *9*, 169–177 (1961)
Parli, C.J., McMahon, R.E.: The mechanism of microsomal deamination: heavy isotope studies. Drug. Metab. Dispos. *1*, 337–341 (1973)
Parli, C.J., Wang, N., McMahon, R.E.: The mechanism of oxidation of d-amphetamine by rabbit liver oxygenase. Oxygen-18 studies. Biochem. Biophys. Res. Commun. *43*, 1204–1209 (1971 a)

Parli, C.J., Wang, N., McMahon, R.E.: The enzymatic N-hydroxylation of an imine. J. Biol. Chem. *246*, 6953–6966 (1971 b)
Perry, T.L.: Urinary excretion of amines in phenylketonuria and mongolism. Science *136*, 879–880 (1962)
Philips, S.R., Durden, D.A., Boulton, A.A.: Identification and distribution of p-tyramine in the rat. Can. J. Biochem. *52*, 366–373 (1974)
Philips, S.R., Davis, B.A., Durden, D.A., Boulton, A.A.: Identification and distribution of m-tyramine in the rat. Can. J. Biochem. *53*, 65–69 (1975)
Philips, S.R., Rezdilsky, B., Boulton, A.A.: Evidence for the presence of m-tyramine, p-tyramine, tryptamine, and phenylethylamine in the rat brain and several areas of the human brain. Biol. Psychol. *13*, 51–57 (1978)
Pinder, R.M., Brogden, R.N., Sawyer, P.R., Speight, T.M., Avery, G.S.: Fenfluramine: a review of its pharmacological properties and therapeutic efficacy in obesity. Drugs *10*, 241–323 (1976)
Placidi, G.F., Masuoka, D.T., Earle, R.W.: Distribution of 14-C amphetamine in mouse brain: an autoradiographic study. Brain Res. *38*, 399–405 (1972)
Richter, D.: Elimination of amines in man. Biochem. J. *32*, 1763–1769 (1938)
Riffee, W.H., Ludden, R.E., Wilcox, R.E., Gerald, M.C.: Brain and plasma concentration of amphetamine isomers in mice. J. Pharmacol. Exp. Ther. *206*, 586–594 (1978)
Rommelspracher, H., Honecker, H., Schulze, G., Strauss, S.M.: The hydroxylation of d-amphetamine by liver microsomes of the male rat. Biochem. Pharmacol. *23*, 1065–1071 (1974)
Ross, S.B., Renyi, A.L., Brunefelter, B.: Cocaine sensitive uptake of sympathomimetic amines in nerve tissue. J. Pharm. Pharmacol. *20*, 283–288 (1968)
Rossum, J.M. van: Mode of action of psychomotor stimulant drugs. Int. Rev. Neurobiol. *12*, 307–383 (1970)
Rossum, J.M. van: Kinetics of drug action. Berlin, Heidelberg, New York: Springer 1977
Rowland, M.: Amphetamine blood and urine levels in man. J. Pharm. Sci. *58*, 508–511 (1969)
Seiler, K.U., Wassermann, O.: Evidence for an unusual distribution of chlorphentermine in vivo: an autoradiographic study in mice. Naunyn. Schmiedebergs Arch. Pharmacol. *282*, 113–122 (1974)
Sever, P.S., Dring, L.G., Williams, R.T.: The metabolism of hydroxy-amphetamines in man and animals: 4-hydroxy C-14-amphetamine (paredrine). Biochem. Soc. Trans. *1*, 1158–1159 (1973)
Sever, P.S., Dring, L.G., Williams, R.T.: The metabolism of (−) ephedrine in man. Eur. J. Clin. Pharmacol. *9*, 193–198 (1975)
Sever, P.S., Dring, L.G., Williams, R.T.: Urinary metabolites of p-hydroxyamphetamine in man, rat, and guinea-pig. Xenobiotica *6*, 345–353 (1976)
Sinsheimer, J.E., Dring, L.G., Williams, R.T.: Species differences in the metabolism of norephedrine in man, rabbit, and rat. Biochem. J. *136*, 763–771 (1973)
Smith, I., Kellow, A.H.: Aromatic amines and Parkinson's disease. Nature *221*, 1261 (1969)
Smith, I., March, S.E.: Tyramine metabolism. A method for the quantitative extraction of radioactive tyramine and its metabolites from urine. Clin. Chim. Acta *40*, 415–419 (1972)
Smith, I., Mitchell, P.D.: The effect of oral inorganic sulphate on the metabolism of 4-hydroxyphenylethylamine (tyramine) in man: tyramine-O-sulphate measurement in human urine. Biochem. J. *142*, 189–191 (1974)
Smith, I., Kellow, A.H., Mullen, P.E., Hanington, E.: Dietary migraine and tyramine metabolism. Nature *230*, 246–248 (1971)
Spector, S., Melmon, K., Lovenberg, W., Sjoerdsma, A.: The presence and distribution of tyramine in mammalian tissues. J. Pharmacol. Exp. Ther. *140*, 229–235 (1963)
Steinberg, M.I., Smith, C.B.: Uptake, retention, and metabolism of H^3-tyramine in rat atria. J. Pharmacol. Exp. Ther. *176*, 139–148 (1971)
Struyker-Boudier, H.A.J.: Physiological approaches to drug design. In: Drug design. Ariëns, E.J. (ed.), Vol. 10. New York: Academic Press (in press) (1979)
Sum, C.Y., Cho, A.K.: Properties of microsomal enzyme systems that reduce N-hydroxyphentermine. Drug Metab. Dispos. *4*, 436–441 (1976)
Tacker, M.M., McIsaac, W.M., Creaven, P.J.: Metabolism of tyramine-1-^{14}C by the rat. Biochem. Pharmacol. *19*, 2763–2775 (1970)

Tacker, M.M., Creaven, P.J., McIsaac, W.M.: Preliminary observations on the metabolism of (1-^{14}C) tyramine in man. J. Pharm. Pharmacol. *24*, 247–250 (1972)
Tallman, J.F., Saavedra, J.M., Axelrod, J.: A sensitive enzymatic-isotopic method for the analysis of tyramine in brain and other tissues. J. Neurochem. *27*, 465–469 (1976a)
Tallman, J.F., Saavedra, J.M., Axelrod, J.: Biosynthesis and metabolism of endogenous tyramine and its normal presence in sympathetic nerves. J. Pharmacol. Exp. Ther. *199*, 216–221 (1976b)
Thiercelin, J.F., Jacquot, C., Rapin, J.R., Cohen, Y.: Pharmacocinétique de la DL-noréphédrine 14-C chez le rat. Arch. Int. Pharmacodyn. Ther. *220*, 153–163 (1976)
Thoenen, H., Hürlimann, A., Gey, K.F., Haefely, W.: Liberation of p-hydroxynorephedrine from cat spleen by sympathetic nerve stimulation after pretreatment with amphetamine. Life Sci. *5*, 1715–1725 (1966)
Udenfriend, S.: Arene oxide intermediates in enzymatic hydroxylation and their significance with respect to drug toxicity. Ann. N.Y. Acad. Sci. *179*, 295–302 (1971)
Vree, T.B.: Pharmacokinetics and metabolism of amphetamines. Nijmegen. Ph.D. Thesis, 1973
Vree, T.B., Rossum, J.M. van: Kinetics of metabolism and excretion of amphetamines in man. In: Amphetamines and related compounds. Costa, E., Garattini, S. (eds.), pp. 165–190. New York: Raven Press 1970
Vree, T.B., Muskens, A.Th.J.M., Rossum, J.M. van: Some physicochemical properties of amphetamine and related drugs. J. Pharm. Pharmacol. *21*, 774–777 (1969)
Vree, T.B., Gorgels, J.P.M.C., Muskens, A.Th.J.M., Rossum, J.M. van: Deuterium isotope effects in the metabolism of N-alkyl substituted amphetamines in man. Clin. Chim. Acta *34*, 333–344 (1971)
Vree, T.B., Muskens, A.Th.J.M., Rossum, J.M. van: Metabolism of N-alkyl substituted aminopropiophenones in man in comparison to amphetamines and ephedrines. Arch. Int. Pharmacodyn. Ther. *197*, 392–395 (1972)
Wan, S.H., Matin, S.B., Azarnoff, D.L.: Kinetics, salivary excretion of amphetamine isomers, and effect of urinary pH. Clin. Pharmacol. Ther. *23*, 585–590 (1978)
Weischer, M.L., Opitz, K.: Bestimmung von Chlorphentermin, Fenfluramin und verwandten Substanzen im Harn. Arzneim. Forsch. *17*, 625–627 (1967)
Wesley-Hadzija, B.: Absorption and urinary excretion of fenfluramine and ethylamphetamine in subjects on different diets. Can. J. Pharm. Sci. *8*, 101–106 (1973)
Wilkinson, G.R., Beckett, A.H.: Absorption, metabolism, and excretion of the ephedrines in man. I. The influence of urinary pH and urine volume output. J. Pharmacol. Exp. Ther. *162*, 139–147 (1968a)
Wilkinson, G.R., Beckett, A.H.: Absorption, metabolism, and excretion of the ephedrines in man. II. Pharmacokinetics. J. Pharm. Sci. *57*, 1933–1938 (1968b)
Williams, R.T., Caldwell, J., Dring, S.G.: Comparative metabolism of some amphetamines in various species. In: Frontiers in catecholamine research. Usdin, E., Snyder, S. (eds.), pp. 927–932. New York: Pergamon Press 1973
Wong, D.T., Van Frank, R.M., Hoing, J.S., Fuller, R.W.: Accumulation of amphetamine and p-chloroamphetamine into synaptosomes of rat brain. J. Pharm. Pharmacol. *24*, 171–173 (1972)
Wright, J., Cho, A.K., Gal, J.: The metabolism of amphetamine in vitro by rabbit liver preparations: a comparison of R(−) and S(+) enantiomers. Xenobiotica *7*, 257–266 (1977a)
Wright, J., Cho, A.K., Gal, J.: The role of N-hydroxyamphetamine in the metabolic deamination of amphetamine. Life Sci. *20*, 467–474 (1977b)
Wu, P.H., Boulton, A.A.: Distribution, metabolism, and disappearance of intraventricularly injected p-tyramine in the rat. Can. J. Biochem. *52*, 374–381 (1974)
Youdim, M.B.H., Carter, S.B., Sandler, M., Hamington, E., Wilkinson, M.: Conjugation defect in tyramine-sensitive migraine. Nature *230*, 127–128 (1971)
Young, R.L., Gordon, M.W.: The disposition of 14 C-amphetamine in rat brain. J. Neurochem. *9*, 161–167 (1962)

CHAPTER 3

Kinetics and Biotransformation of Adrenergic Inhibitors *

A.J. Smith and G.T. Tucker

Introduction

Any attempt to review the current state of knowledge in rapidly changing fields of pharmacology is faced with the common problem of all expanding areas – knowledge has advanced so fast in such a short time that good work completed as little as 10 years ago may now be rendered completely out of date. Although concepts change fairly rapidly, it is supremely technological advance that has transformed our understanding of the biotransformation and kinetics of drugs in all species. Twenty years ago the ability to detect very small quantities of drugs in biological fluids was strictly limited. The developments in gas–liquid and high pressure liquid chromatography and the application of the mass spectrometer to the identification of drug metabolites has now put certainty into many areas that were previously uncertain. With technological advance comes inevitable conceptual change. Perhaps one of the best examples of this in the context of adrenergic inhibitory drugs is the change in our appreciation of the handling of reserpine. Twenty years ago, reserpine was categorically a "hit and run" drug, that is, it could be detected, whether in humans or in animals, only for a very brief while after administration, yet its pharmacological effects clearly were prolonged. Dogma stated that the drug affected its target organ by dealing a lightning blow but the recovery from that onslaught had to continue for days or weeks after the drug had left the organism. It is clear now in retrospect that techniques for measuring both reserpine and its metabolites were simply not adequate, that reserpine enters a deep store in adrenergic vesicles and that there is no need to postulate persistence of action beyond the physical presence of the drug in the biological system. In a similar way, the significance of plasma half-lives of drugs is fraught with hazard if detection of the drug in plasma is virtually impossible after a few hours from administration. Some drugs may disappear rapidly from plasma but persist, perhaps covalently bound, in selected loci. The ability to measure minute amounts of drug or metabolites is the key to cause and effect in this situation.

Criteria for Selection of Drugs

The term "adrenergic inhibitor," if interpreted widely, could include many compounds not normally utilised primarily to alter adrenergic function. We have confined ourselves to agents conventionally used, either experimentally or in therapy, to modify

* This review covers the literature up to April/May, 1978

adrenergic activity by a direct action on the sympathetic nervous system at some point. For example, while compounds modifying α-receptor function are included, direct vasodilators which alter adrenergic function indirectly are not considered.

Definitions

We take "kinetics" to involve the mathematical description and prediction of the time-course of the absorption and disposition (distribution and elimination) of drugs in the organism. Aspects of the "local kinetics" of drugs at sites of action are outside the scope of this article. "Biotransformation" involves metabolic modification of drugs in the biological system, normally, but not always, rendering them more readily eliminated from the organism.

Each drug is considered under a set of standard sub-headings. Absence of such headings and associated discussion for a particular compound implies that we have been unable to find appropriate data.

We have also been careful to make a distinction between the terms "bioavailability" and "systemic availability", although this is not always done in the literature. The former refers to the fraction of an oral dose reaching the systemic circulation as intact drug and is defined as the ratio of the area under the plasma drug concentration versus time curve after an oral dose to the area after a reference i.v. dose or defined as the ratio of the fract ion of the dose excreted unchanged in the urine (f_u) after oral administration to that excreted after i.v. injection. Systemic availability is defined as the fraction of the amount of unchanged drug entering the portal vein after oral administration that reaches the systemic circulation intact. As such, this definition does not encompass the possibility of drug metabolism in the gut wall. (This is a simplifying assumption that allows the use of the equations indicated below). Hence, bioavailability becomes the product of the dose that reaches the portal circulation as intact drug (defined as f, the fraction of the dose absorbed) and the systemic availability. The latter is derived by calculation, either from i.v. or from oral blood drug concentration data by assuming a value for hepatic blood flow.

Thus, from i.v. data, systemic availability is given by $(1-Cl_h/Q)$ and from oral data by $fQ/(Q+f\cdot\text{dose/area})$ (GIBALDI et al., 1971), where Q is hepatic blood flow and Cl_h is hepatic drug clearance (i.e., dose $_{\text{i.v.}}$/area$_{\text{i.v.}}$). These equations are corrected, when necessary, for renal drug clearance.

As a crude indication of drug absorption rate after oral administration the time to maximum plasma drug concentration, $t_{\max}$, is quoted. The elimination half-life ($t_{1/2}$) has been described also in terms of the fast or "distribution" half-life ($t_{1/2\alpha}$) and the slow or "elimination" half-life ($t_{1/2\beta}$). The term V_I is the apparent volume of the central compartment; Vd_{ss} is the volume of distribution at steady state, and Vd_β is the apparent volume of distribution after pseudo distribution equilibrium. The fraction of total drug in plasma that is bound to plasma proteins is designated by f_p and λ represents the ratio of whole blood to plasma drug concentration.

I. Methyldopa

L-3,4-Dihydroxy-α-methylphenylalanine

1. Absorption

a) Extent. Values for fraction absorbed are shown in Table 1.

b) Rate. Values of t_{max} after single oral doses of 250–1,000 mg range from 2 to 4 h (GILLESPIE et al., 1962; SJOERDSMA et al., 1963; BARNETT et al., 1977; STENBAEK et al., 1977).

c) Mechanism. Methyldopa is an L-α-amino acid. The urinary excretion of oral D-methyldopa was 20% that of the L-isomer in rats although no difference in excretion occurred after i.p. dosing (YOUNG and EDWARDS, 1964). Two human subjects excreted less than 16% of an oral dose of D-α-methyldopa but 39% and 41%, respectively, of L-α-methyldopa (AU et al., 1972). These findings suggest stereoselective intestinal absorption which may utilise an active transport process for amino acids. The early results of SJOERDSMA et al. (1963) are compatible with this hypothesis.

Table 1. α-Methyldopa – extent of absorption[a]. Minimum values for fraction (f) absorbed (^{14}C-studies[b] or assays of drug plus metabolites)

Authors	Oral dose (mg)	f (range or mean)	No. of subjects	Duration of Study (h)
GILLESPIE et al. (1962)	1,000	0.07–0.19	6	24
SJOERDSMA et al. (1963)	500	0.12–0.17	3	24
BUHS et al. (1964)	–[c]	0.23–0.46	5	48
PRESCOTT et al. (1966)	500	0.15–0.74	6	48
AU et al. (1972)	250	0.39–0.60	14	24
STENBAEK et al. (1977)	500	≃0.40	5	48

[a] Interpretation of these data may be complicated as authors have not always stated whether L-Methyldopa or the racemic mixture was administered. D-Methyldopa is very poorly absorbed (see e.g., AU et al., 1972)

[b] Included only if faecal plus urinary recovery of label ≧80%

[c] ^{14}C-Labelled drug interpolated in maintenance regime

2. Distribution

a) Blood. Radiolabelled methyldopa in plasma was completely dialysable through a cellulose membrane suggesting negligible plasma binding (BUHS et al., 1964). No protein binding was found by MYHRE et al. (1972).

b) Tissues. In rats after i.p. [^{14}C]methyldopa, radioactivity was distributed early to the kidneys, small amounts were found in lung, heart, and muscle. After 24 h, amounts in all tissues had declined but both kidney and liver maintained detectable quantities (PORTER and TITUS, 1963). It seems probable that there is a stereoselective transport mechanism determining the access of i.p. α-methyldopa to the rat brain. The D-isomer is neither a substrate for brain decarboxylases nor does it readily enter brain tissue (AMES et al., 1977).

3. Biotransformation

a) Sites. Sulphation to α-methyldopa-mono-O-sulphate probably occurs during absorption in the intestinal wall (SAAVEDRA et al., 1975). Peripheral decarboxylation is not essential for the hypotensive action of α-methyldopa in man (KERSTING et al.,

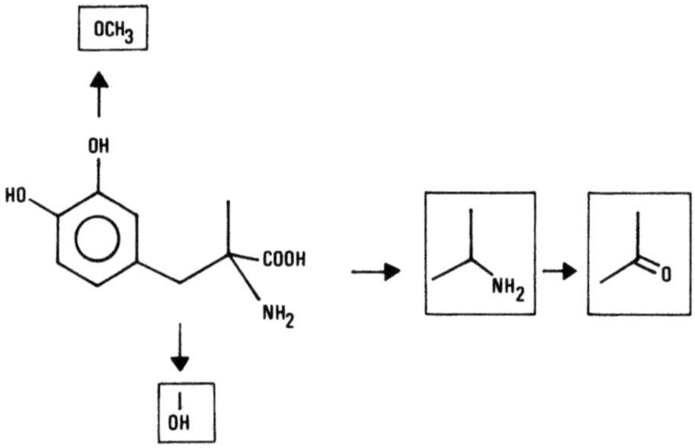

Fig. 1. Structure of α-methyldopa and metabolic products

1977; PLANZ et al., 1977) but stereospecific decarboxylation occurs in the brain of rats (AMES et al., 1977). The hepatotoxicity of methyldopa may relate to its oxidation in liver to a semiquinone and/or quinone derivative (DYBING, 1977). The ability of both rat and human liver microsomes to metabolise α-methyldopa to a covalently binding oxidative product has been demonstrated in vitro (DYBING et al., 1976).

b) Routes. Metabolism occurs through the pathway common to the catecholamines (Fig. 1) utilising Dopa decarboxylases and dopamine β-hydroxylase (CARLSSON and LINDQVIST, 1962). Decarboxylation is stereospecific (SJOERDSMA et al., 1963; AMES et al., 1977). O-Methylation (catechol-O-methyltransferase) and sulphation are quantitatively important routes (AU et al., 1972). The phenyl-ketone metabolite (3-4-dihydroxyphenylacetone) has been identified both in the rat (PORTER and TITUS, 1963) and in human subjects (AU et al., 1972).

c) Activity of Metabolites. α-Methyldopa is believed to produce its hypotensive effect through its centrally active metabolites, α-methyldopamine and α-methylnoradrenaline (GILLESPIE et al., 1962; FINCH and HÄEUSLER, 1973). α-Methyldopamine, when given orally or intramuscularly to hypertensive patients, failed to reduce blood pressure (BUHS et al., 1964), but may not gain access readily to the central nervous system. MYRHE et al. (1972) have suggested that methyldopa-O-sulphate may be pharmacologically active as a hypotensive agent. The possibility of the hepatic production of arylating metabolites responsible for hepatotoxicity has been referred to above. Methyldopa and methylnoradrenaline may inhibit melanocyte-stimulating hormone activity in the frog – an effect antagonised by pretreatment with phentolamine (PETTINGER, 1977).

4. Excretion

a) Routes. Virtually all the radioactivity of an i.v. dose of [^{14}C]methyldopa was recovered from human urine in 48 h, approximately 50% as unchanged drug (STENBAEK et al., 1977) (Table 2). The renal clearance of total radioactivity averaged 0.15 l/min and of unconjugated methyldopa 0.12 l/min. These clearances were slightly greater than creatinine clearance in four out of the five volunteer subjects. These data contradict those obtained by the same group earlier (MYRHE et al., 1972) when they studied renal clearance after intravenous dosing and suggested substantial extra-renal clear-

Table 2. Principal urinary derivatives detectable after administration of [C^{14}] α-methyldopa

Study	Species	Method	α-MD[a]	α-MD-SO_4[b]	3-O-Me-α-MD[c]	Phenyl-acetone and conjugates	α-MDA[d]	3-O-Me-α-MDA[e]	Conjugates (uncharac-terised)
GILLESPIE et al. (1962)	Man	Unlabellec, oral	+				+		+
SJOERDSMA et al. (1963)	Man	C^{14}+ unlabelled	+		+		+	+	+
PORTER and TITUS (1963)	Rat	C^{14}, i.p.	+	Likely	+	+	+	+	
YOUNG and EDWARDS (1964)	Rat	Unlabellec, i.p.	+		+		+	+	
BUHS et al. (1964)	Man	C^{14}, oral	+	+	+		+		
PRESCOTT et al. (1966)	Man	C^{14}, oral	+	+	+				
AU et al. (1972)	Man	C^{14}, oral	+	?	+	+	+	+	

[a] α-MD = α-Methyldopa
[b] α-MD-SO_4 = α-Methyldopa-mono-O-sulphate
[c] 3-o-Me-α-MD = 3-O-Methyl-alpha-methyldopa
[d] α-MDA = α-Methyldopamine
[e] 3-o-Me-α-MDA = 3-O-Methyl-alpha-methyldopamine
+ = Derivatives positively identigied in urine

ance of methyldopa. KWAN et al. (1976) found the mean proportions of unchanged drug plus conjugate excreted after i.v. doses in 12 subjects to be 66% of that administered, with less than 2% in the conjugated form – a finding that would be expected if the mono-O-sulphate is generated during absorptive transit through the gut wall. These authors argue, from evidence of prolonged absorption of methyldopa and of greater fractional recovery of conjugates after repeated dosing, that there is probably significant biliary (?gut) excretion of methyldopa with an enterohepatic (?entero-entero) circulation. Billiary excretion of methyldopa and a metabolite has been demonstrated in the rat (YOUNG and EDWARDS, 1964).

b) Mechanisms. Renal clearance rates close to glomerular filtration rate do not demand specialised tubular transport systems for methyldopa. However, amino-aciduria occurred consistently in rats given L-methyldopa (and not with D-methyldopa; YOUNG and EDWARDS, 1964). This may indicate competition by methyldopa (or its metabolites) for tubular reabsorption sites for natural amino acids.

5. Pharmacokinetics

a) Intravenous. BARNETT et al. (1977) fitted plasma data for five normal subjects to a biexponential function. They found a total plasma clearance rate of 11.2±0.6 l/h, $t_{1/2\beta}$ of 2.84±1.3 h, and V_1 ("central" compartment) of 20.2±1.5 l. KWAN et al. (1976) using the same model in 12 subjects found a mean plasma clearance of 13.2 l/h (renal clearance 5.7 l/h), $t_{1/2\beta}$ 1.77±0.2 h and V_1 of 15.7±3.5 l. STENBAEK et al. (1977) measured a mean plasma clearance of 13.7 l/h renal clearance 7.9 l/h and V_1 19.3 l (three subjects).

b) Oral. BARNETT et al. (1977) recorded a mean terminal half-life for methyldopa of 2.12±0.71 h in four normal subjects after oral administration of a 500 mg dose. A mean renal clearance of 7.95 l/h was calculated by KWAN et al. (1976).

c) Effects of Disease. Linear correlations were found between the α-methyldopa elimination rate constant and glomerular filtration rate (positive) and serum creatinine level (negative) in patients with renal failure (SCHRADER et al., 1971).

6. Concentration–Effect Relationships

It might not be expected that a correlation would exist between effect and plasma concentration of a drug presumed to act through a centrally active metabolite. BARNETT et al. (1977) in a steady-state study and AU et al. (1972) found no such correlation and the latter authors could offer no explanation for failure of hypotensive effect in the presence of normal plasma concentrations of α-methyldopa. One contrary report describes a good correlation between the steady-state concentration of continuously infused α-methyldopa in conscious monkeys and a fall in mean systolic blood pressure (WALSON et al., 1976).

II. Clonidine

2-(2,6-Dichlorophenylamino)-2-imidazoline

1. Absorption

a) Extent. Calculated bioavailability averaged 0.75 in the study of DAVIES et al. (1977) in five normal subjects. Between 65% and 95% of the administered radioactivity was excreted after oral [^{14}C]clonidine in human subjects and high recoveries were also obtained in monkey, dog, guinea pig and rat (REHBINDER, 1970). An average 72% of administered radioactivity was excreted in the urine of nine subjects over 4 days after a single oral dose (DARDA, 1975).

b) Rate. Time to peak plasma concentration was $1^1/_2$ h in both normotensive and hypertensive fasting subjects (DOLLERY et al., 1976; WING et al., 1977), but 3 h in 10 normal volunteers who received single doses of 300 µg after food (DARDA, 1975). Peak concentrations were reached 30 min after oral dosing in fasting rats (DARDA, 1975).

2. Distribution

a) Blood. The f_p ranges from 0.56 to 0.38 in vitro with an apparent concentration dependence (CHO and CURRY, 1969).

b) Tissues. Uptake of radioactivity is higher in cat salivary gland than in muscle or heart and is pH dependent (CHO and CURRY, 1969). Rat brain concentrates clonidine after oral, intravenous, and i.c. injection, highest concentrations appearing between 1 and 2 h after the oral dose (DARDA, 1975).

3. Biotransformation

a) Routes. HODGES (1976) reported 2-6-dichlorophenylguanidine as a metabolite in the urine of rat and dog – a product formed by bis-n-dealkylation (Fig. 2). REHBINDER (1970) demonstrated the presence of 17 separate chromatographic spots which may be metabolites in urine from monkey, rat, and man. Parahydroxyclonidine and its conjugates were positively identified.

Six radioactive substances isolated from the urine of dog, rat and man have been identified as unchanged clonidine, parahydroxyclonidine, and 2-6-dichlorophenylguanidine as principal compounds and in addition 1-(2,6-dichloro-4-hydroxyphenyl)-guanidine, 2-[(2,6-dichlorophenyl)-imino]-imidazoline-4-one and 2-[(2,6-dichloro-4-hydroxyphenyl)-imino]-imidazoline-4-one (DARDA, 1975; DARDA et al., 1978). Cleavage of the imidazolidine ring and hydroxylation of the phenyl ring are thus the two principal metabolic routes. Unchanged clonidine is the preponderant compound in human urine.

b) Activity of Metabolites. 2,6-Dichlorophenylguanidine possesses weak antihypertensive activity in the dog and rat (JEN et al., 1975). Parahydroxyclonidine also may have hypotensive activity (ERHARDT, 1972).

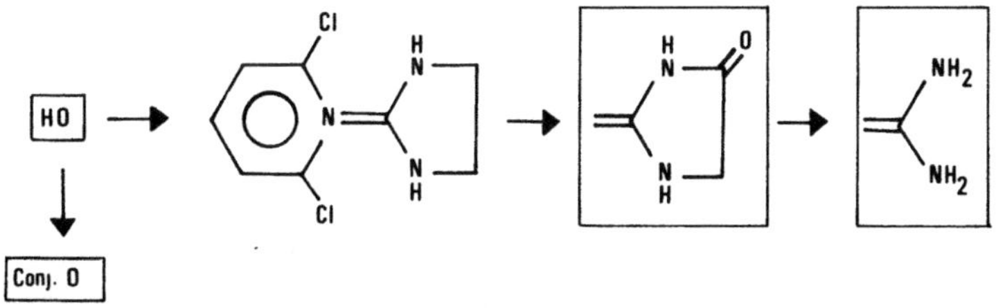

Fig. 2. Structure of clonidine and metabolic products

4. Excretion

a) Routes. A major route of elimination is renal (REHBINDER, 1970; DARDA, 1975) but biliary excretion and enterohepatic recirculation occur in rats (GUNDERT-REMY and WEBER, 1976) and non-renal clearance was approximately 40% of total body plasma clearance in normal human subjects.

b) Mechanism. Renal excretion of clonidine appears to be unrelated to urinary pH and in some normal subjects exceeded glomerular filtration rate suggesting tubular secretion as well as filtration (DAVIES et al., 1977).

5. Pharmacokinetics

a) Intravenous. DAVIES et al. (1977) used a two-compartment open model to derive a $t_{1/2\beta}$ of 8.5±0.9 h, a Vd_{ss} of 2.09±0.19 l/kg and a total plasma clearance of 3.05±0.54 ml/min/kg in normal subjects given i.v. clonidine. Renal (plasma) clearance averaged 1.82±0.34 ml/min/kg.

b) Oral. The $t_{1/2\beta}$ after oral dosing was 8.6±1.5 h. In five hypertensive patients, $t_{1/2\beta}$ was 10.0±0.8 h after oral clonidine (WING et al., 1977). A similar elimination $t_{1/2}$ was described by DARDA (1975).

6. Concentration–Effect Relationships

Reduced salivary flow, believed to be a central effect (RAND et al., 1969), correlated with plasma clonidine concentrations in normal and hypertensive subjects. Sedation correlated only in trained normal subjects. Fall in blood pressure correlated with plasma clonidine concentration up to approximately 2 ng/ml. At higher levels the relationship was lost – possibly due to peripheral postsynaptic α-agonist effects (DAVIES et al., 1977; WING et al., 1977).

III. 6-Hydroxydopamine

Recent comprehensive reviews of the pharmacology of 6-hydroxydopamine (6-OH-DA) have been prepared by THOENEN and TRANZER (1973), KOSTRZEWA and JACOBOWITZ (1974), and SACHS and JONSSON (1975). This compound and the related 6-hydroxydopa and 6-aminodopamine have been used almost exclusively as experimental tools. Most of the reports available deal with the pharmacodynamics of the compounds which are usually administered i.v., i.p., i.c. or into the cerebral ventricles. For this reason data are not available under many of the headings used for other compounds in this review.

1. Distribution

a) Tissues. Selective uptake into adrenergic neurones has been recorded by many authors (TRANZER and THOENEN, 1968; SIGGINS and BLOOM, 1970). 6-OHDA competes with noradrenaline at its uptake site (JONSSON and SACHS, 1971) and may be prevented from gaining access to its site of action by compounds including tricyclic antidepressants, chlorpromazine, and cocaine (STONE et al., 1964; CREVELING et al., 1967; BREESE and TRAYLOR, 1971). Inside the neurone, 6-OHDA is concentrated in the amine-storage granules and noradrenaline content falls rapidly – a process which, together with the ultrastructural lesions, is dose-dependent (JONSSON and SACHS, 1971). There is a decreasing order of tissue susceptibility to 6-OHDA from cardiac ventricles through salivary gland, spleen, atria, and blood vessels to adrenal glands whose noradrenaline content is virtually unaffected (KOSTRZEWA and JACOBOWITZ, 1974).

The rate of 6-OHDA uptake varies with tissue and species but functional effects were noted as early as 30 min after i.v. injection in cats (HÄEUSLER, 1971). Uptake of ^{14}C-labelled 6-OHDA into rat heart was rapid after i.v. injection with evidence of continuing concentration of label/gm tissue to six times that in plasma after 60 min. Brain concentrations were low over the period, suggesting poor brain penetrability of 6-OH-DA from the systemic circulation (GARVER et al., 1975). Uptake outside neuronal tissue (muscle and gland cells in octopus salivary gland, adrenocortical cells of lizards and rats) has been recorded (MARTIN and BARLOW, 1975; UNSICKER et al., 1976).

2. Biotransformation

a) Sites. As 6-OHDA is selectively and almost exclusively taken up into noradrenergic neurones, this is the site of almost all of its metabolic transformation.

b) Routes. 6-OHDA appears to be a substrate for both catechol-o-methyl transferase and monoamine oxidases (JONSSON et al., 1972) but their levels are little altered after its administration (URETSKY and IVERSEN, 1970). Much work has been directed to establishing through which metabolites 6-OHDA exerts its destructive action on adrenergic neurones (Fig. 3).

Two alternative hypotheses are current. 6-OHDA may form highly reactive quinones which can undergo covalent, irreversible binding to nucleophilic groups of proteins (ADAMS et al., 1972; SANER and THOENEN, 1971). Binding between the 1,4-p-quinone and sulphydryl groups may produce protein cross-linking (ROTMAN et al., 1976). The time-course of binding in adrenergic nerves parallels the neurotoxic action of 6-OHDA expressed as inhibition of [^{3}H]noradrenaline uptake (JONSSON, 1976). The reaction product of oxidized 6-OHDA and glutathione has been characterised in the laboratory and also identified in rat brain after injection of 6-OHDA (LIANG et al., 1977). The alternative (or complementary) hypothesis postulates that hydrogen peroxide and superoxide and hydroxyl radicals formed during oxidation of 6-OHDA damage the tissues (HEIKKILA and COHEN, 1972, 1973). Evidence weakening this case

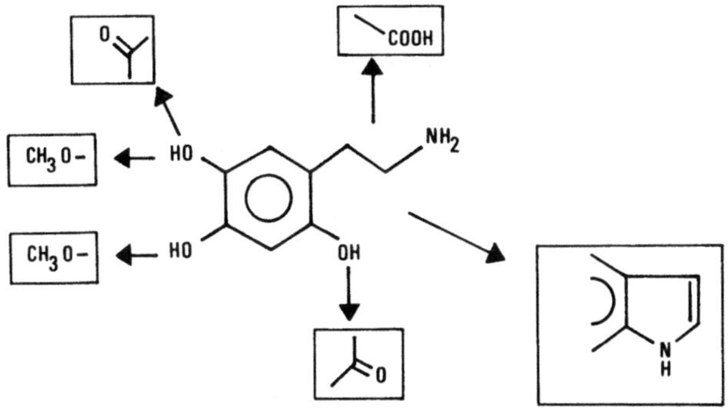

Fig. 3. Structure of 6-hydroxydopamine and metabolic products

was presented by LIANG et al. (1977) but protection from the action by thiourea derivatives (COHEN et al., 1976) would appear to be compatible with either a hydroxyl radical scavenging function or binding of 6-OHDA paraquinone. Intracyclisation of the initial oxidative reaction products of 6-OHDA occurs readily to yield 5,6-dihydroxyindole. This process may be one of the limiting factors to tissue toxicity (BLANK et al., 1976).

IV. Reserpine

3,4,5-Trimethoxybenzoyl-methyl reserpate

A recent full review of the biological fate of reserpine was prepared by STITZEL (1977).

1. Absorption

a) Extent. The very slow elimination of reserpine and metabolites in the urine after oral dosing makes estimates of absorption from such data minimum values only. Between 30%–40% of oral [^{14}C]reserpine given to mice was recovered in urine in 4 h and 93% in 24 h (NUMEROF et al., 1955). In six normal male volunteers, an estimated 30% of administered reserpine was observed (assuming distribution throughout extracellular water); this figure correlating with a mean faecal recovery of 62% radiolabel over 96 h in the same group (MAASS et al., 1969).

b) Rate. Maximum rat tissue concentrations occurred at 2–4 h (GLAZKO et al., 1956). A t_{max} value of 2–4 h was found in psychiatric patients (NUMEROF et al., 1958) and of 1–3 h in normal male volunteers (MAASS et al., 1969). Similar values were found in two subjects by TRIPP et al. (1975).

2. Distribution

a) Blood. A λ value of 1.6 was found at peak plasma concentrations which increased to more than 5 at 70 h as a result of persistent binding of radiolabel to erythrocytes (MAASS et al., 1969). Tight binding to mouse erythrocytes was reported by NUMEROF et al. (1955). Blood platelets accumulate reserpine apparently by both non-specific and specific processes. Irreversible specific binding occurs to 5-hydroxytryptamine granules and could be used as a marker for platelet survival. Early uptake into platelets can be prevented by imipramine (ENNA et al., 1974).

b) Tissues. Peak concentrations of reserpine and methyl reserpate in rat tissues occurred at 2–4 h after oral dosing. Distribution was highest in lung, liver, kidney, spleen, and heart and lowest in brain and fat: at 30 h, brain concentrations had risen and were of the same order as in other tissues (GLAZKO et al., 1956). Similar findings with slightly different time courses were reported by SHEPPARD et al. (1955, 1957). Reserpine was concentrated to a greater extent in rat peritoneal mast cells than in leucocytes. The binding was localised to amine storage granules (GRIPENBERG and JANSSON, 1971).

3. Biotransformation

a) Sites. Hydrolysis of reserpine may occur in the intestinal wall before absorption and active esterases have been isolated from intestinal mucosa of rat but not of dog

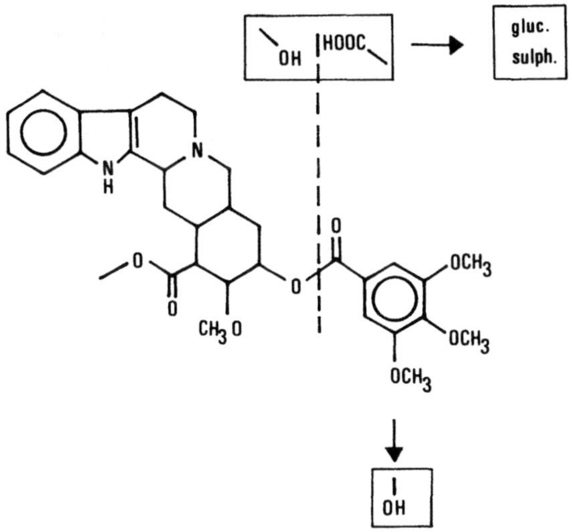

Fig. 4. Structure of reserpine and metabolic products

or monkey. Hydrolysis may be greater in intestine than in liver under aerobic conditions (GLAZKO et al., 1956; SHEPPARD et al., 1957). Esteratic activity was high in guinea-pig liver microsomes but not in rat; oxidative attack (oxidative demethylation of trimethoxybenzoic acid, TMBA) was greater in rat liver than in guinea-pig liver (SHEPPARD and TSIEN, 1955). However, these were in vitro results and relative distribution of reserpine to metabolic sites may be as important in vivo as specific enzyme activities.

b) Routes. Preferred metabolic routes appear to exist for different species (Fig. 4, Table 3). Hydrolysis to TMBA and methyl-reserpate and oxidation of the 4-methyl group of TMBA have both been recognised as primary routes of metabolism in mice, rats, and guinea-pigs (NUMEROF et al., 1955; SHEPPARD et al., 1955; SHEPPARD and TSIEN, 1955; GLAZKO et al., 1956; SHEPPARD et al., 1957). SHEPPARD et al. (1957) detected a urinary metabolite having the characteristic of syringoyl methyl-reserpate suggesting that the rat is capable of oxidizing the 4-methoxy carbon of TMBA before hydrolysis. In man, unchanged reserpine, TMBA and TMBA conjugates (glucuronide and sulphate) have been detected in urine (MAASS et al., 1969; ZSOTÉR et al., 1973) although TMBA administered to rats was excreted unchanged and unconjugated in the study of NUMEROF et al. (1955).

c) Rate. The V_{max} value for hepatic reserpine metabolism was twice as high in adult as in infant rats (MUELLER and SHIDEMAN, 1968).

4. Excretion

a) Routes. Small quantities of unchanged reserpine are excreted by the kidney. After parenteral dosing, faecal excretion of radiolabel amounted to 10% in one study (SHEPPARD et al., 1957), suggesting biliary or intestinal secretion of parent drug or metabolites. In man, a mean 7.9% of oral radiolabel was excreted in the urine of six healthy subjects in 96 h; 61.9% was found in the faeces over the same period (MAASS et al., 1969).

Table 3. Detection of reserpine metabolites

Study	Species: Compound: Route	Samples analysed	Res[a]	MeRes[b]	TMBA[c]	Other
NUMEROF et al. (1955)	Mice: [^{14}C]-reserpine: i.v. and oral	Urine (24 h) Faeces	 + + i.v. > oral		+ + +[d]	
SHEPPARD et al. (1955)	Rat: [^{14}C] reserpine: i.v.	Urine (6 h)	+ +		+	$^{14}CO_2$
SHEPPARD and TSIEN (1955)	Dog/rat/mouse/pigeon/guinea pig: [^{14}C]reserpine: liver slices	Incubation mixture	+ +		+ + +	$^{14}CO_2$
GLAZKO et al. (1956)	Rat: Chronic oral dosing	Urine (4-day)		+ + +		
SHEPPARD et al. (1957)	(a) Guinea pig/rat: [^{14}C]reserpine: i.v. (methoxy- or carboxy-label)	Urine (6 h) Faeces	± + +		+ + +	
	(b) Rat: [^{14}C]reserpine: liver and intestinal slices	Incubation mixture	+ +		+ +	Syringoyl methyl reserpate
MAAS et al. (1969)	Six human subjects: [^{3}H]-reserpine: single oral dose	Urine (24 h)	+		+ + +	
ZSOTÉR et al. (1973)	15 patients – varying renal function: [^{3}H]reserpine: i.m.	Urine and faeces (7 das)	+ (Urine and faeces)		+ +	TMBA glucuronide and sulphate in urine

[a] Res = Reserpine
[b] MeRes = Methylreserpate
[c] TMBA = Trimethoxybenzoic acid
[d] + = Positively identified; + + and + + + indicate relative amount

b) Effect of Disease. A correlation was found between urinary excretion of total radioactivity, plasma $t_{1/2\beta}$ and creatinine clearance in 15 patients with renal function varying from normal to grossly impaired (ZSOTÉR et al., 1973).

5. Pharmacokinetics

The difficulty of assaying unchanged reserpine in plasma has led to estimates of kinetic parameters mainly based on total radioactivity measurements. Plasma elimination $t_{1/2}$ was estimated as 11.5–16 days (MAASS et al., 1969) in normal man, which accords with the finding of detectable plasma radioactivity in the blood of schizophrenic patients up to 6 weeks after administration of labelled drug (NUMEROF et al., 1958). Values from approximately 60–320 h were reported with differing renal function (ZSOTÉR et al., 1973).

V. Bethanidine

1-Benzyl-2,3-dimethylguanidine

1. Absorption

a) Extent. In man, urinary recoveries of unchanged bethanidine after single oral doses are reported as virtually 100% at 24 h from 0.5 mg (DOYLE and MORLEY, 1965), 71%–85% at 4 days from 10 mg (CHREMOS et al., 1976; TURNBULL et al., 1976), 48%–61% at 3–4 days from 25 mg (SHEN et al., 1975), and 48%–79% at 24 h from 30 mg (DRING et al., 1977). Furthermore, on splitting a single 25 mg dose into 6 hourly fractions, the recovery increased to 72%–74% (SHEN et al., 1975). Since bethanidine is not metabolised in man (see below), these data indicate that the extent of oral absorption of the drug decreases with increase in dose.

Estimates of bioavailability based upon a comparison of urinary drug recoveries after 25 mg oral and i.v. doses were 0.52–0.68 and 0.76–0.80 mg for single and divided doses, respectively (SHEN et al., 1975).

In fasting cats, BOURA et al. (1962) recovered 54% of ^{14}C labelled bethanidine in the urine after 7 days, decreasing to 30% in fed animals. Urinary recoveries of radioactivity in rats and dogs were 29%–34% and 83%–89%, respectively, of an oral dose after 4 days (TURNBULL et al., 1976).

b) Rate. Maximum blood drug concentrations after 10 mg oral doses were observed 2–4 h after administration, suggesting relatively rapid absorption (CHREMOS et al., 1976).

2. Distribution

a) Blood. At a concentration of 1 μg/ml, less than 8% of bethanidine is bound to crystalline human albumin (SHEN et al., 1975). Distribution between cellular elements of blood and plasma has not been investigated.

b) Tissues. Consistent with the high polarity of bethanidine, autoradiography and direct estimation of tissue levels of ^{14}C-labelled drug showed that little, if any, penetrates the blood–brain barrier in animals (BOURA et al., 1962; TURNBULL et al., 1976). High drug concentrations are localised in tissues rich in adrenergic nerve terminals.

3. Biotransformation

a) Routes. With the exception of trace amounts of hippuric acid, no metabolites of bethanidine have been detected in man (MCCOUBREY, 1962; SHEN et al., 1975; CHREMOS et al., 1976; TURNBULL et al., 1976; DRING et al., 1977). In contrast, the drug is metabolised in rat and dog to a significant degree (TURNBULL et al., 1976). Thus, in the rat it is mono-N-demethylated, ring-hydroxylated and conjugated and the benzyl group is cleaved off. In the dog, both N-methyl groups are removed as well as the benzyl group, but there is no evidence of ring-hydroxylation (Fig. 5, Table 4).

b) Drug Interactions. An increase in whole rat concentrations of [^{3}H]bethanidine after pretreatment with desipramine observed by MITCHELL et al. (1970) was explained by inhibition of metabolism. However, the same workers could find no evidence of bethanidine metabolism by cell fractions of rat liver in vitro.

4. Excretion

a) Routes. Bethanidine is predominantly excreted unchanged in the urine of man and animals, the remainder appearing unchanged in the faeces (SHEN et al., 1975; CHREMOS et al., 1976; TURNBULL et al., 1976). A low recovery of bethanidine in rat bile suggests

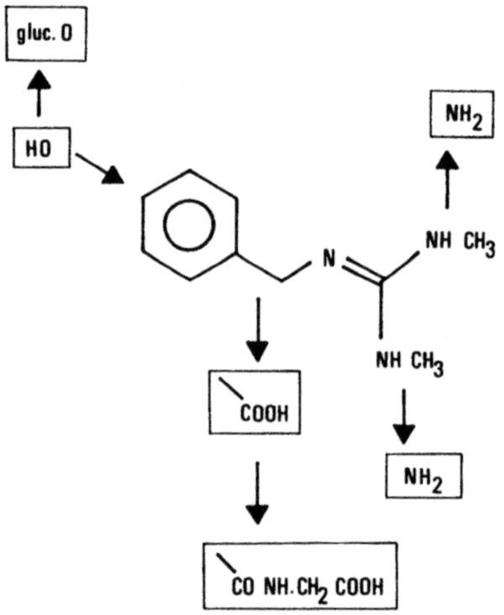

Fig. 5. Structure of bethanidine and metabolic products

Table 4. Urinary metabolites of bethanidine in dog and rat (% of total amount recovered in 24 h – TURNBULL et al., 1976)

	Dog	Rat
Bethanidine	23	48
1-Benzylguanidine	35	–
1-Benzyl-2-methylguanidine	7	9
Benzoic acid	3	–
Hippuric acid	25	9
Hydroxybenzyl-2-methyl-guanidine glucuronide	–	12
Hydroxybenzyl-2,3-dimethyl-guanidine glucuronide	–	25

that faecal drug represents mostly unabsorbed drug (TURNBULL et al., 1976). Renal clearance (blood) values in man indicate that bethanidine is excreted by both glomerular filtration and by tubular secretion. In two hypertensive patients, steady-state urinary drug excretion rates showed a diurnal rhythm, possibly related to diurnal variation of blood pressure and plasma volume (SHEN et al., 1975). DOYLE and MORLEY (1965) found a direct relationship between 24 h urinary recovery of bethanidine and creatinine clearance in 33 patients.

5. Pharmacokinetics

a) Intravenous. After i.v. injection of 25 mg bethanidine in three hypertensive patients, plasma drug concentration versus time and urinary excretion rate versus time curves were described by triexponential equations (SHEN et al., 1975). However, the terminal $t_{1/2}$ from urinary data (7–11 h) was significantly shorter than that from plasma data, reflecting a progressive decrease in renal drug clearance.

b) Oral. After a 10 mg oral dose in three human subjects, terminal $t_{1/2}$ values were found to be 7–11 h from urine data and 17–20 h from blood data (TURNBULL et al., 1976). Again there was evidence of decreasing renal clearance with time, the data suggesting also that the change was independent of drug concentration and unaccompanied by any hypotensive response (TURNBULL et al., 1976; CHREMOS et al., 1976). A possible explanation for this phenomenon may be a decrease in renal blood flow mediated by initial intra-renal release of catecholamines. Steady-state urinary excretion rates of bethanidine were found to be consistent with predictions based upon single oral dose data (SHEN et al., 1975).

c) Drug Interactions. When two patients were given imipramine 2 days prior to a 25 mg oral dose of bethanidine, the terminal $t_{1/2}$ of the urinary excretion rate profiles was 30%–40% shorter than in the same patients when not given imipramine (SHEN et al., 1975). This is consistent with a decrease in the volume of distribution owing to antagonism of bethanidine uptake at adrenergic nerve endings, although effects of imipramine on non-specific tissue uptake and renal clearance cannot be excluded.

6. Concentration–Effect Relationships

DRING et al. (1977) reported an absence of any correlation between the kinetics of bethanidine and hypotensive response after single oral doses. However, noradrenaline release after initial challenge with bethanidine would tend to obscure any relationships, and their conclusion that differences in inter-individual response to the drug are independent of its fate may have to be modified when more extensive studies are done in patients during chronic therapy.

VI. Debrisoquine

3,4-Dihydro-2-(1 *H*)-isoquinolone carboxamidine

1. Absorption

a) Extent. Urinary recoveries of ^{14}C-label over the 24 h after various oral doses of debrisoquine in man range from 70%–90%, indicating extensive absorption (SCHWARTZ and BAUKEMA, 1966; ALLEN et al., 1975; ANGELO et al., 1976; SILAS, 1978).

b) Rate. Maximum plasma debrisoquine concentrations and urinary excretion rates occur at about 2 h after oral administration, indicating rapid absorption. Food delays absorption but does not affect its extent (SILAS et al., 1978 a)

2. Distribution

a) Blood. Human plasma binding of debrisoquine is about 20% at therapeutic concentrations (Roche – personal communication). Debrisoquine has a remarkable affinity for the human platelet in vivo. Thus, platelet/plasma concentration ratios of the drug vary from 400: 1 to 1,600: 1 as plasma drug concentrations decrease, reflecting an avid, saturable uptake process (LENNARD et al., 1977). Accordingly, platelet-rich plasma concentrations of debrisoquine are also much higher than those in platelet-poor plasma, the ratio increasing to 15: 1 at 36 h after dosage (SILAS et al., 1978 a). Erythrocyte/plasma (platelet-poor) concentration ratios of debrisoquine in man are about 0.8, consistent with an f_p value of 0.20 and a lack of significant binding to the red cell (SILAS, 1978). Whole blood concentrations of the drug tend to parallel those in platelet-rich plasma such that λ, determined with respect to normal platelet-poor plasma, increases with time after dose (SILAS et al., 1978 a).

b) Tissues. Uptake of debrisoquine by the brain is negligible but it is localised in the spleen and heart, both of which are particularly well-supplied by adrenergic nerves (MEDINA et al., 1969).

3. Biotransformation

a) Routes. Semiquantitative studies of the metabolism of debrisoquine in man, dog, and rat provided evidence for both alicyclic and aromatic hydroxylation but not for alteration of the amidino group (ALLEN et al., 1975; ANGELO et al., 1976) (Fig. 6). The 4-hydroxy compound was found to be a major metabolite in all three species while traces of each of the possible phenols plus a dihydroxy product were detected in human and rat urine. ALLEN et al. (1976) went on to confirm that about 15%–19% of a dose is excreted as ring-opened carboxylic acids, probably derived via alicyclic 1-

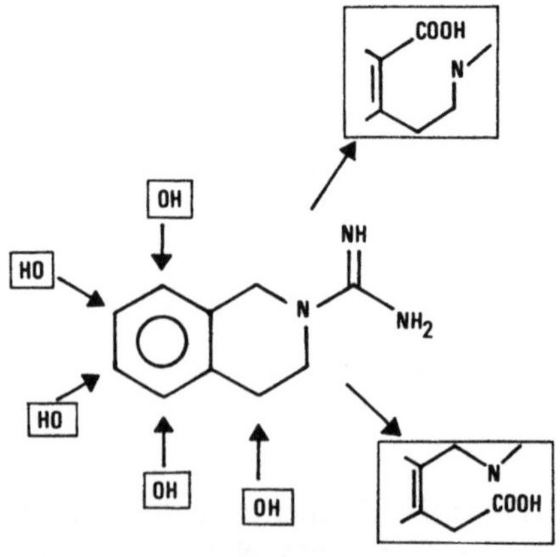

Fig. 6. Structure of debrisoquine and metabolic products

and 3-hydroxylation. Phenols in human urine were measured by ANGELO et al. (1977) who reported a total recovery of 3%–14% of the dose as the 5-, 6-, 7-, and 8-hydroxy compounds in five subjects.

Urinary recoveries and plasma concentrations of debrisoquine and 4-hydroxy-debrisoquine vary widely in man. In a study of 12 compliant patients receiving a 40 mg daily dose of debrisoquine, excretion of unchanged drug varied from 9%–80% of the dose (mean 34%). Excretion of 4-hydroxydebrisoquine was 0–30% (mean 14%), while the total debrisoquine plus 4-hydroxydebrisoquine recovery was 27%–80% (mean 47%). There was a significant inverse correlation between percentage recovery of debrisoquine and that of the hydroxy metabolite (SILAS et al., 1977). Further studies showed that increasing dose and prolonged dosage of debrisoquine are associated with greater percentage urinary recovery of unchanged drug and a lower recovery of 4-hydroxydebrisoquine, suggesting saturation and/or inhibition of the hydroxylation process (SILAS et al., 1978 a).

Two groups have demonstrated that the ratio of the urinary recovery of debrisoquine to that of 4-hydroxydebrisoquine is bimodally distributed, indicating genetic polymorphism in this oxidative pathway (MAGOUB et al., 1977; TUCKER et al., 1977). Thus, although most individuals have a ratio of less than 5, in 7% of the total number of subjects studied it exceeded 21. Further investigation of some of these "poor metabolisers" revealed an unusually high incidence of poor metabolisers amongst their first-degree relatives (MAGOUB et al., 1977). Genetically determined alicyclic hydroxylation of debrisoquine may not be confined to the 4-position. Since less of the total dose could be accounted for as debrisoquine plus 4-hydroxydebrisoquine in the urine of poor metabolisers, it is possible that their production of the ring-opened carboxylic acid metabolites via 1- and 3-hydroxylation might also be deficient (TUCKER et al., 1977).

b) Site. Peak urinary excretion rates and plasma concentrations of both debrisoquine and 4-hydroxydebrisoquine occur simultaneously suggesting pre-systemic metabolism (SILAS et al., 1978 a).

c) Drug Interactions. Inhibition of oxidative metabolism of debrisoquine by desipramine was demonstrated in the rat by MITCHELL et al. (1970), but metabolic products were not measured directly.

d) Activity of Metabolites. Although the phenolic metabolites have antihypertensive activity (British Patent 1,057,280, 1965), their low urinary recoveries after administration of debrisoquine suggests that they do not add materially to the effect of the unchanged drug. Similarly, although 4-hydroxydebrisoquine has some hypotensive action in anaesthetised cats (MALCOLM and MARTEN, 1976), a negative correlation between fall in blood pressure and its urinary recovery after debrisoquine dosage in man indicates that it does not contribute to clinical response (SILAS et al., 1977).

4. Excretion

a) Routes. During chronic therapy, mean renal clearances (plasma) of debrisoquine and of 4-hydroxydebrisoquine of about 0.28 and 0.37 l/min, respectively, were observed, indicating excretion by both glomerular and tubular mechanisms. However, renal clearance of the compounds is not constant with time or concentration. As in the case of bethanidine, a fall in clearance was seen with time after a single dose of debrisoquine and, on multiple dosing, clearance was inversely related to plasma drug concentration. The latter finding may reflect partial saturation of an active tubular transport mechanism. As anticipated for a polar drug having a pK_a of 12.5, the renal excretion of debrisoquine is independent of urinary pH (SILAS et al., 1978a). While urinary excretion and metabolism account for most of the elimination of debrisoquine, the remaining 5%–15% of an oral dose is recoverable in the faeces (ANGELO et al., 1976; SILAS, 1978). This fraction probably represents unabsorbed drug.

5. Pharmacokinetics

a) Oral. When calculated from urinary drug excretion rates between 18 and 66 h after single oral doses, the elimination $t_{1/2}$ of debrisoquine in man is about 15 h. In one subject, terminal $t_{1/2}$ values estimated from measurements of urine, plasma, whole blood, and platelet-rich plasma were 12 h, 17.5 h, 56 h, and 56 h, respectively (SILAS et al., 1978a). The kinetics of formation of 4-hydroxydebrisoquine from debrisoquine are complex since it appears to be eliminated more rapidly from the plasma and in the urine than the parent drug. Thus, calculations on urinary excretion rate data over 18–66 h after dosage of debrisoquine give a mean $t_{1/2}$ of 9.6 h for the metabolite compared to 16.2 h for parent drug. Saturation and/or inhibition of 4-hydroxylation is indicated from incremental and multiple dose studies (SILAS et al., 1978a).

b) Drug Interactions. In man, oral administration of 75 mg of amitriptyline before a 20 mg single dose of debrisoquine was shown to impair metabolism of the latter and to decrease its platelet/plasma concentration ratio (SILAS, 1978). The latter finding is consistent with blockage of the uptake$_1$–pump for biogenic amines and guanidino-hypotensive drugs in the platelet (SOLOMON et al., 1969). Therefore, in this respect the platelet reflects the events at the adrenergic neurone since the clinical combination of tricyclic antidepressants and guanidino-type hypotensive agents is known to cause loss of blood pressure control (LEISHMAN et al., 1963; MITCHELL et al., 1967).

6. Concentration–Effect Relationships

The dose of debrisoquine is poorly related to its hypotensive effect in different patients. However, about 70% of the variance in response has been related to differences in the urinary recovery and plasma concentration of the unchanged drug (ANGELO et al., 1975; SILAS et al., 1977; IDLE et al., 1978). Furthermore, this relationship was found to be independent of biochemical indices of sympathetic blockade and of monoamine oxidase inhibition by debrisoquine (SILAS et al., 1978b; SILAS, 1978). A knowledge of the relationships between urinary debrisoquine and 4-hydroxydebrisoquine recoveries and between urinary debrisoquine recovery and fall in blood pressure has allowed a systematic assessment of the relative importance of non-compliance and resistance to hypotensive therapy with debrisoquine (SILAS et al., 1978c).

VII. Guanethidine

(2-Octahydro-1-azocinyl)-ethyl-guanidine

1. Absorption

a) Extent. The prolonged action and slow elimination of guanethidine make conclusions based on short-term urine collections (after oral or parenteral doses) open to considerable doubt. This is emphasised by the data from five studies in man summarised in Fig. 7 which plots percentage urinary recovery of guanethidine and metabolites against duration of urine collection. RAHN and GOLDBERG (1969) found no plateau in the curve of cumulative excretion of radiolabel in six hypertensive patients until 12 days after a single oral dose. This is the most prolonged study that has been conducted. Estimates of fraction of oral dose absorbed range from 0.05 to 0.50 (DOLLERY et al., 1960; CALESNICK et al., 1961; RAHN and GOLDBERG, 1969; MCMARTIN et al., 1970; MCMARTIN and SIMPSON, 1971).

b) Rate. Peak plasma concentration occurs at 2–4 h after oral guanethidine. Plasma metabolite concentrations peak at the same time (MCMARTIN et al., 1970).

2. Distribution

a) Blood. No plasma binding of guanethidine has been detected (SCHANKER and MORRISON, 1965; RAHN, 1973). Values of λ after intravenous guanethidine rose from 1.8 at 5 min to 4.3 at 72 h (RAHN, 1973). The cellular element in blood concentrating guanethidine was not identified. However, human blood platelets are capable of accumulating guanethidine against a concentration gradient, a process which is energy and sodium dependent and which is inhibited by substances including desipramine, amphetamine, cocaine, and noradrenaline (BOULLIN and O'BRIEN, 1969).

b) Tissues. Specific and non-specific tissue binding of guanethidine has been identified (BRODIE et al., 1965; CHANG et al., 1965). Specific binding is antagonised by amphetamine (DAY and RAND, 1963). Uptake into rat heart is oxygen- (SCHANKER and MORRISON, 1965), pH-, and calcium-dependent (BOULLIN, 1966). Guanethidine possesses two basic centres with pK_{a_1} 8.7 and $pK_{a_2} > 11$. Under normal physiological conditions of acid–base balance it is unlikely that perturbations of pH would significantly affect ionisation and passive uptake, although at pH 8.4 isolated rat heart accumulated guanethidine at a greater initial rate and to higher steady-state levels (BOULLIN, 1966). Uptake, particularly into adrenergically-innervated tissues, probably accounts

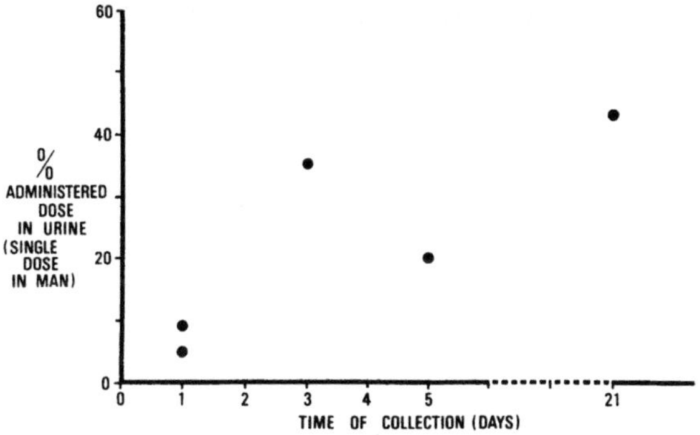

Fig. 7. Percentage urinary recovery of guanethidine and its metabolites in man as a function of duration of urine collection

for the slow elimination of guanethidine. It can be calculated that not less than 45% of an injected dose remains in the body 5 days after dosing (derived from Fig. 3 and 4, MCMARTIN et al., 1970).

3. Biotransformation

a) Sites. The coincidence of peak plasma concentrations of guanethidine and metabolites indicates presystemic metabolism, a conclusion supported by the greater metabolism after oral than after parenteral dosing (MCMARTIN et al., 1970). Rabbit and pig liver homogenates and rat hepatic microsomes metabolise guanethidine (ABRAMSON et al., 1969), by an oxygen-dependent process (FURST, 1967) which can be antagonised by desipramine (MITCHELL et al., 1970).

b) Routes. Two principal metabolites (Fig. 8) have been identified as 2-(6-carboxyhexylamino)-ethyl guanidine and guanethidine-N-oxide (MCMARTIN, 1969; ABRAMSON et al., 1969; MCMARTIN and SIMPSON, 1971). Small amounts of a third metabolite, tentatively identified as 1-(6-carboxyhexyl)-2-iminoimidazolidine, have also been found in human urine (MCMARTIN et al., 1970).

c) Activity of Metabolites. All three identified metabolites of guanethidine possess less than one-tenth of the antihypertensive activity of guanethidine itself in the renal hypertensive rat (Brunner, H., quoted by ABRAMSON et al., 1969; MAITRE et al., 1971).

d) Effects of Disease. Patients with hypertension and impaired renal function excreted more radioactivity in the form of metabolites than did patients with good renal function – an observation which may relate to the slower elimination of total radioactivity in this group (RAHN, 1973).

4. Excretion

a) Routes. Guanethidine and metabolites are mainly excreted by the kidney (DOLLERY et al., 1960). A small amount of drug is excreted in the bile after oral and parenteral injection (CALESNICK et al., 1961; MCMARTIN et al., 1970).

b) Mechanisms. Renal clearance (up to 0.46 l/min) may exceed glomerular filtration rate suggesting tubular excretion as well. Clearance of metabolites is approximately 60% of parent drug but still high enough to demand tubular mechanisms (MCMARTIN et al., 1970).

c) Effect of Disease. Impaired excretion of guanethidine and metabolites was found in patients with impaired renal function (RAHN, 1971).

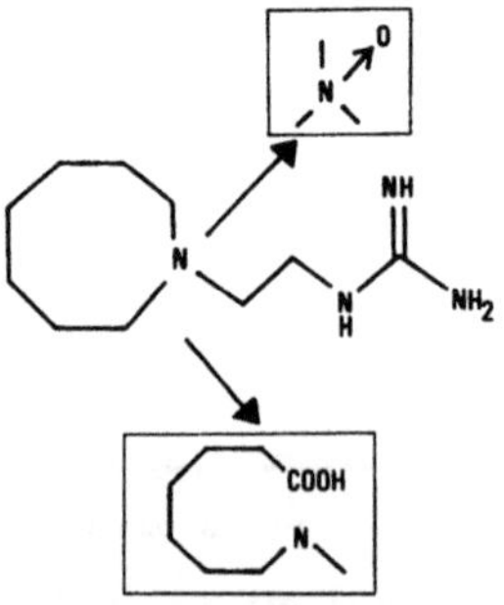

Fig. 8. Structure of guanethidine and metabolic products

5. Pharmacokinetics

Study of two patients given i.m. [^{3}H]guanethidine showed a terminal half life for total radioactivity of 9–10 days. Renal clearance from 0.5 h (patient 1) averaged 0.35 l/min for guanethidine and 0.22 l/min for metabolites. Renal clearance (patient 2) from 2–10 h averaged 0.2 l/min for guanethidine and 0.19 l/min for metabolites (McMARTIN et al., 1970).

Application. OATES et al. (1971) postulated that the late phase of guanethidine elimination ($t_{1/2}$ about 5 days) can be equated with loss when other pools are in equilibrium with guanethidine in the adrenergic neurone. Utilising these data, a loading-maintenance regime has been devised (SHAND et al., 1975c; MCALLISTER, 1975) the safety of which has been attested by WALTER and NIES (1977).

6. Concentration–Effect Relationships

Plasma concentration of guanethidine correlates with inhibition of venous reflex response to Valsalva manoeuvre which in turn correlates with fall in mean standing blood pressure (WALTER et al., 1975).

VIII. Guanoxan

2-Guanidinomethyl-1:4-benzodioxan

1. Absorption

a) Extent. Absorption of guanoxan in man may be quite extensive as no more than 8% of a 20 mg oral dose was recovered in the faeces (JACK et al., 1971).

2. Biotransformation

a) Routes. In dog urine CAÑAS-RODRIGUEZ (1966) identified unchanged guanoxan and hydroxylated guanoxan together with arginine, creatinine, guanidinoacetic acid, creatine, and urea as products of its metabolism. These findings indicated that aromatic ring hydroxylation and alicyclic ring-opening followed by transamidination are significant metabolic pathways, while hydrolysis of the guanidino group is quantitatively small (Fig. 9). The urine of six hypertensive patients receiving oral guanoxan was analysed by JACK et al. (1971) who found only unchanged guanoxan and 7-hydroxyguanoxan, the latter being the preponderant compound in all but one subject. There was no evidence for transformation of the guanidine moiety of guanoxan in man.

IX. Phenoxybenzamine

n-Phenoxyisopropyl-n-benzyl-β-chlorethylamine

1. Absorption

No quantitative studies have been reported but phenoxybenzamine is effective by mouth and was detected in high quantities in the fat of dogs given oral doses (BRODIE et al., 1954).

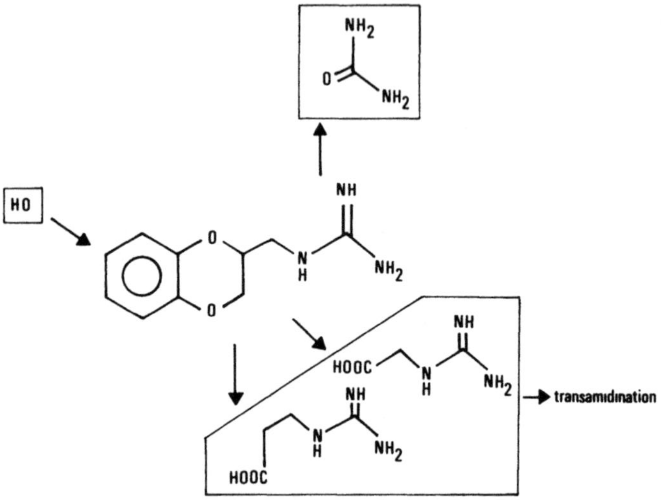

Fig. 9. Structure of guanoxan and metabolic products

2. Distribution

After i.v. infusion to anaesthetized dogs, the concentrations in muscle, liver, and plasma became too low for detection, by a relatively insensitive method, after 2 h. By contrast, in the same experiment, concentrations in fat continued to rise for 12 h and slowly declined to still detectable amounts after 4 days with an apparent $t_{1/2}$ of about 24 h. It was calculated that 20% of the administered dose was in fat at 12 h (BRODIE et al., 1954).

3. Biotransformation

a) Routes. In early studies no phenoxybenzamine was detected in the urine of dogs after i.v. injection. The amine produced by dealkylation was tentatively identified (BRODIE et al., 1954). More recently, KNAPP et al. (1976) have used ^{15}N-labelling to determine metabolic pathways in dog, man, and rat (Fig. 10). The sole metabolite common to the three species was N-benzyl-N-(p-hydroxy-phenoxylisopropyl)-amine, formed by dealkylation and p-hydroxylation of the phenoxy ring. The non-hydroxylated amine precursor was detected in dog and rat. Further metabolism of this amine to 2-benzylamino-propanol was found in the rat and to phenoxyisopropylamine in the dog.

b) Activity of Metabolites. Only N-benzyl-N-phenoxyisopropylamine was found to have α-blocking activity (KNAPP et al., 1976).

4. Concentration–Effect Relationships

The concentration of phenoxybenzamine in fat correlated with the inhibition of blood pressure increase to adrenaline in three dogs. After [^{14}C]phenoxybenzamine, total plasma radioactivity correlated well with inhibition of α-adrenergic activity in dogs. A dose of 110 mg was given i.v. over 24 h and residual α-blocking effects were present at 4, but not at 5, days (BRODIE et al., 1954).

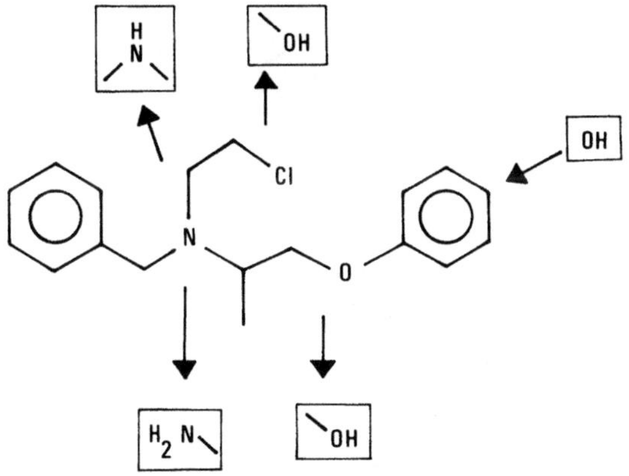

Fig. 10. Structure of phenoxybenzamine and metabolic products

X. Phentolamine

2-(n-p-Tolyl-n-m-hydroxyphenyl-amino-methyl)-imidazoline

1. Absorption

a) Extent. After an oral dose of [^{14}C]phentolamine, a single normal human subject excreted 70% of the carbon label in 24 h (IMHOF et al., 1976).

b) Rate. Peak plasma concentrations appeared between 15 and 30 min in fasting dogs (JONES et al., 1950) and by 30 min in two healthy human subjects. In one subject who received [^{14}C]phentolamine, peak concentrations of unchanged phentolamine were achieved at 30 min but peak plasma radioactivity occurred at 2 h, suggesting rapid and substantial metabolic conversion of phentolamine (IMHOF et al., 1976).

2. Distribution

The persistence of pharmacological effect beyond the point of detection of circulating phentolamine was claimed as evidence for extensive tissue distribution (JONES et al., 1950). However, plasma concentrations below 1 μg/ml could not be detected in this study. IMHOF et al. (1976), with an assay sensitive down to 10 ng/ml, could detect no phentolamine in plasma after 2 h. One explanation of persistent effect beyond this point could be the presence of pharmacologically active metabolites but this has not been examined.

3. Biotransformation

Little more than 10% of unchanged phentolamine could be recovered in dog urine after i.v. doses but hydrolysis of the samples approximately doubled the yield, suggesting the presence of conjugates (JONES et al., 1950). IMHOF et al. (1976) did not characterise metabolites but their study with [^{14}C]phentolamine clearly points to their existence (Fig. 11).

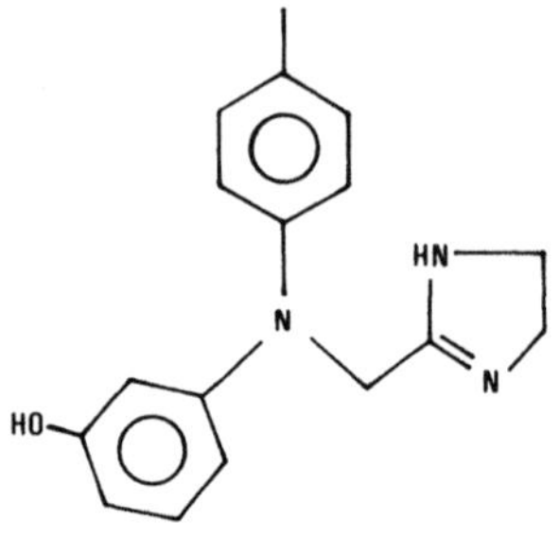

Fig. 11. Structure of phentolamine

4. Concentration–Effect Relationships

Response to i.v. adrenaline (dogs) was antagonised in a dose-dependent manner; a point of maximum blockade being apparent beyond which duration, but not magnitude, of the effect increased.

XI. Prazosin

1-(4-Amino-6,7-dimethoxy-2-quinazolinyl)-4-(2-furoyl)-piperazine

Prazosin, originally thought to be solely a vasodilator drug is now known to have post-synaptic α-blocking activity (CONSTANTINE et al., 1973; GRAHAM et al., 1977). The pharmacology of prazosin has recently been reviewed (BROGDEN et al., 1977).

1. Absorption

a) Extent. High faecal recoveries of ^{14}C-label occur after both oral and i.v. dosing in animals, suggesting extensive oral absorption but rapid elimination via the gastrointestinal tract (TAYLOR et al., 1977).

b) Rate. Reported values for t_{max} in man are 1.5–5 h (mean 3.6 h; hypertensive patients, COLLINS and PEK, 1975), 1–5 h (normal subjects, WOOD, 1975; WOOD et al., 1976), and 2 h (24 volunteers, HOBBS and TWOMEY, 1977). Food had an inconsistent effect on peak plasma concentrations and t_{max} (VERBESSELT et al., 1976).

2. Distribution

a) Blood. An f_p of 0.03 has been reported (HOBBS and TWOMEY, 1977). A λ value of 1.45 was found for human blood by COLLINS and PEK (1975).

b) Tissues. Radioactivity was found particularly in lung, coronary arteries, paw arteries, and heart 30 min after i.v. administration of [^{14}C]prazosin to a dog. Very low concentrations were present in plasma, skeletal muscle, and brain (TAYLOR et al., 1977).

3. Biotransformation

a) Sites. Data quoted by COLLINS and PEK (1975) and TAYLOR et al. (1977) suggest extensive, first-pass metabolism of prazosin in the liver.

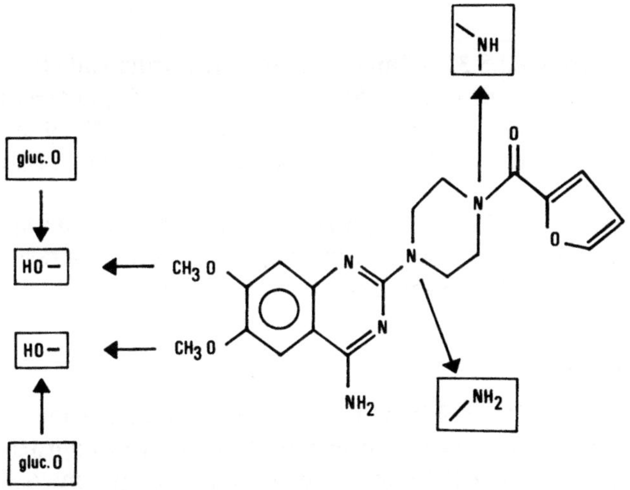

Fig. 12. Structure of prazosin and metabolic products

Table 5. Percentage recovery of prazosin and metabolites in dog and rat. (From TAYLOR et al., 1977)

	Dog			Rat		
	Urine	Bile	Total	Urine	Bile	Total
Prazosin	5	1	6	5	1	6
Metabolite I	1	15	16	1	10	11
Conjugated	–	50	50	–	50	50
Metabolite II	1	5	6	1	2	3
Conjugated	–	15	15	–	10	10
Metabolite III	1	1	2	5	5	10
Metabolite IV	1	1	2		1	1
Total recovery			97%			91%

Metabolite I = 6-O-Methyl prazosin
Metabolite II = 7-O-Methyl prazosin
Metabolite III = 2-(1-Piperazinyl)-4-amino-6,7-dimethoxyquinazoline
Metabolite IV = 2-4-Diamino-6-7-dimethoxyquinazoline

b) Routes. The principal metabolic pathways in rat and dog (and probably man) are O-demethylation at either the 6- or 7-position, followed by glucuronide formation. Hydrolysis of the amide linkage and piperazine ring cleavage with N-dealkylation have both been documented (TAYLOR et al., 1977) but the metabolites constitute only a small fraction of the total recovered (Fig. 12; Table 5).

c) Activity of Metabolites. The free piperazine derivative and 2,4-diamino-6,7-dimethoxy-quinazoline cause hypotension in dogs but have only 10%–25% of the potency of prazosin and can contribute little to the overall pharmacological effect (HESS, 1974).

4. Excretion

a) Routes. Rats excreted 8.3% of an oral dose in the urine and 80.5% in faeces; after i.v. dosing, the proportions were 12.5% in urine and 74.5% in faeces. Similar results were obtained in the dog. A bile-cannulated rat excreted 40% of an i.p. dose in bile over 24 h and 50% of an oral dose was recovered in bile over 72 h in a dog (TAYLOR et al., 1977).

b) Effect of Disease. There is suggestive evidence that renal impairment may affect the handling of prazosin in man yielding higher than average plasma concentrations (COLLINS and PEK, 1975; GRAHAM et al., 1976).

5. Pharmacokinetics

a) Oral. COLLINS and PEK (1975) report a mean terminal plasma $t_{1/2}$ of 3.2 h in five hypertensive patients; they estimated hepatic extraction of approximately 30% and mean hepatic clearance of 0.45 l/min. A mean elimination plasma $t_{1/2}$ of 3.9 h and volume of distribution of 118 l was reported for 10 normal subjects (WOOD, 1975; WOOD et al., 1976). HESS (1974) records a plasma $t_{1/2}$ of 1–2 h in rats and dogs. Distribution volume is quoted as 75 l in another study in man (HOBBS and TWOMEY, 1977)

6. Concentration–Effect Relationships

Plasma concentrations of prazosin are apparently unrelated to fall in blood pressure (CONSTANTINE et al., 1973; WOOD, 1975; WOOD et al., 1976; GRAHAM et al., 1976).

XII. Priscoline

2-Benzyl-imidazoline

1. Absorption

a) Extent. Priscoline is rapidly and almost completely absorbed in the rat, only 15% of the ^{14}C-labelled dose being found in gastro-intestinal contents 1 h after oral dosing. By 5 h, 84% of the radiolabel had appeared in the urine (CENTURY et al., 1953). Urinary priscoline excretion in four human subjects averaged 90% 12 h after oral dosing, with a range of 81%–97%, suggesting rapid and extensive absorption in man (BRODIE et al., 1952).

2. Distribution

a) Blood. The f_p averaged 0.77 at plasma concentrations of 25 and 8 μg/ml (BRODIE et al., 1952). A λ value of 1.0 was found in rats by CENTURY et al. (1953).

b) Tissues. In a dog, priscoline was found in most tissues with a tissue/plasma ratio of approximately 3½ h after i.v. administration. However, neither brain nor fat contained appreciable concentrations (BRODIE et al., 1952). Distribution of ^{14}C-activity was closely similar after both oral and i.v. doses in rats with high concentrations at 1 h in liver and kidneys and only small amounts in brain (CENTURY et al., 1953).

3. Biotransformation

BRODIE et al. (1952) found only unchanged priscoline (Fig. 13) in the urine of dog and man. However, in the rat, while over 90% of the urinary radioactivity extracted with chloroform appeared to be unchanged priscoline, a very small percentage ($\ngtr$7%) appeared as a substance with a slightly different R_f value. This substance was present in greater proportion after oral than after i.v. dosing and may represent a metabolite. Very small amounts of $^{14}CO_2$ were also detected in expired air (CENTURY et al., 1953).

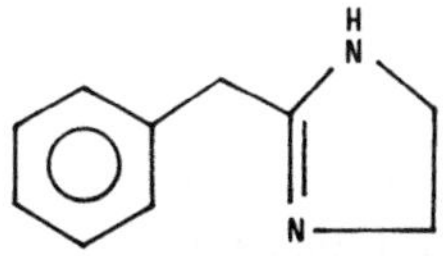

Fig. 13. Structure of priscoline

4. Excretion

Priscoline is excreted virtually quantitatively in urine in dog, man, and rat. Very small amounts of radiolabel appeared in rat faeces after i.v. dosing (<4% of dose) which may indicate limited biliary excretion of parent drug or putative metabolite (CENTURY et al., 1953). In dog, priscoline clearance was virtually the same as renal plasma flow (p-amino-hippurate clearance) at a mean 0.23 l/min (BRODIE et al., 1952).

5. Pharmacokinetics

A plasma elimination rate constant of 0.33 ($t_{1/2}$ = 2.1 h) was calculated after i.v. injection of priscoline to a dog. A graph of the amount of priscoline remaining in the body against time in four human subjects dosed orally produced an almost identical value for the elimination rate constant (BRODIE et al., 1952).

6. Concentration–Effect Relationships

There appeared to be a close relationship between plasma priscoline concentration and degree of adrenergic blockade (pressor response to ephedrine) in the dog (BRODIE et al., 1952).

XIII. Labetalol

2-Hydroxy-5-{1-hydroxy-2-[(methyl-3-phenylpropyl)-amino]-ethyl}-benzamide

1. Absorption

a) Extent. Total mean radioactivity excreted in the urine after oral [^{3}H]- or [^{14}C]labetalol was 72.9% (50 mg/kg, mouse, 72 h), 48.2% (50 mg/kg, rat, 72 h), 61.5% (50 mg/kg, rabbit, 96 h), and 64.3% (20 mg/kg, dog, 48 h). In two men, 55% and 60% of the administered oral dose was excreted in 24 h (MARTIN et al., 1976).

b) Rate. Peak plasma concentration occurred at 1–2 h after oral doses of 100, 200, and 400 mg in five non-fasting healthy subjects (RICHARDS et al., 1977). The t_{max} was 1–2 h in rabbit and 4 h in dog. Radioactivity associated with metabolites peaked at the same time as that of the parent compound (MARTIN et al., 1976).

2. Distribution

a) Blood. The f_p was 0.65 (rabbit), 0.46 (dog), and 0.50 (man) measured over a wide range of plasma concentrations (MARTIN et al., 1976).

b) Tissues. Radioactivity in rabbits after a single oral dose of labelled labetalol was distributed to liver, kidney, lung, and heart with trace amounts only in brain, skeletal muscle, and fat. Very small amounts entered the foetus of pregnant rats (MARTIN et al., 1976). Labetalol is also bound in the uveal tract (POYNTER et al., 1976) but no ocular damage has so far been reported.

3. Biotransformation

a) Sites. The early peak in plasma metabolites, small recovery of metabolites after i.v. dosing, the high uptake of radioactivity in the liver in animals (MARTIN et al., 1976) and the disproportionate increase in area under the plasma labetalol concentration versus time curve with increasing oral dose [100, 200, 400 mg – area under curve ratios 1:2.6:5.6 (RICHARDS et al., 1977)] all suggest extensive presystemic metabolism which may be partly intestinal but is probably mainly hepatic.

b) Routes. Extensive metabolism (Fig. 14) of labetalol occurs in animals and man (HOPKINS et al., 1976; MARTIN et al., 1976). This yields a ring-hydroxylated derivative and its glucuronide in rabbit and rat. In dog, the glucuronide formed by reaction at the secondary alcohol site preponderates. Very small amounts of unchanged labetalol are excreted in man and the O-phenyl glucuronide is the main product currently identified.

4. Excretion

a) Routes. Unchanged labetalol and metabolites are excreted in urine. Biliary excretion has been confirmed in the rabbit. After i.v. dosing 36% appeared in the faeces of the rat and 27% in the dog (MARTIN et al., 1976).

5. Pharmacokinetics

The terminal half-life of labetalol after i.v. dosing was 10 h in the dog and 3.5–4.5 h in man (MARTIN et al., 1976).

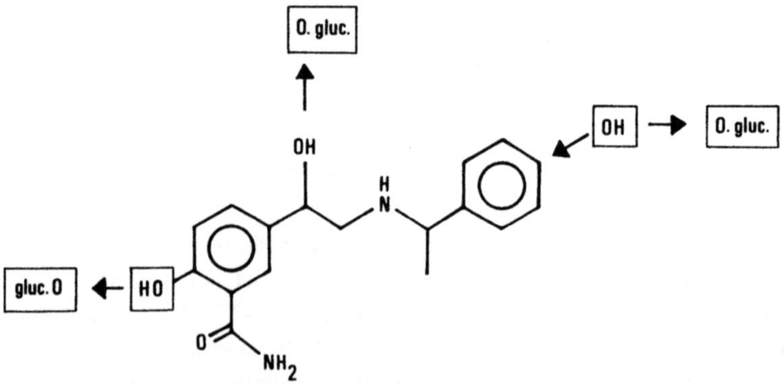

Fig. 14. Structure of labetalol and metabolic products

6. Concentration–Effect Relationships

RICHARDS et al. (1977) showed a linear correlation ($r=0.84$) between log plasma labetalol concentration and reduction in exercise heart rate 2 h after oral dosing. A relationship was also claimed with the reduction in mean systolic pressure after exercise. A significant correlation was observed between steady-state plasma labetalol concentration and isoprenaline dose-ratio -1; no correlation was found with fall in blood pressure in the same 16 hypertensive patients (SANDERS et al., 1978).

Beta-Adrenoceptor Blocking Agents

Several authors have reviewed the metabolism and pharmacokinetics of these drugs (RIESS et al., 1974; REGÅRDH, 1975; PFEIFER and ZIMMER, 1975; JOHNSSON and REGÅRDH, 1976; MEIER, 1977) and we acknowledge the assistance of their analyses in preparing this section. Except when indicated specifically, the discussion of each compound relates to the racemic form.

I. Acebutolol

1-(2-Acetyl-4-n-butyramidophenoxy)-3-isopropylamino-2-propanol

1. Absorption

a) Extent. Published data are limited. Using ^{14}C-labelled acebutolol as a tracer, COLLINS (1975) reported recoveries of total radioactivity of 29% in the urine and 64% in the faeces after a 200 mg oral dose in one patient. It is possible that 30% is a low estimate of net absorption as excretion of parent drug and/or metabolites into the intestine followed by faecal elimination has not been excluded. Unchanged drug accounted for 64% of the urinary recovery. This figure, representing 18.6% of the total dose, is in agreement with an average f_u value of 0.15 found in six patients receiving 300 mg oral doses and using a specific glc assay (MEFFIN et al., 1976). Furthermore, comparing the latter value with the mean found for nine healthy volunteers receiving 0.25–1 mg/kg i.v. doses ($f_u=0.40$) (MEFFIN et al., 1977), would indicate a bioavailability of 0.38 (i.e., 0.15/0.40).

An estimate of the systemic availability of acebutolol can be made from the mean i.v. clearance values reported for Meffin's subjects. Assuming that the mean, non-renal (blood) clearance (0.33 l/min) represents hepatic clearance, that enzymes are not saturated after oral dosage, and that hepatic blood flow is 1.5 l/min, the hepatic extraction should be 0.22, giving a systemic availability of 0.78. If 30% of the dose reaches the portal circulation then this systemic availability would predict a bioavailability of 0.23 (i.e., 0.30×0.78).

b) Rate. Where specific assays have been used, t_{max} values of 1–3 h after oral dosage were found (MEFFIN et al., 1976; MARTIN et al., 1978). Irregularities in the plasma drug concentration time curves of some patients suggest erratic or delayed absorption owing to formulation effects or, possibly, to enterohepatic recycling (MEFFIN et al., 1976).

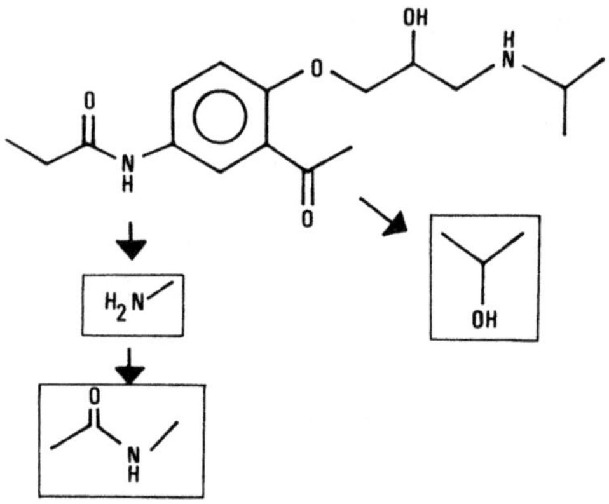

Fig. 15. Structure of acebutolol and metabolic products

2. Distribution

a) Blood. MEFFIN et al. (1977) found mean, concentration-independent f_p and λ values of 0.74 and 0.67, respectively, in healthy subjects.

b) Tissue. Autoradiograms developed 10 min after i.v. injection of 2 mg/kg acebutolol in rats indicated relatively high concentrations of radioactivity in the gastrointestinal wall and relatively low concentrations in the brain (MAXWELL and COLLINS, 1974).

3. Biotransformation

a) Routes. MAXWELL and COLLINS (1974) reported three metabolites in man, dog, and rat, namely a primary amine, an N-acetyl derivative and an alcohol formed via reduction of the 2-acetyl group (Fig. 15). Of these, the N-acetyl compound, presumably formed via acetylation of the primary amine, appears to be quantitatively the most important. MEFFIN et al. (1976) established the presence of the N-acetyl metabolite in human plasma by gas chromatography – mass spectrometry and WINKLE et al. (1977) found that its mean steady-state plasma concentration after oral acebutolol was some 2.7 times greater than that of the parent compound. Renal excretion of the N-acetyl compound accounts for 16%–28% of an oral dose but less of an i.v. dose (13%) (MAXWELL and COLLINS, 1974; MEFFIN et al., 1976, 1977).

Although polymorphic N-acetylation of the primary amine metabolite is a possibility, in common with other drugs so transformed, the overall conversion of acebutolol to the N-acetyl compound does not show a bimodal distribution (GULAID et al., 1978). Individual variation in the rate of the initial hydrolysis step appears to mask any differences in acetylator status.

b) Sites. Differences in the urinary recoveries of acebutolol and its N-acetyl metabolite after oral and i.v. dosage indicate pre-systemic metabolism of the drug. However, although the liver (and/or gut) are, therefore, indicated as major sites of biotransformation, other loci have not been excluded. For example, acetylases are present in blood cells that are capable of metabolising several drugs containing aromatic amino groups (DRAYER et al., 1974). Accordingly, the primary amine metabolite of acebutolol may also be a substrate for these enzymes.

c) Activity of Metabolites. The three metabolites are all claimed to have pharmacological activity (MAXWELL and COLLINS, 1974). All have a β-blocking effect, as measured by inhibition of isoprenaline-induced tachycardia in the cat, the N-acetyl compound being equipota nt with acebutolol but differing in cardiac selectivity (COLLINS, 1975). Only the primary amine appears to have significant antiarrhythmic activity, but this metabolite has not been detected in plasma.

4. Excretion

a) Routes. Using a spectrophotometric method that measured both acebutolol and its N-acetyl metabolite, mean f_u values of 0.6 after i.v. injection and 0.35 after oral administration were obtained in six healthy subjects by KAYE et al. (1976). MEFFIN et al. (1976), using specific glc and hplc assays for acebutolol, found mean f_u values of 0.40 (i.v.) and 0.15 (oral) for unchanged drug. In two patients with T-tubes in their bile ducts, 2.4%–8.5% of a 300 mg oral dose was recovered in the bile after 24 h as equal amounts of unchanged drug and N-acetyl metabolite (KAYE and OH, 1976).

b) Mechanisms. Urinary excretion of acebutolol and the N-acetyl metabolite were found to be independent of urine pH (KAYE and LONG, 1976). Bile: plasma concentration ratios of 60–100: 1 for these compounds suggest an active component in their biliary excretion (KAYE and OH, 1976).

c) Effect of Disease. Urinary 24 h recoveries of acebutolol plus its N-acetyl metabolite after oral acebutolol were 1.8% in patients with severe chronic renal failure compared to 32% in control subjects (KAYE and DUFTON, 1976).

5. Pharmacokinetics

a) Intravenous. The disposition kinetics of acebutolol have been characterised in nine healthy subjects using an hplc assay (MEFFIN et al., 1977). Mean total clearance (plasma) was found to be 0.827 l/min and independent of dose over the range 0.25–1 mg/kg, as was mean renal clearance (plasma) (0.334 l/min). Plasma acebutolol concentration versus time curves were described by a biexponential equation giving a mean $t_{\frac{1}{2}\alpha}$ of 6 min and a $t_{\frac{1}{2}\beta}$ of 157 min. Mean Vd_{ss} was 1.165 l/kg. Reasons for the coincidence of the above figures with those derived from an earlier study by KAYE et al. (1976), but based upon the measurement of combined concentrations of acebutolol and its N-acetyl metabolite, have been discussed by MEFFIN et al. (1977).

b) Oral. The kinetics of acebutolol after oral administration have not been adequately characterised. In patients, the terminal half-life ($t_{\frac{1}{2}\beta}$) is similar to that seen after i.v. injection. The N-acetyl metabolite is eliminated more slowly than the parent compound and its $t_{\frac{1}{2}}$ may be in excess of 10 h in some patients (MEFFIN et al., 1976). An evaluation of oral kinetics from the data of KAYE et al. (1976) is complicated by the use of a non-specific assay. Concentrations of the N-acetyl metabolite in plasma are much higher after oral compared to i.v. administration.

c) Effect of Disease. The half-life of combined acebutolol plus N-acetyl metabolite was found to be four times greater in patients with severe renal failure compared to normal subjects (KAYE and DUFTON, 1976). Haemodialysis, however, reduces the half-life in such patients to nearly normal values (ROUX et al., 1975).

6. Concentration–Effect Relationships

CUTHBERT and COLLINS (1975) showed a direct correlation between the plasma concentration of combined acebutolol plus N-acetyl metabolite and the inhibition of isoprenaline-induced tachycardia after an oral dose of 300 mg acebutolol in three healthy subjects. Plasma concentrations of both acebutolol and the N-acetyl metabolite were separately correlated with degree of β-blockade (assessed by reduction in exercise heart rate) in 11 hypertensive patients receiving daily oral doses of 200–1,200 mg (MARTIN et al., 1978). Although the degree of β-blockade fluctuated with plasma drug concentration within a dosage interval, the reduction in blood pressure from pretreatment value remained constant. In the group as a whole, plasma concentrations of drug and metabolite, separately or together, did not correlate with blood pressure change.

II. Alprenolol

1-(2-Allylphenoxy)-3-isopropylamino-2-propanol

1. Absorption

a) Extent. Urinary recovery of over 90% of tritiated alprenolol indicated essentially complete net oral absorption in man (BODIN et al., 1974). A similar finding was reported using a slow-release form of the drug (JOHANSSON et al., 1971). Considerably lower urinary recoveries were recorded in dogs and rats but comparable faecal recoveries of radioactivity after both oral and i.v. dosage suggests complete absorption in these species also (BODIN et al., 1974). Specific determination of alprenolol by electron-capture gas-liquid chromatography provided estimates of its bioavailability in healthy human subjects ranging from 0.01–0.16 after 100–200 mg oral doses (ABLAD et al., 1974; VON BAHR et al., 1975; ALVAN et al., 1977a). However, the area under the plasma concentration versus time curve increases disproportionately with dose indicating that first-pass removal becomes partially saturated in the therapeutic dose range (ALVAN et al., 1977a).

b) Rate. Maximum plasma concentrations of alprenolol are achieved after 0.5–1.5 h using conventional oral dosage forms (REGÅRDH, 1975). Administration of sustained-release tablets was associated with slightly lower urinary recoveries of unchanged drug despite similar recoveries of total radioactivity compared to ordinary tablets (JOHANSSON et al., 1971). This observation suggests an inverse relationship between absorption rate and systemic availability, consistent with saturable first-pass removal.

2. Distribution

a) Blood. JOHANSSON et al. (1974) found a mean f_p value of 0.85 for human plasma using an ultrafiltration method. Binding was independent of drug concentration over the therapeutic range, but decreased at higher concentrations; it was also shown to be directly related to pH. Alprenolol binds mainly to plasma proteins other than albumin as the fractional binding to the latter was found to be only 0.38 (APPELGREN et al., 1974; JOHANSSON et al., 1974). Recently, PIAFSKY and BORGA (1977) identified the main binding sites to be associated with α_1-acid glycoprotein and showed a direct correlation between plasma binding of alprenolol and the concentration of this acute phase protein in plasma. ALVAN et al. (1977b) reported a mean λ value of 0.98 in healthy subjects.

b) Tissues. Owing to its relatively high lipid-solubility (Table 16), alprenolol distributes rapidly into the brain and other well-perfused tissues. Especially high concentrations of the unchanged drug were observed in rat lung after i.v. injection (BODIN et al., 1974).

3. Biotransformation

a) Routes. BODIN (1974) recovered 23%, 66%, and 61% of a tritiated dose of alprenolol after oral administration in a rat, a dog, and a man, respectively. Of these recoveries, the product of aromatic hydroxylation in the 4-position followed by conjugation accounted for 30% in the rat and 40% in dog and man. In addition, 36% of the total recovery in man and somewhat less in dog and rat was assigned to unidentified conjugates of alprenolol itself and a further 1% to a conjugate of N-desisopropylalprenolol (Fig. 16). Acidic metabolites were also detected but their structures were not elucidated. After oral administration of radiolabelled alprenolol to man, the concentration of labelled metabolites, calculated as alprenolol, was about 100-fold greater than that of the parent drug (JOHANSSON et al., 1971). Alprenolol/4-hydroxyalprenolol plasma concentration ratios are about 10:1 and 1:1 after i.v. and oral administration, respectively (ABLAD et al., 1974). The latter ratio may, however, be significantly greater or less than 1 depending upon the individual; it is also dose- and time-dependent (ALVAN et al., 1977a).

b) Sites. A total blood clearance approaching expected hepatic blood flow (see below) suggests that hepatic metabolism may account entirely for the biotransformation of alprenolol.

c) Activity of Metabolites. 4-Hydroxy alprenolol was found to be equipotent to alprenolol in producing β-blockade in the cat heart (CARLSSON, 1973). Direct i.v. injection of this metabolite in man was also associated with a decrease in exercise heart rate but its relative potency could not be evaluated with the experimental procedure employed (ABLAD et al., 1974).

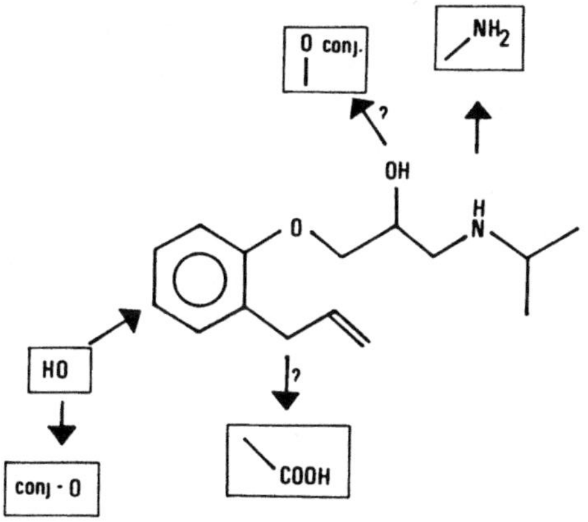

Fig. 16. Structure of alprenolol and metabolic products

d) Drug Interactions. Co-administration of salicylate and alprenolol did not influence the metabolism of either drug indicating that, although salicylate undergoes capacity-limited glucuronide formation, the two drugs do not appear to compete for the same conjugating system (JOHNSSON and REGÅRDH, 1973). Pentobarbitone induces the metabolism of alprenolol in man (ALVAN et al., 1977b). Low concentrations of ethanol stimulate while higher concentrations inhibit the metabolism of alprenolol by isolated rat liver cells. In turn, alprenolol stimulates the metabolism of low but not of high concentrations of ethanol (GRUNDIN, 1975). The clinical significance of these observations is unknown.

4. Excretion

a) Routes. After oral administration of 100 mg alprenolol a mean f_u value of <0.01 was observed in four healthy subjects (JOHNSSON and REGÅRDH, 1973). The corresponding value after i.v. injection was 0.01–0.02 (REGÅRDH, 1975).

As indicated above, dog, and rat, but not man, also excrete about 10% and 50% of a dose, respectively, in the faeces, mostly in the form of metabolites. Similar recoveries were obtained in the bile indicating that this is the major source of faecal drug excretion in these species (BODIN et al., 1974).

5. Pharmacokinetics

a) Intravenous. The disposition kinetics of alprenolol have been determined in 12 healthy subjects after 5 mg i.v. injections (ALVAN et al., 1977a, b). Mean plasma clearance was 1.08 l/min which is equivalent to a blood clearance of 1.10 l/min assuming a λ value of 0.98 (ALVAN et al., 1977b). Plasma alprenolol concentration versus time curves were described by a biexponential equation giving a mean $t_{1/2\beta}$ of 2.78 h. Mean values of Vd_β from different studies range from 3.0 to 3.4 l/kg (REGÅRDH, 1975; BODIN et al., 1974; ALVAN et al., 1977a). After direct i.v. administration of 4-hydroxyalprenolol, its plasma $t_{1/2}$ was found to be 0.3 h, whereas after injection of alprenolol the $t_{1/2}$ of this metabolite is similar to that of the parent drug indicating formation-limited elimination (ABLAD et al., 1974).

b) Oral. Variability in its extensive pre-systemic metabolism largely accounts for the 10–20 fold range of peak plasma concentrations of alprenolol after the same oral dose in different subjects (JOHANSSON et al., 1971; JOHNSSON and REGÅRDH, 1973; ABLAD et al., 1972; BODIN et al., 1974; ALVAN et al., 1977a). Similarly, RAWLINS et al. (1974) found a 25-fold range in mean steady-state plasma concentrations in 30 patients receiving the same chronic dosage. Plasma concentrations of alprenolol will also increase disproportionately with increase in oral dose and absorption rate owing to saturation of the first-pass effect (ALVAN et al., 1977a). The elimination $t_{1/2\beta}$ of alprenolol after oral administration is similar to that after i.v. injection and is independent of dose at least over the range 50–200 mg (ABLAD et al., 1972).

c) Drug Interactions. As predicted by theory for a drug having a high, flow-limited hepatic clearance, enzyme-induction by pentobarbitone did not alter the disposition kinetics of alprenolol after i.v. injection but did significantly reduce the area under the plasma concentration versus time curve after oral dosage (ALVAN et al., 1977b).

6. Concentration–Effect Relationships

ABLAD et al. (1974) observed a linear correlation between log alprenolol plasma concentration and decrease in exercise heart rate in each of four healthy subjects after both i.v. and oral dosage. A parallel displacement towards two to three times higher plasma drug concentrations of the oral dose-response curve compared to the i.v. curve may be explained by a contribution to β-blockade of higher 4-hydroxyalprenolol plasma concentrations with the same $t_{1/2}$ as unchanged drug after oral administration. A threefold difference in plasma levels of unchanged alprenolol was associated with a given degree of β-blockade after oral dosage in one study (ABLAD et al., 1974) but an earlier investigation showed up to a 100-fold variation (ABLAD et al., 1972). COLLSTE et al. (1976a) showed a direct correlation between mean steady-state plasma concentrations of alprenolol and isoprenaline dose-ratio in 16 patients receiving 600 mg alprenolol daily in divided doses. In the same patients there was no correlation between log plasma drug concentration and fall in blood pressure although when three non-responders were excluded a weak relationship did become apparent (COLLSTE et al., 1976b). FRISK-HOLMBERG et al. (1977) have demonstrated negative correlations between plasma alprenolol concentration and change in lactate release from leg muscle and in plasma free fatty acids after exercise.

III. Atenolol

4-(2-Hydroxy-3-isopropylaminopropoxy)phenyl acetamide

1. Absorption

a) Extent. Whereas all of a 50 mg i.v. dose was recovered unchanged in the urine in four normal human subjects, the corresponding recovery of atenolol after 50 mg by mouth in the same individuals was only 44% (BROWN et al., 1976). Others have observed a similar recovery after oral doses of 50–200 mg (KAYE, 1974a; MARLIN et al., 1975; CONWAY et al., 1976; KODA et al., 1977). Therefore, in the absence of significant pre-hepatic metabolism, 44% is an index of both the net absorption and of the bioavailability of this compound. A higher bioavailability of 63% was calculated by BROWN et al. (1976) from the relative areas under the i.v. and oral plasma drug concentration versus time curves, but the discrepancy with the urinary data was not commented upon.

b) Rate. Maximum plasma concentrations of atenolol are achieved between 2–4 h after oral administration (MARLIN et al., 1975; CONWAY et al., 1976; BROWN et al., 1976).

2. Distribution

a) Blood. SCALES and COPSEY (1975) found a λ value of about 1.1 in two subjects. Plasma binding of atenolol occurs to the extent of 40% in man, mostly to albumin (BARBER et al., 1978).

3. Biotransformation

a) Routes. Although the findings of BROWN et al. (1976) indicated no metabolism of atenolol in man (Fig. 17), other data from the same group are in conflict. MCAINSH (1977) reported 12% of a 5 mg ^{14}C-labelled i.v. dose in the form of metabolites in the urine and 10% as unchanged atenolol in the faeces of two subjects. After 100 mg by mouth, 38% appeared in the urine as atenolol with 4% as metabolites; the faeces contained 45% of the dose as atenolol with 7% as metabolites. The identity of the metabolites has not been disclosed. KODA et al. (1977) reported a strikingly lower f_φ value after a 25 mg oral dose (0.22) compared to 50 and 100 mg doses (0.44 and 0.48, respectively). These data are consistent with the hypothesis that atenolol may be metabolised at low doses but saturation of the enzymes responsible occurs readily as the dose is increased.

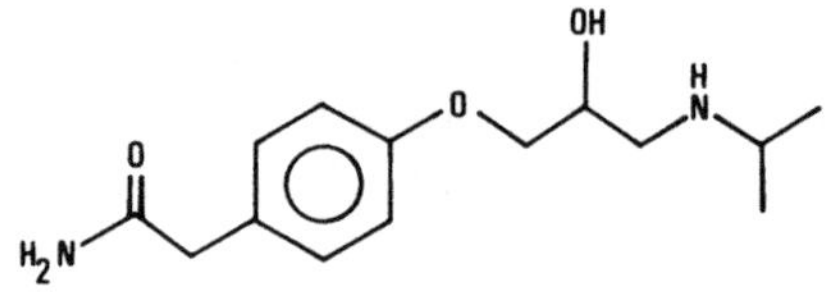

Fig. 17. Structure of atenolol

4. Excretion

a) Routes. As indicated above, the kidney is primarily responsible for the elimination of absorbed atenolol, although the presence of the drug, according to MCAINSH (1977), in the faeces after i.v. injection suggests some biliary or gastro-intestinal secretion.

b) Mechanisms. In keeping with the relatively low lipid-solubility of atenolol, KAYE (1974b) observed that its renal clearance was not dependent upon urinary pH.

5. Pharmacokinetics

a) Intravenous. The disposition kinetics of atenolol were determined in four healthy subjects after 50 mg i.v. injections (BROWN et al., 1976). Mean plasma clearance, synonymous with mean renal clearance, was 0.097 l/min. Plasma atenolol concentration versus time curves were described by a tri-exponential equation giving mean $t_{1/2}$ values for fast, intermediate and slow phases of 0.2 h, 0.94 h, and 6.06 h, respectively. The mean value of Vd_β was 51 l.

b) Oral. After oral doses of 50–200 mg to healthy subjects mean terminal $t_{1/2}$ values of 5.5–9 h have been reported (KAYE, 1974a; CONWAY et al., 1976; KODA et al., 1977). BROWN et al. (1976) found a mean value of 6.36 h after single 200 mg doses changing non-significantly to 6.61 h after eight daily 200 mg doses, with no accumulation of atenolol in the plasma. A relatively short mean $t_{1/2}$ of 2.2 h after a 25 mg dose is consistent with additional metabolic clearance at low atenolol concentrations (KODA et al., 1977).

c) Effect of Disease. A direct correlation between atenolol clearance and inulin clearance was observed in 33 hypertensive patients (SASSARD et al., 1977). Mean terminal $t_{1/2}$ values after single 100 mg oral doses varied from 6.0 h in patients with normal renal function to 22 h in those with severe renal impairment.

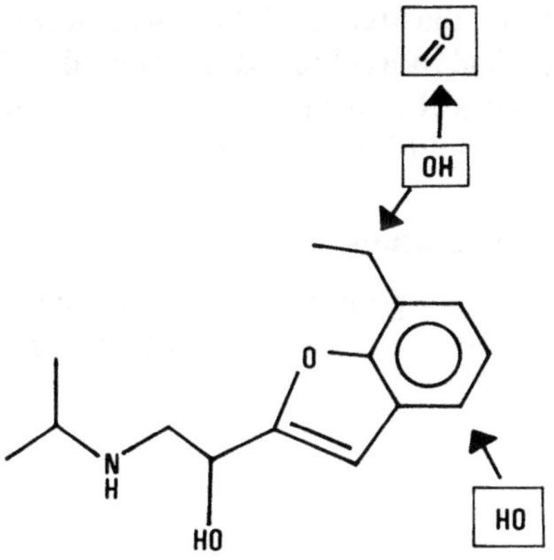

Fig. 18. Structure of bufuralol and metabolic products

6. Concentration–Effect Relationships

McAinsh (1977) has summarised the results of several studies showing a direct correlation between log plasma atenolol concentration and percentage reduction in exercise induced tachycardia. No correlations have been observed between plasma atenolol concentrations and the hypotensive effect of the drug (Dollery et al., 1975; Amery et al., 1977; Sassard et al., 1977).

IV. Bufuralol

7-Ethyl-α[(isopropylamino)-methyl]-2-benzofuran methanol

1. Absorption

a) Rate. After 10–20 mg oral doses to six healthy subjects maximum plasma concentrations of bufuralol occurred at 1–2 h. Food increased t_{max} by about an hour (Kilborn and Turner, 1974).

2. Biotransformation

a) Routes. Three metabolites, a carbinol, a ketone, and a phenol (Fig. 18) have been estimated together with unchanged bufuralol in plasma after a single 20 mg oral dose to one subject (Francis et al., 1976).

b) Activity of Metabolites. The carbinol and ketone derivatives have been synthesised and shown to have β-blocking action in animals comparable to that of the parent drug (Francis et al., 1976). Their relatively long $t_{1/2}$s (estimated at 7 h and 14 h, respectively, in one subject) compared to that of bufuralol (about 4 h) suggests that their accumulation might contribute to pharmacological effects on chronic dosage.

3. Pharmacokinetics

a) Intravenous. In two normal subjects, Balant et al. (1976) found a mean terminal plasma $t_{1/2}$ of 2.4 h, extended to 6.5 h in a further subject.

b) Oral. A mean terminal plasma $t_{1/2}$ of 2.8 h was observed in six normal subjects, extended to 4.2 h in an atypical individual (BALANT et al., 1976). It was suggested that decreased metabolism of bufuralol in the latter subject, who was also the one with a long $t_{1/2}$ after i.v. injection, might have a genetic basis.

4. Concentration–Effect Relationships

In each of five healthy subjects, log plasma bufuralol concentration was highly correlated with exercise heart rate after i.v. injection of 0.15 mg/kg (KILBORN and TURNER, 1974).

V. Bunolol

1-(5,6,7,8-Tetrahydro-5-oxo-1-naphthyl)-3-isopropylamino-2-propanol

The fate of both the DL- and L-forms of this drug has been studied. However, the latter is of greater commercial interest as it is 2.5 times more potent in inhibiting isoprenaline-induced tachycardia in dogs (COMMARATO et al., 1976).

1. Absorption

a) Extent. Urinary recoveries of radioactivity after oral administration of labelled DL-bunolol to dogs and of L-bunolol to man were greater than 75% after 3–4 days, indicating extensive absorption (LEINWEBER et al., 1971 a; DICARLO et al., 1977).

b) Rate. Rapid oral absorption is indicated by the observation of peak levels of radioactivity and of bunolol at 1 h in dogs and man (LEINWEBER et al., 1971 a; DICARLO et al., 1977).

2. Distribution

a) Tissues. At 72 h the highest tissue levels in dogs were 0.6–1.4% of a ^{14}C-labelled dose in the gastrointestinal tract and 0.6–1.1% in the liver (LEINWEBER et al., 1971 a).

3. Biotransformation

a) Routes. Bunolol is extensively metabolised by both oxidative and reductive routes and both acidic and basic products have been demonstrated (Fig. 19). Over 30 metabolites of L-bunolol and 18 metabolites of the DL-form were detected in rat and dog urine, respectively (LEINWEBER et al., 1971 b; 1977; 1978). Of these, the compounds that have been characterised and their recoveries are shown in Table 6. In turn, four of the metabolites listed in the table together with unchanged L-bunolol, have been identified and quantified in human plasma (DICARLO et al., 1977).

The side-chain of bunolol is not subject to N-dealkylation but instead is cleaved to yield *tert*-butylamine and a lactic aldehyde; the latter appearing as a substituted lactic acid. Further chain shortening occurs probably via oxidation of the alcoholic group to a carbonyl followed by decarboxylation of the α-keto acid to an aldehyde which is then oxidised to an acetic acid derivative (Fig. 19). An oxidoreductase appears to be present in various tissues that is capable of interconverting bunolol and its dihydro-metabolite. Hydroxylation of the saturated ring also occurs. Since hydroxybunolol is present in dog but not in rat urine, this suggests that hydroxydihydro-

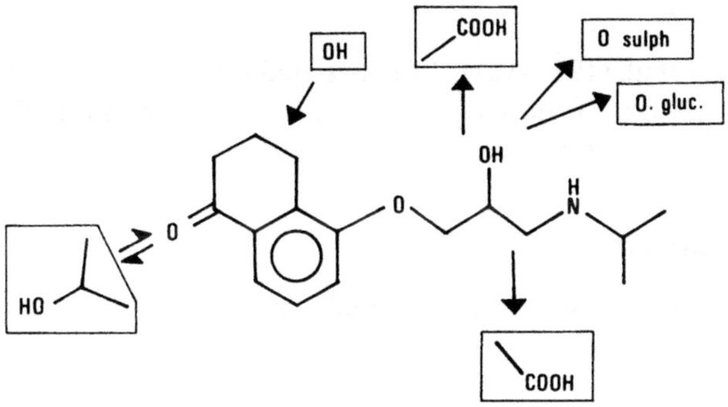

Fig. 19. Structure of bunolol and metabolic products

Table 6. Urinary excretion of bunolol and its metabolites as percentage of dose in 24 h urine (rat, dog) and their presence in plasma (man). (LEINWEBER et al., 1971b, 1977, 1978; DICARLO et al., 1977)

	Species	Unconjugated	Glucuronide	Sulphate
Bunolol	Rat	0.09	1.32	0.02
	Dog[b]	0.43	ND[b]	ND
	Man	+[c]	+	+
Dihydrobunolol	Rat	0.02	0.19	0.03
	Dog	0.30	← 1.71[d] →	
	Man	+	+	ND
Hydroxybunolol	Rat	ND	ND	ND
	Dog	6.10	ND	ND
Hydroxydihydrobunolol	Rat	0.15	ND	ND
	Dog	5.98	–	–
β-(5-Oxytetralonyl) lactic acid	Rat	0.19	ND	ND
	Dog	9.94	ND	ND
(5-Oxytetralonyl) acetic acid	Rat	ND	0.29	ND
	Dog	4.33	ND	ND

[a] Dog data refer to DL-bunolol, p.o.; rat and human data to L-bunolol, p.o.
[b] ND = not detected
[c] A "+" indicates a positive identification
[d] 1.71 refers to the sum of glucuronide plus sulphate

bunolol, found in both, may arise from dihydrobunolol and not from hydroxybunolol (Table 6). Glucuronides and sulphates are formed from bunolol and various of its metabolites but there are species differences (Table 6). It is not known if these conjugates are themselves susceptible to oxidoreductase activity.

b) Sites. Both hepatic and extrahepatic reduction of bunolol to dihydrobunolol have been demonstrated while human and rat erythrocytes are capable of interconversion of these compounds (LEINWEBER et al., 1972; LEINWEBER and DICARLO, 1974).

c) Activity of Metabolites. Dihydrobunolol appears to be equipotent with bunolol as a β-blocker in animals (LEINWEBER et al., 1972), which is not surprising if it is rapidly oxidised to bunolol.

4. Pharmacokinetics

a) Oral. DICARLO et al. (1977) gave 3 mg tritiated L-bunolol by mouth to five healthy subjects and estimated the following $t_{1/2}$ values: bunolol, 6 h; bunolol glucuronide, 9 h; bunolol sulphate, 17 h; dihydrobunolol, 7 h; and dihydrobunolol glucuronide, 8 h.

VI. Dichloroisoprenaline

1-(3,4-Dichlorophenyl)-2-isopropylamino-ethanol

1. Distribution

a) Tissues. The distribution of ^{3}H-labelled dichloroisoprenaline was investigated in dogs and mice after i.v. doses of 7–10 mg/kg (MAYER, 1962). Relatively high counts were observed in lung, liver, and kidney. Unchanged drug appeared to constitute most of the radioactivity in most tissues except kidney. The brain/plasma ratio of radioactivity was 10 after 10 min indicating rapid penetration of the blood–brain barrier.

2. Biotransformation

a) Routes. The only metabolite of dichloroisoprenaline that has been characterised is 3,4-dichloromandelic acid (Fig. 20). The drug is also excreted unchanged in dog urine partly as an unidentified conjugate (MAYER, 1962).

VII. Metoprolol

1-[4-(2-Methoxyethyl)phenoxy]-3-isopropylamino-2-propanol

1. Absorption

a) Extent. Urinary recovery of radioactivity after oral administration of various formulations of tritium-labelled metoprolol to humans was 96% after 72 h, indicating complete absorption of the drug (REGÅRDH et al., 1974, 1975). Similar findings were noted in dog and rat (BORG et al., 1975b). Clearance estimates from i.v. data in humans (see below) suggest an extremely low systemic availability of metoprolol. However, values of bioavailability of the order of 0.45 were found after 50–100 mg oral

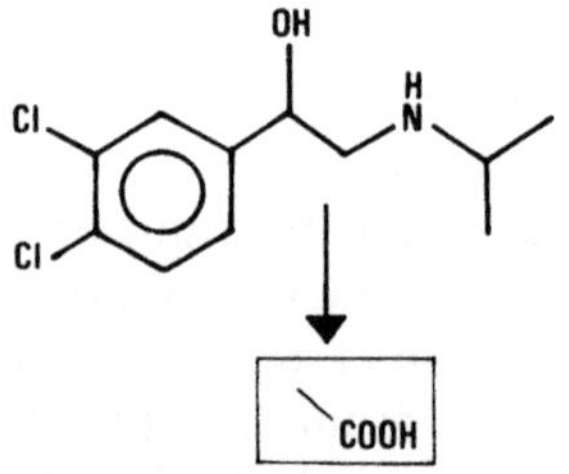

Fig. 20. Structure of dichloroisoprenaline and metabolic product

doses (JOHNSSON et al., 1975) suggesting that some saturation of pre-systemic metabolism of the drug occurs. Although oral bioavailability is relatively constant at therapeutic doses it decreases disproportionately at lower doses. Multiple therapeutic doses and differences in tablet dissolution rate do not significantly influence the bioavailability of metoprolol (BENGTSSON et al., 1975; REGÅRDH et al., 1975) although food increases it (MELANDER et al., 1977). REGÅRDH (1975) indicates a seven-fold variability in oral bioavailability in 20 subjects. Estimates of bioavailability in rat and dog were 0.04 and 0.2–0.4, respectively (BORG et al., 1975b).

b) Rate. Maximum plasma concentrations of metoprolol were observed at 1–2 h after administration of conventional tablets (REGÅRDH, 1975).

2. Distribution

a) Blood. JOHANSSON et al. (1974) reported a mean f_p value of 0.11 for both human plasma and human serum albumin solution. REGÅRDH et al. (1974) found a mean λ value of 1.2 in three healthy subjects.

b) Tissues. Tissue distribution of [^{3}H]metoprolol was studied in the mouse and rat (BODIN et al., 1975). In the pregnant mouse the drug and/or its metabolites readily crossed the placenta to appear in the foetus. A brain: plasma concentration ratio of 3 for unchanged drug was observed in the rat (BODIN et al., 1975); in one human equal concentrations of unbound metoprolol in plasma and cerebro-spinal fluid were indicated (WOOD, 1977).

DAWES et al. (1978) reported saliva: plasma concentration ratios of metoprolol in man greatly in excess of 1 and suggested that the drug gains access to the saliva via an active process. Whereas they found no consistent relationship between salivary and plasma drug concentrations, WAN and MARONDE (1977) indicate a direct proportionality.

3. Biotransformation

a) Routes. The main urinary metabolites of metoprolol in man, dog and rat are formed by oxidative deamination, O-dealkylation with subsequent oxidation and by aliphatic hydroxylation (Fig. 21) (BORG et al., 1975c).

These products account for 85% of the 24-h renal excretion of metoprolol in man and dog and slightly less in the rat. The results of aliphatic hydroxylation of the methoxyethyl group are most evident in the rat although products of degradation of the amine chain are less prominent in this species (Table 7).

b) Sites. Differences in the area under plasma drug concentration versus time curves after i.v. and oral administration indicate significant gut and/or hepatic metabolism (REGÅRDH et al., 1974).

c) Activity of Metabolites. Metabolite III and the presumed alcohol precursor of metabolite I (Table 7, Fig. 21) were shown to have β_1-blocking activity in cats and dogs, but were three to six times less potent than metoprolol itself (BORG et al., 1975c).

4. Excretion

a) Routes. Renal excretion only accounts for the fate of 3%–5% of an oral dose and 10% of an i.v. dose of metoprolol in man (REGÅRDH et al., 1974, 1975).

Table 7. Relative abundances of the main urinary metabolites of metroprolol in man, dog and rat (BORG et al., 1975c)

Species	Relative abundance (% of amount excreted)		
	Metabolite I[a]	Metabolite II[b]	Metabolite III[c]
Man	63	11	10
Dog	33	21	9
Rat	62	1	25

[a] Metabolite I =4-(2-hydroxy-3-isopropylaminopropoxy)-phenylacetic acid
[b] Metabolite II =2-Hydroxy-3-(4-methoxyethylphenoxy)-propionic acid
[c] Metabolite III=1-Isopropylamino-3-[4-(1-hydroxy-2-methoxyethyl)-phenoxy]-2-propanol

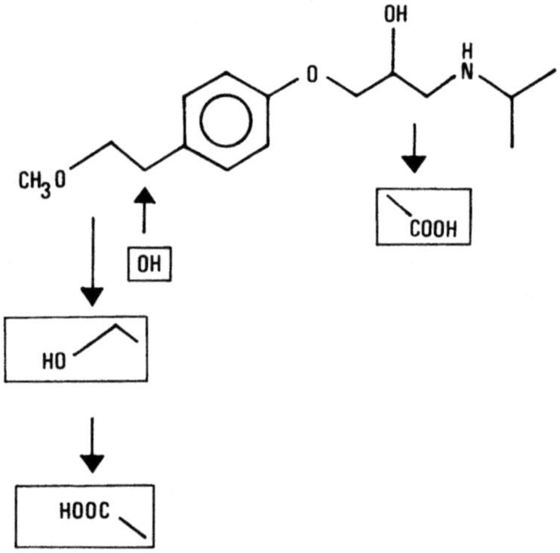

Fig. 21. Structure of metoprolol and metabolic products

5. Pharmacokinetics

a) Intravenous. Disposition kinetics of metoprolol were independent of dose over the range 5–20 mg. The plasma drug concentration versus time curve after i.v. injection in healthy subjects could be described by a biexponential equation giving a mean $t_{1/2\alpha}$ of 0.2 h and a mean $t_{1/2\beta}$ of 3–4 h (REGÅRDH et al., 1974, 1975; JOHNSSON et al., 1975). Mean total (blood) clearance was 1.1 l/min, of w hich 0.109 l/min (corrected for plasma binding) was accounted for by a linear renal clearance. A mean value of 5.6 l/kg was obtained for Vd_β. Terminal plasma elimination half-lives in rats, cats, and dogs were 0.6 h, 1.3 h, and 1.6 h, respectively (BORG et al., 1975a, b). In man, the $t_{1/2}$ of total metabolites in plasma was 5 h (REGÅRDH et al., 1974).

b) Oral. After a solution of metoprolol, the absorption $t_{1/2}$ of the drug was estimated to be 12 min (REGÅRDH et al., 1974). Plasma elimination $t_{1/2\beta}$ values for unchanged drug similar to those after i.v. injection were recorded after various single and multiple oral doses in healthy subjects and hypertensive patients (JOHNSSON et al., 1975; BENGTSSON et al., 1975; REGÅRDH et al., 1975). Total metabolites in plasma after oral metoprolol were eliminated at the same rate as unchanged drug, indicating formation rate-limited kinetics (REGÅRDH et al., 1974). This contrasts with the findings after i.v. injection but the reason for the difference has not been investigated.

c) Effect of Disease. KENDALL et al. (1977) found no statistically significant differences in the areas under plasma drug concentration versus time curves after 100 mg oral doses in young healthy subjects, a group of middle-aged hypertensive patients and a group of elderly non-hypertensive subjects. However, the data for the latter group were more variable, with a trend towards higher areas.

6. Concentration–Effect Relationships

JOHNSSON and REGÅRDH (1976) have summarised the results of a number of studies showing significant correlations between plasma metoprolol concentrations and each of the following: reduction in exercise and isoprenaline-induced tachycardia, reduction in resting heart rate and systolic blood pressure on exercise. However, no correlation was found between plasma drug concentration and resting systolic blood pressure. After i.v. and oral doses, similar plasma drug concentrations were associated with similar degrees of β-blockade – indicating that metoprolol metabolites formed on the "first-pass" do not contribute significantly to pharmacological activity.

VIII. Oxprenolol

1-(2-Allyloxyphenoxy)-3-isopropylamino-2-propanol

1. Absorption

a) Extent. Extensive, but possibly incomplete, absorption of oral oxprenolol in man and dogs is indicated firstly by urinary recoveries of labelled drug between 70%–95% (RIESS et al., 1970, 1974) and secondly by predicted systemic availabilities, based upon i.v. data, equal to or greater than experimental oral bioavailabilities in six healthy subjects (MASON and WINER, 1976). Reported oral bioavailabilities vary from 0.23–0.66 in different subjects but are independent of dose over the range 20–160 mg within a subject (BRUNNER et al., 1975; MASON and WINER, 1976; WEST et al., 1976).

b) Rate. Maximum plasma concentrations of oxprenolol occur at 0.5–1.5 h after conventional oral dosage forms in normal subjects (MASON and WINER, 1976; WEST et al., 1976).

2. Distribution

a) Blood. According to DAWES et al. (1978), Riess and others have found an f_p value of 0.78 for oxprenolol binding to human plasma. MASON and WINER (1976) quote a mean λ value of 0.80 in man.

b) Tissues. Whole body autoradiography indicated a preferential uptake of labelled oxprenolol in mouse lung, kidney, and liver; concentrations in the brain were the lowest of any of the organs examined and equivalent to blood concentrations of radioactivity (RIESS et al., 1970). Salivary and plasma concentrations of oxprenolol were found to be directly proportional to each other in healthy volunteers, with a mean saliva: plasma concentration ratio of 0.42, close to the predicted value for passive diffusion (DAWES et al., 1978).

3. Biotransformation

a) Routes. Analysis of human, dog, and rat urine after oxprenolol administration has indicated several metabolic pathways for the drug, i.e., O-glucuronidation of unchanged drug, N-dealkylation followed by N-methylation, oxidative deamination followed by oxidation to a lactic acid derivative, oxidation of the carbinol group to yield a substituted acetic acid, aromatic hydroxylation, and splitting of both ether linkages to yield phenols (Fig. 22, Table 8) (GARTEIZ, 1971; GARTEIZ and GAFFNEY, 1971; LEESON et al., 1973; RIESS et al., 1970, 1974; WALLE, 1974). Quantitative data on each metabolite are sparse. RIESS et al. (1970) found that most of the urinary recovery in man could be accounted for as oxprenolol glucuronide.

b) Site. Most of the metabolism of oxprenolol appears to occur pre-systemically, presumably in the liver. However, some breakdown in the gastrointestinal wall might account for the incomplete absorption indicated by urinary recoveries (RIESS et al., 1970, 1974). GAFFNEY et al. (1971) detected N-desalkyl oxprenolol and oxprenolol glycol in the perfusate of a dog heart–lung preparation but the extent of this metabolism was not indicated.

4. Excretion

a) Routes. In man, renal excretion of unchanged oxprenolol accounts for less than 5% of the dose (RIESS et al., 1974).

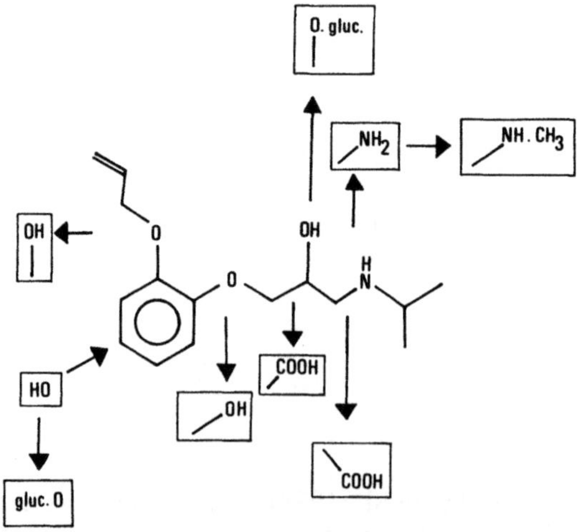

Fig. 22. Structure of oxprenolol and metabolic products

Table 8. Detection of oxprenolol and metabolites in urine (GARTEIZ, 1971; GARTEIZ and GAFFNEY, 1971; LEESON et al., 1973; RIESS et al., 1970, 1974; WALLE, 1974

	Man	Dog	Rat
Oxprenolol[a]	+[b]	+	+
3-(2-Allyloxyphenoxy) lactic acid	+		
2-Allyloxyphenoxy acetic acid	+		
2-Allyloxy phenol	+		+
1-(2-Allyloxyphenoxy)-3-amino-2-propanol[a]	+	+	+
1-(2-Allyloxyphenoxy)-3-methylamino-2-propanol[a]		+	
1-(2-Hydroxyphenoxy)-3-isopropylamino-2-propanol[a]	+	+	+
1-(2-Allyloxy-4-hydroxyphenoxy)-3-isopropylamino-2-propanol[a]			+

[a] Indicates also excreted as a glucuronide
[b] Indicates positive identification of derivative

5. Pharmacokinetics

a) Intravenous. The disposition kinetics of oxprenolol were studied by MASON and WINER (1976) after 10 and 20 mg i.v. doses in six healthy subjects. Plasma concentration versus time profiles of unchanged drug were described by a biexponential equation giving dose-independent mean $t_{1/2\alpha}$ and $t_{1/2\beta}$ values of 17 min and 2.3 h, respectively. Blood clearance averaged 0.4 l/min., mean Vd_β (plasma) was 1.11 l/kg and mean Vd_{ss} (plasma) was 0.86 l/kg.

b) Oral. A mean terminal $t_{1/2}$ of 1.94 h was obtained in six subjects and was independent of dose over the range 20–160 mg (MASON and WINER, 1976). BRUNNER et al. (1975) reported a mean $t_{1/2}$ of 80 min but their data only extended over an 8-h period.

6. Concentration–Effect Relationships

Correlations between the logarithm of plasma oxprenolol concentration and reduction in exercise-induced tachycardia have been reported by several groups (BRUNNER et al., 1975; DAVIDSON et al., 1976; MASON and WINER, 1976). DAVIDSON et al. (1976) also showed a correlation between plasma oxprenolol concentration and reduction in isoprenaline-induced tachycardia. Prolonged-release forms of the drug significantly extend the duration of β-blockade over that observed after conventional tablets or capsules (DAVIDSON et al., 1976; WEST et al., 1976).

IX. Pindolol

1-(1-Indol-4-yloxy)-3-isopropylamino-2-propanol

1. Absorption

a) Extent. Several estimates of the urinary recovery of ^{14}C-labelled pindolol indicate a net absorption of at least 80% of an oral dose (MEIER and NUESCH, 1977). The bioavailability of the drug in healthy subjects averages about 0.92 as determined from the relative areas under plasma drug concentration versus time curves after i.v. and oral dosage (MEIER and NUESCH, 1977) and from the urinary recoveries of unchanged drug after the two routes of administration (GUGLER et al., 1974). Any contribution of the first-pass effect to the metabolism of pindolol is, therefore, quite small. CHAU et al. (1977) estimated a mean oral bioavailability of 0.86 in hypertensive patients with normal renal function.

b) Rate. Mean estimates of t_{max} after conventional oral dosage forms vary from 1.3 to 3 h (GUGLER et al., 1974; ANAVEKAR et al., 1975).

2. Distribution

a) Blood. Using equilibrium dialysis, CHAU et al. (1977) found a mean f_p value of 0.51 for 50 mg/pindolol/ml human plasma, similar to the figure of 0.57 reported by GUGLER et al. (1974) for binding to human serum albumin. CHAU et al. (1977) also quote a mean erythrocyte: plasma concentration ratio of 0.42 for hypertensive patients. Assuming an average haematocrit of 0.42 this gives a mean λ value of 0.76.

3. Biotransformation

a) Routes. OHNHAUS et al. (1974) indicate that over 90% of the urinary metabolites of pindolol in man are glucuronides and sulphates. Nine metabolites have been separated from the urine of rhesus monkeys, rats, cats, and rabbits, suggesting four main pathways (KIECHEL et al., 1975): (1) side-chain conjugation with glucuronic acid; (2) hydroxylation or oxidation and conjugation of the indole ring to give the indolin-2-one analogue of pindolol, 3-hydroxy-pindolol sulphate, 5-hydroxy-pindolol glucuronide and sulphate, 6-hydroxy-pindolol glucuronide and the side-chain glucuronide of an indigotin-like derivative of pindolol; (3) oxidative ring scission to the corresponding anthranilic acid derivative, and (4) side-chain oxidation and deamination to 3-(5-indolyloxy) lactic acid (Fig. 23, Table 9). Relative proportions of these metabolites have not been quantitated.

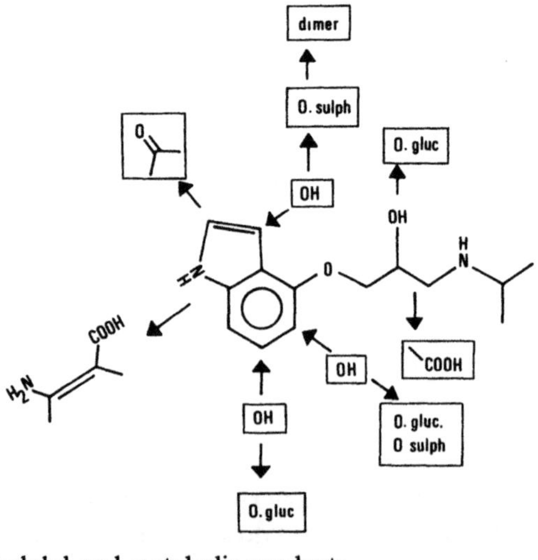

Fig. 23. Structure of pindolol and metabolic products

Table 9. Detection of pindolol and metabolites in urine (KIECHEL et al., 1975)

	Rhesus monkey	Rat	Cat	Rabbit
Pindolol[a]	+[c]			
5-Hydroxy pindolol[a]		+		
6-Hydroxy pindolol[a, b]	+	+		+
Indolin-2-one analogue of pindolol			+	
3-Hydroxy pindolol[b]		+		
Anthranilic acid derivative		+		
Indigotin-like derivative[a]		+		
3-(5-Indolyloxy) lactic acid				+

[a] Indicates found as a glucuronide
[b] Indicates found as a sulphate
[c] + Indicates positive identification of derivative

b) Sites. Direct estimates of hepatic clearance of pindolol in patients with renovascular hypertension are identical to indirect estimates of their non-renal clearance; this shows that the liver is the sole site of metabolism of the drug (LAVENE et al., 1977).

4. Excretion

a) Routes. Data from several studies in healthy subjects indicate mean f_u values of 0.37–0.39 and 0.32–0.36 after i.v. and oral dosage, respectively (MEIER and NUESCH, 1977).

b) Effects of Disease. The f_u value of pindolol after i.v. injection varied from a mean of 0.50 in hypertensive patients with normal renal function to a mean of 0.09 in a group with an average creatinine clearance of 20 ml/min (LAVENE et al., 1977).

5. Pharmacokinetics

a) Intravenous. GUGLER et al. (1974) gave i.v. infusions of 5 mg pindolol to 17 healthy subjects and found a mean plasma elimination $t_{1/2}$ of 3.1 h, a mean plasma clearance of 0.48 l/min, a mean renal (plasma) clearance of 0.22 l/min and a volume of distribution of 2 l/kg.

b) Oral. In the same subjects that received i.v. infusions of pindolol, (see above) the mean plasma elimination $t_{1/2}$ of the drug was found to be 3.6 h after 5 mg oral doses. A four-fold variation was seen in maximum plasma drug concentrations (GUGLER et al., 1974).

c) Effects of Disease. The plasma pindolol concentration versus time course after 0.04 mg/kg i.v. bolus injections in nine hypertensive patients with normal renal function was described by a biexponential equation giving mean $t_{\geqq\beta}$ and $t_{\geqq\beta}$ values of 5 min and 2 h, respectively; the mean plasma clearance was 0.54 l/min and mean renal (plasma) clearance was 0.27 l/min (CHAU et al., 1977). Relatively short terminal $t_{1/2}$ values were measured in this study compared to those found by GUGLER et al. (1974) in healthy subjects and may be explained by a sampling period of only 3 h. CHAU et al. (1977) also found that oral absorption of pindolol in their patients could not be described by a simple first-order process and that their calculations further suggested some back excretion of the drug from blood into the gastrointestinal tract.

Three groups have looked at the kinetics of pindolol in patients with renal disease. Based upon a lack of correlation between plasma $t_{1/2}$ of pindolol and creatinine clearance, OHNHAUS et al. (1974) concluded that there is a compensatory increase in non-renal elimination in patients with renal impairment. This was subsequently challenged by ØIE and LEVY (1975) who demonstrated that although there was a direct relationship between renal clearance of pindolol and creatinine clearance, non-renal clearance of pindolol was independent of renal function. Data obtained by CHAU et al. (1977) endorsed the latter finding and further showed a decrease in total pindolol clearance with decrease in creatinine clearance together with an increase in the initial absorption rate of the drug but a reduction in its bioavailability. Mean bioavailability was 0.52 in patients with creatinine clearances of 7–38 ml/min compared to 0.86 in those with creatinine clearances of 69–120 ml/min. Using antipyrine as a marker of liver function, OHNHAUS et al. (1976) found no correlation between its clearance and that of pindolol. Only in patients with liver failure having antipyrine clearances less than 10 ml/min did the clearance of pindolol decrease. Lower doses of the drug may, therefore, be required in these patients.

6. Concentration–Effect Relationships

Several groups have demonstrated correlations between plasma pindolol concentration and reduction in exercise- and isoprenaline-induced tachycardia (GUGLER et al., 1975; HICKS et al., 1972). In addition, ANAVEKAR et al. (1975) found a significant relationship between maximum plasma drug concentrations and decrease in resting blood pressure after single 20 mg oral doses in 15 hypertensive patients. When a further 99 patients on chronic pindolol therapy were grouped into good, fair, and non-responders, mean plasma drug concentrations at 2–3 h after the morning dose corresponded generally with the degree of blood pressure control.

X. Practolol

1-(4-Aminophenoxy)-3-isopropylamino-2-propanol

1. Absorption

a) Extent. Several studies have shown the oral absorption of practolol to be extensive. Estimates of urinary recovery of radiolabelled drug in man vary from 74%–90% (FITZGERALD and SCALES, 1968; CASE et al., 1978; DRING et al., 1978) and in dogs and rats were in excess of 85% (SCALES and COSGROVE, 1970). Other studies using colorimetric, fluorometric, and glc assays found 92%–97% of oral doses as unchanged practolol in human urine, indicating virtually complete bioavailability (BODEM and CHIDSEY, 1973; CARRUTHERS et al., 1974).

b) Rate. Maximum plasma practolol concentrations occur between 1–3 h after conventional tablets in healthy subjects (CARRUTHERS et al., 1974; HARVENGT et al., 1975; CASTLEDEN et al., 1975).

2. Distribution

a) Blood. Binding of practolol in whole plasma has not been reported but approximately 32% was shown to associate with human serum albumin (GIUDICELLI et al., 1973).

b) Tissues. After i.v., i.p., and oral administration, [^{14}C]practolol was rapidly distributed throughout the tissues of rats, mice, and dogs (SCALES and COSGROVE, 1970). The lowest levels were found in the brain and blood of these species and the highest in some secretory glands of the mouse. Equilibration between plasma and brain concentrations of the drug in dogs occurs very slowly, equal concentrations being achieved only after 24 h.

3. Biotransformation

a) Routes. The metabolism of practolol has been examined in several species including man (Fig. 24, Table 10). In rat, 15% of a ^{14}C-labelled dose was excreted in urine as 18 metabolites, of which only two have been characterised directly (SCALES and COSGROVE, 1970). 3-Hydroxy practolol and its glucuronide were the major products accounting for 3% and 6% of the dose, respectively. Formation of $^{14}CO_2$ and [^{14}C]urea from [^{14}C]acetyl-labelled practolol suggested that about 4% of the dose is metabolised by removal of the acetyl side-chain. Similar findings were obtained in man, mouse, and dog with 5%–14% of the dose recovered as $^{14}CO_2$, although as much as 51% appeared to be deacetylated in the marmoset (CASE et al., 1978). Interestingly, desacetylpractolol has never been detected in animal or human urine (SCALES and COSGROVE, 1970; BODEM and CHIDSEY, 1973; HARVENGT et al., 1975; CASE et al., 1978) indicating that deacetylation must precede or be preceded by a further metabolic breakdown, al-

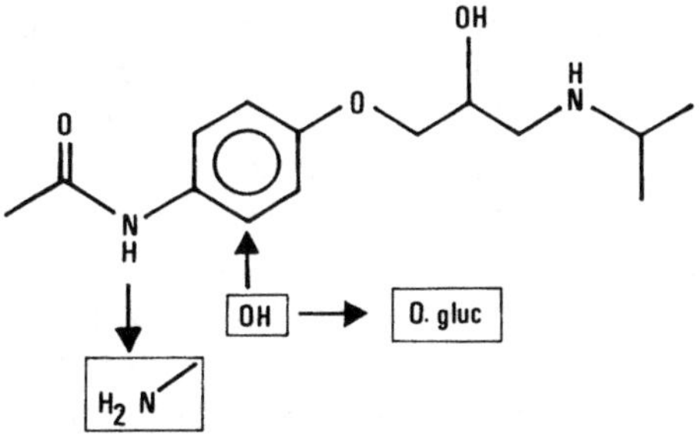

Fig. 24. Structure of practolol and metabolic products

Table 10. Detection of practolol and metabolites in urine (FITZGERALD and SCALES, 1968; SCALES and COSGROVE, 1970; BODEM and CHIDSEY, 1973; KAYE et al., 1973; KAYE and KUMANA, 1974; CASE et al., 1978; DRING et al., 1978)

	Man	Dog	Rat	Marmoset	Hamster
Practolol	+[a]	+	+	+	
3-Hydroxy practolol			+	+	+
CO_2	+	+	+	+	

[a] + Indicates positive identification of derivative

though, as suggested by DRING et al. (1978), deacetylation may be followed by rapid reacetylation. In human urine there is little or no evidence for the presence of conjugates of 3-hydroxy practolol (HARVENGT et al., 1975; DRING et al., 1978).

b) Activity of Metabolites. Development of an oculomucocutaneous syndrome in some patients treated with practolol has focussed interest on the possibility that the side-effects may be mediated by practolol metabolites. Although affected patients do not appear to show gross differences in metabolism of the drug (CASE et al., 1978; DRING et al., 1978), this leaves a possibility that transient, reactive metabolic intermediates might be responsible. Microsomal studies (ORTON and LOWERY, 1977; CASE et al., 1978) have indeed shown that hepatic enzymes from several species produce such compounds, possibly via N-hydroxylation, that are capable of binding irreversibly to proteins. Antibody binding to epithelial tissue was demonstrated in patients with conjunctival damage by AMOS et al. (1975). More recently, antigen prepared by metabolising practolol in a microsomal mixed-function oxidase system has been used to study antibody-binding curves in serum from patients with a history of adverse reaction to practolol. The presence of antibody was found to relate to practolol administration and amounts were increased by challenge doses of the drug (AMOS et al., 1978).

4. Excretion

a) Routes. As indicated above, virtually all of a dose of practolol is excreted unchanged in human urine. The rate of excretion approximates to glomerular filtration rate and is independent of urinary pH (BODEM and CHIDSEY, 1973; KAYE et al., 1973; TILSTONE et al., 1974). Evidence for biliary secretion and enterohepatic recirculation of practolol and its metabolites has been obtained in animals (SCALES and COSGROVE, 1970) and has been suggested to account for the drug's prolonged plasma $t_{1/2}$ and the occurrence of secondary plasma drug peaks after i.v. injection in man (AELLIG et al., 1970; CARRUTHERS et al., 1974). Although KAYE and KUMANA (1974) recovered only 0.02%–0.15% of an i.v. dose as unchanged practolol in the bile of one patient, CARRUTHERS et al. (1976) obtained a mean biliary recovery of 8% after 48 h in six patients who had undergone biliary surgery. In two of these patients, the recoveries were 23% and 41%. Since virtually complete urinary excretion of practolol is found in normal subjects, the presence of these relatively large amounts of drug in the bile suggests that significant enterohepatic recirculation of the drug occurs at least in some patients.

b) Drug Interactions. Frusemide has been shown to increase the renal clearance of practolol in man, presumably via elevation of glomerular filtration rate (TILSTONE et al., 1974). CARRUTHERS et al. (1976) suggested that the relatively high biliary recoveries of practolol in the two patients described above may be accounted for by an absence of concurrent therapy with other drugs. In the other four patients, with smaller quantities of practolol in the bile, they proposed that other drugs may have inhibited practolol secretion.

5. Pharmacokinetics

a) Intravenous. Blood practolol concentration versus time curves after i.v. injection in six hypertensive patients were described by a triexponential equation giving a mean terminal $t_{1/2}$ value of 12 h (AELLIG et al., 1970). However, interpretation of i.v. data is complicated by the appearance of secondary peaks at 2 and 7 h, possibly due to enterohepatic recycling (CARRUTHERS et al., 1974).

b) Oral. Estimates of the mean plasma elimination $t_{1/2}$ of practolol after oral administration in healthy subjects and hypertensive patients are in the range 6–13 h (SCHNECK et al., 1972; BODEM and CHIDSEY, 1973; KAYE and KUMANA, 1974; CARRUTHERS et al., 1974; HARVENGT et al., 1975; CASTLEDEN et al., 1975). It is possible that lower values may have been biased by relatively short sampling times. From plasma practolol data obtained after termination of a continuous oral dosage regimen in hypertensive patients, BODEM and CHIDSEY (1973) calculated a mean value of 0.135 l/min for both total and renal drug clearance and a volume of distribution of 1.6 l/kg.

c) Effect of Age. Although the mean plasma elimination $t_{1/2}$ of practolol was 8.6 h in a group of healthy elderly subjects compared to a mean of 7.1 h in young controls, the difference is probably not of clinical significance and may be related entirely to differences in renal function (CASTLEDEN et al., 1975).

d) Effect of Disease. Plasma practolol concentrations in patients with coeliac disease appeared to lag behind those of normal subjects but peak concentrations were similar (PARSONS and KAYE, 1974). Patients with hypothyroidism were found to have a mean practolol $t_{1/2}$ of 16 h compared to 9.8 h in hyperthyroid subjects (BELL et al., 1977). The mean area under the plasma drug concentration versus time curve was also significantly lower in the latter group, probably as a result of an increased clearance rather than of a reduced absorption. Again, these findings might be explained by differences in glomerular filtration rate. A direct relationship has been shown between the plasma $t_{1/2}$ of practolol and the reciprocal of creatinine clearance in patients with varying degrees of renal impairment (EASTWOOD et al., 1973; BODEM et al., 1974). In those with severe renal failure, the normal $t_{1/2}$ may be prolonged up to seven-fold and in anephric patients $t_{1/2}$ values of up to 166 h have been observed. On average, haemodialysis successfully reduces the elimination $t_{1/2}$ by a factor of four, although plasma drug levels tend to rebound at the end of the procedure (EASTWOOD et al., 1973; HARVENGT et al., 1975).

6. Concentration–Effect Relationships

Plasma concentrations of practolol have been correlated with both exercise- and isoprenaline-induced tachycardia in hypertensive patients (SCHNECK et al., 1972; KUMANA and KAYE, 1974; CARRUTHERS et al., 1974). Relatively high plasma drug concentrations produce a loss of cardioselectivity (KUMANA et al., 1977).

XI. Pronethalol

3-Naphthyl-1-isopropylamino-2-propanol

1. Absorption

a) Extent. In man 100% of a ^{14}C-labelled oral dose was recovered in the urine indicating complete absorption. Small amounts of radiolabel in the faeces of animal species were accounted for by biliary excretion of metabolites (BOND and HOWE, 1967).

2. Distribution

a) Tissues. Highest amounts of radioactivity were found in liver and kidney, with some in the brain, after oral doses of ^{14}C-labelled drug to mice (BOND and HOWE, 1967).

3. Biotransformation

a) Routes. Urinary metabolites isolated from various species indicate both side-chain oxidation and ring-hydroxylation followed by conjugation (Fig. 25, Table 11) (BOND and HOWE, 1967; STILLWELL and HORNING, 1974). Although the primary amine me-

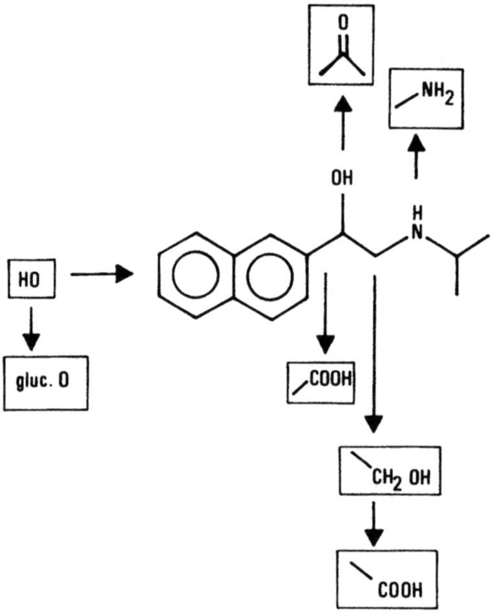

Fig. 25. Structure of pronethalol and metabolic products

Table 11. Pronethalol and metabolites identified in urine (BOND and HOWE, 1967; STILLWELL and HORNING, 1974)

	Man	Rabbit	Mouse	Guinea pig	Rat
Pronethalol[a]	+	+	+	+	+
2-Naphthylglycollic acid	+	+		+	+
2-Naphthylglyoxylic acid	+	+			+
2-Naphthoic acid	+	+		+	+
2-Naphthylethane-1:2-diol[a]			+	+	+
Ring dihydrodiols[a]					+
6-Hydroxy pronethalol[a]			+		+
7-Hydroxy pronethalol[a]	+		+	+	+
Other ring hydroxy compounds[a]			+	+	+

[a] Indicates excreted as a conjugate

tabolite is assumed to be a precursor of further side-chain degradation products, it has only been observed in in vitro experiments. Major acidic metabolites are 2-naphthylglycollic and 2-napthoic acids with 2-naphthylglyoxylic acid as a minor product in rat, rabbit, and human urine. Side-chain metabolism is prominent in the guinea-pig but in the urine of other species, compounds derived via the ring-hydroxylation route are about twice as prevalent. The 6- and 7-hydroxy compounds, mostly present as conjugates, have been demonstrated as well as other phenols, although the positions of the OH group in the latter are not known. Conjugated dihydrodiols, presumably formed via epoxides, have also been detected but their exact structures are uncertain.

b) Activity of Metabolites. Animal data indicate that 7-hydroxy pronethalol is five times more potent as a β-blocker than pronethalol and, since its blood levels in man after oral administration are considerably higher than those of unchanged drug, it may account for most of the pharmacological activity (BOND and HOWE, 1967). The product of pronethalol responsible for thymic tumours and other sarcomas in mice is not likely to be one of the identified metabolites. Suggested candidates include ethylenimine and intermediates associated with the epoxide pathway (BOND and HOWE, 1967; STILLWELL and HORNING, 1974).

XII. Propranolol

3-(1-Naphthoxy)-1-isopropylamino-2-propanol

1. Absorption

a) Extent. Radiotracer studies indicate virtually complete oral absorption of propranolol in all species studied, including man (HAYES and COOPER, 1971; PATERSON et al., 1970). The systemic availability of oral propranolol is relatively low and very variable owing to significant pre-systemic drug elimination. Thus, the average bioavailability after a single 80 mg dose in five healthy subjects ranged from 0.16–0.60 with a mean of 0.32 (SHAND et al., 1970). After doses of 30 mg or less, SHAND and RANGNO (1972) were unable to detect propranolol in the plasma using a fluorometric assay, and suggested this as a "threshold dose" above which hepatic extraction processes become saturated resulting in appreciable availability. More recently, however, GOMENI et al. (1977), using a glc assay, reported bioavailabilities from 0.09–0.38 in three normal subjects after single doses of 10–40 mg. Availability was consistent within a subject and independent of dose over the range studied. The same group also reported a mean systemic availability of 0.19 after a single 40 mg oral dose in five individuals (BIANCHETTI et al., 1976). According to EVANS and SHAND (1973 a), hepatic extraction of propranolol remains saturated throughout a dosage interval of 6 h leading to higher bioavailability of all doses subsequent to the first. Using a different experimental design and a regimen of 80 mg every 8 h, the same group showed a greater accumulation of plasma propranolol than predicted from initial dose data and a mean systemic availability of 0.36 at steady state (KORNHAUSER et al., 1978). At steady state, bioavailability appears to be proportional to dose up to 160 mg/day but a disproportional increase occurs at higher daily dosage (EVANS and SHAND, 1973).

Food intake was shown to be associated with a 1.5-fold increase in the area under the plasma propranolol versus time curve from 0 to 8 h after 80 mg oral doses in healthy subjects (MELANDER et al., 1977). The mechanism of this effect is unclear but it may be related to an increase in splanchnic blood flow (MCLEAN et al., 1978).

b) Rate. Most studies indicate rapid absorption of propranolol after administration of solutions or tablets, maximum plasma drug concentrations occurring after 1–3 h (PATERSON et al., 1970; SHAND et al., 1970; THOMPSON et al., 1972; GOMENI et al., 1977). SHAND et al. (1970) found that food tended to increase t_{max}, but this was not confirmed by MELANDER et al. (1977). Variability in gastric emptying per se was not considered by CASTLEDEN et al. (1978) to be a significant determinant of individual differences in maximum plasma propranolol concentrations after oral administration.

2. Distribution

a) Blood. Mean f_p values between 0.84–0.95 have been reported for healthy subjects and there are some data for plasma binding in various disease states (Table 12). Binding tends to decrease as propranolol concentration is raised above therapeutic levels and it cannot be accounted for entirely by association with albumin (EVANS et al., 1973a; BORGA et al., 1977; BARBER et al., 1978). A significant negative correlation between plasma concentration of α_1-acid glycoprotein and the free fraction of propranolol in plasma suggests that, as in the case of alprenolol, this is the major binding protein (BORGA et al., 1977). Species differences in plasma binding have also been shown. Thus, mean f_p values in man, monkey, dog, and rat were 0.93, 0.99, 0.97, and 0.92, respectively (EVANS et al., 1973a).

Mean estimates of λ in healthy humans, monkeys, dogs, and rats are 0.78–0.81, 0.85, and 0.80, respectively, and were found to be directly related to the free fraction of propranolol in blood (EVANS et al., 1973a; BRANCH et al., 1977; LOWENTHAL et al., 1974). SAWCHUCK et al. (1974) reported a much greater variation in λ in hypertensive patients, with a mean value of 1.33, although it is possible that spuriously high figures might have resulted from the method of blood collection (COTHAM and SHAND, 1975). Patients with cirrhosis appear to have increased λ values owing to reduced plasma drug binding (BRANCH et al., 1977).

b) Tissues. Radiotracer studies in animals show rapid entry of unchanged propranolol from plasma to brain tissue, especially the cerebral cortex (HAYES and COOPER, 1971; MASUOKA and HANSSON, 1967). Furthermore, the drug also leaks back quickly from the cerebro-spinal fluid to the plasma after intracerebroventricular injection, a finding which questions the validity of the use of this route of administration in differentiating between central nervous and peripheral mechanisms contributing to lowering of blood pressure (ANDERSON et al., 1977; MYERS et al., 1975). Preferential uptake of the active L-isomer of propranolol in both brain and heart tissue has been demonstrated after injection of the DL-form by a radioimmunoassay technique employing stereospecific antibodies (LEVY et al., 1976).

The observation of relatively high concentrations of propranolol and of its metabolites in animal lungs in vivo (HAYES and COOPER, 1971) has been extended by studies using an isolated perfused rat lung preparation, lung slices and isolated alveolar macrophages (DOLLERY and JUNOD, 1976; VESTAL et al., 1976). Propranolol uptake by these systems was shown to have active and saturable components, to be independent of the β-receptor and to be subject to competition by other basic drugs. A preliminary study of the clinical implications of these findings was reported by GEDDES et al. (1978)

Table 12. Plasma binding (f_p) of propranolol in man

Reference	Method	Propranolol conc. (μg/ml)	Normals	Hyperten-sives	Liver disease	Renal failure	Crohn's disease	Inflamm. arthritis	Thyroid disease
EVANS et al. (1973a)	ED, RT	1.0	0.93						
MCDEVITT et al. (1976)	ED, RT	1.0	0.93	0.95[a]					
BRANCH et al. (1976)	ED, RT	0.13	0.88		0.82[a]				
BRANCH et al. (1977)	ED, RT		0.93		0.90[a]				
BIANCHETTI et al. (1976)	UF, RT	0.03–0.15	0.95			0.95			
KELLY and MCDEVITT (1977)	ED, 37 °C	0.03–0.42							0.87[b]
BORGA et al. (1977)	ED, 37 °C		0.88		0.85[c]	0.89[c]	0.93[c]	0.93[c]	
BARBER et al. (1978)	ED, 37 °C	0.2–1.6	0.84						

[a] Significantly different from normal control
[b] No difference between hypo- and hyperthyroid patients either before or after treatment
[c] No indication of statistical differences
ED = Equilibrium dialysis UF = Ultrafiltration RT = Room temperature

who showed that "first-pass" lung uptake of propranolol in man may be sufficiently great to provide a "buffer" against high input drug concentrations in the pulmonary artery after i.v. injection and that this protection may be attenuated in patients on chronic therapy owing to saturation of the uptake process.

Experiments using an isolated perfused rat liver preparation have documented the existence of both high affinity–low capacity and low affinity–high capacity tissue binding sites for propranolol in the liver. The former is considered to account in large part for the extensive and dose-dependent first-pass hepatic extraction of the drug (EVANS et al., 1973b; SHAND et al., 1973). Further studies have located the high affinity site in the microsomal fraction of the liver (MCEWAN et al., 1974).

3. Biotransformation

a) Routes. Qualitative aspects of the metabolic fate of propranolol have been studied in man and laboratory animals resulting in the identification of 13 products and their conjugates (Table 13, Fig. 26). Attack on the naphthylene ring occurs as well as oxidation and cleavage of the side-chain (BAKKE et al., 1973; BOND, 1967; HAYES and COOPER, 1971; ISHIZAKI et al., 1974; PATERSON et al., 1970; SAELENS et al., 1974; TINDELL et al., 1972; WALLE and GAFFNEY, 1972; WALLE et al., 1972, 1974).

Although 3- and 4-hydroxypropranolol are listed in Table 13 as the products of ring hydroxylation of propranolol, recent in vitro observations have extended the possibilities to two dihydroxy metabolites (one of which may be catechol-like) and four monophenols (TINDELL et al., 1978). The evidence suggests that one of the dihydroxy compounds may be the 3,4-product, formed via an epoxide (WALLE, 1977). Although this compound has not been isolated, identification of two isomeric methoxy-hydroxypropranolols in man suggests the formation of a dihydroxypropranolol also in vivo with subsequent O-methylation similar to catecholamine metabolism (TINDELL et al., 1978). Unequivocal evidence for the position of the ring OH group in any of

Table 13. Identification of propranolol and its metabolites in various species

Compound	Man	Monkey	Dog	Rabbit	Mouse	Guinea pig	Rat
Propranolol[a]	+	+	+	+	+	+	+
N-Desisopropylpropranolol[a]	+		+				
Naphthoxylactic acid	+	+	+	+	+	+	+
Naphthoxyacetic acid	+		+				
4-Hydroxynaphthoxylactic acid							+
Propranolol glycol[a]	+		+				
4-Hydroxy propranolol glycol[a]	+		+				
4-Hydroxy propranolol[a]	+	+	+	+	+	+	+
3-Hydroxy propranolol[a]	+						+
α-Naphthol[a]	+		+				
Dihydroxynaphthalene[a]	+		+				
Acetone							+
CO_2							+
Isopropylamine			+				+

[a] Indicates that the compound is also excreted as conjugates (glucuronides or etheral sulphates)

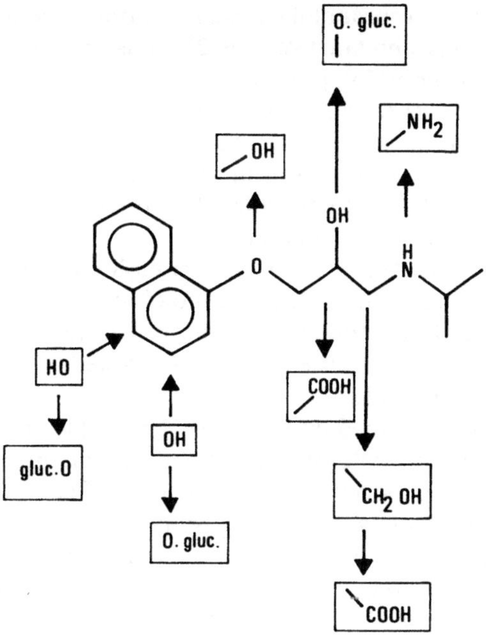

Fig. 26. Structure of propranolol and metabolic products

the phenols is lacking. The compound designated as 4-hydroxypropranolol was only found in the plasma of animals and man after oral and not after i.v. administration of propranolol; relatively little is excreted in the urine (PATERSON et al., 1970; HAYES and COOPER, 1971). Peak plasma 4-hydroxy propranolol/propranolol concentration ratios were about 0.4 and 0.8 in two subjects after a single 40 mg oral dose (PATERSON et al., 1970) and about 0.25 in four patients during chronic therapy with a 40 mg dose every 6 h (WALLE et al., 1975).

Propranolol is deaminated both directly to yield isopropylamine and via the primary amine formed from initial N-dealkylation (WALLE et al., 1972; BAKKE et al., 1973). The first route seems to be quantitatively less important, however, as only 1.4% of an i.p. dose of propranolol given to rats was excreted as isopropylamine in the urine and isopropylamine when given as such is rapidly excreted in unchanged form (BAKKE et al., 1973). A major urinary metabolite of propranolol is naphthoxylactic acid which accounts for about 20% and 40% of oral and i.v. doses, respectively, in man (PATERSON et al., 1970). The diastereomeric O-glucuronides of DL-propranolol were recently identified by gc-ms (EHRSSON, 1975) and they are present in human plasma in concentrations up to 10 t imes that of unchanged drug (MURPHY et al., 1976; WALLE et al., 1976). In urine, propranolol-O-glucuronide accounts for 2.5%–25% of a daily propranolol dose (WALLE et al., 1976).

b) Sites. A dominant role of hepatic metabolism of propranolol is indicated by studies employing portal vein injection, hepatic vein catheterisation, and isolated perfused rat livers (SHAND et al., 1971, 1972; SUZUKI et al., 1974). In dogs, GEORGE et al. (1976) estimated that the liver accounts for 75% and 91% of the total clearance of D- and L-propranolol, respectively.

Some metabolism of propranolol has been demonstrated in an isolated dog heart–lung preparation (WALLE and GAFFNEY, 1972). Thus, the lung was capable of producing N-desisopropyl propranolol, propranolol glycol, naphthyloxylactic acid and isopropylamine, although heart and blood were unable to metabolise propranolol they could deaminate the primary amine metabolite through to the glycol. Regrettably, no quantitative information was obtained in these studies but similar investigations by DOLLERY and JUNOD (1976) with an isolated perfused dog lung preparation showed very little net metabolism of propranolol.

c) Activity of Metabolites. 4-Hydroxypropranolol was shown to possess β-blocking properties equivalent to those of propranolol in dogs (FITZGERALD and O'DONNELL, 1971) and a significant contribution to the β antagonism seen after single oral doses of propranolol in man has been strongly suggested (COLTART and SHAND, 1970; CLEAVLAND and SHAND, 1972).

Many of the other identified and putative metabolites of propranolol have also been shown to have pharmacological activity but few quantitative data are available to assess their biological importance in relation to the effects of the parent drug. Thus, N-desisopropyl propranolol has β-blocking properties (CROWTHER and SMITH, 1968), 5-hydroxy propranolol is said to be more potent than propranolol as an antihypertensive agent (RAM et al., 1976) and the other ring-hydroxy products are also suggested to be β-blockers (WALLE et al., 1976). When injected into dogs, isopropylamine influences the heart and the peripheral vasculature (WALLE et al., 1972; ISHIZAKI et al., 1974), but the findings of BAKKE et al. (1973) (op. cit.) argue against a significant contribution from this metabolite to the effects of propranolol.

Both propranolol glycol and N-desisopropyl propranolol, a metabolic intermediate between propranolol and propranolol glycol, protect against strychnine and pentylenetetrazole seizures in mice (SAELENS et al., 1974, 1976). Propranolol also has anticonvulsant activity in this model and the delayed onset plus the presence of propranolol glycol in the brain at the peak of effect, suggest that its action may be mediated via the formation of the glycol. A tentative link has also been made between propranolol glycol and both cardiac depression and sedation in rats receiving propranolol (SAELENS et al., 1974). Propranolol glucuronide is probably inactive as the decline in β-blockade after [^{14}C]propranolol correlates with plasma concentrations of unconjugated drug rather than with total levels of radioactivity (PATERSON et al., 1970).

d) Drug Interactions. Propranolol metabolism in the isolated perfused rat liver is inhibited competitively by SKF 525 A while phenobarbitone pre-treatment increases both the V_{max} for metabolism and the capacity of the high affinity propranolol binding site (EVANS et al., 1973b). Phenothiazines and tricyclic antidepressants have been shown to inhibit the metabolism of propranolol by rat liver microsomes (SHAND and OATES, 1971), and propranolol inhibits amphetamine metabolism and tolerance in intact rats (SHOEMAN et al., 1974). The clinical significance of the latter observations is not known.

4. Excretion

a) Routes. Although KAYE et al. (1973) have shown that the renal excretion of propranolol varies with urinary pH, very little of the dose is eliminated via this route as unchanged drug. Faecal excretion accounts for 20%–25% of a radiolabelled dose of propranolol in rat and dog after both i.v. and oral administration, but less than 5% in monkey and man (PATERSON et al., 1970; HAYES and COOPER, 1971). However, a considerable amount of radioactivity was found in the bile of monkeys suggesting that enterohepatic re-circulation of propranolol metabolites may be significant. Compared to normal subjects, patients with renal failure eliminate proportionately more of a radiolabelled dose in the faeces (THOMPSON et al., 1972). Results of studies in two nursing mothers given single oral doses of propranolol showed that it is excreted in breast milk in a dose-dependent manner (KARLBERG et al., 1974).

5. Pharmacokinetics

a) Intravenous. The plasma drug concentration versus time curve after i.v. injection of propranolol has been described by a biexponential equation, giving mean $t_{1/2\alpha}$ and $t_{1/2\beta}$ values of 6–9 min and 2–4 h, respectively (SHAND et al., 1970; EVANS et al., 1973 a; MCALLISTER, 1976; GOMENI et al., 1977). Total clearance (blood) varies relatively little about 0.95–1.2 l/min approaching and, therefore, depending upon hepatic blood flow (SHAND and RANGNO, 1972). This is consistent with hepatic extraction ratios of 0.90 and 0.74–0.79 demonstrated directly in dogs and in hypertensive patients, respectively (SHAND et al., 1972; WEISS et al., 1978). Propranolol itself can lower hepatic blood flow by some 30%, thereby reducing its own clearance. This effect is a consequence of β-blockade and hence of reduction in cardiac output by the L-isomer, a property not shared by the D-form. Accordingly, the latter was shown to be cleared more efficiently than racemic propranolol in the monkey (NIES et al., 1973). That this difference was the result of differential haemodynamic effects rather than of any difference in the intrinsic hepatic clearance of the isomers was demonstrated by KAWASHIMA et al. (1976) who, using a stereospecific radioimmunoassay, found that the isomers had similar clearances when measured after injection of the racemate in rats. A longer elimination $t_{1/2}$ for the L-isomer reflects stereoselective distribution processes (op. cit.). In dogs, EHRSSON (1976) found no difference in the enantiomeric ratio in urine using a gaschromatographic procedure to separate the isomers.

The Vd_{β} value for propranolol in man ranges from 182–281 l and the variance is largely determined by plasma drug binding, such that the volume decreases as binding increases (EVANS et al., 1973 a). Because hepatic drug extraction is so avid, it is unaffected by blood propranolol binding so that $t_{1/2}$ is prolonged in individuals with relatively low binding owing to their large volumes of distribution and, therefore, reduced rate of drug delivery to the liver. By the same token, when allowances are made for differences in clearance, variability in plasma binding also accounts for species differences in Vd_{β} and $t_{1/2}$ (EVANS et al., 1973 a). A relatively low hepatic extraction (about 50%) of propranolol in the monkey compared to other species is rationalised by a perfusion model that predicts binding-limited hepatic extraction when binding exceeds a critical limit (SHAND et al., 1976).

b) Oral. During oral dosage, and particularly chronic oral administration of propranolol, SHAND and co-workers found longer elimination $t_{1/2}$ values (3–6 h) than after i.v. injections. This was explained by "first-pass" saturation of both the high affinity binding sites in the liver and of drug metabolising enzymes (SHAND et al., 1970; SHAND and RANGNO, 1972; EVANS and SHAND, 1973 a). However, recent data of GOMENI et al. (1977) indicate more complexities since they observed much longer $t_{1/2}$s after a single 10 mg oral dose (mean 9.4 h) compared to 20 and 40 mg doses in the same subjects (mean 3.6 and 3.2 h, respectively).

According to theoretical predictions based upon a particular perfusion model of the liver, hepatic blood flow is not a determinant of the area under the plasma propranolol concentration versus time curve after oral dosage. Assuming complete absorption of drug from the gut and only hepatic elimination, this is controlled only by the intrinsic activity of the metabolising enzymes and by blood drug binding (EVANS and SHAND, 1973a; SHAND et al., 1975a). Therefore, variability in these may account for the range of plasma propranolol concentrations seen after the same oral dose in different subjects. Estimates of this range vary from 20-fold (SHAND, 1974; ESLER et al., 1977) to less than three-fold (WALLE et al., 1978). In contrast to total blood drug concentrations, theoretical considerations indicate that the area under the concentration of unbound drug in the circulation versus time curve is independent of blood binding (WILKINSON and SHAND, 1975).

At steady-state during chronic oral dosing, mean plasma concentrations of propranolol and its $t_{1/2}$ are unrelated. Although both depend upon systemic drug clearance, $t_{1/2}$ is also inversely related to the fraction of unbound drug in the circulation which can vary independently of systemic clearance (EVANS and SHAND, 1973b). The kinetics of formation of 4-hydroxy propranolol from propranolol are curious and poorly understood. It has only been detected in the systemic circulation after oral administration or portal vein injection of propranolol; its elimination $t_{1/2}$ may be shorter than that of the parent drug; and, unlike propranolol, it does not accumulate when the latter is given chronically (PATERSON et al., 1970; HAYES and COOPER, 1971; WALLE et al., 1975). A satisfactory explanation for these phenomena awaits further investigation using a reliable assay for 4-hydroxy propranolol.

c) Drug Interactions. Apart from affecting its own clearance by decreasing liver blood flow, propranolol may also reduce the elimination rate of other drugs via this haemodynamic mechanism (NIES et al., 1973a, b). Thus, when propranolol was given to dogs simultaneously with lignocaine, the clearance of the latter was reduced by an amount approximately equal to the reduction in hepatic blood flow (BRANCH et al., 1973a). In a similar experiment, the clearance of oxyphenbutazone was changed much less, as predicted for a drug with a relatively low hepatic extraction ratio (BRANCH et al., 1973b). Similar to oxyphenbutazone, antipyrine is also subject to essentially flow-independent hepatic elimination. However, observations in man indicate that propranolol can significantly decrease the clearance of this agent, possibly in this case via direct enzyme inhibition (GREENBLATT, 1977). The kinetics of quinidine and morphine – drugs with intermediate and high hepatic extraction ratios, respectively – are apparently unaltered by propranolol in man (OCHS et al., 1978; BRUNK et al., 1974). Results of studies on the effects of propranolol on ethanol metabolism are variable. Whereas SVENDSEN et al. (1976) found no difference in blood ethanol concentration before and after β-blockade with propranolol in man, WAGNER et al. (1976) showed a 26% reduction in steady-state blood ethanol concentrations following an i.v. bolus of propranolol in cats. Significant inhibition of ethanol metabolism in intact rats and by rat liver slices was related to an effect of propranolol specifically on mitochondrial oxidising enzymes (ISSELBACHER and CARTER, 1976).

Enhanced clearance of D-propranolol in the monkey by phenobarbitone treatment was accounted for by both enzyme induction and by a stimulatory effect of the barbiturate on hepatic blood flow (BRANCH et al., 1974). The latter mechanism alone explained increased D-propranolol clearance after i.v. infusion of glucagon (BRANCH et al., 1973c). In man, halofenate also increases the clearance of propranolol but in this case the mechanism has not been determined (HUFFMAN et al., 1976). Chlorpromazine can inhibit propranolol metabolism in man but the extent of its influence seems to be highly variable in different individuals (VESTAL et al., 1977).

d) Effect of Age. SHAND et al. (1970) measured plasma propranolol levels in four children (aged 8 weeks to 3 yr) and concluded that a dose intermediate between that based upon body weight and that based upon body surface area is required to approximate average drug concentrations in adults given an equivalent dose. Another seven children were studied by WILSON et al. (1976) who found no relation between dose corrected for body weight and plasma drug concentration. CASTLEDEN et al. (1975) found that the mean peak plasma concentration of propranolol was about four times higher in elderly patients (mean age 77 yr) compared with young patients (mean age 27 yr) after a single 40 mg oral dose, an observation presumably related to a reduced "first-pass" effect. WOOD et al . (1978) indicate that the systemic clearance of propranolol declines with age, as does hepatic blood flow, but that there is a significant decrease in the activity of the enzymes responsible for metabolism of the drug with age only in smokers.

e) Effect of Disease. Since hepatic blood flow, hepatic enzyme activity and plasma protein binding are the major determinants of propranolol kinetics, their perturbation by disease should have predictable effects. Thus, in patients with chronic liver disease, decreases in these variables conspire to reduce propranolol clearance and increase its $t_{1/2}$ and volume of distribution (BRANCH and SHAND, 1976; BRANCH et al., 1976). In addition, such patients will have abnormally high oral availability of propranolol when pre-systemic elimination is bypassed by naturally developed or surgically induced porto-caval shunts (SHAND and RANGNO, 1972; BRANCH et al., 1977). The development of ascitic fluid is also associated with a further increase in volume of distribution of propranolol (BRANCH et al., 1976). In patients with untreated coeliac disease, reduced pre-systemic drug elimination associated with liver involvement presumably accounts for abnormally elevated plasma propranolol concentrations after oral dosage (PARSONS et al., 1976; SCHNEIDER et al., 1976). Patients with crohn's disease also show considerably enhanced systemic availability of propranolol (SCHNEIDER et al., 1976).

Analysis of single oral dose data from patients in chronic renal failure indicates a three-fold increase in the systemic availability of propranolol compared to healthy controls, associated with a decrease in clearance and impaired hepatic extraction; $t_{1/2}$, volume of distribution and f_p values are not altered significantly (LOWENTHAL et al., 1974; BIANCHETTI et al., 1976). Dialysis reduces systemic availability by about half and there is evidence to suggest that prolonged oral dosage is associated with a significant shortening of propranolol $t_{1/2}$ (LOWENTHAL and MUTTERPERL, 1976). These studies by LOWENTHAL et al. (1974) and BIANCHETTI et al. (1976) did not confirm an earlier report from THOMPSON et al. (1972) indicating delayed absorption of propranolol in renal failure and shorter single dose $t_{1/2}$ values directly related to creatinine clearance.

Three groups have looked at propranolol kinetics in thyroid disease. BELL et al. (1977) found delayed t_{max} values in hypothyroid compared to hyperthyroid patients but otherwise no significant differences in drug kinetics after single oral doses. In contrast, FEELY et al. (1978), studying hypo- and hyperthyroid patients during chronic oral therapy reported significantly higher steady-state plasma propranolol concentrations in the former, indicating differences in drug clearance. Furthermore, steady-state plasma propranolol was related to serum thyroxine and the return to euthyroid status was associated with converging changes in plasma drug concentration in the two groups. RUBENFELD et al. (1978) reported average increases in clearance of 43% and in *Vd* of 31% in thyrotoxic patients compared to normal controls, after i.v. injection of propranolol. However, they did not observe significant differences in the oral kinetics of the drug in their two groups.

Enhanced cardiac output and its distribution to the liver was shown to account for increased propranolol clearance and decreased $t_{1/2}$ in patients with labile hypertension (characterised by a high basal cardiac output) compared to permanent hypertensives (with normal or slightly reduced cardiac output) (WEISS et al., 1976).

6. Concentration–Effect Relationships

Numerous studies have demonstrated relationships between plasma propranolol concentration and reduction in exercise-, isoprenaline-, and glyceryltrinitrate-induced tachycardia in healthy subjects and in patients after both acute and chronic drug administration (JOHNSSON and REGÅRDH, 1976). Furthermore, MCDEVITT et al. (1976) have shown much better correlations when unbound rather than total plasma drug concentrations are used and, therefore, that individual variations in β-receptor sensitivity are relatively small compared to individual variations in bioavailability.

Formation of the active 4-hydroxy metabolite after single oral doses of propranolol causes the regression line for β-blockade versus plasma propranolol concentration 2 h after the dose to be shifted to the left compared to that after i.v. injection (COLTART and SHAND, 1970). However, at 6 h after a single oral dose and throughout a dosage interval during chronic oral dosage, the effects of propranolol were attributed entirely to circulating levels of the parent drug (CLEAVELAND and SHAND, 1972). In contrast, others have suggested that active metabolites of propranolol might contribute to β-blockade during chronic therapy. Thus, ZACEST and KOCH-WESER (1972) observed two sub-groups of hypertensive patients, one of which had substantially lower plasma propranolol levels but the same degree of β-blockade and proposed that this group might have had correspondingly higher levels of active metabolite. Preliminary findings reported by WALLE et al. (1975) indicate, however, that the ratio of 4-hydroxy propranolol to propranolol in the plasma may be remarkably consistent in different individuals during chronic dosage despite large variations in plasma propranolol concentration. In confirming that the time-course of β-blockade due to propranolol and its plasma concentrations after i.v. injection are entirely compatible with classical drug receptor theory of competitive antagonism, MCDEVITT and SHAND (1975) emphasised that correlations with the decrease in isoprenaline-induced tachycardia must be linear with respect to drug concentration but logarithmic when percentage reduction of exercise-induced tachycardia is used as a measure of β-blockade.

Significant correlations between plasma propranolol concentration and antihypertensive effect have been described by three groups. Two of these have reported linear relationships between log plasma propranolol and fall in blood pressure (HANSSON et al., 1974; LEONETTI et al., 1975) whereas ESLER et al. (1977) found a biphasic relationship. Thus, a plateau of effect between 3 and 30 ng/ml was associated with clinically small falls in blood pressure, high sympathetic cardiovascular tone and elevated plasma renin activity, although the latter was not causally, related to the reduction in pressure. Above 100 ng/ml, the blood pressure response appeared to plateau again but in this region was unrelated to sympathetic tone or plasma renin activity. It has been suggested that blood pressure responses to propranolol at relatively high plasma drug concentrations are related to its central effects (SHAND et al., 1975b). ESLER et al. (1977) also observed that patients with relatively low plasma propranolol levels for a given dose responded to a greater extent. This may reflect variation in receptor sensitivity, in plasma drug binding or, as suggested by ZACEST and KOCH-WESER (1972) in relation to β-blockade, differences in the production of active metabolite(s).

XIII. Sotalol

4-(2-Isopropylamino-1-hydroxyethyl)-methanesulphonamide

1. Absorption

a) Extent. After oral administration to man and dog 60%–90% of the dose was recovered in the urine indicating extensive but perhaps incomplete absorption and bioavailability (LISH et al., 1967; SCHNELLE and GARRETT, 1973; BROWN et al., 1976; TJANDRAMAGA et al., 1976).

b) Rate. Maximum plasma concentrations of sotalol were observed 2–3 h after conventional tablet dosage forms (BROWN et al., 1976; TJANDRAMAGA et al., 1976).

2. Distribution

a) Blood. While high concentrations (54%) of sotalol were claimed to be bound to human serum albumin (GIUDICELLI et al., 1973), SCHNELLE and GARRETT (1973) found no evidence of any binding to dog plasma. Similarly, a low degree of protein binding was indicated by equal concentrations of drug in haemodialysis ultrafiltrate and human plasma in vivo (TJANDRAMAGA et al., 1976). In dogs a mean λ value of 1 was reported by SCHNELLE and GARRETT (1973).

3. Biotransformation

a) Routes. Several authors report no evidence for any sotalol (Fig. 27) metabolites in plasma or urine (LISH et al., 1967; TJANDRAMAGA et al., 1976; SCHNELLE and GARRETT, 1973).

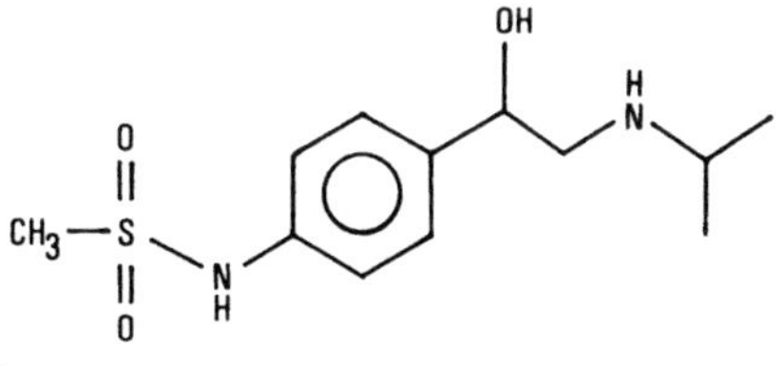

Fig. 27. Structure of sotalol

4. Excretion

a) Routes. Fluorometric assays indicate that sotalol is excreted predominantly unchanged in the urine (SCHNELLE and GARRETT, 1973; BROWN et al., 1976; TJANDRAMAGA et al., 1976; McDEVITT and SHANKS, 1977).

5. Pharmacokinetics

a) Intravenous. Plasmsa drug concentration versus time curves after i.v. injection in three dogs were described by a biexponential equation giving a mean terminal $t_{1/2}$ of 4.8 h and a renal clearance consistent with glomerular filtration (SCHNELLE and GARRETT, 1973).

b) Oral. The absorption $t_{1/2}$ of sotalol after administration of oral solutions to dogs was found to be 11–17 min (SCHNELLE and GARRETT, 1973). BROWN et al. (1976) and McDEVITT and SHANKS (1977) reported mean terminal plasma elimination $t_{1/2}$ values of 13–15 h after oral doses in man with no change on multiple dose administration over 8 days. TJANDRAMAGA et al. (1976) found a lower value of 5 h but this was based upon sampling only up to 12 h.

c) Effect of Disease. TJANDRAMAGA et al. (1976) described prolonged elimination of sotalol in six patients with chronic renal failure (creatinine clearance <2 ml/min). A mean plasma $t_{1/2}$ of 42 h was reduced to about 7 h during haemodialysis and plasma drug concentrations post-dialysis were some 20% lower than those pre-dialysis. Recovery of sotalol in urine over 48 h was only about 9% of the dose in these patients.

6. Concentration–Effect Relationships

Correlations between plasma sotalol concentrations and decreases in both exercise- and isoprenaline-induced tachycardia have been demonstrated in dog and man (LISH et al., 1967; BROWN et al., 1976; McDEVITT and SHANKS, 1977).

XIV. Timolol

3-[(4-Morpholino-1,2,5-thiadiazole-3-yl)oxy]-1-isopropylamino-2-propanol

1. Absorption

a) Extent. Oral absorption of timolol in man occurs to the extent of at least 66% of the dose, as indicated by urinary recoveries of ^{14}C-labelled drug and metabolites (TOCCO et al., 1975). However, systemic availability, estimated at 0.48, is considerably lower as a result of a moderate "first-pass" effect (VERMEIJ et al., 1977). Hence, bioavailability may be of the order of 30% of an oral dose.

b) Rate. Oral absorption of timolol is rapid from both aqueous solution and from tablets since maximum plasma drug concentrations occur at 1–2 h (TOCCO et al., 1975; VERMEIJ et al., 1977).

2. Distribution

a) Tissues. Brain tissue had the lowest concentrations of radioactivity after i.v. injection of [^{14}C]timolol in rats (TOCCO et al., 1975). As well as binding non-specifically to heart, lung, and brain tissue, the L-isomer of timolol binds to stereospecific sites in these organs (TOCCO et al., 1976).

3. Biotransformation

a) Routes. Identification of urinary metabolites in various species indicates that timolol undergoes extensive oxidation and cleavage of both the isopropylamino side-chain and of the morpholino group (Fig. 28) (Tocco et al., 1975).

A major metabolite in dogs, but relatively minor in rats and man, is the lactic acid derivative. Thus, in one dog, 50% of urinary radioactivity was identified as this compound whereas in rat and man only 6% and 10%, respectively, were observed by electrophoresis. Electrophoretograms also suggested the presence of small quantities of the acetic acid metabolite (4%–15%) in all three species.

Cleavage of the morpholino ring constitutes the major pathway in man; the ethanolamine, 3-[4-(2-hydroxyethylamino)-1,2,5-thiadiazole-3-yloxy]-1-isopropylamino-2-propanol, comprises 10% of urinary radioactivity and 3-[4-(N-2-hydroxyethylglycolamido)-1,2,5-thiadiazole-3-yloxy]-1-isopropylamino-2-propanol accounts for 30%. A minor metabolite, apparently resulting from hydroxylation of the terminal methyl of the isopropylamino group, accounted for an additional 3% of the radioactivity in human urine.

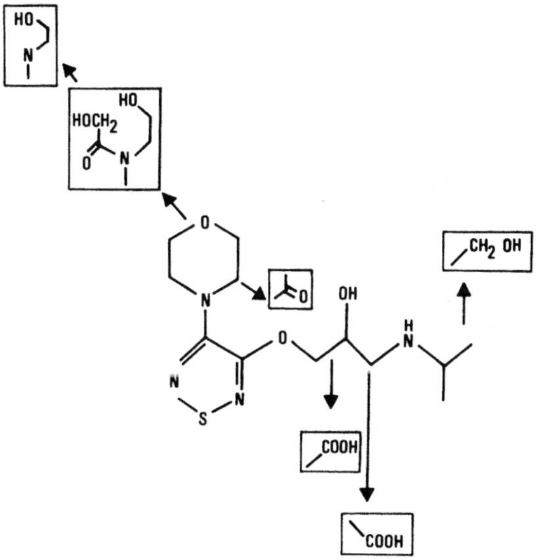

Fig. 28. Structure of timolol and metabolic products

4. Excretion

a) Routes. After oral administration, 20% of the dose is excreted unchanged in human urine whereas the corresponding figure for rat and dog is only 2%. Faecal recoveries of 20%–30% of both i.v. and oral doses in rat and dog suggest extensive biliary excretion of timolol and/or its metabolites in these species (Tocco et al., 1975).

5. Pharmacokinetics

a) Intravenous. The plasma timolol concentration versus time curve, determined by ec–glc assay, after i.v. infusion of 0.1 mg/kg in two normal subjects was described by a biexponential equation giving $t_{1/2\alpha}$ and $t_{1/2\beta}$ values of 4–7 min and 1.8–2.6 h, respectively (VERMEIJ et al., 1977).

b) Oral. The terminal plasma $t_{1/2}$ values of timolol in five normal subjects ranged from 2.0–2.5 h and no significant differences were noted between aqueous solution or tablet dosage forms. Estimated absorption $t_{1/2}$ was about 5 min after the aqueous solution (VERMEIJ et al., 1977).

c) Effect of Disease. PITONE et al. (1977) found no significant effect of chronic renal disease on the kinetics of oral timolol except a slight delay in the time of peak plasma drug concentrations. Mean terminal plasma drug $t_{1/2}$ values were 3.4 h in 10 healthy subjects compared to 2.96 h in seven azotemic patients.

6. Concentration–Effect Relationships

Significant correlations between plasma timolol concentration and the degree of β-blockade or antihypertensive effect were not found in a group of 20 hypertensive patients. Lack of correlation with reduction in exercise or isoprenaline-induced tachycardia may have been due to the relatively high degree of β-blockade achieved with the lowest dose (20 mg) used (SIMON et al., 1978).

XV. Tolamolol

4-[2-(2-Hydroxy-3-o-tolyloxypropylamino)-ethoxy]-benzamide

1. Absorption

a) Extent. Oral bioavailability in man averaged 30% of the dose in six healthy subjects, consistent with a high first-pass effect predicted from i.v. clearance data (FAULKNER et al., 1975). No differences in bioavailability were found between tablets and capsules (FAULKNER et al., 1976).

b) Rate. Rapid oral absorption of tolamolol is indicated by a t_{max} of about 2 h (FAULKNER et al., 1975).

2. Distribution

a) Blood. Using an ultrafiltration technique, FAULKNER et al. (1975) found a mean f_p value for human plasma of 0.90 at a drug concentration of 100 ng/ml. They also reported a mean λ value of 0.74 in man.

3. Biotransformation

a) Routes. WOOD et al. (1975) investigated the metabolism of tolamolol in various species and found evidence of hydrolysis of the amino group and of hydroxylation in the 4-position of the o-tolyl ring followed by both O-glucuronide and O-sulphate formation (Fig. 29) (Table 14).

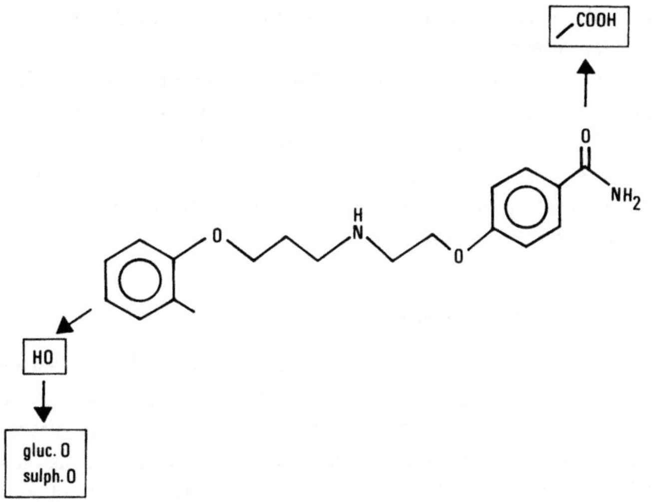

Fig. 29. Structure of tolamolol and metabolic products

Table 14. Species variation in urinary plus faecal recoveries[a] of tolamolol and metabolites (Wood et al., 1975)

	Mouse	Rat	Guinea pig	Rabbit	Dog
Tolamolol	10	7	20	10	15
Hydroxytolamolol	45	65	35	12	
Hydroxytolamolol glucuronide	3	3	5	22	1
Hydroxytolamolol sulphate	2	3		18	
Tolamolol acid	5	7	10	2	45
Hydroxytolamolol acid sulphate					10

[a] Recovery is expressed as an approximate percentage of the dose

b) Activity of Metabolites. 4-Hydroxy tolamolol is known to possess about half of the β-blocking activity of tolamolol but it has only been found in low concentration in the plasma of two of six subjects after oral administration of the parent drug (Faulkner et al., 1975; Monro et al., 1976).

4. Excretion

a) Routes. Little unchanged tolamolol is excreted in human urine (Faulkner et al., 1975).

5. Pharmacokinetics

a) Intravenous. Plasma tolamolol concentration versus time curves after i.v. injection of 20 mg in six healthy subjects were described by a biexponential equation giving mean $t_{1/2\alpha}$ and $t_{1/2\beta}$ values of 7 min and 2.5 h, respectively, and a clearance (blood) of 1.0 l/min (Faulkner et al., 1975).

In two subjects, BALANT et al. (1976) observed a $t_{1/2}$ of 2.4 h but this was extended to 6.5 h in a third subject.

b) Oral. A mean terminal $t_{1/2}$ of 1.8 h was noted in six healthy subjects after 100 mg doses. After ten 8-hourly doses, the $t_{1/2}$ remained unchanged and there was no accumulation of plasma tolamolol (FAULKNER et al., 1975).

BALANT et al. (1976) found a mean $t_{1/2}$ of 2.8 h in six subjects. The individual with the relatively long i.v. $t_{1/2}$ showed the same phenomenon when dosed orally with both tolamolol and bufuralol (op. cit.).

6. Concentration–Effect Relationships

FAULKNER et al. (1975) found a significant positive correlation between reduction in maximum exercise heart rate and log of plasma tolamolol concentration after both i.v. and oral administration in healthy subjects. Although they observed no relationship between mean steady state plasma concentrations of tolamolol in 15 hypertensive patients and lying mean blood pressure response, ROUTLEDGE et al. (1977) reported a significant correlation with fall in standing blood pressure.

XVI. Toliprolol

3-(3-Methylphenoxy)-1-isopropylamino-2-propanol

1. Absorption

a) Extent. A comparison of the recoveries of ^{3}H-labelled drug in urine and faeces after i.v. and oral administration in man, dog, and rat indicated complete oral absorption (ARNDTS and POLLMANN, 1973).

b) Rate. Oral absorption in man is probably complete within 2 h (ARNDTS and POLLMANN, 1973).

2. Distribution

a) Tissues. Using a fluorometric assay for unchanged drug, STOCK and WESTERMANN (1965) found a rapid distribution throughout rat tissues with a particularly high concentration in the lungs.

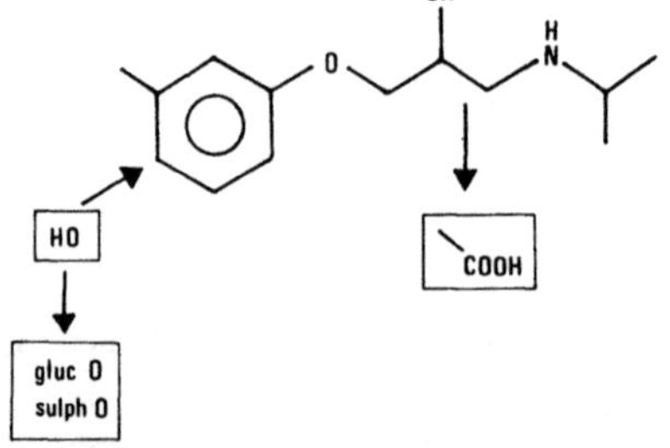

Fig. 30. Structure of toliprolol and metabolic products

3. Biotransformation

a) Routes. About 30% of the urinary metabolites in man and dog was accounted for as methylphenoxy lactic acid, a product of side-chain oxidation. Ring-hydroxylation in the 4-position accounted for the rest; 20% as the free phenol and 50% as conjugates. Only glucuronides were observed in human urine but the dog excreted equal amounts of glucuronide and sulphate (ARNDTS and POLLMANN, 1973) (Fig. 30).

Table 15. Absorption characteristics of some β-blockers in man

Agent	t_{max} (h)	f	BA	Dose-dependent BA
Acebutolol	1–3	>0.30	0.37	No
Alprenolol	0.5–1.5	>0.90	0.01–0.16	Yes
Atenolol	2–4	0.44	0.44/0.63[a]	No
Bufuralol	1–2			
Bunolol	1	>0.75		
Metoprolol	1–2	>0.96	0.45	Yes[b]
Oxprenolol	0.5–1.5	0.70–0.95	0.23–0.66	No
Pindolol	1.3–3.0	>0.90	0.92	No
Practolol	1–3	0.74–0.97	0.92–0.97	No
Pronethalol		1.00	1.00	No
Propranolol	1–3	>0.90	~0.30	Yes
Sotalol	2–3	0.60–0.90	0.60–0.90	No
Timolol	1–2	>0.66	~0.30	
Tolamolol	2		0.30	
Toliprolol	2	1.00		

[a] Urinary/plasma estimates
[b] But not in therapeutic dose range
f = Fraction of dose absorbed from the gut; BA = Biovailability

Table 16. Distribution characteristics of some β-blockers in man

Agent	Partition coefficient[a]	f_P	λ	$t_{1/2}(\alpha)$ (min)	$V_{D\beta}$[b] (l/kg)	$V_{D_{ss}}$[b] (l/kg)
Acebutolol		0.74	0.67	6		1.2
Alprenolol	3.27	0.85	0.98		3.2	
Atenolol		0.40	1.10	12	0.8	
Bufuralol						
Bunolol						
Metoprolol	0.18	0.11	1.20	12	5.6	
Oxprenolol	0.43	0.78	0.80	17	1.1	0.86
Pindolol	0.12	0.51	0.76		2	
Practolol	0.009					
Pronethalol						
Propranolol	5.39	0.84–0.95	0.80	6–10	3.6	
Sotalol	0.011	0		5		
Timolol						
Tolamolol		0.90	0.74	7		
Toliprolol						

[a] Octanol/water pH 7 (RIESS et al. 1974)
[b] Based upon plasma concentrations of bound plus free drug

Table 17. Elimination characteristics of some β-blockers in man

Agent	$t_{1/2}$ (h)	Cl[a] (l/min)	fu[b]	Active metabolite(s)[c]
Acebutolol	2.6	1.23	0.6	Yes
Alprenolol	2.8	1.10	0.01–0.02	Yes
Atenolol	6.1	0.09	1.0	No
Bufuralol	2.4			Yes
Bunolol	~6			
Metroprolol	3–4	1.10	0.1	Yes[d]
Oxprenolol	2.3	0.5	<0.05	
Pindolol	3.1	0.63	0.38	
Practolol	12	0.13	0.92–0.97	
Pronethalol				Yes
Propranolol	2–4	1.0	<0.01	Yes
Sotalol	13–15		≧0.60–0.90	No
Timolol	1.8–2.6		0.20	
Tolamolol	2.5	1.0	Low	Yes[d]
Toliprolol			Low	

[a] Blood clearance
[b] Fraction of an i.v. dose extracted unchanged in the urine
[c] β-Blocking activity
[d] Probable do not contribute significantly to activity of drug

Table 18. Correlations between plasma drug concentrations of β-blocker and effect

Agent	Reduction in exercise-induced tachycardia	Isoprenaline-induced tachycardia	Blood pressure
Acebutolol	+	+	–
Alprenolol	+	+	– ?
Atenolol	+		–
Bufuralol	+		
Bunolol			
Metoprolol	+	+	+[a]
Oxprenolol	+	+	
Pindolol	+	+	+[b]
Practolol	+	+	
Pronethalol			
Propranolol	+	+	±[b]
Sotalol	+	+	
Timolol	–	–	–
Tolamolol	+		+[c]
Toliprolol			

[a] Exercise
[b] Resting
[c] Standing
– Indicates no correlation
+ Indicates significant correlation

4. Excretion

a) Routes. Negligible amounts of the drug are excreted unchanged in human urine and faeces. Faecal recoveries of 8% and 10%–18% after both i.v. and oral doses in dogs and rats suggests that toliprolol metabolites are also eliminated via the bile (ARNDTS and POLLMANN, 1973).

Summary

Salient features of each of the agents with respect to absorption, distribution, and elimination characteristics and relationships between concentration and effect are collated in Tables 15–18.

The diversity of the aromatic ring system and its substituents in the series of marketed compounds precludes a detailed analysis of relationships between structure and pharmacokinetic properties. Nevertheless, some general trends are apparent. For example, there is a strong inverse correlation between partition coefficient and the contribution of renal excretion to overall drug elimination (Fig. 31). The significance of lipid solubility in drug metabolism is also indicated by a positive relationship between oral bioavailability and the fraction of an i.v. dose excreted unchanged in the urine (Fig. 32). Atenolol and acebutolol deviate somewhat in the latter plot indicating perhaps that extensive output via the kidney may sometimes be offset by reduced input through the gut wall.

Although the isopropylaminoalcohol side-chain is common to all of the β-blockers, the extent to which products of its oxidative degradation have been identified

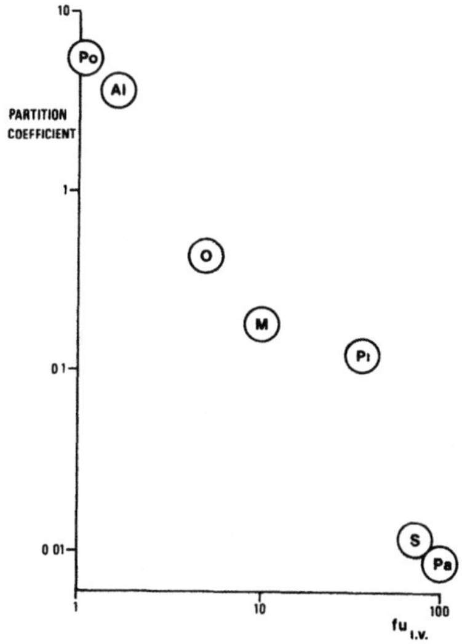

Fig. 31. Relationship between octanol/water partition coefficients of some β-blocking agents and the extent of renal excretion of unchanged drug after i.v. injection in man (f_u). (Al = alprenolol; M = metoprolol; O = oxprenolol; Po = propranolol; Pa = practolol; S = sotalol; Pi = pindolol)

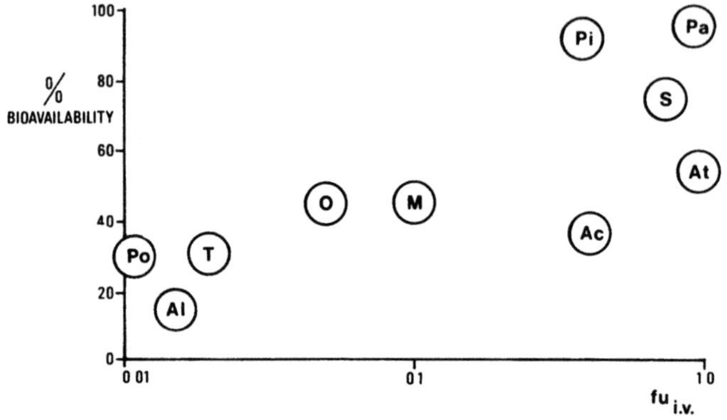

Fig. 32. Relationship between oral bioavailability of some β-blocking agents and the extent of renal excretion of unchanged drug after i.v. injection in man. (Ac = acebutolol; Al = alprenolol; At = atenolol; M = metoprolol; O = oxprenolol; Pi = pindolol; Pa = practolol; Po = propranolol; S = sotalol; T = timolol)

varies considerably. In some cases, especially where the ring moiety is relatively water-soluble, as in atenolol, practolol, and sotalol, this may protect the side-chain from metabolic attack. However, it is difficult to conceive, for example, that alprenolol does not share many side-chain reactions in common with oxprenolol whose fate has been investigated in rather more detail.

Acknowledgements. We would like to thank for their help in preparation of this manuscript: Ms. I. RUDOLPH, Ms. J. BRICE, JOHN SINGLE, BRUCE TURNBULL, STEPHEN MCINALLY – all of the University of Newcastle, New South Wales: and Ms. J. HILDITCH of Ciba-Geigy Australia Limited.

References

Ablad, B., Ervik, M., Hallgren, J., Johnsson, G., Solvell, L.: Pharmacological effects and serum levels of orally administered alprenolol in man. Eur. J. Clin. Pharmacol. *5*, 44–52 (1972)

Ablad, B., Borg, K.O., Johnsson, G., Regårdh, C.-G., Solvell, L.: Combined pharmacokinetic and pharmacodynamic studies on alprenolol and 4-hydroxy-alprenolol in man. Life Sci. *14*, 693–704 (1974)

Abramson, F.B., Furst, C.I., McMartin, C., Wade, R.: The isolation, identification and synthesis of two metabolites of guanethidine formed in pig and rabbit liver homogenates. Biochem. J. *113*, 143–155 (1969)

Adams, R.N., Murrill, E., McCreery, R., Blank, L., Karolczak, M.: 6-hydroxydopamine, a new oxidation mechanism. Eur. J. Pharmacol. *17*, 287–292 (1972)

Aellig, W.H., Prichard, B.N.C., Scales, B.: Blood levels of practolol following intravenous administration. Br. J. Pharmacol. *48*, 573 (1970)

Allen, J.G., East, P.B., Francis, R.J., Haigh, J.L.: Metabolism of debrisoquine sulfate. Identification of some urinary metabolites in rat and man. Drug Metab. Dispos. *3*, 332–337 (1975)

Allen, J.G., Brown, A.N., Marten, T.R.: Metabolism of debrisoquine sulphate in rat, dog, and man. Xenobiotica *6*, 405–409 (1976)

Alvan, G., Lind, M., Hellström, B., von Bahr, C.: Importance of "first-pass elimination" for interindividual differences in steady-state concentrations of the adrenergic β-receptor antagonist alprenolol. J. Pharmacokinet. Biopharm. *5*, 193–205 (1977a)

Alvan, G., Piafsky, K., Lind, M., von Bahr, C.: Effect of pentobarbitone on the disposition of alprenolol. Clin. Pharmacol. Ther. *22*, 316–321 (1977b)

Amery, A., de Plaen, J.-F., Lijnen, P., McAinsh, J., Reybrouck, T.: Relationship between blood level of atenolol and pharmacological effect. Clin. Pharmacol. Ther. *21*, 691–699 (1977)

Ames, M.M., Melmon, K.L., Castagnoli, N.: Stereochemical course in vivo of alpha-methyldopa decarboxylation in rat brains. Biochem. Pharmacol. *26*, 1757–1762 (1977)

Amos, H.E., Brigden, W.D., McKerron, R.A.: Unwanted effects associated with practolol: demonstration of antibody binding to epithelial tissue. Br. Med. J. *1975 I*, 598–600

Amos, H.E., Lake, B.G., Artis, J.: Possible role of antibody specific for a practolol metabolite in the pathogenesis of oculomucocutaneous syndrome. Br. Med. J. *1978 I*, 402–407

Anavekar, S.N., Louis, W.J., Morgan, T.O., Doyle, A.E., Johnston, C.I.: The relationship of plasma levels of pindolol in hypertensive patients to effects on blood pressure, plasma renin and plasma noradrenaline levels. Clin. Exp. Pharmacol. Physiol. *2*, 203–212 (1975)

Anderson, W.P., Korner, P.I., Bobik, A., Chalmers, J.P.: Leakage of DL-propranolol from cerebrospinal fluid to the blood stream in the rabbit. J. Pharmacol. Exp. Ther. *202*, 320–325 (1977)

Angelo, M., Dring, L.G., Lancaster, R., Latham, A., Smith, R.L.: A correlation between the response to debrisoquine and the amount of unchanged drug excreted in urine. Br. J. Pharmacol. *55*, 264 P (1975)

Angelo, M., Dring, L.G., Lancaster, R., Smith, R.L.: The metabolism of debrisoquine in rat and man. Biochem. Soc. Trans. *4*, 704–706 (1976)

Angelo, M., Dring, L.G., Idle, J.R., Lancaster, R., Mahgoub, A., Smith, R.L.: Defective alicyclic hydroxylation of debrisoquine in man. Br. J. Clin. Pharmacol. *4*, 725 P (1977)

Appelgren, C., Borg, K.O., Elofsson, R., Johansson, K.A.: Binding of adrenergic beta-receptor antagonists to human serum albumin. Acta Pharm. Suec. *11*, 325–332 (1974)

Arndts, D., Pollmann, W.: The pharmacokinetics and metabolism of Kö 592 in man, dog, and rat. Arch. Pharmacol. *277*, 349–362 (1973)

Au, W.Y.W., Dring, L.G., Grahame-Smith, D.G., Isaac, P., Williams, R.T.: The metabolism of ^{14}C-labelled α-methyldopa in normal and hypertensive human subjects. Biochem. J. *129*, 1–10 (1972)

Bakke, O.M., Davies, D.S., Davies, L., Dollery, C.T.: Metabolism of propranolol in rat: The fate of the N-isopropyl group. Life Sci. *13*, 1665–1675 (1973)

Balant, L., Gorgia, A., Tschopp, J.-M., Revillard, C., Fabre, J.: Pharmacocinetique de deux medicaments beta-bloquants: detection d'une anomalie pharmacogenetique. Schweiz. Med. Wochenschr. *106*, 1403–1407 (1976)

Barber, H.E., Hawkesworth, G.M., Kitteringham, N.R., Petrie, J.C., Swann, J.M., Petersen, J.: Protein binding of atenolol and propranolol to human serum albumin and human plasma. Proc. Br. Pharmacol. Soc. Meeting, Univ. of London, Jan. 1978

Barnett, A.J., Bobik, A., Carson, V., Korman, J.S., McLean, A.J.: Pharmacokinetics of methyldopa: plasma levels following single intravenous, oral, and multiple oral dosage in normotensive and hypertensive subjects. Clin. Exp. Pharmacol. Physiol. *4*, 331–339 (1977)

Bell, J.M., Russell, C.J., Nelson, J.K., Kelly, J.G., McDevitt, D.G.: Studies of the effect of thyroid dysfunction on the elimination of β-adrenoceptor blocking drugs. Br. J. Clin. Pharmacol. *4*, 79–81 (1977)

Bengtsson, C., Johnsson, G., Regårdh, C.-G.: Plasma levels and effects of metoprolol on blood pressure and heart rate in hypertensive patients after an acute dose and between two doses during long term treatment. Clin. Pharmacol. Ther. *17*, 400–408 (1975)

Bianchetti, G., Graziani, G., Brancaccio, D., Morganti, A., Leonetti, G., Manfrin, M., Sega, R., Gomeni, R., Ponticelli, C., Morselli, P.L.: Pharmacokinetics and effects of propranolol in terminal uraemic patients and in patients undergoing regular dialysis treatment. Clin. Pharmacokinet. *1*, 373–384 (1976)

Bisson, G.M., Muscholl, E.: Die Beziehung zwischen der Guanethidin Konzentration im Rattenherzen und der Noradrenalingehalt. Naunyn Schmiedebergs Arch. Pharmakol. *244*, 185 (1962)

Blank, C.L., McCreery, R.L., Wightman, R.M., Chey, W., Adams, R.N.: Intracyclization rates of 6-hydroxydopamine and 6-aminodopamine analogs under physiological conditions. J. Med. Chem. *19*, 178–180 (1976)

Bodem, G., Chidsey, C.A.: Pharmacokinetic studies of practolol, a beta-adrenergic antagonist, in man. Clin. Pharmacol. Ther. *14*, 26–29 (1973)

Bodem, G., Grieser, H., Eichelbaum, M., Gugler, R.: Pharmacokinetics of practolol in renal failure. Eur. J. Clin. Pharmacol. *7*, 249–252 (1974)
Bodin, N-O.: Identification of the major urinary metabolite of alprenolol in man, dog and rat Life Sci. *14*, 685–692 (1974)
Bodin, N-O., Borg, K.O., Johansson, R., Obianwu, H., Svensson, R.: Absorption, distribution, and excretion of alprenolol in man, dog and rat. Acta Pharmacol. Toxicol. (Kbh.) *35*, 261–269 (1974)
Bodin, N-O., Borg, K.O., Johansson, R., Ramsay, R.-H., Skanberg, I.: Tissue distribution of metoprolol-(^{3}H) in the mouse and the rat. Acta Pharmacol. Toxicol. (Kbh.) *36* (suppl. 5), 116–124 (1975)
Bond, P.A.: Metabolism of propranolol ("Inderal"), a potent specific β-adrenergic receptor blocking agent. Nature *213*, 721 (1967)
Bond, P.A., Howe, R.: The metabolism of pronethalol. Biochem. Pharmacol. *16*, 1261–1280 (1967)
Borg, K.O., Carlsson, E., Ek, L., Johansson, R.: Combined pharmacokinetic and pharmacodynamic studies of metoprolol in the cat and the dog. Acta Pharmacol. Toxicol. (Kbh.) *36* (suppl. 5), 24–30 (1975a)
Borg, K.O., Fellenius, E., Johansson, R., Wallborg, M.: Pharmacokinetic studies of metoprolol-(^{3}H) in the rat and the dog. Acta Pharmacol. Toxicol. (Kbh.) *36* (suppl. 5), 104–115 (1975b)
Borg, K.O., Carlsson, E., Hoffmann, K.-J., Johnsson, T.-E., Thorin, H., Wallin, B.: Metabolism of metoprolol-(^{3}H) in man, the dog, and the rat. Acta Pharmacol. Toxicol. (Kbh.) *36* (suppl. 5), 125–135 (1975c)
Borga, O., Odar-Cederlöf, I., Piafsky, K.M., Sjöqvist, F.: Plasma protein binding of propranolol in disease states. Br. J. Clin. Pharmacol. *4*, 627–628 (1977)
Boullin, D.J.: Reduction of ^{14}C-guanethidine levels in rat heart and diaphragm by excess calcium. Br. J. Pharmacol. Chemother. *28*, 289–295 (1966)
Boullin, D.J., O'Brien, R.A.: The accumulation of guanethidine by human blood platelets. Br. J. Pharmacol. *35*, 90–102 (1969)
Boura, A.L.A., Duncombe, W.G., Robson, R.D., McCoubrey, A.: The distribution and excretion by cats of a new hypotensive drug, N-benzyl-N′, N″-dimethylguanidine. J. Pharm. Pharmacol. *14*, 722–726 (1962)
Branch, R.A., Shand, D.G.: Propranolol disposition in chronic liver disease: A physiological approach. Clin. Pharmacokinet. *1*, 264–279 (1976)
Branch, R.A., Shand, D.G., Wilkinson, G.R., Nies, A.S.: The reduction of lidocaine clearance by DL-propranolol: An example of hemodynamic drug interaction. J. Pharmacol. Exp. Ther. *184*, 515–519 (1973a)
Branch, R.A., Shand, D.G., Nies, A.S.: Hemodynamic drug interactions: The reduction of oxyphenbutazone clearance by DL-propranolol in the dog. J. Pharmacol. Exp. Ther. *187*, 133–137 (1973b)
Branch, R.A., Shand, D.G., Nies, A.S.: Increase in hepatic blood flow and D-propranolol clearance by glucagon in the monkey. J. Pharmacol. Exp. Ther. *187*, 581–587 (1973c)
Branch, R.A., Shand, D.G., Wilkinson, G.R., Nies, A.S.: Increased clearance of antipyrine and D-propranolol after phenobarbital treatment in the monkey. J. Clin. Invest. *53*, 1101–1107 (1974)
Branch, R.A., James, J., Read, A.E.: A study of factors influencing drug disposition in chronic liver disease using the model drug (+)-propranolol. Br. J. Clin. Pharmacol. *3*, 243–249 (1976)
Branch, R.A., Kornhauser, D.M., Shand, D.G., Wilkinson, G.R., Wood, A.J.J.: Biological determinants of propranolol disposition in normal subjects and patients with cirrhosis. Br. J. Clin. Pharmacol. *4*, 630 (1977)
Breese, G.R., Traylor, T.D.: Depletion of brain noradrenaline and dopamine by 6-hydroxydopamine. Br. J. Pharmacol. *42*, 88–99 (1971)
Brodie, B.B., Aronow, L., Axelrod, J.: The fate of benzazoline (Priscoline) in dog and man and a method for its estimation in biological material. J. Pharmacol. Exp. Ther. *106*, 200–207 (1952)
Brodie, B.B., Aronow, L., Axelrod, J.: The fate of dibenzyline in the body and the role of fat in its duration of action. J. Pharmacol. Exp. Ther. *111*, 21–29 (1954)

Brodie, B.B., Chang, C.C., Costa, E.: On the mechanism of action of guanethidine and bretylium. Br. J. Pharmacol. Chemother. *25*, 171–178 (1965)

Brogden, R.N., Heel, R.C., Speight, T.M., Avery, G.S.: Prazosin: a review of its pharmacological properties and therapeutic efficacy in hypertension. Drugs *14*, 163–197 (1977)

Brown, H.C., Carruthers, S.G., Kelly, J.G., McDevitt, D.G., Shanks, R.G.: Observations on the efficacy and pharmacokinetics of sotalol after oral administration. Eur. J. Clin. Pharmacol. *9*, 367–372 (1976)

Brown, H.C., Carruthers, S.G., Johnston, G.D., Kelly, J.G., McAinsh, J., McDevitt, D.G., Shanks, R.G.: Clinical pharmacologic observations on atenolol, a beta-adrenoreceptor blocker. Clin. Pharmacol. Ther. *20*, 524–534 (1976)

Brunk, S.F., Delle, M., Wilson, W.R.: Effect of propranolol on morphine metabolism. Clin. Pharmacol. Ther. *16*, 1039–1044 (1974)

Brunner, L., Imhof, P., Jack, D.: Relation between plasma concentrations and cardiovascular effects of oral oxprenolol in man. Eur. J. Clin. Pharmacol. *8*, 3–9 (1975)

Buhs, R.P., Beck, J.L., Speth, O.C., Smith, J.L., Trenner, N.R., Cannon, P.J., Laragh, J.H.: The metabolism of methyldopa in hypertensive human subjects. J. Pharmacol. Exp. Ther. *143*, 205–214 (1964)

Calesnick, B., Sheppard, H., Bowen, M., Kandar, J.: Direct comparison of ^{14}C-guanethidine (Ismelin) excretion following oral and subcutaneous administration. Biochem. Pharmacol. *8*, 49 (1961)

Cañas-Rodriguez, A.: Preliminary studies of the metabolism of 2-guanidinomethyl-1:4-benzodioxan sulphate (Guanoxan) Experientia *22*, 472–473 (1966)

Carlsson, A., Lindqvist, M.: In vivo decarboxylation of α-methyl DOPA and α-methyl metatyrosine. Acta Physiol. Scand. *54*, 87–94 (1962)

Carlsson, E.: In: Samband mellan farmakokinetik och farmakodynamik for olika lakemedel. Johnsson, G., Lundborg, P., Roos, B-E., Svedmyr, N. (eds.), p. 146. Molndal: Lindgren and Soner 1973

Carruthers, S.G., Kelly, J.G., McDevitt, D.G., Shanks, R.G.: Blood levels of practolol after oral and parenteral administration and their relationship to exercise heart rate. Clin. Pharmacol. Ther. *15*, 497–509 (1974)

Carruthers, S.G., Kelly, J.G., Johnson, G.W., McDevitt, D.G.: Biliary excretion and enterohepatic recirculation of practolol in man. Ir. J. Med. Sci. *145*, 187–194 (1976)

Case, D.E., Lindup, W.E., Lowery, C., Orton, T.C., Reeves, P.R., Whittaker, S.L.: Metabolism studies with practolol. Br. J. Pharmacol. *63*, 352–353 (1978)

Castleden, C.M., Kaye, C.M., Parsons, R.L.: The effect of age on plasma levels of propranolol and practolol in man. Br. J. Clin. Pharmacol. *2*, 303–306 (1975)

Castleden, C.M., George, C.F., Short, M.D.: Contribution of individual differences in gastric emptying to variability in plasma propranolol concentrations. Br. J. Clin. Pharmacol. *5*, 121–122 (1978)

Century, B., Ellinwood, L.E., Kohli, J.D., Coon, J.M.: Distribution and excretion of C^{14}-labelled priscoline HCl in rats. J. Pharmacol. Exp. Ther. *109*, 318–327 (1953)

Chang, C.C., Costa, E., Brodie, B.B.: Interaction of guanethidine with adrenergic neurons. J. Pharmacol. Exp. Ther. *147*, 303–312 (1965)

Chau, N.P., Weiss, Y.A., Safar, M.E., Lavene, D.E., Georges, D.R., Milliez, P.L.: Pindolol availability in hypertensive patients with normal and impaired renal function. Clin. Pharmacol. Ther. *22*, 505–510 (1977)

Cho, A.K., Curry, S.H.: The physiological disposition of 2-(2,6-dichlorophenylamino)-2-imidazoline. Biochem. Pharmacol. *18*, 511–520 (1969)

Chremos, A.N., Shen, D., Gibaldi, M., Proctor, J.D., Newman, J.H.: Time-dependent change in renal clearance of bethanidine in humans. J. Pharm. Sci. *65*, 140–142 (1976)

Cleavland, C.R., Shand, D.G.: Effect of route of administration on the relationship between β-adrenergic blockade and plasma propranolol level. Clin. Pharmacol. Ther. *13*, 181–185 (1972)

Cohen, G., Heikkila, R.E., Allis, B., Cabbat, F., Dembiec, D., MacNamee, D., Mytilineou, C., Winston, B.: Destruction of sympathetic nerve terminals by 6-hydroxy-dopamine: protection by 1-phenyl-3(2-thiazolyl)-2-thiourea, diethyldithiocarbamate, methimazole, cysteamine, ethanol, and n-butanol. J. Pharmacol. Exp. Ther. *199*, 336–352 (1976)

Collins, I.S., Pek, P.: Pharmacokinetics of prazosin, a new antihypertensive compound. Clin. Exp. Pharmacol. Physiol. *2*, 445–446 (1975)
Collins, R.F.: Pharmacocinétique de l'acebutolol. Nouv. Presse Med. *4*, 3223–3228 (1975)
Collste, P., Haglund, K., Frisk-Holmberg, M., Rawlins, M.: Pharmacokinetics and pharmacodynamics of alprenolol in the treatment of hypertension. I. Relationship between plasma concentration and adrenergic β-receptor blockade. Eur. J. Clin. Pharmacol. *10*, 85–88 (1976a)
Collste, P., Haglund, K., Frisk-Holmberg, M., Orme, M.L., Rawlins, M., Ostman, J.: Pharmacokinetics and pharmacodynamics of alprenolol in the treatment of hypertension. II. Relationship to its effect on blood pressure and plasma renin activity. Eur. J. Clin. Pharmacol. *10*, 89–95 (1976b)
Coltart, D.J., Shand, D.G.: Plasma propranolol levels in the quantitative assessment of β-adrenergic blockade in man. Br. Med. J. *1970 III*, 731–734
Commarato, M.A., Giardino, E.C., Kopia, G.A., Kaplan, H.R.: Levobunolol and propranolol: Further evaluation of β-blocking activity in conscious dogs. Pharmacologist *18*, 227 (1976)
Constantine, J.W., McShane, W.K., Scriabine, A., Hess, H.J.: In: Hypertension: mechanisms and management. Onesti, G., Kim, K.E., Moyer, J.H. (eds.), Vol. VI, p. 429. New York: Grune and Stratton 1973
Conway, F.J., Fitzgerald, J.D., McAinsh, J., Rowlands, D.J., Simpson, W.T.: Human pharmacokinetic and pharmacodynamic studies on atenolol (ICI 66082), a new cardioselective beta-adrenoreceptor blocking drug. Br. J. Clin. Pharmacol. *3*, 267–272 (1976)
Cotham, R.H., Shand, D.G.: Spuriously low plasma propranolol concentrations resulting from blood collection methods. Clin. Pharmacol. Ther. *18*, 535–538 (1975)
Creveling, C.R., Daly, J.W., Witkop, B.: The depletion of cardiac norepinephrine by 3,5-dihydroxy-4-methoxyphenethylamine and related compounds. J. Pharmacol. Exp. Ther. *158*, 46–54 (1967)
Crowther, A.F., Smith, L.H.: Beta adrenergic blocking agents II. Propranolol and related 3-amino-1-naphthoxy-2-propranolols. J. Med. Chem. *11*, 1009–1013 (1968)
Cuthbert, M.F., Collins, R.F.: Plasma levels and β-adrenoreceptor blockade with acebutolol, practolol, and propranolol in man. Br. J. Clin. Pharmacol. *2*, 49–55 (1975)
Darda, S.: Pharmacokinetics of clonidine. In: Recent advances in hypertension – proceedings of an International Symposium. Milliez, P., Safar, M. (eds.), pp. 375–388. Ingelheim: Laboratoires Boehringer 1975
Darda, S., Förster, H.-J., Stähle, H.: Metabolischer Abbau von Clonidin. Arzneim. Forsch. Drug Res. *28*, 255–259 (1978)
Davidson, R., Thadani, U., Taylor, S.H., Hess, H., Riess, W.: Pharmacological studies with slow-release formulations of oxprenolol in man. Eur. J. Clin. Pharmacol. *10*, 189–195 (1976)
Davies, D.S., Wing, L.M.H., Reid, J.L., Neill, E., Tippett, P., Dollery, C.T.: Pharmacokinetics and concentration effect relationships of intravenous and oral clonidine. Clin. Pharmacol. Ther. *21*, 593–601 (1977)
Dawes, C.P., Kendall, M.J., John, V.A.: Comparison of plasma and saliva levels of metoprolol and oxprenolol. Br. J. Clin. Pharmacol. *5*, 217–221 (1978)
Day, M.D., Rand, M.J.: Evidence for a competitive antagonism of guanethidine by dexamphetamine. Br. J. Pharmacol. Chemother. *20*, 17–28 (1963)
Di Carlo, F.J., Leinweber, F.J., Szpiech, J.M., Davidson, I.W.F.: Metabolism of L-bunolol. Clin. Pharmacol. Ther. *22*, 858–863 (1977)
Dollery, C.T., Junod, A.F.: Concentration of ($\pm$)-propranolol in isolated perfused lungs of rat. Br. J. Pharmacol. *57*, 67–71 (1976)
Dollery, C.T., Emslie Smith, D., Milne, M.D.: Clinical and pharmacological studies with guanethidine in the treatment of hypertension. Lancet *1960 II*, 381–387
Dollery, C.T., Lewis, G., Myers, M.G.: Clinical evaluation of a new beta-adrenoceptor antagonist ICI 66082 in essential hypertension. Br. J. Clin. Pharmacol. *2*, 185–186 (1975)
Dollery, C.T., Davies, D.S., Draffan, G.H., Dargie, H.J., Dean, C.R., Reid, J.L., Clare, R.A., Murray, S.: Clinical pharmacology and pharmacokinetics of clonidine. Clin. Pharmacol. Ther. *19*, 11–17 (1976)

Doyle, A.E., Morley, R.H.: Studies on the absorption and excretion of ^{14}C-bethanidine in man. Br. J. Pharmacol. *24*, 701–704 (1965)

Drayer, D.E., Strong, J.M., Jones, B., Sandler, A., Reidenberg, M.M.: In vitro acetylation of drugs by human blood cells. Drug Metab. Dispos. *2*, 499–505 (1974)

Dring, L.G., Kamanyiro, G.H., Lancaster, R., Smith, R.L.: Absence of correlation between the oral pharmacokinetics and response to bethanidine. Br. J. Clin. Pharmacol. *4*, 390P (1977)

Dring, L.G., Gorchein, A., Mahgoub, A.A., Smith, R.L.: The elimination of practolol in two human subjects. Br. J. Clin. Pharmacol. *5*, 262–265 (1978)

Dybing, E.: Activation of α-methyldopa, paracetamol, and furosemide by human liver microsomes. Acta Pharmacol. Toxicol. (Kbh.) *41*, 89–93 (1977)

Dybing, E., Nelson, S.D., Mitchell, J.R., Sasame, H.A., Gillette, J.R.: Oxidation of α-methyldopa and other catechols by cytochrome P-450-generated superoxide anion: possible mechanism of methyldopa hepatitis. Mol. Pharmacol. *12*, 911–920 (1976)

Eastwood, J.B., Curtis, J.R., Smith, R.B.: Pharmacodynamics of practolol in chronic renal failure. Br. Med. J. *1973 IV*, 320–322

Ehrsson, H.: Identification of diastereomeric propranolol-O-glucuronides by gas chromatography-mass spectrometry. J. Pharm. Pharmacol. *27*, 971–973 (1975)

Ehrsson, H.: Simultaneous determination of (−)- and (+)-propranolol by gas chromatography-mass spectroscopy using a deuterium labelling technique. J. Pharm. Pharmacol. *28*, 662–663 (1976)

Enna, S.J., Da Prada, M., Pletscher, A.: Subcellular distribution of reserpine in blood platelets: evidence for multiple pools. J. Pharmacol. Exp. Ther. *191*, 164–171 (1974)

Erhardt, J.D.: Métabolism du Catapresan: Action hypotensive du 4-hydroxycatapresan. Therapie *27*, 947–954 (1972)

Esler, M., Zweifler, A., Randall, O., de Quattro, V.: Pathophysiologic and pharmacokinetic determinants of the antihypertensive response to propranolol. Clin. Pharmacol. Ther. *22*, 299–308 (1977)

Evans, G.H., Shand, D.G.: Disposition of propranolol V. Drug accumulation and steady-state concentrations during chronic oral administration in man. Clin. Pharmacol. Ther. *14*, 487–493 (1973a)

Evans, G.H., Shand, D.G.: Disposition of propranolol. VI. Independent variation in steady-state circulating drug concentrations and half-life as a result of plasma drug binding in man. Clin. Pharmacol. Ther. *14*, 494–500 (1973b)

Evans, G.H., Nies, A.S., Shand, D.G.: The disposition of propranolol III. Decreased half-life and volume of distribution as a result of plasma binding in man, monkey, dog, and rat. J. Pharmacol. Exp. Ther. *186*, 114–122 (1973a)

Evans, G.H., Wilkinson, G.R., Shand, D.G.: The disposition of propranolol IV. Dominant role for tissue uptake in the dose-dependent extraction of propranolol by the perfused rat liver. J. Pharmacol. Exp. Ther. *186*, 447–454 (1973b)

Faulkner, J.K., Stopher, D.A., Walden, R., Singleton, W., Taylor, S.H.: Pharmacokinetic and pharmacological studies with tolamol in man. Br. J. Clin. Pharmacol. *2*, 423–428 (1975)

Faulkner, J.K., Stopher, D.A., Walden, R., Singleton, W., Taylor, S.H.: Bioavailability of tolamolol. Eur. J. Clin. Pharmacol. *9*, 315–317 (1976)

Feely, J., Crooks, J., Stevenson, I.H.: Alterations in plasma propranolol steady-state concentration in thyroid disease. Clin. Pharmacol. Ther. *23*, 112–113 (1978)

Finch, L., Häeusler, G.: Further evidence for a central hypotensive action of alpha-methyldopa in both the rat and cat. Br. J. Pharmacol. *47*, 217–228 (1973)

Fitzgerald, J.D., O'Donnell, S.R.: Pharmacology of 4-hydroxypropranolol, a metabolite of propranolol. Br. J. Pharmacol. *43*, 222–235 (1971)

Fitzgerald, J.D., Scales, B.: Effect of a new adrenergic beta-blocking agent (ICI 50,172) on heart rate in relation to its blood levels. Int. J. Clin. Pharmacol. *16*, 467–474 (1968)

Francis, R.J., East, P.B., McLaren, S.J., Larman, J.: Determination of bufuralol and its metabolites in plasma by mass fragmentography and by gas chromatography with electron capture detection. Biomed. Mass Spectrom. *3*, 281–285 (1976)

Frisk-Holmberg, M., Jorfeldt, L., Juhlin-Cannfeldt, A.: Influence of alprenolol on hemodynamic and metabolic responses to prolonged exercise in subjects with hypertension. Clin. Pharmacol. Ther. *21*, 675–683 (1977)

Furst, C.I.: Studies on the metabolism in vitro of (^{14}C)-guanethidine including polarographic measurements of oxygen uptake. Biochem. J. *104*, 1P (1967)
Gaffney, T.E., Walle, T., Garteiz, D., Whitnack, E.: The catabolism of β-blocking drugs by the dog heart-lung preparation. Pharmacologist *13*, 268 (1971)
Garteiz, D.A.: Metabolism of a beta-blocking drug, oxprenolol. J. Pharmacol. Exp. Ther. *179*, 354–358 (1971)
Garteiz, D.A., Gaffney, T.E.: Determination of the metabolic fate of oxprenolol in rats and man by gas chromatography – mass spectrometry. Pharmacologist *13*, 221 (1971)
Garver, D.L., Cedarbaum, J., Maas, J.W.: Blood-brain barrier to 6-hydroxydopamine: uptake by heart and brain. Life Sci. *17*, 1081–1084 (1975)
Geddes, D.M., Nesbitt, K., Traill, T.: First-pass uptake of ^{14}C-propranolol by the lung in man. Br. J. Clin. Pharmacol. *5*, 354–355 (1978)
George, C.F., Orme, M.L'E., Buranapong, P., Macerlean, D., Breckenridge, A.M., Dollery, C.T.: Contribution of the liver to overall elimination of propranolol. J. Pharmacokinet. Biopharm. *4*, 17–27 (1976)
Gibaldi, M., Boyes, R.N., Feldman, S.: Influence of first-pass effect on availability of drugs on oral administration. J. Pharm. Sci. *60*, 1338–1340 (1971)
Gillespie, L., Oates, J.A., Crout, J.R., Sjoerdsma, A.: Clinical and chemical studies with α-methyldopa in patients with hypertension. Circulation *25*, 281–291 (1962)
Giudicelli, J.-F., Tillement, J.-P., Boissier, J.-R.: Activite β-adrenalytique compare in vitro et in vivo et fixation proteique. J. Pharmacol. (Paris) *4*, 129–136 (1973)
Glazko, A.J., Dill, W.A., Wolf, L.M., Kazenko, A.: Studies on the metabolism of reserpine. J. Pharmacol. Exp. Ther. *118*, 377–387 (1956)
Gomeni, R., Bianchetti, G., Sega, R., Morselli, F.L.: Pharmacokinetics of propranolol in normal healthy volunteers. J. Pharmacokinet. Biopharm. *5*, 183–192 (1977)
Graham, R.M., Thornell, I.R., Gain, J.M., Bagnoli, C., Oates, H.E., Stokes, G.S.: Prazosin: the first-dose phenomenon. Br. Med. J. *1976 II*, 1293–1249
Graham, R.M., Oates, H.E., Stoker, L.M., Stokes, G.S.: Alpha blocking action of the antihypertensive agent, prazosin. J. Pharmacol. Exp. Ther. *201*, 747–750 (1977)
Greenblatt, D.J.: Impairment of antipyrine clearance in humans by propranolol. Clin. Pharmacol. Ther. *21*, 104 (1977)
Gripenberg, J., Jansson, S.-E.: Preliminary report on the incorporation of guanethidine and reserpine into rat peritoneal mast cells in vitro. Experentia *27*, 1451–1452 (1971)
Grundin, R.: Metabolic interaction of ethanol and alprenolol in isolated liver cells. Acta Pharmacol . Toxicol. (Kbh.) *37*, 185–200 (1975)
Gugler, R., Herold, W., Dengler, H.J.: Pharmacokinetics of pindolol in man. Eur. J. Clin. Pharmacol. *7*, 17–24 (1974)
Gugler, R., Hobel, W., Bodem, R., Dengler, H.J.: The effect of pindolol on exercise-induced cardiac acceleration in relation to plasma levels in man. Clin. Pharmacol. Ther. *17*, 127–133 (1975)
Gulaid, A., James, I.M., Kaye, C.M., Lewellen, O.R.W., Roberts, E., Sankey, M., Smith, J., Templeton, R., Thomas, R.J.: Lack of correlation between acetylator status and the production of the acetyl metabolite of acebutolol in man. Br. J. Clin. Pharmacol. *5*, 261–262 (1978)
Gundert-Remy, U., Weber, E.: Different pattern of excretion of ^{14}C-Clonidin in rats after interruption of enterohepatic circulation. Naunyn Schmiedebergs Arch. Pharmacol. *293*, Supplement 247, p. R 47 (1976)
Häeusler, G.: Early pre- and post-junctional effects of 6-hydroxydopamine. J. Pharmacol. Exp. Ther. *178*, 49–62 (1971)
Hansson, L., Zweifler, A.J., Julius, S., Ellis, C.N.: Propranolol therapy in essential hypertension. Observations on predictability of therapeutic response. Int. J. Clin. Pharmacol. *10*, 78–79 (1974)
Harvengt, C., Desager, J.P., Muschart, J.M., Tjandramaga, T.B., Verbeeck, R., Verberckmoes, R.: Influence of the hemodialysis on the half-life of practolol in patients with severe renal failure. J . Clin. Pharmacol. *15*, 605–610 (1975)
Hayes, A., Cooper, R.G.: Studies on the absorption, distribution, and excretion of propranolol in rat, dog, and monkey. J. Pharmacol. Exp. Ther. *176*, 302–311 (1971)

Heikkila, R., Cohen, G.: Further studies on the generation of hydrogen peroxide by 6-hydroxydopamine: potentiation by ascorbic acid. Mol. Pharmacol. *8*, 241–248 (1972)
Heikkila, R., Cohen, G.: 6-hydroxydopamine: evidence for superoxide radical as an oxidative intermediate. Science *181*, 456–457 (1973)
Hess, H.J.: Biochemistry and structure-activity studies with prazosin. In: Prazosin, evaluation of a new anti-hypertensive agent. Cotton, D.W.K. (ed.), pp. 3–13. Amsterdam: Excerpta Medica 1974
Hicks, D.C., Arbab, A.G., Turner, P., Hills, M.: A comparison of intravenous pindolol and propranolol in normal man. J. Clin. Pharmacol. *12*, 212–216 (1972)
Hobbs, D.C., Twomey, T.M.: Quoted by Brogden et al. *vide supra* (1977)
Hodges, P.: Identification of 2-6-dichlorophenyl-guanidine as a metabolite of clonidine. J. Pharm. Pharmacol. *28*, 61–62 (1976)
Hopkins, R., Martin, L.E., Bland, R.: The metabolism of labetalol in animals and man. Biochem. Soc. Trans. *4*, 726–729 (1976)
Huffman, D.H., Azarnoff, D.L., Shoeman, D.W., Dujovna, C.A.: The interaction between halofenate and propranolol. Clin. Pharmacol. Ther. *19*, 807–812 (1976)
Idle, J.R., Mahgoub, A., Lancaster, R., Smith, R.L.: Hypotensive response to debrisoquine and hydroxylation phenotype. Life Sci. *22*, 979–984 (1978)
Imhof, P.R., Garnier, B., Brunner, L., Keller, G., Rohrer, T.: Human pharmacology of orally administered phentolamine. In: Phentolamine in heart failure and other cardiac disorders. Taylor, S.H., Gould, L.A. (eds.), p. 11. Bern: Hans Huber 1976
Ishizaki, T., Privitera, P.J., Walle, T., Gaffney, T.E.: Cardiovascular actions of a new metabolite of propranolol: isopropylamine. J. Pharmacol. Exp. Ther. *189*, 626–632 (1974)
Isselbacher, K.J., Carter, E.A.: Effect of propranolol on ethanol metabolism – evidence for the role of mitochondrial NADH oxidation. Biochem. Pharmacol. *25*, 169–174 (1976)
Jack, D.B., Stenlake, J.B., Templeton, R.: Metabolism and excretion of guanoxan in man. J. Pharm. Pharmacol. *23*, 222S–223S (1971)
Jen, T., Vanhoeven, H., Groves, W., McLean, R.A., Loev, B.: Amidines and related compounds. 6. Studies on structure-activity relationships of anti-hypertensive and antisecretory agents related to Clonidine. J. Med. Chem. *18*, 90–99 (1975)
Johansson, K.A., Appelgren, C., Borg, K.O., Elofsson, R.: Binding of two adrenergic beta-receptor antagonists, alprenolol, and H 93/26, to human serum proteins. Acta Pharm. Suec. *11*, 333–346 (1974)
Johansson, R., Regårdh, C.-G., Sjogren, J.: Absorption of alprenolol in man from tablets with different rates of release. Acta Pharm. Suec. *8*, 59–70 (1971)
Johnsson, G., Regårdh, C.-G.: Lack of biological interaction between alprenolol and salicylate. Eur. J. Clin. Pharmacol. *6*, 9–14 (1973)
Johnsson, G., Regårdh, C.-G.: Clinical pharmacokinetics of β-adrenoreceptor blocking drugs. Clin. Pharmacokinet. *1*, 233–263 (1976)
Johnsson, G., Regårdh, C.-G., Solvell, L.: Combined pharmacokinetic and pharmacodynamic studies in man of the adrenergic beta$_1$-receptor antagonist metoprolol. Acta Pharmacol. Toxicol. (Kbh.) *36* (suppl. 5), 31–44 (1975)
Jones, P.S., Walker, H.A., Richardson, A.P.: Relationship between physiological disposition and adrenolytic action of 2-(N-p-tolyl-N-m-hydroxyphenyl-amino-methyl)-imidazoline hydrochloride (C-7337). Proc. Soc. Exp. Biol. Med. *73*, 366–370 (1950)
Jonsson, G.: Studies on the mechanisms of 6-hydroxydopamine cytotoxicity. Med. Biol. *54*, 406–420 (1976)
Jonsson, G., Sachs, C.H.: Uptake and accumulation of ^{3}H-6-hydroxydopamine in adrenergic nerves. Eur. J. Pharmacol. *16*, 55–62 (1971)
Jonsson, G., Malmfors, T., Sachs, C.H.: Effects of drugs on the 6-hydroxydopamine induced degeneration of adrenergic nerves. Res. Commun. Chem. Pathol. Pharmacol. *3*, 543–556 (1972)
Karlberg, B., Lundberg, D., Aberg, H.: Excretion of propranolol in human breast milk. Acta Pharmacol. Toxicol. (Kbh.) *34*, 222–224 (1974)
Kawashima, K., Levy, A., Spector, S.: Stereospecific radioimmunoassay for propranolol isomers. J. Pharmacol. Exp. Ther. *196*, 157–523 (1976)

Kaye, C.M.: A simple spectrophotofluorometric method for the measurement of ICI 66082 in plasma and urine. Br. J. Clin. Pharmacol. *1*, 84–86 (1974a)
Kaye, C.M.: The influence of urine pH on the renal excretion of ICI 66082 in man. Br. J. Clin. Pharmacol. *1*, 513–514 (1974b)
Kaye, C.M., Dufton, J.F.: Preliminary observations on the elimination of acebutolol in severe chronic renal failure. Br. J. Clin. Pharmacol. *3*, 198–199 (1976)
Kaye, C.M., Kumana, C.R.: Enterohepatic circulation of practolol in man. Br. J. Clin. Pharmacol. *1*, 169–172 (1974)
Kaye, C.M., Long, A.D.: The influence of pH on the buccal absorption and plasma and renal elimination of acebutolol. Brit. J. Clin. Pharmacol. *3*, 196–197 (1976)
Kaye, C.M., Oh, V.M.S.: The biliary excretion of acebutolol in man. J. Pharm. Pharmacol. *28*, 449–450 (1976)
Kaye, C.M., Robinson, D.G., Turner, P.: The influence of urinary pH on the renal excretion of practolol and propranolol. Br. J. Pharmacol. *49*, 155–156 (1973)
Kaye, C.M., Kumana, C.R., Leighton, M., Hamer, J., Turner, P.: Observations on the pharmacokinetics of acebutolol. Clin. Pharmacol. Ther. *19*, 416–420 (1976)
Kelly, J.G., McDevitt, D.G.: Plasma protein binding of drugs in thyroid dysfunction. Br. J. Clin. Pharmacol. *4*, 628 (1977)
Kendall, M.J., Brown, D., Yates, R.A.: Plasma metoprolol concentrations in young, old and hypertensive subjects. Br. J. Clin. Pharmacol. *4*, 497–499 (1977)
Kersting, F., Reid, J.L., Dollery, C.T.: Clinical and cardiovascular effects of alpha methyldopa in combination with decarboxylase inhibitors. Clin. Pharmacol. Ther. *21*, 547–555 (1977)
Kiechel, J.R., Nicklaus, P., Schreier, E., Wagner, H.: Metabolites of pindolol in different animal species. Xenobiotica *5*, 741–754 (1975)
Kilborn, J.R., Turner, P.: Ro 3-4787 m a new β-adrenoceptor blocking agent: Studies in normal volunteers. Br. J. Clin. Pharmacol. *1*, 143–149 (1974)
Knapp, D.R., Holcombe, N.H., Krueger, S.A., Privitera, P.J.: Qualitative metabolic fate of phenoxybenzamine in rat, dog, and man. Drug Metab. Dispos. *4*, 164–168 (1976)
Koda, R.T., Maronde, R.F., Wan, S.H., Malbion, J., Lesky, W.: Kinetics of absorption and excretion of atenolol (ICI 66082) from single intravenous and oral doses in humans. Clin. Pharmacol. Ther. *21*, 108 (1977)
Kornhauser, D.M., Wood, A.J.J., Vestal, R.E., Wilkinson, G.R., Branch, R.A., Shand, D.G.: Biological determinants of propranolol disposition in man. Clin. Pharmacol. Ther. *23*, 165–174 (1978)
Kostrzewa, R.M., Jacobowitz, D.M.: Pharmacological actions of 6-hydroxydopamine. Pharmacol. Rev. *26*, 199–288 (1974)
Kumana, C.R., Kaye, C.M.: An investigation of the relationship between β-adrenoceptor blockade and plasma practolol concentration in man. Eur. J. Clin. Pharmacol. *7*, 243–248 (1974)
Kumana, C.R., Kaye, C.M., Leighton, M., Martin, G.E.: An investigation of "absolute plasma level effect relationships" and "absolute cardioselectivity with respect to beta-adrenoceptor blockade". Eur. J. Clin. Pharmacol. *12*, 7–13 (1977)
Kwan, K.C., Foltz, E.L., Breault, G.O., Baer, J.E., Totaro, J.A.: Pharmacokinetics of methyldopa in man. J. Pharmacol. Exp. Ther. *198*, 264–277 (1976)
Lavene, D., Weiss, Y.A., Safar, M.E., Loria, Y., Agorus, N., Georges, D., Milliez, P.L.: Pharmacokinetics and hepatic extraction ratio of pindolol in hypertensive patients with normal and impaired renal function. J. Clin. Pharmacol. *17*, 501–508 (1977)
Leeson, G.A., Garteiz, D.A., Knapp, W.C., Wright, G.J.: N-methylation, a newly identified pathway in the dog for the metabolism of oxprenolol, a beta-receptor blocking agent. Drug Metab. Dispos. *1*, 565–568 (1973)
Leinweber, F.J., Di Carlo, F.J.: Bunolol metabolism by human and rat red blood cells and extrahepatic tissues. J. Pharmacol. Exp. Ther. *189*, 271–277 (1974)
Leinweber, F.J., Haynes, L.J., Crew, M.C., Di Carlo, F.J.: Absorption, tissue distribution, and excretion of bunolol-^{14}C by dogs. J. Pharm. Sci. *60*, 1512–1515 (1971a)
Leinweber, F.J., Greenough, R.C., Schwender, C.F., Haynes, L.J., Di Carlo, F.J.: Bunolol metabolism by dogs: Isolation and identification of two acidic metabolites. J. Pharm. Sci. *60*, 1516–1519 (1971b)

Leinweber, F.J., Greenough, R.C., Schwender, C.F., Kaplan, H.R., Di Carlo, F.J.: Bunolol metabolism by cell-free preparation of human liver: Biosynthesis of dihydrobunolol. Xenobiotica *2*, 191–202 (1972)
Leinweber, F.J., Greenough, R.C., Di Carlo, F.J.: Bunolol metabolism by dogs: Identification of basic metabolites and their conjugates. J. Pharm. Sci. *66*, 1570–1575 (1977)
Leinweber, F.J., Szpiech, J.M., Di Carlo, F.J.: L-bunolol metabolism in rats: Identification of urinary metabolites. J. Pharm. Sci. *67*, 128–130 (1978)
Leishman, A.W.D., Matthews, H.L., Smith, A.J.: Antagonism of guanethidine by imipramine. Lancet *1963 I*, 112
Lennard, M.S., Silas, J.H., Smith, A.J., Tucker, G.T.: Concentration of debrisoquine by human platelets in vivo: Relationship to hypotensive response. Br. J. Clin. Pharmacol. *4*, 635P (1977)
Leonetti, G., Mayer, G., Morganti, A., Terzoli, L., Zanchetti, A., Bianchetti, G., Di Salle, E., Morselli, P.L., Chidsey, C.A.: Hypotensive and renin-suppressing activities of propranolol in hypertensive patients. Clin. Sci. Mol. Med. *48*, 491–499 (1975)
Levy, A., Ngai, S.H., Finck, A.D., Kawashima, K., Spector, S.: Disposition of propranolol isomers in mice. Eur. J. Pharmacol. *40*, 93–100 (1976)
Liang, Y-O., Plotsky, P.M., Adams, R.N.: Isolation and identification of an in vivo reaction product of 6-hydroxydopamine. J. Med. Chem. *20*, 581–583 (1977)
Lish, P.M., Shalanski, M.V., La Budde, J.A., Williams, W.R.: Inhibition of cardiac chronotropic action of isoproterenol by sotalol (MJ 1999) in rat, dog, and man. Curr. Ther. Res. *9*, 311–324 (1967)
Lowenthal, D.T., Mutterperl, R.: The pharmacokinetics of multiple-dose propranolol in chronic renal disease. Clin. Pharmacol. Ther. *19*, 111 (1976)
Lowenthal, D.T., Briggs, W.A., Gibson, T.P., Nelson, H., Cirksena, W.J.: Pharmacokinetics of oral propranolol in chronic renal disease. Clin. Pharmacol. Ther. *16*, 761–769 (1974)
Maass, A.R., Jenkins, B., Shen, Y., Tannenbaum, P.: Studies on absorption excretion and metabolism of ^{3}H-reserpine in man. Clin. Pharmacol. Ther. *10*, 366–371 (1969)
Magoub, A., Idle, J.R., Dring, L.G., Lancaster, R., Smith, R.L.: Polymorphic hydroxylation of debrisoquine in man. Lancet *1977 II*, 584–586
Maitre, L., Staehelin, M., Brunner, H.: Antihypertensive and noradrenaline-depleting effects of guanethidine metabolites. J. Pharm. Pharmacol. *23*, 327–331 (1971)
Malcolm, S.L., Marten, T.R.: Determination of debrisoquine and its 4-hydroxy metabolite in plasma by gas chromatography/mass spectrometry. Anal. Chem. *48*, 807–809 (1976)
Marlin, G.E., Kumana, C.R., Kaye, C.M., Smith, D.M., Turner, P.: An investigation into the cardiac and pulmonary β-adrenoceptor blocking activity of ICI 66082 in man. Br. J. Clin. Pharmacol. *2*, 151–157 (1975)
Martin, L.E., Hopkins, R., Bland, R.: Metabolism of labetolol by animals and man. Br. J. Clin. Pharmacol. *3* (Suppl. 3), 695–710 (1976)
Martin, M.M., Phillips, F., Smith, A.J., Tucker, G.T.: Acebutolol in hypertension – relationship between plasma concentration and effect. Proc. 5th Scientific Meeting Int. Soc. Hypertension, Paris, July 1978
Martin, R., Barlow, J.J.: Muscle and gland cell degeneration in the octopus posterior salivary gland after 6-hydroxydopamine administration. J. Ultrastruct. Res. *52*, 167–178 (1975)
Mason, W.D., Winer, N.: Pharmacokinetics of oxprenolol in normal subjects. Clin. Pharmacol. Ther. *20*, 401–412 (1976)
Masuoka, D., Hansson, E.: Autoradiographic distribution studies of adrenergic blocking agents II. ^{14}C-propranolol, a β-receptor-type blocker. Acta Pharmacol. Toxicol. (Kbh.) *25*, 447–455 (1967)
Maxwell, D.R., Collins, R.F.: Acebutolol (Sectral): Review of the pharmacology and pharmacokinetics. Clin. Trials J. *2*, 9–18 (1974)
Mayer, S.E.: The physiological disposition of ^{3}H-dichloroisoproteronol. J. Pharmacol. Exp. Ther. *135*, 204–212 (1962)
McAinsh, J.: Clinical pharmacokinetics of atenolol. Postgrad. Med. J. *53* (Suppl. 3), 74–78 (1977)
McAllister, R.G.: Guanethidine in antihypertensive therapy: experience with an oral loading regime. J. Clin. Pharmacol. *15*, 771–778 (1975)

McAllister, R.G.: Intravenous propranolol administration: a method for rapidly achieving and sustaining desired plasma levels. Clin. Pharmacol. Ther. *20*, 517–523 (1976)
McCoubrey, A.: The estimation of N-benzyl-N′-N″-dimethylguanidine (BW 467 C 60) in urine and some observations on its reaction with hypobromite. J. Pharm. Pharmacol. *14*, 798–802 (1962)
McDevitt, D.G., Shand, D.G.: Plasma concentrations and the time-course of beta blockade due to propranolol. Clin. Pharmacol. Ther. *18*, 708–713 (1975)
McDevitt, D.G., Shanks, R.G.: Evaluation of once daily sotalol administration in man. Br. J. Clin. Pharmacol. *4*, 153–156 (1977)
McDevitt, D.G., Frisk-Holmberg, M., Hollifield, J.W., Shand, D.G.: Plasma binding and the affinity of propranolol for a beta receptor in man. Clin. Pharmacol. Ther. *20*, 152–157 (1976)
McEwan, J., Shand, D.G., Wilkinson, G.R.: High-affinity hepatic microsomal binding of propranolol: its relationship to metabolism and to the first-pass effect. Br. J. Pharmacol. *52*, 140–141 (1974)
McLean, A.J., McNamara, P., du Seuch, P., Gibaldi, M., Lalka, D.: Food, splanchnic blood flow and bioavailability of drugs subject to first pass metabolism. Clin. Res. *26*, 291 A (1978)
McMartin, C.: The separation and detection of metabolites of guanethidine. Biochem. Pharmacol. *18*, 238–243 (1969)
McMartin, C., Simpson, P.: The absorption and metabolism of guanethidine in hypertensive patients requiring different doses of the drug. Clin. Pharmacol. Ther. *12*, 71–77 (1971)
McMartin, C., Rondel, R.K., Vinter, J., Allan, B.R., Humberstone, P.M., Leishman, A.W.D., Sandler, G., Thirkettle, J.L.: The fate of guanethidine in two hypertensive patients. Clin. Pharmacol. Ther. *11*, 423–431 (1970)
Medina, M.A., Giachetti, A., Shore, P.A.: On the physiological disposition and possible mechanism of the antihypertensive action of debrisoquine. Biochem. Pharmacol. *18*, 891–901 (1969)
Meffin, P.J., Harapat, S.R., Harrison, D.C.: Quantitation in plasma and urine of acebutolol and a major metabolite with preliminary observations on their disposition kinetics in man. Res. Commun. Chem. Pathol. Pharmacol. *15*, 31–52 (1976)
Meffin, P.J., Winkle, R.A., Peters, F.A., Harrison, D.C.: Acebutolol disposition after intravenous administration. Clin. Pharmacol. Ther. *22*, 557–567 (1977)
Meier, J.: Pindolol: A pharmacokinetic comparison with other beta-adrenoceptor blocking agents. Curr. Med. Res. Opin. *4* (suppl. 5), 31–38 (1977)
Meier, J., Nuesch, E.: Pindolol, a β-adrenoceptor blocking agent with a negligible first-pass effect. Br. J. Clin. Pharmacol. *4*, 371–372 (1977)
Melander, A., Danielson, K., Schersten, B., Wahlin, E.: Enhancement of the bioavailability of propranolol and metoprolol by food. Clin. Pharmacol. Ther. *22*, 108–112 (1977)
Mitchell, J.R., Arias, L., Oates, J.A.: Antagonism of the antihypertensive action of guanethidine by desipramine. J. Am. Med. Assoc. *202*, 973–976 (1967)
Mitchell, J.R., Cavanaugh, J.H., Dingell, J.V., Oates, J.A.: Guanethidine and related agents II. Metabolism by hepatic microsomes and its inhibition by drugs. J. Pharmacol. Exp. Ther. *172*, 108–114 (1970)
Monro, A.M., Faulkner, J.K., Stoperh, D.A., Wood, B.A.: The pharmacokinetics of tolamolol in man. In: Clinical experiences with tolamolol, a cardioselective beta-blocking drug. Amsterdam: Excerpta Medica 1976
Mueller, R.A., Shideman, F.E.: A comparison of the absorption distribution and metabolism of reserpine in infant and adult rats. J. Pharmacol. Exp. Ther. *163*, 91–97 (1968)
Murphy, P.J., Bellamy, G., Williams, T.L., Molloy, B.B.: Glucuronide formation and stereospecificity in metabolism of D,L-propranolol and Lilly 112092 (D,L-1-(isopropylamino)-4,4-diphenyl-2-butanol). Pharmacologist *18*, 114 (1976)
Myers, M.G., Lewis, P.J., Reid, J.L., Dollery, C.T.: Brain concentration of propranolol in relation to hypotensive effect in the rabbit with observations on brain propranolol levels in man. J. Pharmacol. Exp. Ther. *192*, 327–335 (1975)
Myrhe, E., Brodwall, E.K., Stenbaek, Ö., Hansen, T.: The renal excretion of methyldopa. Scand. J. Clin. Lab. Invest. *29*, 201–204 (1972a)

Myrhe, E., Brodwall, E.K., Stenbaek, Ö., Hansen, T.: Plasma turnover of methyldopa in advanced renal failure. Acta Med. Scand. *191*, 343–347 (1972b)

Myrhe, E., Stenbaek, Ö., Brodwall, K., Hansen, T.: Conjugation of methyldopa in renal failure. Scand. J. Clin. Lab. Invest. *29*, 195–199 (1972c)

Nies, A.S., Evans, G.H., Shand, D.G.: Regional hemodynamic effects of beta-adrenergic blockade with propranolol in the unanesthetized primate. Am. Heart. J. *85*, 97–102 (1973a)

Nies, A.S., Evans, G.H., Shand, D.G.: The hemodynamic effects of beta-adrenergic blockade on the flow-dependent hepatic clearance of propranolol. J. Pharmacol. Exp. Ther. *184*, 716–720 (1973b)

Numerof, P., Gordon, M., Kelly, J.M.: The metabolism of reserpine I studies in the mouse with ^{14}C-labelled reserpine. J. Pharmacol. Exp. Ther. *115*, 427–431 (1955)

Numerof, P., Virgona, A.J., Cranswick, E.H., Cunningham, T., Kline, S.: The metabolism of reserpine: II Studies in schizophrenic patients. Psychiatry *9*, 139–142 (1958)

Oates, J.A., Mitchell, J.R., Feagin, O.T., Kauffman, J.S., Shand, D.G.: Distribution of guanidinium antihypertensives – mechanism of their selective action. Ann. N.Y. Acad. Sci. *179*, 302–308 (1971)

Ochs, H.R., Greenblatt, D.J., Woo, E., Franke, K.: Effect of propranolol on quinidine pharmacokinetics. Clin. Pharmacol. Ther. *23*, 123 (1978)

Ohnhaus, E.E., Nuesch, E., Meier, J., Kalberer, F.: The pharmacokinetics of unlabelled and ^{14}C-labelled pindolol in uraemia. Eur. J. Clin. Pharmacol. *7*, 25–29 (1974)

Ohnhaus, E.E., Munch, U., Meier, J.: Vergleichende Untersuchung zur Elimination von Pindolol (Visken) und Antipyrin bei Patienten mit Lebererkrankungen. Schweiz. Med. Wochenschr. *106*, 1748–1750 (1976)

Øie, S., Levy, G.: Relationship between renal function and elimination kinetics of pindolol in man. Eur. J. Clin. Pharmacol. *9*, 115–116 (1975)

Orton, T.C., Lowery, C.: Irreversible protein binding of ^{14}C-practolol metabolite(s) to hamster liver microsomes. Br. J. Pharmacol. *60*, 319 (1977)

Parsons, R.L., Kaye, C.M.: Plasma propranolol and practolol in adult coeliac disease. Br. J. Clin. Pharmacol. *1*, 348 (1974)

Parsons, R.L., Kaye, C.M., Raymond, K., Trounce, J.R., Turner, P.: Absorption of propranolol and practolol in coeliac disease. Gut *17*, 139–143 (1976)

Paterson, J.W., Conolly, M.E., Dollery, C.T., Hayes, A., Cooper, R.G.: The pharmacodynamics and metabolism of propranolol in man. Pharmacologia Clin. *2*, 127–133 (1970)

Pettinger, W.A.: Unusual alpha adrenergic receptor potency of methyldopa metabolites on melanocyte function. J. Pharmacol. Exp. Ther. *201*, 622–626 (1977)

Pfeifer, S., Zimmer, C.: Biotransformation und pharmakokinetik von β-rezeptorenblockern. Pharmazie *10*, 625–633 (1975)

Piafsky, K.M., Borga, O.: Plasma protein binding of basic drugs II. Importance of α_1-acid glycoprotein for inter-individual variation. Clin. Pharmacol. Ther. *22*, 545–549 (1977)

Pitone, J.M., Lowenthal, D.R., Onesti, G., Affrime, M.B., Nancarrow, J.F., Swartz, C.: Timolol maleate pharmacokinetics in chronic renal disease. Clin. Pharmacol. Ther. *21*, 114 (1977)

Planz, G., Gierlichs, H.W., Hawlina, A., Planz, R., Stephany, W., Rahn, H.K.: Influence of the decarboxylase inhibitor bensarazide on the antihypertensive effect and metabolism of alpha-methyldopa in patients with essential hypertension. Eur. J. Clin. Pharmacol. *12*, 241–245 (1977)

Porter, C.C., Titus, D.C.: Distribution and metabolism of methyldopa in the rat. J. Pharmacol. Exp. Ther. *139*, 77–87 (1963)

Poynter, D., Martin, L.E., Harrison, C., Cook, J.: Affinity of labetalol for ocular melanin. Br. J. Clin. Pharmacol. *3* Suppl. 3, 711–720 (1976)

Prescott, L.F., Buhs, R.P., Beattie, J.O., Speth, O.C., Trenner, N.R., Lasagna, L.: Combined clinical and metabolic study of the effects of alpha-methyldopa on hypertensive patients. Circulation *34*, 308–321 (1966)

Rahn, K.H.: Plasma levels and renal excretion of guanethidine in hypertensive patients. Arzneim. Forsch. *21*, 1487–1489 (1971)

Rahn, K.H.: The influence of renal function on plasma levels, urinary excretion, metabolism and antihypertensive effect of guanethidine (Ismelin) in man. Clin. Nephrol. *1*, 14–23 (1973)

Rahn, K.H., Goldberg, L.I.: Studies on the intestinal absorption of guanethidine in hypertensive patients. Pharmacologist *10*, 167 (1968)
Rahn, K.H., Goldberg, L.I.: Comparison of antihypertensive efficacy, intestinal absorption and excretion of guanethidine in hypertensive patients. Clin. Pharmacol. Ther. *10*, 858–866 (1969)
Ram, N., Bauer, E.W., Heilman, R.D.: The antihypertensive effects of ORF 12592 (an analog of propranolol) in dogs. Fed. Proc. *35*, 318 (1976)
Rand, M.J., Rush, M., Wilson, J.: Some observations on the inhibition of salivation by St 155 (2-(2,6-dichloro-phenylamino)-2-imidazolin hydrochloride (Catapres, Catapresan). Eur. J. Pharmacol. *5*, 158–172 (1969)
Rawlins, M., Collste, P., Frisk-Holmberg, M., Lind, M., Ostman, J., Sjoqvist, F.: Steady-state plasma concentrations of alprenolol in man. Eur. J. Clin. Pharmacol. *7*, 353–356 (1974)
Regårdh, C.-G.: Pharmacokinetics and biopharmaceutics of some adrenergic beta-receptor antagonists with special emphasis on alprenolol and metoprolol. Acta Pharmacol. Toxicol. [Suppl. 1] (Kbh) *37*, (1975)
Regårdh, C.-G., Borg, K.O., Johansson, R., Johnsson, G., Palmer, L.: Pharmacokinetic studies on the selective beta-receptor antagonist metoprolol in man. J. Pharmacokinet. Biopharm. *2*, 347–364 (1974)
Regårdh, C.-G., Johnsson, G., Jordo, L., Solvell, L.: Comparative bioavailability and effect studies on metoprolol administered as ordinary and slow-release tablets in single and multiple doses. Acta Pharmacol. Toxicol. (Kbh.) *36* (suppl. 5), 45–58 (1975)
Rehbinder, D.: The metabolism of clonidine (Catapres, St 155). In: Catapres in hypertension. Connolly, M.E. (ed.), pp. 227–233. London: Butterworth 1970
Richards, D.A., Maconochie, J.G., Bland, R.E., Hopkins, R., Woodings, E.P., Martin, L.E.: Relationship between plasma concentrations and pharmacological effects of labetalol. Eur. J. Clin. Pharmacol. *11*, 85–90 (1977)
Riess, W., Rajagopalan, T.G., Imhof, P., Schmid, K., Keberle, H.: Metabolic studies on oxprenolol in animals and man by means of radio-tracer techniques and glc-analysis. Postgrad. Med. J. *46* (suppl.), 32–40 (1970)
Riess, W., Hurzeler, R., Raschdorf, F.: The metabolites of oxprenolol (Trasicor) in man. Xenobiotica *4*, 365–373 (1974)
Riess, W., Brechbühler, S., Brunner, L., Imhoff, P.R., Jack, D.B.: The metabolism of betablockers in relation to their pharmacokinetic and pharmacodynamic behaviour. In: Betablockers – present status and future prospects. Schweizer, W. (ed.), pp. 276–289. Bern, Stuttgart, Vienna: Hubert 1974
Rotman, A., Daly, J.W., Creveling, C.R.: Oxygen-dependent reaction of 6-hydroxydopamine, 5,6-dihydroxy-tryptamine and related compounds with proteins in vitro: A model for cytotoxicity. Mol. Pharmacol. *12*, 887–899 (1976)
Routledge, P.A., Davies, D.M., Rawlins, M.D.: Pharmacokinetics of tolamolol in the treatment of hypertension. Eur. J. Clin. Pharmacol. *12*, 171–174 (1977)
Roux, A., Aubert, P., Guedon, J., Flouvat, B.: Study of acebutolol dialysis and pharmacokinetics data concerning patients with renal insufficiency undergoing haemodialysis. Nouv. Presse Med. *4*, 3228–3233 (1975)
Rubenfeld, S., Silverman, V.E., Weich, K.M.A., Mallette, L.E., Kohler, P.C.: Propranolol pharmacokinetics in thyrotoxicosis. Clin. Res. *26*, 295 A (1978)
Saavedra, J.A., Reid, J.L., Jordan, W., Rawlins, M.D., Dollery, C.T.: Plasma concentration of α-methyldopa and sulphate conjugate after oral administration of methyldopa and intravenous administration of methyldopa and methyldopa hydrochloride ethyl ester. Eur. J. Clin. Pharmacol. *8*, 381–386 (1975)
Sachs, C., Jonsson, G.: Mechanisms of action of 6-hydroxydopamine. Biochem. Pharmacol. *24*, 1–8 (1975)
Saelens, D.A., Walle, T., Privitera, P.J., Knapp, D.R., Gaffney, T.: Central nervous system effects and metabolic disposition of a glycol metabolite of propranolol. J. Pharmacol. Exp. Ther. *188*, 86–92 (1974)
Saelens, D.A., Walle, T., Privitera, P.J.: Quantitative determination of propranolol, propranolol glycol, and N-desisopropyl-propranolol in brain tissue by electron capture gas chromatography. J. Chromatogr. *123*, 185–192 (1976)

Sanders, G.L., Ward, A., Davies, D.M., Rawlins, M.D.: Multiple dose kinetics of labetalol in the treatment of hypertension. Br. J. Clin. Pharmacol. *5*, 358–359 (1978)

Saner, A., Thoenen, H.: On the molecular mechanism of action of 6-hydroxydopamine. Mol. Pharmacol. *7*, 147–154 (1971)

Sassard, J., Pozet, N., McAinsh, J., Legheand, J., Zech, P.: Pharmacokinetics of atenolol in patients with renal impairment. Eur. J. Clin. Pharmacol. *12*, 175–180 (1977)

Sawchuck, R.J., Robayo, J., Miller, K.W.: The distribution of propranolol between blood and plasma in hypertensive patients. Br. J. Clin. Pharmacol. *1*, 440–442 (1974)

Scales, B., Copsey, P.B.: The gas chromatographic determination of atenolol in biological samples. J. Pharm. Pharmacol. *27*, 430–433 (1975)

Scales, B., Cosgrove, M.B.: The metabolism and distribution of the selective adrenergic beta-blocking agent, practolol. J. Pharmacol. Exp. Ther. *175*, 338–347 (1970)

Schanker, L.S., Morrison, A.S.: Physiological disposition of guanethidine in the rat and its uptake by heart slices. Int. J. Neuropharmacol. *4*, 27–39 (1965)

Schneider, R.E., Babb, J., Bishop, H., Mitchard, M., Hoare, A.M., Hawkins, C.F.: Plasma levels of propranolol in treated patients with coeliac disease and patients with Crohn's disease. Br. Med. J. *1976 II*, 794–795

Schnelle, K., Garrett, E.R.: Pharmacokinetics of the β-adrenergic blocker sotalol in dogs. J. Pharm. Sci. *62*, 362–375 (1973)

Schrader, K., Brass, H., Renner, D.: Zur Pharmakokinetic von α-Methyldopa bei Nieren-Insuffizienz. Klin. Wochenschr. *49*, 1329–1334 (1971)

Schwartz, M.A., Baukema, J.: Quoted by Kitchen, A.M., Turner, R.W.D.: Studies on debrisoquine sulphate. Br. Med. J. *1966 II*, 728–731

Shand, D.G.: Individualization of propranolol therapy. Med. Clin. North Am. *58*, 1063–1069 (1974)

Shand, D.G., Oates, J.A.: Metabolism of propranolol by rat liver microsomes and its inhibition by phenothiazines and tricyclic antidepressant drugs. Biochem. Pharmacol. *20*, 1720–1723 (1971)

Shand, D.G., Rangno, R.E.: The disposition of propranolol I: Elimination during oral absorption in man. Pharmacology *7*, 159–168 (1972)

Shand, D.G., Nuckolls, E.M., Oates, J.A.: Plasma propranolol levels in adults with observations in four children. Clin. Pharmacol. Ther. *11*, 112–120 (1970)

Shand, D.G., Evans, G.H., Nies, A.S.: The almost complete hepatic extraction of propranolol during intravenous administration in the dog. Life Sci. *10*, 1417–1421 (1971)

Shand, D.G., Rangno, R.E., Evans, G.R.: The disposition of propranolol II. Hepatic elimination in the rat. Pharmacology *8*, 344–352 (1972)

Shand, D.G., Branch, R.A., Evans, G.H., Nies, A.S., Wilkinson, G.R.: The disposition of propranolol VII. The effects of saturable hepatic tissue uptake on drug clearance by the perfused rat liver. Drug Metab. Dispos. *1*, 679–686 (1973)

Shand, D.G., Kornhauser, D.M., Wilkinson, G.R.: Effects of route of administration and blood flow on hepatic drug elimination. J. Pharmacol. Exp. Ther. *195*, 424–432 (1975a)

Shand, D.G., Frisk-Holmberg, M., McDevitt, D.G., Sherman, K., Hollifield, J.: A dual antihypertensive mechanism for propranolol based on plasma level/response relationships. In: Pathophysiology and management of arterial hypertension. Berglund, G., Hansson, L., Werka, L. (eds.), pp. 175–182. Mölndal: Lindgren and Söner 1975b

Shand, G., Nies, A.S., McAllister, R.G., Oates, J.A.: A loading-maintenance regime for more rapid initiation of the effect of guanethidine. Clin. Pharmacol. Ther. *18*, 139–144 (1975c)

Shand, D.G., Cotham, R., Wilkinson, G.R.: Perfusion-limited effects of plasma drug binding on hepatic drug extraction. Life Sci. *19*, 125–130 (1976)

Shen, D., Gibaldi, M., Throne, M., Bellwood, G., Cunningham, R., Israili, Z., Dayton, P., McNay, J.: Pharmacokinetics of bethanidine in hypertensive patients. Clin. Pharmacol. Ther. *17*, 363–373 (1975)

Sheppard, H., Tsien, W.H.: Metabolism of reserpine-^{14}C. II. Species differences as studied in vitro. Proc. Soc. Exp. Biol. Med. *90*, 437–440 (1955)

Sheppard, H., Lucas, R.C., Tsien, W.H.: The metabolism of reserpine-^{14}C. Arch. Int. Pharmacodyn. *103*, 256–259 (1955)

Sheppard, H., Tsien, W.H., Sigg, E.B., Lucas, R.A., Plummer, A.J.: The metabolism of Reserpine-^{14}C. III. ^{14}C-concentration vs. time in the brains and other tissues of rats and guinea-pigs. Arch. Int. Pharmacodyn. *113*, 160–168 (1957)
Shoeman, D.W., Sirtori, C.R., Azarnoff, D.L.: Inhibition of amphetamine tolerance and metabolism by propranolol. J. Pharmacol. Exp. Ther. *191*, 68–71 (1974)
Siggins, G.R., Bloom, F.E.: Cytochemical and physiological effects of 6-hydroxydopamine on periarteriolar nerves of frogs. Circ. Res. *27*, 23–38 (1970)
Silas, J.H.: Factors affecting variability in response to oral debrisoquine. M.D. Thesis, University of Sheffield 1978
Silas, J.H., Lennard, M.S., Tucker, G.T., Smith, A.J., Malcolm, S.L., Marten, T.R.: Why hypertensive patients vary in their response to oral debrisoquine. Br. Med. J. *1977 I*, 422–425
Silas, J.H., Lennard, M.S., Tucker, G.T., Smith, A.J., Malcolm, S.L., Marten, T.R.: The disposition of debrisoquine in hypertensive patients. Br. J. Clin. Pharmacol. *5*, 27–34 (1978a)
Silas, J.H., Tucker, G.T., Townshend, M.M., Phillips, C.A., Smith, A.J.: Dissociation of biochemical and hypotensive effects of debrisoquine in hypertensive patients. Proc. 7th Int. Congr. Pharmacol. Paris, July 1978 (1978b)
Silas, J.H., Tucker, G.T., Smith, A.J.: Compliance, response, and resistance to hypotensive therapy with debrisoquine. Clin. Sci. Mol. Med. (in press) (1978c)
Simon, G., Kiowski, W., Julius, S.: Antihypertensive and β-adrenoceptor action of timolol. Clin. Pharmacol. Ther. *23*, 152–157 (1978)
Sjoerdsma, A., Vendsalu, A., Engelman, K.: Studies on the metabolism and mechanism of action of methyldopa. Circulation *28*, 492–502 (1963)
Solomon, H.M., Ashley, C., Spirit, N., Abrams, W.B.: The influence of debrisoquin on the accumulation and metabolism of biogenic amines by the human platelet, *in vivo* and *in vitro*. Clin. Pharmacol. Ther. *10*, 229–238 (1969)
Stenbaek, Ö., Myhre, E., Rugstad, H.E., Arnold, E., Hansen, T.: Pharmacokinetics of methyldopa in healthy man. Eur. J. Clin. Pharmacol. *12*, 117–123 (1977)
Stillwell, W.G., Horning, M.G.: Metabolism of pronethalol in the rat, guinea-pig, and the mouse. Res. Commun. Chem. Pathol. Pharmacol. *9*, 601–617 (1974)
Stitzel, R.E.: The biological fate of reserpine. Pharmacol. Rev. *28*, 180–205 (1977)
Stock, K., Westermann, E.: Quantitative estimation and tissue distribution of K8 592, 1-(3-methylphenoxy)-3-isopropylamino propanol (2)-hydrochloride, a new sympathetic beta-receptor blocking agent. Biochem. Pharmacol. *14*, 227–236 (1965)
Stone, C.A., Porter, C.C., Stavorski, J.M., Ludden, C.T., Totaro, J.A.: Antagonism of certain effects of catecholamine-depleting agents by antidepressant and related drugs. J. Pharmacol. Exp. Ther. *144*, 196–204 (1964)
Suzuki, T., Isozaki, S., Ishida, R., Saitoh, Y., Nakagawa, F.: Drug absorption and metabolism studies by use of portal vein infusion in the rat. II. Influence of dose and infusion rate on the bioavailability of propranolol. Chem. Pharm. Bull. (Tokyo) *22*, 1639–1645 (1974)
Svendsen, T.L., Hartling, O., Trap-Jensen, J.: Ethanol metabolism before and during beta-receptor blockade in man. Acta Physiol. Scand. suppl. 440 Abstract 177 (1976)
Taylor, J.A., Twomey, T.M., Schach von Wittenau, M.: The metabolic fate of prazosin. Xenobiotica *7*, 357–364 (1977)
Thoenen, H., Tranzer, J.P.: The pharmacology of 6-hydroxydopamine. Annu. Rev. Pharmacol. *13*, 169–180 (1973)
Thompson, F.D., Joekes, A.M., Foulkes, D.M.: Pharmacodynamics of propranolol in renal failure. Br. Med. J. *1972 II*, 434–436
Tilstone, W.J., Semple, P.F., Boyle, J.A.: The renal clearance of practolol in man. J. Pharm. Pharmacol. *26*, 66–67 (1974)
Tindell, G.L., Walle, T., Gaffeney, T.E.: Rat liver microsomal metabolism of propranolol: Identification of seven metabolites by gc-ms. Life Sci. *11*, 1029–1036 (1972)
Tindell, G.L., Walle, T., Knapp, D.R.: Formation of catechol-like and monophenolic metabolites of propranolol by the rat liver 9000 G supernatant. Res. Commun. Chem. Pathol. Pharmacol. *19*, 11–22 (1978)
Tjandramaga, T.B., Thomas, J., Verbeek, R., Verbesselt, R., Verberckmoes, R., de Schepper, P.J.: The effect of end-stage renal failure and haemodialysis on the elimination kinetics of sotalol. Br. J. Clin. Pharmacol. *3*, 259–265 (1976)

Tocco, D.J., Duncan, A.E.W., de Luna, F.A., Hucker, H.B., Gruber, V.F., Van den Heuvel, W.J.A.: Physiological disposition and metabolism of timolol in man and laboratory animals. Drug Metab. Dispos. *3*, 361–370 (1975)

Tocco, D.J., Hooke, K.F., de Luna, F.A., Duncan, A.E.W.: Stereospecific binding of timolol, a beta-adrenergic blocking agent. Drug Metab. Dispos. *4*, 323–329 (1976)

Tranzer, J.P., Thoenen, H.: An electron microscopic study of selective acute degeneration of sympathetic nerve terminals after administration of 6-hydroxydopamine. Experientia *24*, 155–156 (1968)

Tripp, S.L., Williams, E., Wagner, W.E., Lukas, G.: A specific assay for subnanogram concentration of reserpine in human plasma. Life Sci. *16*, 1167–1178 (1975)

Tucker, G.T., Silas, J.H., Iyun, A.O., Lennard, M.S., Smith, A.J.: Polymorphic hydroxylation of debrisoquine. Lancet *1977 II*, 718

Turnbull, L.B., Teng, L., Newman, J., Chremos, A.N., Bruce, R.B.: Disposition of bethanidine, N-benzyl-N′-N″-dimethylguanidine, in the rat, dog, and man. Drug Metab. Dispos. *4*, 269–275 (1976)

Unsicker, K., Allan, I.J., Newgreen, D.F.: Extraneuronal effects of 6-hydroxydopamine and extraneuronal uptake of noradrenaline. In-vivo and in-vitro studies on adrenocortical cells of lizards and rats. Cell Tissue Res. *173*, 45–69 (1976)

Uretsky, N.J., Iversen, L.L.: Effects of 6-hydroxydopamine on catecholamine-containing neurones in the rat brain. J. Neurochem. *17*, 269–278 (1970)

Verbesselt, R., Mullie, A., Tjandramarga, T.B., de Schepper, P.J., Dessain, P.: The effect of food intake on the plasma kinetics and toleration of prazosin. Acta Ther. *2*, 27–30 (1976)

Vermeij, P., el Sherbini-Schepers, M., Van Zwieten, P.A.: The disposition of timolol in man. J. Pharm. Pharmacol. *30*, 53–55 (1977)

Vestal, R.E., Kornhauser, D.M., Shand, D.G.: Active uptake of ^{3}H-propranolol by isolated alveolar macrophages. Clin. Res. *24*, 259 A (1976)

Vestal, R.E., Kornhauser, D.M., Hollifield, J.W., Shand, D.G.: Interaction between chlorpromazine and propranolol in man. Clin. Res. *25*, 277 A (1977)

Von Bahr, C., Alvan, G., Lind, M., Mellström, B., Sjöqvist, F.: "First-pass" effect and dose dependent availability as factors contributing to interindividual differences in equilibrium concentrations of alprenolol in man. Acta Pharm. Seuc. *11*, 649–650 (1975)

Wagner, J.G., Weidler, D.J., Lin, Y.J.: New method for detecting and quantitating drug-drug interactions applied to ethanol-propranolol. Res. Commun. Chem. Pathol. Pharmacol. *13*, 9–18 (1976)

Walle, T.: Glc determination of propranolol, other β-blocking drugs and metabolites in biological fluids and tissues. J. Pharm. Sci. *63*, 1885–1891 (1974)

Walle, T.: Methylthio incorporation in the naphthalene ring system of propranolol in vivo. Fed. Proc. *36*, 961 (1977)

Walle, T., Gaffney, T.E.: N-dealkylation and oxidative deamination of propranolol in the cardio-pulmonary circuit of dogs. Proc. 5th Int. Congr. Pharmacol. San Francisco 1972, p. 245

Walle, T., Ishizaki, T., Gaffney, T.E.: Isopropylamine, a biologically active deamination product of propranolol in dogs. Identification of deuterated and unlabeled isopropylamine by gas chromatography-mass spectrometry. J. Pharmacol. Exp. Ther. *183*, 508–512 (1972)

Walle, T., Morrison, J.I., Tindell, G.L.: Isomeric ring hydroxylated metabolites of propranolol in rats, man, and dogs. Res. Commun. Chem. Pathol. Pharmacol. *9*, 1–9 (1974)

Walle, T., Morrison, J., Walle, K., Conradi, E.: Simultaneous determination of propranolol and 4-hydroxypropranolol in plasma by mass fragmentography. J. Chromatogr. *114*, 351–359 (1975)

Walle, T., Conradi, E.C., Walle, U.K., Gaffney, T.E.: Steady-state plasma concentrations and urinary excretion of propranolol-O-glucuronide and propranolol in patients during chronic oral propranolol therapy. Fed. Proc. *35*, 665 (1976)

Walle, T., Conradi, E., Walle, K., Fagan, T., Gaffney, T.E.: Steady-state kinetics of the active propranolol metabolite 4-hydroxy-propranolol and its glucuronic acid conjugate in patients with hypertension and coronary artery disease. Clin. Res. *25*, 10 A (1977)

Walle, T., Conradi, E., Walle, K., Fagan, T., Gaffney, T.: A small between-patient variation in plasma propranolol: Implications. Clin. Pharmacol. Ther. *23*, 133 (1978)

Walson, P.D., Pesout, J., Forsyth, R.P., Castagnoli, N., Melmon, K.L.: Hypotensive action of S-α-methyldopa during long-term (steady-state) intravenous infusions. J. Pharmacokinet. Biopharm. *4*, 389–394 (1976)

Walter, I.E., Nies, A.S.: Safety of single large oral doses of guanethidine. Clin. Pharmacol. Ther. *21*, 706–708 (1977)

Walter, I.E., Khandelwal, J., Falkner, F., Nies, A.S.: The relationship of plasma guanethidine levels to adrenergic blockade. Clin. Pharmacol. Ther. *18*, 571–580 (1975)

Wan, S.K., Maronde, R.F.: Correlations of the blood and salivary levels of the beta-one blocker metoprolol. Clin. Pharmacol. Ther. *21*, 122 (1977)

Weiss, Y.A., Safer, M.E., Chevillard, C., Frydman, A., Simon, A., Lemaire, P., Alexandre, J.M.: Comparison of the pharmacokinetics of intravenous DL-propranolol in borderline and permanent hypertension. Eur. J. Clin. Pharmacol. *10*, 387–393 (1976)

Weiss, Y.A., Safer, M.E., Lehner, J.P., Levenson, J.A., Simon, A., Alexandre, J.M.: (+)-propranolol clearance, an estimation of hepatic blood flow in man. Br. J. Clin. Pharmacol. *5*, 457–460 (1978)

West, M.J., Kendall, M.J., Mitchard, M., Faragher, E.B.: A comparison of slow release with conventional oxprenolol: plasma concentrations and clinical effects. Br. J. Clin. Pharmacol. *3*, 349–443 (1976)

Wilkinson, G.R., Shand, D.G.: A physiological approach to hepatic drug clearance. Clin. Pharmacol. Ther. *18*, 377–390 (1975)

Wilson, J.T., Atwood, G.F., Shand, D.G.: Disposition of propoxyphene and propranolol in children. Clin. Pharmacol. Ther. *19*, 264–270 (1976)

Wing, L.M.H., Reid, J.L., Davies, D.S., Neill, E.A.M., Tippett, P., Dollery, C.T.: Pharmacokinetics and concentration-effect relationships of clonidine in essential hypertension. Eur. J. Clin. Pharmacol. *12*, 463–469 (1977)

Winkle, R.A., Meffin, P.J., Ricks, W.B. , Harrison, D.C.: Acebutolol metabolite plasma concentration during chronic oral therapy. Br. J. Clin. Pharmacol. *4*, 519–522 (1977)

Wood, A.J.: Pharmacokinetics of prazosin in man. Clin. Exp. Pharmacol. Physiol. *2*, 446 (1975)

Wood, A.J.: Cerebrospinal fluid concentration of metoprolol in a hypertensive patient. Br. J. Clin. Pharmacol. *4*, 240–241 (1977)

Wood, A.J., Bolli, P., Simpson, F.O.: Prazosin in normal subjects: plasma levels, blood pressure, and heart rate. Br. J. Clin. Pharmacol. *3*, 199–201 (1976)

Wood, A.J., Vestal, R.E., Branch, R.A., Wilkinson, G.R., Shand, D.G.: Age related effects of smoking on elimination of propranolol, antipyrine, and indocyanine green. Clin. Res. *26*, 297 A (1978)

Wood, B.A., Stopher, D.A., Monro, A.M.: The metabolism of tolamolol in the mouse, rat, guinea-pig, rabbit, and dog. Xenobiotica 5, 183–195 (1975)

Young, J.A., Edwards, K.D.G.: Studies on the absorption, metabolism, and excretion of methyldopa and other catechols and their influence on amino acid transport in rats. J. Pharmacol. Exp. Ther. *145*, 102–112 (1964)

Zacest, R., Koch-Weser, J.: Relation of propranolol plasma levels to β-blockade during oral therapy. Pharmacology 7, 178–184 (1972)

Zsotér, T.T., Johnson, G.E., de Veber, G.A., Paul, H.: Excretion and metabolism of reserpine in renal failure. Clin. Pharmacol. Ther. *14*, 325–330 (1973)

CHAPTER 4

Toxic Effects of Adrenergic Nerve-End Inhibitors, Neural-Transmitter Depleting Agents and False Transmitters

P. JUUL

A. Introduction

During more than thirty years numerous compounds have been developed in the search for efficient antihypertensive drugs with qualitatively and quantitatively acceptable adverse reactions. The *unwanted effects* of hypotensive drugs constitute the main reason for the continuous development of new drugs and for changes in recommended therapy since many antihypertensives including the compounds dealt with here may generally be considered drugs of *sufficient antihypertensive efficacy*.

Although there are other indications for the drugs dealt with here, their main field of clinical use is arterial hypertension. Thus the information concerning unwanted effects mainly originates from investigations concerning patients treated for arterial hypertension.

The value of lowering elevated arterial blood pressure in certain patients has been demonstrated beyond doubt, at least in males (Veterans Administration Cooperative Study Group on Antihypertensive Agents, 1960, 1970, 1972). However, a general principle of normalizing the blood pressure at all costs in every patient with arterial hypertension is highly debatable. First of all an improvement of the prognosis of patients with only moderately elevated blood pressure has not been demonstrated beyond doubt. Secondly, lowering of the elevated blood pressure in itself involves a risk of aggravating the patient's condition, e.g. by precipitating ischaemia of the central nervous system, myocardium, and kidneys (CUNNINGHAM, 1967; DOUGLAS, 1964; GOLDBERG and RAFTERY, 1976; GORMSEN et al., 1961). The increase in death rate from myocardial infarction, however, cannot at present be related to the effect of antihypertensive therapy, since hypertensive patients now survive longer and have more chance of developing a myocardial infarct (BRECKENRIDGE et al., 1970). Thirdly, every hypotensive drug possesses inherent toxic properties that must be weighed against the desired hypotensive effect.

Despite the development of several drugs within the three pharmacological groups discussed here, an increasing tendency towards the use of other groups of antihypertensives has developed within recent years. Thus, in many countries particularly the β-receptor blocking agents and peripheral vasodilators are replacing the "classical" antihypertensives, e.g. reserpine, methyldopa, and guanethidine. However, the latter drugs are still considered of some value by many authors (BROWN and BROWN, 1975; CHIDELL and WHITESIDE, 1969; DUNN and FREEMAN, 1975; FERGUSON et al., 1976; STUART et al., 1972; TARPLEY, 1974; WOOSLEY and NIES, 1976), and they furthermore constitute an important era in the history of pharmacotherapeutics. However frequent the unwanted effects of these drugs are, the majority of the effects may be considered acceptable to the patients, may diminish upon continuation of therapy, may be reduced by the employment of combination therapy, and, finally, may be regarded as reversible upon dicontinuation of therapy. A clinical evaluation comparing the various groups of antihypertensive drugs is too involved to be treated here, and for this reason the reader is referred to a few recent monographs: [GROSS (ed.), 1977; LARAGH (ed.), 1973; SIMPSON (ed.), 1976; WOLLAM et al., 1977].

The three groups of drugs whose adverse reactions shall be considered all interfere with the function of the postganglionic sympathetic neurone, resulting in a pharmacological inhibition of the quantity of noradrenaline released from the sympathetic nerve terminals. The drugs in part exert their effects by interference with the biosynthesis of noradrenaline and through the formation of false transmitters (methyldopa), by depletion of the stores of noradrenaline in the granules of the sympathetic terminals (rauwolfia alkaloids), or by inhibition of the release of noradrenaline from the terminals (guanidine derivatives). However, some of the drugs mentioned possess profound actions in the central nervous system, and certain compounds, e.g. reserpine and methyldopa, presumably exert their main sympatholytic effect via central mechanisms (cf. SMITH, 1976).

Main emphasis shall be given to drugs in current clinical use, particularly to guanethidine, reserpine, and methyldopa. Ganglionic blocking agents, monoamine oxidase inhibitors, and clonidine, all of which influence the function of the postganglionic sympathetic neurone, will not be considered.

Main emphasis shall be given to the description of organotoxic effects of the drugs observed in humans during ordinary use. No distinction is made between toxic effects, adverse reactions, and side effects.

Proper treatment of patients with arterial hypertension requires a more intensive monitoring of the patients than may be necessary in many other fields of therapy. Although an elevated blood pressure may in a few cases be permanently normalized during antihypertensive treatment, allowing a reduction of the dose of antihypertensives and in some cases even a cessation of therapy (PAGE and DUSTAN, 1962; SPACH et al., 1974), antihypertensive therapy must generally be considered purely symptomatic requiring life-long administration. Unwanted effects caused by the treatment are frequent and in many trials are reported for more than two-thirds of the patients. These facts have resulted in an immense literature concerning both therapeutic efficiency and toxic effects of antihypertensives. Within the space allotted to the present section it is only possible to include a limited numer of references. Further references are found in other chapters of this volume and in surveys and monographs on adverse reactions: (FROHLICH, 1974; JANDHYALA et al., 1974; KELLAWAY, 1976; NIES, 1975; TESTER-DALDERUP, 1976, 1977) and on drug interactions involving antihypertensive drugs (BRATER and MORRELLI, 1977; DOLLERY, 1965b; KOCH-WESER, 1975; NIES, 1975; OATES, 1973).

Despite the extensive literature on antihypertensive therapy, a qualitative and quantitative evaluation of the unwanted effects of hypotensive drugs is often difficult and in some cases impossible. There are many reasons for this difficulty. a) Carefully controlled investigations of unwanted effects are rare. b) Different authors often use different definitions of "unwanted effects". c) The selection of patients for treatment with a new drug is often inappropiate, e.g. inclusion criteria comprising patients with an unsatisfactory response to previous therapy. d) The majority of studies are short-term investigations of a few weeks' duration, which is insufficient to detect many types of adverse reactions. e) Many investigations are carefully controlled but for practical reasons involve only a limited number of patients, thus leaving little possibility of disclosing rare adverse reactions. f) The methods employed for the detection of possible unwanted effects differ considerably between different studies, e.g. intensive monitoring in hospitalized patients and self-questionnaires in outpatients; types, methods, and frequency of biochemical blood analyses performed, etc. Some antihypertensives may even interfere with the clinical chemical analyses. g) Certain "toxic effects" ascribed to the medication occur spontaneously, sometimes even more frequently in patients suffering from arterial hypertension. h) Some unwanted effects may not be recognized by the patient until discontinuation of medication. i) The majority of patients investigated has been treated with two or more antihypertensive drugs administered simultaneously, sometimes in fixed-ratio combinations (DOLLERY, 1977; GLAZER, 1972). j) Finally, the problem of noncompliance, resulting in drug-defaulting and sometimes very high drop-out rates, may invalidate any conclusions (ABERNATHY, 1976; BULPITT and DOLLERY, 1973; KELLAWAY and MCCRAE, 1975). These conditions must be taken into consideration when evaluating wanted as well as unwanted effects of the individual antihypertensive drugs (PRICHARD, 1971).

B. Adrenergic Nerve-End Inhibitors

"Adrenergic nerve-end inhibitors" comprise drugs interfering with the release of noradrenaline from the sympathetic nerve terminals. The term is used here synonymously with "adrenergic neurone blocking agents", a term that is used by some authors to comprise also inhibitors of the synthesis of noradrenaline and catecholamine-depleting agents.

The development of several drugs within this group of antihypertensives is mainly caused by rather frequent adverse reactions. Thus, acetylcholine-like actions of xylocholine developed by HEY and WILLEY (1954) prohibited its clinical application. Tolerance and parotid pain hampered the long-term use of bretylium introduced by BOURA et al. (1959a). Similarly adverse reactions led to the withdrawal from clinical investigation of the precursor of guanethidine, hexahydro-1-azepinyl-propionamidoxime, developed by MULL et al. (1957). Guanethidine was the first postganglionic neurone blocking agent to gain widespread use in arterial hypertension (MAXWELL et al., 1959; PAGE and DUSTAN, 1959), followed by a long series of guanidine derivatives (COSTA et al., 1962; CURWAIN et al., 1971; MULL and MAXWELL, 1967; SCHLITTER et al., 1962; WOLLWEBER et al., 1971).

A survey of the pharmacokinetics of guanethidine has been published by FURST (1967), and the relationship between plasma concentration and adrenergic blockade has been investigated by WALTER et al. (1975). Guanethidine as well as other guanidine antihypertensives are actively taken up into the entire postganglionic sympathetic neurone by means of the amine pump (survey by JUUL, 1974), and although the molecular mechanism of action is still unknown, it seems likely that the very high concentration obtained results in a stabilization of the membrane potential (HAEUSLER et al., 1969). The intraneuronally located gunethidine may be bound extravesicularly (GIACHETTI and HOLLENBECK, 1976). The kinetics of guanethidine and other guanidine derivatives with respect to the sympathetic ganglia have been investigated by JUUL (1974) and by JUUL and SAND (1973).

The majority of guanidine derivatives does not pass the blood-brain barrier. Exceptions to this rule exist, e.g. concerning guanoxan (DAVEY and REINERT, 1965) and guanabenz, the latter drug even partially exerting its hypotensive effect via central mechanisms (MACMAHON et al., 1977; NASH, 1973; SILVA et al., 1976).

Certain guanidine derivatives, e.g. guancydine, exert a direct effect on vascular smooth muscle (RUSSO and MENDLOWITZ, 1972). Some guanidinium compounds, e.g. debrisoquine, possess a monoamine oxidase inhibitory effect (KUNTZMAN and JACOBSON, 1963; PETTINGER et al., 1969). The postganglionic neurone blocking drugs generally deplete peripheral catecholamine stores (except the adrenal medulla) and exert various effects on the amine pump, ganglionic and neuromuscular transmission (reviews by BOURA and GREEN, 1965; JUUL, 1974). Guancydine and debrisoquine do not deplete peripheral catecholamine stores.

The various guanidine derivatives differ with respect to pharmacokinetics, the recent derivatives mainly characterized by a shorter half-life than that of guanethidine. With regard to adverse reactions, the drugs may differ quantitatively and even qualitatively depending upon the different pharmacological properties mentioned above. Generally the unwanted effects of the guanethidine analogues that have been marketed are less frequent than those of guanethidine, and the dosing schedule is easier due to their shorter half-lives. These advantages should be weighed against the assumed better patient compliance with guanethidine, which is administered in single daily doses. Among investigations comparing the unwanted effects of different postganglionic neurone blocking agents, a few references are: ADI et al. (1975); BATH et al. (1967); BLOOMFIELD and CANGIANO (1970); BULPITT and DOLLERY (1973); CHRYSANT and FROHLICH (1976); HANSSON et al. (1973); PASCUAL and JULIUS (1972); PRICHARD et al. (1968); RUEDY and DAVIES (1967); STUART et al. (1972); TALBOT et al. (1975); VEJLSGAARD et al. (1967).

A few references to papers comparing the unwanted effects of postganglionic neurone blocking agents with other groups of antihypertensives are: BATH et al. (1967); BULPITT and DOLLERY (1973); CHIDELL and WHITESIDE (1969); DUNN and FREEMAN (1975); FERGUSON et al. (1976); GLAZER (1975); HARVALD and SCHAUMBURG (1976); JOHNSON et al. (1966); LEVI et al. (1970); MATTS (1975); MERCERON et al. (1973); OATES et al. (1965); PRICHARD et al. (1968); ROSENBLOOM et al. (1963); SAFAR et al. (1975); SILVA et al. (1976); TARPLEY (1974); VEJLSGAARD et al. (1967); WEISS et al. (1973).

The usual daily dose of guanethidine is 10–100 mg.

I. General Toxicity

The acute LD_{50} of guanethidine following i.v. administration is 22 mg/kg in the mouse (Ciba Pharmaceutical Company Information, 1973), and 23 mg/kg in the rat (MAXWELL et al., 1960). Dogs have tolerated 15 mg/kg i.v. (HARRISON et al., 1963). The LD_{50} following i.p. administration in the mouse is 115 mg/kg (YEN et al., 1970), and rats have been reported to survive 600 mg/kg (CLEMENTI, 1965). Perorally the LD_{50} in rats is above 1000 mg/kg (MAXWELL et al., 1960).

The LD_{50} following prolonged i.p. administration is within the range of 120–180 mg/kg (JUUL, 1974). Rats treated chronically with guanethidine up to 20 mg/kg i.p. have been reported to have a normal growth rate (BLASZKOWSKI et al., 1970; ERÄNKÖ and ERÄNKÖ, 1971 b; JUUL, 1974; ZAIMIS, 1966), whereas higher doses reduce the weight gain (JUUL, 1974). During long-term administration of guanethidine at high doses some animals devolop diarrhoea, and a few animals develop a hyperexcitation shortly after the individual i.p. injections (JUUL, 1974). The cervical, thoracic, and abdominal lymph nodes and the thymus are enlarged following prolonged i.p. adminstration of guanethidine at 20 mg/kg (JENSEN-HOLM, 1974). Apart from the sympatholytic effects, e.g. miosis and ptosis, and the effects described below, no organ toxicity is encountered following even prolonged parenteral administration at high doses.

In humans large doses may be tolerated without signs of organ toxicity. Although the usual daily dose of guanethidine is below 100 mg, requirement of 300 mg or more ist not uncommon; even doses above 600 mg daily are some times necessary (e.g. STOCKS and ROBERTSON, 1967). Single oral doses of 100 mg or more, e.g. as used in oral load regimes, are well tolerated (MCALLISTER, 1975; SHAND et al., 1972, 1975; WALTER and NIES, 1977).

More than forty different unwanted effects have been ascribed to the use of the postganglionic neurone blocking agents [survey by KELLAWAY (1976)]. The frequency of adverse reactions varies between different reports. Thus unwanted effects were reported among 63% of patients treated with guanethidine, 83% with guanoxan (VEJLSGAARD et al., 1967), 52% on debrisoquine (ROSENDORFF et al., 1968), and 30% on bethanidine (SMIRK, 1963 b). Up to 30% of patients treated with guanethidine discontinued treatment (LOWTHER and TURNER, 1963), and 73% on guanochlor (VEJLSGAARD et al., 1967), mainly due to unwanted effects. In many trials, however, the frequency of unwanted effects is reported lower – the differences probably to a large extent being due to different definitions of "unwanted effects" and different techniques of their detection.

II. Cardiovascular System

The most common unwanted vascular effects of the postganglionic neurone blocking agents are to be expected when considering their mechanism of action, their haemodynamic effects, and their pharmacokinetics.

The haemodynamic response to a single i.v. injection of guanethidine is triphasic: After a transient fall in arterial blood pressure, a period of moderate hypertension caused by release of noradrenaline from the sympathetic terminals occurs, followed by a gradual and long-lasting decline (COHN et al., 1963; HARRISON et al., 1963; MAXWELL et al., 1960). The decreased blood pressure is caused by a substantial reduction of the cardiac output and by a minor reduction of the peripheral resistance (BREST, 1965; NOWACK, 1961; ONESTI et al., 1966).

Following prolonged administration, the haemodynamic effects underlying the hypotension seem to shift from a reduction of cardiac output to a lowering of the peripheral resistance. This has been described by CHAMBERLAIN and HOWARD (1964), SANNERSTEDT and CONWAY (1970), and by VILLAREAL et al. (1964). Other investigators consider a decreased cardiac output with a nearly unchanged peripheral resistance responsible for the hypotensive effect even during long-term administration (Brest et al., 1970; Merceron et al., 1973; Onesti et al., 1966; Richardson and Wyso, 1960). These differences may largely be due to different dose regimens, different duration of administration, and to differences of the techniques used for the determination of haemodynamic changes.

The elimination data concerning guanethidine fit best with a 3 compartment model (Rahn and Rupp, 1971), the therapeutic point of attack being located in a peripheral compartment. The half-life of the slow elimination phase is 4–10 days (McMartin et al., 1970; Oates, 1970). Thus the very slow onset of hypotensive action upon repeated administration and the slow rise following discontinuation can be predicted.

The doses of guanethidine necessary for the control of the blood pressure vary considerably, and some cases of hypertension are almost resistant to guanethidine. This resistance may be of kinetic origin since a 6-fold interindividual variation in the plasma levels resulting from any given dose has been reported, whereas the adrenergic neuronal blockade occurs when the plasma levels exceed 8 ng/ml (Walter et al., 1975). Patients with guanethidine-resistant hypertension on the other hand have been reported to have an increased sensitivity to catecholamines (Sandler et al., 1968).

In many patients the dose of guanethidine has to be increased to obtain a satisfactory response, particularly during the initial period of treatment. This phenomenon by many authors is referred to as development of "tolerance," although this may not be the appropriate term. The tolerance cannot be explained pharmacokinetically, e.g. by hepatic enzyme induction, but may be caused by fluid retention, by the development of denervation hypersensitivity to endogenous catecholamines, or by a progression of the disease. Tolerance has been reported in 0%–63% of the patients treated with guanethidine (Dollery et al., 1960 b; Galskov et al., 1961; Lowther and Turner, 1963; Page et al., 1961; Pascual and Julius, 1972; Stocks and Robertson, 1967), the differences in frequency being probably in part due to different definitions of tolerance. Similarly tolerance may develop towards bethanidine (Smirk, 1963 b), towards debrisoquine (Jackson, 1972; Kitchin and Turner, 1966; Rosendorff et al., 1968), and towards other guanidinium compounds. The majority of patients treated with bretylium develops resistance towards the drug within a few months (Dollery et al., 1960 a; Hurley et al., 1960; Soloff, 1961; Soloff et al., 1960).

Fluid retention occurs in up to one-third of the patients treated with guanethidine (Galskov et al., 1961; Leishman et al., 1961; Smith, 1965 a). In 5 patients responding poorly to combined adrenergic blockade and diuretic treatment the plasma volume was either expanded or normal, whereas 11 patients responding well to treatment had a plasma volume below normal (Dustan et al., 1972). Changes in blood volume during the day may account for part of the diurnal changes in arterial blood pressure during treatment with long-acting autonomic blocking agents (Cranston and Brown, 1963). Fluid retention caused by postganglionic neurone blocking agents can induce heart failure in patients with a reduced margin of compensation (Dollery et al., 1960 b; Guazzi et al., 1973 a, b; Lauler et al., 1963; Ronnov-Jessen, 1963). Antihypertensive drugs as a rule do not induce fluid retention, but may induce a changed equilibrium in fluid compartments (Leth, 1976). The postganglionic neurone blocking agents induce an increased plasma volume (often of the order of 10%) with or without sodium retention (Leth and Ibsen, 1976; Merceron et al., 1973; Muelheims and Brown, 1962; Rønnov-Jessen and Hansen, 1969; Smith, 1965 b; Weil and Chid-

SEY, 1968). The increased plasma volume is caused by a decreased sympathetic tone and venodilation, a derangement of volume control mechanisms relating to the distribution of fluids between intravascular and interstitiel compartments, and in some cases probably by a long-lasting failure of renal mechanisms (DUSTAN et al., 1972; LETH and IBSEN, 1976).

During administration of postganglionic neurone blocking drugs a hypersensitivity towards directly acting sympathomimetics may occur, the mechanism of action being probably presynaptic (inhibition of the amine pump) as well as postsynaptic. The impaired neuronal uptake may result in a diminished response to indirectly acting sympathomimetics. These findings have been reported in animals as well as in man (BOURA and GREEN, 1962; GOKHALE et al., 1967; GREEN and ROBSON, 1965; LAURENCE and NAGLE, 1961; MUELHEIMS et al., 1965; NIELSEN, 1977a; PAGE and DUSTAN, 1959; PETTINGER et al., 1969; ZIMMERMANN and HARRIS, 1963).

Orthostatic or exertional hypotension of varying frequency and intensity occurs during treatment with all postganglionic neurone blocking agents. The differences in frequency between different reports (varying between a few and almost a hundred percent) mainly depend upon the evaluation of the effect as being an inevitable side effect or an adverse reaction (BATH et al., 1967; BREST et al., 1961; BREST and MOYER, 1961; BREST et al., 1962; BULPITT and DOLLERY, 1973; CHAMBERLAIN and HOWARD, 1964; FROHLICH and FREIS, 1959; GIFFORD, 1965; HEFFERNAN et al., 1971; HURLEY et al., 1960; JACKSON, 1972; LEISHMAN et al., 1961; LEVI et al., 1970; LOWTHER and TURNER, 1963; LUOMANMÄKI et al., 1975; MATTS, 1975; MERCERON et al., 1973; OATES et al., 1965; PAGE et al., 1961; PEART and MACMAHON, 1964; PRICHARD et al., 1968; RICHARDSON et al., 1960; ROSENDORFF et al., 1968; SMIRK, 1963b; TALBOT et al., 1975; TALBOT and SMITH, 1975; VEJLSGAARD et al., 1967). Failure of splanchnic resistance to rise during exercise following postganglionic sympathetic blockade is an important factor contributing to orthostatic and exercise-induced hypotension (GOLDBERG and RAFTERY, 1976; KHATRI and COHN, 1968; KISIN and YAZHAKOV, 1976). It has been suggested that a negative chronotropic effect of the postganglionic neurone blocking drugs may potentiate hypotensive symptoms in patients with cardiovascular, renal, or cerebrovascular disease (TALBOT and SMITH, 1975). In atherosclerotic cockerels the combination of exercise and guanethidine contrary to the above mentioned findings produced a significant tachycardia and hypertension, the cardiac output being reduced and the total peripheral resistance increased (WONG et al., 1975). The acute sympathomimetic response following i.v. guanethidine is due to release of endogenous noradrenaline (e.g. HARRISON et al., 1963; KOPIA and CONDOURIS, 1977).

Prolonged administration of guanacline may result in a partial, but persistent impairment of sympathetic function as shown in animals (GERKENS, 1974b) as well as in man (BOCK and HEIMSOTH, 1969; DAWBORN et al., 1969; SAMEE et al., 1970). The possible mechanism behind this apparently irreversible effect shall be discussed in the section concerning effects on the peripheral nervous system. Up to one year after the discontinuation of debrisoquine a pronounced augmentation of the chlorthalidone-reserpine-induced antihypertensive effect in approximately half of 32 patients has been reported (BRYANT et al., 1964), an effect that has not been further investigated. Although persistent normotension in a few previously hypertensive patients has been claimed following discontinuation of guanethidine (SPACH et al., 1974), it can be stated that all sympatholytic effects of guanethidine are fully reversible upon discontinuation of medication. Thus reversibility of side effects caused by guanethidine has been demonstrated in 28 patients after treatment at daily doses from 12.5–150 mg for up to more than 10 years (BAUER et al., 1973). Continuous administration to dogs of guanethidine at 2.5 mg/kg for up to 8 months resulted in a complete restoration of cardiac and lumbar sympathetic neuronal function that could not be explained on the basis of an altered sensitivity of adrenoceptors (JANDHYALA and BUCKLEY, 1974).

Mitochondrial changes have been reported in the myocardial cells of dogs following a single i.v. injection of guanethidine 15 mg/kg (WILCKEN et al., 1967a). However, other investigations in animals and man rule out any direct cardiotoxic effect of guanidinium compounds (e.g. BALAZS et al., 1975; JANDHYALA et al., 1975; KÁLDOR and JUVANCZ, 1969; WALTER and NIES, 1977).

III. Respiratory System

Nasal stuffiness is observed at varying frequency during treatment with postganglionic neurone blocking drugs. The frequency and intensity of this side effect are smaller than during rauwolfia therapy, but 20%–40% of the patients may complain of nasal stuffiness during guanethidine therapy, less commonly on guanoxan and debrisoquine, and more commonly on bretylium (ADI et al., 1975; BAUER et al., 1961, 1973; BOURA et al., 1959b; FERGUSON et al., 1976; FROHLICH and FREIS, 1959; LOWTHER and TURNER, 1963; PEART and MACMAHON, 1964).

IV. Blood

Haematologic effects are not observed during treatment with the postganglionic neurone blocking agents, not even during long-term administration (BLOOMFIELD and CANGIANO, 1969; CHRYSANT and FROHLICH, 1976; FROHLICH and FREIS, 1959; HARVALD and SCHAUMBURG, 1976; OATES et al., 1965; VEJLSGAARD et al., 1967).

V. Liver

Among the postganglionic neurone blocking agents only guanoxan has been suspected of possessing hepatotoxic properties. A few cases of impairment of hepatic function were reported by COTTON and MONTUSCHI (1966) and by MONTUSCHI and LOVEL (1964). Subsequently COTTON and MONTUSCHI (1967) reported that 26 out of 96 patients treated with guanoxan for 2–27 months had some derangement of liver function, out of which 10 were considered severe abnormalities (4 had frank jaundice, and one patient died). Other investigations comprising a total of 175 patients treated with guanoxan for 1–12 months did not reveal any impairment of hepatic function (PEART and MACMAHON, 1964; RUEDY and DAVIES, 1967; VEJLSGAARD, 1968; VEJLSGAARD et al., 1967).

VI. Gastrointestinal System

Parotid pain is a frequent complaint during treatment with bretylium, arising in up to 75% of the patients (HURLEY et al., 1960). With other postganglionic neurone blocking agents parotid tenderness may also appear, but much less frequently, e.g. following guanethidine (DOLLERY et al., 1960b; PAGE et al., 1961). Experimental studies have indicated a guanethidine-induced reversible peripheral neurogenic sialoadenosis (ARGLEBE et al., 1975; CHILLA et al., 1975). Following guanacline administration, parotid pain may persist up to 5 years after discontinuation of medication (BOCK and HUEP, 1971). Biopsies of the parotid gland from patients during long-term treatment with guanacline have demonstrated a neurovegetative sialoadenosis resembling the effect of postganglionic sympathectomy. Axons containing granular vesicles were almost completely absent, and some of the remaining axons appeared empty and with an accumulation of dense bodies. Some Schwann cells contained degenerated nerve fibres. The myoepithelial cells and glandular cells also were abnormal (DONATH et al., 1973; PIRSIG et al., 1973). Experiments in animals on chronic guanacline have demonstrated a destruction of the granular vesicles of the terminal axons in the parotid gland as well as a degeneration of the mitochondria and an appearance of lysosome-like bodies in axons as well as in Schwann cells. The catecholamines of the sympathetic nerve fibres were depleted (DONATH and SEIFERT, 1973). In the acinar cells of the rat parotid gland a massive accumulation of secretory granules and lesions in the cytoplasm were observed, probably due to a degeneration of the secretory granules (DONATH, 1973).

Occasional nausea and vomiting have been reported, e.g. during treatment with guanabenz (SILVA et al., 1976) and with guanadrel (BLOOMFIELD and CANGIANO, 1969).

Diarrhoea is a frequent unwanted effect during guanethidine therapy occurring in 10%–60% of the patients (BAUER et al., 1961, 1973; BLOOMFIELD and CANGIANO, 1970; BREST et al., 1961, 1962; BREST and MOYER, 1961; BULPITT and DOLLERY, 1973; DOLLERY et al., 1960b; FERGUSON et al., 1976; FROHLICH and FREIS, 1959; GALSKOV et al., 1961; LEISHMAN et al., 1959, 1961; LOWTHER and TURNER, 1963; MATTS, 1975; OATES et al., 1965, PAGE et al., 1961; ROSENBLOOM et al., 1963; TALBOT et al., 1975). Similar findings have been reported with guanoxan (MONTUSCHI and LOVEL, 1964; PEART and MACMAHON, 1964). Diarrhoea has been reported in only a few percent of patients treated with bethanidine (LEVI et al., 1970; TALBOT et al., 1975), whereas a laxative effect was not observed in other investigations (BATH et al., 1967; GIFFORD, 1965; JOHNSTON et al., 1964). A similar low incidence of diarrhoea is observed following debrisoquine (ATHANASSIADIS et al., 1966; HARVALD and SCHAUMBURG, 1976; JACKSON, 1972; KITCHIN and TURNER, 1966; ROSENDORFF et al., 1968; TALBOT, 1965; TALBOT et al., 1975) and following guanadrel (BLOOMFIELD and CANGIANO, 1969, 1970; HANSSON et al., 1973; PASCUAL and JULIUS, 1972).

The mechanism behind the laxative effect of postganglionic neurone blocking agents is obscure. It is often ascribed to the sympatholytic effect per se, but this is unlikely to be the case when the great differences in frequency of diarrhoea between different sympatholytic drugs of similar sympatholytic efficacy are considered.

VII. Genitourinary System

The postganglionic neurone blocking agents are not nephrotoxic per se. Based upon the haemodynamic changes induced by these drugs comprising a reduced renal blood flow, long-term administration might be expected to induce an impairment of renal function (NOWACK, 1961; ONESTI et al., 1966; SANNERSTEDT and CONWAY, 1970; VIL-

LAREAL et al., 1964). A reduced glomerular filtration is observed in acute experiments with guanethidine (NOWACK, 1961; VILLAREAL et al., 1964). Various investigations deal with the influence of guanethidine on the tubular reabsorption of sodium and water (GILL and BARTTER, 1966; GILL et al., 1964; WILLIAMS et al., 1971). The fluid retention caused by postganglionic neurone blocking drugs has previously been mentioned.

Using a combination of guanethidine, hydralazine, and a thiazide diuretic WOODS et al. (1974) concluded that aggressive reduction of the blood pressure does not necessarily result in a deterioration of renal function. Using methyldopa, clonidine, propranolol, resperine, and guanethidine SAFAR et al. (1975) found that a reduced renal function at the beginning of therapy partly or totally diminished in course of time (47 patients treated for 2 years). BROWN and BROWN (1975) in a retrospective study concerning guanethidine found that out of 9 patients with elevated blood urea nitrogen at the start of therapy, 7 patients revealed only minor changes whereas in 2, a marked change for the worse was observed. The study comprised 70 patients treated for 4 months to 11 years, and the authors conclude that guanethidine is well suited for long-term use, even in the presence of impaired renal function.

No impairment of renal function was found during treatment with debrisoquine (HARVALD and SCHAUMBURG, 1976), guanadrel (CHRYSANT and FROHLICH, 1976), and with guanabenz (BOSANEC et al., 1976).

Disturbed sexual function is often encountered during prolonged treatment with guanethidine. Most often a failure of ejaculation with preserved orgasm is observed. The frequency of impaired ejaculation varies between 6%–84% in different reports; the higher frequencies are probably more accurate because they were based on thorough questioning of the patients (BAUER et al., 1973; BLOOMFIELD and CANGIANO, 1970; BREST et al., 1961, 1962; BREST and MOYER, 1961; BROWN and BROWN, 1975; BULPITT and DOLLERY, 1973; CHIDELL and WHITESIDE, 1969; DOLLERY et al., 1960b; FERGUSON et al., 1976; FROHLICH and FREIS, 1959; GALSKOV et al., 1961; HANSSON et al., 1973; LEISHMAN et al., 1959, 1961; LOWTHER and TURNER, 1963; MATTS, 1975; OATES et al., 1965; PAGE et al., 1961; RICHARDSON and WYSO, 1960; RICHARDSON et al., 1960; ROSENBLOOM et al., 1963; RUEDY and DAVIES, 1967). The effect is dose-dependent and reversible, and BAUER et al. (1973) states that a history of normal ejaculation during guanethidine treatment is an indication of inadequate drug dosage or frequent treatment default.

The ejaculatory failure may be caused by absent contraction of the seminal vesicles, ampulla, and ductus deferens rather than retrograde ejaculation (KEDIA and MARKLAND, 1975), and aspermia may also be caused by a total, but reversible impairment of the sperm liquor secretion (KIESSLING and HUHNSTOCK, 1963). Animal experiments have demonstrated a profound interference of guanethidine with the function of the short postganglionic sympathetic neurones to the internal male genital organs (EVANS et al., 1972; GANNON et al., 1971), as shall be discussed in the section on effects on the peripheral nervous system. The isolated vas deferens may function normally despite lowering of the tissue catecholamines (JOHNSON and O'BRIEN, 1976; JOHNSON et al., 1975). Eight weeks following discontinuation of guanethidine 25 mg/kg for 8 weeks in male rats, all males were able to deposit sperm in the vagina, whereas fertility at that time had returned in only 2 out of 9 of the males (HEPP and KREYE, 1973). Four months after the discontinuation of guanethidine 5 mg/kg i.p. for 19 weeks to rats, spermatic granulomata of the epididymis were found in all animals, which was not the case following similar dose regimens of quanacline (BHATHAL et al., 1974).

With bethanidine, ejaculation failure is reported in 8%–40% of the patients (BULPITT and DOLLERY, 1973; GIFFORD, 1965; JOHNSTON et al., 1964; LEVI et al., 1970; VEJLSGAARD, 1968), with guanoxan in 30%–88% (PEART and MACMAHON, 1964; RUEDY and DAVIES, 1967), with debrisoquine in 6%–20% (JACKSON, 1972; ROSENDORFF et al., 1968; TALBOT, 1965), and with guanadrel in 0%–53% (BLOOMFIELD and CANGIANO, 1969, 1970; HANSSON et al., 1973). The frequency of impotence is much lower. Thus RUEDY and DAVIES (1967) reporting failure of ejaculation in 22 out of 25 of males on guanoxan and 21/25 on guanethidine in a double blind cross-over study found impotence in 4/25 and 5/25 of the males respectively.

Clinical studies on guancydine were terminated due to the development of a few mammary carcinomas in rats treated with the combination of guancydine and propranolol. Guancydine administered alone did not induce tumors. The clinical implication of the finding is unknown (Cyanamid Overseas Corporation Information, 1975).

VIII. Central Nervous System

The majority of postganglionic neurone blocking agents does not pass the blood-brain barrier and thus does not exert a direct central effect. Mental depression has been described with guanethidine (BAUER et al., 1961; DOLLERY et al., 1960b), and with bethanidine (GIBB et al., 1970; GIFFORD, 1965), but the effects are probably coincidental. Guanabenz, which passes the blood-brain barrier, may induce sedation in one-fifth to one-third of the patients (NASH, 1973; SILVA et al., 1976).

IX. Peripheral Nervous System

Destruction of the postganglionic sympathetic neurone may be accomplished by surgical axotomy (reviews by BARRON et al., 1971; COLE, 1968; CRAGG, 1970; LIEBERMAN, 1971; MATTHEWS and RAISMAN, 1972), by immunosympathectomy induced by administration of nerve growth factor antiserum (reviews by LEVI-MONTALCINI and ANGELETTI, 1966; STEINER and SCHÖNBAUM, 1972; ZAIMIS, 1972), by administration of 6-hydroxydopamine (reviews by KOSTRZEWA and JACOBOWITZ, 1974; MALMFORS and THOENEN, 1971; THOENEN and TRANZER, 1973), and by long-term administration of guanethidine and guanacline (review by JUUL, 1974). Comparisons between surgical, immunologic, and chemical sympathectomy have been undertaken by THOENEN (1972a, b) and by JUUL (1974).

In 1967, JENSEN-HOLM demonstrated that prolonged administration of guanethidine at large doses (20 mg/kg i.p. for 6–14 days) induced an increase in the size and protein content, and a pronounced reduction in the activities of the ganglionic cholinesterases of the rat superior cervical ganglion. Subsequent investigations have shown that these changes are the result of a destruction of the ganglionic nerve cells accompanied by an infiltration of small cells, mainly lymphocytes (BITTIGER et al., 1977; BURNSTOCK et al., 1971b; JENSEN-HOLM and JUUL, 1968, 1970a, b; JUUL and MCISAAC, 1973; NIELSEN, 1977b, c). Electronmicroscopically the most severe changes have been shown to involve the mitochondria (HEATH et al., 1972; HEATH and SOBELS,

1977; JENSEN-HOLM and JUUL, 1971). Parenteral doses above 10 mg/kg for more than one week are necessary to induce morphologic changes; perorally the doses must be much larger – 180 mg/kg for several weeks (BITTIGER et al., 1977). The changes to a large extent are reversible upon discontinuation, and a near total sympathectomy may require the i.p. administration of 40 mg/kg for 3 months (BITTIGER et al., 1977; NIELSEN, 1977c). Newborn animals are much more sensitive to the neurotoxic effects of guanethidine (ANGELETTI et al., 1972; ERÄNKÖ and ERÄNKÖ, 1971a, b; JOHNSON et al., 1975, 1976). Guanethidine does not destroy the sympathetic neurones of cat, rabbit, or hamster (JOHNSON et al., 1977), or of guinea pig (O'DONNELL and SAAR 1974). Short adrenergic neurones innervating the internal male genital organs are more sensitive than long adrenergic neurones (BITTIGER et al., 1977; EVANS et al., 1972; GANNON et al., 1971; GERKENS, 1974a). Axon retraction has been reported to occur prior to the degeneration of the sympathetic nerve cell bodies (HEATH et al., 1973b, 1974). Large concentrations of guanethidine exert toxic effects in cultures of sympathetic ganglia of newborn rats (HEATH et al., 1973a, 1974; HILL et al., 1973). Sympathetic ganglia in culture may develop an increased capacity for amine storage (BROWN et al., 1977), which may explain the lack of toxicity reported following low concentrations of guanethidine (ERÄNKÖ et al., 1972) since the cytotoxic properties of guanethidine have been ascribed to the intraneuronal, but extragranular concentrations (JUUL, 1973b, 1974; JUUL and SAND, 1973). Extragranular binding of guanethidine has also been reported by GIACHETTI and HOLLENBECK (1976). The active uptake of guanethidine into the postganglionic sympathetic neurone probably accounts for the selective toxicity; other tissues including nonsympathetic ganglia are unaffected by doses inducing sympathectomy (JENSEN-HOLM and JUUL, 1971). The cytotoxic effect in itself is probably nonspecific, since glial cells of ganglia form newborn rats also showed degenerative changes following addition to the vehicle of high concentrations of guanethidine (HILL et al., 1973); mitochondrial changes may be provoked in the adrenal medulla by very high doses – 600 mg/kg (CLEMENTI, 1965). Administration to newborn animals may induce neurotoxic effects in some catecholamine-containing neurones in the central nervous system, probably due to an incomplete function of the neonatal blood-brain barrier (BARTOLOMÉ et al., 1976a; LUIZZI et al., 1974).

Administration of guanethidine does not change the number of small intensely fluorescent cells in the adult rat superior cervical ganglion (ERÄNKÖ and ERÄNKÖ, 1971; JENSEN-HOLM and JUUL, 1970b), whereas the number is greatly increased after administration to newborn animals (ERÄNKÖ and ERÄNKÖ, 1971b) and after the addition of guanethidine to cultures of ganglia from newborn animals (ERÄNKÖ et al., 1972; HEATH et al., 1973a).

Nerve growth factor suppresses the cytotoxicity of guanethidine in vitro and in vivo (JOHNSON and ALOE, 1974; LEVI-MONTALCINI et al., 1973). Similarly concomitant vinblastine prevents the destruction of sympathetic neurones of neonatal rats, suggesting that guanethidine induces cell death by depriving the sympathetic neurone of the trophic nerve growth factor from the periphery (JOHNSON, 1977).

Methylprednisolone at high doses exerts a protective effect against the cytotoxicity of guanethidine (JUUL, 1974, 1977).

The histologic picture dominated by the infiltration of lymphocytes resembles the picture of autoimmune diseases, and the hypothesis has been put forward, that the infiltration of small cells is the result of an immunologic response to the damaged ganglion cells (JENSEN-HOLM and JUUL, 1970b; JUUL, 1974). An enlargement of the thymus and cervical, thoracic, and abdominal lymph nodes has been described by JENSEN-HOLM (1974). On the other hand, an involution of thymus and suppression of immune responses have been observed in rats treated with guanethidine (DRAŠKOCI and JANKOVIČ, 1964).

The molecular point of attack concerning the cytotoxic effect of guanethidine is unknown, but it has been suggested that the drug may primarily interfere with the mitochondrial oxidative phosphorylation that is known to be inhibited by postganglionic neurone blocking agents (JOHNSON and ALOE, 1974; MALMQUIST and OATES, 1968).

Guanacline may induce a destruction of the postganglionic sympathetic neurone (BURNSTOCK et al., 1970, 1971a; JENSEN-HOLM and JUUL, 1971; JUUL, 1973a) although the morphologic changes are different from those resulting from the administration of guanethidine (review by JUUL, 1974). The ultrastructural changes appear to be identical to the lipidosis-like alterations in various tissues induced by other catamphiphilic drugs (LÜLLMANN et al., 1973). Similar changes have been observed in sympathetic nerves of the parotid gland in animals as well as in patients following treatment with guanacline.

Several other guanidine derivatives have been investigated but none of these possessed neurotoxic properties. These drugs are: debrisoquine, guanoxan, guanadrel, bethanidine, guanochlor, guanisoquine, guanoctine, guancydine, guanidine, and n-(β-guanidinoethyl)-hexahydrobenzo-[D]-azocine (Ph 881/7) administered at high doses for long periods (HAEUSLER et al., 1974; JOHNSON and ALOE, 1974; JUUL, 1973a, 1977; LOREZ and KETTLER, 1975). Bretylium does not induce sympathectomy in adult rats (JUUL, 1973a), but may induce morphologic lesions in developing sympathetic neurones (CARAMIA et al., 1972).

Numerous other drugs with known or suspected influence on sympathetic neurones have been investigated in single experiments, and none of the following drugs possessed cytotoxic properties with regard to the superior cervical ganglion: xylazine, morphine, mecamylamine, physostigmine, clonidine, desmethylimipramine, amipramazide, atropine, methyldopa, pentolinium, furosemide, phentolamine, and reserpine (JENSEN-HOLM and JUUL, 1970a; JUUL, 1974).

The cytotoxic effects of guanethidine results in quantitative, but not qualitative changes in the ganglionic transmission (DOWNING and JUUL, 1973).

In animal experiments the dose regimens of guanethidine and guanacline producing a partial sympathectomy may cause a partial and persistent impairment of sympathetic function that, however, is counteracted by the development of denervation hypersensitivity (BOUQUET et al., 1969; GERKENS, 1974a, b; GOKHALE et al., 1975; JOHNSON and O'BRIEN, 1976; NIELSEN, 1977a, b, c). However, varying sensitivity is observed in different sympathetically innervated areas, and a denervation hypersensitivity is not always observed (CLARKE et al., 1974; JANDHYALA and BUCKLEY, 1974). After guanethidine was administered (25 mg/kg i.p.) for several weeks to rats an increased cardiac turnover of noradrenaline was observed (LEMMER et al., 1974). The attenuation of the sympathetic nervous system vasoconstrictor reflex to general body cooling was not statistically significant in 12 normal subjects following guanethidine 40–60 mg daily for 2–3 weeks, indicating that functional sympathetic neurotransmitter is not absent (COFFMAN, 1967).

Pharmacological doses of the postganglionic neurone blocking agents result in a denervation hypersensitivity to directly acting sympathomimetic amines in animals (BOURA and GREEN, 1962; GREEN and ROBSON, 1965; STONE et al., 1962; TRENDELENBURG, 1972; ZIMMERMANN and HARRIS, 1963) as well as in man (COFFMAN, 1967, DOLLERY, 1965b; DOLLERY et al., 1963; LAURENCE and NAGLE, 1961; MUELHEIMS et al., 1965; PETTINGER et al., 1969; SMULYAN et al., 1963; SNEDDON and TURNER, 1969a, b; STEVENS, 1966).

Persistent orthostatic hypotension and irreversible parotid pain may result from long-term therapy with guanacline (BOCK and HEIMSOTH, 1969; BOCK and HUEP, 1971; DAWBORN et al., 1969; DONATH, 1973; DONATH et al., 1973; SAMEE et al., 1970). Following even large therapeutic doses of guanethidine for long periods, however, wanted as well as unwanted effects are fully reversible (ARGLEBE et al., 1975; BAUER et al., 1973; CHILLA et al., 1975).

X. Other Adverse Reactions

During treatment with the postganglionic neurone blocking agents, up to two-thirds of the patients complain of one or more of the following subjective side effects: fatigue, muscle weakness, blurring of vision (ADI et al., 1975; BATH et al., 1967; BLOOMFIELD and CANGIANO, 1969, 1970; BREST and MOYER, 1961; BROWN and BROWN, 1975; GALSKOV et al., 1961; GIBB et al., 1970; GIFFORD, 1965; JACKSON, 1972; LEISHMAN et al., 1959, 1961; LOWTHER and TURNER, 1963; MONTUSCHI and LOVEL, 1964; OATES et al., 1965; PEART and MACMAHON, 1964; ROSENBLOOM et al., 1963; VEJLSGAARD et al., 1967). Generally the symptoms are reported more frequently with guanethidine than with the more recent guanidinium compounds guanoxan, guanadrel, debrisoquine, and bethanidine.

Three cases resembling polyarteritis nodosa have been reported during treatment with guanethidine (DEWAR and PEASTON, 1964), but similar reactions have not been published since then. One case of systemic lupus erythematosus has been published as a possible effect of guanoxan (BOARDMAN et al., 1967), and a few cases of fever and weight gain have been ascribed to guanoxan (PEART and MACMAHON, 1964).

The guanidinium compounds are surprisingly devoid of other unwanted effects including skin reactions and allergic reactions.

XI. Effects on Foetus

Although conflicting results of the benefits of antihypertensive therapy of severe toxaemia of pregnancy have been published, the majority of investigators report a considerable lowering of the number of eclamptic episodes and a lowered maternal and fetal death rate (e.g. ANSELMINO, 1960).

The postganglionic neurone blocking agents do not possess teratogenic effects (e.g. ATHANASSIADIS et al., 1966; WEST, 1962).

XII. Drug Interactions

Numerous compounds interfering with the sympathetic terminal transport mechanisms concerning catecholamines and the postganglionic neurone blocking agents antagonize the sympatholytic effects of the drugs described, resulting in clinically important drug interactions. The groups of compounds comprise tricyclic antidepressants, cocaine, chlorpromazine, certain antihistamines, and indirectly acting sympathomimetics (DAY, 1962; DAY and RAND, 1962, 1963; FANN et al., 1971, 1972; GOKHALE et al., 1966; GULATI et al., 1966; HANAHOE et al., 1969; JANOWSKY et al., 1972, 1973; LAURENCE and ROSENHEIM, 1960; LEISHMAN et al., 1963; MCQUEEN, 1974; MEYER et al., 1970; MISAGE and MACDONALD, 1970; MITCHELL et al., 1967, 1970; MITCHELL and OATES, 1970; OATES, 1973; OBER and WANG, 1973; SKINNER et al., 1969; STOCKS and ROBERTSON, 1967; STONE et al., 1964; WILLIAMS and SHERTER, 1971; WILSON and LONG, 1960; WOOSLEY et al., 1976). In a series of hypertensive patients on guanethidine, bethanidine, and debrisoquine, 34% of the patients were considered exposed to theoretically potential drug interactions (sympathomimetics, tricyclic antidepressants, and chlorpromazine), but only 3 out of 22 potential interactions were documented: two concerning ephedrine, and one concerning imipramine (STARR and PETRIE, 1972). Debrisoquine, which possesses a monoamine oxidase inhibitory effect, may increase the sensitivity to tyramine and phenylephrine (ALLUM et al., 1974; AMINU et al., 1970; PETTINGER et al., 1969), and a case of considerable rise of arterial blood pressure has been reported in a debrisoquine-treated patient after the ingestion of 50 g of Gruyère cheese (AMERY and DÊLOOF, 1970).

An adequate sympathetic drive to the heart during general anaesthesia may be reduced by antihypertensives. The hypersensitivity to directly acting sympathomimetics and the decreased sensitivity to indirectly acting sympathomimetics have been previously discussed. These effects may be of clinical importance, e.g. under anaesthesia (survey by BALMER, 1965). The minimum alveolar anaesthetic requirement was unchanged following guanethidine (MILLER et al., 1968). The interaction between sympathomimetics and local guanethidine in the human eye has previously been mentioned (SNEDDON and TURNER, 1969a, b).

Guanethidine possesses an antidiabetic effect of unknown mechanism (GUPTA, 1969; GUPTA and LILLICRAP, 1969), and a few cases of hypoglycaemia during simultaneous treatment with sulfonylurea antidiabetics and guanethidine have been suspected of being drug interactions (BERGER, 1971).

The dose of guanethidine has to be reduced in patients in simultaneously treated with L-Dopa (HUNTER et al., 1970).

C. Neural Transmitter-Depleting Agents

Drugs whose mechanism of action is believed to be mainly dependent upon their depleting effect on various biogenic amines are alkaloids of *rauwolfia serpentina*. Although rauwolfia was investigated in the nineteenth century and a hypotensive activity was claimed in the early 1930s, the paper by VAKIL (1949) describing the antihypertensive activity of rauwolfia extracts in man is regarded as the starting point of modern rauwolfia research.

Reserpine is the most important member of this group of compounds and was isolated by MÜLLER et al. (1952). Numerous genuine and synthetic rauwolfia alkaloids have been tried in the treatment of arterial hypertension; this research was mainly due to the unwanted central nervous system depressant action of reserpine.

The pharmacokinetics of reserpine have been reviewed by STITZEL (1976). The rauwolfia alkaloids exert many pharmacological effects apart from the peripheral noradrenaline depletion (review by BEIN, 1956; PLUMMER et al., 1955, 1959), and presumably the most important actions are exerted via central nervous system mechanisms (e.g. SMITH, 1976).

There may be quantitative differences with regard to unwanted effects of the different rauwolfia alkaloids. However, when compared at equipotent doses, none of the drugs seems to possess significant advantages compared with reserpine. The following references represent a few of the investigations comparing different rauwolfia alkaloids: ACHOR et al. (1955); LOCKET (1955); SIMPSON (1961); SMIRK and MCQUEEN (1955). Reports comparing reserpine with other groups of antihypertensives are: AGNEW et al. (1963); BULPITT and DOLLERY (1973); CHIDELL and WHITESIDE (1969); FERGUSON et al. (1976); FORRESTER and SHERIFFS (1967); GROOVER et al. (1974); LEVI et al. (1970); MERCERON et al. (1973); SAFAR et al. (1975); SHAPIRO and TENG (1957); SMITH et al. (1966); WEISS et al. (1973).

The dose of reserpine recommended for antihypertensive therapy is below 0.5 mg daily, usually 0.25 mg daily.

I. General Toxicity

The acute LD_{50} of reserpine administered i.v. to rats is 18 mg/kg (PLUMMER et al., 1959), and to dogs 0.5 mg/kg (Ciba Pharmaceutical Company Information, 1973). The i.p. LD_{50} in mice is 70 mg/kg (CARMINATI, 1969). Dogs have been reported to survive 3 mg/kg i.v. (HARRISON et al., 1963). The oral LD_{50} in mice is 500 mg/kg (TRIPOD et al., 1954). Orally monkeys tolerate single doses of 400 mg/kg, and rats 1000 mg/kg (PLUMMER et al., 1955).

In mice, chronic reserpine administration results in a mortality within 8–10 days of 10% following 0.1 mg/kg, and 100% following 3 mg/kg (MARINO, 1962). Prolonged administration of even small doses to animals results in diarrhoea and weight loss, and the animals develop signs of central nervous system depression, rigidity, and akinesia ("reserpine catalepsy") (ADAMS et al., 1971; BEIN, 1956; POZOS and HOLBROOK, 1971; WITHRINGTON and ZAIMIS, 1967).

The acute toxicity in humans is low. Up to 25 mg i.m. have been administered in the treatment of hypertensive crisis (GIFFORD, 1963; GRENFELL, 1971), and this dose was well tolerated apart from somnolence and parkinsonian-like rigidity. A 20-months-old baby weighing 32 pounds was reported to survive a single dose of reserpine of 200 mg orally (PLUMMER et al., 1955). Intra-arterial injection of reserpine (1–2 mg) in the treatment of Raynaud's phenomenon is well tolerated (ROMEO et al., 1970). The frequency of unwanted effects during long-term reserpine therapy varies considerably between different trials, e.g. adverse reactions in 11% of 231 reserpine-treated hospitalized patients (PFEIFER et al., 1975) and 80% side effects in 75 patients; of the latter, 27% of the patients had so severe side effects that treatment had to be discontinued (KROGSGAARD, 1958).

There seems to be only quantitative differences between the various rauwolfia alkaloids with respect to unwanted effects.

II. Cardiovascular Effects

The numerous central and peripheral effects caused by reserpine make a prediction of the unwanted cardiovascular effects difficult. Mainly due to the adverse reactions of the central nervous system, reserpine has usually been administered in rather small doses and therefore possible adverse reactions caused by prolonged administration of high doses in humans have not been investigated.

Although minor discrepancies are found between various reports on the haemodynamic effects of reserpine following single and chronic administration, the majority of reports point to a reduced total peripheral resistance as being mainly responsible for the hypotensive effect with a nearly unchanged cardiac output (MERCERON et al., 1973; REUSCH, 1962; SANNERSTEDT et al., 1962, 1963). A fall in cardiac output was reported by COHEN et al. (1968), and a depressed myocardial contractility by ROLAND et al. (1977).

Tolerance to reserpine does not seem to occur even during prolonged treatment (WILKINS and JUDSON, 1953).

As has been described concerning guanethidine and methyldopa, a decreased resistance of the gastrointestinal vascular region may play a basic role in the hypotensive effect of reserpine (KISIN and YUZHAKOV, 1976). However, contrary to the findings with the postganglionic neurone blocking agents and methyldopa, treatment with reserpine does not result in any significant orthostatic or exertional hypotension (MERCERON et al., 1973; WEISS et al., 1973).

Fluid retention may occur in some patients, and in case of a reduced margin of compensation this fluid retention may result in overt heart failure (GROOVER et al., 1974; GUAZZI et al., 1973a, b; MARLEY and PARE, 1956; PERERA, 1955). However, MELICK and MCGREGOR (1957) and KROGSGAARD (1957b) did not observe any constant or pronounced fluid retention during reserpine treatment for up to 4 months.

Hypersensitivity to noradrenaline, adrenaline, and isoprenaline, but a decreased effect of indirectly acting sympathomimetic amines have been reported in animals as well as in man, although most often to a moderate extent (CAIROLI et al., 1962; EGER and HAMILTON, 1959; FLEMING, 1962; FLEMING and TRENDELENBURG, 1961; HESTER and CARRIER, 1973; MOORE and MORAN, 1962; SMITH, 1976; SMULYAN et al., 1963; STONE et al., 1962; TRENDELENBURG and WEINER, 1962; WESTFALL, 1977; WITHRINGTON and ZAIMIS, 1967; ZIMMERMANN and HARRIS, 1963). An increase of both the positive chronotropic and inotropic effect of noradrenaline and adrenaline was reported by WITHRINGTON and ZAIMIS (1967) whereas MOORE and MORAN (1962) found a potentiation of the chronotropic effects, but not of the positive inotropic effects of noradrenaline and adrenaline following chronic reserpine administration. The sensitivity of the rat isolated perfused mesenteric arteries to noradrenaline was found unchanged following chronic reserpine administration (FINCH, 1974), and similar findings were obtained in the response of vessels of the forearm to sympathomimetic amines in humans following chronic administration (ABBOUD and ECKSTEIN, 1964; PARKS et al., 1961).

Although the sympatholytic effects of reserpine may persist for long periods following discontinuation of medication, irreversible effects caused by rauwolfia alkaloids have not been described.

Various cardiac effects caused by reserpine administration to animal and man have been interpreted as indications of a cardiotoxic action: reduced intrinsic heart rate, prolonged atrioventricular-conduction time, various forms of cardiac arrhythmias, and a decreased ventricular contractility (COHEN et al., 1968; FLEMING, 1962; HENSLER, 1953; INNES et al., 1958; KÁLDOR and JUVANCZ, 1969; NAYLER, 1963; ROBERTS and MODELL, 1961; SCHREADER and ETZL, 1956; WILSON and WIMBERLEY, 1955; WITHRINGTON and ZAIMIS, 1961, 1967; ZAIMIS, 1961). Progressive myocardial damage was observed by electrocardiography in mouse and guinea pig during prolonged administration (MARINO, 1962). Mitochondrial damage accompanied by a derangement in lipid and glycogen metabolism and a depression of mitochondrial oxidative phosphorylation has been observed in animal myocardial cells (SUN et al., 1968; WILCKEN et al., 1967b). Focal necrosis of the heart of cat and guinea pig following reserpine administration was reported by SCOTT and ZAIMIS (1962), and following administration during the last trimester or pregnancy in guinea pigs a significant increase in the size and number of lipid droplets was observed in both fetal and adult myocardium (LIFRAK et al., 1976). HESS (1965) found a diffuse fatty infiltration of cat heart muscle fibres with no changes in enzyme activity. Other investigators did not observe impairment of cardiac performance following reserpine (CAIROLI et al., 1962; SPANN et al., 1966) or signs of myocardial necrosis (BALAZS et al., 1975). The possible qualitative and quantitative significance of the above mentioned effects during prolonged use of reserpine at therapeutic dose levels in hypertensive patients is still unknown.

III. Respiratory System

Nasal stuffiness is a frequent side effect during rauwolfia therapy, in most trials encountered in 10%–40% of the patients, in occasional reports up to more than 80% (ACHOR et al., 1955; GROOVER et al., 1974; HILDEN et al., 1955; LOCKET, 1955; MURR, 1976; SMITH et al., 1966; WILKINS and JUDSON, 1953). The nasal obstruction is due to vasodilation, and investigations in rabbits have shown that reserpine does not induce changes in the subepithelial glands (MURR, 1976).

IV. Blood

In dogs treated with reserpine at 26 μg/kg for 1–12 months the haematocrit, haemoglobin content, and total leukocyte counts decreased (ADAMS et al., 1971). Similar findings in patients during prolonged administration of rauwolfia alkaloids have not been reported.

V. Liver

No indications of a possible hepatotoxic effect of the rauwolfia alkaloids have been published.

VI. Gastrointestinal System

Treatment with rauwolfia alkaloids does not induce parotid pain, and any interference by reserpine of the function or morphology of the salivary glands has not been reported. An investigation in rats has shown that daily reserpine administration at 1 mg/kg induces changes in the pancreatic acinar cells with mitochondrial damage (RICHTER, 1975).

Nausea may occur during treatment with rauwolfia alkaloids, however, infrequently (HENSLER, 1953). Reserpine may cause epigastric distress (FERGUSON et al., 1976), and in some patients gastric ulver has been ascribed to reserpine (DENNEY et al., 1955; GELFAND and GOODKIN, 1958; HAVERBACK et al., 1955; KERT et al., 1955; PFEIFER et al., 1976; SCHROEDER and PERRY, 1955; WEST, 1958). Haematemesis without evidence of peptic ulcer occurred in a patient following intra-arterial administration of reserpine for Raynaud's phenomenon (SHARON et al., 1972). In the study by the Veterans Administration Cooperative Study Group on Antihypertensive Agents (1972), 6 cases of peptic ulcer were encountered in 186 patients during treatment with reserpine, hydralazine, and hydrochlorothiazide in combination; this is compared to 4 cases in 194 controls. BACHRACH (1959) considered it unlikely that reserpine at daily doses of 0.5–1 mg could provoke symptoms and signs of gastric ulcer. Intravenous administration of reserpine (20 µg/kg) in man induces a pronounced increase in the total acidity of the gastric secretion and a less pronounced rise in the volume of the secretion (KROGSGAARD, 1957a). Similarly reserpine can induce an increased acidity of the gastric secretion in dogs (BARRETT et al., 1955; PLUMMER et al., 1955). Reserpine (5 mg/kg i.m.) to rats results in gastric ulcers in 100% of the animals within 20 h, whereas a dose of 250 µg/kg intracerebroventricularly did not induce ulcers. The development of ulcers was antagonized by α-receptor blocking agents, by atropine, and by 6-hydroxydopamine. These results indicate a peripheral point of attack involving both α-receptors and cholinergic mechanisms (GUPTA et al., 1974). Brompheniramine did not protect against the reserpine induced gastric ulcers in the rat, whereas this was the case with glycopyrrolate (ALPHIN and WARD, 1969). The influence of age, sex, and cold exposure on the susceptibility to reserpine-induced gastric lesions has been studied by REILLY et al. (1969).

A laxative effect is observed in 8%–28% of the patients treated with reserpine (ACHOR et al., 1955; GROOVER et al., 1974; HENSLER, 1953; HILDEN et al., 1955; LOCKET, 1955; PFEIFER et al., 1976). Diarrhoea was not observed following deserpidine (SIMPSON, 1961) or following methoserpidine (HOLT, 1961).

VII. Genitourinary System

During prolonged administration of reserpine the renal blood flow is unchanged, and there are no indications of drug-induced impaired renal function or reserpine nephrotoxicity (MOYER, 1954; MOYER et al., 1954; REUSCH, 1962; SANNERSTEDT and CONWAY, 1970).

Rauwolfia alkaloids do not induce failure of ejaculation whereas libido may be impaired (GLAZER, 1972).

In 1974 three retrospective investigations initiated by the Boston Collaborative Drug Surveillance Program were published indicating an increased risk of breast cancer in women exposed to reserpine (and certain other rauwolfia alkaloids), whereas no association between breast cancer and the use of other antihypertensives or other drugs known to enhance the pituitary prolactin release was found (ARMSTRONG et al., 1974; Boston Collaborative Drug Surveillance Program, 1974; HEINONEN et al., 1974).

These reports aroused a series of critical comments particularly concerning the selection of patients, selection of control groups, and the statistical calculations. A history of high blood pressure in itself does not appear to be related to breast cancer (DEWAARD and HALEWIJN, 1974; DYER et al., 1975; GARFINKEL and HAMMOND, 1974). ARMSTRONG et al. (1976) based on a retrospective analysis of death certificates similarly found an increased risk of breast cancer in hypertensive women treated with reserpine. Four studies failed to reveal any correlation between rauwolfia and breast cancer (CHRISTOPHER et al., 1977; LASKA et al., 1975; MACK et al., 1975; O'FALLON et al., 1975). Similarly AROMAA et al. (1976) concluded that it is unlikely that the use of rauwolfia alkaloids should increase the risk of cancer. LILIENFELD et al. (1976) probably states the most reasonable conclusion at present, that it does not appear that reserpine is strongly associated with breast cancer. However, a possible small overall relationship cannot be definitely excluded. The relative risks reported from different centres are: 0.93, 0.99, 0.99, 1.03, 1.20, 1.24, 1.64, 2.0, 2.04, and 3.5.

The problems of a possible relation between reserpine and breast cancer have revived the interest in the stimulation by reserpine of the pituitary prolactin secretion. Lactation and gynaecomastia have been reported as rare unwanted effects during rauwolfia treatment (PETTINGER et al., 1963a; PLATT and SEARS, 1956; ROBINSON, 1957; SOMLYO and WAYE, 1960). Increased serum prolactin levels are observed in patients during reserpine treatment (LEE et al., 1976; TURKINGTON, 1972). Intrahypothalamic implantation of reserpine initiated milk secretion and depleted the hypophysis of prolactin in the estrogen-primed ovariectomized rabbit, whereas implantation into the hypophysis had no effect (KANEMATSU and SAWYER, 1963). Marked ultrastructural changes in the neural lobes of the rat pituitary induced by reserpine that consisted of a depletion of the neurosecretory granules and of changes in the pituicytes have been reported (RECHARDT and HERVONEN, 1975). In the rat reserpine at 0.3 mg/kg induced a significant development of the mammary gland epithelium in female juvenile rats, and furthermore a positive effect could be observed on the epithelium of the uterus, the uterine glands, and on the adrenal cortex (NEUHAUS, 1974). WELSCH and MEITES (1970) found that reserpine increased the development and growth of mammary tumors in female rats induced by 7,12-dimethylbenzanthracene; NEWBALL and BYAR (1973) found no evidence that reserpine in therapeutic doses exacerbates cancer of the prostate. Interestingly reserpine originally was reported to possess antitumor effects. However, this proved to be a nonspecific effect probably dependent on depression and reduction of food intake (WEST et al., 1961).

VIII. Central Nervous System

Some of the most serious adverse reactions following reserpine therapy are of central nervous system origin. Sedation occurs frequently, in different reports varying between 17%–75% of the patients (ACHOR et al., 1955; ADAMS et al., 1971; FERGUSON et al., 1976; HENSLER, 1953; HILDEN et al., 1955; HOLT, 1961; LOCKET, 1955; WILKINS and JUDSON, 1953).

Mental depression of varying intensity is reported in 5%–28% of patients treated with reserpine, in some cases leading to suicide. The depression is at least partly dose-dependent and often appears within the first 6 months of treatment (ACHOR et al., 1955; AMBROSINO, 1974; BERNSTEIN and KAUFMAN, 1960; FERGUSON et al., 1976; FREIS,

1954; GROOVER et al., 1974; HILDEN et al., 1955; HOLT, 1961; KROGSGAARD, 1958, 1961; LEMIEUX et al., 1956; LOCKET, 1955; MULLER et al., 1955; PFEIFER et al., 1976; PLATT and SEARS, 1956; QUETSCH et al., 1959; SCHROEDER and PERRY, 1955; WALLACE, 1955). In a large proportion of patients a psychic predisposition existed; in some reports more than half of the depressed patients were predisposed (AYD, 1958; QUETSCH et al., 1959). Some authors have questioned the induction of depression by reserpine and found no relation between antihypertensive medication and the occurrence of depression (AYD, 1958; SNAITH and MCCOURBRIE, 1974). Other rauwolfia alkaloids have been claimed to be more or less devoid of central nervous system adverse reactions: rescinnamine (SMIRK and MCQUEEN, 1955) and methoserpidine (JONES et al., 1961), but these drugs have not been tested in large populations using equipotent antihypertensive doses.

Numerous animal experiments have been undertaken to investigate the "reserpine-depression" and serve as a model system for the endogenous depression in man. Apart from a depletion of various biogenic amines, the behavioral effects have been studied, e.g. in monkeys (MCKINNEY et al., 1971).

Reserpine induces in animals as well as in man dose-dependent extrapyramidal symptomes: tremors, rigidity, akinesia (ADAMS et al., 1971; BEIN, 1956; DUVOISIN and MARSDEN, 1974; MCGEER et al., 1961; MORRISON and WEBSTER, 1973a). Histologically, alterations of the nerve cells in the substantia nigra are observed consisting of swelling of the endoplasmic reticulum, cytoplasmic vacuolization, nuclear lobulation, and disappearance of the catecholamine-containing granules (BAK, 1965; POZOS and HOLBROOK, 1971). The rigidity may be caused by a loss of brain dopamine, by an increase in deaminated metabolites, or both (MORRISON and WEBSTER, 1973b). The reserpine-induced catalepsy is not antagonized by L-Dopa (e.g. MCGEER et al., 1961), whereas methyldopa in mice reversed the reserpine-induced bradykinesia (DUVOISIN and MARSDEN, 1974).

Dreaming or nightmares are frequently reported during reserpine therapy (ACHOR et al., 1955), and in man as well as in animals reserpine has been shown to increase the REM-sleep (COULTER et al., 1971; HARTMANN, 1966; HOFFMAN and DOMINO, 1969; STERN and MORGANE, 1973; TISSOT, 1965).

IX. Peripheral Nervous System

In adult animals reserpine does not exert any neurotoxic effects in the postganglionic sympathetic neurone (JUUL, 1973a). However, prenatal reserpine administration induces long-lasting changes in the central nervous system and in the adrenal medulla that persist into adulthood and may be interpreted as results from permanently increased sympathoadrenal stimulation (BARTOLOMÉ and SLOTKIN, 1975; BARTOLOMÉ et al., 1976b). Early postnatal reserpine administration produces an acute depletion of catecholamines that is not dependent upon either blockade of granular uptake or on reflex actions of the drug and that may account for the more intense and longer-lasting effects of the drug in neonates (BARTOLOMÉ and SLOTKIN, 1976). Reserpine has been shown to retard the growth of sympathetic ganglia from newborn rats (ANGELETTI and LEVI-MONTALCINI, 1972).

Prolonged administration of reserpine to animals produces a denervation hypersensitivity towards directly acting sympathomimetic amines, whereas the effect of indirectly acting sympathomimetics is decreased (CAIROLI et al., 1962; EGER and HAMILTON, 1959; FLEMING, 1962; FLEMING and TRENDELENBURG, 1961; HESTER and CARRIER, 1973; MOORE and MORAN, 1962; SMITH, 1976; SMULYAN et al., 1963; STONE et al., 1962; TRENDELENBURG and WEINER, 1962; WESTFALL, 1977; WITHRINGTON and ZAIMIS, 1967; ZIMMERMANN and HARRIS, 1963). However, unchanged sensitivity to noradrenaline of the isolated perfused mesenteric arteries following prolonged reserpine administration to rats has been reported (FINCH, 1974), and no changes in the sensitivity to noradrenaline of the human forearm vessels was found following reserpine (ABBOUD and ECKSTEIN, 1964; PARKS et al., 1961).

X. Other Adverse Reactions

Tiredness is not frequently reported during the use of rauwolfia alkaloids (GIBB et al., 1970; KROGSGAARD, 1961), but the reason may well be that such symptoms are classified as the "sedation" that occurs frequently with these drugs.

Excessive appetite and weight gain are frequent unwanted effects occurring in up to 75% of patients treated with reserpine (ACHOR et al., 1955; HILDEN et al., 1955; KROGSGAARD, 1958; LOCKET, 1955; SIMPSON, 1961; WILKINS and JUDSON, 1953). In 35% of the patients a weight gain above 2 kg has been reported (KROGSGAARD, 1961), and in one patient the weight gain amounted to 33 kg (JØRSTAD, 1956).

In the rat reserpine may induce hypothermia (TAYLOR and FREGLY, 1962). The rauwolfia alkaloids are devoid of skin reactions and allergic reactions.

XI. Effects on Foetus

Various effects of reserpine on pregnancy and newborns have been recorded. Impairment of implantation (depending on the dose and time of administration), an increased fetal resorption rate, and disturbed last stages of pregnancy have been observed in animals (BOVET-NITTI and BOVET, 1959; KEHL et al., 1956; WEST, 1962). Other investigations failed to observe any impairment of implantation (ARNAUD and GIROD, 1963). Large doses of reserpine administered to pregnant rats on the ninth and tenth days of gestation are highly teratogenic, and pretreatment with reserpine increases salicylate teratogenicity (GOLDMAN and YAKOVAC, 1965). A low incidence of malformations following rauwolfia alkaloids was found by TUCHMANN-DUPLESSIS and MERCIER-PAROT (1956, 1961).

Administration of reserpine during pregnancy in rats results in an increased neonatal mortality, a reduced body weight gain, and alterations of behavior and learning ability, which may persist through adulthood (DÖRNER et al., 1976; HOFFELD et al., 1967; LEWIS et al., 1977; LIFRAK et al., 1976; WERBOFF and DEMBICKI, 1962; WERBOFF and HAVLENA, 1962; WERBOFF and KESNER, 1963; WERBOFF et al., 1961). Other investigations did not reveal any behavioral modifications of the offspring (JEWETT and NORTON, 1966).

In humans no teratogenic effect of reserpine has been observed (GAUNT et al., 1959; HOCHULI and WEICHE, 1972; RAVINA, 1964; SOBEL, 1960). On the other hand in some investigations reserpine failed to improve foetal salvage in toxaemia of pregnancy (FRIEDBERG, 1964; LANDESMAN et al., 1957). Reserpine administration during the last part of pregnancy results in reserpine effects in approximately 10% of the newborn infants: nasal congestion for as long as 6 days, lethargy for usually less than 24 h, cyanosis, and retraction. The majority of side effects are considered mild, but in a few cases they may be severe, and in one case death was ascribed to reserpine toxicity. The symptoms were not closely related to the dose (BUDNICK et al., 1955; DESMOND et al., 1957). Neonatal cold injury ascribed to maternal reserpine medication has been observed (ANAGNOSTAKIS and MATSANIOTIS, 1974). Maternally administered reserpine may lower the bilirubin concentration in the newborn infant (DREW and KITCHEN, 1976).

XII. Drug Interactions

Reserpine treatment does not significantly interfere with general anaesthetics, although the hypotension and bradycardia induced by reserpine may be more pronounced, and the previously discussed changes in sensitivity to directly and indirectly acting sympathomimetics may be observed (BAGWELL et al., 1964a, b; BALMER, 1965; KATZ et al., 1964). In dogs reserpine reduces the minimum alveolar anaesthetic requirement of halothane (MILLER et al., 1968).

The central nervous system effects of reserpine occur more frequently in patients also receiving barbiturates; this suggests additive effects (PFEIFER et al., 1976).

Simultaneous administration to animals of reserpine and monoamine oxidase inhibitors may result in sympathomimetic effects and excitation, which can be blocked by chlorpromazine (CHESSIN et al., 1957; SHORE and BRODIE, 1957), and in humans psychotic reactions may result from this combination (GRADWELL, 1960).

Pretreatment with reserpine has been reported to increase the toxicity of digitalis glycosides in humans (DICK et al., 1962; LOWN et al., 1961), whereas a reduced digitalis toxicity was observed in cats during reserpine administration (ROBERTS et al., 1963).

Rauwolfia alkaloids have been reported to increase the hypoglycaemia produced by sulfonylurea antidiabetics (BERGER, 1971). Rauwolfia alkaloids enhance the analgesia produced by morphine (e.g. DANDIYA and MENON, 1963).

D. False Transmitters

"False transmitters" comprise compounds (other than the physiologic neurotransmitter noradrenaline) that fulfill the following criteria: presence in the granules of the noradrenergic terminals and release by adrenergic nerve stimulation and noradrenaline-depleting drugs. The false transmitter is usually less potent than noradrenaline at the adrenoceptors (KOPIN, 1968).

Certain adrenergic nerve-end inhibitors are released into perfusates of organs during sympathetic nerve stimulation, e.g. bretylium (FISCHER et al., 1966) and guanethidine (BOUILLIN, 1966), but here only alpha-methyldopa is dealt with; its mechanism of action is believed to be due at least partly to the formation of the false transmitter α-methylnoradrenaline, as shown by MUSCHOLL and MAÎTRE (1963). Apart from this mechanism of action methyldopa interferes with the synthesis of noradrenaline and depletes the stores of noradrenaline. Methyldopa exerts peripheral as well as central effects (SMITH, 1976). Since simultaneous administration of a peripheral dopa decarboxylase inhibitor, benserazide, did not modify the hypotensive effect of methyldopa, a central nervous site of action can be considered the more important (KERSTING et al., 1976).

The pharmacology of methyldopa has been reviewed by EULER (1972) and by MUSCHOLL (1972). Only the L-form of methyldopa is active (GILLESPIE et al., 1962; WEIL et al., 1963). The kinetics of methyldopa in man has been described by KWAN et al. (1976). The discovery by OATES et al. (1960) of the antihypertensive action of methyldopa forms the basis for its use in the treatment of arterial hypertension. The following references compare the unwanted effects of methyldopa with those of other groups of antihypertensives: AGNEW et al. (1963); BATH et al. (1967); BULPITT and DOLLERY (1973); CHIDELL and WHITESIDE (1969); DUNN and FREEMAN (1975); FORRESTER and SHERIFFS (1967); GLAZER (1975); GROOVER et al. (1966); MERCERON et al. (1973); MROCZEK et al. (1972); OATES et al. (1965); PRICHARD et al. (1968); SAFAR et al. (1975); SMITH et al. (1966); TARPLEY (1974); VEJLSGAARD et al. (1967); WEISS et al. (1973).

The usual dosage is 500–1000 mg daily in 2–4 divided doses.

I. General Effects

The acute LD_{50} of methyldopa in the mouse following i.v. injection is 1900 mg/kg, i.p. 406 mg/kg, orally 5300 mg/kg; in the rat i.p. 647 mg/kg, orally 7490 mg/kg; and in the rabbit orally 713 mg/kg (Merck Institute Information, 1973).

The acute toxicity in humans is relatively low. Treatment of hypertensive crisis may involve 500 mg every 2 h up to a total dose of 2 g (GRENFELL, 1971). However, adverse reactions are frequent during long-term use. More than sixty different unwanted effects have been ascribed to methyldopa (survey by KELLAWAY, 1976). Methyldopa is the ninth most frequently reported drug registered by the WHO program for International Monitoring of Drugs, constituting 1.9% of the reports received (HELLING, 1976). As examples of the various frequencies of unwanted effects reported during methyldopa therapy can be mentioned: 33% (VEJLSGAARD et al., 1967), 84% (MATHISEN, 1963), and 72% (JOHNSON et al., 1966). Methyldopa is not tolerated by 10%–24% of the patients (DOLLERY, 1965a; HILDEN and NILSSON, 1968; LEONARD et al., 1965; PRICHARD et al., 1968). Methyldopa belongs to the group of drugs with a reported higher rate of toxicity in patients with elevated blood urea nitrogen level (JICK, 1977).

II. Cardiovascular System

The hypotensive effect of methyldopa by some authors is considered due to a decreased total peripheral resistance (MERCERON et al., 1973; ONESTI et al., 1964; SANNERSTEDT et al., 1962); others found a decreased peripheral resistance and a fall in cardiac output (DOLLERY et al., 1963); and still others, a fall in cardiac output with little effect on the total peripheral resistance (LUND-JOHANSEN, 1972, 1973). As is the case concerning other antihypertensives, these discrepancies may at least partly be due to different dose regimens, different duration of therapy, and different techniques employed for the measurement of the haemodynamic changes.

Although tolerance has been reported in up to approximately 50% of the patients treated with methyldopa the majority of clinical trials report a much lower frequency (GILMORE and FREIS, 1965; HAMILTON and KOPELMAN, 1963; SANNERSTEDT et al., 1963; TARPLEY, 1974), and in some reports tolerance was not observed (MATHISEN, 1963; WEIL et al., 1963).

Fluid retention, mainly observed as an increased plasma volume without changes in extracellular fluid volume and with insignificant changes in exchangeable sodium and body weight, may account for the variability in drug response and also contribute to the development of drug resistance (DOLLERY and HARINGTON, 1962; FINNERTY et al., 1970; GROOVER et al., 1974; HAMILTON and KOPELMAN, 1963; HANSEN, 1968; LETH and IBSEN, 1975; MORIN et al., 1964; SHEPS et al., 1963; WEIL et al., 1963). In some patients edema and precipitation of heart failure have been observed (DOLLERY and HARINGTON, 1962).

A minor hypersensitivity to directly and indirectly acting sympathomimetics has been observed in patients receiving methyldopa (DOLLERY et al., 1963), whereas animal experiments did not reveal any hypersensitivity to directly acting sympathomimetics (SMITH et al., 1976; STONE et al., 1962) and did reveal a diminished response to indirectly acting sympathomimetics (STONE et al., 1962).

Postural or exertional hypotension is reported by most investigators, but it is usually of less intensity and frequency than following the administration of postganglionic neurone blocking agents (CHAMBERLAIN and HOWARD, 1964; GILMORE and FREIS, 1965; HORWITZ et al., 1967; OATES et al., 1965; PRICHARD et al., 1968; SMIRK, 1963a; VEJLSGAARD et al., 1967). In some trials orthostatic hypotension was not observed (e.g. MORIN et al., 1964).

Intravenous administration of methyldopa may induce a hypertensive response in patients (LEVINE and STRAUCH, 1966). Following acute methyldopa withdrawal, rebound hypertension has been described (BURDEN and ALEXANDER, 1976; SCOTT and McDEWITT, 1976). Raynaud's phenomenon which is rather common among patients treated with β-blocking agents has been described in 1 of 21 patients during long-term treatment with methyldopa (MARSHALL et al., 1976).

After treatment with methyldopa for 7 days, a prolongation of the pre-ejection period and left ventricular ejection time has been observed. This suggests a possible impairment of left ventricular performance and a depressed myocardial contractility (ROLAND et al., 1977). The unwanted cardiovascular effects of methyldopa are usually reversible, but a few cases of fatal myocarditis associated with methyldopa therapy have been described. The patients had been treated with methyldopa for a period of a few weeks to several months and died suddenly without clinical suspicion of myocarditis. At autopsy, an acute inflammatory reaction of the myocardium including many eosinophils was observed. The inflammatory changes were most consistent with a hypersensitivity reaction, and in 5 of 6 reported cases inflammatory reaction of the liver was also observed (CONSTON, 1974; MULLICK and MCALLISTER, 1977).

III. Respiratory System

Nasal stuffiness may be observed in patients on methyldopa, but it is generally of a low frequency and intensity compared to the effect of reserpine and guanethidine (BAUER et al., 1973; LEONARD et al., 1965; SMITH et al., 1966).

IV. Blood

In 1966, six years after the introduction of methyldopa, the first report on methyldopa-induced haemolytic anaemia appeared (CARSTAIRS et al., 1966b). Subsequent investigations have demonstrated that a positive direct Coombs' test occurs in 10%–36% of Caucasian patients treated with methyldopa [CANTOR and BARNETT, 1967; CARSTAIRS et al., 1966a; CHIDELL and WHITESIDE, 1969; DUNN and FREEMAN, 1975; HAMILTON, 1968; HILDEN and NILSSON, 1968; HUNTER et al., 1971; MACKAY et al., 1968; PERRY et al., 1971; PETZ and FUDENBERG (survey), 1975]. A higher incidence is found in females compared to males. In Africans, Chinese, and Indian patients this effect of methyldopa is not observed at all or at a very low frequency (BURNS-COX, 1970; CHAN et al., 1971; PERRY et al., 1971; SEEDAT and VAWDA, 1968, 1972). The development of a positive Coombs' test is dose-dependent and may occur after treatment lasting for a few months up to several years, but most commonly after 3–12 months [CARSTAIRS et al. (1966a); HUNTER et al. (1971); PETZ and FUDENBERG (survey), (1975)]. In a few cases the positive Coombs' test is only transitory (HUNTER et al., 1971). The antibody disappears upon discontinuation of therapy, although it may last for up to two years, and it reappears on reexposition to the drug (survey by PETZ and FUDENBERG, 1975). The antibodies react directly with normal erythrocytes in vitro in the absence of methyldopa and are indistinguishable from those found in patients with idiopathic warm antibody autoimmune haemolytic anaemia. A similar type of autoimmunity has been described with other drugs, e.g. L-Dopa and mefenamic acid. The warm-active antibody is of the IgG class and shows specificity for the Rh-locus. In a large proportion of the patients, various other immunologic abnormalities outside the erythrocyte antibody system have also been noted: antinuclear antibodies, elevated levels of IgG, IgA, or IgM immunoglobulins, positive rheumatoid factor, and LE cells (EYSTER and JENKINS, 1970; HUNTER et al., 1971; MACKAY et al., 1968; PERRY et al., 1971; SHERMAN et al., 1967). A high proportion of patients with a positive Coomb's test during methyldopa therapy has been shown to have a typical hydralazine toxicity (PERRY et al., 1971). The mechanism behind the described changes has not been completely clarified. It has been suggested that methyldopa may alter the Rh-protein of the erythrocytes so as to make it antigenic (LOBUGLIO and JANDL, 1967), that the drug may alter a portion of the immune system leading to a state of intolerance to certain self-antigens (DAMESHEK, 1967), and that the effect may be a response of basically normal lymphoid tissue to some antigenic properties brought about by methyldopa (BAKEMEIER and LEDDY, 1968). Experimental studies have been performed in rabbits (VYAS et al., 1969). Several surveys have been published on the possible mechanisms behind the immunologic changes induced by methyldopa (CHAPLIN and AVIOLI, 1977; NEELY and KRAUS, 1972; NYDEGGER and MIESCHER, 1975; PERRY et al., 1971; PETZ and FUDENBERG, 1975). The immunologic changes may create difficulties in cross-matching blood (GILLIES, 1974).

Several cases of haemolytic anaemia have been described, but the frequency is rather low, less than 1% of patients with a positive Coombs' test revealing overt haemolysis (BÖTTIGER and WESTERHOLM, 1973; DJALDETTI et al., 1974; GILDER, 1975; HAMILTON, 1968; HILDEN and NILSSON, 1968; MACKAY et al., 1968; MCQUEEN, 1974; SHERMAN et al., 1967; Swedish Adverse Reactions Committee, 1977; WORLLEDGE et al., 1966). These patients had been treated with methyldopa for 3 months to several years, the majority being treated for less than 1½ years (WORLLEDGE et al., 1966; Swedish Adverse Reactions Committee, 1977). In three patients with methyldopa-induced haemolytic anaemia, the incorporation of ^{3}H-uridine in proerythroblasts was impaired, which was not the case concerning ^{3}H-thymidine (DJALDETTI et al., 1974).

Reversible thrombocytopenia has been described in a few patients during methyldopa therapy, in some cases proved upon rechallenge (ALKALAY, 1975; BENRAAD and SCHOENAKER, 1965; BLAHJCHMAN et al., 1972; MANOHITHARAJAH et al., 1971; MARCUS et al., 1975; SMIRK, 1963b; TEN PAS et al., 1966). In one case, methyldopa-induced platelet antibodies were detected (MARCUS et al., 1975), and in another case a positive complement fixation test for platelet and leukocyte antibodies was found that became negative following discontinuation of methyldopa (MANOHITHARAJAH et al., 1971).

Reversible leukopenia has been described in a few patients on methyldopa (GREENE and SPENCE, 1967; HALLWRIGHT, 1961; TEN PAS et al., 1966). Eosinophilia may occur during treatment with methyldopa (BONKOWSKY and BRISBANE, 1976; COLWILL et al., 1964).

V. Liver

During the initial clinical trials with methyldopa no indications of hepatotoxicity were encountered (e.g. DOLLERY and HARINGTON, 1962; MATHISEN, 1963). However, subsequent investigations have revealed hepatotoxic changes varying from slight and transient increases in serum transaminases, lactate dehydrogenase, and phosphatases to fatal submassive hepatic necrosis. In a review by HOYUMPA and CONNELL (1973) comprising 2604 patients treated with methyldopa, a total of 2.8% had hepatic reactions. In the majority of trials the frequency of liver function impairment has been low (CANNON and LARAGH, 1963; COLWILL et al., 1964; DOLLERY, 1965a; GILLESPIE et al., 1962; GILMORE and FREIS, 1965; HORWITZ et al., 1967; HORWITZ and SJOERDSMA, 1963; MORIN et al., 1964; SHEPS et al., 1963; SMITH et al., 1966; VEDIN et al., 1973). In some investigations the frequency of elevated transaminases was up to 35% of the patients treated with methyldopa (FORRESTER and SHERIFFS, 1967; IRVINE et al., 1962; LEONARD et al., 1965; SMITH et al., 1966). Often the elevation of the transaminases was transient and subsided spontaneously without interruption of therapy (SMITH et al., 1966). Some of the abnormal laboratory analyses may be caused by interference of methyldopa with the clinical chemical methods employed (PEARSON et al., 1972; SINGH et al., 1972). Furthermore abnormal liver function tests have been found in 16% of males and 6% of females with arterial hypertension not treated with methyldopa (RAMSAY, 1977).

In some cases symptoms recurred upon rechallenge with methyldopa (ELIASTAM, 1971; GILMORE and FREIS, 1965; GOLDSTEIN et al., 1973; HORWITZ and SJOERDSMA, 1963; REHMAN et al., 1973; SCHWEITZER and PETERS, 1974; TOGHILL et al., 1974; TYSELL and KNAUER, 1971). Fever has been observed in several patients with methyldopa-induced impairment of hepatic function (BONKOWSKY and BRISBANE, 1976; GILLESPIE et al., 1962; GILMORE and FREIS, 1965; GLONTZ and SASLAW, 1968). Immunologic disturbances, e.g. positive LE phenomenon and positive Coombs' test have been observed in some patients (ELIASTAM, 1971; HOYUMPA and CONNELL, 1973; SCHWEITZER and PETERS, 1974), indicating a possible hypersensitivity reaction (ZIMMERMAN,

1975). However, BOUCHIER et al. (1964) reported that antinuclear antibodies and "rheumatoid factors" were often present in certain types of cirrhosis of patients not treated with methyldopa. DYBING et al. (1976) in investigations of rat and human liver microsomes found that methyldopa was oxidized to a reactive semiquinone and/or quinone, which was possibly responsible for the methyldopa-induced hepatic dysfunction.

Serious hepatic adverse reactions are assumed to occur in less than 0.1% of patients treated with methyldopa (CACACE and COHEN, 1976; ELKINGTON et al., 1969). CACACE and COHN (1976) reviewed 122 cases of hepatic cell injury reported in the literature, of which 52 were considered serious and life-threatening. Five deaths occurred.

Fatal cases have been reported by HOYUMPA and CONNELL (1973), MADDREY and BOITNOTT (1975), RODMAN et al. (1976), THOMAS et al. (1976), and by TOGHILL et al. (1974). One of the patients died following re-exposition to methyldopa (HOYUMPA and CONNELL, 1973). Liver biopsy has revealed nonspecific changes with mononuclear infiltrates and focal centrilobular necrosis indistinguishable from the pathologic picture of viral hepatitis (BROUILLARD and BARRETT, 1973; GOLDSTEIN et al., 1973; REHMAN et al., 1973; TOGHILL et al., 1974; ZARDAY et al., 1967). Some cases have shown the picture of intrahepatic cholestasis (HOFFBRAND et al., 1974; SATALINE and LOWELL, 1975 b). The majority of patients were treated with methyldopa for 1–12 months, some patients, however, for several years (BROUILLARD and BARRETT, 1973; CACACE and COHEN, 1976; GOLDSTEIN et al., 1973; SATALINE and LOWELL, 1975 a, b; Swedish Adverse Reactions Committee, 1977). One case of granulomatous hepatitis after two days' treatment with methyldopa has been described (MILLER, 1976). Hepatocellular injury is reported more commonly in female than in male patients. It does not seem to be dose-dependent. In 21 consecutive cases of active chronic hepatitis, 14 were considered drug-induced, 5 of which were caused by methyldopa (GOLDSTEIN et al., 1973).

VI. Gastrointestinal System

Dry mouth is a frequent complaint of patients during methyldopa treatment and is reported in 10%–63% of the patients (BECKER-CHRISTENSEN et al., 1971; COLWILL et al., 1964; IGLOE, 1964; JOHNSON et al., 1966; LAUWERS et al., 1963; LEONARD et al., 1965; OATES et al., 1965; SMIRK, 1963 a; SMITH et al., 1966).

Parotid pain does not appear during treatment with methyldopa. However, three cases of sialadenitis following treatment with methyldopa have been reported (MÅRDH et al., 1974).

Nausea may be induced by methyldopa (DOLLERY, 1965 a; OATES et al., 1965). The symptoms are usually mild, and epigastric pain and gastric ulcer are not observed.

Diarrhoea following methyldopa occurs with a frequency of 4%–6% of the patients, although higher frequencies have been reported by some authors (BECKER-CHRISTENSEN et al., 1971; COLWILL et al., 1964; HAMILTON and KOPELMAN, 1963; HILDEN and NILSSON, 1968; HORWITZ et al., 1967; JOHNSON et al., 1966; LAUWERS et al., 1963; LEONARD et al., 1965; OATES et al., 1965). One case of reversible colitis and hepatitis was reported in a patient, which was accompanied by fever skin rash and eosinophila (BONKOWSKY and BRISBANE, 1976).

VII. Genitourinary System

Methyldopa does not reduce renal blood flow or glomerular filtration rate and is considered well suited for treatment of arterial hypertension in patients with impaired renal function (HANSEN, 1968; LUKE and KENNEDY, 1964; MOHAMMED et al., 1968; MORIN et al., 1964; ONESTI et al., 1964; WEIL et al., 1963). Methyldopa belongs to the group of drugs with higher rates of toxicity in the presence of elevated blood urea nitrogen levels (JICK, 1977).

Failure of ejaculation and impotence are reported rarely during methyldopa therapy (e.g. GILLESPIE et al., 1962; HORWITZ and SJOERDSMA, 1963; LAUWERS et al., 1963; OATES et al., 1965). However, on thorough questioning of the patients NEWMAN (1974) found sexual dysfunction in 7 out of 27 males during methyldopa therapy: decrease of libido, inability to maintain an erection, and difficulty in ejaculation. Similarly ALEXANDER and ALEXANDER and EVANS (1975) found erection failure in 53% of the males treated.

Methyldopa can induce lactation (HORWITZ et al., 1967) caused by release of pituitary prolactin, serum prolactin levels being three- to fourfold increased (HORWITZ et al., 1967; STEINER et al., 1976; TURKINGTON, 1972). No association has been found between the use of methyldopa and breast cancer.

VIII. Central Nervous System

Sedation is a common unwanted effect of methyldopa. During the initial 24–72 h of therapy nearly all patients become drowsy (BAYLISS and HARVEY-SMITH, 1962; GILLESPIE et al., 1962; HAMILTON and KOPELMAN, 1963; OATES et al., 1960). During chronic administration of methyldopa sedation is reported in 18%–60% of the patients and is a rather common reason for discontinuation (ALEXANDER and EVANS, 1975; BECKER-CHRISTENSEN et al., 1971; BREST et al., 1961; BULPITT and DOLLERY, 1973; DOLLERY, 1965a; HILDEN and NILSSON, 1968; HORWITZ et al., 1967; IGLOE, 1964; JOHNSON et al., 1966; LAUWERS et al., 1963; LEONARD et al., 1965; MATHISEN, 1963; MROCZEK et al., 1972; OATES et al., 1965; SANNERSTEDT et al., 1963; SHEPS et al., 1963; SMIRK, 1963a; SMITH et al., 1966; WEIL et al., 1963).

Mental depression of varying intensity (in a few cases leading to suicide) has been reported in 3%–20% of patients treated with methyldopa; in the majority of trials 3%–4% of the patients. The depression tends to appear early in the course of treatment and is reversible – usually within one or two days – upon discontinuation of medication (BAUER et al., 1973; BECKER-CHRISTENSEN et al., 1971; COLWILL et al., 1964; DOLLERY, 1965a; DOLLERY and HARINGTON, 1962; FULLERTON and MORTON-JENKINS, 1963; GIBB et al., 1970; GILLESPIE et al., 1962; GLAZER, 1975; HORWITZ and SJOERDSMA, 1963; JOHNSON et al., 1966; LAUWERS et al., 1963; MCKINNEY and KANE, 1967; SMIRK, 1963a). As is the case concerning reserpine, a few authors doubt the causal relationship between methyldopa therapy and depression (AYD, 1958; SNAITH and MCCOURBRIE, 1974).

Methyldopa has been reported to interfere with mental acuity, e.g. inducing lack of concentration ability, amnesia, difficulty in single calculations, and problems in reading (ADLER, 1974), forgetfulness (FERNANDEZ, 1976), temporary derangement of memory (GHOSH, 1976), prolongation of reaction time (BAYLISS and DUNCAN, 1975), and even dementia (THORNTON, 1976). Nightmares have been reported in a few patients (DOLLERY, 1965a; JOHNSON et al., 1966).

Extrapyramidal symptoms may occur during treatment with methyldopa (GRODEN, 1963; PEASTON, 1964), and one case of abnormal involuntary movements indistinguishable from those of Huntington's chorea was reported in a patient with bilateral cerebrovascular disease (YAMADORI and ALBERT, 1972).

IX. Peripheral Nervous System

Methyldopa does not exert cytotoxic effects in the superior cervical ganglion of the rat (JENSEN-HOLM and JUUL, 1970a). Experiments in newborn animals have not been undertaken. Prolonged administration of methyldopa by some investigators has been reported to induce a moderate hypersensitivity to directly acting sympathomimetic amines (DOLLERY et al., 1963), whereas other investigators did not observe a denervation hypersensitivity (SMITH, 1976; STONE et al., 1962).

X. Other Adverse Reactions

Subjective side effects of methyldopa including muscle weakness and fatigue are frequent (BULPITT and DOLLERY, 1973; HEFFERNAN et al., 1971; JOHNSON et al., 1966; OATES et al., 1965).

Up to two-thirds of the patients may gain weight, particularly during the initial weeks of treatment with methyldopa, part of the weight gain being caused by fluid retention (BAYLISS and HARVEY-SMITH, 1962; HAMILTON and KOPELMAN, 1963; JOHNSON et al., 1966; WILSON et al., 1963).

Three to fourteen percent of the patients on methyldopa develop hyperpyrexia. In some cases the fever has been proved to be drug-induced by rechallenge, in others the patients have become afebrile despite continued treatment with methyldopa. The majority of febrile reactions occurs within a few weeks of treatment. In approximately one-third of the cases impairment of liver function has been observed, and in some patients a positive direct Coombs' test (BRUHN-PETERSEN, 1967; COLWILL et al., 1964; GILMORE and FREIS, 1965; GLONTZ and SASLAW, 1968; HAMILTON and KOPELMAN, 1963; IGLOE, 1964; KLEIN and KAMINSKY, 1973; LEONARD et al., 1962, 1965; PUGSLEY, 1972; Swedish Adverse Reactions Committee, 1977; TALLGREN and SERVO, 1969). One case of hypothermia has been described (MOHAN and JOHNSON, 1975).

Skin reactions during methyldopa therapy occur, although rarely: rash (JOHNSON et al., 1966), eczema (CHURCH, 1974), seborrhoic dermatitis-like eruption (CHURCH, 1973), granulomatous skin lesion (WELLS et al., 1974), and ulcerative lichenoid eruption (BURRY, 1976; BURRY and KIRK, 1974).

One case of retroperitoneal fibrosis has been described during treatment with methyldopa (IVERSEN et al., 1975).

XI. Effects on Foetus

Methyldopa does not possess teratogenic properties and does not adversely affect the newborn infant (HAMILTON, 1968; HANS and KOPELMAN, 1964; KINCAID-SMITH et al., 1966; REDMAN et al., 1976; WEST, 1962).

XII. Drug Interactions

The effects of methyldopy on the response to sympathomimetic amines have previously been discussed. Methyldopa increased the tyramine response and restores the reserpine-induced depression of the tyramine response (PETTINGER et al., 1963 b). Severe hypertension has been produced by phenylpropanolamine in a patient treated with methyldopa and oxprenolol (MCLAREN, 1976).

In dogs methyldopa reduces the minimum alveolar anaesthetic requirement of halothane (MILLER et al., 1968).

Amitriptyline has been reported to antagonize the effect of methyldopa (WHITE, 1965), whereas desmethylimipramine did not antagonize the effect of methyldopa (MITCHELL et al., 1970).

Hallucinations may arise from the combined administration of methyldopa and monoamine oxidase inhibitors (PAYKEL, 1966), whereas other investigators did not find any untoward interactions (e.g. GILLESPIE et al., 1962).

Possible interaction between methyldopa and lithium carbonate has been reported. It was suggested that methyldopa might interfere with the renal excretion of lithium, but the symptoms of lithium overdosage persisted when the serum lithium concentrations were low (0.5–0.7 meq/l) (BYRD, 1975; O'REGAN, 1976).

Methyldopa has been used as an adjunct to L-Dopa treatment of Parkinson's disease (SWEET et al., 1972).

References

Abboud, F.M., Eckstein, J.W.: Effects of small oral doses of reserpine on vascular responses to tyramine and norepinephrine in man. Circulation *9*, 219–223 (1964)

Abernathy, J.D.: The problem of non-compliance in long-term antihypertensive therapy. Drugs *11*, Suppl. 1, 89–90 (1976)

Achor, R.W.P., Hanson, N.O., Gifford, R.W.: Hypertension treated with rauwolfia serpentina (whole root) and with reserpine. J. Am. Med. Assoc. *159*, 841–845 (1955)

Adams, H.R., Smookler, H.H., Clarke, D.E., Jandhyala, B.S., Dixit, B.N., Ertel, R.J., Buckley, J.P.: Clinicopathologic effects of chronic reserpine administration in mongrel dogs. J. Pharm. Sci. *60*, 1134–1138 (1971)

Adi, F.C., Eze, C.J., Anwunah, A.: Comparison of debrisoquine and guanethidine in treatment of hypertension. Br. Med. J. *1*, 482–485 (1975)

Adler, S.: Methyldopa-induced decrease in mental activity. J. Am. Med. Assoc. *230*, 1428–1429 (1974)

Agnew, T.M., Irvine, R.O.H., North, J.D.K.: Methyldopa and hydrochlorothiazide compared with reserpine and hydrochlorothiazide. Br. Med. J. *2*, 781–783 (1963)

Alexander, W.D., Evans, J.I.: Side effects of methyldopa. Br. Med. J. *2*, 500 (1975)

Alkalay, L.: Thrombocytopenia due to methyldopa. Harefuah *89*, 261–262 (1975)

Allum, W., Aminu, J., Bloomfield, T.H., Davies, C., Scales, A.H., Vere, D.W.: Interaction between debrisoquin and phenylephrine in man. Br. J. Clin. Pharmacol. *1*, 51–57 (1974)

Alphin, R.S., Ward, J.W.: An investigation of antihistaminic activity and gastric ulceration. Eur. J. Pharmacol. *6*, 61–66 (1969)

Ambrosino, S.V.: Depressive reactions associated with reserpine. N.Y. State J. Med. *74*, 860–864 (1974)

Amery, A., Deloof, W.: Chesse reaction during debrisoquine treatment. Lancet *2*, 613 (1970)

Aminu, J., D'Mello, A., Vere, D.W.: Interaction between debrisoquine and phenylephrine. Lancet *2*, 935–936 (1970)

Anagnostakis, D., Matsaniotis, N.: Neonatal cold injury and maternal reserpine administration. Lancet *2*, 471 (1974)

Angeletti, P.U., Levi-Montalcini, R.: Growth inhibition of sympathetic cells by some adrenergic blocking agents. Proc. Natl. Acad. Sci. USA *69*, 86–88 (1972)
Angeletti, P.U., Levi-Montalcini, R., Caramia, F.: Structural and ultrastructural changes in developing sympathetic ganglia induced by guanethidine. Brain. Res. *43*, 515–525 (1972)
Anselmino, K.J.: Die Behandlung der hypertensiven Spätgestose mit blutdrucksenkenden Mitteln unter besonderer Berücksichtigung der Eklampsie. Geburtshilfe Frauenheilkd. *20*, 1097–1110 (1960)
Arglebe, C., West, J., Chilla, R.: Sialoadenosis produced by drug-treatment of hypertonicity. II. Experimental studies on the effects of guanethidine (ismelin) on the submaxillary glands of the rat. Arch. Otorhinolaryngol. (NY) *211*, 259ö–265 (1975)
Armstrong, B., Stevens, N., Doll, R.: Retrospective study of the association between use of Rauwolfia derivatives and breast cancer in English women. Lancet *2*, 672–675 (1974)
Armstrong, B., Skegg, D., White, G., Doll, R.: Rauwolfia derivative and breast cancer in hypertensive women. Lancet *2*, 8–12 (1976)
Arnaud, G., Girod, C.: Nouvelles recherces concernant l'influence de la réserpine sur la gestation de la lapine. C.R. Soc. Biol. (Paris) *157*, 1585–1586 (1963)
Aromaa, A., Hakama, M., Hakulinen, T., Saxén, E., Teppo, L., Idanpaan-Heikkila, J.: Breast cancer and use of rauwolfia and other antihypertensive agents in hypertensive patients: a nationwide case-control study in Finland. Int. J. Cancer *18*, 727–738 (1976)
Athanassiadis, D., Cranston, W.I., Juel-Jensen, B.E., Oliver, D.O.: Clinical observations on the effects of debrisoquine sulphate in patients with high blood-pressure. Br. Med. J. *2*, 732–735 (1966)
Ayd, F.D.: Drug-induced depression – fact or fallacy. N.Y. State J. Med. *58*, 354–356 (1958)
Bachrach, W.H.: Reserpine, gastric secretion, and peptic ulcer. Am. J. Dig. Dis. *4*, 117–124 (1959)
Bagwell, E.E., Woods, E.F., Durst, G.G.: Influence of reserpine on cardiovascular and sympatho-adrenal responses to cyclopropane anesthesia in the dog. Anesthesiology *25*, 148–155 (1964a)
Bagwell, E.E., Woods, E.F., Linker, R.P.: Influence of reserpine on cardiovascular and sympatho-adrenal responses to ether anesthesia in the dog. Anesthesiology *25*, 15–24 (1964b)
Bak, I.J.: Electron microscopic observations in the substantia nigra of mouse during reserpine administration. Experientia *21*, 568–570 (1965)
Bakemeier, R.F., Leddy, J.P.: Erythrocyte autoantibody associated with alpha-methyldopa: heterogeneity of structure and specificity. Blood *32*, 1–14 (1968)
Balazs, T., Herman, E.H., Earl, F.L., Wolff, F.W.: Cardiotoxicity studies with diazoxide, reserpine, guanethidine and combinations of diazoxide and propranolol in dogs. Toxicol. Appl. Pharmacol. *33*, 498–504 (1975)
Balmer, V.G.: Antihypertensive drugs and general anaesthesia. Med. J. Aust. *1*, 143–148 (1965)
Barrett, W.E., Earl, A.E., Rogie, B.: Effect or reserpine on gastric secretion in the dog. J. Pharmacol. Exp. Ther. *113*, 3 (1955)
Barron, K.D., Chang, T.Y., Daniels, A.C., Doolin, P.F.: Subcellular accompaniments of axon retraction in cervical motoneurones of the cat. In: Progress in neuropathology. Zimmerman, H.M. (ed.). New York-London: Grune & Stratton, Vol. 1, 255–280 (1971)
Bartolomé, J., Bartolomé, M., Seidler, F.J., Anderson, T.R., Slotkin, T.A.: Effects of early postnatal guanethidine administration on adrenal medulla and brain of developing rats. Biochem. Pharmacol. *25*, 2387–2390 (1976a)
Bartolomé, J., Seidler, F.J., Anderson, T.R., Slotkin, T.A.: Effects of prenatal reserpine administration on development of the rat adrenal medulla and central nervous system. J. Pharmacol. Exp. Ther. *197*, 293–302 (1976b)
Bartolomé, J., Slotkin, T.A.: Prenatal reserpine administration: Permanent changes in adrenal tyrosine hydroxylase and dopamine-β-hydroxylase. Psychopharmacol. Commun. *1*, 465–472 (1975)
Bartolomé, J., Slotkin, T.A.: Effects of postnatal reserpine administration on sympatho-adrenal development in the rat. Biochem. Pharmacol. *25*, 1513–1519 (1976)
Bath, J., Pickering, D., Turner, R.: Clinical experience with bethanidine in treatment of hypertension. Br. Med. J. *4*, 519–521 (1967)
Bauer, G.E., Croll, F.J.T., Goldrich, R.B., Jeremy, D., Raftos, J., Whyte, H.M., Young, A.A.: Guanethidine in treatment of hypertension. Br. Med. J. *2*, 410–415 (1961)

Bauer, G.E., Hull, R.D., Stokes, G.S., Raftos, J.: The reversibility of side effects of guanethidine. Med. J. Aust. *1*, 930–933 (1973)

Bayliss, P.F.C., Duncan, S.M.: The effects of atenolol (tenormin) and methyldopa on simple tests of central nervous function. Br. J. Clin. Pharmacol. *2*, 527–531 (1975)

Bayliss, R.I.S., Harvey-Smith, E.A.: Methyldopa in the treatment of hypertension. Lancet *1*, 763–768 (1962)

Becker-Christensen, F., Bang, H.O., Ditzel, J.: Treatment of severe hypertension with catapres (ST 155). A comparative study of the effect of catapres and methyldopa in a series of hypertensive outpatients (WHO stage III). Acta Med. Scand. *190*, 21–26 (1971)

Bein, H.J.: The pharmacology of rauwolfia. Pharmacol. Rev. *8*, 435–483 (1956)

Benraad, A.H., Schoenaker, A.H.: Thrombopenia after use of methyldopa. Lancet *2*, 292 (1965)

Berger, W.: 88 schwere Hypoglykämiezwischenfälle unter der Behandlung mit Sulfunylharnstoffen. Schweiz. Med. Wochenschr. *101*, 1013–1022 (1971)

Bernstein, S., Kaufman, M.R.: A psychological analysis of apparent depression following Rauwolfia therapy. J. Mt. Sinai Hosp. *27*, 525–530 (1960)

Bhathal, P.S., Gerkens, J.F., Mashford, M.L.: Spermatic granuloma of the epididymis in rats treated with guanethidine. J. Pathol. *112*, 19–26 (1974)

Bittiger, H., Maitre, L., Krinke, G., Schnider, K., Hess, R.: A study of long-term effects of guanethidine on peripheral noradrenergic neurones of the rat. Toxicology *8*, 63–78 (1977)

Blahjchman, M.A., Pineo, G.G., Shimizu, A.G.: Methyldopa induced thrombocytopenia. Abstr. XIII Congr. Int. Soc. Blood Transf. p. 62 (1972)

Blaszkowski, T.P., Defeo, J.J., Guarino, A.M.: Central vs. peripheral catecholamines in rats during adaptation to chronic restraint stress. Pharmacology *4*, 321–333 (1970)

Bloomfield, D.K., Cangiano, J.L.: Clinical experience with a new antihypertensive agent, guanadrel sulfate. Curr. Ther. Res. *11*, 727–735 (1969)

Bloomfield, D.K., Cangiano, J.L.: Guanadrel and guanethidine in hypertension. Clin. Pharmacol. Ther. *11*, 200–204 (1970)

Boardman, P.L., Robinson, K.C., Hart, F.D.: Guanoxan and systemic lupus erythematosus. Br. Med. J. *1*, 111 (1967)

Bock, K.D., Heimsoth, V.: Persistierende orthostatische Hypotonie nach Behandlung mit Guanaclin. Dtsch. Med. Wochenschr. *94*, 265–270 (1969)

Bock, K.D., Huep, W.W.: Irreversibler Parotisschmerz nach Verabreichung von Guanaclin. Dtsch. Med. Wochenschr. *96*, 1649–1650 (1971)

Bonkowsky, H.L., Brisbane, J.: Colitis and hepatitis caused by methyldopa. J. Am. Med. Assoc. *236*, 1602–1603 (1976)

Bosanec, P., Dubb, J., Walther, B., Goldberg, M., Agus, Z.S.: Renal effects of guanabenz: A new antihypertensive. J. Clin. Pharmacol. *16*, 631–636 (1976)

Boston Collaborative Drug Surveillance Program: Reserpine and breast cancer. Lancet *2*, 669–671 (1974)

Böttiger, L.E., Westerholm, B.: Drug-induced blood dyscrasias in Sweden. Br. Med. J. *3*, 339–343 (1973)

Bouchier, I.A.D., Rhodes, K., Sherlock, S.: Serological abnormalities in patients with liver disease. Br. Med. J. *1*, 592–596 (1964)

Bouillin, D.J.: A calcium requirement for release of ^3H-guanethidine by sympathetic nerve stimulation. J. Pharm. Pharmacol. *18*, 709–712 (1966)

Bouquet, J., Kroon, M.C., Rees, H. v., Stakenburg, J., Wolff, F.A. de, Noachi, E.L.: Influence of guanethidine on contractions of isolated seminal vesicles of the rat. Arch. Int. Pharmacodyn. Ther. *182*, 402 (1969)

Boura, A.L.A., Green, A.F.: Comparison of bretylium and guanethidine: tolerance, and effects on adrenergic nerve function and responses to sympathomimetic amines. Br. J. Pharmacol. *19*, 13–41 (1962)

Boura, A.L.A., Green, A.F.: Adrenergic neuron blocking agents. Ann. Rev. Pharmacol. Toxicol. *5*, 183–212 (1965)

Boura, A.L.A., Copp, F.C., Green, A.F.: New antiadrenergic compounds. Nature (Lond.) *184*, 70–71 (1959a)

Boura, A.A.L., Green, A.F., McCourbrey, A., Laurence, D.R., Moulton, R., Rosenheim, M.L.: Darenthin. Hypotensive agent of a new type. Lancet *2*, 17–21 (1959b)

Bovet-Nitti, F., Bovet, D.: Action of some sympatholytic agents on pregnancy in the rat. Proc. Soc. Exp. Biol. Med. *100*, 555–557 (1959)
Brater, D.C., Morrelli, H.F.: Cardiovascular drug interaction. Annu. Rev. Pharmacol. Toxicol. *1*, 293–309 (1977)
Breckenridge, A., Dollery, C.T., Parry, E.H.O.: Prognosis of treated hypertension. Q. J. Med. *39*, 411–429 (1970)
Brest, A.N.: Hemodynamic response to antihypertensive drug therapy. J. Am. Med. Assoc. *192*, 41–44 (1965)
Brest, A.N., Moyer, J.H.: Therapeutic use of guanethidine. In Brest, A.N., Moyer, J.H. (eds.): Hypertension – recent advances. Philadelphia: Lea & Fibiger, 449–454 (1961)
Brest, A.N., Kodama, R., Naso, F., Moyer, J.H.: Guanethidine in the treatment of hypertension. Postgrad. Med. *30*, 260–264 (1961 a)
Brest, A.N., Seller, R., Onesti, G., Sekine, G., Moyer, J.H.: Preliminary observations on the antihypertensive effectiveness of alpha-methyl dopa, a decarboxylase inhibitor, In Brest, A.N., Moyer, J.H. (eds.): Hypertension – recent advances. Philadelphia, Lea & Fibiger, 424–429 (1961 b)
Brest, A.N., Novack, P., Kasparian, H., Moyer, J.H.: Guanethidine. Dis. Chest. *42*, 359–363 (1962)
Brest, A.N., Onesti, G., Swartz, C., Seller, R., Kim, K.E., Chinitz, J.: Mechanisms of antihypertensive therapy. J. Am. Med. Assoc. *211*, 480–484 (1970)
Brouillard, R.P., Barrett, O.: Methyldopa associated hepatitis. J. Am. Med. Assoc. *224*, 904 (1973)
Brown, W.J., Brown, F.K.: The use of guanethidine and hydrochlorothiazide in the long-term treatment of essential hypertension. Curr. Ther. Res. *17*, 544–554 (1975)
Brown, J.H., Nelson, D.L., Molinoff, A.: Organ culture of rat superior cervical ganglia. J. Pharmacol. Exp. Ther. *201*, 293–311 (1977)
Bruhn-Petersen, F.: Methyldopum-drug fever. Ugeskr. Laeger *129*, 639–641 (1967)
Bryant, J.M., Schwartz, N., Fertig, H., Fletcher, L., Quan, R.B.F.: Prolonged antihypertensive drug potentiation following isocaramidine withdrawal: A new therapeutic effect. J. New Drugs *4*, 221 (1964)
Budnick, I.S., Leikin, S., Hoeck, L.E.: Effect in the newborn infant of reserpine administration ante partum. Am. J. Dis. Child. *90*, 286–289 (1955)
Bulpitt, C.J., Dollery, C.T.: Side effects of hypotensive agents evaluated by a self-administered questionnaire. Br. Med. J. *3*, 485–490 (1973)
Burden, A.C., Alexander, C.P.T.: Rebound hypertension after acute methyldopa withdrawal. Br. Med. J. *1*, 1056–1057 (1976)
Burns-Cox, C.J.: Negative Coombs test in Chinese on methyldopa. Lancet *2*, 673–674 (1970)
Burnstock, G., Doyle, A.E., Gannon, B.J., Gerkens, J.F., Iwayama, T., Mashford, M.L.: Prolonged hypotension and ultrastructural changes in sympathetic neurons following guanacline treatment. Eur. J. Pharmacol. *13*, 175–187 (1971 a)
Burnstock, G., Evans, B., Gannon, B.J., Heath, J.W., James, V.: A new method of destroying adrenergic nerves in adult animals using guanethidine. Br. J. Pharmacol. *43*, 295–301 (1971 b)
Burnstock, G., Gannon, B., Iwayama, T.: Sympathetic innervation of vascular smooth muscle in normal and hypertensive animals. Circ. Res. *26–27*, Suppl. 2, 5–21 (1970)
Burry, J.N.: Ulcerative lichenoid eruption from methyldopa. Arch. Dermatol. *112*, 880 (1976)
Burry, J.N., Kirk, J.: Lichenoid drug reaction from methyldopa. Br. J. Dermatol. *91*, 475–476 (1974)
Byrd, G.J.: Methyldopa and lithium carbonate: Suspected interaction. J. Am. Med. Assoc. *233*, 320 (1975)
Cacace, L.G., Cohen, M.: Alpha-methyldopa (Aldomet) hepatitis. Drug. Intell. Clin. Pharmacol. *10*, 144–152 (1976)
Cairoli, V.J., Reilly, J.F., Roberts, J.: Effect of reserpine pretreatment on the response of isolated papillary muscle to ephedrine. Br. J. Pharmacol. *18*, 588–594 (1962)
Cannon, P.J., Laragh, J.H.: Treatment of hypertension with alpha-methyl-dopa. Pharmakotherapia *1*, 171–184 (1963)
Cantor, S., Barnett, A.J.: Haematological effects of methyldopa. Lancet *1*, 625 (1967)

Caramia, F., Angeletti, P.U., Levi-Montalcini, R., Carratelli, L.: Mitochondrial lesions of developing sympathetic neurons induced by bretylium tosylate. Brain Res. *40*, 237–246 (1972)

Carminati, G.M.: Attività comparata di svariati farmaci in alcuni tests sperimentali di syudio del comportamento. Arch. Int. Pharmacodyn. Ther. *181*, 68–93 (1969)

Carstairs, K.C., Breckenridge, A., Dollery, C.T., Worlledge, S.M.: Incidence of a positive direct Coombs test in patients on α-methyldopa. Lancet *2*, 133–135 (1966a)

Carstairs, K.C., Worlledge, S., Dollery, C.T., Breckenridge, A.: Methyldopa and haemolytic anaemia. Lancet *1*, 201 (1966b)

Chamberlain, D.A., Howard, J.: Guanethidine and methyldopa: A haemodynamic study. Br. Heart. J. *26*, 528–536 (1964)

Chan, C.S., Chan, T.K., Lee, S.K.: Direct Coombs test and methyldopa. Lancet *2*, 881 (1971)

Chaplin, H., Avioli, L.V.: Autoimmune hemolytic anemia. Arch. Intern. Med. *137*, 346–351 (1977)

Chessin, M., Kramer, E.R., Scott, C.C.: Modifications of the pharmacology of reserpine and serotonin by iproniazid. J. Pharmacol. Exp. Ther. *119*, 453–460 (1957)

Chidell, M.P., Whiteside, J.D.: A hypertension clinic. Four years' experience in a provincial hospital. Practitioner *202*, 542–552 (1969)

Chilla, R., Rieger, R., Arglebe, C.: Sialoadenosis produced by drug-treatment of hypertonicity. I. Experimental studies on the effects of guanethidine (ismelin) on the parotid gland of the rat. Arch. Otorhinolaryngol. (NY) *211*, 185–192 (1975)

Christopher, L.J., Crooks, J., Davidson, J.F., Erskine, Z.G., Gallon, S.C., Moir, D.C., Weir, R.D.: A multicentre study of rauwolfia derivatives and breast cancer. Eur. J. Clin. Pharmacol. *11*, 409–417 (1977)

Chrysant, S.G., Frohlich, E.D.: Comparison of the antihypertensive effectiveness of guanadrel and guanethidine. Curr. Ther. Res. *19*, 379–385 (1976)

Church, R.: Methyldopa causing seborrhoic dermatitis-like eruption. Br. J. Dermatol. *89*, Suppl. 9, 10 (1973)

Church, R.: Eczema provoked by methyl dopa. Br. J. Dermatol. *91*, 373–378 (1974)

Ciba Pharmaceutical Company Information. In Barnes, C.D., Eltherington, L.G.: Drug dosage in laboratory animals. Berkeley-Los Angeles-London: University of California Press, (1973), p. 112 and 234

Clarke, D.E., Jandhyala, B.S., Cavero, I., Dixit, B.N., Buckley, J.P.: A differential effect of chronically administered guanethidine on sympathetic neurotransmission to the dog heart and mesenteric arterial blood vessels. Can. J. Physiol. Pharmacol. *52*, 641–648 (1974)

Clementi, F.: Modifications ultrastructurelles provoquées par quelques médicaments sur les terminaisons nerveuses adrénergiques et sur la médullaire surrénale. Experientia (Basel) *21*, 171–176 (1965)

Coffman, J.D.: Persistence of reflex sympathetic nervous system activity in man on guanethidine or reserpine. Circulation *35*, 339–346 (1967)

Cohen, S.I., Young, M.W., Lau, S.H., Haft, J.I., Damato, A.N.: Effects of reserpine therapy on cardiac output and atrioventricula conduction during rest and controlled heart rates in patients with essential hypertension. Circulation *37*, 738–746 (1968)

Cohn, J.N., Liptake, T.E., Freis, E.D.: Hemodynamic effects of guanethidine in man. Circ. Res. *12*, 298–307 (1963)

Cole, M.: Retrograde degeneration of axon and soma in the nervous system. In: Bourne, G.H. (ed.): The structure and function of nervous tissue. New York-London: Academic Press, (1968), pp. 269–300

Colwill, J.M., Dutton, A.M., Morrissey, J. Yu, P.N.: Alpha-methyldopa and hydrochlorothiazide. A controlled study of their comparative effectiveness as antihypertensive agents. N. Engl. J. Med. *271*, 696–703 (1964)

Conston, A.S.: Hypersensitivity myocarditis: A fatal reaction. J. Med. Soc. N. J. *71*, 61 (1974)

Costa, E., Kuntzman, R., Gessa, H.L., Brodie, B.B.: Structural requirements for bretylium and guanethidine-like activity in a series of guanidine derivatives. Life Sci. *3*, 75–80 (1962)

Cotton, S.G., Montuschi, E.: Side-effects of guanoxan. Br. Med. J. *1*, 51 (1966)

Cotton, S.G., Montuschi, E.: Guanoxan. Br. Med. J. *3*, 174 (1967)

Coulter, J.D., Lester, B.K., Williams, H.L.: Reserpine and sleep. Psychopharmacology *19*, 134–147 (1971)

Cragg, B.G.: What is the signal for chromatolysis? Brain Res. *23*, 1–21 (1970)
Cranston, W.I., Brown, W.: Diurnal variation in plasma volume in normal and hypertensive subjects. Clin. Sci. Mol. Med. *25*, 107–114 (1963)
Cunningham, J.A.K.: Hypertension and cardiovascular disease, adverse effects of guanethidine. N. Z. Med. J. *66*, 373–378 (1967)
Curwain, B.P., Fake, C.S., Gordon, J.L., Mehta, M.D., Miller, D., Poyser, R.H., Wates, E.A.: Synthesis and antihypertensive properties of some *N*-(guanidinoalkyl)pyrrolidines. J. Med. Chem. *14*, 737–742 (1971)
Dameshek, W.: Alpha-methyldopa red cell antibody: cross reaction or forbidden clones. N. Engl. J. Med. *276*, 1382 (1967)
Dandiya, P.C., Menon, M.K., Studies on central nervous system depressants. (III) Influence of some tranquilizing agents on morphine analgesia. Arch. Int. Pharmacodyn. Ther. *141*, 223–232 (1963)
Davey, M.J., Reinert, H.: Pharmacology of the antihypertensive guanoxan. Br. J. Pharmacol. *24*, 29–48 (1965)
Dawborn, J.K., Doyle, A.E., Ebringer, A., Howqua, J., Jerums, C., Johnston, C.I., Mashford, M.L., Parkin, J.D.: Persistent postural hypotension due to guanacline. Pharmacol. Clin. *2*, 1–5 (1969)
Day, M.D.: Effect of sympathomimetic amines on the blocking action of guanethidine, bretylium, and xylocholine. Br. J. Pharmacol. *18*, 421–439 (1962)
Day, M.D., Rand, M.J.: Antagonism of guanethidine ande bretylium by various agents. Lancet *2*, 1282–1283 (1962)
Day, M.D., Rand, M.J.: Evidence for a competitive antagonism of guanethidine by dexamphetamine. Br. J. Pharmacol. *20*, 17–28 (1963)
Denney, J.L., Frasher, W.G., Hoytt, D.D.: Clinical evaluation of drug therapy in hypertension. Am. J. Med. Sci. *230*, 269–281 (1955)
Desmond, M.M., Rogers, S.F., Lindley, J.E., Moyer, J.H.: Management of toxemia of pregnancy with reserpine. II. The newborn infant. Obstet. Gynecol. *10*, 140–145 (1957)
Dewaard, F., Halewijn, E.A.B. van: A prospective study in general practice of breast-cancer risk in postmenopausal women. Int. J. Cancer *14*, 153–160 (1974)
Dewar, H.A., Peaston, M.J.T.: Three cases resembling polyarteritis nodosa arising during treatment with guanethidine. Br. Med. J. *2*, 609–611 (1964)
Dick, H.L.H., McCawley, E.L., Fischer, W.A.: Reserpine-digitalis toxicity. Arch. Intern. Med. *109*, 503–506 (1962)
Djaldetti, M., Bessler, H., Lewinski, U., Mandel, E.M.: Inhibition of uridine incorporation in proerythroblasts of patients with α-methyldopa induced haemolytic anaemia. Br. J. Haematol. *27*, 579–586 (1974)
Dollery, C.T.: Methyldopa in the treatment of hypertension. Prog. Cardiovasc. Dis. *8*, 278–289 (1965a)
Dollery, C.T.: Physiological and pharmacological interactions of antihypertensive drugs. Proc. R. Soc. Med. *58*, 983–987 (1965b)
Dollery, C.T.: Pharmacological basis for combination therapy of hypertension. Annu. Rev. Pharmacol. Toxicol. *17*, 311–323 (1977)
Dollery, C.T., Harington, M.: Methyldopa in hypertension, Clinical and pharmacological studies. Lancet *1*, 759–763 (1962)
Dollery, C.T., Emslie-Smith, D., McMichael, J.: Bretylium tosylate in the treatment of hypertension. Lancet *2*, 261–262 (1960a)
Dollery, C.T., Emslie-Smith, D., Milne, M.D.: Clinical and pharmacological studies with guanethidine in the treatment of hypertension. Lancet *2*, 381–387 (1960b)
Dollery, C.T., Harington, M., Hodge, J.V.: Haemodynamic studies with methyldopa: Effects on cardiac output and responses to pressor amines. Br. Heart J. *25*, 670–676 (1963)
Donath, K.: Ultrastrukturelle Acinusveränderungen der Rattenparotis unter der Einwirkung von Antihypertensiva (Guanacline). Arch. Otorhinolaryngol. (NY) *206*, 77–90 (1973)
Donath, K., Seifert, G.: Veränderungen des vegetativen Nervensystems der Parotis nach Einwirkung von Antihypertensiva (Guanacline). Virchows Arch. [Pathol. Anat.] *361*, 109–120 (1973)

Donath, K., Seifert, G., Pirsig, W.: Parotis-Sialadenosis nach Langzeittherapie mit Antihypertensiva (Guanacline). Virchows Arch. [Pathol. Anat.] *360,* 33–44 (1973)

Dörner, G., Hecht, K., Hinz, G.: Teratopsychogenetic effects apparently produced by nonphysiological neurotransmitter concentrations during brain differentiation. Endokrinologie *68,* 1–5 (1976)

Douglas, R.M.: Hypertensive cerebrovascular damage: considered in relation to treatment with hypotensive drugs. Med. J. Aust. *2,* 525–533 (1964)

Downing, O.A., Juul, P.: The effect of guanethidine pretreatment on transmission in the superior cervical ganglion. Acta Pharmacol. Toxicol. (Kbh) *32,* 369–381 (1973)

Draškoci, M., Jankovič, B.D.: Involution of thymus and suppression of immune responses in rats treated with guanethidine. Nature *202,* 408–409 (1964)

Drew, J.H., Kitchen, W.H.: The effect of maternally administered drugs on bilirubin concentrations in the newborn infant. J. Pediatr. *89,* 657–661 (1976)

Dunn, M.I., Freeman, J.: Moderate hypertension: Treatment with guanethidine and methyldopa. Curr. Ther. Res. *18,* 285–291 (1975)

Dustan, H.P., Tarazi, R.C., Bravo, E.L.: Dependence of arterial pressure on intravascular volume in treated hypertensive patients. N. Engl. J. Med. *286,* 861–866 (1972)

Duvoisin, R.C., Marsden, C.D.: Reversal of reserpine-induced bradykinesia by α-methyldopa – new light on its modus operandi. Brain Res. *71,* 178–182 (1974)

Dybing, E., Nelson, S.D., Mitchell, J.R., Sasame, H.A., Gillette, J.R.: Oxidation of α-methyldopa and other catechols by cytochrome P-450-generated superoxide in man: Possible mechanism of methyldopa hepatitis. Mol. Pharmacol. *12,* 911–920 (1976)

Dyer, A.R., Stamler, J., Berkson, D.M., Lindberg, H.A., Stevens, E.: High blood-pressure: A risk factor for cancer mortality, Lancet *1,* 1051–1056 (1975)

Eger, E.I., Hamilton, W.K.: The effect of reserpine on the action of various vasopressors. Anesthestiology *20,* 641–645 (1959)

Eliastam, M.: Hepatitis, arthritis and lupus cell phenomena caused by methyldopa. Digest. Dis. *16,* 1014–1018 (1971)

Elkington, S.G., Schreiber, W.M., Conn, H.O.: Hepatic injury caused by L-alpha-methyldopa. Circulation *40,* 589–595 (1969)

Eränkö, O., Eränkö, L.: Histochemical evidence of chemical sympathectomy by guanethidine in newborn rats. Histochem. J. *3,* 451–456 (1971 a)

Eränkö, L., Eränkö, O.: Effect of guanethidine on nerve cells and small intensely fluorescent cells in sympathetic ganglia of newborn and adult rats. Acta Pharmacol. Toxicol. (Kbh) *30,* 403–410 (1971 b)

Eränkö, L., Hill, C., Eränkö, O., Burnstock, G.: Lack of toxic effect of guanethidine on nerve cells in cultures of sympathetic ganglia of newborn rats. Brain Res. *43,* 501–513 (1972)

Euler, U.S. v.: Synthesis, uptake, and storage of catecholamines in adrenergic nerves, the effect of drugs. In: Blaschko, H. and Muscholl, E. (eds.): Catecholamines. Handbook of experimental pharmacology, vol. 33. Berlin-Heidelberg-New York, Springer Verlag, 186–230 (1972)

Evans, B., Gannon, B.J., Heath, J.W., Burnstock, G.: Long-lasting damage to the internal male genital organs and their adrenergic innervation in rats following chronic treatment with the antihypertensive drug guanethidine. Fertil. Steril. *23,* 657–667 (1972)

Eyster, M.E., Jenkins, D.E.: Gamma G erythrocyte auto-antibodies: Comparison of in vivo complement coating and in vitro "Rh" specificity. J. Immunol. *105,* 221–226 (1970)

Fann, W.E., Janowsky, D.S., Davis, J.M., Oates, J.A.: Chlorpromazine reversal of the antihypertensive action of guanethidine. Lancet *2,* 436–437 (1971)

Fann, W.E., Cavanaugh, J.H., Kaufmann, J.S., Griffith, J.D., Davis, J.M., Janowsky, D.S., Oates, J.A.: Doxepin: effects on transport of biogenic amines in man. Psychopharmacologia *22,* 111–125 (1972)

Ferguson, R.K., Rothenburg, R.J., Nies, A.S.: Patient acceptance of guanethidine as therapy for mild to moderate hypertension. A comparison with reserpine. Circulation *54,* 32–37 (1976)

Fernandez, P.G.: Alpha methyldopa and forgetfulness. Ann. Intern. Med. *85,* 128 (1976)

Finch, L.: Vascular reactivity in hypertensive rats after treatment with anti-hypertensive agents. Life Sci. *15,* 1827–1836 (1974)

Finnerty, F.A., Davidov, M., Mroczek, W.J., Gavrilovich, L.: Influence of extracellular fluid volume on response to antihypertensive drugs. Circ. Res. *27*, Suppl. 1, 71–80 (1970)
Fischer, J.E., Weise, V.K., Kopin, I.J.: Release of tritiated bretylium by sympathetic nerve stimulation. Nature (Lond.) *209*, 778–779 (1966)
Fleming, W.W.: Supersensitivity of the cat heart to catecholamine-induced arrhythmias following reserpine. Proc. Soc. Exp. Biol. Med. *111*, 484–486 (1962)
Fleming, W.W., Trendelenburg, U.: Development of supersensitivity to norepinephrine after pretreatment with reserpine. J. Pharmacol. Exp. Ther. *133*, 41–51 (1961)
Forrester, T.M., Sheriffs, G.G.: Methyldopa and methoserpidine in hypertension. A double-blind trial. Lancet *1*, 141–142 (1967)
Freis, E.D.: Mental depression in hypertensive patients treated for long periods with large doses of reserpine. N. Engl. J. Med. *251*, 1006–1008 (1954)
Friedberg, V.: Über die perinatale Sterblichkeit bei Neugeborenen bei Präeklampsien. Geburtshilfe Frauenheilkd. *24*, 649–660 (1964)
Frohlich, E.D.: Inhibition of adrenergic function in the treatment of hypertension. Arch. Intern. Med. *133*, 1033–1048 (1974)
Frohlich, E.D., Freis, E.D.: Clinical trial of guanethidine, a new type of antihypertensive agent. Medical Annals, District of Columbia *28*, 419–422 (1959)
Fullerton, A.G., Morton-Jenkins, D.: Methyldopa and depression. Br. Med. J. *1*, 538–539 (1963)
Furst, C.I.: The biochemistry of guanethidine. Adv. Drug Res. *4*, 133–161 (1967)
Galskov, Å., Clausen, E., Hilden, T., Krogsgaard, A.R.: Guanethidine in the ambulatory treatment of arterial hypertension. Acta Med. Scand. *170*, 31–42 (1961)
Gannon, B.J., Iwayama, T., Burnstock, G., Gerkens, J., Mashford, M.L.: Prolonged effects of chronic guanethidine treatment on the sympathetic innervation of the genitalia of male rats. Med. J. Aust. *2*, 207–208 (1971)
Garfinkel, L., Hammond, E.C.: Breast cancer and hypertension. Lancet *2*, 1381 (1974)
Gaunt, R., Renzi, A.A., Antonchak, N., Miller, G.J.: Endocrine aspects of the pharmacology of reserpine. Ann. N. Y. Acad. Sci. *59*, 22–35 (1959)
Gelfand, M.L., Goodkin, L.: Drug-induced gastrointestinal bleeding. N. Y. J. Med. *58*, 2381–2384 (1958)
Gerkens, J.F.: Guanethidine and guanacline on the rat vas deferens. Br. J. Pharmacol. *52*, 191–195 (1974a)
Gerkens, J.F.: Effect of long-term treatment with guanacline or guanethidine on sympathetic function. Eur. J. Pharmacol. *26*, 143–150 (1974b)
Ghosh, S.K.: Methyldopa and forgetfulness. Lancet *1*, 202–203 (1976)
Giachetti, A., Hollenbeck, R.A.: Extra-vesicular binding of noradrenaline and guanethidine in the adrenergic neurones of the rat heart: A proposed site of action of adrenergic neurone blocking agents. Br. J. Pharmacol. *58*, 497–504 (1976)
Gibb, W.E., Malpas, J.S., Turner, P., White, R.J.: Comparison of bethanidine, α-methyldopa, and reserpine in essential hypertension. Lancet *2*, 275–277 (1970)
Gifford, R.W.: Management of hypertensive emergencies. Postgrad. Med. *34*, 145–149 (1963)
Gifford, R.W.: Bethanidine sulfate – a new antihypertensive agent. J. Am. Med. Assoc. *193*, 901–905 (1965)
Gilder, J.E.V.: Alpha-methyldopa-induced immune hemolytic anemia. W. Va. Med. J. *71*, 327–332 (1975)
Gill, J.R., Bartter, F.C.: Adrenergic nervous system in sodium metabolism. N. Engl. J. Med. *275*, 1466–1471 (1966)
Gill, J.R., Mason, D.T., Bartter, F.C.: Adrenergic nervous system in sodium metabolism: Effects of guanethidine and sodium-retaining steroids in man. J. Clin. Invest. *43*, 177–184 (1964)
Gillespie, L., Oates, J.A., Crout, J.H., Sjoerdsma, A.: Clinical and chemical studies with α-methyl-dopa in patients with hypertension. Circulation *25*, 281–291 (1962)
Gillies, J.D.: A complication of alpha-methyldopa therapy. Anaesth. Intensive Care *2*, 179–181 (1974)
Gilmore, B.L., Freis, E.D.: Methyldopa in the treatment of hypertension. Med. Ann. D. C. *34*, 13–18 (1965)

Glazer, N.: Reserpine, hydralazine, hydrochlorothiazide combination (ser-ap-es) in essential hypertension. Curr. Ther. Res. *14*, 561–572 (1972)
Glazer, N.: Comparison of guanethidine and methyldopa in essential hypertension: A controlled study. Curr. Ther. Res. *17*, 249–256 (1975)
Glontz, G.E., Saslaw, S.: Methyldopa fever. Arch. Intern. Med. *122*, 445–447 (1968)
Gokhale, S.D., Gulati, O.D.; Udwadia, B.P.: Antagonism of the adrenergic neuron blocking action of guanethidine by certain antidepressants and antihistaminic drugs. Arch. Int. Pharmacodyn. Ther. *160*, 321–329 (1966)
Gokhale, S.D., Gulati, O.D., Kelkar, V.V.: Supersensitivity to catecholamines following guanethidine. Br. J. Pharmacol. *30*, 445–462 (1967)
Goldberg, A.D., Raftery, E.B.: Patterns of blood-pressure during chronic administration of postganglionic sympathetic blocking drugs for hypertension. Lancet *2*, 1052–1054 (1976)
Goldman, A.S., Yakovac, W.C.: Teratogenic action in rats of reserpine alone and in combination with salicylate and immobilization. Proc. Soc. Exp. Biol. Med. *118*, 857–862 (1965)
Goldstein, G.B., Lam, K.C., Mistilis, S.P.: Drug-induced active chronic heptatitis. Am. J. Dig. Dis. *18*, 177–184 (1973)
Gormsen, J., Dyrbye, M., Eiken, M., Rønnov-Jessen, V.: Acute cerebral infarct. Extracerebral genesis with particular reference to cardiovascular status. Acta Med. Scand. *169*, 455–466 (1961)
Gradwell, B.G.: Psychotic reactions and phenelzine. Br. Med. J. *2*, 1018 (1960)
Green, A.F., Robson, R.D.: Adrenergic neurone blocking agents: Tolerance and hypersensitivity to adrenaline and noradrenaline. Br. J. Pharmacol. *25*, 497–506 (1965)
Greene, R. Spence, A.W.: Neutropenia caused by methyldopa. Br. Med. J. *4*, 618 (1967)
Grenfell, R.F.: Treatment of hypertensive crisis. Chest *59*, 212–213 (1971)
Groden, B.M.: Parkinsonism occurring with methyldopa treatment. Br. Med. J. *1*, 1001 (1963)
Groover, M.E., Fulghum, J.E., Simpson, W.G.: Arterial hypertension – Northwest Florida Health Survey. II. Diagnosis and treatment. Curr. Ther. Res. *16*, 1203–1213 (1974)
Gross, F. (ed.): Antihypertensive agents. Handbook of experimental pharmacology, Vol. 39. Berlin-Heidelberg-New York: Springer Verlag (1977)
Guazzi, M., Magrini, F., Fiorentini, C., Polese, A.: Role of the sympathetic nervous system in supporting cardiac function in essential arterial hypertension. Br. Heart J. *35*, 55–64 (1973a)
Guazzi, M., Polese, A., Fiorentini, C., Magrini, F.: Importance of the adrenergic nervous system in the support of cardiac function in patients with arterial hypertension. Clin. Sci. Mol. Med. *45*, Suppl. 1, 1515–1545 (1973b)
Gulati, O.D., Dave, S.D., Gokhale, S.D., Shah, K.M.: Antagonism of adrenergic neuron blockade in hypertensive subjects. Clin. Pharmacol. Ther. *7*, 510–514 (1966)
Gupta, K.K.: The anti-diabetic action of guanethidine. Postgrad. Med. J. *45*, 455–456 (1969)
Gupta, K.K., Lillicrap, C.A.: Guanethidine and diabetes. Br. Med. J. *2*, 697–698 (1968)
Gupta, M.B., Tangri, K.K., Bhargava, K.P.: Mechanism of ulcerogenic action of reserpine in albino rats. Eur. J. Pharmacol. *27*, 269–271 (1974)
Haeusler, G., Haefely, W., Huerliman, A.: On the mechanism of the adrenergic blocking action of bretylium and guanethidine. Arch. exp. Path. Pharmak. *264*, 241–243 (1969)
Haeusler, G., Lorez, H.P., Bartholini, G., Kettler, R., Tranzer, J.P.: Absence of degeneration of adrenergic neurons after prolonged treatment with debrisoquin. J. Pharmacol. Exp. Ther. 189, 646–658 (1974)
Hallwright, G.P.: Agranulocytosis caused by methyl dopa (Aldomet). N. Z. Med. J. *60*, 567–570 (1961)
Hamilton, M.: Some aspects of the long-term treatment of severe hypertension with methyldopa. Postgrad. Med. J. *44*, 66–69 (1968)
Hamilton, M., Kopelman, H.: Treatment of severe hypertension with methyldopa. Br. Med. J. *1*, 151–155 (1963)
Hanahoe, T.H.P., Ireson, J.D., Large, B.J.: Interactions between guanethidine and inhibitors of noradrenaline uptake. Arch. Int. Pharmacodyn. Ther. *182*, 349–353 (1969)
Hans, S.F., Kopelman, H.: Methyldopa in treatment of severe toxaemia of pregnancy. Br. Med. J. *1*, 736–739 (1964)

Hansen, J.: Alpha-methyl-dopa (Aldomet) in the treatment of hypertension. Acta Med. Scand. *183*, 323–327 (1968)
Hansson, L., Pascual, A., Julius, S.: Comparison of guanadrel and guanethidine. Clin. Pharmacol. Ther. *14*, 204–208 (1973)
Harrison, D.C., Chidsey, C.A., Goldman, R., Braunwald, E.: Relationships between the release and tissue depletion of norepinephrine from the heart by guanethidine and reserpine. Circ. Res. *12*, 256–263 (1963)
Hartmann, E.: Reserpine: Its effect on the sleep-dream cycle in man. Psychopharmacologia *9*, 242–247 (1966)
Harvald, B., Schaumburg, E.: Debrisokin som led i kombineret antihypertensiv terapi. Ugeskr. Laeger *138*, 420–422 (1976)
Haverback, B.J., Stevenson, T.D., Sjoerdsma, A., Terry, L.L.: The effect of reserpine and chlorpromazine on gastric secretion. Am. J. Med. Sci. *230*, 601–604 (1955)
Heath, J.W., Sobels, G.: Intracellular site of action of guanethidine on adrenergic neurons. In: Drug design and adverse reactions. Bundgaard, H., Juul, P., Kofod, H. (eds.): Copenhagen: Munksgaard, (1977), pp. 52–60
Heath, J.W., Evans, B.K., Gannon, B.J., Burnstock, G., James, V.B.: Degeneration of adrenergic neurons following guanethidine treatment: An ultrastructural study. Virchows Arch. [Cell Pathol.] *11*, 182–197 (1972)
Heath, J., Eränkö, O., Eränkö, L.: Effect of guanethidine on the ultrastructure of the small, granule-containing cells in cultures of rat sympathetic ganglia. Acta Pharmacol. Toxicol. (Kbh) *33*, 209–218 (1973a)
Heath, J.W., Evans, B.K., Burnstock, G.: Axon retraction following guanethidine treatment. Z. Zellforsch. *146*, 439–451 (1973b)
Heath, J.W., Hill, C.E., Burnstock, G.: Axon retraction following guanethidine treatment: Studies of sympathetic neurons in tissue culture. J. Neurocytol. *3*, 263–276 (1974)
Heffernan, A., Carty, A., O'Malley, K., Bugler, J.: A within-patient comparison of debrisoquin and methyldopa in hypertension. Br. Med. J. *1*, 75–78 (1971)
Heinonen, O.P., Shapiro, S., Tuominen, L., Turunen, M.I.: Reserpine use in relation to breast cancer. Lancet *2*, 675–677 (1974)
Helling, M.: Experience with World Health Organization. In: Gouveia, W.A., Tognoni, G., Kleijn, E.v.d. (eds): Clinical pharmacy and clinical pharmacology. Amsterdam-New York-Oxford: North-Holland, (1976), pp. 141–151
Hensler, L.: Hypertonietherapie mit Serpasil, einem Alkaloid der Rauwolfia serpentina. Schweiz. Med. Wochenschr. *83*, 1162–1166 (1953)
Hepp, R., Kreye, V.A.W.: Effect of long-term treatment with high doses of guanethidine on sperm transport and fertility in rats. Br. J. Pharmacol. *48*, 30–35 (1973)
Hess, R.: Functional interpretation of drug-induced morphological changes. In: Advances in toxicological methodology. Proc. Eur. Soc. Study Drug Tox. Amsterdam-New York-London-Milan-Tokyo-Buenos Aires: Excerpta Medica, 130–140 (1965)
Hester, R.K., Carrier, O.: Reserpine supersensitity four hours after pretreatment of rabbits. Fed. Proc. *32*, 405 (1973)
Hey, P., Willey, G.L.: Choline 2:6-xylyl ether bromide; an active quaternary local anaesthetic. Br. J. Pharmacol. *9*, 471–475 (1954)
Hilden, T., Krogsgaard, A.R., Godtfredsen, E.: Behandling af hypertension med reserpin (Serpasil). Ugeskr. Laeger *117*, 572–575 (1955)
Hilden, T., Nilsson, R.: Metyldopa i behandlingen af hypertension. T. Norsk. Laegeforen. *88*, 1416–1420 (1968)
Hill, C.E., Mark, G.E., Eränkö, O., Eränkö, L., Burnstock, G.: Use of tissue culture to examine the actions of guanethidine and 6-hydroxydopamine. Eur. J. Pharmacol. *23*, 162–174 (1973)
Hochuli, E., Weiche, V.: Zur Dauermedikation mit hypotensiven Substanzen in Graviditate. Geburtshilfe Frauenheilkd. *32*, 32–39 (1972)
Hoffbrand, B.I., Fry, W., Bunton, G.L.: Cholestatic jaundice due to methyldopa. Br. Med. J. *3*, 559 (1974)
Hoffeld, D.R., Webster, R.L., McNew, J.: Adverse effects on offspring of tranquilizing drugs during pregnancy. Nature (Lond.) *215*, 182–183 (1967)

Hoffman, J.S., Domino, E.: Comparative effects of reserpine on the sleep cycle of man and cat. J. Pharmacol. Exp. Ther. *170*, 190–198 (1969)
Holt, M.C.: Methoserpidine, A non-depressant isomer of reserpine. Br. Med. J. *2*, 415–418 (1961)
Horwitz, D., Sjoerdsma, A.: Use of two enzyme inhibitors in hypertension therapy. Postgrad. Med. *34*, 140–144 (1963)
Horwitz, D., Pettinger, W.A., Orvis, H., Thomas, R.E., Sjoerdsma, A.: Effects of methyldopa in fifty hypertensive patients. Clin. Pharmacol. Ther. *8*, 224–234 (1967)
Hoyumpa, A.M., Connell, A.M.: Methyldopa hepatitis. Report of three cases. Am. J. Dig. Dis. *18*, 213–222 (1973)
Hunter, E., Raik, E., Gordon, S.: Incidence of positive Coombs' test, LE cells and antinuclear factor in patients on alpha-methyldopa (Aldomet) therapy. Med. J. Aust. *2*, 810–812 (1971)
Hunter, K.R., Stern, G.M., Laurence, D.R.: Use of levodopa with other drugs. Lancet *2*, 1283–1285 (1970)
Hurley, R.E., Page, I.H., Dustan, H.P.: Bretylium tosylate as an antihypertensive drug. J. Am. Med. Assoc. *172*, 2081–2083 (1960)
Igloe, M.C.: Effects of methyldopa in hypertension. J. Am. Med. Assoc. *189*, 188–190 (1964)
Innes, I.R., Krayer, O., Wand, D.R.: The action of rauwolfia alkaloids on the heart rate and on the functional refractory period of atrio-ventricular transmission in the heart-lung preparation of the dog. J. Pharmacol. Exp. Ther. *124*, 324–332 (1958)
Irvine, R.O.H., O'Brien, K.P., North, J.D.K.: Alpha-methyldopa in treatment of hypertension. Lancet *1*, 300–303 (1962)
Iversen, B.M., Johannesen, J.W., Nordahl, E., Ofstad, J., Thunold, S., Willassen, Y.: Retroperitoneal fibrosis during treatment with methyldopa. Lancet *2*, 302–304 (1975)
Jackson, W.B.: Tolerance and side effects during long term treatment of hypertension with debrisoquine. Aust. N. Z. J. Med. *4*, 357–365 (1972)
Jandhyala, B.S., Buckley, J.P.: Autonomic and cardiovascular effects of guanethidine in dogs. Circulation *50*, Suppl. 3, 37 (1974)
Jandhyala, B.S., Cavero, I., Buckley, J.P.: Effects of chronic guanethidine administration on cardiovascular function of dogs. Res. Commun. Chem. Pathol. Pharmacol. *11*, 523–532 (1975)
Jandhyala, B.S., Clarke, D.E., Buckley, J.P.: Effects of prolonged administration of certain antihypertensive agents. J. Pharm. Sci. *63*, 1497–1513 (1974)
Janowsky, D.S., El-Yousef, M.K., Davis, J.M., Fann, W.E.: Antagonism of guanethidine by chlorpromazine. Am. J. Psychiatry *130*, 808–812 (1973)
Janowsky, D.S., El-Yousef, M.K., Davis, J.M., Fann, W.E., Oates, J.A.: Guanethidine antagonism by antipsychotic drugs. J. Tenn. Med. Assoc. *65*, 620–622 (1972)
Jensen-Holm, J.: Cholinesterases and protein changes in sympathetic ganglia after guanethidine. Acta Pharmacol. Toxicol. [Suppl. 4] (kbn) *25*, 74 (1967)
Jensen-Holm, J.: The influence of guanethidine and ascorbic acid on the rat lymph nodes and thymus (weight, histology and cholinesterases). Acta Pharmacol. Toxicol. [Suppl. 1] (Kbh) *35*, 33 (1974)
Jensen-Holm, J., Juul, P.: Changes of the rat superior cervical ganglion induced by guanethidine (histology and cholinesterase histochemistry). Br. J. Pharmacol. *34*, 211 P (1968)
Jensen-Holm, J., Juul, P.: The effects of guanethidine, pre- and postganglionic nerve division on the rat superior cervical ganglion: Cholinesterases and protein. Acta Pharmacol. Toxicol. (Kbh) *28*, 270–282 (1970a)
Jensen-Holm, J., Juul, P.: The effects of guanethidine, pre- and postganglionic nerve division on the rat superior cervical ganglion: Cholinesterases and catecholamines (histochemistry), and histology. Acta Pharmacol. Toxicol. (Kbh). *28*, 283–298 (1970b)
Jensen-Holm, J., Juul, P.: Ultrasructural changes in the rat superior cervical ganglion following prolonged guanethidine administration. Acta Pharmacol. Toxicol. (Kbh) *30*, 308–320 (1971)
Jewett, R.E., Norton, S.: Effect of tranquilizing drugs on postnatal behavior. Exp. Neurol. *14*, 33–43 (1966)
Jick, H.: Adverse drug effects in relation to renal function. Am. J. Med. *62*, 514–517 (1977)

Johnson, E.M.: Destruction of the sympathetic nervous system of neonatal rats by vinblastine: Preventing by concomitant administration of nerve growth factor (NGF). Fed. Proc. *36*, 956 (1977)
Johnson, E.M., Aloe, L.: Suppression of the in vitro and in vivo cytotoxic effects of guanethidine in sympathetic neurons by nerve growth factor. Brain Res. *81*, 519–532 (1974)
Johnson, E.M., O'Brien, F.: Evaluation of the permanent sympathectomy produced by the administration of guanethidine to adult rats. J. Pharmacol. Exp. Ther. *196*, 53–61 (1976)
Johnson, P., Kitchin, A.H., Lowther, C.P., Turner, R.W.D.: Treatment of hypertension with methyldopa. Br. Med. J. *1*, 133–137 (1966)
Johnson, E.M., Cantor, E., Douglas, J.R.: Biochemical and functional evaluation of the sympathectomy produced by the administration of guanethidine to newborn rats. J. Pharmacol. Exp. Ther. *193*, 503–512 (1975)
Johnson, E.M., O'Brien, F., Werbitt, R.: Modification and characterization of the permanent sympathectomy produced by the administration of guanethidine to newborn rats. Eur. J. Pharmacol. *37*, 45–54 (1976)
Johnson, E.M., Macia, R.A., Yellin, T.O.: Marked difference in the susceptibility of several species to guanethidine-induced chemical sympathectomy. Life Sci. *20*, 107–112 (1977)
Johnston, A.W., Prichard, B.N.C., Rosenheim, M.L.: The use of bethanidine in the treatment of hypertension. Lancet *2*, 659–661 (1964)
Jones, D.L.B.H., Michael, A.M., Ommer, J.P.: Clinical trial of methoserpidine in general practice. Br. Med. J. *2*, 1738–1741 (1961)
Jørstad, J.: Reserpin ved psykoser. Nord. Med.*55*, 794–798 (1956)
Juul, P.: Effects of various antihypertensive guanidine derivatives on the adult rat superior cervical ganglion: Histology, ultrastructure, and cholinesterase histochemistry. Acta Pharmacol. Toxicol. (Kbh) *32*, 500–512 (1973a)
Juul, P.: Accumulation of guanethidine by sympathetic ganglia of reserpinized rats. Acta Pharmacol. Toxicol. (Kbh) *33*, 79–80 (1973b)
Juul, P.: Guanethidine and sympathetic ganglia. (Thesis). Copenhagen (1974)
Juul, P.: Cytotoxicity of a series of guanidine derivatives. In: Drug design and adverse reactions. Bundgaard, H., Juul, P., Kofod, H. (eds.). Copenhagen: Munksgaard, (1977), pp. 63–73
Juul, P., McIsaac, R.L.: The effect of guanethidine on the noradrenaline content of the adult rat superior cervical ganglion. Acta Pharmacol. Toxicol. (Kbh) *32*, 382–389 (1973)
Juul, P., Sand, O.: Determination of guanethidine in sympathetik ganglia. Acta Pharmacol. Toxicol. (Kbh) *32*, 487–499 (1973)
Kaldor, A., Juvancz, P.: Effect of antihypertensive drugs on the "intrinsic" heart rate. Br. Med. J. *2*, 486–487 (1969)
Kanematsu, S., Sawyer, C.H.: Effects of intrahypothalamic implants of reserpine on lactation and pituitary prolactin content in the rabbit. Proc. Soc. Exp. Biol. Med. *113*, 967–969 (1963)
Katz, R.L., Weintraub, H.D., Papper, E.M.: Anesthesia, surgery and rauwolfia. Anesthesiology *25*, 142–147 (1964)
Kedia, K., Markland, C.: The effect of pharmacological agents on ejaculation. J. Urol. *114*, 569–573 (1975)
Kehl, R. Audibest, A., Gage, C., Amarger, J.: Action de la réserpine à différentes périodes de la gestation chez la lapine. C. R. Soc. Biol. (Paris) *150*, 2196–2199 (1956)
Kellaway, G.S.M.: Adverse drug reactions during treatment of hypertension. Drugs *11*, suppl. 1, 91–99 (1976)
Kellaway, G.S.M., McCrae, E.: Non-compliance and errors of drug administration in patients discharged from acute medical wards. N. Z. Med. J. *81*, 508–512 (1975)
Kersting, F., Reid, J.L., Dollery, C.T.: Clinical and cardiovascular effects of alpha methyldopa in combination with decarboxylase inhibitors. Clin. Pharmacol. Ther. *21*, 548–555 (1976)
Kert, M.J., Carleton, H.G., Nordyke, R.A., Roth, S.I., Smith, L.A., Westgart, J.P.: Clinical experiences with reserpine (Serpasil) in hypertension. Angiology *6*, 138–143 (1955)
Khatri, I.M., Cohn, J.N.: Effect of sympathetic blockade on exercise-induced splanchnic vasoconstriction. Circulation *28*,, Suppl. 6, 114 (1968)
Kiessling, W., Huhnstock, K.: Aspermatismus nach peroralen Gaben von Guanethidin. Klin. Wochenschr. *41*, 948–952 (1963)

Kincaid-Smith, P., Bullen, M., Mills, J.: Prolonged use of methyldopa in severe hypertension in pregnancy. Br. Med. J. *1*, 274–276 (1966)

Kisin, I., Yuzhakov, S.: Effects of reserpine, guanethidine and methyldopa on cardiac output and its distribution. Eur. J. Pharmacol. *35*,253–260 (1976)

Kitchin, A.H., Turner, R.W.D.: Studies on debrisoquine sulphate. Br. Med. J. *2*, 728–731 (1966)

Klein, H.O., Kaminsky, N.: Methyldopa fever. Recurrence of symptoms with resumption of therapy. N. Y. State J. Med. *73*, 448–451 (1973)

Koch-Weser, J.: Drug interactions in cardiovascular therapy. Am. Heart. J. *90*, 93–116 (1975)

Kopia, G.A., Condouris, G.A.: Guanethidine-induced cardiac arrhythmias in cats anesthetized with halothane. Fed. Proc. *36*, 1013 (1977)

Kopin, I.J.: False adrenergic transmitters. Annu. Rev. Pharmacol. Toxicol. *8*, 377–394 (1968)

Kostrzewa, R.M., Jacobowitz, D.M.: Pharmacological actions of 6-hydroxydopamine. Pharmacol. Rev. *26*, 199–288 (1974)

Krogsgaard, A.R.: Reserpine and gastric secretion in man. Acta Med. Scand. *158*, 1–11 (1957a)

Krogsgaard, A.R.: The effect of reserpine on the electrolyte and fluid balance in man. Acta Med. Scand. *159*, 127–132 (1957b)

Krogsgaard, A.R.: Side-effects of reserpine in the treatment of essential hypertension. Acta Med. Scand. *162*, 465–474 (1958)

Krogsgaard, A.R.: On reserpine with particular reference to its use in hypertension. (Thesis). Copenhagen, Munksgaard (1961)

Kuntzman, R., Jacobson, M.M.: Monoamine oxidase inhibition by a series of compounds structurally related to bretylium and guanethidine. J. Pharmacol. Exp. Ther. *141*, 166–172 (1963)

Kwan, K.C., Foltz, E.L., Breault, G.O., Baer, J.E., Totaro, J.A.: Pharmacokinetics of methyldopa in man. J. Pharmacol. Exp. Ther. *198*, 264–277 (1976)

Landesman, R., McLarn, W.D., Ollskin, R.N., Mendelsohn, B.: Reserpine in toxemia of pregnancy. Obstet. Gynecol. *9*, 377–383 (1957)

Laragh, J.H. (ed.): Hypertension manual. New York, Dun-Donnelley (1973)

Laska, E.M., Siegel, C., Meisner, M., Fischer, S., Wanderling, J.: Matched pairs study of reserpine use and breast cancer. Lancet *2*, 296–300 (1975)

Lauler, D.P., Vagnucci, A.I., Hickler, R.B., Thorn, G.W.: Clinical features of sodium retention induced by antihypertensive therapy. Circulation *28*, 754–755 (1963)

Laurence, D.R., Nagle, R.E.: The interaction of bretylium with pressor agents. Lancet *1*, 593–594 (1961)

Laurence, D.R., Rosenheim, M.L.: Clinical effects of drugs which prevent the release of adrenergic transmitter. In: Vane, J.R. (ed.): Adrenergic mechanisms. CIBA symposium. London: Churchill, 201–208 (1960)

Lauwers, P., Verstraete, M., Joossens, J.V.: Methyldopa in the treatment of hypertension. Br. Med. J. *1*, 295–300 (1963)

Lee, P.A., Kelly, M.R., Wallin, J.D.: Increased prolactin levels in patients during reserpine treatment of hypertensive patients. J. Am. Med. Assoc. *235*, 2316–2317 (1976)

Leishman, A.W.D., Matthews, H.L., Smith, A.J.: Guanethidine. Hypotensive drug with prolonged action. Lancet *2*, 1044–1048 (1959)

Leishman, A.W.D., Matthews, H.L., Smith, A.J.: Further experience with guanethidine. Lancet *2*, 4–7 (1961)

Leishman, A.W.D., Matthews, H.L., Smith, A.J.: Antagonism of guanethidine by imipramine. Lancet *1*, 112 (1963)

Lemieux, G., Davignon, A., Genest, J.: Depressive states during Rauwolfia therapy for arterial hypertension. Can. Med. Assoc. J. *4*, 522–526 (1956)

Lemmer, B., Saller, R., Grobecker, H.: Increased cardiac turnover of noradrenaline after chronic administration of guanethidine in the rat. Experientia (Basel) *30*, 379–381 (1974)

Leonard, J. W., Gifford, R.W., Humphrey, D.C.: Febrile reactions to L-alpha-methyl-dopa. Cleve. Clin. Q. *29*, 144–147 (1962)

Leonard, J.W., Gifford, R.W., Humphrey, D.C.: Treatment of hypertension with methyldopa alone or combined with diuretics and/or guanethidine. Am. Heart J. *69*, 610–618 (1965)

Leth, A.: Body fluid compartments in essential hypertension. (Thesis). Copenhagen (1976)
Leth, A., Ibsen, H.: Changes in plasma and extracellular fluid volume during long-term treatment with alpha-methyldopa in 11 thiazide-treated patients with essential hypertension. Acta Med. Scand. *198,* 45–48 (1975)
Leth, A., Ibsen, H.: Changes in the ratio of plasma to interstitial fluid volume during long-term antihypertensive therapy. J. Lab. Clin. Med. *87,* 781–791 (1976)
Levi, J., Robson, M., Rosenfeld, J.: The treatment of hypertension. Comparative trial of bethanidine (Esbatal) and bethanidine with reserpine. Clinical Trials Journal *17,* 263–270 (1970)
Levi-Montalcini, R., Angeletti, P.U.: Immunosympathectomy. Pharmacol. Rev. *18,* 619–628 (1966)
Levi-Montalcini, R., Aloe, L., Johnson, E.M.: Interaction between the nerve growth factor (NGF) and adrenergic blocking agents in sympathetic neurons. Front. Catecholamine Res. 267–276 (1973)
Levine, R.J., Strauch, B.S.: Hypertensive response to methyldopa. N. Engl. J. Med. *275,* 946–948 (1966)
Lewis, P.D., Patel, A.J., Béndek, G., Balázs, T.: Do drugs acting on the nervous system affect cell proliferation in the developing brain. Lancet *1,* 399 (1977)
Lieberman, A.R.: The axon reaction: A review of the principal features of perikaryal responses to axon injury. In: International review of neurobiology. Pfeffer, C.C., Smythies, J.R. (eds.). London: Academic Press, (1971), Vol. 14, pp. 49–124
Lifrak, I.L., Strebel, R., Settles, H.: The effect of reserpine on the cardiac muscle of pregnant and fetal guinea pigs. Fed. Proc. *35,* 611 (1976)
Lilienfeld, A.M., Chang, L., Thomas, D.B., Levin, M.L.: Rauwolfia derivatives and breast cancer. John Hopkins Med. J. *139,* 41–50 (1976)
Lobuglio, A.F., Jandl, J.H.: The nature of the alpha-methyldopa red-cell antibody. N. Engl. J. Med. *276,* 658–665 (1967)
Locket, S.: Oral preparations of Rauwolfia serpentina in treatment of essential hypertension. Br. Med. J. *1,* 809–813 (1955)
Lorez, H.-P., Kettler, R.: Absence of degeneration of adrenergic neurons after prolonged treatment of newborn rats with debrisoquin. Acta Pharmacol. Toxicol. (Kbh) *36,* 132–144 (1975)
Loumanmäki, K., Heikkila, J., Härtel, G.: Bretylium tosylate. Adverse effects in acute myocardial infarction. Arch. Intern. Med. *135,* 515–518 (1975)
Lown, B., Ehrlich, L., Lipschulz, B., Blake, J.: Effect of digitalis in patients receiving reserpine. Circulation *24,* 1185–1191 (1961)
Lowther, C.P., Turner, R.W.D.: Guanethidine in the treatment of hypertension. Br. Med. J. *2,* 776–781 (1963)
Luizzi, A., Foppen, F.H., Angeletti, P.U.: Adrenaline, noradrenaline and dopamine levels in brain and heart after administration of 6-hydroxydopamine and guanethidine to newborn mice. Biochem. Pharmacol. *23,* 1041–1044 (1974)
Luke, R.G., Kennedy, A.C.: Methyldopa in treatment of hypertension due to chronic renal disease. Br. Med. J. *1,* 27–30 (1964)
Lüllmann, H., Lüllmann-Rauch, R., Wassermann, O.: Arzneimittelinduzierte Phospholipidspeicherkrankheit. Dtsch. Med. Wochenschr. *98,* 1616–1625 (1973)
Lund-Johansen, P.: Hemodynamic changes in long-term alpha-methyldopa therapy of essential hypertension. Acta Med. Scand. *192,* 221–226 (1972)
Lund-Johansen, P., Hemodynamic changes in long-term therapy of essential hypertension: A comparative study of diuretics, α-methyldopa and clonidine. Clin. Sci. Mol. Med. *45,* Suppl. 1, 199S–203S (1973)
Mack, T.M., Henderson, B.E., Gerkins, V.R., Arthur, M., Baptista, J., Pike, M.: Reserpine and breast cancer in a retirement community. N. Engl. J. Med. *292,* 1366–1371 (1975)
Mackay, I.R., Cowling, D.C., Hurley, T.H.: Drug-induced autoimmune disease: Haemolytic anaemia and lupus cells after treatment with methyldopa. Med. J. Aust. *2,* 1047–1050 (1968)
Macmahon, F.G., Ryan, J.R., Jain, A.K., Vargas, R., Vanov, S.K.: Guanabenz in essential hypertension. Clin. Pharmacol. Ther. *21,* 272–277 (1977)

Maddrey, W.C., Boitnott, J.K.: Severe hepatitis from methyldopa. Gastroenterology *68*,351–360 (1975)
Malmfors, T., Thoenen, H. (eds.): 6-hydroxydopamine and catecholamine neurons. Amsterdam-London: North-Holland, (1971)
Malmquist, J., Oates, J.A.: Effects of adrenergic neuron-blocking guanidine derivatives on mitochondrial metabolism. Biochem. Pharmacol. *17*, 1845–1854 (1968)
Manohitharajah, S.M., Jenkins, W.J., Roberts, P.D., Clarke, R.C.: Methyldopa and associated thrombocytopenia. Br. Med. J. *1*, 494 (1971)
Marcus, G.J., Stevenson, M., Brown, T.: Alpha-methyldopa-induced immune thrombocytopenia. Am. J. Clin. Path. *64*, 113–115 (1975)
Mårdh, P.A., Belfrage, I., Naversten, E.: Sialadenitis following treatment with α-methyldopa. Acta Med. Scand. *195*, 333–335 (1974)
Marino, A.: Ricerche sperimentali su elcuni effetti psichici e cardiaci dell' 1-fenil-2-pirrolodinopentano e della stricnina. Rass. med. Sper. *9*, 1–33 (1962)
Marley, E., Pare, C.M.B.: Cardiac failure with reserpine. Br. Med. J. *1*, 267–269 (1956)
Marshall, A.J., Roberts, C.J.C., Barritt, D.W.: Raynaud's phenomenon as side effect of betablockers in hypertension. Br. Med. J. *1*, 1498–1499 (1976)
Mathisen, H.J.: Clinical studies with methyl-dopa (Aldomet) in patients with hypertension during two years. Acta Med. Scand. *174*, 183–192 (1963)
Matthews, M.R., Raisman, G.: A light and electron microscopic study of the cellular response to axonal injury in the superior cervical ganglion of the rat. Proc. R. Soc. Lond. [Biol.] *181*, 43–79 (1972)
Matts, S.G.F.: A comparative trial of clonidine (Catapres) and guanethidine (Ismelin) in the treatment of hypertension. J. Int. Med. Res. *3*, 21–25 (1975)
Maxwell, R.A., Mull, R.P., Plummer, A.J.: [2-octahydro-(1-azocinyl)-ethyl]-guanidine sulfate (CIBA 5864-SU), a new synthetic antihypertensive agents. Experientia (Basel) *15*, 267 (1959)
Maxwell, R.A., Plummer, A.J., Schneider, F., Povalski, H., Daniel, A.I.: Pharmacology of [2-(octahydro-1-azocinyl)-ethyl] guanidine sulfate (SU-5864). J. Pharmacol. Exp. Ther. *128*, 22–29 (1960)
McAllister, R.G.: Guanethidine in antihypertensive therapy: Experience with an oral loading regimen. J. Clin. Pharmacol. *15*, 771–778 (1975)
McGeer, P.L., Boulding, J.E., Gibson, W.C., Foulkes, R.G.: Drug-induced extrapyramidal reactions. J. Am. Med. Assoc. *177*, 665–670 (1961)
McKinney, W.T., Kane, F.J., Depression with the use of alpa-methyldopa. Am. J. Psychiat. *124*, 80–81 (1967)
McKinney, W.T., Eising, R.G., Moran, E.C., Suomi, S.J.: Effects of reserpine on the social behavior of rhesus monkeys. Dis. Nerv. Syst. *32*, 735–741 (1971)
McLaren, E.H.: Severe hypertension produced by interaction of phenylpropanolamine with methyldopa and oxprenolol. Br. Med. J. *2*, 283–284 (1976)
McMartin, C., Rondel, R.K., Vinter, J., Allan, B.R., Humberstone, P.M., Leishman, A.W.D., Sandler, G., Thirkette, J.L.: The fate of guanethidine in two hypertensive patients. Clin. Pharmacol. Ther. *11*, 423–431 (1970)
McQueen, E.G.: New Zealand Committee on Adverse Drug Reactions: Ninth annual report 1974. N. Z. Med. J. *80*, 305–311 (1974)
Melick, R., McGregor, M.: Reserpine and extracellular-fluid volume. N. Engl. J. Med. *256*, 1000–1002 (1957)
Merceron, R., Weiss, Y., Safar, M., Milliez, P.: Comparaison des effets hémodynamiques de la clonidine, de l'alpha méthyl dopa, de la guanéthidine, et de la réserpine: Etude preliminaire. Thérapie *28*, 93–101 (1973)
Merck Institute Information. In: Barnes, C.D., Eltherington, L.G. Drug dosage in laboratory animals. Berkeley-Los Angeles-London: University California Press, (1973), p. 162
Meyer, J.F., McAllister, C.K., Goldberg, L.I.: Insidious and prolonged antagonism of guanethidine by amitriptyline. J. Am. Med. Assoc. *213*, 1487–1488 (1970)
Miller, A.C.: Methyldopa-induced granulomatous hepatitis. J. Am. Med. Assoc. *235*, 2001–2002 (1976)

Miller, R.D., Way, W.L., Eger, E.I.: The effects of alpha-methyldopa, guanethidine and iproniazid on minimum alveolar anesthetic requirement (MAC). Anestesiology *29*, 1153–1158 (1968)
Misage, J.R., McDonald, R.H.: Antagonism of hypotensive action of bethanidine by "common cold" remedy. Br. Med. J. *4*, 347 (1970)
Mitchell, J.R., Oates, J.A.: Guanethidine and related agents. I. Mechanism of the selective blockade of adrenergic neurons and its antagonism by drugs. J. Pharmacol. Exp. Ther. *172*, 100–107 (1970)
Mitchell, J.R., Arias, L., Oates, J.A.: Antagonism of the antihypertensive action of guanethidine sulfate by desipramine hydrochloride. J. Am. Med. Assoc. *202*, 973–975 (1967)
Mitchell, J.R., Cavanaugh, J.H., Arias, L., Oates, J.A.: Guanethidine and related agents. III. Antagonism of drugs which inhibit the norepinephrine pump in man. J. Clin. Invest. *49*, 1596–1604 (1970)
Mohammed, S., Hanenson, I.B., Magenheim, H.G., Gaffney, T.E.: The effects of alpha-methyldopa on renal function in hypertensive patients. Am. Heart J. *76*, 21–27 (1968)
Mohan, M.C., Johnson, E.S.: Hypothermia during treatment with alpha methyl dopa (a case report). J. Assoc. Physicians India *23*, 221–225 (1975)
Montuschi, E., Lovel, T.W.I.: Guanoxan in hypertension. Lancet *2*, 1339–1340 (1964)
Moore, J.I., Moran, N.C.: Cardiac contractile force responses to ephedrine and other sympathomimetic amines in dogs after pretreatment with reserpine. J. Phamacol. Exp. Ther. *136*, 89–96 (1962)
Morin, Y., Turmel, L., Fortier, J.: Methyldopa: Clinical studies in arterial hypertension. Am. J. Med. Sci. *248*, 633–639 (1964)
Morrison, A.B., Webster, R.A.: Drug-induced experimental parkinsonism. Neuropharmacology *12*, 715–724 (1973a)
Morrison, A.B., Webster, R.A.: Reserpine rigidity and adrenergic neurones. Neuropharmacology *12*, 725–733 (1973b)
Moyer, J.H.: Cardiovascular and renal hemodynamic responses to reserpine and clinical results of using this agent for the treatment in hypertension. Ann. N. Y. Acad. Sci. *59*, 82–94 (1954)
Moyer, J.H., Hughes, W., Huggins, R.: The cardiovascular and renal hemodynamic response to the administration of reserpine (Serpasil). Am. J. Med. Sci. *227*, 640–648 (1954)
Mroczek, W.J., Leibel, B.A., Finnerty, F.A.: Comparison of clonidine and methyldopa in hypertensive patients receiving a diuretic. Am. J. Cardiol. *29*, 712–717 (1972)
Muelheims, G.H., Brown, G.O., Effect of guanethidine therapy on total blood volume in patients with essential hypertension. Proc. Soc. Exp. Biol. Med. *109*, 613–615 (1962)
Muelheims, G.H., Entrup, R.W., Paiewonsky, D., Mierzwiak, D.S.: Increased sensitivity of the heart to catecholamine-induced arrhythmias following guanethidine. Clin. Pharmacol. Ther. *6*, 757–762 (1965)
Mull, R.P., Maxwell, R.A.: Guanethidine and related adrenergic neuronal blocking agents. In: Antihypertensive agents. Schlitter, E. (ed.). New York-London: Academic Press, (1967), pp. 115–149
Mull, R.P., Maxwell, R.A., Plummer, A.J.: Antihypertensive activity of hexahydro-1-azepine-propionamidoxime. Nature (Lond.) *180*, 1200–1201 (1957)
Müller, J.C., Pryor, W.W., Gibbons, J.E., Organ, E.S.: Depression and anxiety occurring during rauwolfia therapy. J. Am. Med. Assoc. *159*, 836–839 (1955)
Müller, J.M., Schlitter, E., Bein, H.J.: Reserpin, der sedative Wirkstoff aus Rauwolfia serpentina Benth. Experientia (Basel) *8*, 338 (1952)
Mullick, F.G., McAllister, H.A.: Myocarditis associated with methyldopa therapy. J. Am. Med. Assoc. *237*, 1699–1701 (1977)
Murr, G.: Einfluß des Reserpins auf die Nasenschleimhaut. Laryngol. Rhinol. Otol. (Stuttg.) *55*, 178–185 (1976)
Muscholl, E.: Adrenergic false transmitters. In: Catecholamins. Blaschko, H., Muscholl, E. (eds.): Handbook of experimental pharmacology, Vol. 33, Berlin-Heidelberg-New York: Springer Verlag, (1972), pp. 618–660
Muscholl, E., Maître, L.: Release by sympathetic stimulation of α-methyl-noradrenaline stored in the heart after administration of α-methyldopa. Experientia (Basel) *19*, 658–659 (1963)

Nash, D.T.: Clinical trial with guanabenz, a new antihypertensive agent. J. Clin. Pharmacol. *13,* 416–421 (1973)
Nayler, W.G.: A direct effect of reserpine on ventricular contractility. J. Pharmacol. Exp. Ther. *139,* 222–229 (1963)
Neely, C.L., Kraus, A.P.: Mechanisms of drug-induced hemolytic anemia. Adv. Intern. Med. *18,* 59–76 (1972)
Neuhaus, A.W.: Nebenwirkungen psychotroper Substanzen an den Epithelien der Milchdrüse, des Uterus unter der Nebenniere bei der Ratte. Acta Anat. (Basel) *90,* 101–116 (1974)
Newball, H.H., Byar, D.P.: Does reserpine increase prolactin and exacerbate cancer of prostate. Urology *11,* 525–529 (1973)
Newman, R.J.: Sexual dysfunction due to methyldopa. Br. Med. J. *4,* 106 (1974)
Nielsen, G.D.: Guanethidine induced acute hypersensitivity to noradrenaline in anaesthetized rats. Acta Pharmacol. Toxicol. (Kbh) *40,* 273–279 (1977a)
Nielsen, G.D.: Guanethidine induced sympathectomy in the adult rat. I. Functional effects following subacute administration. Acta Pharmacol. Toxicol. (Kbh) *41,* 203–208 (1977b)
Nielsen, G.D.; Guanethidine induced sympathectomy in the adult rat. II. Functional effects following chronic administration. Acta Pharmacol. Toxicol. (Kbh) *41,* 209–217 (1977c)
Nies, A.S.: Adverse reactions and interactions limiting the use of antihypertensive drugs. Am. J. Med. *58,* 495–503 (1975)
Nowack, P.: The effect of guanethidine on renal, cerebral and cardiac hemodynamics. In: Hypertension – recent advances. Brest, A.N., Moyer, J.H. (eds.): Philadelphia: Lea & Fibiger, (1961) pp. 444–448
Nydegger, U., Miescher, P.A.: Immunological mechanisms in drug-induced blood dyscrasias. J. Clin. Path. *28,* Suppl. 9, 46–49 (1975)
Oates, J.: Distribution of guanidinium antihypertensives – mechanism of their selective action. Drug Intelligence and Clinical Pharmacy *4,* 349 (1970)
Oates, J.A.: Drug interactions in man. A critical appraisal of their relative role in interindividual variations in drug response. In: Pharmacology and the future of man. Problems of therapy. Okita, T., Acheson, G.H. (eds.). Basel: Karger, Vol. 3, 1973 pp. 191–199
Oates, J.A., Gillespie, L., Udenfriend, S., Sjoerdsma, A.: Decarboxylase inhibition and blood pressure reduction by α-methyl-3,4-dihydroxy-DL-phenylalanine. Science *131,* 1890–1891 (1960)
Oates, J.A., Seligman, A.W., Clark, M.A., Rousseau, P., Lee, R.E.: The relative efficacy of guanethidine, methyldopa and pargyline as antihypertensive agents. N. Engl. J. Med. *273,* 729–734 (1965)
Ober, K.F., Wang, R.I.H.: Drug interactions with guanethidine. Clin. Pharmacol. Ther. *14,* 190–195 (1973)
O'Donnell, S.R., Saar, N.: The effects of 6-hydroxydopamine and guanethidine on peripheral adrenergic nerves in the guinea pig. Eur. J. Pharmacol. *28,* 251–256 (1974)
O'Fallon, W.M., Labarthe, D.R., Kurland, L.T.: Rauwolfia derivatives and breast cancer. Lancet *2,* 292–296 (1975)
Onesti, G., Brest, A.N., Nowack, P., Kasparian, H., Moyer, J.H.: Pharmacodynamic effects of alpha-methyl dopa in hypertensive subjects. Am. Heart. J. *67,* 32–38 (1964)
Onesti, G., Laschiazza, D., Brest, A.N., Moyer, J.H.: Cardiac and renal hemodynamic effects of debrisoquin sulfate in hypertensive subjects. Clin. Pharmacol. Ther. *7,* 17–20 (1966)
O'Regan, J.B.: Adverse interaction of lithium carbonate and methyldopa. Can. Med. Assoc. J. *115,* 385–386 (1976)
Page,I.H., Dustan, H.P.: A bew, potent antihypertensive drug. Preliminary study of [2-(octahydro-1-azocinyl)-ethyl]-guanidine sulfate (guanethidine). J. Am. Med. Assoc. *170,* 1265–1271 (1959)
Page, I.H., Dustan, H.P.: Persistence of normal blood pressure after discontinuing treatment in hypertensive patients. Circulation *25,* 433–436 (1962)
Page, I.H., Hurely, R.E., Dustan, H.P.: The prolonged treatment of hypertension with guanethidine. J. Am. Med. Assoc. *175,* 543–549 (1961)
Parks, V.J., Sandison, A.G., Skinner, S.L., Whelan, R.F.: The mechanism of the vasodilator action of reserpine in man. Clin. Sci. Mol. Med. *20,* 289–295 (1961)

Pascual, A.V., Julius, S.: Short term effectiveness and hemodynamic actions of guanadrel, a new sympatholytic drug. Curr. Ther. Res. *14,* 333–342 (1972)
Paykel, E.S.: Hallucinosis on combined methyldopa and pargyline. Br. Med. J. *1,* 803 (1966)
Pearson, M., Meerkin, M., Baird, C.: Aldomet interference with the Babson method of SGOT analysis. Med. J. Aust. *2,* 84–85 (1972)
Peart, W.S., MacMahon, M.T.: Clinical trial of 2-guanidinomethyl (1,4) benzodioxan (compound 1003). Br. Med. J. *1,* 398–402 (1964)
Peaston, M.J.T.: Parkinsonism associated with alpha-methyldopa therapy. Br. Med. J. *2,* 168 (1964)
Perera, G.A.: Edema and congestive failure related to administration of rauwolfia serpentina. J. Am. Med. Assoc. *159,* 439 (1955)
Perry, H.M., Chaplin, H., Carmody, S., Haynes, C., Frei, C.: Immunologic findings in patients receiving methyldopa: A prospective study. J. Lab. Clin. Med. *78,* 905–917 (1971)
Pettinger, W.A., Horwitz, D., Sjoerdsma, A.: Lactation due to methyldopa. Br. Med. J. *1,* 146/ (1963 a)
Pettinger, W.A., Horwitz, D., Spector, S., Sjoerdsma, A.: Enhancement by methyldopa of tyramine sensitivity in man. Nature (Lond.) *200,* 1107–1108 (1963 b)
Pettinger, W.A., Korn, A., Spiegel, H., Solomon, H.M., Pocelinko, R., Abrams, W.B.: Debrisoquin, a selective inhibitor of intraneuronal monoamine oxidase in man. Clin. Phamacol. Ther. *10,* 667–674 (1969)
Petz, L.D., Fudenberg, H.H.: Immunologic mechanisms in drug-induced cytopenias, Progr. Hematol. *9,* 185–206 (1975)
Pfeifer, H.J., Greenblatt, D.J., Koch-Weser, J.: Clinical toxicity of reserpine in hospitalized patients: A report from the Boston Collaborative Drug Surveillance Program. Am. J. Med. Sci. *271,* 269–276 (1976)
Pirsig, W., Proescher, K., Donath, K.: Zur Ultrastruktur geschädigter Nerven in der Parotis bei Guanacline-therapierten Hypertonikern: morphologische Substrate zum Parotisschmerz. Arch. klin. exp. Ohren Nasen Kehlkopfheilk. *205,* 103–109 (1973)
Platt, R., Sears, H.T.N.: Reserpine in severe hypertension. Lancet *1,* 401–403 (1956)
Plummer, A.J., Earl, A., Schneider, A.E., Trapold, J., Barrett, W.: Pharmacology of rauwolfia alkaloids, including reserpine. Ann. N. Y. Acad. Sci. *59,* 8–21 (1955)
Plummer, A.J., Barrett, W.E., Maxwell, R.A., Finocchio, D., Lucas, R.A., Earl, A.E.: Hypotensive properties of syrosingopine, SU-3118, an ester of methyl reserpate. Arch. Int. Pharmacodyn. Ther. *119,* 245–257 (1959)
Pozos, R.S., Holbrook, J.R.: Tremoregenesis: Effects of reserpine on the substantia nigra. Exp. Neurol. *32,* 317–330 (1971)
Prichard, B.N.C.: Aspects of the evaluation of antihypertensive drugs. Arch. int. Pharmacodyn. Ther. *192,* suppl., 193–208 (1971)
Prichard, B.N.C., Johnston, A.W., Hill, I.D., Rosenheim, M.L.: Bethanidine, guanethidine, and methyldopa in treatment of hypertension: A within-patient comparison. Br. Med. J. *1,* 135–144 (1968)
Pugsley, E.B.: Adverse reactions to methyldopa. Can. Med. Assoc. J. *106,* 1064 (1972)
Quetsch, R.M., Achor, R.W.P., Litin, E.M., Faucett, R.L.: Depressive reactions in hypertensive patients. Circulation *19,* 366–375 (1959)
Rahn, K.H., Rupp, W.: Plasma levels and urinary excretion of guanethidine in hypertensive patients. Acta Pharmacol. Toxicol (Kbh) *29,* suppl. 4, 46 (1971)
Ramsay, L.E.: Liver dysfunction in hypertension. Lancet *2,* 111–114 (1977)
Ravina, J.H.: Les thérapeutiques dangereuses chez la femme enciente. Presse Med. *72,* 3057 (1964)
Rechardt, L., Hervonen, H.: Ultrastructural changes in the neural lobe of the rat pituitary induced by reserpine treatment. Experientia (Basel) *31,* 1205–1207 (1975)
Redman, C.W.G., Beilin, L.J., Bonnar, J., Ounsted, M.K.: Fetal outcome in trial of antihypertensive treatment in pregnancy. Lancet *2,* 753–756 (1976)
Rehman, O.U., Keith, T.A., Gall, E.A.: Methyldopa-induced submassive hepatic necrosis, J. Am. Med. Assoc. *224,* 1390–1392 (1973)
Reilly, J.F., Ahlstrom, A.P., Watts, J.S., Cassidy, P.S., Lusky, L.M.: Influence of age, sex, and cold exposure on susceptibility to reserpine-induced gastric lesions. Toxicol. Appl. Pharmacol. *15,* 97–105 (1969)

Reusch, C.S.: The cardiorenal hemodynamic effects of antihypertensive therapy with reserpine. Am. Heart. J. *64,* 643–649 (1962)
Richardson, D.W., Wyso, E.M.: Human pharmacology of guanethidine. Ann. N. Y. Acad. Sci. *88,* 944–955 (1960)
Richardson, D.W., Wyso, E.M., Magee, J.H., Cavell, G.C.: Circulatory effects of guanethidine. Circulation *22,* 184–190 (1960)
Richter, K.: Einfluß des Reserpins auf das exokrine Pankreas der Ratte. Zentralbl. Allg. Pathol. *119,* 329 (1975)
Roberts, J., Modell, W.: Pharmacological evidence for the importance of catecholamines in cardiac rhythmicity. Circ. Res. *9,* 171–176 (1961)
Roberts, J., Ito, R., Reilly, J., Cairoli, V.J.: Influence of reserpine and βTM10 on digitalis-induced ventricular arrhytmia. Circ. Res. *13,* 149–158 (1963)
Robinson, B.: Breast changes in the male and female with chlorpromazine or reserpine therapy. Med. J. Aust. *2,* 239–241 (1957)
Rodman, J.S., Deutsch, D.J., Gertman, S.I.: Methyldopa hepatitis. A report of six cases and review of the literature. Am. J. Med. *60,* 941–948 (1976)
Roland, E.Q., Safar, M.E., Lelquen, C.E., Aboras, Y.A., Weiss, Y.A., Milliez, P.M.: Effect of certain antiadrenergic agents an systolic time intervals in essential hypertension. Eur. J. Clin. Pharmacol. *11,* 423–427 (1977)
Romeo, S.G., Whalen, R.E., Tindall, J.P.: Intra-arterial administration of reserpine. Arch. Intern. Med. *125,* 825–829 (1970)
Rønnov-Jessen, V.: Blood-volume during treatment of hypertension. Acta. Med. Scand. *174,* 307–310 (1963)
Rønnov-Jessen, V., Hansen, J.: Blood volume and exchangeable sodium during treatment of hypertension with guanethidine and hydrochlorothiazide. Acta Med. Scand. *186,* 255–263 (1969)
Rosenbloom, S.E., Shapera, R.P., Goldbloom, R.S., Sheps, M.C., Shapiro, A.P.: Technic of controlled drug assay. III. Comparison of guanethidine, mecamylamine and a placebo in the hypertensive patient. N. Engl. J. Med. *268,* 797–803 (1963)
Rosendorff, C., Marsden, C.D., Cranston, W.I.: Clinical evaluation of debrisoquin in the treatment of hypertension. Arch. J. Intern. Med. *122,* 487–490 (1968)
Ruedy, J., Davies, R.O.: A comparative clinical trial fo guanoxan and guanethidine in essential hypertension. Clin. Pharmacol. Ther. *8,* 38–47 (1967)
Russo, C., Mendlowitz, M.: The effect of guancydine on blood pressure, vascular reactivity, and norepinephrine uptake in essential hypertension. Clin. Pharmacol. Ther. *13,* 875–878 (1972)
Safar, M., Simon, A., Maiz, H.B., Weiss, Y., Milliez, P.: Hypertensions artérielles sévères traitées médicalement. Nouv. Presse Med. *4,* 1403 1406 (1975)
Samee, H.J., Klug, P., Zalandek, G., Sterz, H.: Orthostatische Hypotonie nach Cyclazenin-Medikation. Wien Med. Wochenschr. *120,* 56–60 (1970)
Sandler, G., Leishmann, A.W.D., Humberstone, P.M.: Guanethidine-resistent hypertension. Circulation *38,* 542–551 (1968)
Sannerstedt, B., Bojs, G., Varnauskas, E., Werkö, L.: Alpha-methyldopa in arterial hypertension. Clinical, renal, and hemodynamic studies. Acta Med. Scand. *174,* 53–67 (1963)
Sannerstedt, R., Conway, J.: Hemodynamic and vascular responses to antihypertensive treatment with adrenergic blocking agents: A review. Am. Heart J. *79,* 122–127 (1970)
Sannerstedt, R., Varnauskas, E., Werkö, L.: Hemodynamic effects of methyldopa (Aldomet) at rest and during exercise in patients with arterial hypertension. Acta Med. Scand. *171,* 75–82 (1962)
Sataline, L., Lowell, D.: Delayed hepatotoxicity from methyldopa. Conn. Med. *39,* 775–776 (1975a)
Sataline, L., Lowell, D.: Methyldopa toxicity. Gastroenterology *70,* 148–149 (1957b)
Schlitter, E., Druey, J., Marxer, A.: Antihypertensive agents. In: Progress in drug research. Jucker, E. (ed.): Basel-Stuttgart: Birkhäuser Verlag, Vol. 4, (1962) pp. 297–351
Schreader, C.J., Etzl, M.M.: Premature ventricular contractions due to Rauwolfia therapy. J. Am. Med. Assoc. *162,* 1256 (1956)
Schroeder, H.A., Perry, H.M.: Psychosis apparently produced by reserpine. J. Am. Med. Assoc. *159,* 839–841 (1955)

Schweitzer, I.L., Peters, R.L.: Acute submassive hepatic necrosis due to methyldopa. Gastroenterology *66*, 1203–1211 (1974)
Scott, J.N., McDevitt, D.G.: Rebound hypertension after acute methyldopa withdrawal. Br. Med. J. *2*, 367 (1976)
Scott, M.G., Zaimis, E.: Histological changes in the heart following treatment with reserpine. J. Physiol. (Lond.) *162*, 8P (1962)
Seedat, Y.K., Vawda, E.I.: The Coombs test and methyldopa. Lancet *1*, 427 (1968)
Seedat, Y.K., Vawda, E.I.: Direct Coombs test and methyldopa. Lancet *1*, 97 (1972)
Shand, D.G., Nies, A.S., McAllister, R.G., Oates, J.A.: An improved method for treating severe hypertension with guanethidine. Clin. Res. *20*, 413 (1972)
Shand, D.G., Nies, A.S., McAllister, R.G., Oates, J.A.: A loading-maintenance regimen for more rapid initiation of the effect of guanethidine. Clin. Pharmacol. Ther. *18*, 139–144 (1975)
Shapiro, A.P., Teng, H.C.: Technic of controlled drug assay illustrated by a comparative study of Rauwolfia serpentina, phenobarbital and placebo in the hypertensive patient. N. Engl. J. Med. *256*, 970–975 (1957)
Sharon, E., Paolino, J.S., Kaplan, D.: Hematemesis after reserpine for Raynaud's phenomenon. Ann. Intern. Med. *77*, 479 (1972)
Sheps, S.G., Schirger, A., Osmundson, P.J., Fairbairn, J.F.: Methyldopa for treatment of hypertension. J. Am. Med. Assoc. *184*, 616–621 (1963)
Sherman, J.D., Love, D.E., Harrington, J.F.: Anemia, positive lupus and rheumatoid factors with methyldopa. Arch. Intern. Med. *120*, 321–326 (1967)
Shore, P.A., Brodie, B.B.: LSD-like effects elicited by reserpine in rabbits pretreated with iproniazid. Proc. Soc. Exp. Biol. Med. *94*, 433–435 (1957)
Silva, J.A.F. de, Capaceia, J.P. de O., Cohen, I.: Assessment of a new antihypertensive agent, 2,6-dichlorbenzylidene amino guanidine acetate (guanabenz). A double-blind, crossover trial against placebo. Pharmatherapeutica *1*, 1–7 (1976)
Simpson, F.O.: Deserpidine: A controlled trial of a Rauwolfia alkaloid. Med. J. Aust. *2*, 821–823 (1961)
Simpson, F.O. (ed.): Symposium on hypertension. Drugs *11*, Suppl. 1, 1–204 (1976)
Singh, H.P., Hebert, M.A., Gault, M.H.: Effect of some drugs on clinical laboratory values as determined by the Technicon SMA 12/60. Clin. Chem. *18*, 137–144 (1972)
Skinner, C., Coull, D.C., Johnston, A.W.: Antagonism of the hypotensive action of bethanidine and debrisoquine by tricyclic antidepressants. Lancet *2*, 564–566 (1969)
Smirk, H.: Hypotensive action of methyldopa. Br. Med. J. *1*, 146–151 (1963a)
Smirk, H.: The hypotensive action of B. W. 467C60. Lancet *1*, 743–746 (1963b)
Smirk, F.H., McQueen, E.G.: Comparison of rescinnamine and reserpine as hypotensive agents. Lancet *2*, 115–116 (1955)
Smith, A.J.: Clinical features of fluid retention complicating treatment with guanethidine. Circulation *31*, 485–489 (1965a)
Smith, A.J.: Fluid retention produced by guanethidine. Circulation *31*, 490–496 (1965b)
Smith, C.: Effects of reserpine and alpha-methyldopa upon adrenergic nerve function in the guinea pig heart. In: The nervous system in arterial hypertension. Julius, S., Esler, M.D. (eds.): Springfield-Illinois: Charles C. Thomas, (1976) pp. 442–453
Smith, W.M., Bachman, B., Galante, J.G., Hanowell, E.G., Johnson, W.P., Koch, C.E., Korfmacher, S.D., Thurm, R.H., Broomer, L.: Co-operative clinical trial of alpha-methyldopa. III. Double-blind control comparison of alpha-methyldopa and chlorothiazide and chlorothiazide and Rauwolfia. Ann. Intern. Med. *65*, 657–671 (1966)
Smulyan, H., Markason, C.R., Keighley, M., Cuddy, R.P., Eich, R.H., Lyons, R.H.: Effects of reserpine on the circulation and on the circulatory responses to tilting and norepinephrine. Am. J. Cardiol. *11*, 743–756 (1963)
Snaith, R.P., McCourbrie, M.: Antihypertensive drugs and depression. Psychol. Med. *4*, 393–398 (1974)
Sneddon, J.M., Turner, P.: Ephedrine mydriasis in hypertension and the response to treatment. Clin. Pharmacol. Ther. *10*, 64–71 (1969a)
Sneddon, J.M., Turner, P.: The interaction of local guanethidine and sympathomimetic amines in the human eye. Arch. Ophthal. *81*, 622–627 (1969b)

Sobel, D.E.: Fetal damage due to ECT, insulin coma, chlorpromazine, or reserpine. Arch. gen. Psychiatry. *2*, 606–611 (1960)
Soloff, L.A.: Clinical pharmacology and therapeutic use of bretylium tosylate. In: Hypertension – recent advances. Brest, A.N., Moyer, J.H. (eds.): Philadelphia: Lea & Fibiger, (1961) pp. 432–436
Soloff, L.A., Reidenberg, M., Winters, W.L., Bello, C.T.: Clinical experiences with bretylium tosylate. Ann. N. Y. Acad. Sci. *88*, 1003–1010 (1960)
Somlyo, A.P., Waye, J.D.: Abnormal lactation. Report of a case induced by reserpine and a brief review of the subject. J. Mt. Sinai Hosp. *27*, 5–9 (1960)
Spach, M.O., Bloch, R., Velly, J., Imbs, J.L., Bousquet, P., Schwartz, J.: Guérison apparante de l'hypertension artérielle. Nouv. Presse Med. *3*, 241–243 (1974)
Spann, J.F., Sonnenblick, E.H., Cooper, T., Chidsey, C.A. William, V.L., Braunwald, E.: Cardiac norepinephrine stores and the contractile state of heart muscle. Circ. Res. *19*, 317–325 (1966)
Starr, K.J., Petrie, J.C.: Drug interactions in patients on long-term oral anticoagulant and antihypertensive adrenergic neuron-blocking drugs. Br. Med. J. *4*, 133–135 (1972)
Steiner, J., Cassar, J., Mashiter, K., Dawes, I., Fraser, T.R., Breckenridge, A.: Effects of methyldopa on prolactin and growth hormone. Br. Med. J. *1*, 1186–1188 (1976)
Steiner, G., Schönbaum, E. (eds): Immunosympathectomy. Amsterdam-London-New York: Elsevier (1972)
Stern, W.C., Morgane, P.J.: Effects of reserpine on sleep and brain biogenic amine levels in the cat. Psychopharmacology *28*, 275–286 (1973)
Stevens, F.R.T.: A danger of sympathomimetic drugs. Med. J. Aust. *2*, 576 (1966)
Stitzel, R.E.: The biological fate of reserpine. Pharmacol. Rev. *28*, 179–205 (1976)
Stocks, A.E., Robertson, A.: The long-term therapy of severe hypertension with guanethidine. Am. Heart J. *73*, 569–570 (1967)
Stone, C.A., Ross, C.A., Wenger, H.C., Ludden, C.T., Blessing, J.A., Totaro, J.A., Porter, C.C.: Effect of α-methyl-3,4-dihydrocyphenylalanine (methyldopa), reserpine and related agents on some vascular responses in the dog. J. Pharmacol. Exp. Ther. *136*, 80–88 (1962)
Stone, C.A., Porter, C.C., Stavorski, J.M., Ludden, C.T., Totaro, J.A.: Antagonism of certain effects of catecholamine-depleting agents by antidepressants and related drugs. J. Pharmacol. Exp. Ther. *144*, 196–204 (1964)
Stuart, K.L., MacIver, C., Nicholson, J.A.: Outpatient treatment trial of mild and severe hypertension. Br. Med. J. *2*, 21–24 (1972)
Sun, S.-C., Sohal, R.S., Colcolough, H.L., Burch, G.E.: Histochemical and electron microscopic studies of the effects of reserpine on the heart muscle of mice. J. Pharmacol. Exp. Ther. *161*, 210–221 (1968)
Swedish Adverse Reactions Committee: Biverkninger av metyldopa under 10 år. Communication no. 26, may (1977)
Sweet, R.D., Lee, J.E., McDowell, F.H.: Methyldopa as an adjuvant to levodopa treatment of Parkinson's disease. Clin. Pharmacol. Ther. *13*, 23–27 (1972)
Talbot, F.J.: Clinical evaluation of the antihypertensive effects of debrisoquin, a new postganglionic vasodepressor agent. Med. Ann. D.C. *34*, 580–583 (1965)
Talbot, S., Smith, A.J.: Factors predisposing to postural hypotensive symptoms in the treatment of high blood pressure. Br. Heart J. *37*, 1059–1063 (1975)
Talbot, S., O'Malley, B.C., Bing, R.F.: Debrisoquine, guanethidine, and bethanidine in hypertension. Br. Med. J. *2*, 278 (1975)
Tallgren, L.G., Servo, C.: Hyperpyrexia in association with L-alpha methyl dopa. A report of two cases. Acta Med. Scand. *186*, 223–226 (1969)
Tarpley, E.L.: Controlled trial of guanethidine and methyldopa in moderate hypertension. Curr. Ther. Res. *16*, 1187–1196 (1974)
Taylor, R.E., Fregly, M.J.: Effect of reserpine on body temperature regulation of the rat. J. Pharmacol. Exp. Ther. *138*, 200–207 (1962)
Ten Pas, A., de Leeuw, N.K.M., Stacey, C.H.: Methyldopa-induced thrombocytopenia. Can. Med. Assoc. J. *95*, 322 (1966)
Tester-Dalderup, C.B.M.: Hypotensive drugs. In: Meyler's side effects of drugs. Dukes, M.N.G. (ed.): Vol. 8. Amsterdam-Oxford: Excerpta Medica, (1976) pp. 461–482

Tester-Dalderup, C.B.M.: Hypotensive drugs. In: Side effects of drugs, annual 1. Dukes, M.N.G. (ed.) Amsterdam-Oxford: Excerpa Medica, (1977) pp. 164–179
Thoenen, H.: Surgical, immunological and chemical sympathectomy. In: Catecholamines. Blaschko, H., Muscholl, E. (eds.): Handbook of experimental pharmacology, Vol. 33. Berlin-Heidelberg-New York: Springer Verlag. (1972a) pp. 813–844
Thoenen, H.: Chemical sympathectomy: A new tool in the investigation of the physiology and pharmacology of peripheral and central adrenergic neurons. In: Perspectives in neuropharmacology. Snyder, S.H. (ed.) New York-London-Toronto: Oxford University Press, (1972b) pp. 301–338
Thoenen, H., Tranzer, J.P.: The pharmacology of 6-hydroxydopamine. Annu. Rev. Pharmacol. Toxicol. *13*, 169–180 (1973)
Thomas, E., Bhula, S., Rosenthal, W.S.: Methyldopa-induced liver injury. Rapid progression to fatal postnecrotic cirrhosis. Arch. Pathol. Lab. Med. *100*, 132–135 (1976)
Thornton, W.E.: Dementia induced by methyldopa with haloperidol. N. Engl. J. Med. *294*, 1222 (1976)
Tissot, R.: The effect of certain drugs on the sleep cycle in man. In: Progress in brain research. Sleep mechanisms. Akert, K., Bally, C., Schadé, J.P. (eds.) Vol. 18, Amsterdam: Elsevier (1965) pp. 175–177
Toghill, P.J., Smith, P.G., Benton, P., Brown, R.C., Matthews, H.L.: Methyldopa liver damage. Br. Med. J. *3*, 545–548 (1974)
Trendelenburg, U.: Factors influencing the concentration of catecholamines at the receptors. In: Catecholamines. Blashcko, H., Muscholl, E. (eds.) Handbook of experimental pharmacology, Vol. 33. Berlin-Heidelberg-New York: Springer Verlag, (1972) pp. 726–761
Trendelenburg, U., Weiner, N.: Sensitivity of the nictitating membrane after various procedures. J. Pharmacol. Exp. Ther. *136*, 152–161 (1962)
Tripod, J., Bein, H.J., Meier, R.: Characterization of central effects of serpasil (reserpin, a new alkaloid of rauwolfia serpentina B) and of their antagonistic reaction. Arch. Int. Pharmacodyn. Ther. *96*, 406–425 (1954)
Tuchmann-Duplessis, H., Mercier-Parot, L.: Repercussions de la réserpine sur la gestation chez la ratte. C. R. Acad. Sci. (Paris) *243*, 410–412 (1956)
Tuchmann-Duplessis, H., Mercier-Parot, L.: Malformation foetales chez le rat traité par de fortes doses de deserpidine. C. R. Soc. Biol. (Paris) *155*, 2291 (1961)
Turkington, R.W.: Prolactin secretion in patients treated with various drugs. Arch. Intern. Med. *130*, 349–354 (1972)
Tysell, J.E., Knauer, C.M.: Hepatitis induced by methyldopa (Aldomet). Am. J. Dig. Dis. *16*, 849–855 (1971)
Vakil, R.J.: A clinical trial of Rauwolfia serpentina in essential hypertension. Br. Heart J. *2*, 350–355 (1949)
Vedin, J.A., Wilhelmsson, C.-E., Werkö, L.: Comparative study of alprenolol and methyldopa in previously untreated essential hypertension. Br. Heart J. *35*, 1285–1292 (1973)
Vejlsgaard, V.: Betanidin (Esbatal, Regulin) ved behandling af hypertension. Ugeskr. Laeger *130*, 134–136 (1968)
Vejlsgaard, V., Christensen, M., Clausen, E.: Double-blind trial of four hypotensive drugs (methyldopa and three sympatholytic agents). Br. Med. J. *2*, 598–600 (1967)
Veterans Administration Cooperative Study Group on Antihypertensive Agents: A double-blind control study of antihypertensive effectiveness of reserpine and hydralazine, and three ganglionic blocking agents. Arch. Intern. Med. *106*, 81–96 (1960)
Veterans Administration Cooperative Study Group on Antihypertensive Agents: Effects of treatment on morbidity in hypertension. II. Results in patients with diastolic blood pressure averaging 90 through 114 mm Hg. J. Am. Med. Assoc. *213*, 1143–1152 (1970)
Veterans Administration Cooperative Study Group on Antihypertensive Agents: Effects of treatment on morbidity in hypertension. III. Influence of age, diastolic pressure, and prior cardiovascular disease; further analysis of side effects. Circulation *45*, 991–1004 (1972)
Villareal, H., Exaire, J.E., Rubio, V., Dávila, H.: Effect of guanethidine and bretylium tosylate on systemic and renal hemodynamics in essential hypertension. Am. J. Cardiol. *14*, 633–640 (1964)

Vyas, G.N., Sassetti, R.J., Petz, L.D., Fudenberg, H.H.: Experimental study of aldomet-induced positive antiglobulin reaction. Br. J. Haematol. *16*, 137–143 (1969)

Wallace, D.C.: Treatment of hypertension. Hypotensive drugs and mental changes. Lancet *2*, 116–117 (1955)

Walter, I.E., Nies, A.S.: Safety of single large doses of guanethidine. Clin. Pharmacol. Ther. *21*, 706–708 (1977)

Walter, I.E., Khandelwal, J., Falkner, F., Nies, A.S.: The relationship of plasma guanthidine levels to adrenergic blockade. Clin. Pharmacol. Ther. *18*, 571–580 (1975)

Weil, M.H., Barbour, B.H., Chesne, R.B.: Alpha-methyl dopa for the treatment of hypertension. Circulation *28*, 165–174 (1963)

Weil, J.V., Chidsey, C.A.: Plasma volume expansion resulting from interference with adrebergic function in normal men. Circulation *37*, 54–61 (1968)

Weiss, Y., Merceron, R., Safar, M., Milliez, P.: Action anti-hypertensive de quatre drogues inhibant le système nerveux sympathique. Coeur Med. Interne *12*, 425–429 (1973)

Wells, J.D., Kurtay, M., Lochner, J.C., George, W.L.: Granulomatous skin lesions and alphamethyldopa. Ann. Intern. Med. *81*, 701–702 (1974)

Welsch, C.W., Meites, J.: Effects of reserpine on development of 7,12-dimethylbenzantracene induced mammary tumors in female rats. Experientia (Basel) *26*, 1133–1134 (1970)

Werboff, J., Dembicki, E.L.: Toxic effects of tranquilizers administered to gravid rats. J. Neuropsychiatry *4*, 87–91 (1962)

Werboff, J., Havlena, J.: Postnatal behavioral effects of tranquilizers administered to the gravid rat. Exp. Neurol. *6*, 263–269 (1962)

Werboff, J., Kesner, R.: Learning deficits of offspring after administration of tranquilizing drugs to the mothers. Nature (Lond.) *197*, 106–107 (1963)

Werboff, J., Gottlieb, J.S., Havlena, J., Word, T.J.: Behavioral effects of prenatal drug administration in the white rat. Pediatrics *27*, 318–324 (1961)

West, G.B.: Drugs and rat pregnancy. J. Pharm. Pharmacol. *14*, 828–830 (1962)

West, W.O.: Perforation and hemorrhage from duodenal ulcer during administration of rauwolfia serpentina: Report of five cases. Ann. Intern. Med. *48*, 1033–1039 (1959)

West, W.L., Baird, G.M., Steward, J.D., Pradhan, S.N.: Some studies on the anti-tumor effect of reserpine in mice. J. Pharmacol. Exp. Ther. *131*, 171–178 (1961)

Westfall, D.P.: The effects of denervation, cocaine, 6-hydroxydopamine and reserpine on the characteristics of drug-induced contractions of the depolarized smooth muscle of the rat and guinea-pig vas deferens. J. Pharmacol. Exp. Ther. *201*, 267–275 (1977)

White, A.G.: Methyldopa and amitriptyline, Lancet *2*, 441 (1965)

Wilcken, D.E.L., Brender, D., Shorey, D., MacDonald, G.J.: Reserpine: Effect on structure of heart muscle. Science *157*, 1332–1334 (1967a)

Wilcken, D.E.L., MacDonald, G.J., Brender, D.: Mitochondrial changes following pharmacological depletion of myocardial catecholamines. Aust. Ann. Med. *16*, 364–365 (1967b)

Wilkins, R.W., Judson, W.E.: The use of rauwolfia serpentina in hypertensive patients. N. Engl. J. Med. *248*, 48–53 (1953)

Williams, R.L., Maines, J.E., Pearson, J.E.: Direct und systemic effects of guanethidine on renal function. J. Pharmacol. Exp. Ther. *177*, 69–77 (1971)

Williams, R.B., Sherter, C.: Cardiac complications of tricyclic antidepressant therapy. Ann.Intern. Med. *74*, 395–398 (1971)

Wilson, R., Long, C.: Action of bretylium antagonised by amphetamine. Lancet *2*, 262 (1960)

Wilson, W.R., Okun, R., Tetreault, L., Fallis, N.: Methyldopa and hydrochlorothiazide in primary hypertension. J. Am. Med. Assoc. *185*, 819–825 (1963)

Wilson, B.N., Wimberley, N.A.: Production of premature ventricular contractions by Rauwolfia. J. Am. Med. Assoc. *159*, 1363–1364 (1955)

Withrington, P., Zaimis, E.: The reserpine-treated cat. Br. J. Pharmacol. *17*, 380–391 (1961)

Withrington, P., Zaimis, E.: Cardiovascular effects produced in cats by the chronic administration of small doses of reserpine. Carciovasc. Res. *1*, 52–62 (1967)

Wollam, G.L., Gifford, R.W., Tarazi, R.C.: Antihypertensive drugs: Clinical pharmacology and therapeutic use. Drugs *14*, 420–460 (1977)

Wollweber, H., Wilms, H., Hiltmann, R., Stoepel, K., Kroneberg, G.: Guanidinoalkyl-aza-cycloalkane: Chemische Struktur und antihypertensive Wirkung. Arzneim. Forsch. *21,* 2089–2100 (1971)

Wongs, H.Y.C., Nightingale, T.E., David, S.N., Orimlikwe, S.O., Reinshagen, J.A.: Effects of exercise, guanethidine or its combination on hemodynamic changes in atherosclerotic cockerels. Physiologist *18,* 455 (1975)

Woods, J.W., Blythe, W.B., Huffines, W.D.: Management of malignant hypertension complicated by renal insufficiency. N. Engl. J. Med. *291,* 10–14 (1974)

Woosley, R.L., Nies, A.S.: Guanethidine. N. Engl. J. Med. *295,* 1053–1057 (1976)

Woosley, R.L., Walter, I., Oates, J.A., Nies, A.S.: Antagonism of the antihypertensive and sympathoglegic effects of guanethidine by ephedrine in man. Clin. Res. *24,* 259A (1976)

Worlledge, S.M., Carstairs, K.C., Dacie, J.V.: Autoimmune haemolytic anaemia associated with α-methyldopa therapy. Lancet *2,* 135–139 (1966)

Yamadori, A., Albert, M.L.: Involuntary movement disorder caused by methyldopa. N. Engl. J. Med. *286,* 610 (1972)

Yen,H.C.Y., Katz, M.H., Krop, S.: Effects of various drugs on 3,4-dihydroxyphenylalanine (DL-DOPA)-induced excitation (aggressive behavior) in mice. Toxicol. Appl. Pharmacol. *17,* 597–604 (1970)

Zaimis, E.: Reserpine-induced circulatory failure. Nature (Lond.) *192,* 521–523 (1961)

Zaimis, E.: Functional, biochemical, and morphological changes produced by hypotensive drugs. In: Antihypertensive therapy. Gross, F. (ed.) Berlin-Heidelberg-New York: Springer Verlag, (1966) pp. 59–70

Zaimis, E. (ed): Nerve growth factor and its antiserum. Athlone Press of the University of London (1972)

Zarday, Z., Rosenthal, W.S., Wolff, F.W.: Severe liver toxicity after methyldopa. N. Y. State J. Med. *2,* 1897–1899 (1967)

Zimmermann, A.M., Harris, L.S.: Microcirculation: Effects of guanethidine and reserpine. J. Pharmacol. Exp. Ther. *142,* 76–82 (1963)

Zimmerman, H.J.: Liver disease caused by medical agents. Med. Clin. North. Am. *59,* 897–907 (1975)

CHAPTER 5

Clinical Features of Adrenergic Agonists and Antagonists

B.N.C. PRICHARD, C.W.I. OWENS, and J. TUCKMAN

A. Alpha- and Beta-Adrenoceptor Agonists

I. Introduction

LANGLEY (1905) first suggested that adrenergic receptors contained inhibitory and excitatory receptor substances. This concept was supported by DALE's (1906) observations that, while the excitatory actions of adrenaline were blockaded by ergot, the inhibitory ones were not, which suggested the existence of two types of adrenergic receptors. AHLQUIST (1948) extended this concept when he studied the effect of six sympathomimetic amines on a variety of adrenergic responses. Their order of potency had two distinct sequences. One sequence, involving predominantly excitatory actions, was termed "α-effects". Adrenaline was the most potent stimulant of the α-receptor, followed by noradrenaline. The second sequence was called "β-effects"; these were predominantly inhibitory, but included cardiac stimulation. At the β-site, isoprenaline was most active, L-adrenaline was second in activity, adrenaline was the third most active and noradrenaline the least potent.

Stimulation of α-receptors leads to vasoconstriction in the coronary and peripheral vasculature whilst β-receptors mediate cardiac (β_1) or peripheral vascular activity and metabolism (β_2) (LANDS et al., 1967). More recently the α-receptors have also been subdivided into α_1 (postsynaptic) and α_2 (presynaptic) according to the action of various drugs (LANGER, 1974) 8 reently but the exact anatomical location has been disputed. For example, clonidine and possibly ergometrine stimulate the α_2-receptor (MARSHALL et al., 1977b) whilst phenoxybenzamine is an inhibitor. Prazosin inhibits the α_1-receptor.

The immediate precursor of noradrenaline and putative transmitter dopamine, also activates specific receptors of clinical relevance especially in the kidney but also in the mesentery and brain (GOLDBERG et al., 1978).

The distribution of adrenergic receptors are listed in Table 1, whilst the structures and pharmacological characteristics of the naturally occurring and synthetic α- and β-adrenoceptor stimulants discussed in this section are shown in Table 2.

II. Mode of Action

1. Non-Selective

The pharmacology of the catecholamines, the naturally occurring sympathomimetics, is comprehensively summarised by INNES and NICKERSON (1975). *Adrenaline* activates both α- and β-receptors with greater potency than noradrenaline, but it has less effect on the β-receptor than isoprenaline. There is (Table 1) a dilatation of vessels in

Table 1. Tissue distribution of some α- and β-adrenoceptors and the effects produced by their stimulation

Tissue	Alpha-receptors	Beta-receptors
Heart		
Sino-atrial node		Increased rate (automaticity)
Atria		Increased contractility and conduction velocity
Atrioventricular node		Increased conduction velocity, decreased refractory period, increased automaticity
His-Purkinje fibres		Increased automaticity
Ventricles		Increased contractility
Coronary blood vessels	Vasoconstriction	Vasodilatation
Cardiac metabolism		Glycogenolysis
Blood vessels		
Skin	Vasoconstriction	
Kidney	Vasoconstriction	
Skeletal muscle		Vasodilatation
Veins	Vasoconstriction	Vasoconstriction
Lung		
Bronchial muscle		Relaxation
Uterus		
Uterine muscle		Relaxation
Pancreas	? Inhibition of insulin release	Enhancement of insulin release
Insulin stores		
Muscle and liver		
Glycogen stores	? Glycogenolysis	Glycogenolysis

skeletal muscle and constriction of those in the kidney and skin. At lower doses, through its combined effect on the α- and β_1-receptors, heart rate and force of contraction increase and peripheral resistance falls. At larger doses α-stimulation starts to predominate and peripheral resistance rises especially in the kidney. Probably at most doses, renal blood flow decreases.

Adrenaline half-life is less than 1 min; the catecholamine ring is unsubstituted and the molecule is therefore prone to rapid degradation by catechol-o-methyl transferase.

Noradrenaline increases peripheral resistance, blood pressure therefore rises, there is a vagal bradycardia, and, in normal man a slight fall in cardiac output. In the failing heart there is a particular need to balance the improvement in organ perfusion against the disadvantage of increased left ventricular after-load and oxygen consumption. These considerations limit the therapeutic value of this agent, even in the treatment of circulatory collapse.

Dopamine is the immediate precursor of noradrenaline and at a low dose it preferentially stimulates the dopamine receptor. As doses increase, first β- and finally α-stimulatory effects become more important, but it has become clear that there is enormous variation in patient response. Dopamine's pharmacology and potential clinical application has been reviewed by GOLDBERG (1972) and GOLDBERG et al. (1977). An

Table 2. Structure and relative stimulatory actions of clinically useful α- and β-stimulants

Stimulant			α	β_1	β_2	Dopamine
Catecholamine derivatives						
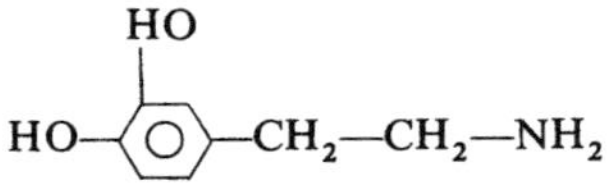	Dopamine	High dose	+++	++	−	++
		Low dose	±	++	−	++
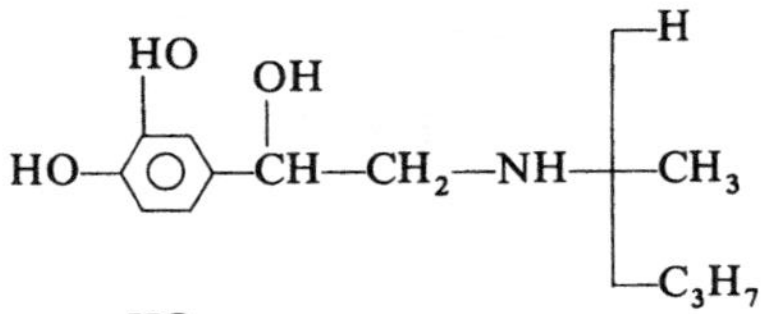	Noradrenaline		+++	+	−	−
	Adrenaline	High dose	++	+++	±	−
		Low dose	±	+++	++	−
	Isoprenaline		−	+++	+++	−
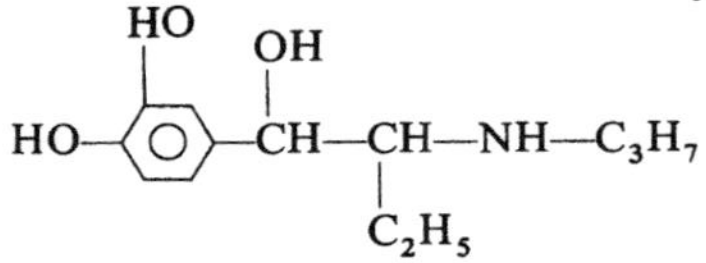	Isoetharine		−	+	++	−
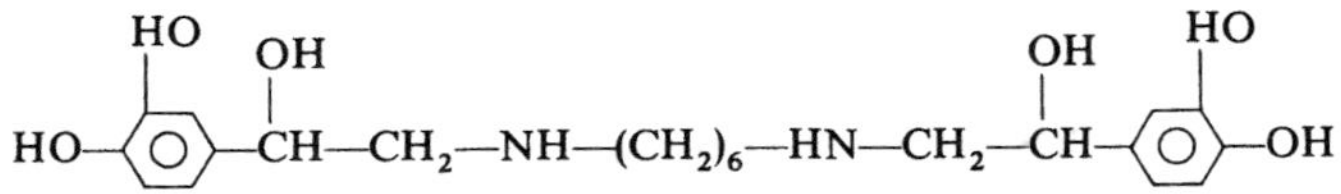	Hexoprenaline		−	−	++	−
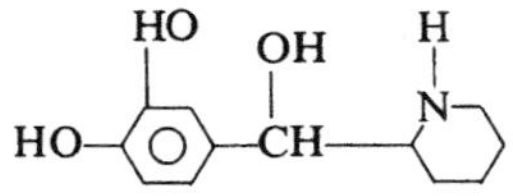	Rimiterol		−	−	++	−
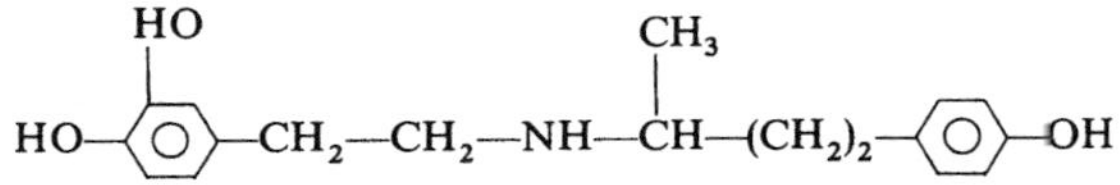	Dobutamine		±	+++	±	−

Table 2 (continued)

Stimulant		α	β_1	β_2	Dopamine
Resorcinol derivatives					
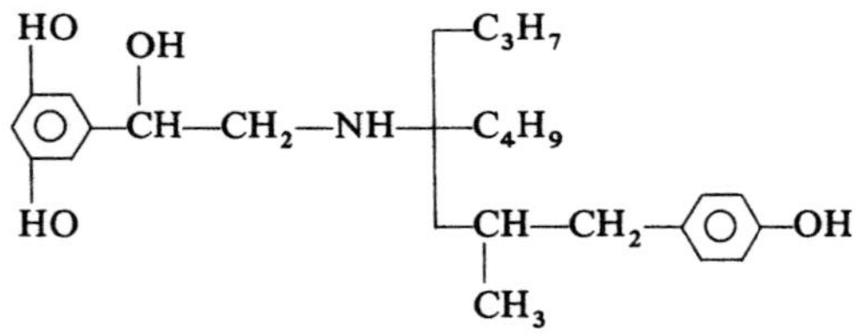	Orciprenaline	–	+	++	–
	Terbutaline	–	–	++	–
	Fenoterol	–	±	++	–
Phenol derivatives					
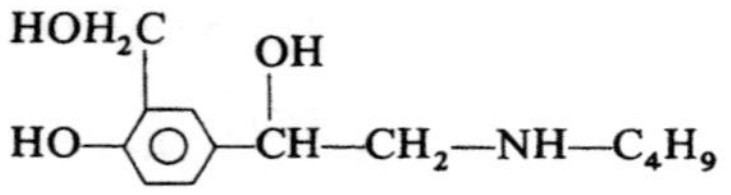	Salbutamol	–	±	++	–
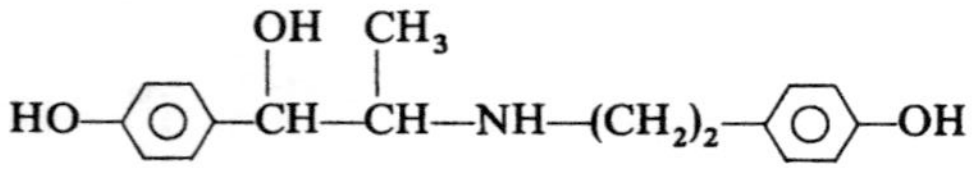	Ritodrine	–	–	++	–
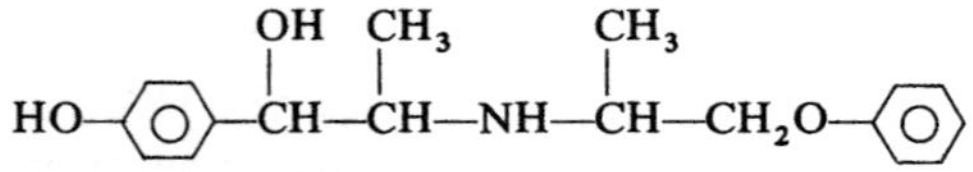	Isoxsuprine	–	±	++	–
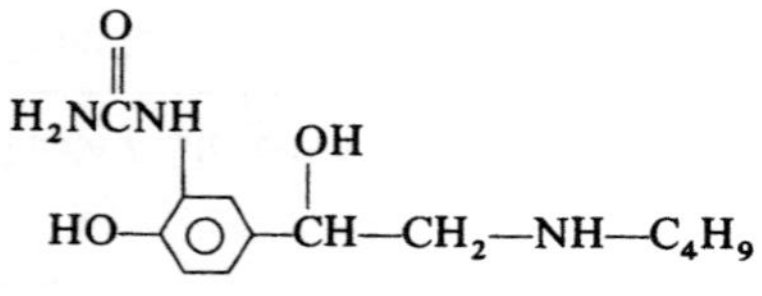	Carbuterol	–	–	++	–

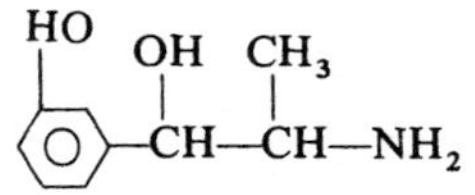	Metaraminol	+++	+	–	–
Phenyl derivatives					
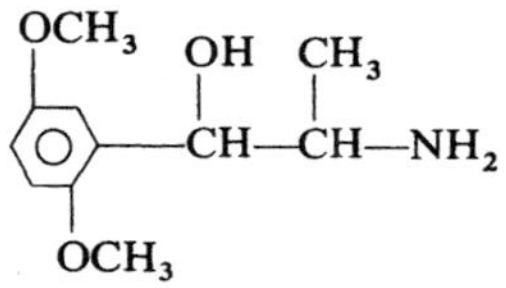	Methoxamine	+++	–	–	–
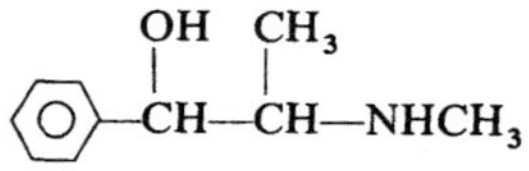	Ephedrine	+	++	++	–

initially unexpected finding, but subsequently found to be due to its effects on dopamine receptors (GOLDBERG et al., 1978), was that doses of 0.5–2.0 μg/kg/min produce arteriolar vasodilatation in the kidney (MCNAY et. al., 1965) and mesentery, and also arterial dilatation in the heart and brain. At 2–10 μg/kg/min, β-effects start to appear and there is an increase in cardiac output, stroke volume and contractility. In the normal heart a 20%–30% increase in cardiac output is achieved almost entirely by increases in stroke volume rather than heart rate (MCDONALD et al., 1964; HORWITZ et al., 1962). Peripheral resistance does fall but rather less than with isoprenaline and adrenaline. Diastolic blood pressure and heart rate are normally affected, but once above 10 μg/kg/min peripheral resistance starts to rise, and by 20–50 μg/kg/min α-effects predominate. The virtual absence of any increase in heart rate (GOLDBERG, 1972) augments the benefit derived from any reflex increase in coronary blood flow, secondary to the increased myocardial oxygen consumption (BROOKS et al., 1969). A further indirect advantage is that dopamine releases stored noradrenaline from sympathetic nerve endings (NASH et al., 1968). This, in the absence of any marked β_2 activity, leads to a degree of vasoconstriction in skeletal muscle and skin and unlike isoprenaline, favours a more advantageous distribution of blood to vital organs if there is an increase in cardiac output from the failing heart.

Disadvantages of dopamine include a tendency towards ventricular ectopic activity, tachycardia, and even angina. However, in its favour it produces fewer tachyarrhythmias than adrenaline, but prolonged use in high doses has caused peripheral gangrene and local extravasation can result in tissue necrosis. The appropriate antidote in this situation is local infiltration of 5–10 mg phentolamine in 10 ml saline. Its use is contra-indicated in the presence of phaeochromocytoma or uncontrolled tachyarrhythmias, and monoamine oxidase inhibitors markedly potentiate the action of the drug.

Dopamine has a biological half-life of approximately 2 min, which is an advantage it shares with other catecholamines; manipulation of inotropic therapy is therefore much more rapid than for example with digoxin. Its potency and rapid metabolism means that a metering pump is necessary for intravenous delivery and at present its use is confined to the treatment of circulatory failure. Because the renal and mesenteric vasodilatation is mediated specifically through the dopamine receptor, β-adrenergic blocking drugs do not inhibit this action, in contrast to the dopaminergic receptor blocking action of phenothiazines and haloperidol.

As a synthetic catecholamine, *isoprenaline* is a potent and almost pure β-stimulator with little action on the α-receptor. It consequently has positive inotropic and chronotropic effects, producing increases in the force and velocity of myocardial contraction, heart rate and consequently the rate of myocardial oxygen consumption. It increases coronary arterial flow by direct action on the β_1-receptors and indirectly through heart rate and increased oxygen consumption (SONNENBLICK et al., 1968; SARNOFF et al., 1965) which produces a reflex increase in coronary blood flow (LOMBARDO et al., 1953). A normal or increased stroke volume is delivered in a shortened ejection time (KRASNOW et al., 1964). Through its action on the β_2-receptors it produces vasodilatation in the kidney, brain, and pulmonary vascular beds with relaxation of bronchial muscle in the lung. Through these effects it tends to promote peripheral run-off, which means that any rise in arterial pressure during its use in circulatory collapse represents an improvement in myocardial contractility.

Disadvantages are that much of the peripheral flow may be directed through relatively unimportant vascular beds such as those in muscle, skin, and the mesentery. Furthermore, improved organ perfusion is difficult to assess accurately at the bedside in the short term, and excessive falls in peripheral resistance lead to decreased diastolic pressure and coronary perfusion. Renal blood flow and the fraction of the cardiac output delivered to the kidneys may also be reduced (ROSENBLUM et al., 1968). These peripheral effects may be particularly disadvantageous in the presence of narrowed vessels and further aggravated by failure of the normal autoregulation of coronary blood flow such as is seen in the presence of ischaemic heart disease. Of all the catecholamines in use, isoprenaline is the most potent stimulator of cardiac output but also is known to cause arrhythmias. Despite this, it has been used parenterally in circulatory failure and remains of some value if a degree of tachycardia can be tolerated during the correction of hypotension (GOLDBERG and TALLEY, 1971; TALLEY et al., 1969).

The isopropyl substitution of the terminal nitrogen increases β_2-stimulatory activity but because the catechol ring is unmodified, destruction by catechol-o-methyl transferase is rapid. Its half-life by the intravenous route is 3–4 min (CONWAY et al., 1968). It has been used orally and sublingually in the treatment of atrioventricular block, bradycardia and Stokes-Adams attacks and it is particularly well established in the treatment of asthma by aerosol inhalation.

Dobutamine was first synthesised with a view to providing inotropic activity without the disadvantages of noradrenaline and isoprenaline, namely, increased heart rate, myocardial oxygen requirement and peripheral vasoconstriction. It has been shown to have this desired increase in inotropic/chronotropic ratio in man (LOEB et al., 1975). It acts primarily on the β_1-receptors with some α-stimulating properties, but only affects the β_2-receptor weakly. It has no indirect effect through the release of noradrenaline, it does not bring about alteration in renal blood flow, and it does not seem to stimulate the dopamine receptor (ROBIE and GOLDBERG, 1975). In isolated atria there was less effect on sino-atrial node activity than with isoprenaline (TUTTLE, 1974). It consequently increases myocardial contractility without greatly changing heart rate or peripheral resistance (TUTTLE and MILLS, 1975).

Mean arterial pressure, heart rate, and ventricular volumes change little at doses under 20 µg/kg/min (TUTTLE and MILLS, 1975; ROBIE and GOLDBERG, 1975; VATNER et al., 1974). Cardiac output is increased by dobutamine more than by dopamine (ROBIE and GOLDBERG, 1975). The slight increase in systolic pressure generates a reflex increase in vagal tone, which helps attenuate the tachycardia that might be expected from β_1-stimulation. The more prominent inotropic action of dobutamine appears to indicate inotropic selectivity (TUTTLE et al., 1976). By direct injection arterial vasodilatation can be demonstrated (ROBIE et al., 1974), but it is less pronounced in the mesenteric and renal vessels, where effects are partly offset by α-mediated vasoconstriction (VATNER et al., 1974).

An informative comparison has recently been made between the haemodynamic responses at two dose levels of dopamine, dobutamine and isoprenaline in patients with ischaemic heart disease but normal ejection fractions (STEPHENS et al., 1979). All these drugs increased cardiac output – isoprenaline was associated with increased heart rate, while dopamine and dobutamine by increased stroke volume.

Dopamine and isoprenaline decreased peripheral resistance, dobutamine did not and there was therefore a rise in mean arterial pressure. As expected, mean myocardial oxygen consumption rose with all three drugs. Extraction fell or remained constant for isoprenaline and dobutamine, but it tended to rise with dopamine. It is suggested that this could be due to a coronary vasoconstrictive influence partially limiting the coronary vasodilatation in response to increased oxygen demand. This suggestion might help account for increased ST changes following the use of dopamine in experimental coronary occlusion (STEMPLE et al., 1976).

A disadvantage of dobutamine is that the increase in cardiac output is deflected from kidney to muscle, but it has the advantage that there is a decreased propensity towards the production of tachyarrhythmias, especially in the presence of halogenated hydrocarbon anaesthetics (HOLLOWAY and FREDERICKSON, 1974). In the presence of β-blockade, dobutamine can, by virtue of its α-stimulating properties, decrease cardiac output and increase total peripheral resistance. It should therefore be used with caution in a patient who has also received a β-adrenergic blocking drug.

2. Alpha-Selective

Metaraminol is a synthetic compound which releases stored noradrenaline from postsynaptic sympathetic nerve endings (HARRISON et al., 1963). Its effects are therefore indirect and similar to those of noradrenaline. However, it is less potent but lasts longer. Eventually potency decreases as noradrenaline stores run out. It predominantly acts as an α-stimulator without any significant direct β_1-action on the heart.

It increases systolic and diastolic blood pressures and produces a vagal-mediated fall in heart rate. Some authors considered it to have marginal advantages over noradrenaline in the treatment of cardiogenic shock in that it was longer-acting and could be given intramuscularly without local adverse effects (MUNE and NORREGAARD, 1959).

Methoxamine was discovered during a systematic appraisal of aromatic-substituted alkyl amines. It has a strong direct α-stimulatory action and produces intense vasoconstriction (ZAIMIS, 1968). It has no β-effects and the pulse rate tends to slow by vagal reflex and cardiac output is reduced. Despite this, because there are relatively few vascular α-adrenoceptors in the brain and the heart, blood flow to these organs is not necessarily decreased and may even increase. Its clinical application has been limited to restoration of blood pressure during hypotensive episodes following epidural anaesthesia. Its use in correcting hypotension associated with halothane or cyclopropane anaesthesia is contra-indicated because of its tendency to precipitate ventricular arrhythmias.

3. Beta$_2$-Selective

Salbutamol has tertiary butyl substitution of the terminal nitrogen atom and 3-methanol substitution in the catechol ring prevents rapid enzymatic degradation. It is primarily a β_2-stimulant (CULLUM et al., 1969) but has some slight β_1-activity (BRITTAIN, 1971). However, increases in the pulse rate in, for example, the failing heart, during infusion of up to 40 μg/min have been modest (TIMMIS et al., 1979) and although there is slightly increased oxygen demand, blood pressure falls and there is no effect on the velocity of contraction.

The metabolism in man is complex. There are significant plasma levels of metabolites after oral doses (EVANS et al., 1973b), and there is probably a substantial first pass effect in the liver. This in part explains the large variation in response between individuals which is frequently observed. There is considerable dissociation between plasma concentrations and physiological effects. EVANS et al. (1973b) find peak plasma levels at 3 h, while FREDHOLM et al. (1978) describe several metabolic parameters which change within 30–90 min. Some effects probably are shorter-lived than the drug itself. There are also reports of metabolic tolerance developing during long-term treatment of asthmatics (CONOLLY et al., 1971); nevertheless it is a well-established and effective bronchodilator in asthmatic subjects, whether given orally (LEGGE et al., 1971; O'DONNELL et al., 1971), sublingually, intravenously or by aerosol (SCHUMANN and HERXHEIMER, 1971; PATERSON, 1971).

Terbutaline has the same terminal nitrogen substitution as salbutamol and it therefore has β_2-stimulatory properties. It does not produce contraction of rabbit aortic strips (25 µg/ml) (SORENBY, 1975) or rat vas deferens smooth muscle (1 ng/ml) (MALTA and RAPER, 1974) and is therefore considered not to have any α-stimulatory properties, but it does have partial agonist activity on cardiac muscle (WASSERMAN and LEVY, 1974). The relaxing effect of terbutaline on mouse ileum (β_1-mediated) was only 1/100th that of isoprenaline. Its β_1-activity is therefore considered slight (OLSSON, 1972).

The resorcinol dihydroxy substitution of the aromatic ring resembles that of orciprenaline and confers protection against catechol-o-methyl transferase activity (PERSSON and PERSSON, 1972), which normally destroys the catecholamines (HERTTING, 1964), and the relatively large terminal nitrogen substitution increases its β-selectivity (BERGMAN et al., 1969; PERSSON and JOHNSON, 1970). This has been confirmed in man by THIRINGER and SVEDMYR (1976) who constructed intravenous dose-response curves for increases in forced expiratory volume in 1 s (FEV_1) and heart rate. The greatest separation was in the dose range of 0.25 mg/kg/min, when the FEV_1 had increased by 32% but the heart rate by only 12%. The estimated selectivity ratio of approximately 5:1 is considerably less than that found in vitro. The reason for this discrepancy has not yet been established.

The action of terbutaline is relatively long; most reports describe bronchospasmolytic activity lasting up to 8 h. By the oral route this is in excess of orciprenaline but about the same as equipotent doses of salbutamol. Peak effect from oral use is at 2–3 h while subcutaneously 0.5 mg is an effective dose which has an onset of action within 10 min and lasts up to 4 h. Only parenteral administration is associated with marked side-effects and there is some evidence that isoprenaline-induced tachycardia and muscle tremor may be attenuated by its prolonged use (SVEDMYR et al., 1974).

Like other β_2-stimulants, terbutaline relaxes carbachol-excited rat uterus (OLSSON and PERSSON, 1971). The effect is antagonised by propranolol, as is the action of terbutaline on decreasing the frequency and amplitude of spontaneous contractile activity in isolated human uterine strips obtained at caesarean section (ANDERSSON et al., 1973). Terbutaline has also been investigated for its effect on tracheal mucous velocity and mucociliary activity. By watching Teflon particles with a fibroscope or detecting the movement of radioactive particles, terbutaline has been shown to increase speed of mucous movement in chronic obstructive airway disease (SANTA CRUZ et al., 1974) and cystic fibrosis (WOOD et al., 1975), where this movement is usually subnormal. Particle velocity was increased from 2.6 to 5.5 mm/min with 0.25 mg terbutaline administered subcutaneously (normal: 20.1 mm/min). Lesser effects have been seen in asthma.

This property which is shared by isoprenaline and carbuterol (SACKNER et al., 1976) remains of possible, but as yet unproven, clinical value.

Fenoterol is a resorcinol related to orciprenaline but topographically similar to other non-resorcinol β_2-agonists such as salbutamol. The particularly large aromatic substitution on the terminal nitrogen, whilst conferring β_2 -selectivity, may also hinder enzymatic cleavage at the α-carbon–NH bond. It is a potent oral bronchodilator producing maximal effects within 2 h (GEUMEI et al., 1976) and with some effects lasting up to 10 h. Intravenous studies in animals indicate that there is some agonist activity on the heart (BRITTAIN et al., 1976), but in vitro studies with isolated atria and trachea indicate that it is more selective than isoprenaline but less so than salbutamol or terbutaline (APPERLEY et al., 1976). Other studies in vivo show that it is probably more powerful than salbutamol in inhibiting reagin-mediated mast cell degranulation (FÜGNER, 1973) or protecting against passive peritoneal anaphylaxis (FÜGNER, 1977). Like salbutamol and terbutaline it exerts its maximun effect by aerosol at 60–120 min, which is somewhat later than, for example, isoprenaline (AVERY, 1971; BROGDEN et al., 1973), but because of its structure it is longer-lasting (MINETTE, 1970; POWLES, 1975). Its properties and clinical evaluation have been reviewed in detail by HEEL et al. (1978), and because of its bronchodilatory powers and prolonged duration of action LEIFER and WITTIG (1975) consider it one of the better agents available.

Carbuterol is related to salbutamol and terbutaline in having tertiary butyl substitution of the terminal nitrogen. Its individual property is in having a urea group replacing the 3-hydroxyl group in the catechol ring which lengthens its duration of action to about 4 h. In keeping with the postulate that enlargement of the alkyl group attached to the side-chain nitrogen increases β_2-selectivity (BRITTAIN et al., 1970), carbuterol is found to be a selective β_2-stimulant and consequently a bronchodilator (BEALE and STEPHENSON, 1972; SALEEBY and ZISKIND, 1975; FUNAHASHI and HAMILTON, 1976; MINETTE et al., 1976).

Orciprenaline has an isopropyl substitution at the terminal nitrogen and 3,5-dihydroxy substitution in the aromatic ring, which confers β_2-selectivity and resistance to enzymic destruction. It has medium duration of action with peak bronchodilatation at 30–60 min and effects lasting for 3–4 h. It has been reviewed by LEIFER and WITTIG (1975) and MILLER (1967). Its principal clinical use has been in the treatment of asthma, where it has the particular advantage of minimal side-effects when given by aerosol. When given parenterally there is a tendency for β_2-selectivity to be lost as more widespread β-stimulation occurs and side-effects appear. Its efficacy by mouth is somewhat variable.

Isoetharine was the first of the synthetic catechols produced with β_2 activity. Ethyl substitution of the α-carbon atom and isopropyl substitution of the terminal nitrogen conferred this property. α- and β_1-Mediated side-effects are minimal, but because the catechol ring is unsubstituted, enzymatic degradation is rapid and the duration of action is only 2 h. Experience has not revealed convincing evidence of superiority in terms of lung function, arterial oxygen saturation or ventilation status in the treatment of asthma (THIRINGER et al., 1971). Despite limited advantages over orciprenaline and its marginally fewer side-effects, it has largely been superseded by more recent additions.

Rimiterol has a cyclised structure around the α-carbon atom and is structurally related to isoetharine. It is highly selective for the β_2-receptor, but because it has an unmodified catecholamine ring, it has a relatively short half-life (CARNEY et al., 1971; GRIFFIN et al., 1973; EVANS et al., 1973a). Its duration of action is about 1.5–2 h, and it is therefore similar to isoprenaline but has fewer α- and β_1-mediated side-effects. It is effective intravenously and by aerosol (SVEDMYR et al., 1972), but by mouth it is inactive. Its clinical application has been in the treatment of asthma and it probably does not represent any great advance.

Hexoprenaline comprises two "adrenaline moieties" linked by a six-membered saturated carbon chain. It has effects lasting up to 4 h, which is rather difficult to explain in terms of structure unless the molecule folds upon itself to hinder access of catechol-o-methyl transferase as the two aromatic rings become adjacent.

Reproterol is a β-phenyl ethyl amino alkyl xanthine and is a bronchodilator with relatively few undesirable cardiac effects. It was one of a series of 90 compounds described by HABERSANG et al. (1977). It has an interesting structure, with the xanthine moiety perhaps being expected to augment β-stimulation by inhibiting the breakdown of the synthesised intracellular cyclic AMP.

Salmefamol is structurally similar to fenoterol but with different ring substitutions. Like salbutamol it is β_2-specific and resists degradation. It produces little in the way of side-effects when given parenterally, and animal studies suggest that it is equipotent to isoprenaline (SHENFIELD and PATERSON, 1973; LAL et al., 1974).

III. Clinical Uses

The principal uses of α- and β-adrenoceptor stimulants in cardiovascular medicine have been for the acute treatment of circulatory failure, and long-term β-stimulants have been used in the treatment of heart block and cerebral and peripheral ischaemia. In respiratory medicine the β_2-stimulants have been extensively used intravenously, orally and by inhalation for the treatment of bronchospasm and more recently in obstetrics by intravenous infusion for the control of premature labour.

1. Cardiovascular Medicine

a) Introduction

When organs of the body cease to be adequately perfused for reasons other than obstruction to blood flow then circulatory failure is present.

The most important acute cardiac cause is the sudden loss of functioning left ventricular mass, as occurs in myocardial infarction. Chronically there is the insidious depression of intrinsic myocardial muscle function in congestive heart failure. A possible mechanism is disturbance of calcium transport interfering with excitation-contraction coupling. There is a fall of stroke volume at rest and a rise in the left ventricular end-diastolic pressure. Peripheral causes include hypovolaemia – absolute or relative. The former occurs secondary to contraction of the circulating intravascular fluid volume, as in haemorrhage, dehydration, and excessive use of diuretics. The latter is associated with expansion of the intravascular space or reduction of peripheral resistance. This is seen in vasodilatation, e.g., during halothane or cyclopentane anaesthesia, in endotoxin shock or when normal vasoconstrictive responses are suppressed, e.g. during spinal anaesthesia.

It remains the underlying principle in treatment of circulatory failure that absolute hypovolaemia is excluded as a major contributary factor and, where feasible, repair of any mechanical defects is attempted as soon as possible. It is mandatory to insert a central venous pressure line and establish that there is an adequate filling pressure for the right ventricle (16–19 cm H_2O) before embarking upon treatment with inotropic pressor agents. The American literature favours also the insertion of a Swan-Ganz catheter (JAHRE et al., 1975; JOHNSON and GUNNAR, 1977) for serial assessment of pulmonary wedge pressure. Once clearly established that inotropic agents are an appropriate interim measure, scrupulous attention should be paid to the correction of arterial oxygen tension, arrhythmias, electrolyte imbalance and pH, so to take full advantage of beneficial effects and minimise their toxicity. Even the most modern agents have a tendency towards beneficial effects on the heart, being counteracted by adverse peripheral actions. In excess they all have adverse effects on the heart, most commonly the production of tachyarrhythmias.

b) Cardiogenic Shock

When they became available for clinical use there was a strong inclination to use pressor amines in the treatment of hypotension following myocardial infarction. Particularly noradrenaline, first utilised in 1948, and later metaraminol, with its marginal advantages, were favoured. Consideration of the physiological forces operating indicate that the treatment principle is complex and that neither is truly appropriate, and with the alternatives now available, noradrenaline should only be used as a last resort.

Cardiogenic shock is a physiological response to sudden loss of functional left ventricular mass. α- and β-Stimulation become maximal following the release of endogenous catecholamines and consequently any exogenous contribution is unlikely to contribute extra benefit. In particular, α-stimulants can only produce more intense vasoconstriction and further increase left ventricular after-load. Furthermore it transpires that if there is more than 40% loss of ventricular mass then inotropic agents are unlikely to be of any use in any case. This, in part, explains why probably less than 10% of patients suffering cardiogenic shock derive any dramatic benefit from their use. Even if the systolic pressure rises, the heart rate falls through the vagal reflex and there is decreased oxygen supply at a cost of increased myocardial oxygen consumption and left ventricular work. It should also be noted that all sympathomimetic drugs have the ability to increase cardiac work. Oxygen demand could eventually outstrip supply and cause extension of infarction.

By a similar argument it is uneconomical and in most cases counter-productive to aim for systolic pressures in excess of 95 mm Hg. Ideally stimulation of myocardial contractility should be accompanied by decreased peripheral resistance, enabling better organ perfusion at lower work cost to the left ventricle.

Intravenous adrenaline, enough to maintain systolic pressures of 80–100 mm Hg initially through its β-effect increases heart rate and force of contraction. However, although peripheral resistance falls, unfortunately blood flow is to dilated vessels in skeletal muscle at the expense of the kidney where vessels remain constricted. Increasing the dose only causes α-effects to predominate with further vasoconstriction. In this context there is little to recommend it.

Similarly isoprenaline is far from an ideal, particularly since it increases ventricular irritability and eventually through vasodilatation promotes a fall in blood pressure with decreases in coronary artery perfusion and heart muscle oxygenation under circumstances of increased demand. Isoprenaline can increase infarct size following experimental coronary occlusion (MAROKO et al., 1971) and intensify myocardial hypoxia in patients with cardiogenic shock (MUELLER et al., 1970). Having said this however, there are two circumstances where its use may be considered. In patients with aortic or mitral incompetence any α-receptor-mediated increase in peripheral resistance, however small, must be avoided since it will only increase regurgitation. Secondly, in cardiogenic shock JAHRE et al. (1975) have suggested that if the heart rate remains below 120 beats/min then isoprenaline, particularly if it is the only alternative, may be of some value in restoring a reasonable blood pressure. It has also been effective in patients in whom dopamine did not increase cardiac output (TALLEY et al., 1969).

At the present time, dopamine, which has less vasodilating action than isoprenaline and a slightly greater ability to increase mean arterial pressure, has proved valuable when hypotension is not profound and where peripheral vasoconstriction and oliguria persist. It has the added advantage of producing haemodynamic effects without creating undue myocardial hypoxia (CREXELLS et al., 1973). When used with isoprenaline, the two drugs combined improve cardiac output and urine flow more effectively than either drug alone (TALLEY et al., 1969). Although dopamine enhances cardiac output and stroke index (LEVINE et al., 1975), it does not predispose towards undue increases in heart rate (ROBIE and GOLDBERG, 1975; ROSENBLUM et al., 1972) at doses below 5.0 μg/kg/min. This is a potential advantage in minimising oxygen demand, which is known to be related to heart rate (SONNENBLICK and SKELTON, 1971). There can, however, be a reduction in diastolic blood pressure, presumably secondary to decreased peripheral resistance in the mesentery and kidneys.

Dobutamine, with its favourable inotropic/chronotropic ratio, would appear to have certain advantages in this situation in that it is also thought to mediate against extension of infarct size (TUTTLE et al., 1973), whereas dopamine appears to increase ST elevation in experimental animals after coronary occlusion. The precise reason for this is not clear (STEMPLE et al., 1976).

Salbutamol, a relatively specific β_2-stimulant and consequently a vasodilator, has been successfully used to reduce after-load and to treat shock following myocardial infarction (TIMMIS et al., 1979). Its relatively long half-life makes fine adjustment to therapy difficult, and because it increases heart rate, oxygen demand almost certainly rises. As a vasodilator nitroprusside probably has the more favourable characteristics (POOLE-WILSON et al., 1977). However, following cardiac surgery salbutamol has been found to increase cardiac output (YACOUB and BOYLAND, 1973; WYSE et al., 1974) and promote tissue perfusion without undue increases in oxygen uptake. With isoprenaline, oxygen requirement was almost tenfold greater immediately after operation (WYSE et al., 1974). There was no control group.

c) Heart Failure

The optimal treatment of the more prolonged loss of myocardial contractility associated with chronic heart failure remains primarily that of diuretics and long-acting inotropic agents such as the cardiac glycosides. With time, considerable effort has been made to recruit the assistance of the adrenoceptor stimulants to improve cardiac performance especially when low cardiac output is a troublesone feature.

Isoprenaline has improved cardiac performance (ELLIOTT and GORLIN, 1966; TALLEY et al., 1969) but adverse reactions have usually included tachycardia or falls in blood pressure which necessitated discontinuation of treatment (GUNNAR et al., 1967; SMITH et al., 1967).

Dopamine can also increase cardiac output without significantly increasing heart rate or diastolic blood pressure (HORWITZ et al., 1962), but in the failing heart improvement in output is usually made at the expense of increased left ventricular filling pressure (LOEB et al., 1977; LEIER et al., 1978). Most of the benefit seen in congestive heart failure is centred around increasing sodium excretion (GOLDBERG et al., 1963), (MCDONALD et al., 1964; BEREGOVICH et al., 1974). Comparison of dopamine (2–16 μg/kg/min) with dobutamine (10 μg/kg/min) during short infusions in patients with severe heart failure secondary to ischaemic disease or cardiomyopathy showed that while both drugs increased cardiac index and to some extent heart rate, with dopamine the systolic pressure also rose and there was no decrease in left ventricular end-diastolic pressure. Dobutamine lowered the end-diastolic pressure (STONER et al., 1977).

Dobutamine produced similar results in another group of patients with chronic low-output cardiac failure (LOEB et al., 1977). When doses were adjusted to give similar incremental increases in cardiac output to dopamine, dobutamine reduced left ventricular filling pressure whilst dopamine increased it and in nearly half the patients caused the arterial oxygen saturation to fall below 90%.

Dobutamine has been further studied since it is known to increase contractility and cardiac output and decrease pulmonary wedge pressure without increasing blood pressure or heart rate significantly both in patients with heart failure and in patients without (STONER et al., 1977; BEREGOVICH et al., 1975; AKHTAR et al., 1975; ANDY et al., 1977). LEIER et al. (1977) have studied 25 patients with left ventricular failure (Class IV) secondary to cardiomyopathy (21) or valvular disease (4). Following dobutamine in doses up to 15 μg/kg/min for 72 h there was clinical improvement to Class II or III for at least a week after the infusion. During the actual treatment there were significant ($p<0.05$) increases in cardiac output, urine flow and urinary sodium concentration and a fall in pulmonary wedge pressure. There was no increase in heart rate, blood pressure or ventricular irritability and tachyphylaxis was not a problem. DURAIRAJ and HAYWOOD (1978) found similar improvements with dopamine amongst 12 cases of congestive heart failure resistant to diuretics and digoxin. In addition they noted improvement in stroke volume index and stroke work index and a decrease in total systemic and pulmonary arteriolar resistance. Five patients subsequently died and the favourable outcome was then seen to be towards patients with ischaemic heart disease as opposed to valvular disease. Comparison between dobutamine and isoprenaline has been attempted in patients with heart failure following cardiac surgery. Dobutamine produced a greater increase in cardiac index per unit increase in heart rate

(SAKAMOTO and YAMADA, 1977). Others (KERSTIN et al., 1976) found both drugs effective.

In 12 patients with severe congestive heart failure secondary to ischaemic disease or cardiomyopathy, dobutamine and nitroprusside increased cardiac output almost identically but dobutamine gave significantly higher mean arterial pressures and heart rates with less impressive falls in pulmonary wedge pressure. Best results were obtained by using both drugs together (MIKULIC et al., 1977). In low-output failure, nitroprusside reduced systolic and diastolic pressures. Taken together this evidence suggests that dobutamine may be the preferred agent, once coronary perfusion is jeopardised (BERKOWITZ et al., 1977). Favourable features of dobutamine used after myocardial infarction include the absence of increase in the extent of injury (GILLESPIE et al., 1977), and there being no exacerbation of arrhythmias after surgery (SAKAMOTO and YAMADA, 1977). It also has a theoretical advantage in that the failing heart has a reduced content of noradrenaline (CHIDSEY et al., 1965) and to some extent the beneficial effects of dopamine are dependent on its ability to release this stored catecholamine (TUTTLE and MILLS, 1975).

Salbutamol also improves haemodynamic parameters such as cardiac index and end-diastolic pressure without altering heart rate in congestive cardiomyopathy (SHARMA and GOODWIN, 1978) and in left ventricular failure following myocardial infarction (LAL et al., 1972). Recently (TIMMIS et al., 1979) have infused up to 40 μg/kg/min and found a substantial improvement in cardiac output and a fall in systemic resistance. Arrhythmias were not a problem, but over the time of the infusion there was no beneficial effect on the increased end-diastolic pulmonary pressure.

d) Endotoxin (Septic) and Hypovolaemic (Traumatic) Shock

Once these diagnoses are made (LEES, 1976) fluid replacement and adequate ventilation become prime priorities. Shock is accompanied by increases in peripheral resistance (DIETZMAN and LILLEHEI, 1968) with increases in sympathetic tone of the veins, heart, and arterioles (KELMAN, 1971); this reduces circulatory capacity, which helps to maintain cardiac output. Consequently in this situation it is colloid and not crystalloid solution that is appropriate for resuscitation (FAKUDA et al., 1969). The use of colloid further protects against the onset of pulmonary oedena. In cases of endotoxin shock, appropriate consideration must also be given to antibiotic and steroid therapy.

The early literature recorded benefit derived from isoprenaline (KARDOS, 1966; MACLEAN et al., 1965) originally when low cardiac output was accompanied by increased peripheral resistance.

However, if vasoconstriction is intense and persists after appropriate restoration of the right ventricular filling pressure, then α-blockade, with e.g. phentolamine, may also be useful. If hypotension predominates, judicious use of adrenoceptor stimulants can be made. If the pulse rate is greater than 120 beats/min or there is evidence of ventricular irritability, then α-agonists such as noradrenaline or dopamine in the high dose range are probably the most appropriate. If the pulse rate remains below 120 beats/min or there is no sign of ventricular irritability, then isoprenaline or low-dose dopamine with their predominantly β-actions are probably the best choice. The dose of isoprenaline can be increased until the heart rate is 150 beats/min, provided the blood pressure does not fall below a mean arterial pressure of 60 mm Hg. Above this rate cardiac output falls and there is an increasing tendency towards dysrhythmias, especially as arterial oxygen saturation and pH fall. Noradrenaline will improve blood pressure, but it will be at the expense of tissue perfusion and even here noradrenaline is probably best avoided.

Dobutamine has not been formally validated in the treatment of shock but it may well have advantages over isoprenaline in that it maintains a better perfusion pressure.

2. Obstetric Medicine

a) Introduction

The myometrium contains α- and β_2-adrenoceptors; stimulation of the β_2-site causes myometrial relaxation almost certainly initiated by receptor-mediated activation of adenylate cyclase (KAUMANN and BIRNBAUMER, 1974). The discovery of compounds which selectively stimulate the β_2-receptor has meant that the observed effect of a decreased frequency and force of contraction in the gravid uterus can be turned to therapeutic advantage in the treatment of pre-term labour with minimal effects on the maternal (and fetal) cardiovascular system. Gradually since 1964, the idea of β_2-adrenoceptor stimulation for the control of pre-term labour has gained acceptance especially once relatively selective stimulants became available which were well tolerated. These compounds had the advantage of not appearing to cause unfavourable effects, as do, for examle, the steroids which, when given in early pregnancy, are associated with appearance of congenital defects, and ethanol which may delay circulatory and respiratory adaption of the new-born (SEPPALA et al., 1971) or give raise to the well-described fetal alcohol syndrome (CHRISTOFFEL and SALAFSKY, 1975).

However, despite the efficacy and obvious advantages of this approach its final clinical role in the delay of pre-term labour ist not yet finally proven. Well-designed trials have been organised with the appropriate theoretical considerations, but most have been uncontrolled because the onset of true labour is difficult to define and once detected it is, in the view of some, unethical not to commence treatment. LIU and BLACKWELL (1978) have tried to overcome the inherent difficulty of assessing the severity of pre-term labour, the stage at which it is being treated (RICHTER, 1977) and the outcome that might be expected. They describe a scoring system based on membrane integrity, "mucoid show", uterine contractions, cervical dilatation and other contributory factors such as the presence of twins or cervical incompetence. In general, it seems that when only contractions are present then labour is likely to be delayed effectively. Once cervical effacement has occurred or the membranes ruptured then progress to delivery is almost inevitable, irrespective of treatment. Non-specific forms of care such as bed rest, as judged from the success of placebo in some trials, also make a distinct contribution which further confuses the situation. Despite this, however, the use of β_2-stimulants has become part of the standard obstetric practice (RICHTER, 1977), albeit based on little hard evidence regarding any advantage to the new-born. The sympathomimetic agents that have been used include isoxsuprine (HENDRICKS et al., 1961), orciprenaline (BAILLIE et al., 1970), ritodrine (WESSELIUS et al., 1971), salbutamol (LIGGINS and VAUGHAN, 1973), and terbutaline (INGEMARSSON, 1976); a useful review of the numerous trials has been provided by HEMMINKI and

STARFIELD (1978). These authors have critically surveyed 18 controlled trials; 6 concerning isoxsuprine, 3 ritodrine, 1 terbutaline, and others involving the steroid hormones and ethanol. Thirteen were considered to be without obvious drawbacks which might have impaired the quality of conclusions and two drugs have been convincingly shown to be therapeutically better than placebo, namely long-term ethanol (ZLATNIK and FUCHS, 1972) and terbutaline (INGEMARSSON, 1976). Ritodrine has been found to be more effective than ethanol, but the trial did not formally establish whether it was better than no treatment at all (LAUERSEN et al., 1977). In a randomised single-blind trial of oral isoxsuprine against placebo, the investigation was discontinued because a clear-cut prophylactic benefit was lacking. The situation was further complicated by the fact that it is clear that the therapeutic half-life of some of the substances investigated varies from 2 h (ritodrine) to 6 h (salbutamol); this makes timing of oral doses particularly critical.

That uterine contractility can be inhibited and labour delayed for a time is now beyond doubt, but that there is clear benefit to the children that are born has only been shown in the trials involving terbutaline (INGEMARSSON, 1976) and progesterone (JOHNSON et al., 1975). It is probably still fair to adhere to the original principle that even a few hours' delay gives time for steroids to be administered in order to counteract the onset of respiratory distress syndrome.

b) Clinical Applications

Practical possibilities include oral and intravenous therapy. Both have been assessed and it seems that the quicker a therapeutic result is established the better. Initial intravenous treatment followed by oral maintenance has the best properties, with the initial intravenous phase providing tight control of the clinical situation.

α) Intravenous Therapy. LIPSHITZ and BAILLIE (1976) have compared the effect of intravenous fenoterol (2.5 μg/min), hexoprenaline (0.38 μg/min), ritodrine (300 μg/min), and salbutamol (10 μg/min) on uterine activity during elective induction of labour by oxytocin. All drugs reduced activity to less than 30% of the initial level ($p < 0.001$). Hexoprenaline achieved the greatest effect, but once treatment was stopped the slowest return to pretreatment activity was after ritodrine. This long-term effect of ritodrine was secondary to a prolonged slowing in the frequency of contractions. Fenoterol was the shortest-acting drug and may be the best agent for rapid relief of fetal distress before Caesarean section. The longer duration of action by ritodrine favours oral use and the minimal cardiovascular side-effects of hexoprenaline confers advantages for the patient where tachycardia is best avoided. Salbutamol in this context had no distinctive features. It should also be remembered that the various β_2-stimulants vary in their intravenous potency, e.g., ritodrine has probably a fifth of the potency of salbutamol.

Intravenous terbutaline (between 5 and 20 μg/min for 40 min) also inhibits basal uterine activity produced by both prostaglandin $F_{2\alpha}$ and hypertonic saline in patients undergoing therapeutic abortions (ANDERSSON et al., 1975 b). Similar doses of terbutaline inhibited particularly the amplitude but also the frequency of uterine activity in normal-term labour (ANDERSSON et al., 1975 a). In the control of premature labour (5–10 μg terbutaline/min for 8 h followed by oral therapy), 12 of 15 patients had delivery delayed until the 37 th week, whereas this was only achieved in three patients in a similar-sized control group on placebo (VARGAS-GARCIA et al., 1974). Intravenous (1 week) followed by oral therapy in a heterogeneous group of 135 patients (RICHTER, 1977) did not reveal any real difference between fenoterol (1–3 μg/min, 30–50 mg daily) and ritodrine (100–300 μg/min, 20–40 mg daily) in the delaying of labour. There was no control group, but it seemed again that the more advanced the labour, the less were the chances of success, the outcome most effectively being related to a prolongation index.

In a randomised comparison of salbutamol with ethanol (SIMS et al., 1978), 46 patients were treated with intravenous ethanol and 42 with up to 50 μg/min of intravenous salbutamol (mean dose 26 μg/min). Responses were very varied and although salbutamol acted more rapidly, effects were less well sustained. There was no real difference between the two drugs: neither was truly effective in that only 27% of the patients continued their pregnancy to 37 weeks, and there was no difference in the number of babies surviving the neonatal period. However, it should be pointed out that patients with ruptured membranes and cervical dilatation were not excluded from study. There has also been comparison with intravenous aminophylline in 64 patients but with no control group (LIU and BLACKWELL, 1978). Salbutamol was effective in suppressing uterine activity early in treatment, but again overall there was no significant difference between the two drugs.

The sympathomimetic amines not only modify uterine activity but also influence changes in hormone concentrations. For example, salbutamol has been given in doses of between 4 and 32 μg/min intravenously followed by oral therapy (8 mg, 8-hourly) to stabilise uterine activity (BIBBY et al., 1978). During treatment oestradiol and progesterone levels fell independently but significantly ($p < 0.05$) by about 20% within 1 h. Once again, responses varied enormously with some decreases of up to 82% in the first 4 h. Progesterone levels returned to pretreatment levels within 6 h and oestradiol within 40 h of ceasing treatment, but it was not ascertained that these effects were physiologically independent of the control of pre-term labour. It was, however, considered that they were not secondary to changes in uterine blood flow.

It has been reported that ritodrine infusions decrease uterine blood flow in pregnant sheep (EHRENKRANZ et al., 1976), but according to data which include an unaltered production of placental lactogen this does not seem to be the case in humans with salbutamol (BIBBY et al., 1978). In fact, contrary to the findings in sheep, blood flow may actually increase – at least with ritodrine – possibly through an increase in cardiac output (BIENIARZ et al., 1974; BRETTES et al., 1976).

β) Oral Therapy. In a retrospective study (TAMBYRAJA, 1978) the outcome for 50 patients carrying twins and who were treated with 6–12 mg oral salbutamol daily, according to the pulse rate, were compared with 42 women who were treated with variable periods of bed rest. The mean gestational period for the treated and control groups were 271 and 258 days ($p < 0.001$) respectively with a birth weight of 2.73 kg and 2.33 kg. From the treated mothers there were four babies less than 2 kg and only one was stillborn. In the control group there were ten such babies, six of whom died before or immediately after birth. HASTWELL et al. (1978) have attempted to show that the oral route is as effective but more practical than the intravenous. They used doses up to 12 mg 6-hourly, suggesting that 4 mg 6-hourly was inadequate, but in this range 68% of their patients experienced tremor and 21% had pulse rates of more than 110 beats/min.

It was these authors who commented on the low incidence of postpartum haemorrhage (2%), pre-eclampsia (1%), and respiratory distress syndrome (4%) in their series of 208 treated patients who had experienced painful contractions (more than one per 10 min) between the 20 th and 36 th weeks of gestation. In a retrospective study (HASTWELL and LAMBERT, 1978) a group of 26 patients with premature labour including some with antepartum haemorrhage were treated with either bed rest (5), or ritodrine 10 mg thrice daily (4) or salbutamol 16–32 mg daily (17). The number of days elapsing until delivery were 1.2, 26.8, and 24.5 days respectively, and the mean Apgar score at 1 min was similarly 2.6, 5.3, and 4.4. Estimates of blood loss from continuing haemorrhage averaged 420, 75, and 70 ml, but it must be pointed out that the matching of the treatment groups was not good. Despite this it would seem that contrary to earlier opinion, β_2-agonists are not necessarily contra-indicated in antepartum haemorrhage. They may well slow cervical effacement and reduce the shearing effects at the placental edge and therefore confer actual benefit when it is placenta praevia causing haemorrhage. In abruptio placentae β-sympathomimetics may increase blood flow and predispose towards continued bleeding and possible exsanguination of the fetus. Ritodrine, which is not effective orally, as expected, did not delay labour when given in doses of 10 mg every 6 h (WALTERS and WOOD, 1977).

c) Toxicity

The agents described in this section do not have a blemish-free record when administered to the pregnant woman. One report (DAUBERT et al., 1978) described the intravenous use over 5 months of approximately 30 g isoxsuprine to stabilise a pregnancy in a 32-year-old who had been noted to have what was considered a benign systolic murmur at the age of 6. After the sixth month of treatment, asthenia, hypoproteinaemia, dyspnoea, and peripheral vasodilatation were marked. At 8 months β-stimulation was stopped and there was sudden onset of pulmonary oedema during the ensuing labour. ECG evidence included an abnormal repolarisation pattern, various conduction defects and ventricular ectopic activity. Phonocardiography and catheter studies indicated a non-obstructive cardiomyopathy which took some 6 months to recover. Another patient (DHAINAUT et al., 1978), receiving an unspecified amount of salbutamol and isoxsuprine, suffered the acute onset of left ventricular failure with extrasystoles, abnormal repolarisation, and left anterior hemiblock at the commencement of delivery. This patient recovered within 1 month.

In a third case treated with ritodrine and salbutamol, heart failure occurred 5 days after delivery. It remains to be answered whether with high doses of β_2-agonists selectivity is lost and increased stimulation of the heart creates a mimic of adrenergic myocarditis (MAGNUSSON and HANSSON, 1973) more usually associated with chronic catecholamine stimulation from, e.g., phaeochromocytoma. Such a situation might well be worsened critically by the additional burden of labour.

Although significant falls in plasma potassium (SMITH and THOMPSON, 1977) and increases in plasma glucose and insulin (THOMAS et al., 1977) are seen after intravenous salbutamol, HASTWELL and LAMBERT (1978) found no consistent hypokalaemia or hyperglycaemia during long-term control of labour with oral therapy. They conclude that at least with oral therapy changes are minor and should be monitored but not treated since they tend to revert to normal within 48 h and 96 h for potassium and glucose, respectively, on cessation of treatment.

3. Respiratory Medicine

a) Introduction

Tone in bronchial smooth muscle is influenced by activation of β_2- and possibly α-adrenoceptors found in the bronchial tree. Compounds which stimulate β_2-receptors decrease this tone and are therefore of clinical importance in the treatment of diseases associated with bronchospasm. At first, non-specific drugs such as adrenaline were used successfully in bronchial asthma, but more recently the stimulants selective for the β_2-receptor have been found to be more effective and probably safer. They are widely used in the treatment of various forms of asthma and bronchospasm associated with chronic obstructive airway disease, where they produce virtually maximal bronchodilatation with minimum effect on the cardiovascular system.

They are catecholamine, resorcinol or phenol derivatives with an ethanolamine side chain. The more bulky the substitution of the side-chain nitrogen atom, the better the β_2-selectivity and the less the stimulatory effects on the β_1-and α-receptors (BRITTAIN et al., 1970; BRITTAIN et al., 1976). Substitution of the aromatic ring slows enzymic cleavage (catechol-o-methyl transferase) of the side chain between the α-carbon and terminal nitrogen atoms, and it is generally agreed that the biological effect of stimulation continues for as long as the drug-receptor complex is stable. Ring substitution, therefore, partly determines the duration of drug action. The stimulants are probably allosteric activators of the adenyl cyclase enzyme system within the cell wall, and increase intracellular concentration of cyclic AMP. The relation between structure and β-stimulatory activity has been reviewed by HARTLEY and JACK (1978).

So intense has interest been that practically within a decade of the first suggestion of β_2-receptors, some 14 stimulant aerosols were in clinical use (LEIFER and WITTIG, 1975).

b) Evaluation of Clinical Trials

As the study of treatment for bronchospastic conditions has evolved, so a number of shortcomings have become apparent in some of the methods used for the clinical assessment of bronchodilators.

It is inherently difficult to compare the results of various trials when there is insufficient attention paid to the true comparability of doses employed for comparison. It is also clear that during validation of aerosols, for example, it is especially important to include placebo treatment, since this alone can cause marked changes in FEV_1 and maximum expiratory flow (RUFFIN et al., 1977). It is imperative to standardise background therapy, as far as possible the time of year and certainly the time of day for assessment, the inhalation technique and the possibilities of allergic reactions. Treatment groups should be truly matched and randomised treatment should preferably be given on different days. Long-term trials are bedevilled with variations in the response of individuals over a period of time and the effects of ill-defined extraneous factors. Particularly bronchodilatory activity in a given subject depends on basal levels of bronchoconstriction (HUME and GANDEVIA, 1957) which means that this must be assessed before each treatment. The enormous variations amongst and within patients tends to create a need for large numbers and makes within-patient comparative studies more preferable. Whole-body plethysmograhy probably represent the best measurement of airway resistance but it is clearly not practical for the majority of studies.

Routine spirometry has to provide the mainstay of assessment and it is best that measurements are recorded over a number of hours with up to the largest tolerated dose being evaluated in order to produce well-defined clinical side-effects. Only when all these factors have received due consideration is it possible to compare the efficacy of one treatment against another and assess the effect of optimal doses, and thus ensure the results are relevant to everyday clinical practice.

c) Asthma

In this disease the major physiological component, bronchospasm, is accompanied by a varying degree of mucosal oedema and mucus plugging (DUNNILL, 1971). It is essential that stimulation of β_2-receptors to relieve bronchospasm should not cause further deterioration of the hypoxia frequently associated with the asthmatic attack and in particular it should not predispoe towards carbon dioxide retention, which is normally regarded as a serious prognostic sign. There was unterstandable concern after the introduction of aerosols when it was thought that there could be actual deterioration of the perfusion/ventilation ratio in the lungs following their use. LEIFER and WITTIG (1975), however, concluded that most reports of decreases in arterial oxygen tension were confined to patients who had particularly high baseline values. It appeard that in many cases blood sampling techniques were not optimal and that there was not a single case where the partial pressure of oxygen fell below 40 mm Hg after use of an aerosol. On the other hand, subcutaneous and inhaled terbutaline and oral terbutaline and salbutamol have been compared against placebo in spasm-free asthmatics with special reference to blood gases. They did not cause any changes other than an unexpected slight increase in oxygen tension (HOLTEN, 1974; LEGGE et al., 1971).

Adrenaline was first given subcutaneously in the treatment of asthma in 1903 and 7 years later by aerosol (BARGER and DALE, 1910). It was not until 1940 that a synthetic catecholamine (isoprenaline) was used (KONZETT, 1940). The decrease in side-effects was encouraging and led to the trial of isoetharine (HERSCHFUS et al., 1951), which was followed 10 years later with further improvement regarding side-effects by orciprenaline (GUNTHNER, 1962). Once LANDS and co-workers (1967) raised the possibility of β_2-stimulation, major advances came with selective activators such as salbutamol (BRITTAIN, et al., 1968; PALMER et al., 1970) and terbutaline (FORMGREN, 1970; FREEDMAN, 1971).

Whilst the value of β-stimulation is clear in the relief of bronchospasm, it must not be forgotton that steroids have an important role in the relief of the oedema and they are probably still underused (COCHRANE and CLARK, 1975; Editorial, 1978). Adrenaline, used little in routine treatment of asthma (Editorial, 1978), remains the first-line drug in the acute life-threatening situation, in otherwise healthy young subjects (HUTCHISON, 1975). Above all, it cannot be emphasised too often that any failure to respond to treatment should prompt a vigorous search for medical attention.

α) Routes of Drug Administration. β_2-Stimulants can be administered orally, sublingually, intravenously, subcutaneously, and by inhalation from metered aerosols or nebulisers.

The efficiency of the various routes is illustrated, for example, with terbutaline. Subcutaneously 0.25 mg will produce an increase in FEV_1 of 0.40–0.48 l (HOLTEN, 1974; GLASS and DULFANO, 1973); from metered aerosol (0.5 mg) (FORMGREN, 1970;

HUHTI, 1972), 0.57–0.60 l; from an intermittent positive-pressure respirator (5 mg) (SIMONSSON et al., 1976), 0.51 l; and orally 5 mg, an increase of 0.45 l (DULFANO and GLASS, 1973). About one-tenth the dose is needed with direct inhalation from an aerosol, compared with the oral dose.

Subcutaneously, effects are seen within 5 min; they peak at 30 min and have a duration of some 4 h or more (HOLTEN, 1974; GLASS and DULFANO, 1973). Orally peak effects are seen at about 2–3 h, lasting up to 5 h (DULFANO and GLASS, 1973).

Most evidence suggests both the dose-response characteristics and effect/side-effect ratios are best if β_2-stimulants are taken properly by inhalation (DUBI et al., 1974; SCHWITTER et al., 1975), despite the fact that it is well known that only a small proportion of the administered dose reaches the smaller airways (SHENFIELD et al., 1973). Radiotracers and detection of metabolites suggest that only approximately 10% of isoprenaline (DAVIES, 1975), salbutamol (SHENFIELD et al., 1973) and terbutaline (NILSSON et al., 1976) reaches lung tissue. This route, has the advantage in that it allows direct access for stimulants to lessen the effect of mediators released from mast cells on the mucosal surface or in the lumen of the airways (KALINER and AUSTEN, 1975) as the antigen-antibody reaction proceeds. The aerosol route is also dramatically more effective at prophylactically blocking exercise-induced asthma in children than is the oral route (ANDERSON et al., 1975; GODFREY and KÖNIG, 1976; ANDERSON et al., 1976). In a series of 23 children (LENNEY and MILNER, 1978 a) aged between 3.1 and 5.2 years with recurrent wheeze, 20 were found to have abnormal postexercise bronchoconstriction. All responded well to nebulised salbutamol. In ten older patients (14–29 years) with a 20% fall in PEFR following exercise, oral salbutamol (16 mg daily) did not prevent the onset of postexercise bronchoconstriction (SEALE et al., 1977).

Metered aerosols can be used by children, but under the age of 5 (or 9 during an attack) it is unlikely that they will be used effectively. Nebulisers have the advantage of effective delivery and easily controlled maximum doses (BLOOMFIELD et al., 1979 a), but most important of all, synchronisation with the respiratory cycle is not required. This is of particular value if there is lack of co-ordination, ability or understanding and is as much true for the elderly as it is for children.

The effect of nebulisation does not appear to be enhanced further by use of a delivery system involving intermittent positive pressure. The same benefits in flow rate and volumes were achieved after salbutamol and isoprenaline (400 μg) using the patient's own chest muscles. However, though the patients assessed were all symptom-free and not obviously severely bronchoconstricted, they had FEV_1/FVC ratios of $63 \pm 8\%$ (GUPTA et al., 1978). Furthermore, nebulised salbutamol can be as effective as that given intravenously (LAWFORD et al., 1978) but has the added advantage of fewer metabolic and symptomatic side-effects. In children aged between 2 and 11 (BACON, 1978) it was as effective as intravenous aminophylline. Nebulised particles (2 μm in diameter) containing sympathomimetics can create immediate beneficial effects, presumably by direct action, since bronchodilatation occurs before drugs can be detected in the plasma, and it is interesting to note how it has become accepted that effective doses by nebuliser are 20–25 times those of aerosol, e.g., 5–10 mg and 200 μg respectively for salbutamol (SHENFIELD et al., 1973) – the lower effective doses having never really been determined. RUFFIN et al. (1978 b) studied nine salbutamol-responsive asthmatics in a double-blind fashion with placebo and five different doses of salbutamol. First, they found that by a radiotracer technique, only 2%–10% of the dose reaches the lung in normal subjects – the larger the breath, the less the dose. Significant responses occurred in a dose-related fashion down to 1 mg in asthmatics. The effect was not as long-lasting as 5 mg but it was nevertheless definite. It would seem that, in the absence of particularly high respiratory flow rates, starting doses of 1 mg may be more appropriate than the higher doses currently in use.

RUFFIN et al. (1978 a) found that of a dose of fenoterol from an ultrasonic generator (median droplet diameter 3.5 μm) 86% reached the lungs on average and maximal changes in FEV_1 and peak flow at 50% vital capacity could be achieved with doses as low as 3 μg. A calculated dose of 5.6 μg produced effects about half-way between those of placebo and a dose of 32.7 μg, but they were shorter-lived and indistinguishable from placebo at 4 h. The trial was carried out on 22 isoprenaline-responsive ambulatory asthmatics with the doses given in a randomised double-blind fashion as far as possible on consecutive days.

More recently, salbutamol has been prepared in powder form specifically for use in the "Rota Haler". The dry powder inhaler has the advantages of an easily fixed maximum dose and less co-ordination being required for its use. A disadvantage is that the apparatus tends to need careful assembly, which may be difficult for the elderly with arthritic disease or tremor or for the very young. It is of particular value for children and the elderly and it has been shown that children down to the age of 6 years can manage quite adequately. In a trial of ten children, peak expiratory flow rates (PEFR) 10 min after 200 μg powder increased by a mean of 20.2%. Ten minutes later 200 μg aerosol produced a further 6.6% increase in PEFR. When the control was conducted the other way round, the aerosol first produced an increase of 14.7% and the powder a further 10.4%. This suggests that the powder is as effective if not better than aerosol, a result that has also been noted in adults (HETZEL and CLARK, 1977). The powder produced significantly greater increases in PEFR (55%) than placebo (3.7%). Between 3 and 5 years of age, the benefit is still present but not as great (LENNEY et al., 1978).

Formal comparison between the long-term use of the commonest routes, oral, and metered aerosol, has not yet been reported. However, there have been comparisons between intravenous administration and aerosol. For example, terbutaline and salbutamol are equipotent by either route but intravenously there are more symptomatic side-effects (NEVILLE et al., 1977; THIRINGER and SVEDMYR, 1976). It may be anticipated the same will be found with oral administration when compared with aerosol. Parenteral adminstration of a bronchodilator ought to have slightly more effect on smaller airways, especially in the presence of extensive mucous plugging, but its remains to be demonstrated that important gains are to be made on selective improvement of ventilation and gas exchange through effect on small airways from the use of oral preparations.

Oral therapy does have practical advantages over aerosol in, for example, children, the elderly and those who may be embarrassed by using an aerosol in public. Severe bronchospasm and mucous plugging might limit access of nebulised particles, so for those with expectoration difficulties or severe bronchospasm oral treatment combined with aerosol might have distinct therapeutic advantages, most likely if given at separate times. If tablets and inhalation are used at the same time, there is no benefit from using a combination (LAHDENSUO and ALANKO, 1976). If side-effects become troublesome with combined routes of administration then it would appear most reasonable to reduce the oral component. Small doses given frequently are likely to be more beneficial than large doses given spasmodically, but again formal validation of this point has not been made.

Inhalation has been compared with intravenous administration in a carefully constructed randomised double-blind cross-over trial (BLOOMFIELD et al., 1979b) of 22 life-threatening episodes of asthma using salbutanol. Intravenous injection (500 μg) improved PEFR to the same extent as a 0.5% solution given by nebuliser for 3 min but it produced a tachycardia which masked the decrease in heart rate during-early clinical improvement seen with nebuliser treatment. Furthermore, the decrease in pulsus paradoxus was less impressive with the intravenous route and it was these patients who noted cardiovascular side-effects. Intravenous salbutamol compared with aerosol tends to produce tremor and cardiovascular side-effects without corresponding benefit, even in the relief of stable asthma (HETZEL and CLARK, 1976). Side-effects were not reported when using a nebuliser in severely ill patients (LAWFORD et al., 1978), however, it still stands that if mucous plugging is excessive then nebulised preparations may fail. Under these circumstances, the intravenous route is probably more effective (WILLIAMS and SEATON, 1977).

The advantages of intravenous therapy are that doses are easily controlled and that the onset of action is rapid. Disadvantages, however, include the fact that the agent gains wider distribution to create side-effects by stimulation of other β_2-receptors. The nebulised routes of administration have been shown to be highly effective and it is probably becoming true to say that the intravenous therapy should be reserved for resistant cases, unresponsive to nebulisers, or for when the necessary apparatus is not available.

Finally the relative potency of β_2-stimulants is influenced by their route of administration. Salbutamol, when given either orally or by aerosol is equipotent to, or a little more potent than isoprenaline (WARRELL et al., 1970) but when given intravenously it is about one-seventh as potent (MARLIN and TURNER, 1975). Similarly, rimiterol, taken by aerosol, is equipotent to isoprenaline in normal and asthmatic subjects (GRIFFIN and TURNER, 1971; SHENFIELD and PATERSON, 1973), but intravenously isoprenaline is about seven times more potent. This is partly explained by oral isoprenaline being rapidly taken into tissues and being inactivated by sulphatases and catechol-o-methyl transferases in different tissues, particularly the gut wall. This explains why rimiterol is inactive when taken by mouth. The enzymes also account for the short half-lives and relatively short durations of action when given intravenously or by aerosol (CONOLLY et al., 1972; EVANS et al., 1973b; GRIFFIN et al., 1973; BLACKWELL et al., 1974).

β) Clinical Evaluation. Aerosol Therapy. Inhalation of β-sympathomimetic agents produces rapid symptomatic improvement. Bronchodilatation occurs rapidly, mucociliary clearance increases (CAMNER et al., 1976) and intrabronchial mast cells are probably stabilised (SORENBY, 1974). Retrospective studies suggest benefit is greater with regular rather than intermittent use (AYRES et al., 1974; FORMGREN, 1975).

Isoprenaline given by aerosol gives excellent bronchodilatation within 2–5 min with a relatively short duration of action lasting 1–2 h. There is a tendency to produce side-effects such as tachycardia (WARRELL et al., 1970). A large dose (1 mg) produced effects on FEV_1 and FVC at 15 min, indistinguishable from 200 μg salbutamol (PAL-

MER, 1971) with a small but significant fall in arterial oxygen tension. Orciprenaline is similarly effective but with a longer duration of action. (MILLER, 1967).

Salbutamol (AVERY, 1971) produces peak effects within 30–60 min of inhalation, and has some benefit remaining at 6 h (WARRELL et al., 1970). It improves FEV_1 and FVC without decreasing arterial oxygen tension (PALMER and DIAMENT, 1969; PATERSON et al., 1971). The median effective dose (ED_{50}) by nebuliser is 110 μg (WILDBOLZ et al., 1978). The normal recommended dose of 5 drops of 0.5% salbutamol in 2 ml saline (1,250 μg) produces 85% of the maximal response, and marginal advantages of using higher doses are likely to be outweighed by the appearance of side-effects. Salbutamol (100 μg) and terbutaline (250 μg) produce similar changes in FEV_1 over 90 min, but thereafter effects are significantly more pronounced with terbutaline (FREEDMAN, 1972).

HUHTI and POUKKULA (1978) compared the newer drug, fenoterol (400 μg), with salbutamol (200 μg) in a placebo-controlled randomised double-blind cross-over. For the first 2 h the two active agents produced similar increases in FEV_1 (46–48%) and peak expiratory flow (47%–48%). Thereafter fentoerol was confirmed as having significantly greater effects than salbutamol on FEV_1 and peak expiratory flow but less on FVC. From the first 5 min the heart rate was significantly faster with fenoterol, but only because the salbutamol group showed an unexpected and unexplained fall in heart rate.

In a double-blind study of 20 asthmatic patients, 400μg fenoterol was statistically more effective than 1,500 μg orciprenaline at improving airway function and its action was maintained for over 3 h. The dose of 800 μg however was indistinguishable from 3,000 μg orciprenaline. Furthermore at the higher dose, heart rate was increased by 10%, and it took 120 min to return to normal (BEARDSHAW et al., 1974). The effect of orciprenaline on heart rate at the higher dose was less (2.1% increase) and it only lasted 30 min. Orciprenaline and fenoterol in lower doses (200–800 μg) produced similar increases in FEV_1, but the latter, weight for weight, appeared more potent. Doses of fenoterol above 400 μg do not further improve respiratory function (TWEEL, 1971).

In children between the ages of 7 and 13, fenoterol 200 μg and salbutamol 100 μg were indistinguishable, both producing rapid increases in FEV_1 and vital capacity with peak values at 120 and 60 min respectively and some effects lasting 6 h (GRAFF-LONNEVIG, 1976). In two studies with nebulisers in children between 6 and 14.5 years, fenoterol (1 and 2 mg) was compared with placebo, and salbutamol (1 and 2 mg), orciprenaline (2.5 and 5 mg), and isoprenaline (5 and 10 mg) were compared with each other in a randomised manner. There was no difference fenoterol (2 mg) and salbutamol (2 mg) or between either dose of fenoterol. There was no difference in the increase of FEV_1 and PEFR between fenoterol, orciprenaline and isoprenaline, but salbutamol gave higher maximal values and isoprenaline produced a tachycardia (BLACKHALL et al., 1976).

In chronic studies over 3 months in 31 isoprenaline-responsive asthmatics, fenoterol (400 μg; 17 patients) appeared to have a greater and more lasting effect on FEV_1 and specific airway conductance than isoprenaline (150 μg; 14 patients) (STEEN et al., 1977). BRANDON (1978) also found a slight progressive improvement of baseline FEV_1 with fenoterol (400 μg thrice daily) over 90 days but not with isoprenaline (150 μg thrice daily). Areas under the dose-response curve were significantly greater in the former group but they remained unchanged throughout the study. Tolerance did not appear to develop. Fenoterol improved FEV_1 and forced expiratory flow for 6 and 4 h respectively whereas isoprenaline had effects for 2 and 1,5 h. The clinical use of fenoterol has been extensively reviewed by HEEL et al. (1978); it is superior to placebo with a longer time to maximum effect than isoprenaline but with a longer duration of action. In general there are few demonstrations of any real difference from salbutamol, orciprenaline or terbutaline except that its action is more prolonged. It may have a slightly larger maximal effect on FEV_1.

Terbutaline is longer-acting than either isoprenaline or orciprenaline. In a double-blind cross-over study, two puffs of terbutaline (500 μg) had the same effect in increasing FEV_1 as orciprenaline (1.5 mg) (FORMGREN, 1970). The effect of terbutaline was still marked after 5 h, as was also seen in a comparison with isoprenaline (160 μg) (HUHTI, 1972). Similar changes in the peak expiratory flow rate were seen 1 h after salbutamol, total dose 300 μg, and terbutaline (750 μg) given cumulatively over half an hour. At 5 h there was still significant improvement with terbutaline whereas with salbutamol flow rates were approximating to pretreatment levels (SIMONSSON et al., 1972a).

Rimiterol was equipotent to isoprenaline in a human histamine bronchospasm model and in asthmatic subjects (GRIFFIN and TURNER, 1971; SHENFIELD and PATERSON, 1973) but it is shorter acting and clearly more β_2-selective, as shown in a study of 15 asthmatics who received salbutamol (0.5%) or rimiterol (0.5%–1.0%). No increase in heart rate was observed with rimiterol despite an equal but shorter-lived bronchodilating action (COOKE et al., 1974).

Hexoprenaline (100 μg) produces a 60% increase in maximum voluntary ventilation within 15 min which is still 40% above baseline at 3 h (VAN AS et al., 1973). Neither in this study nor following oral (SCHINDL, 1970) or intravenous use has there been any significant adverse effect on blood gases (BENJAMIN and VAN AS, 1972).

Oral Therapy. Terbutaline is effective orally. Single doses (5 mg) have been found in double-blind studies on patients with chronic bronchitis and asthma to be significantly more effective at increasing FEV_1 than orciprenaline (20 mg) (FORMGREN, 1970) and ephedrine (25 mg) (GEUMEI et al., 1975). In adults 15 mg daily taken over 12 months remained effective, there was no shift in the isoprenaline/FEV_1 dose-response curves, tolerance did not develop and the addition of an aerosol to oral treatment produced a further increment of benefit (SVEDMYR et al., 1976). In children 0.075 mg/kg produced a 55% increase in PEFR after 2 h with a 20% increase still persisting at 5 h (LEEGAARD and FJULSRUD, 1973).

Milligram for milligram, salbutamol and terbutaline produce similar improvements in FEV_1 and over a similar time course and without altering arterial oxygen tension (LEGGE et al., 1971). In 24 patients with chronic obstructive lung disease, terbutaline (5 mg) was more effective than fenoterol (5 mg), the time course suggesting this to be related to dose rather than a different mechanism of action. Maximum benefit in peak flow, forced expiratory volume and vital capacity is usually apparent at 3 h and lasts up to 8 h. Earliest benefits are seen within half an hour (GEUMEI et al., 1975) and increases in heart rate are less than those seen with orciprenaline (20 mg) (GEUMEI et al., 1976). No deterioration was seen in changing from mainly theophylline and ephedrine to thrice daily terbutaline, but steroid requirements were significantly reduced. In another group there were reductions in the number of days spent in hospital (30%) and average sick leave (63%) for each patient (FORMGREN, 1971).

SEALE et al. (1977) have looked for prophylactic effects in exercise-induced asthma with oral salbutamol (4 mg, 6-hourly), theophylline (125 mg, 6-hourly) or placebo given up to 48 h before an 8-min treadmill exercise test. Resting peak flow rates were increased by salbutamol and theophylline when compared with placebo but neither agent significantly prevented a fall of between 30% and 40% in flow during exercise. This agrees with the findings of ANDERSON et al. (1975), who found that oral terbutaline was similarly ineffective in the prevention of exercise-induced asthma, and supports the concept that exercise-induced asthma (SILVERMAN et al., 1973) is best treated by β-stimulants given by aerosol (GODFREY and KÖNIG, 1976).

Oral fenoterol is more effective than placebo and probably better than either ephedrine or orciprenaline, and it compares well with salbutamol and terbutaline. Single-blind assessment of ten isoprenaline-responsive asthmatics with fenoterol (5–20 mg) and orciprenaline (20 mg) were better than placebo in terms of FEV_1, FVC, and forced midexpiratory flow. Maximal effects were seen 120 min after fenoterol and 90 min after orciprenaline (GEUMEI et al., 1976). At 6 h, 25% and 5% increases in the parameters described above were present for 10 mg fenoterol and 20 mg orciprenaline respectively. There was a dose-related increase in heart rate for the fenoterol. It may be anticipated that 10 mg fenoterol, 4 mg salbutamol, and 5 mg terbutaline would have indistinguishable effects in single-dose comparative studies.

In longer-term studies fenoterol and terbutaline (and by implication, salbutamol), are effective and superior to ephedrine. In asthmatics double-blind comparison of fenoterol (up to 40 mg daily) with ephedrine (up to 96 mg daily) over 12 weeks showed fenoterol to be superior (SIMI and MILLER, 1977) at improving respiratory function but not the number of asthmatic attacks. Fenoterol and terbutaline (15 mg daily) under double-blind conditions produced a 15% rise in baseline FEV_1 over 6 weeks in moderate airway obstruction (CHERVINSKY, 1977).

Carbuterol (up to 12 mg daily) has been compared with ephedrine (up to 140 mg daily) in a double-blind fashion over 6 months in aged-matched isoprenaline-responsive bronchitic asthmatics who kept to their usual oral theophylline and aerosol therapy (MILLER et al., 1977). In a group receiving carbuterol, baseline values of FEV_1, FVC, and maximum midexpiratory flow increased significantly over 4 months. The percentage response 3 h after a challenge dose of carbuterol (3 mg) decreased, there was a large standard deviation and not all patients completed the trial but all were included in the data analysis. Baseline changes with ephedrine were not consistent (this group had the highest drop-out rate) but they may have improved over the first 2 months. Carbuterol challenge was associated with tachycardia, but ephedrine challenge was not. MINETTE et al. (1976) studied 30 chronic bronchitics responsive to orciprenaline. They compared in random fashion oral carbuterol (3 mg), salbutamol (3 mg), terbutaline (3 mg), orciprenaline (20 mg), and placebo. Fenoterol was included in doses of either 5 or 12 mg. FEV_1 and specific airway conductance were measured for up to 7 h after morning doses taken on different days. In the doses used, which can be criticised for not being equipotent, carbuterol, like terbutaline, had maximal effects on FEV_1 at 2 h, with a steady fall over the next 5 h. They were both significantly more effective than orciprenaline after 2 h. Salbutamol had maximal effect within 1 h, with little fall over the next 6 h. The effects of fenoterol (12 mg and 5 mg) were not convincingly different from carbuterol (3 mg). Specific airway conductance at 1 h was significantly ($p < 0.05$) increased above that of placebo by carbuterol, orciprenaline, and salbutamol, but not by terbutaline. By 3 h all agents showed significant increases, with terbutaline and carbuterol continuing to cause improvement whereas the effects of salbutamol and especially orciprenaline were wearing off. Fenoterol (12 mg) mimicked carbuterol, but the 3 mg dose was only half as effective at 3 h. Carbuterol, orciprenaline and the higher dose of fenoterol produced increases in heart rate. Weight for weight, carbuterol was the most potent agent and although the heart rate was increased by only 10 beats/min over 3 h, in two patients, ECG changes were noted which might urge caution in patients with ischaemic heart disease.

Reproterol, having an alkyl xanthine substitution of the terminal nitrogen, has been shown to be superior to orciprenaline orally (NOLTE et al., 1977; TABORI et al., 1977), intravenously it was better tolerated than aminophylline (PINES et al., 1978) and by aerosol more efficacious in improving specific airway conductance than orciprenaline (MÁNDI et al., 1977). However, in a two-centre placebo-controlled double-blind cross-over comparison in 38 patients with reversible obstructive airway disease due to asthma, salbutamol (4 mg thrice daily) was accompanied by slightly better values for morning peak flow rate (292 ± 18.7 litres/min as opposed to 273 ± 18 l/min) for reproterol (20 mg thrice daily). All other parameters, including side-effects and heart rate, showed no difference. At best the drug can only be considered as an alternative to salbutamol (BATEMAN et al., 1979).

Hexoprenaline has been used orally and the use of the drug in 1,400 asthmatics has shown it to be comparable but having no distinctive advantages over orciprenaline or salbutamol (SCHINDL, 1970).

Intravenous Therapy. KLAUSTERMEYER et al. (1975) compared the effect of different doses of intravenous isoprenaline in several adults with acute exacerbation of asthma but who were not in status asthmaticus. Doses of 0.04–0.225 μg/kg/min were given in a graded stepwise fashion over 20–25 min intervals with serial assessment of respiratory function. The infusion was followed by 5% dextrose. Tachycardia and a fall in diastolic blood pressure were noted in all the patients assessed; the bronchodilator effect was seen within 2–5 min and was dose-related. Hypotension necessitated cessation of the treatment in one case and pulsus paradoxus was seen in another. Arterial oxygen tension (mean values) tended to fall in the lower dose range but response of individuals was not disclosed. It was considered that underperfused lungs may have contributed, since the minute ventilation increased. In view of evidence from aninals where isoprenaline toxicity is enhanced by hypoxia (COLLINS et al., 1969), the frequency of hypoxia in severe asthma and the tendency for there to be slight further falls in oxygen tension with isoprenaline would suggest it is not the first drug of choice. However, it has been used intravenously in children in status asthmaticus successfully for up to 48 h (WOOD et al., 1972). In other work on clinically stable adult asthmatics, intravenous salbutamol (up to 10.8 μg/min) tended to increase arterial tension but isoprenaline (up to 2.2 μg/min) did not (PATERSON et al., 1971).

Salbutamol's relatively long therapeutic half-life is an advantage in the treatment of asthma when compared with the situation in obstetrics and cardiovascular medicine, where finer adjustment of therapy is indicated. It is as effective as aminophylline but less likely to cause nausea and vomiting (WILLIAMS et al., 1975) and it is between one-fifth and one-tenth as potent as isoprenaline (WARRELL et al., 1970).

Single high and low doses (0.5 and 0.05 μg/kg/min) of rimiterol given intravenously, have been compared with high and low doses of intravenous salbutamol (0.3 and 0.03 μg/kg/min), isoprenaline (0.05 and 0.005 μg/kg/min), and placebo in histamine-induced bronchospasm (MARLIN and TURNER, 1975). The trial was conducted over 7 days in a double-blind randomised Latin square fashion and it was seen that high doses of rimiterol, salbutamol, and isoprenaline produced 98%, 96%, and 69% protection respectively and the lower doses were not different from placebo although significant improvement was noted in subjects receiving rimiterol. At the higher dose, least tremor was seen with rimiterol but the increases in both heart rate and blood pressure were not significantly different from those with salbutamol. A dose-response relationship was seen for all parameters with each drug. On an equimolar basis, intravenous rimiterol is about one-seventh as potent a bronchodilator as isoprenaline and five-sevenths as potent as salbutamol. By inhalation, rimiterol and isoprenaline were equipotent in normal and asthmatic subjects (GRIFFIN and TURNER, 1971; SHENFIELD and PATERSON, 1973).

Terbutaline is effective intravenously but it is not generally administered by this route. Formal validation has concentrated on the subcutaneous route. In a double-blind cross-over trial in 15 patients with stable asthma, terbutaline (0.25 mg subcutaneously) produced significant increases in mean expiratory flow rate without increasing pulse rate. The effects were similar to those produced by 0.25 mg adrenaline but less than those with 0.5 mg terbutaline, which produced increases in heart rate (GLASS and DULFANO, 1973). In a cross-over study, terbutaline (0.5 mg), adrenaline (0.5 mg), and fenoterol (0.16 mg) were assessed single-blind in 14 asthmatic patients. They produced almost identical increases in peak expiratory flow rate at 30 min but the effect lasted up to 3 h with terbutaline. In contrast to the aerosol route, fenoterol seems to be short-acting and this may represent an increased rate of destruction. At these doses, palpitations were most pronounced after fenoterol (DA COSTA and GOH, 1973). Comparison with adrenaline (AMORY et al., 1975) in reversible airway obstruction has confirmed the prolonged action of terbutaline.

γ) Side-effects. In general the duration and nature of symptomatic side-effects with β_2-stimulants salbutamol, terbutaline, and fenoterol are probably much the same (LEIFER and WITTIG, 1975). They include tachycardia, palpitations, tremor, various manifestations of anxiety and less obvious metabolic disturbances.

Tremor, although not always severe, is frequently reported but seldom quantified (FORMGREN, 1975; LEGGE et al., 1971; SCHUMANN and HERXHEIMER, 1971; SVEDMYR et al., 1972). It appears to be dose-dependent and is consequently associated more frequently with intravenous or oral use than positive-pressure ventilation or aerosol (WALKER et al., 1972; SHENFIELD et al., 1973). The suggestion that tremor accompanying β_2-stimulation is due to the direct effect on the β-receptors of skeletal muscle (MARSDEN and MEADOWS, 1970; BOWMAN and NOTT, 1969) has been supported by the fact that isoprenaline- and adrenaline-induced tremor can be blocked by propranolol (MARSDEN et al., 1967) but not by the β_1-selective practolol (BOWMAN and NOTT, 1970) or the inactive *d*-propranolol (MARSDEN and MEADOWS, 1970). Rimiterol and salbutamol have about one-eighth the potency of isoprenaline in producing tremor in cat soleus muscle (BOWMAN and NOTT, 1970; BOWMAN and RODGER, 1972). Quantitative assessment has been attempted by WATSON and RICHENS (1974), and MARLIN and

TURNER (1975) found increases in tremor after intravenous injection: 140% for rimiterol (0.5 μg/min/kg), 164% for salbutamol (0.3 μg/min/kg), and 222% for isoprenaline (0.05 μg/min/kg). Subjective increases in tremor were also noted for rimiterol and isoprenaline given by aerosol to patients with obstructive lung disease (SVEDMYR et al., 1972).

The onset of tremor and other side-effects with parenteral administration is thought to be due to higher doses of the drug reaching a wider distribution of receptors. However, there is an inconsistency that both rimiterol (COOKE et al., 1974) and salmefamol when given by aerosol maintain their β_2-selectivity with no changes in heart rate, blood pressure or objective side-effects. One explanation is that orciprenaline, terbutaline, and salbutamol are partially degraded by transmethylases in the liver which reduces the size of the terminal nitrogen substitution with subsequent loss of β_2-specificity.

Depending on how much various drugs or their metabolites stimulate receptors to which they gain access, so side-effects will depend on the parent substance and its route of administration, as is illustrated by the following examples. Fenoterol 7.5–10 mg daily (MINETTE, 1970) had no cardiac effects during 6 months of treatment in 20 patients with chronic obstructive airway disease. However, 20% of patients complained of nervousness and 10% of shakiness (STEEN et al., 1975). Tachycardia only became pronounced with doses above 10 mg daily (GEUMEI et al., 1976; MINETTE et al., 1976). Two hours after an oral dose of terbutaline (5 mg) there was a 14.1% increase in heart rate as opposed to a 6.4% increase following the same dose of fenoterol; however, this became insignificant with prolonged use (CHERVINSKY, 1977).

The aerosol route is accompanied by the least number of side-effects, which was highlighted when salbutamol from aerosol used by a collected series was accompanied by 3% of cases complaining of tremor. This rose to 25%–35% if oral doses above 16 mg daily or the intravenous route were used. Orciprenaline used by 1173 patients collected from various trials using aerosols caused tachycardia in only 3.7% and other symptoms in less than 1% of the patients (LEIFER and WITTIG, 1975).

The intravenous route is frequently associated with tachycardia. For example, heart rate rose by 40%–50% with doses between 0.001 and 0.1 μg/kg/min with isoprenaline and salbutamol. Isoprenaline was about ten times more potent than salbutamol (WARRELL et al., 1970). Similarly for an equal degree of bronchodilatation, intravenous isoprenaline puts up heart rate between 2 and 2.5 times more than rimiterol and salbutamol respectively secondary to direct β_1-stimulation. With β_2-stimulation heart rate may increase indirectly through reflex following vasodilatation and the fall in diastolic blood pressure. In absolute terms, isoprenaline is about 14 times as potent at increasing heart rate as rimiterol and ten times as potent as salbutamol.

PALMER (1978) briefly reports that salbutamol (4 mg thrice daily) in 50 patients was accompanied by muscle cramps in 46%, with tremor and palpitations noted in 42% and 20% respectively. Side-effects such as these are minimised if not abolished by the use of aerosol. With single doses of carbuterol (3 mg) and fenoterol (12 mg) tremor, palpitations and dizziness were all noted, but with terbutaline (3 mg), fenoterol (5 mg), and salbutamol (3 mg) few side-effects are seen (MINETTE et al., 1976). It is therefore suggested that the doses be kept within these levels.

Metabolic effects of β_2-stimulation have been studied in bronchial asthma, where it was found that a single injection of salbutamol (300 µg) produced a transient but significant hypokalaemia within 10 min, accompanied by, as expected, a significant increase in peak flow. Continuous infusion (10 µg/min for 30 min) produced a significant fall ($p<0.01$) from 4.4 ± 0.5 to 3.3 ± 0.4 mEq/l potassium within 20 min with only partial recovery 3½ h after cessation of infusion. Even with doses to give significant bronchodilatation there was no significant hyperglycaemia. From the electrolyte point of view, bolus injections seemed preferable to prolonged infusion (ELEGBELYE et al., 1978). In further work with consecutive doses, salbutamol (0.1, 0.4, and 0.7 µg/kg/min) and rimiterol (0.15, 0.30, and 0.60 µg/kg/min) were infused for 90 and 60 min respectively, in four fasting subjects on totally separate occasions. There was a significant dose-related increase in heart rate and plasma glucose and a fall in potassium. Only for the increase in glucose concentration was salbutamol significantly more potent. Other phenomena include transient hyperinsulinaemia, a decrease in growth hormone, increases in renin activity as potassium concentration falls, a significant hyperlactaemia and changes in phosphate calcium and magnesium levels (PHILLIPS et al., 1978).

δ) Tolerance. The existence of this phenomenon remains contentious. Early reports included a diminished response to ephedrine following long-term use (HERXHEIMER, 1946) but this was not confirmed in more carefully controlled trials amongst children treated with 12.5–25 mg ephedrine daily for 6 days (TAYLOR et al., 1965). SIMS (1974) found that 16 mg oral salbutamol daily for 1 month did not cause a decrease in response to 200 µg inhaled salbutamol in a placebo-controlled trial. Similarly, treatment with 15 mg terbutaline daily by mouth (WILSON et al., 1976b) and 75 mg ephedrine did not decrease the response to inhaled doses after 1 year. LARSSON et al. (1977) sought a slight shift in the dose-response curve as a sensitive indication of tolerance. Prolonged use of terbutaline (5 mg thrice daily) over 12 months, produced no shift in the isoprenaline/FEV_1 dose-response curve. Interestingly there were shifts which indicated apparent tolerance developing for heart rate and, curiously enough, tremor. Pulmonary function tended to improve over the 12 months.

No convincing demonstration of tolerance has been seen in the following trials with orciprenaline (CHERVINSKY and CHERVINSKY, 1975), salbutamol (PARKER et al., 1971), terbutaline (TRAUTLEIN et al., 1976), or fenoterol (STEEN et al., 1977).

The weight of evidence suggests that despite some reports in animals, true tolerance per se of clinical relevance does not develop, certainly for the β_2-stimulants, although some doubt remains regarding the less specific agents.

Supportive evidence is to be found in several studies (AYRES et al., 1974; SMITH and DAVIES, 1973; FORMGREN, 1975; LIGHT et al., 1975; SIMS, 1974; LARSSON et al., 1977; TABORI et al., 1977).

There remains, however, the fact that under certain circumstances, which are not yet clearly defined, asthma can deteriorate following the prolonged use of aerosols (REISMAN, 1970; SIMS, 1974; KEIGHLEY, 1966). The whole subject has recently been reviewed by PATEL (1979), where evidence is summarised that suggests that there is decreased adrenoceptor responsiveness in asthma and that this, in part, may be brought about by prolonged exposure to endogenous and, more particularly within this context, exogenous β-stimulants. In the presence of diminished β-receptor function the bronchial muscle is increasingly sensitive to α-stimulation or overtone and therefore bronchoconstriction is potentiated. This is in accord with the original suggestions (CONOLLY et al., 1971) and seems relevant in the pathogenesis of death associated with overuse of aerosols.

ε) Toxicity. Aerosol Deaths. In general, it seems that the β_2-stimulants are safe, but this cannot be said with total confidence for all sympathomimetic aerosols. Data has been assembled which, although not conclusive, suggests that overuse of non-selective aerosols can precede sudden death. An association was noted between an increasing number of asthma deaths and the rise in the sale of pressurised aerosols (INMAN and ADELSTEIN, 1969), which naturally drew considerable attention (SPEIZER et al., 1968; Editorial, 1972). However, it was GANDEVIA (1973) who pointed out that the sale and use of aerosols had also increased in the United States and Australia without a closely linked increase in asthma deaths. It turned out that one difference was that aerosols available in the United Kingdom were providing, for example, doses of isoprenaline some five times greater than those used in other parts of the world. PATERSON et al. (1968) then suggested that isoprenaline resistance was playing an important part after prolonged overuse. Studies in normal subjects, and this may be particularly relevant, indicate that this is not so, at least for the β_1-receptor, as was confirmed by KINGSLEY et al. (1972). They found that dose-response curves repeated at various intervals over a few hours in the same subject were identical. At the end of the experiments, heart rates were higher than before the isoprenaline was given and there was no difference in heart rate response before and after a 45-min infusion of 0.75 µg/isoprenaline/min. This does not preclude resistance developing in the β_2-receptor, and CONOLLY et al. (1971) argued this was so in cases of severe asthma when the patients relied heavily on aerosols and eventually showed "therapeutic resistance". It could have been also said that oedema and plugging limited access, but this could not have been so when it transpired that some patients actually improved upon cessation of use of aerosols (CAPLIN and HAYNES, 1969; EISENSTADT and NICHOLAS, 1969; REISMAN, 1970). Rebound and idiosyncratic bronchoconstriction can occur after adrenaline and isoprenaline (RIDING et al., 1970; SPECTOR et al., 1975). Further considerations of this phenomenon revealed that it only appeared to occur after the use of less selective β-stimulants (FRASER et al., 1971). In this context, isoprenaline, orciprenaline, and adrenaline all have some α-stimulatory activity and this potentiates bronchoconstriction (SIMONSSON et al., 1972b). It may be relevant that when isoprenaline is repeatedly applied to rat aortic smooth muscle eventually there is less β-sensitivity and unmasking of α-mediated contraction (FLEISCH and TITUS, 1972). In the lung this may be further augmented by bacterial endotoxin from infection and endogenous catecholamines from fear and hypoxia increasing α-mediated bronchoconstriction (SIMONSSON et al., 1972b).

Aerosol Asthma. This is a described but rare entity which should be suspected when asthma is severe and unresponsive to steroids and where the use of aerosols is excessive. Its relevance to the above discussion is not yet established since the mechanism by which it is produced is not clear. Suggestions have included allergy to the propellants (AVIADO, 1975) or their breakdown products. If these postulates are true, improvement should be anticipated when aerosols are withdrawn, a fact which has been observed (VAN METRE, 1969; REISMAN, 1970). Many of these patients will be detected when they show a diminished response to isoprenaline 1 h after previous aerosol treatment.

ζ) *Beta-Stimulants and Children.* It has been noticed that β_2-stimulation with isoprenaline, salbutamol, and orciprenaline appears to be ineffective in wheezy children under the age of 1 year (PHELAN and WILLIAMS, 1969; RADFORD, 1975; RUTTER et al., 1975) and yet by the age of 5 years the children become responsive. LENNEY and MILNER (1978 b) examined this further among 32 patients aged between 7 months and 3 years 7 months. The children had audible wheeze and certain airway obstruction. It was found that significant decreases in total respiratory resistance only occurred above the age of 20 months, despite tachycardia (indicating absorption) being generated in both age groups. One child was resistant to treatment at the age of 17 months but had become responsive 11 months later. The reason for this or its relationship to maturity of bronchial muscle or numbers of β_2-receptors is as yet undetermined. In children above 2 years it has been shown that for the treatment of the acute attack nebulised salbutamol has been found to be as effective as intravenous and is a preferred route of administration (GODFREY, 1977).

d) Bronchiectasis

A study of 16 patients with bronchographically confirmed bronchiectasis were assessed randomly with placebo or nebulised (5 mg) salbutamol. Nine were studied, presumably on the same day, with intravenous (4 µg/kg) salbutamol. There was a significant ($p<0.05$) percentage increase in PEFR (26%) and FEV_1 (16%) between placebo and nebuliser, with slightly lower values (insignificant) after intravenous use. The authors were unable to detect responders from non-responders on immunological or clinical criteria (NOGRADY et al., 1978). Despite their having no history of asthma, salbutamol (400 µg) from an aerosol produced significant improvement in respiratory function amongst 20 patients with radiological evidence of emphysema. Thirteen, however, had also chronic bronchitis. In a placebo-controlled double-blind cross-over study, 400 µg salbutamol produced a significant increase in FEV_1 and, in particular, FVC. Parameters of ventilation during exercise were also improved by salbutamol (BELLAMY et al., 1978).

e) Chronic Bronchitis

In 24 patients with MRC criteria for bronchitis and no evidence of asthma, salbutamol aerosol (200 µg) produced significant ($p<0.001$) rises in FEV_1, FVC, and a 12-min walking distance (LEITCH et al., 1978). Clinical detection of patients who will respond is difficult and it should remain that such persons be given the facility of laboratory investigation to determine whether or not β_2-stimulants are likely to be of benefit.

f) Childhood Bronchospasm

Salbutamol (0.2–0.3 mg/kg/24 h) in syrup produced significant clinical relief in 16 of 18 children under the age of 2 suffering from presumed viral infection (non-asthmatic acute dyspnoeic bronchopneumopathy) or clinical asthma.

It was well tolerated and produced no increase in heart rate (FOURNET and DUPARD, 1978). Although it was suggested that a more dilute form should be prepared for babies under the age of 3 years, it should be remembered that there is evidence (LENNEY et al., 1978 b) that children under the age of 20 months may not be responsive.

4. Psychiatry

The discovery of a central adenyl cyclase system stimulated by isoprenaline (BOCKAERT et al., 1977) and the demonstration of uptake by cerebral tissue of β-blockers (BYLUND et al., 1977) lend support to the existence of β-adrenoceptors in the central nervous system. This is further strengthened by the central side-effects produced by some adrenergic blocking drugs and several hints that they are anxiolytic in themselves (OWENS, 1978). SIMON et al. (1978 b) gave up to 6 mg salbutamol daily to 49 depressive patients in an uncontrolled open manner. The drug was given for up to 10 days and it was noted that 18 of the 22 endogenous depressives responded well, mostly within 3 days. The effect was not as clear with the less serious psychopathologic states with a depressive element.

IV. The Future

A number of possibilities exist for future improvements. They centre around the design of new β-stimulants which are effective and ideally released at the required site of action. More potent substances have been developed such as clenbuterol (VON ENGELHARDT, 1972) but 10 µg thrice daily was indistinguishable in terms of effects and side-effects from salbutamol (SALORINNE et al., 1975). Others, which included imolin (IWASAWA and KIYOMOTO, 1967), are analogues of catecholamines with the ring structures held rigidly in the preferred conformational state of the natural transmitters. These tetrahydronaphthalenes are extremely potent, but this could be a disadvantage in terms of possible overdose.

Because β_2-stimulants are selective and not specific it is tempting to suggest that increased selectivity will minimise side-effects. This seems unlikely because tremor, for example, is also β_2-mediated. Another possibility is to ensure that they are released or activated at the preferred site of action. Ibuterol is a lipid-soluble ester of terbutaline and is activated by tissue-bound esterases (OLSSON et al., 1974). This could be turned to therapeutic advantage if lung tissue esterase activity exceeded that of muscle. Following parenteral administration, the active substance would be preferentially released in the lung.

Relative drug affinity for the bronchial β_2-receptor may be another area to exploit (LARSEN and HERMANSEN, 1977) and the advantage of physically placing the stimulant at the required site of action is already clear. One only has to compare side-effects of oral and aerosol therapy.

More recently attention has turned to combining β-stimulants, which increase cellular cyclic AMP concentration through stimulation of the receptor, with methyl xanthines which inhibit its breakdown. In preliminary studies of ten asthmatics, LEOPOLD and HANDSLIP (1979) found no change in the gradient of a salbutamol/FEV_1 dose-response curve prepared 30 min after pretreatment with 30 µg/kg intravenous aminophylline. They conclude that effects are simply additive and not synergistic, which has been borne out in practice.

The principle of sustained release has been extended to β_2-stimulants. Salbutamol (16 mg twice daily) and aminophylline (450 mg twice daily) have been compared in a double-blind cross-over trial against placebo in 12 asthmatics with nocturnal wheeze and low morning expiratory flow rates. Morning and evening PEFR readings were improved against placebo but the subjective quality of the night's rest did not improve nor did the requirement for auxiliary use of aerosol bronchodilators. A significant reduction in the morning dip of peak expiratory flow was only noted with the sustained-release aminophylline. Side-effects were experienced with both drugs but in different individuals, suggesting that changes to alternative compounds may be a useful therapeutic manoeuvre if side-effects are troublesome (MILLEDGE and MORRIS, 1979). In 18 chronic bronchitics a Wilcoxon's sum of ranks test showed that the aminophylline preparation (450 mg twice daily) produced a greater increase in peak expiratory flow rate than salbutamol (16 mg twice daily) (MANEKSHA, 1979). It is not surprising therefore that sustained-release aminophylline (450 mg daily) produced significantly greater improvement in FEV_1 and FVC/FEV_1 than conventional oral salbutamol (12 mg) and that the two preparations combined provided more than either alone (BOYD and CLARK, 1979). Further evidence of this additive effect is shown where the addition of 800 μg salbutamol daily from aerosol to 450 mg aminophylline twice daily produced further improvement. This is presumably due to different modes of action (SAHAY and CHATTERJEE, 1979).

B. Clonidine

The use of clonidine was reported in the treatment of hypertension in 1966 (BOCK et al., 1966). It was clear that the drug's mechanism of action was different from those of other antihypertensive agents then in use, and this stimulated a large number of basic investigations. It was hoped that study of the drug's properties might lead to the development of a new class of antihypertensive compounds. Research into the manner in which clonidine reduced centrally mediated sympathetic nervous system activity led to renewed interest in the role of the central nervous system in hypertension (HAEUSLER, 1975; HENNING, 1975).

I. Mode of Action

Clonidine does not block the sympathetic ganglia, nor does it inhibit release of noradrenaline from the terminals of postganglion neurons (VON HOEFKE and KOBINGER, 1966; RAND and WILSON, 1968), neither do large doses deplete noradrenergic neurons of noradrenaline as do large amounts of guanethidine or reserpine (VON HOEFKE and KOBINGER, 1966). Clonidine does not cause blockade of either the α- or the β-receptors of the cardiovascular system (RAND and WILSON, 1968), in fact it stimulates α-adrenoceptors and this produces an initial pressor response after intravenous administration (RAND and WILSON, 1968; KOBINGER and KLUPP, 1975). Cases of failure to reduce the blood pressure with large doses of oral clonidine may also be due to stimulation of peripheral α-receptors (WING et al., 1977). The mechanism of the clonidine pressor response is different from that associated with intravenous administration of guanethidine or debrisoquine. The elevations of blood pressure in those cases are caused by release of noradrenaline from the terminals of postganglionic sympathetic neurons and are abolished in animals after pretreatment with reserpine. Pretreatment with resperine does not block the initial direct α-adrenoceptor-mediated stimulatory pressor response to intravenous clonidine (KOBINGER and WALLAND, 1967; NAYLER et al., 1968).

There is general agreement that clonidine lowers arterial pressure primarily by its direct action on the brain and the resultant diminution of sympathetic activity to the cardiovascular system (HAEUSLER, 1975; HENNING, 1975). However, some workers have proposed that the drug, in addition, has peripheral sites of action which reduce vascular resistance and cardiac work. Some investigators have concluded from in vitro experiments that it stimulates presynapatic α-receptors of postganglionic sympathetic nerves and in this manner reduces the amount of noradrenaline released by the action potentials (WERNER et al., 1972; STARKE and MONTEL, 1973; LANGER, 1974). They also concluded from experiments with rat cerebral slices that the drug acted in the brain in a similar way by stimulating presynaptic α-receptors of central noradrenergic neurons. This hypothesis has not been supported by in vivo experiments, which showed that stimulation of peripheral sympathetic nerves caused normal release of noradrenaline and sympathetic responses in animals treated with clonidine (VON HOEFKE and KOBINGER, 1966; RAND and WILSON, 1968). Further results have clearly demonstrated that the stimulation of presynaptic α-receptors of noradrenergic neurons is not a significant effect of clonidine's central action. Clonidine still produces marked reduction of sympathetic neuro-electrical activity (HAEUSLER, 1974; FINCH, 1975) in animals whose hind-brain is depleted of noradrenaline by reserpine or 6-hydroxydopamine and in which its synthesis is inhibited by α-methyl-p-tyrosine.

Other groups of workers have interpreted their results to indicate that clonidine reduces peripheral vascular resistance by some type of direct postsynaptic vascular effect (ZAIMIS and HANINGTON, 1969; SHAW et al., 1971). They are not supported by results from investigations which reported that intra-arterial injections of clonidine in man caused vasoconstriction (VON EHRINGER, 1966), or that vascular responses, in muscle and skin, to intravenous injections of adrenaline, noradrenaline, and angiotensin were essentially unchanged in subjects who were pretreated with intravenous clonidine (MERGUET et al., 1968). In any event, we are unaware of evidence which shows that clonidine causes the strong local vasodilatation comparable to the postsynaptically acting antihypertensive drugs hydrallazine, minoxidil, and guancydine.

The antihypertensive effect of clonidine appears to be due to the drug's direct stimulation of α-receptors in the hind-brain. When it is administered orally or intravenously, or when it is given in much smaller doses into a vertebral artery or the ventricular systems of the hind-brain, or applied directly to the "vasometer centers" of the medulla oblongata, the subsequent fall of heart rate and blood pressure is associated with a fall in activity of the sympathetic nerves (KOBINGER, 1967; SATTLER and VAN ZWIETEN, 1967; SCHMITT et al., 1967; HÄUSLER, 1975; KOBINGER and KLUPP, 1975; SCHMITT, 1975). At the same time there is an increase of efferent vagal activity (KOBINGER and KLUPP, 1975; ROBSON and ANTONACCIO, 1975; SINHA et al., 1975). The administration of these small amounts of the drug to the brain does not result in the initial pressor response which is associated with the use of larger intravenous doses as there is no stimulation of the peripheral α-receptors (KOBINGER and WALLAND, 1967; SATTLER and VON ZWIETON, 1967). These centrally mediated cardiovascular responses, and changes in autonomic activity are blocked by pretreatment with α-blocking drugs (KOBINGER and WALLAND, 1971; SCHMITT et al., 1971). When noradrenaline is applied to the hind-brain it also reduces heart rate, blood pressure, and sympathetic nervous system activity and presumably also acts by stimulating α-adrenoceptors (KRONEBERG and HEISE, 1975).

Clonidine not only brings about reductions in sympathetic activity and an increased vagal activity but it also facilitates the autonomic changes resulting from stimulation of the carotid sinus and aortic arch baroreceptors (KOBINGER and PICHLER, 1975; ROBSON and ANTONACCIO, 1975). Animal experiments have demonstrated an increase of sympathetic nervous system activity caused by hypoxia (SHAW et al., 1971), common carotid artery occlusion (decreased carotid sinus pressure combined with increased carotid chemoreceptor stimulation) (SCHMITT, 1975), and stimulation of "hypertensive areas" of the hypothalamus (HÄUSLER, 1974). The observation that clonidine greatly inhibits the increase of sympathetic tone caused by decreased baroreceptor stimulation (common carotid artery occlusion) is difficult to extrapolate to man, as one of the principal advantages of clonidine in antihypertensive treatment, compared with other drugs which influence sympathetic activity, is that it seldom produces any significant postural hypotension (GIFFORD, 1969; SMET et al., 1969; AMERY et al., 1970; HOOBLER and SAGASTUME, 1971; RAFTOS et al., 1973). As it appears that decreased carotid sinus stimulation is an important factor (TUCKMAN et al., 1968) in the mechanism that causes the compensatory vasoconstriction on changes from supine to upright positions (TUCKMAN and SHILLINGFORD, 1966) it is assumed that clonidine permits the evoked increase of sympathetic tone which is necessary to prevent symptoms of orthostatic hypotension. Relevant to this, it has been shown that the central inhibition of sympathetic responses by clonidine is less effective when there are higher levels of afferent stimulation.

At greater degrees of hypoxia and chemoreceptor stimulation, in animals, there is a break through the central clonidine block and normal cardiovascular responses result (SHAW et al., 1971), and in man treated with clonidine exercise produces normal increases of cardiac output and blood pressure and elevations of peripheral vascular resistance in non-exercising areas of the body (BARNETT and CANTOR, 1968; MUIR et al., 1969).

The effect of clonidine, in contrast to that of α-methyldopa, is to stimulate the α-adrenoceptors directly and is not dependent on the interposition of noradrenergic neurons. This has been demonstrated in animals in which the hind-brains were depleted of noradrenaline by reserpine or 6-hydroxydopamine and noradrenaline synthesis was inhibited by α-methyl-p-tyrosine (HAEUSLER, 1974; KOBINGER and PICHLER, 1974; HAEUSLER, 1975; KOBINGER and PICHLER, 1975). This does indicate, of course, that the noradrenergic neurons which are abundantly present in the medulla oblongata (DAHLSTROM and FLUXE, 1964, 1965) do not normally, in the absence of clonidine, mediate sympathetic and vagal tone. These noradrenergic neurones may indeed have a close "functional proximity" to the autonomic α-receptors and this has been demonstrated in experiments with α-methyldopa.

There are observations to indicate that tricyclic antidepressant drugs interfere with the action of clonidine on the central nervous system and inhibit its antihypertensive effect (BRIANT and REID, 1972; BRIANT et al., 1973; REID et al., 1973; VAN ZWIETEN et al., 1975). VAN ZWIETEN et al. (1975) suggested that this was due to the α-blocking property of the antidepressants which results when they are used in high doses. Others

(BRIANT and REID, 1972; BRIANT et al., 1973; DOLLERY and REID, 1973; REID et al., 1973), however, attributed this inhibition to a presynaptic interaction between the two drugs. They found that using tricyclic antidepressants in doses which were insufficient to block the α-receptors still reduced the hypotensive action of clonidine in animals in which the central neurons were depleted of noradrenaline. However, others have demonstrated that the hypotensive action of clonidine does not depend on intact central noradrenergic neurons nor that there is this type of interaction between clonidine and tricyclic antidepressants in animals (SCHOLTYSIK and SALZMANN, 1973; FINCH, 1974; HAEUSLER, 1974; HOEFKE and WARNKE-SACHS, 1974; KOBINGER and PICHLER, 1974; FINCH, 1975) or in man (RAFTOS et al., 1973).

II. Haemodynamic and Renal Effects

It appears that clonidine lowers arterial pressure by reducing sympathetic traffic to the heart and blood vessels and by increasing efferent vagal activity to the heart. Evidence from specialised animal preparations (NAYLER et al., 1968) show that the drug has little or no direct effect on myocardial function. These results seem applicable to man as patients receiving clonidine have normal increases in blood pressure and cardiac work during exercise (BARNETT and CANTOR, 1968; MUIR et al., 1969). It is possible, therefore, that clonidine could act on the cardiovascular capacity vessels (thus increasing peripheral venous pooling and reducing cardiac filling pressure), decreasing cardiac output, and reducing arteriolar resistance.

There have however been relatively few studies of the haemodynamic effects of clonidine in man and a number of these have not published sufficient details of the experiments to allow full analysis. It appears that they have all been concerned with effects of acute intravenous or oral administrations of the medication.

BROD et al. (1972) gave intravenous clonidine to 17 normotensive and hypertensive subjects. The studies were presumably done in the supine position and the fall in mean arterial pressure was associated with a 24% reduction of cardiac output. Total peripheral resistance was unchanged in nine subjects and decreased in the other eight by unspecified amounts, although comparison of the average mean arterial pressure and cardiac output show that those changes in vascular resistance were small. The superior vena cava and right atrial pressures decreased by an average of 2.3 mm Hg. DAVIDOV et al. (1967) studied six hypertensive patients after single oral doses of clonidine. The experiment was probably performed with the subjects sitting, there was a decrease in mean arterial pressure of 18%, an insignificant increase in cardiac output of 10% and a decrease in vascular resistance of 25%. ONESTI et al. (1969) reported the most detailed results and they studied the acute oral administration to seven hypertensive patients. There were reductions in mean supine arterial pressure of 17% and in cardiac output of 21%, while vascular resistance did not change significantly (+1%). Mean arterial pressure decreased 33%, cardiac output fell 15% and there was a reduction of 21% in vascular resistance in the 45° tilt position after clonidine compared with values in the same position before the drug.

Hence the fall in supine blood pressure was associated with a moderate reduction in cardiac output and insignificant changes of vascular resistance. The results also indicate that the drug prevented the expected compensatory increase in arteriolar resistance which would have occurred in untreated subjects with this decrease in cardiac output. In the sitting and 45° tilt positions the antihypertensive effect of clonidine was associated with moderately large decreases of peripheral resistance. The studies of ONESTI et al. (1969) indicate that not only is the usual compensatory vasoconstriction of approximately 30% which is associated with changes of posture (TUCKMAN and SHILLINGFORD, 1966) largely abolished but the drug in addition caused a moderate decrease of the cardiac output which was already reduced by the orthostatic change. Because of these simultaneous reductions of cardiac output and peripheral resistance clonidine produced a considerable degree of postural hypotension of 33%; however, these findings are not in accord with the relative absence of postural hypotension in normal clinical use of clonidine.

BROD et al. (1972) suggested that their results indicated that the reduction in cardiac output was secondary to the increased venous distensibility after clonidine and decreased cardiac filling pressure. This is supported by investigations in man (VON EHRINGER, 1966) which showed that the drug decreased venous tone in the limbs and by animal studies with heart-lung preparations (NAYLER et al., 1968) where the clonidine was found to cause large shifts of blood volume to the capacitance vessels.

Exercise is associated with increased levels of sympathetic tone and it was therefore possible that clonidine might influence the haemodynamic changes caused by physical activity. However, it has been shown (MACDOUGALL et al., 1970; RAFTOS et al., 1973) that an advantage of clonidine in the treatment of hypertension, compared with α-methyldopa or the adrenergic neuron inhibiting drugs, is that exercise hypotension rarely occurs. There are two studies on the haemodynamic changes caused by exercise and both investigated the influence of acute intravenous administration. In one (BARNETT and CANTOR, 1968), normotensive subjects were studied during supine exercise and had normal increases in cardiac output and either no changes or increases in mean arterial pressure. In the other study (MUIR et al., 1969), six hypertensive patients were studied during supine and two during walking exercise. Clonidine did not alter the per cent increases of mean arterial pressure and of cardiac output which occurred during exercise. As it also did not change the per cent decrease in peripheral resistance it suggested that clonidine did not inhibit vasoconstriction in the non-exercising parts of the body.

Clonidine does not cause conspicuous elevations of serum creatinine even in patients with advanced renal impairment (MACDOUGALL et al., 1970; HOOBLER and SAGASTUME, 1971; ONESTI et al., 1971 a). The results from several investigations (DAVIDOV et al., 1967 b; ONESTI et al., 1969; BROD et al., 1972) indicate that intravenous or oral administration of clonidine lowered blood pressure in both normotensive and hypertensive subjects in the supine, sitting, and 45° tilt positions, and failed to lower renal blood flow or glomerular filtration rate. The renal vascular resistance was therefore necessarily reduced. ONESTI et al. (1971 a) measured the effect of chronic clonidine treatment given between 10 and 110 days in seven hypertensive patients. Blood pressure was reduced in all subjects but there was no change in renal plasma flow or glomerular filtration rate. These results are particularly important as four of the seven patients had advanced renal impairment with glomerular filtration rates between 9 and 23 ml/min/1.7 m^2 prior to the administration of clonidine. It appears therefore that the use of clonidine in antihypertensive treatment tends to preserve renal blood flow and glomerular filtration, similar to the use of α-methyldopa (ONESTI et al., 1971 b). On the other hand, acute administration of the drug causes retention of sodium and water (DAVIDOV et al., 1967b; ONESTI et al., 1969) and others have shown that when clonidine is used alone during chronic treatment it can cause important increases in weight (DAVIDOV et al., 1967b; GIFFORD, 1969).

III. Clinical Use

The intravenous use of clonidine lowers blood pressure fairly rapidly and has ben tried in hypertensive emergencies (ONESTI et al., 1971b; BROD et al., 1972; RAFTOS et al., 1973). A rapid intravenous injection produces an initial moderate elevation of pressure of between 5 and 20 mm Hg which occurs within 1 min and lasts between 30 s and 5 min. The antihypertensive effects commence within 5–10 min after administration, reaches its peak within an hour and may persist for several hours (BROD et al., 1972; RAFTOS et al., 1973). The initial pressor response is not seen if clonidine is given by the intramuscular or subcutaneous route (ONESTI et al., 1971b).

The rises in blood pressure can also be largely avoided if the intravenous injection is given slowly over 5–10 min or if they are preceded by 5 mg injections of the α-blocker phentolamine (RAFTOS et al., 1973). A convenient starting dose is 300 μg and subsequent intravenous or intramuscular injections of 150–300 μg can be given every 1–6 h (ONESTI et al., 1971a). A total daily dose of 5–6 mg has been used without untoward effects (ONESTI et al., 1971a). As large injections of 2–3 mg can cause dangerous prolonged hypertensive reactions it has been strongly recommended that those large amounts should not be used to treat accelerated hypertension or other types of more urgent hypertensive emergencies (ONESTI et al., 1971b).

Intravenous clonidine does not lower pressure adequately in a sufficiently high proportion of patients and therefore it is not the drug of choice for use in acute hypertensive emergencies. Its principal use is for the chronic treatment of hypertension. Some investigators have suggested that clonidine is a more effective antihypertensive agent than α-methyldopa (AMERY et al., 1970; ONESTI et al., 1971b). However, unlike α-methyldopa (PRICHARD et al., 1968), clonidine rarely controls blood pressure unless it is used with a diuretic (DAVIDOV et al., 1967b; GIFFORD, 1969; SMET et al., 1969; ONESTI et al., 1971b).

The use of clonidine with a diuretic controls the blood pressure in as many as 80% of patients (ONESTI et al., 1971b). Following oral administration it begins to lower blood pressure within 30–60 min, reaches its peak action within 2–4 h and has a significant effect for approximately 6–12 h (DAVIDOV et al., 1967b; NG et al., 1967; SMET et al., 1969; ONESTI et al., 1969). The drug therefore is given in divided daily doses, usually three times a day. There is wide dosage variation between 75 μg and 6 mg/day (DAVIDOV et al., 1967b; GIFFORD, 1969; AMERY et al., 1970; MACDOUGALL et al., 1970; ONESTI et al., 1971b).

IV. Side-Effects

Clonidine rarely causes clinically significant postural or exercise hypotension; however, it does occasionally produce troublesome postural hypotension in patients with severe renal impairment (VORBURGER, 1970; TUCKMAN, unpublished observations) and this could be due to accumulation of the drug because the kidneys are a major pathway of its excretion (REHBINDER, 1970).

Unfortunately clonidine produces sedation (drowsiness and tiredness), dryness of the mouth and constipation in the majority of patients (Davidov et al., 1967b; Gifford, 1969; Amery et al., 1970; Onesti et al., 1971a, b; Mroczek et al., 1972). These side-effects are dose-dependent and diminish with time (Davidov et al., 1967b; Smet et al., 1969; Hoobler and Sagastume, 1971; Onesti et al., 1971b; Mroczek et al., 1972) and therefore it is best, whenever possible, to increase the dose of the drug gradually at intervals of 1 or 2 weeks, in order to increase acceptance of it by the patient. Sedation is the most commonly troublesome side-effect that often prevents administration of adequately high doses to obtain blood pressure control. It is not easy to judge the frequency and severity of sedation because appreciation of its importance obviously varies greatly between different investigators. Awareness of the side-effects is likely to be greater in those patients who are engaged in intellectually demanding occupations. As sedation and the antihypertensive effects of clonidine are probably mediated in different areas of the brain, several newer imidazoline derivatives have been developed in the hope that they may cause less drowsiness; as yet this has not met with success.

Dry mouth can be relieved by measures which increase salivary secretion, for instance the application of lemon juice on the tongue, sucking citrus sweets, etc. Patients may often try to minimise the dry mouth by drinking large amounts of water but this causes an inconvenient frequent diuresis and is usually ineffective. Constipation is usually only minor; however, one instance of paralytic ileus has been reported (Davidov et al., 1967b). The condition was promptly corrected within 24 h after the drug was stopped.

The use of clonidine is associated with another important side-effect which appears unique in antihypertensive treatment. If the drug is abruptly stopped the patient may experience within 8–24 h an exaggerated elevation of blood pressure, tachycardia, palpitations, sweating, agitation and a feeling of anxiety (Hunyor et al., 1973). These symptoms are associated with elevations of plasma and urinary catecholamines (Hunyor et al., 1973; Geyskes et al., 1979). Plasma renin does not alter (Geyskes et al., 1979). The withdrawal syndrome has been treated by intravenous phentolamine and propranolol to lower blood pressure (Hunyor et al., 1973) or oral thymoxamine and propranolol (Goldberg et al., 1976). More effective treatment is probably provided by intravenous injections of clonidine, 300 μg (Tuckman, unpublished observations). Oral clonidine also provides effective treatment, 300–600 μg, but the onset of action is slower (Raftos et al., 1973). Another approach is to use intravenous labetalol (Brown et al., 1976). The incidence of the withdrawal syndrome is difficult to assess, it did not seem to occur in cross-over studies (clonidine to a placebo or other antihypertensive drugs) of the drug (Amery et al., 1970; Mroczek et al., 1972; Hunyor et al., 1973). In a prospective study in 20 patients who were not receiving a diuretic, clonidine was stopped in hospital after 3 days' treatment (average dose 0.5 mg daily) and after 30 days (average dose 0.62 mg daily). Blood pressures were measured every 2 h (Arteriosonde) and in neither case was an overshoot seen (Whitsett et al., 1978). There was an increase in noradrenaline levels that approached the upper limit of normal. However, Goldberg et al. (1976) found an abrupt rise of blood pressure in nine of 15 patients. Pressure increased 12 h after withdrawal and in those patients taking 0.6 mg/day or more to high levels within 24 h of the last dose. In one of three patients on 0.9 mg/day a gradual reduction in dosage over 3 days still resulted in a severe rise of blood pressure. It was not clear in this study whether or not patients were receiving a diuretic, but in another study (STRAUSS et al., 1977) all three patients showing a pressor response on withdrawal of clonidine were receiving a diuretic. In another study of 14 patients on 0.9 mg clonidine with no other drugs, only one patient had no rise in blood pressure when clonidine was stopped (GEYSKES et al., 1979). Twelve patients, from a mean pressure of 110 mm Hg, showed an average rise to 141 mm Hg by the third day after clonidine was stopped ($p < 0.001$); in the remaining two patients pressures exceeded 160 mm Hg the day after stopping clonidine, so the study was terminated in these.

The syndrome does not occur if the drug is gradually discontinued during 1–2 weeks. Patients should be advised against stopping the drug abruptly and they should always carry with them several tablets in case they are separated from their source of supply. Also, this complication should be foreseen in circumstances that will require that the drug be abruptly discontinued, such as surgical operations. If clonidine cannot be discontinued gradually, an oral dose should be given as close as possible to the intervention (RAFTOS et al., 1973) and the anaesthetist or other personnel concerned should have a supply of intravenous medication where this is available.

The occurrence of severe vomiting has been reported to follow abrupt withdrawal of clonidine (HOPKIRK et al., 1975) and it was relieved by parenteral administration of the drug.

A bradycardia occurs from the administration of clonidine, but the degree is unpredictable and is often only a reduction of several beats per minute and seldom as much as 20 beats/min (NG et al., 1967; GIFFORD, 1969; RAFTOS et al., 1973). The drug seldom, if ever, causes cardiac arrhythmias (HOOBLER and SAGASTUME, 1971). Clonidine does not often disturb sexual function in the male and the complication may occur about as often as in treatment with α-methyldopa (AMERY et al., 1970; MROCZEK et al., 1972) or less frequently (RAFTOS et al., 1973).

A number of rarer side-effects have been reported. These include rashes, parotid pain, shivering, sleep reversal, exceptionally gynaecomastia (ONESTI et al., 1971 a) Raynaud's phenomenon (RAFTOS et al., 1973), visual blurring (NG et al., 1967), and one case of suspected toxic hepatitis (GIFFORD, 1969). The use of clonidine has been associated with de novo episodes or exacerbations of pre-existing psychological disturbances in hypertensive patients (NG et al., 1967; MACDOUGALL et al., 1970; RAFTOS et al., 1973). The incidences are rare and have been difficult to document with certainty. In five patients with severely impaired renal function, semicoma occurred during 2–5 days' treatment with large doses of propranolol and clonidine (KINCAID-SMITH et al., 1975). Recovery was rapid when clonidine was withdrawn.

It has been observed that the tricyclic antidepressants inhibit the antihypertensive action of clonidine (BRIANT and REID, 1972; DOLLERY and REID, 1973; REID et al., 1973; VAN ZWIETEN et al., 1975). Other investigators have failed to confirm this interaction or a theoretical basis for its existence (RAFTOS et al., 1973; SCHOLTYSIK and SALZMANN, 1973; FINCH, 1974; HAEUSLER, 1974; HOEFKE and WARNKE-SACHS, 1974; KOBINGER and PICHLER, 1974; FINCH, 1975).

Clonidine's place in antihypertensive treatment today is probably best considered as a substitute for α-methyldopa or the adrenergic inhibiting drugs (ANIDs) in patients in whom the last two mentioned medications cannot be changed to a β-blocker alone or some combination of diuretic, β-blocker and a vasodilating drug. When clonidine, α-methyldopa and/or ANIDs provide similar blood pressure control, the drug of choice will be the one which causes the fewest untoward side-effects.

Clonidine can be substituted for ANIDs in many patients, and in others in whom it is added to ANIDs the dose of the latter required to control blood pressure is greatly reduced and side-effects from it diminished (SMET et al., 1969; HOOBLER and SAGASTUME, 1971; ONESTI et al., 1971 b; RAFTOS et al., 1973). As ANIDs frequently cause disagreeable side-effects, clonidine may be preferable to them provided it does not cause unacceptable sedation.

It is not so easy to compare clonidine with α-methyldopa. It appears that clonidine is sometimes a more effective antihypertensive agent than α-methyldopa (AMERY et al., 1970; ONESTI et al., 1971 b). However, because of side-effects some patients prefer α-methyldopa (SEEDAT et al., 1969; AMERY et al., 1970) and others clonidine (HOOBLER and SAGASTUME, 1971; ONESTI et al., 1971 b). There is little to be gained by giving α-methyldopa and clonidine together and the incidence of side-effects is increased (HOOBLER and SAGASTUME, 1971; RAFTOS et al., 1973).

C. Alpha-Methyldopa

I. Mode of Action

The way that α-methyldopa acts has been a matter of debate, but the evidence is now accepted as being in favour of a central mode of action (LAVERTY, 1973; DAY et al., 1973; HAEUSLER, 1975; HENNING, 1975; KRONEBERG and HEISE, 1975).

Methyldopa inhibits dopa decarboxylase, reducing the rate of catecholamine synthesis, however, other inhibitors of the enzyme are not antihypertensive (LEVINE and SJOERDSMA, 1964). It has been shown that α-methyldopa is metabolised to α-methyldopamine and then to α-methylnoradrenaline. It was suggested by DAY and RAND (1963) that α-methyldopa exerted its hypotensive action by being converted to α-methylnoradrenaline which then acts as a false transmitter when liberated at sympathetic nerve endings. However, α-methylnoradrenaline is about equipotent to noradrenaline in the cat and dog, where α-methyldopa exerts a hypotensive effect (TRINKER, 1971), and in man it is only slightly less potent than noradrenaline on human smooth muscle (COUPAR and TURNER, 1970). Moreover although the acute administration of α-methyldopa depresses the function of sympathetic nerves, depressing the response of the cat nictitating membrane to nerve stimulation (DAY and RAND, 1964) no effect was seen on the responses after chronic treatment (HAEFELY et al., 1967).

It has long been apparent that α-methyldopa exerts a number of central effects, and several observations have suggested that the central nervous system is probably the site of its antihypertensive action. HENNING and VAN ZWIETEN (1968) observed that a small dose of α-methyldopa injected into the vertebral artery produced a fall of blood pressure, while intravenous administration produced no effect. Secondly, INGENITO et al. (1970) found the administration of α-methyldopa into the vascularly isolated perfused cat brain caused a fall in blood pressure in the rest of the animal. Thirdly, BAUM et al. (1972) have demonstrated a reduction of sympathetic nerve traffic following the administration of methyldopa to renal hypertensive rats.

α-Methyldopa is converted into α-methylnoradrenaline in the brain (CARLSSON and LINDQVIST, 1962; HENNING and RUBENSON, 1971), which then stimulates the central α-adrenergic receptors. The resultant hypotensive effect is blocked by α-adrenoceptor blocking drugs (HEISE and KRONEBERG, 1972). The prevention of the metabolism of methyldopa and thus the formation of α-methylnoradrenaline by the administration of a centrally active dopa decarboxylase inhibitor abolishes the antihypertensive effect of α-methyldopa, but this does not occur when a dopa-decarboxylase inhibitor which does not penetrate the brain is given (HENNING and RUBENSON, 1971). Similarly the prevention of α-methylnoradrenaline synthesis by the destruction of central adrenergic neurons by intraventricular 6-hydroxydopamine also prevented the hypotensive effect of α-methyldopa, whereas intravenous 6-hydroxydopamine reduced, but did not prevent the hypotensive effect (FINCH and HAEUSLER, 1973). That the hypotensive effect of α-methyldopa is also abolished by intraventricular phentolamine serves to support the concept of a central α-adrenergic site of action. Lastly, it was also found that hypotensive doses of α-methyldopa failed to reduce the pressor response that is seen when the entire sympathetic outflow is stimulated (FINCH and HAEUSLER, 1973).

The hypotensive effect of methyldopa appears to be unrelated to its renin-suppressing action (LEONETTI et al., 1977).

II. Cardiovascular Effects

The administration of intravenous α-methyldopa reduces blood pressure chiefly by reducing peripheral resistance. There was a small average reduction in cardiac output for both supine and erect position but the changes were not significant (ONESTI et al., 1964; COHEN et al., 1967). Following the short-term oral administration there was no change in the supine cardiac output accompanying the fall in blood pressure (SANNERSTEDT et al., 1962; DOLLERY et al., 1963). CHAMBERLAIN and HOWARD (1964) did not observe any reduction in cardiac output from short-term doses of 0.75–3 g α-methyldopa daily; the fall in blood pressure in the supine position was associated with a reduction in peripheral resistance. There was an increased fall in blood pressure on standing and on exercise that was associated with a failure of the peripheral resistance to rise as it did prior to the administration of α-methyldopa. There was no evidence to indicate any increased venous pooling on standing as the fall of cardiac output on adopting the erect position was not enhanced after α-methyldopa. The blood pressures in many of these patients were relatively high even after treatment with α-methyldopa and hence these results may not be fully applicable to patients when blood pressure is adequately controlled, although all except one patient showed at least some postural hypotension. When there is more adequate control of the blood pressure, venous pooling may play some part, as a venodepressor effect has been demonstrated after oral administration of α-methyldopa (2.0–5.0 g daily) over periods between 21 and 49 days (MASON and BRAUNWALD, 1964). However, LUND-JOHANSEN (1972) studied a series of 13 mild hypertensives before and after treatment with α-methyldopa for 1 year (500–1,500 mg/day, average 896 mg/day), and it was found that the fall in blood pressure at rest, standing and on exercise was associated with a fall in cardiac output; no change in peripheral resistance was observed. There was no postural drop in blood pressure, and the blood pressures after α-methyldopa were supine 139/84, standing 150/93 mm HG. There appears to be little effect on heart rate following intravenous administration (ONESTI et al., 1964) whereas after oral administration there is a modest reduction, supine, standing and after exercise (CHAMBERLAIN and HOWARD, 1964; LUND-JOHANSEN, 1972). α-Methyldopa results in less of a reduction in heart rate than bethanidine or guanethidine for a similar antihypertensive effect (PRICHARD et al., 1968).

It is quite clear that larger doses of α-methyldopa used in the treatment of hypertension are associated with postural and exercise hypotension, although less than that seen with sympathetic inhibiting drugs, bethanidine or guanethidine (OATES et al., 1965; PRICHARD et al., 1968). There is an alteration of the cardiovascular response to Valsalva's manoeuvre, in a way characteristic of inhibition of vasoconstriction, overshoot is abolished (DOLLERY et al., 1963) and the rise in blood pressure during the effort phase is inhibited in contrast to the lack of effect seen from cardiac inhibition by means of β-adrenergic blockade (PRICHARD et al., 1970b). Intravenous α-methyldopa has been found to reduce vascular resistance in the skin (MENDLOWITZ et al., 1965) and in the coronary circulation (COHEN et al., 1967).

ONESTI et al. (1964) observed an insignificant fall in renal blood flow following intravenous α-methyldopa in the supine position (8%) but a significant fall in glomerular filtration rate of 13% ($p<0.05$). As there was relatively greater fall in arterial blood pressure, calculated renal vascular resistance was decreased. The short-term oral administration of methyldopa produced a fall in renal vascular resistance but no reduction in renal blood flow or glomerular filtration (SANNERSTEDT et al., 1962). This was confirmed by MOHAMMED et al. (1968) in patients with renal insufficiency.

MEYER et al. (1968) observed a slight increase in cerebral flow in spite of a reduced blood pressure after 2 weeks' administration of α-methyldopa to hypertensive patients with cerebrovascular disease.

III. Clinical Use

The antihypertensive effect of α-methyldopa was first observed by OATES et al. (1960). If a level of a standing diastolic pressure of 100 mm Hg is taken as reasonable control, α-methyldopa has been found to control about half the hypertensive patients to this degree, for instance 42% of 33 patients (CANNON et al., 1962), 54% of 59 patients (DOLLERY and HARINGTON, 1962), 67% of 69 patients (HAMILTON and KOPELMAN, 1963), 49% of 100 patients (JOHNSON et al., 1966). JOHNSON et al. found that the fall in blood pressure in 37 patients on α-methyldopa was similar to that seen in 66 patients of similar severity on guanethidine. This confirmed a previous within-patient study in 19 patients by OATES et al. (1965), who found α-methyldopa, guanethidine and pargyline produced similar blood pressure control. Likewise PRICHARD et al. (1968) in a within-patient study in 30 patients found α-methyldopa produced similar control to bethanidine and guanethidine, although six of these patients could not tolerate α-methyldopa. In another study ($n=17$) it has been confirmed that α-methyldopa produces similar control of the standing blood pressure to bethanidine, and also to propranolol (PRICHARD et al., 1976).

The differences that exist between α-methyldopa and other antihypertensive drugs reside in the effect on cardiovascular responses and the nature of side-effects. As has been discussed, the control of the blood pressure with methyldopa is associated with less postural and exercise fall in blood pressure than that seen with adrenergic neuron inhibitory drugs.

The usual starting dose of methyldopa is 250 mg two to three times daily, occasionally half this dose. Increments of 250 mg per dose may be made. Some physicians only use up to 2 g/day, others have used higher doses, e.g., 6 g/day (HAMILTON and KOPELMAN, 1963). A diuretic should be used in addition if any side-effects, such as sedation, occur and most usually would be added in any case if a daily dosage of 2 g is reached. The development of tolerance is not uncommon, but it can usually be overcome by increasing the dose (SMIRK, 1963b).

IV. Side-Effects

The most common side-effect from α-methyldopa is tiredness and it is also the most common factor limiting dosage. It may occur in about half of the patients treated, occurring in 41% of the patients of JOHNSON et al. (1966), and more frequently than seen with other drugs (OATES et al., 1965). PRICHARD et al. (1968) found tiredness occurred in 75% of their patients on methyldopa, compared with 10% on bethanidine, and 17% on guanethidine. There may be generally impaired mental activity – of particular trouble to professional people (ADLER, 1974). Other central nervous system side-effects occur, such as dreams (JOHNSON et al., 1966; PRICHARD et al., 1968), and depression – in 2 of 59 patients (DOLLERY and HARINGTON, 1962), 3 of 69 patients (HAMILTON and KOPELMAN, 1963), 4 of 100 patients (JOHNSON et al., 1966), 5 of 47 patients (SMIRK, 1963b), and 2 severe and 3 mild out of 30 patients (PRICHARD et al., 1968). Others, however, have found a lower incidence of central nervous system side-effects (LAWSON et al., 1978). Weight gain is another common side-effect, and has even been reported in 64% of cases (JOHNSON et al., 1966).

Diarrhoea may occur with α-methyldopa in about 4% (JOHNSON et al., 1966) to 8% of patients (PRICHARD et al., 1968) but is much less frequent than with guanethidine. Symptoms of postural or exertional hypotension are relatively unusual on α-methyldopa (JOHNSON et al., 1966; PRICHARD et al., 1968), a number of trials not reporting these symptoms (SMIRK, 1963b). Excessive hypotension from methyldopa, however, has been reported, particularly in younger patients under 55 years with elevated blood urea levels (LAWSON et al., 1978).

There have been reports of various skin rashes, urticaria, eczema, particularly in patients with previous skin disorders (CHURCH, 1974).

An incidence of 20% of positive Coombs' test in patients receiving α-methyldopa in periods of over 6 months has been found (CARSTAIRS et al., 1966), but an auto-immune haemolytic anaemia only develops in about 0.02% of patients receiving α-methyldopa (WORLLEDGE et al., 1966). Haemolysis may be more likely to occur in women (FURHOFF, 1978). Rarely, reversible leucopenia (CLARK, 1967) or thrombocytopenia may occur (BENRAAD and SCHOENAKER, 1965). A positive reaction for antinuclear factor has been reported in just under 15% of patients on α-methyldopa (BRECKENRIDGE et al., 1967).

α-methyldopa may rarely cause a number of other untoward effects, hepatotoxicity, most often a hepatic syndrome (TOGHILL et al., 1974), more common among women (FURHOFF, 1978), hyperpyrexia (GLONTZ and SASLAW, 1968; FURHOFF, 1978), lactation and parkinsonism. SOTANIEMI et al. (1977) found α-methyldopa liver damage occurred either acutely within months after starting treatment, or chronically years after starting treatment. The acute type recovered more quickly when the drug was stopped. There was evidence of impaired drug metabolism and a suggestion of genetic predisposition as a few cases occurred in one family. Finally a paradoxical pressor response has been reported with methyldopa (LEVINE and STRAUCH, 1966), and there has been a report of a case of rebound hypertension after methyldopa withdrawal (BURDEN and ALEXANDER, 1976).

D. Adrenergic Neuron Inhibiting Drugs (ANIDs)

I. Mode of Action

Bethanidine, debrisoquine and guanethidine are the most extensively used hypotensive drugs in this group. They are selectively concentrated in the terminals of postganglionic sympathetic nerves and lower blood pressure by inhibiting the release of noradrenaline evoked by the action potentials; however, the drugs vary in their effects on catecholamine metabolism.

Noradrenaline is synthesised in postganglionic neurons from tyrosine, via dopa and dopamine, and it is stored there in morphologically distinct vesicles (IVERSEN, 1973; LIVETT, 1973; SMITH, 1973). These axons also contain mitochondrial monoamine oxidase (MAO) and that deaminates free intraneuronal noradrenaline to vanilmandelic acid. When noradrenaline is released by postganglionic action potentials its principal pathways include direct stimulation of the adrenergic cardiovascular receptors, metabolism by extraneuronal catechol-o-methyl transferase to normetanephrine, or uptake back into the nerves by an energy-dependent membrane pump (IVERSEN, 1973). The amount of uptake of noradrenaline is an important factor which limits receptor stimulation; less uptake provides more transmitter at the receptors and vice versa. The adrenergic neuron inhibiting drugs (ANIDs) are also taken up into the sympathetic nerves through the same membrane pump and are competitive antagonists of noradrenaline at this site. Therefore, ANIDs can dangerously enhance the pressor response to intravenously administered noradrenaline or to the endogenous release of the amine in patients with phaeochromocytoma. Similarly, amphetamine, tricyclic antidepressants, and chlorpromazine affect the neuronal pump and by that means block the entry of ANIDs into the sympathetic nerves and reduce their antihypertensive action (MITCHELL et al., 1970; JANOWSKY et al., 1973).

Bethanidine, debrisoquine, and guanethidine lower blood pressure by reducing the amount of noradrenaline liberated during stimulation of sympathetic nerves. Guanethidine was the first of these drugs used and it was quickly established in animals that single injections of what was by clinical standards a large dose depleted the neurons of their stores of noradrenaline. Later, investigations showed that this did not occur when bethanidine or debrisoquine were given (BOURA and GREEN, 1963; MOE et al., 1964). These results from animal investigation led some workers to propose that the antihypertensive effect of guanethidine in man was due to depletion of noradrenaline from the sympathetic nerves and that of the other drugs was dependent on inhibition of the "physiological release" of the transmitter (ABRAMS et al., 1964). In addition as guanethidine depleted the heart of its noradrenaline stores in those studies and the other two drugs did not, it was suggested that guanethidine was more likely to cause heart failure during the treatment of hypertension. However, it has been shown that bethanidine also greatly reduced the catecholamine content in the heart and spleen of animals after 6 months of large daily injections (BOURA et al., 1961). Unfortunately, measurements were not done after short periods of administration (BOURA and GREEN, 1963; BOURA and GREEN, 1965) and we are not aware of comparable experiments with debrisoquine.

These drugs are also concentrated in postganglionic sympathetic nerve cell bodies. When large amounts of guanethidine are given to rats for 6 weeks it is cytotoxic and produces a widespread sympathectomy (BURNSTOCK et al., 1971). Large injections of bethanidine and debrisoquine have been given to rats for 2 and 3 weeks and although they caused only minor and variable histological changes in the cell bodies, compared with guanethidine administered for a similar time, the two drugs significantly disturbed several basic intracellular metabolic processes (MALMQVIST and OATES, 1968; JENSEN-HOLM and JUUL, 1970; PETTINGER and HORST, 1971; JUUL, 1973). It is possible that if large doses of bethanidine or debrisoquine were given for longer periods these disturbances might lead to severe histological damage of the cell bodies besides the loss of tissue catecholamines (BOURA et al., 1961).

Experimental work strongly suggests that the clinical effects of the ANIDs are not dependent on depletion of the transmitter. First, in animals, guanethidine inhibits noradrenaline release during sympathetic stimulation long before it depletes nerves of noradrenaline (BOURA and GREEN, 1965; ABBS and DODD, 1974). Secondly, the doses of ANIDs used in man are much smaller than those needed to deplete animals of noradrenaline. Thirdly, effective antihypertensive treatment with ANIDs does not produce a complete sympathectomy. The patients are not incapacitated by postural hypotension and exercise causes substantial increase in cardiac work (DOLLERY et al., 1961; TAYLOR et al., 1962; CHAMBERLAIN and HOWARD, 1964; KHATRI and COHN, 1970). Fourthly, the intravenous administration of tyramine to patients on long-term guanethidine therapy causes obvious pressor responses (COHN et al., 1963), from the presumed release of endogenous noradrenaline. And fifthly, the side-effects of ANIDs which are due to sympathetic inhibition quickly disappear when the drugs are stopped, even after they have been given for as long as 12 years (BAUER et al., 1973). This quick reversal could not have been predicted from animal experiments in which the administration of large doses of guanethidine during several weeks caused extensive histological destruction of sympathetic nerves and the organs they innervated (see above).

The intravenous injections of ANIDs first release noradrenaline from the sympathetic nerves and produce a pressor response prior to a reduction in blood pressure. The intravenous administration of debrisoquine causes a moderate to large increase in pressure over 1 or 2 h (ABRAMS et al., 1964; KAKAVIATOS et al., 1964), guanethidine induces a moderate increase for several minutes (DOLLERY et al., 1960), while bethanidine is only associated with a minimal elevation of blood pressure (FEWINGS et al., 1964; JOHNSTON et al., 1964). Since these initial pressor effects are not combined with an important decrease of the transmitter in the sympathetic nerves, it is not immediately apparent how the three drugs differentially change the balance between neuronal noradrenaline synthesis, release, uptake, storage, and monoamine deamination during this period. It may be relevant that bethanidine (BOURA and GREEN, 1965) and debrisoquine (PETTINGER et al., 1969) are MAO inhibitors and guanethidine is not (FURST, 1967). As ANIDs are concentrated in the sympathetic nerve terminals, MAO inhibition would prevent inactivation of free intraneuronal noradrenaline and in this way increase the pressor response. This could explain the greater hypertensive effect of debrisoquine compared with guanethidine, and of debrisoquine compared with bethanidine if the former had greater MAO inhibitory activity, however, it does not explain the larger rise of pressure caused by guanethidine compared with bethanidine. Large *oral* doses of debrisoquine cause severe elevations of blood pressure which can last several hours (LURIA and FREIS, 1965). This definitely occurs when a patient first receives the drug, but it has not been reported during chronic treatment after an abrupt increase in dose. Evidence of MAO inhibition from debrisoquine has been found in man. Subjects given debrisoquine showed increased pressor responses to oral and intravenous tyramine and that they experienced serious hypertensive reactions after eating gruyère cheese and oral administration of phenylephrine (ABRAMS et al., 1964; PETTINGER et al., 1969; AMERY and DELOOF, 1970; AMINU et al., 1970).

II. Haemodynamic Effects

The reduction of sympathetic nervous system stimulation to the veins, heart, and arterioles from ANIDs could lead to the lowering of arterial pressure by three mechanisms. First by increasing the distensibility of postarteriolar capacity vessels (increased peripheral venous pooling and decreased cardiac filling pressure), second by reducing cardiac output, and third by decreasing arteriolar resistance. There have not been many haemodynamic studies of these drugs in man and the majority of these have been with guanethidine. The reduction of arterial pressure when resting supine was associated with either average decreases in cardiac output or peripheral resistance or with simultaneous reductions of both measurements (RICHARDSON et al., 1960; NOVACK, 1961; COHN et al., 1963; ABRAMS et al., 1964; VILLAREAL et al., 1964; ONESTI et al., 1966; CHRYSANT et al., 1974). This apparent variation in results has led some authors to conclude that the antihypertensive effect of ANIDs is due to a decrease in cardiac output and others that it is rather caused by a reduction of peripheral resistance. However, as a fall in cardiac output would normally (in normotensive subjects or untreated hypertensive subjects) cause a reflex rise in peripheral resistance and, conversely, a decrease in peripheral resistance would produce an elevation of cardiac output, the above results indicate that ANIDs lower blood pressure by a combined inhibition of cardiac output and arteriolar vasoconstriction. Whether cardiac output or peripheral resistance fell below ANID pretreatment values in the various investigations cannot be taken as necessarily meaning that different haemodynamic mechanisms were responsible for the antihypertensive action. It solely indicates that under the conditions of the studies there was a relative difference between the decreases of the two variables from their expected levels. The haemodynamic studies also suggest that when ANIDs reduced cardiac output in supine subjects this was probably secondary to increased peripheral venous pooling (WALSH et al., 1969) and not to cardiac failure. When patients treated with ANIDs exercise there is a large increase in cardiac output showing that they possess good cardiac reserve (DOLLERY et al., 1961; TAYLOR et al., 1962; CHAMBERLAIN and HOWARD, 1964; KHATRI and COHN, 1970).

There is a greater lowering of arterial pressure from bethanidine, debrisoquine, and guanethidine when patients are erect than when they are supine, i.e., the drugs characteristically cause postural hypotension. There is also controversy whether ANIDs produce this postural effect by decreasing cardiac output or peripheral resistance. Many investigations have been inadequate because the upright haemodynamic measurements have usually been compared with those obtained in the supine position. When untreated hypertensive patients or normotensive subjects change from a supine to erect position there is peripheral pooling of blood in the dependent veins, leading to a reduction in cardiac output of 20%–25% and there is a compensatory reflex increase in peripheral resistance of approximately 30% (TUCKMAN and SLATER, 1964; TUCKMAN and SHILLINGFORD, 1966; TUCKMAN et al., 1966). Hence any analysis of the antihypertensive action of ANIDs which fails to take into account the fact that cardiac output is much less and peripheral resistance much higher in untreated erect subjects overemphasises the drugs' effect on cardiac output and underestimates their influence on peripheral resistance.

The results from haemodynamic studies of ANIDs when these parts are considered in upright subjects at rest indicate that they usually produce their postural effect on blood pressure largely by reducing peripheral resistance (RICHARDSON et al., 1960; ABRAMS et al., 1964; CHAMBERLAIN and HOWARD, 1964; VILLAREAL et al., 1964; ONESTI et al., 1966; KHATRI and COHN, 1970; HANSSON et al., 1973). There is only a slight exaggeration of the normal orthostatic fall in cardiac output, but an inhibition of part or all of the usual 30% postural compensatory increase of peripheral resistance. The evidence also suggests that ANIDs do not cause excessive peripheral venous pooling in upright patients at doses which produce tolerable degrees of postural hypotension. The small reduction of cardiac output that occurs in upright patients at rest after administration of ANIDs is not due to cardiac failure, for these patients also have a large increase in cardiac output during exercise (DOLLERY et al., 1961; CHAMBERLAIN and HOWARD, 1964; KHATRI and COHN, 1970).

Exercise is associated with high levels of adrenergic stimulation to the cardiovascular system and the haemodynamic changes caused by physical activity are altered by ANIDs. Initial clinical observations of the drugs quickly established that they sometimes caused hypotension during exercise (LEISHMAN et al., 1959; DOLLERY et al., 1960). Exercise in untreated subjects produces a large fall of vascular resistance in the active limbs and adequate blood flow is assured to this area and to the heart and brain by the increased sympathetic activity which causes arteriolar and venous vasoconstriction in other regions and a large increase in cardiac output. Normally, this results in a small increase in mean arterial pressure in spite of the large reduction in total peripheral resistance. Only an approximate assessment can be made of the effects that ANIDs have on the above haemodynamic changes because the relevant investigations were performed under different conditions, e.g. they involved different levels of efforts, supine or upright subjects, and the measurements were obtained during or after exercise. Exercise was associated with small increases or decreases of mean arterial pressure in both supine and upright positions (TAYLOR et al., 1962; CHAMBERLAIN and HOWARD, 1964; KHATRI and COHN, 1970), except in the study of a group of patients who were selected because they had moderate to large degrees of exertional hypotension, even when supine (DOLLERY et al., 1961). All results showed large average increases in cardiac output on exercise, even in the subjects who had the large falls of arterial pressure. The evidence is not detailed enough to assess whether those patients with significant falls in pressure had smaller increases in cardiac output and/or greater decreases of peripheral resistance. It does indicate that patients treated with ANIDs still possess considerable cardiac reserve and can increase their cardiac work (cardiac output × mean arterial pressure) by at least 100%.

III. Clinical Use

These drugs are very effective antihypertensive drugs but unfortunately they also cause important side-effects. Some authors have reported that one or another of them is better tolerated. However, the differences are clearly marginal, except that guanethidine often causes severe diarrhoea (BATH et al., 1967; PRICHARD et al., 1968; ADI et al., 1975; TALBOT et al., 1975).

There are major differences between the ANIDs in the speed of onset and duration of their antihypertensive effect following their oral use. The lowering of arterial pressure from guanethidine takes until 3 days after treatment is started and it takes another 2 or 3 days before a given dose reaches its maximum effect. This delay and the wide range of patients' sensitivities to the drug, which is between 10 and 1,050 mg/day (DOLLERY et al. 1960; MCMARTIN and SIMPSON, 1971), means that it may require a considerable period to determine an individual's correct antihypertensive dose. If there is an attempt to shorten this time by rapid elevations of dosage it carries the risk of producing an exaggerated response and incapacitating hypotension lasting several days. Guanethidine has a prolonged duration of action that does not decline until about 3 days after the drug is discontinued. On the other hand, the maximum antihypertensive action of oral bethanidine and debrisoquine is usually produced within 4 h and subsides several hours later (ABRAMS et al., 1964; JOHNSTON et al., 1964). Thus, these two rapidly acting drugs can gain control of blood pressure within a day, when necessary, and also because of their short effect they have to be given in divided daily doses, three or even four times a day. The longer-acting guanethidine, of course, has the advantage that it need only be given as a single daily dose.

The range of dosage with bethanidine is also large and varies between 10 and 1,000 mg/day (JOHNSTON et al., 1964). The range reported for debrisoquine has been between 10 and 360 mg/day (ABRAMS et al., 1964; LURIA and FREIS, 1965; ATHANASSIADIS et al., 1966; KITCHIN and TURNER, 1966; JACKSON, 1972). The doses of bethanidine and debrisoquine may have to be increased during the initial months of treatment to maintain the same degree of control of blood pressure (MONTUSCHI and PICKENS, 1962; JACKSON, 1972). With respect to patients' sensitivities to bethanidine and debrisoquine it should be noted that both are primarily excreted by the kidneys and that single oral doses can produce severe hypotensive episodes that may be prolonged for 1 or 2 days in subjects with poor renal function (MONTUSCHI and PICKENS, 1962; DOYLE and MORLEY, 1965; ROCHE, 1975).

In addition to showing a postural effect, patients on ANIDs have lower pressures in the morning and then they gradually rise during the rest of the day (DOLLERY et al., 1960; CRANSTON and BROWN, 1963; ATHANASSIADIS et al., 1966). Indeed, the highest dose of guanethidine that can be given is usually limited to that amount which produces the lowest tolerated level of standing and postexercise blood pressures in the morning, and consequently patients have substantially higher arterial pressures later in the day. In theory, varied doses of bethanidine and debrisoquine could provide smoother antihypertensive control (ATHANASSIADIS et al., 1966). The smallest dose of the drug would be given in the evening to prevent excessive morning postural hypotension, and the later elevation of blood pressure would be mitigated by a larger dose in the morning and the largest dose in the afternoon, e.g. 10 mg in the evening, 25 mg on the following morning, and 35 mg in the afternoon. However, this approach is often too complicated to be of use for the treatment of most patients.

If the criterium of a standing diastolic pressure is that 100 mm Hg or less is taken as satisfactory, then an estimate of the efficacy of ANIDs often used in combination with diuretics is provided by the following results. This level of blood pressure was obtained by different investigators with bethanidine in 44% (MONTUSCHI and PICKENS, 1962), 58% (JOHNSTON et al., 1964), 46% (SMIRK, 1963a), and 77% (PRICHARD et al., 1968) of their patients. Similar levels were achieved with guanethidine in 44% (LEISHMAN et al., 1959), 43% (DOLLERY et al., 1960), 64% (BAUER et al., 1961), 40% (LOWTHER and TURNER, 1963), and 87% (PRICHARD et al., 1968) of treated subjects. Debrisoquine attained this level of control in 42%–67% (KITCHIN and TURNER, 1966), approximately 70% (JACKSON, 1972), and 88% (ADI et al., 1975) of the patients studied.

IV. Side-Effects and Precautions

The most important and debilitating symptoms are from postural and exercise hypotension (PRICHARD et al., 1968; TALBOT and SMITH, 1975) and these are aggravated by hot climates and working environments. Postural symptoms from guanethidine tended to occur early in the morning, but from bethanidine and debrisoquine at any time in the day and particularly 1–2 h after injection of the drug (TALBOT and SMITH, 1975). Patients should be warned to avoid rapid changes from supine or sitting positions to one of standing, and in particular dizziness and sometimes syncope may happen on getting up in the night to go to the toilet or on rising in the morning. Special care should also be taken when standing up after a hot bath and patients should be encouraged to empty the bath before doing so. They should avoid prolonged periods of quiet standing and should be aware that symptoms of postural hypotension might occur particularly in the morning, for instance when shaving. Symptoms are also commonly associated with activities that cause pooling of blood in the dependent limbs after a Valsalva manoeuvre, or similar physiological events, for instance on standing after defecation or micturition. Patients soon learn that climbing stairs and other types of effort may produce hypotensive side-effects. They should be advised to avoid types of exercise in which dizziness and syncope could have dangerous consequences. Patients who do heavy manual labour are best not treated with ANIDs, they must not be given if dizziness and syncope at those jobs might cause catastrophic accidents. Finally, it should be foreseen that the dose of an ANID may have to be reduced when a patient in a northern climate goes on holiday in the winter to hot regions. The 24-h monitoring of blood pressure has confirmed the occurrence of marked exercise hypotension on bethanidine and guanethidine (GOLDBERG and RAFTERY, 1976).

Another troublesome side-effect of ANIDs is that they disturb sexual functions in a majority of male patients (PRICHARD et al., 1968; A.M.A. Committee on Hypertension, 1972; BAUER et al., 1973; ADI et al., 1975). They abolish ejaculation by inhibiting constriction of the internal uretheral sphincter, which causes semen to take a retrograde course. The drugs may also produce impotence and they sometimes decrease libido, perhaps secondary to the effect on ejaculation. It therefore follows that ANIDs should only be used in young males when absolutely necessary and with particular understanding in older men in whom sexual activity is still of significance.

A particular disadvantage of guanethidine is that it causes loose stools in as many as two-thirds of patients (PRICHARD et al., 1968). In most instances this is only a nuisance but in others the bowel movements are so frequent, urgent, and explosive that the drug is intolerable. Diarrhoea rarely occurs with bethanidine or debrisoquine and, indeed, bethanidine may cause constipation (SMIRK, 1963a; KITCHIN and TURNER, 1966; PRICHARD et al., 1968).

ANIDs cause other side-effects, usually of minor importance. Guanethidine produces an obvious bradycardia (PRICHARD et al., 1968; TALBOT and SMITH, 1975), but this is rarely of clinical significance. Fluid retention that may occur with the use of all three ANIDs can be easily prevented or reversed in patients with adequate renal function by adding a diuretic to the antihypertensive regimen. The drugs can also cause muscle weakness and stuffiness of the nose (KITCHIN and TURNER, 1966; PRICHARD et al., 1968; A.M.A. Committee on Hypertension, 1972; JACKSON, 1972).

There are other precautions which should be observed when using ANIDs. As they reduce glomerular filtration rate (RICHARDSON et al., 1960; NOVACK, 1961; VILLAREAL et al., 1964), they can aggravate uraemia in patients with advanced renal impairment, although it is nearly always reversible when the drugs are discontinued. Secondly, blood pressure will usually increase to near pretreatment levels within a day if bethanidine or debrisoquine are abruptly stopped and this rapid elevation might present a danger to patients who take their medications in an undisciplined manner. However, under other circumstances it would be advantageous, for instance when the drugs are stopped or the dosages reduced during the episodes of hypotension which might be associated with haemorrhage, myocardial infarction, infection or trauma.

Finally amphetamine, tricyclic antidepressants, and chlorpromazine inhibit the antihypertensive action of ANIDs and, on the other hand, a serious hypotension could occur when these psychotropic agents are discontinued (see above).

E. Alpha-Receptor Inhibitory Drugs

α-Adrenoceptor inhibitory drugs have been available for very much longer than β-adrenergic blocking drugs. Attempts have been made to use them in the treatment of hypertension initially with little success but more recently with the advent of long-acting orally active competitive blocking agents some success has been achieved. Recently, new uses outside the field of hypertension have been reported.

I. Hypertension

1. Mode of Action

The basic mode of action of α-receptor inhibitory drugs in the treatment of hypertension is readily understood. Peripheral vascular tone is under control of the sympathetic innervating alpha vasoconstrictor receptors. The inhibition of this tone reduces peripheral resistance and reduces blood pressure. Inhibition of α-mediated tone to the veins reduces venous return, thus lowering cardiac output which also can contribute to the fall in blood pressure. A reduction in cardiac output may not necessarily be seen as the reduced peripheral resistance, speeds blood flow and thus may enhance venous return.

There are certain physiological events (see above, discussion of β-blocking drugs in hypertension) that demand increased sympathetic vasoconstrictor activity to α-receptors in order to maintain blood pressure such as the erect posture, exercise or a hot environment. It is possible therefore that an α-receptor inhibitory drug producing sufficient lowering of blood pressure in the supine position may produce too great an inhibitory action at high rates of sympathetic traffic, e.g. standing and standing plus exercise, and so produce postural or exercise hypotension, as does indeed occur. Ideally an α-receptor blocking drug is required that produces an inhibitory effect at low rates of sympathetic traffic, e.g. in the supine position, but that allows sufficient impulses through at high rates of sympathetic traffic, e.g. the standing position. This is more likely to be achieved with a competitive rather than a non-competitive inhibitory drug. Practical experience indicates that this indeed is the case.

2. Prazosin

a) Mode of Action

Prazosin lowers the blood pressure by postsynaptic α-receptor blockade (CAMBRIDGE et al., 1977; BROGDEN et al., 1977). It had been suggested that prazosin had a direct vasodilator action but experiments in rats demonstrated that it had no hypotensive effect in animals where sympathetic tone had been abolished by ganglionic blockade with pentolinium or the other α-receptor blocker phentolamine, in contrast to the persistence of a hypotensive effect from the vasodilator hydrallazine (GRAHAM et al., 1977). The observation that prazosin fails to modify the pressor response to angiotensin unlike hydrallazine or diazoxide also suggests the absence of a direct vasodilator component to the action of prazosin (GRAHAM et al., 1977).

Experiments in dogs (CONSTANTINE et al., 1973) indicated that prazosin reduced arterial resistance without affecting veins. However, investigations in man have suggested prazosin has a greater dilator action on veins than arteries (COLLIER et al., 1978).

Unlike conventional α-blocking drugs, prazosin does not cause tachycardia or renin release in dogs (MASSINGHAM and HAYDEN, 1975). Investigations have suggested a reduction in plasma renin activity (HAYES et al., 1976).

b) Haemodynamic Effects

Intravenously prazosin reduces arterial pressure and peripheral resistance. There is some increase in heart rate, changes in cardiac output are inconsistent (ONESTI et al., 1974), and long-term oral administration up to 2 months (KOSHY et al., 1977) or up to a year at rest and on exercise (LUND-JOHANSEN, 1974) have yielded similar results.

Prazosin may increase plasma volume. This has been observed in patients showing a poor response to prazosin (KOSHY et al., 1977) and when prazosin was added to patients already receiving propranolol (IBSEN et al., 1977). Prazosin does not adversely affect renal function (KOSHY et al., 1977, IBSEN et al., 1977).

c) Pharmacokinetics

Peak concentration occurs about 2 h after the administration of prazosin (VERBESSELT et al., 1976; WOOD et al., 1976). Food has a variable effect, in some patients increasing, in some decreasing prazosin absorption (VERBESSELT et al., 1976).

Prazosin follows first-order kinetics with a mean half-life of 2.5–4 h (COLLINS and PEK, 1975; WOOD et al., 1976) although a longer half-life may occur in patients on long-term treatment, 5–8 h (SIMPSON et al., 1977). It is highly protein-bound, about 97% (HOBBS and TOWNEY, cited by BROGDEN et al., 1977), with an apparent volume of distribution of about 75 l.

Prazosin is exclusively metabolised in rats and dogs, less than 10% being excreted unchanged. Preliminary experiments in man indicate similar findings. (TAYLOR et al., 1977).

d) Effect in Hypertension

Studies of prazosin versus placebo using a between-patient (MROCZEK and FINNERTY, 1974; SCHNAPER and OBERMAN, 1975), and a within-patient design (BOLLI et al., 1976b) have all indicated that prazosin is superior to placebo. The falls in standing blood pressure tended to be greater than in the supine in all three studies. A dose range of 1.5–38 mg daily was used.

Investigations in mild and moderate hypertension have been performed comparing methyldopa and prazosin. When each drug is individually titrated, within-patient studies indicate that there is little difference in degree of blood pressure control and incidence of side-effects (BLOOM et al., 1975; SMITH et al., 1975). Similar findings have been found with between-patient studies, while numerous fixed-dose studies have revealed less useful information (BROGDEN et al., 1977).

Prazosin may be used in combination with other antihypertensive drugs. Studies with thiazides indicate that the addition of the diuretic may allow the dose of prazosin to be halved (ROUGIER et al., 1974) or in more resistant cases enable a larger number of patients to be controlled that did not respond satisfactorily to prazosin alone (DE LA PAZ et al., 1976).

Studies of hydrallazine or prazosin in combination with a β-adrenoceptor blocking drug and a diuretic have indicated similar blood pressure control with both agents, with fewer side-effects from prazosin (HUA et al., 1977). RASMUSSEN and JENSEN (1976) found an average dose of 5.46 mg prazosin produced a similar effect to an average dose of 163 mg hydrallazine when given in combination with propranolol. In a within-patient study in severe hypertension inadequately controlled by β-blockade alone, the addition of prazosin (6–15 mg daily) gave a 16% average fall of mean standing blood pressure, bendrofluazide (5 or 10 mg) an average fall of 13% (MARSHALL et al., 1976b). Prazosin has been used with a number of other agents, including clonidine and adrenergic neuron blocking agents (STOKES et al., 1977b; TURNER et al., 1977).

e) Side-Effects

Dizziness and faintness is common early in treatment with prazosin in about 10% (ROUGIER et al., 1974) to 58% of patients (TURNER, 1976; TURNER et al., 1977). There have been several studies where syncope has occurred related to the initial dosage. This occurred in 16% of cases after 2 mg, but rechallenging with an initial dose of 0.5 mg suggested an incidence of mild dizziness of less than 5% (ROSENDORFF, 1976). Other studies have indicated that this first dose effect is dose-dependent (VERBESSELT et al., 1976). A considerable initial fall in blood pressure may occur with doses as low as 0.25 mg in patients also taking a diuretic and a β-adrenoceptor blocking drug (SIMPSON et al., 1977). STOKES et al. (1977b) have shown that falls in blood pressure in response to the first dose are reduced by a 250 mmol daily sodium intake and symptoms abolished in contrast to the response seen on a 100 mmol diet.

Among other side-effects that have been reported is the suggestion that prazosin may aggravate angina pectoris (SIMPSON et al., 1977).

3. Labetalol

a) Mode of Action

Labetalol competitively inhibits both β- and α-adrenoceptors (FARMER et al., 1972); this was confirmed in man (BOAKES et al., 1971; COLLIER et al., 1972). RICHARDS et al., (1976) found that a single dose of 400 mg oral labetalol produced a rightward shift in the isoprenaline dose response curve to increases in heart rate and the fall in diastolic pressure. There was no difference in the effect on either of these parameters, suggesting that labetalol is a non-selective β-adrenoceptor inhibitor. Log dose-response curves of phenylephrine-induced rises of systolic pressure also showed a rightward parallel displacement. It was found that the ratio of α:β antagonism was approximately 1:3. When labetalol was given intravenously, the ratio was 1:6.9 (RICHARDS, et al., 1977b). The dose-response curve of increase in cardiac output produced by graded doses of isoprenaline is also shifted to the right by isoprenaline. (RICHARDS et al., 1978).

b) Haemodynamic Effects

Labetalol given intravenously in the supine position reduces blood pressure and peripheral resistance, without reducing the cardiac output or stroke volume (PRICHARD et al., 1975; KOCH, 1977). On standing or on exercise, blood pressure, heart rate and both cardiac output and peripheral resistance are modestly reduced (KOCH, 1977). Pulmonary arterial pressures are lowered at rest, supine and standing, but were unchanged on exercise (KOCH, 1977). With continuous oral administration there is a reduction of blood pressure, heart rate and peripheral resistance, with no change in cardiac output, supine and standing (EDWARDS and RAFTERY, 1976; MEHTA and COHN, 1977). Heart rate and blood pressure are reduced on exercise. At lower levels of exercise (350 kpm/min) cardiac output was maintained, peripheral resistance fell, whereas at high levels of exercise (700 kpm/min) there was some reduction in cardiac output (EDWARDS and RAFTERY, 1976). The response to intravenous labetalol, at rest, is similar to the combination of intravenous propranolol and hydrallazine (PRICHARD et al., 1975).

c) Other Effects

While labetalol is a non-selective β-adrenoceptor blocking drug, its α-blocking activity may be responsible for it producing less bronchoconstriction than propranolol. This has been observed in normal subjects (RICHARDS et al., 1977c) and in asthmatic patients (SKINNER et al., 1975).

Labetalol reduces plasma renin and angiotensin II levels after acute intravenous and long-term oral use (TRUST et al., 1976; KOCH, 1976).

d) Pharmacokinetics

Autoradiographic studies and radiochemical analysis of the tissues obtained from rats, rabbits and dogs given large doses of ^{14}C-labetalol have shown that the radioactivity was quickly taken up into the tissues and then rapidly cleared from the body via both the kidney and the bile (MARTIN et al., 1976). Labetalol is well absorbed but extensively metabolised during its passage through the gut and liver, i.e. there is considerable first-pass metabolism. It is only about 50% bound to human plasma protein and therefore is rapidly cleared from the plasma. The half-life of elimination of labetalol in man is 3½–4½ h.

The lipophilicity of labetalol (partition coefficient 1.2 between chloroform and pH 7 buffer) is much less than that of propranolol (partition coefficient 9) or oxprenolol (partition coefficient 10). These latter two compounds have a high uptake into the brain (REISS et al., 1970; BAKER and FOULKES, 1973) Radioautography and radiochemical analysis of the brains from rats and rabbits given oral and intravenous doses of up to 200 mg ^{14}C-labetalol have shown that the concentration of radioactivity in the brain was negligible. Studies carried out in pregnant rats and rabbits given oral and intravenous doses of up to 200 mg ^{14}C-labetalol/kg have shown that there is negligible penetration of radioactivity into the fetus (MARTIN et al., 1976).

Experiments in man have shown that the concentration of plasma labetalol increased with increasing doses of from 100 to 400 mg labetalol, and concentration of drug correlated with the pharmacological activity as measured by the inhibition of exercise-induced tachycardia (RICHARDS et al., 1977a).

From radiochemical analysis of the urine it has been shown that man excretes 60% of the orally administered dose of radioactivity in the urine, the remainder in the faeces. Labetalol is extensively metabolised with only 5% or less excreted as the unchanged drug, with no evidence of an active metabolite being formed (MARTIN et al., 1976).

In both animals and man, labetalol is extensively conjugated. In every case, the major metabolites are glucuronides. The site of conjugation varies with the species. In the mouse, rat and rabbit the major metabolite ist the o-phenyl glucuronide of labetalol. This metabolite is also present in dog and human urine. In the urine of these two species two other major glucuronides are also present. These metabolites have been isolated by chromatographic techniques and their structure determined. The major one of the two is formed by conjugation at the secondary alcohol group of labetalol. The other conjugate which is present to a lesser extent is labile and has been tentatively identified as the *N*-glucuronide (MARTIN et al., 1976).

e) Duration of Action

Labetalol has a plasma half-life of 3½–4½ h (MARTIN et al., 1976), and this is not altered in patients with renal insufficiency (THOMPSON et al., 1977). Duration of action studies using inhibition of an exercise tachycardia showed that about 75% of the maximum effect obtained was present 6 h after the oral administration of a single dose of 400 mg, with the suggestion that about 40%–50% remained at 8 h (RICHARDS et al., 1974).

f) Use in Hypertension

PRICHARD and BOAKES (1976) reported a long-term study largely in patients already under treatment with existing antihypertensive drugs. They used an average dose of 889 mg (range 75–3,200 mg) but in the 11 patients not previously treated who were generally a more mildly affected group, the average dose was 529 mg. Blood pressure control on labetalol was similar to treatment with methyldopa and to sympathetic inhibitory drugs, bethanidine, debrisoquine and guanethidine. Long-term follow-up for over 3 years in 13 patients indicated that tolerance to labetalol did not develop. PRICHARD and BOAKES (1976) found no significant fall in blood pressure on standing in 26 patients receiving less than 1,800 mg labetalol a day, but a significant fall in mean pressure from 122 mm Hg supine to 111 mm Hg standing ($p<0.002$). BOLLI et al. (1967a) found some postural effect with a lower dosage (200–1,200 mg, average 585 mg) in contrast to patients previously treated with β-adrenergic blocking drugs. All but one of these patients were receiving a diuretic with labetalol, in contrast to the study of PRICHARD and BOAKES (1976), in which only five of the 26 patients not showing a postural fall in pressure used a diuretic.

Further evidence to support the suggestion of PRICHARD et al. (1975) that labetalol was a drug that could control the blood pressure in patients previously needing large doses of methyldopa was provided by the work of DARGIE et al. (1976). They treated a group of 16 very severely hypertensive patients whose outpatient blood pressures averaged 172/108 mm Hg supine, 155/102 mm Hg standing, while being treated with bendrofluazide (10 mg) plus a mixture of other drugs: propranolol, average dose 892 mg, in 13 patients; methyldopa, average 4,560 mg, in 8 patients; clonidine, average 2.53 mg, in 7; bethanidine, average 62 mg, in 7; hydrallazine, average 300 mg, in 4; and guanethidine, 70 mg, in 1 patient. The diuretic was continued but labetalol, average 3,091 mg (range 1,200–8,000 mg), was substituted for the other drugs; blood pressures were 150/98 mm Hg supine, 131/91 mm Hg standing.

Other recent reports have confirmed that labetalol is a highly effective agent (LOUIS et al., 1978).

PUGSLEY et al. (1976) performed a formal between-patient double-blind trial of labetalol and propranolol in 18 patients, with all patients receiving hydrochlorothiazide (100 mg daily) and amiloride (10 mg daily) (Moduretic, 2 tablets). Pressures were reduced to a similar degree by labetalol (average 763 mg) and propranolol (average 532 mg) in the supine position. Pressures on standing and after exercise tended to fall on labetalol, but the difference from propranolol only reached statistical significance for the postexercise diastolic pressure. The ratio of doses of labetalol to propranolol in this study was 1.44:1. In patients whose blood pressure control had been inadequate on β-blocking drugs when tansferred to labetalol, adequate control was achieved in all patients (DENT and KELLAWAY, 1977).

JENNINGS and PARSONS (1976) also found a satisfactory response to labetalol in white patients but not in African or West Indian patients; however, the compliance of the latter was suspect; we have not observed this racial difference (PRICHARD and BOAKES, unpublished). HANSSON and HÄNEL (1976) used labetalol average 273 mg (range 100–600 mg) in 12 mild hypertensives, reducing standing blood pressure from an average of 168/112 mm Hg to 140/95 mm Hg. Double-blind trials comparing labetalol with placebo have demonstrated significant falls in blood pressure with individually titrated doses (BOLLI et al., 1976a) or fixed doses (FRICK and PÖRSTI, 1976; KANE et al., 1976).

A double-blind comparative study in mild to moderately severe hypertensives found labetalol (600 mg, twice daily) was approximately equivalent to pindolol (15 mg twice daily) plus hydrallazine (50 mg twice daily) (BARNETT et al., 1978).

g) Acute Use

The intravenous use of labetalol has been reported to control the blood pressure of severely hypertensive patients, in phaeochromocytoma and hypertensive reactions after clonidine withdrawal, as well as an adjunct to produce hypotensive anaesthesia.

TRUST et al. (1976) reported a series of 20 severely hypertensive patients given 1–2 mg/kg intravenous labetalol, in four as a rapid bolus injection, in the remaining 16 slowly over 10 min. All patients showed a fall in blood pressure within 5 min of the end of the injection. The largest fall seen was 188/142 mm Hg to a trough of 90/64 mm Hg, 10 min after 100 mg labetalol. Two other patients complained of nausea and faintness even while remaining recumbent. The pressures of these three patients averaged 229/140 mm Hg, heart rate 99 beats/min before labetalol, and 100/77 mm Hg, heart rate 60 beats/min after labetalol. Another approach by the same group of investigators has been to given graded infusions of labetalol in order to improve the smoothness of the fall of blood pressure. A preliminary report has appeared describing an infusion technique for labetalol. The infusion was commenced at 20 mg for the first hour, 40 mg for the second hour, 80 mg for the third and 160 mg during the fourth hour. This resulted in a smooth reduction from a diastolic blood pressure level of 160–170 mm Hg to levels between 90 and 100 mm Hg (BROWN et al., 1977).

ROSEI et al. (1976) report one case where 150 mg labetalol intravenously was used to control the blood pressure after a hypertensive crisis from clonidine withdrawal.

ROSEI et al. (1976) reported that in four of five patients with phaeochromocytoma, labetalol successfully controlled the blood pressure. In the other patient, intravenous labetalol lowered the blood pressure but subsequent oral administration up to 1,600 mg four times a day failed to control hypertensive attacks. Dosage could not be further increased because of nausea, but attacks were controlled by a mixture of propranolol and phenoxybenzamine.

Labetalol has been used in single oral doses to control blood pressure in nine patients whose diastolic blood pressures were persistently in excess of 130 mm Hg (GHOSE and SAMPSON, 1977), using 200 mg (two patients), 300 mg (four patients), 400 mg (three patients). Two of these patients required additional doses 2–4 h later because of inadequate response, but otherwise significant reductions in blood pressure occurred without symptoms or complications. A considerable part of the hypotensive response is seen within 2 h of drug administration.

There have been reports of labetalol being used in combination with halothane anaesthesia to produce controlled hypotension. A synergistic effect was observed between the labetalol and halothane with good circulatory and operating conditions. Blood pressure rose to near normal when halothane was withdrawn (SCOTT et al., 1976; KAUFMANN and RICHARDS, unpublished observations).

h) Side-Effects

Labetalol interferes with the innervation of the α-receptor, and therefore symptoms of postural hypotension might be expected to occur. These however are uncommon with labetalol; there are two factors that might be responsible: firstly labetalol also lowers the blood pressure because of its β-blocking action, and secondly as the inhibition is of the competitive type, the increased alpha sympathetic activity associated with the erect posture might be expected to at least partly overcome any partial blockade. When the non-competitive α-blocker phenoxybenzamine is added to propranolol, the additional antihypertensive effect was entirely postural (BEILEN and JUEL-JENSEN, 1972). Postural effects tend to occur more frequently with higher doses of labetalol (DARGIE et al., 1976; PRICHARD and BOAKES, 1976). Postural effects occurring with lower dosages have been seen in series where a diuretic was used in all or most of the patients (BOLLI et al., 1976 a; PUGSLEY et al., 1976). Diuretics produce a chronic reduction in blood volume (PRICHARD and TUCKMAN, 1977) and this will increase sensitivity to α-adrenoceptor inhibition under physiological stresses such as the erect posture. Another reason for postural hypotension with lower dosages might be the abrupt administration of moderate doses, e.g. 400 mg and 800 mg, in double-blind trials (KANE et al., 1976).

Side-effects in general appear to be more frequent early in treatment with labetalol than later (PUGSLEY et al., 1976). This is possibly a function of the initial effects of lowering of the blood pressure, and diminution of side-effects with time has been reported, regardless of the drug administered, when bethanidine, guanethidine and methyldopa were examined (PRICHARD et al., 1968).

Transient tiredness in three patients and transient calf muscle pain in two patients were reported in a series of 17 patients by ANDERSSON et al. (1976). Urinary retention due to labetalol has been reported in one patient (DARGIE et al., 1976) as there has been an isolated report of one patient suffering from vivid dreams that could possibly have been due to labetalol (HANSSON and HÄNEL, 1976). BOLLI et al. (1976) in a series of 17 patients reported two patients with mild constipation and one patient with angina, whose angina was worsened when labetalol was substituted for metoprolol. Although labetalol does have significant anti-anginal action, it may be less effective than β-blocking agents in normotensive patients (BOAKES and PRICHARD, 1973).

DARGIE et al. (1976) reported that sedation and dry mouth were less common than on methyldopa and clonidine, and BOLLI et al. (1967 a) found that two patients experiencing Raynaud's phenomenon on β-blocking drugs were improved on labetalol.

The two side-effects in susceptible subjects, heart failure and asthma, associated with the administration of β-adrenergic blocking drugs, have not been reported with labetalol. However, we have seen one hypertensive patient develop subjective symptoms and objective signs of airway obstruction in labetalol that were reversed on dosage reduction, without loss of blood pressure control (PRICHARD, 1979). There have not been any reports of heart failure being precipitated by labetalol, but the drug is probably best avoided in patients crucially dependent on their sympathetic drive to maintain cardiac output.

Overall, labetalol produces only modest side-effects; in some instances they have been less than on previous treatment.

II. Heart Failure Following Myocardial Infarction

The pathophysiological basis for the use of agents to reduce after-load in patients with congestive heart failure has recently been discussed (MASON, 1978). When arterial impedance reduction occurs as a result of arterial vasodilatation in patients with normal hearts there is a minimal effect on stroke output and thus a fall in blood pressure with a reflex tachycardia. However, arterial resistance is increased and cardiac output is low in the presence of left ventricular insufficiency. The cardiac output is very dependent on arterial resistance, and after-load reduction from arterial vasodilatation results in a considerable increase in cardiac output with little change in heart rate and blood pressure (COHN and FRANCOISA, 1977; ROSS, 1976).

MAJID et al. (1971) demonstrated that phentolamine infusions in post-myocardial-infarction patients reduced the elevated vascular resistance and the raised pulmonary arterial pressure, and increased the cardiac output, without changing systemic blood pressure or heart rate. These findings have been confirmed (KELLY et al., 1973; GOULD et al., 1974). Further studies indicated that phentolamine infusions had a greater effect in patients with increased left ventricular filling pressure than in those with normal pressures (WALINSKY et al., 1974).

In a study of nine patients with congestive failure due to coronary heart disease, oral prazosin (2–7 mg) reduced forearm venous tone from 58.9 to 18.5 mm Hg/ml, forearm vascular resistance from 88.9 to 47.9 mm/Hg/ml/100 g/min and arterial pressure from a mean of 99.7 to 77.7 mm Hg and decreased left ventricular filling pressure from 32.0 to 17.6 mm Hg, but there was a rise of cardiac index from 1.95 to 2.89 min/m^2. Two weeks' oral treatment (2–7 mg four times a day resulted in a reduction in end-diastolic size as measured by the echocardiogram, with an increase in treadmill exercise tolerance and a reduction of symptoms (AWAN et al., 1978). In a further study in 16 patients with heart failure from various causes despite the administration of digitalis and diuretic, prazosin, and the similar drug trimazosin, were found to prolong exercise tolerance (ARONOW and DANAHY, 1978).

III. Asthma

It has been demonstrated that α-receptors play a part in bronchial smooth muscle tone. Stimulation of α-receptors causes bronchial constriction and this is prevented by α-adrenergic blockade (ANTHRACITE et al., 1971; KAMBUROFF, 1976).

A number of α-receptor inhibitory drugs have been shown to reduce histamine-induced bronchospasm. This has been shown with phenoxybenzamine (KERR, et al., 1970), which has strong antihistaminic properties, and thymoxamine (BIANCO et al., 1972; GADDIE et al., 1972).

It has been shown that the α-adrenergic blocking drug indoramin can prevent exercise-induced asthma (BIANCO et al., 1974).

F. Beta-Adrenergic Inhibitory Drugs

The β-adrenoceptor blocking drugs have now become widely used in therapeutics. These drugs were first used in the treatment of angina pectoris, arrhythmias and phaeochromocytoma, but many uses have been found that were not originally predicted from an understanding of the pharmacology of these agents. This includes their ability to lower the blood pressure in hypertension, which now represents the major indication for the use of these compounds. Other situations in which their use has been explored include thyrotoxicosis, anxiety, schizophrenia, drug addiction withdrawal syndromes, migraine, obstruction of the outflow tract of the heart and glaucoma. The largest clinical experience has been gained with propranolol but uses that have also been demonstrated with this drug are likely to be shared by the newer β-adrenoceptor blocking drugs. The associated properties which some of these drugs have do not seem to be over-important in their therapeutic efficacy.

I. Hypertension

1. Introduction

Blood pressure changes little after acute administration of β-blocking agents at rest, but the rise of blood pressure on exercise (SHINEBOURNE et al., 1967; THADANI et al., 1973) or in the overshoot after Valsalva's manoeuvre (PRICHARD and GILLAM, 1966), is markedly reduced.

The hypotensive effect of β-adrenoceptor blocking drugs was first reported in 1964 (PRICHARD, 1964) and the use of propranolol in hypertension was described later that year (PRICHARD and GILLAM, 1964). Then, after some initial delay, the value of the β-adrenoceptor blocking drugs in hypertension became widely accepted (SIMPSON, 1974).

This slow acceptance of β-blocking drugs may have been due first to conservatism because β-receptor antagonists inhibit cardiac contraction. This was considered basically undesirable and in addition was thought to have been associated with untoward reactions in acutely ill patients. Secondly, this effect had not been seen in animals and the mechanism of the hypotensive action was still unknown. Thirdly, antihypertensive effects are not seen immediately and peripheral resistance increases, properties which both seemed disadvantageous. A further reason was the use of inadequate doses. Early investigators tended to fix doses at suboptimal levels despite original reports (PRICHARD and GILLAM, 1964, 1966) emphasising the importance of variable dosage regimes. These fixed and low doses often produced unimpressive results. The misgivings about dosage arose from erroneous concepts of complete β-adrenoceptor blockade, where a relatively small dose of propranolol had been observed to block the effect of a dose of isoprenaline which had previously given a maximal tachycardia. Considerably larger doses were needed to produce maximum inhibition of exercise-induced tachycardia or even the supine or standing resting heart rate (BOAKES et al., 1973). It is these larger doses that are often needed to given an adequate antihypertensive effect.

These misconceptions also led to the belief that the use of large doses had a "direct depressing action" ("quinidine-like effect", "membrane action", local anaesthetic effect) on the heart. Indeed a membrane action is seen with large doses in animals (FITZGERALD, 1972) and it causes a depression of myocardial function independent of β-blockade. It is, however, a pharmacological curiosity with no relevance to the treatment of hypertension, and it is not responsible for the haemodynamic effects of β-blocking drugs. It is inhibition of sympathetic activity per se that produces the negative inotropic and chronotropic effect on the heart in man. The use of the term "negative inotropic effect" is probably best avoided but if applied to β-receptor blocking drugs, it should refer to their sympathetic blocking action.

2. Mode of Action

The antihypertensive effect of a β-adrenoceptor blocking drug seems to be a function of its β-receptor inhibitory action. Blood pressure is lowered regardless of the presence or absence of properties such as membrane stabilisation, intrinsic sympathomimetic activity or cardioselectivity. However, molecular configuration is important since the D(+) optical isomer of propranolol contrasts with standard DL-propranolol in having no antihypertensive action (WAAL-MANNING 1970a, 1976; PRICHARD, 1970; PRICHARD and BOAKES, 1977).

Proposals to explain the hypotensive effect of β-adrenergic blocking drugs have included direct actions on the central nervous system, adrenergic neuron blocking, antirenin activity, effects secondary to reduced cardiac output, and resetting of baroreceptors secondary to reduced pressor peaks from reduced cardiac activity.

a) Effect on Central Nervous System

Animal observations have suggested a possible central mode of action. Propranolol (0.1 mg/kg) injected into either the carotid or the vertebral artery in the anaesthetised dog produced a fall in blood pressure that was of more rapid onset than when the drug was administered via the femoral artery (STERN et al., 1971). However, OFFERHAUS and VAN ZWIETEN (1974) found that the non-β-blocking isomers of alprenolol and propranolol were as effective as the racemic mixtures when injected into the vertebral arteries of the chloralose-anaesthetised cat. This hypotensive effect of D(+) and racemic mixtures alike was abolished by reserpinisation (KELLIHER and BUCKLEY, 1970) and must be regarded as non-specific since the D(+) isomer is devoid of an antihypertensive effect in man.

β-Receptor antagonists (propranolol, alprenolol, pindolol, practolol, atenolol, sotalol and oxprenolol) when injected into the cerebral ventricles of conscious normotensive cats produce a transient rise before a fall in blood pressure. The non-β-blocking D(+) isomers of propranolol and alprenolol, showed only the initial pressor response (DAY and ROACH, 1974) with no hypotensive effect. Intraventricular propranolol in doses giving concentrations in brain of conscious rabbits comparable to those following intravenous infusion of 1.0–2.0 mg/kg/h for 1–2 h also produced a hypotensive effect (MYERS et al., 1975). These authors also demonstrated brain penetration by propranolol in man.

GARVEY and RAM (1975a) found that oral or subcutaneous propranolol and pindolol given for 14 days reduced blood pressure and heart rate in hypertensive and normotensive conscious rats. Propranolol was concentrated particularly in the hippocampus and pindolol in the septum. Sotalol, however, failed to reduce blood pressure and significant concentrations were not found in the central nervous system. All three drugs were given in sufficient amounts to produce persistent peripheral β-adrenergic blockade. Direct injection of propranolol into the hippocampus, and of pindolol into the septum, produced maximal effects on the blood pressure and heart rate in chloralose-anaesthetised cats and dogs, with less effect being seen at other brain sites (GARVEY and RAM, 1975b). These manoeuvres also produced reductions in efferent sympathetic and increases in parasympathetic nerve activity. The injection of sotalol at various brain sites had no effect. Intravenous infusion of racemic propranolol into the conscious rabbit (LEWIS and HAEUSLER, 1975) produced a significant fall of blood pressure and splanchnic efferent nerve activity after 2 h whereas the (+) isomer did not. In contrast, practolol in conscious rabbits did not reduce sympathetic nerve activity but rather when pressures fell after larger doses there was a rise in sympathetic nerve activity (LEWIS and HAEUSLER, cited by DOLLERY and LEWIS, 1976).

Further experiments in chloralose cats showed that racemic propranolol, (+)-propranolol and pindolol were more effective in producing a fall in blood pressure when given into the lateral ventricle than intravenously. The decline in blood pressure was associated with a decrease in sympathetic nerve activity following sciatic nerve stimulation. Sotalol had no such effect (KLEVANS et al., 1976).

Acutely, pindolol did not reduce plasma noradrenaline concentration (ANAVEKAR et al., 1975) but chronically it did, with levels finally reaching those seen in normotensives (BRECHT et al., 1976). The pretreatment plasma noradrenaline levels were found to correlate with diastolic blood pressure, as reported by LOUIS et al. (1973), but other workers (REID et al., 1977) have not found consistent relationships between arterial pressure and plasma noradrenaline. Similarly the decline in plasma noradrenaline caused by pindolol did not correlate with falls in blood pressure (BRECHT et al., 1976) and hypertensive patients on long-term penbutolol therapy maintained their plasma noradrenaline despite reduction of blood pressure (HANSSON and HÖKFELT, 1975). Indeed the cardioselective agent atenolol increased plasma noradrenaline both at rest and after exercise (DISTLER et al., 1978). However, they also found that the ratio of exercise to resting plasma noradrenaline before treatment correlated well with the subsequent fall in blood pressure. IRVING, et al. (1974) concur on the postexercise catecholamine levels, particularly of noradrenaline, but they did not observe any effects on resting levels. During long-term treatment with metoprolol, plasma noradrenaline did not alter although blood pressure fell; in fact, standing concentrations were higher on metoprolol (HANSSON et al., 1977 a). It should be noted that although some reports suggest a decline in supine resting noradrenaline levels with chronic treatment, there is no fall in the rise on standing or on exercise (HANSSON and HÖKFELT, 1975; BRECHT et al., 1976).

Undoubtedly most β-adrenoceptor blocking drugs administered systemically penetrate the central nervous system. Concentrations rapidly achieve a steady state. In cats, for example, there was no evidence of accumulation in the cerebrospinal fluid following 2 weeks' administration of alprenolol, as compared with acute administration (OFFERHAUS and VAN ZWIETEN, 1974).

Although it appears that β-receptor blocking drugs can influence central sympathetic activity, it is unlikely that this is the explanation for their antihypertensive action in man. First, β-adrenergic blocking drugs that do not penetrate the central nervous system such as practolol (SCALES and COSGROVE, 1970) and sotalol (GARVEY and RAM, 1975 a) still have an effective antihypertensive action in man. Secondly, with the exception of the observations of GARVEY and RAM (1975 a), the effects described in animals are of acute onset, but those in man are not. (PRICHARD and GILLAM, 1969; PRICHARD and BOAKES, 1974).

b) Adrenergic Neuron Blocking Effects

Racemic propranolol has an adrenergic neuron inhibiting effect in rats and rabbits, but so does the (+) isomer (BARRETT and NUNN, 1970) which is devoid of antihypertensive effects in man. The racemic compound also inhibited nerve stimulation in cats but the (+) isomer did not (ABLAD et al., 1970). In man there is no evidence that α-receptor innervation is inhibited. The rise in blood pressure during the effort phase of Valsalva's manoeuvre is not inhibited by β-receptor blocking drugs (PRICHARD and GILLAM, 1966, PRICHARD et al., 1970 b), and more direct measurements did not find evidence of inhibition of vasoconstriction (KORNER et al., 1976). No depression of the cold pressor test was seen after 3 weeks' oral propranolol in male hypertensive patients, again suggesting that the innervation of the α-receptor was not impeded (GUAZZI et al., 1976). The fact that propranolol (and other β-adrenergic blocking drugs) control the blood pressure in man without producing the postural hypotension characteristic of adrenergic neuron inhibiting drugs (PRICHARD and GILLAM, 1969) confirms that this action is not important.

c) Renin

Blockade of the β-adrenoceptor in normal subjects (WINER et al., 1969) and hypertensives (BUHLER et al., 1972; MICHELAKIS and MCALLISTER, 1972) lowers plasma renin; although the β-adrenergic system is important in the release of renin it is not the only factor (BRAVO et al., 1974).

BUHLER et al. (1972) divided their patients before treatment into high, normal and low renin groups according to their ambulant peripheral renin levels, and daily urinary sodium excretion. The three groups were similar as regards age and severity of hypertension and they were treated with up to 540 mg propranolol daily. The 12 patients with high renin levels showed the greatest falls of pressure, those with low renin (14 patients) showed only a very small effect, while those with normal renin levels (23 patients) were intermediate. There was good overall correlation between the fall in blood pressure and plasma renin activity. DRAYER et al. (1978) using propranolol also found slightly greater decreases in renin levels in patients who showed a good response to blood pressure, but falls in aldosterone levels were far greater in responders than in non-responders (DRAYER et al., 1978). Propranolol, oxprenolol, LL21945, and the cardioselective agents atenolol and metoprolol were studied in a further series of 137 patients (BUHLER et al., 1975) and again high renin patients showed the largest fall in blood pressure, which was poor in the low and intermediate in normal renin patients. Similarly during treatment with alprenolol, falls in diastolic blood pressure correlated with reduction in plasma renin (CASTENFORS et al., 1973). In hypertensive patients receiving acebutolol, FOURNIER et al. (1976) found a greater fall in blood pressure when plasma renin activity was normal as opposed to low, although overall fall of blood pressure did not significantly correlate with initial plasma renin activity.

There is, however, evidence against effects on renin being central to the antihypertensive qualities of β-adrenergic blocking drugs, because frequently there appears to be no correlation between the fall in blood pressure and pretreatment levels of plasma renin for propranolol (HANSSON, 1973; STOKES et al., 1974; LEONETTI et al., 1975; MORGAN et al., 1975; ZWEIFLER and ESLER, 1976; NIELSEN et al., 1978), pindolol (MORGAN et al., 1975; LANCASTER et al., 1976; STUMPE et al., 1976), alprenolol (PEDERSEN and KORNERUP, 1977), sotalol (VERNIORY et al., 1974), metoprolol (GENEST et al., 1976; HANSSON et al., 1977a), atenolol (AMERY et al., 1976b) or timolol (SIMON et al., 1978a).

MORGAN et al. (1975) divided their patients as described by BUHLER et al. (1972), but in contrast they found equal falls in blood pressure with low, normal and high renin patients. Relatively small doses of propranolol which suppress plasma renin levels have little effect on blood pressure (MICHELAKIS and MCALLISTER, 1972; LEONETTI et al., 1975; ZWEIFLER and ESLER, 1976). LEONETTI et al. (1975) found 40 mg daily produced almost maximal suppression of supine and frusemide-stimulated renin levels, and 60% of the fall in standing renin levels. The further fall in standing levels brought about by up to 160 mg propranolol daily was significant. In contrast, only a small fall in blood pressure was seen at 40 mg daily, the reduction in diastolic pressure being only significant between 40 and 160 mg propranolol daily.

No relationship was found between the fall in blood pressure and change in renin when propranolol was added to patients on diuretics for their hypertension; indeed, in some, renin increased (BRAVO et al., 1975). CHALMERS et al. (1976) found while timolol alone lowered plasma renin when hydrochlorothiazide was added, plasma renin levels were not different from those seen on placebo, although there was the additive antihypertensive effect.

Additional evidence of the dissociation of renin and antihypertensive effect is found where intravenous propranolol lowers plasma renin without lowering blood pressure (BRAVO et al., 1974; MORGAN et al., 1975), although it can still be argued that the fall in blood pressure, although delayed, was secondary to an antirenin effect.

STOKES et al. (1974) found propranolol lowered plasma renin, but substitution of pindolol for propranolol in nine patients for 48 h allowed plasma renin to reach control levels although the hypotensive effect was maintained.

Similarly STUMPE et al. (1976) found that pindolol and propranolol produced similar falls in blood pressure both in patients with borderline and patients with established hypertension, but the fall in renin was greater with propranolol. Falls in blood pressure and renin correlated with propranolol but not with pindolol. Other work has also indicated that fall in blood pressure after pindolol is not correlated with changes in plasma renin (LANCASTER et al, 1976; ANAVEKAR et al., 1975). Likewise, AMERY et al. (1976a) found that when they altered treatment from propranolol (480 mg) to atenolol (600 mg) the hypotensive effect continued but renin levels rose and were no longer significantly different from placebo.

Finally STUMPE et al. (1976) took four patients who showed a fall in blood pressure with propranolol and a drop in renin levels and found that the angiotensin antagonist sar^1 – ala^8 – angiotensin II failed to lower blood pressure.

d) Effect on Plasma Volume

TARAZI et al. (1971) reported a reduction in plasma volume by propranolol in a series of 14 hypertensive patients; however, this did not correlate with the fall in blood pressure. In some patients blood pressure fell without any fall in plasma volume. JULIUS et al. (1972) observed a fall in plasma volume after intravenous propranolol but, as others had shown before, there was no fall in blood pressure.

On the other hand SEDENBERG-OLSEN and IBSEN (1972), using higher doses of propranolol than TARAZI et al. (1971), found that after 4 months of treatment hypertensive patients had an unchanged plasma volume but significantly increased extracellular fluid volume. As in previous reports (PRICHARD and GILLAM, 1969), body weight did not increase and it was seen that changes in extracellular fluid volume did not correlate with the hypotensive effect of propranolol or other hypotensive drugs (RONNOV-JESSEN and HANSEN, 1969). Similarly pindolol did not affect plasma volume in hypertensive patients (PARVING and GYNTELBERG, 1973), but HANSSON et al. (1977a) found a small but significant increase after the use of metoprolol.

Smaller doses of pindolol (15 mg/day) and propranolol (30 mg/day) increased plasma volume after 1 month despite a fall in blood pressure GORDON (1976). Larger doses of propranolol (40 mg thrice daily) produced inconsistent effects with a fall in plasma volume in seven, and no change or an increase in the remaining six patients. Pindolol (10 mg thrice daily) in three of four patients reduced plasma volume. In patients using diuretics with a plasma volume 93% of normal, the addition of propranolol restored it to 99% of normal (BRAVO et al., 1975). These changes did not correlate with the further fall of blood pressure seen with propranolol, which taken with the other evidence suggests that changes in plasma volume are not likely to be important in the hypotensive action of β-blocking drugs.

Although total blood volume may be reduced by propranolol, the cardiopulmonary volume appears unaltered (TARAZI et al., 1974) and this is compatible with systemic vasoconstriction. TARAZI et al. (1974) using the ratio of cardiac output to control pulmonary volume as an index of cardiac performance found that after intravenous propranolol there was a fall from 6.03 to 4.65 ($p < 0.0001$); isoprenaline increased the ratio.

β-blockade produced by propranolol (EPSTEIN and BRAUNWALD, 1966) and sotalol (RICE et al., 1970) appeared to alter the kidney's ability to eliminate sodium in the normal subject. Daytime sodium excretion fell but nocturnal sodium clearance increased, so that overall sodium retention did not occur. Normal subjects taking propranolol were slow to re-equilibrate after being given added sodium each day, although after a lag of several days urinary sodium output increased to balance the increased load. These workers also found that sodium retention with fluid overload was precipitated only in those patients who were dependent on high adrenergic tone to avoid cardiac failure. GIBSON et al. (1970) confirmed sodium retention after 5 days of propranolol but this was not seen with a lower β-blocking dose of practolol. SINGH et al. (1971) found that oxprenolol up to 240 mg/day, like propranolol, did not cause sodium retention when given for 4–10 days to patients with moderately severe cardiac disease. A fall in renal blood flow may be part of the overall systemic adaption to counteract β-blockade which reduces peritubular blood flow and enhances sodium reabsorption (NIES et al., 1971) although local arterial injection of propranolol had no effect on sodium handling. The micropuncture studies of BLENDIS et al. (1972) supported these findings.

e) Delayed Response to Blood Pressure and Role of Cardiac Output

The immediate and long-term haemodynamic effects of β-adrenergic blockade have frequently been found to differ. Although acute and long-term drug administration usually reduces cardiac output to a similar extent (GIBSON, 1974) it is only after long-term administration that blood pressure falls along with a decline in peripheral resistance (TARAZI and DUSTAN, 1972; HANSSON, 1973).

VAUGHAN-WILLIAMS and RAINE (1974) found chronic administration of propranolol or practolol to young rabbits produced a reduction in heart weight without altering the inotropic response to isoprenaline. The relative volume of mitochondria was reduced and the ratio of vascular elements to interfibrillar volume increased, so narrowing the gap between capillary and cell wall (VAUGHAN-WILLIAMS et al., 1977); relative volumes of myofibrils and nuclei were unchanged. Whether these observations are relevant to adult hypertensives is at present unknown; data in man is not available.

When propranolol was added to a diuretic acutely, blood pressure did not fall, but cardiac output and renin did, with a rise in peripheral resistance. One month later blood pressure was reduced with an adaptive fall of peripheral resistance (TARAZI and DUSTAN, 1972; NIARCHOS et al., unpublished, cited by TARAZI et al., 1976). Lowering of cardiac output per se does not generally appear to be the reason for the hypotensive effect of β-adrenergic blocking drugs, except when one is given to a patient receiving a vasodilator. For example, when propranolol was added to minoxidil, a further fall in blood pressure occurred with a fall in cardiac output but there was no change in peripheral resistance (TARAZI et al., 1976).

Some earlier investigators thought that an elevated pretreatment cardiac output might be a reliable guide to the hypotensive response to β-receptor blocking drugs, but later experience with propranolol indicated that there was no correlation between it and reduction in blood pressure (BIRKENHÄGER et al., 1971; TARAZI and DUSTAN, 1972).

f) Resetting the Baroreceptors

The antihypertensive effect of β-adrenoceptor blocking drugs in mild hypertension in seen rapidly. In more severely affected patients there may be some delay, although the greater part of the effect is achieved in the first 2 weeks (PRICHARD and GILLAM, 1969). In standardised clinic conditions (PRICHARD and GILLAM, 1969) the blood pressure in patients receiving propranolol fell significantly between the visit after stabilisation and a month later. The visit after stabilisation of dosage was on average 3 weeks after adjustment of the dosage. There was no further drop after another 2 months and the average heart rate was constant throughout. No such fall after dose stabilisation occurred in patients treated with bethanidine, methyldopa or guanethidine in 1 or up to 3 months. A similar delay in full hypotensive effect has been observed under double-blind conditions with sotalol (PRICHARD and BOAKES, 1974). Because arterial pressure is a function of cardiac output and peripheral resistance, as cardiac output falls so should the blood pressure. However, after intravenous propranolol although cardiac output falls peripheral resistance rises and consequently there is little effect on arterial pressure (SHINEBOURNE et al., 1967; ULRYCH et al., 1968). Perhaps more important is inhibition of cardiac sympathetic activity which reduces the cardiac contribution and so attenuates pressor events. There is, for instance, as discussed above, a reduction in the rise of blood pressure on exercise, of the pressor overshoot in Valsalva's manoeuvre and of the pressor effect of some stresses, but the response to painful stimuli is not reduced.

It has been suggested (PRICHARD and GILLAM, 1964, 1969) that attenuation of pressor responses to various stimuli leads to the baroreceptors generating their inhibitory impulses at lower level of blood pressure, consequently mean pressure falls. Similar conditions exist when a hypertensive patient is put to bed; there is reduction of sensory input and hence pressor events, which allows the baroreceptors over a few days to lower blood pressure by a variable amount.

Experiments in dogs showed that chronic propranolol therapy blunted the pressor response to carotid occlusion (DUNLOP and SHANKS, 1969). Short-term administration was without effect. If chronic propranolol administration enhanced baroreceptor sensitivity then acute reduction in carotid sinus pressure (from carotid occlusion) should leave more inhibitory impulses remaining than if it was not given. It then becomes possible that with higher afferent inhibitory traffic, occlusion would result in a reduced rise in blood pressure. ANGEL-JAMES and BOBIK (1978) recorded action potentials in aortic baroreceptor fibres and reported an increase in activity in hypertensive rabbits treated with propranolol for 2 weeks and even more in those treated for 15 weeks. Baroreceptor reflexes in response to pressor effects may be blunted in hypertension, but the reflex is enhanced modestly by propranolol in normals (PICKERING et al., 1972) and in patients with borderline hypertension (TAKESHITA et al., 1978). In contrast, others do not find any significant increase in baroreceptor sensitivity in hypertensive patients treated with long-term timolol or acutely with propranolol (SIMON, et al., 1978a).

A drug with such wide actions as a β-receptor inhibitor probably lowers blood pressure by more than one mechanism. In some cases one of the many effects may be of overriding importance, e.g. reducing plasma renin in patients with a high renin, whilst in others one of its other effects may be all-important.

3. Classification and Clinical Evaluation

The treatment of hypertension is now a principal application for β-adrenergic blocking drugs and agents with all the permutations of associated properties have been found effective.

a) Division I: Non-Selective

α) Group I These substances possess both membrane stabilising action and intrinsic sympathomimetic action (ISA). Original observations were made with pronethalol (PRICHARD, 1964) but other members of the group have an anti-hypertensive effect.

Oxprenolol. LEISHMAN et al. (1970) found pressures on placebo in 19 patients were 173/102 mm Hg supine and 165/106 mm Hg standing in a double-blind phase. With up to 430 mg oxprenolol/day, the pressures were 160/99 and 151/99 mm Hg respectively. No side-effects were noted but five patients were withdrawn prior to the double-blind part of the trial because of inadequate pressure control, hence those assessed were necessarily preselected. TUCKMAN et al. (1972) reported an open trial in 17 patients of oxprenolol in doses of 60–600 mg/day (mean 374 mg/day), which did not produce orthostatic hypotension. An open study showed it to be similar in efficacy to propranolol, pindolol and practolol (WAAL-MANNING, 1976). Under double-blind conditions, oxprenolol (mean 580 mg/day; range 160–1,280 mg) was found to have a similar effect to propranolol 540 mg/day (160–1,280 mg), practolol 720 mg (400–1,600 mg/day), tolamolol 480 mg (200–800 mg/day) and metoprolol 380 mg (100–800 mg/day) (DAVIDSON et al., 1976).

Alprenolol. Double-blind cross-over testing of alprenolol up to 400 mg/day in 12 patients showed a statistically significant fall in systolic pressure from 180/111 mm Hg on placebo to 162/104 on atenolol after 12 weeks (FURBERG and MICHAELSON (1969). This has been confirmed elsewhere (TIBLIN and ABLAD, 1969; BENGTSSON, 1972; NID-AKHTAR et al., 1975; HARTIKAINEN and HEIKKILA, 1976).

β) Group II This group of drugs have membrane activity but no intrinsic sympathomimetic action.

Propranolol. It was propranolol that established the value of β-receptor blocking agents in hypertension (PRICHARD and GILLAM, 1964, 1966; BACZKO et al., 1967;

FROHLICH et al., 1968; TEWARI and GRANT, 1968; ZACHARIAS and COWEN, 1970; KARLBERG and HORNKVIST, 1971; ZACHARIAS et al., 1972). PRICHARD and GILLAM (1969) reported the first large study, 109 patients treated for up to 4 years.

Propranolol appears to produce similar control to that obtained with bethanidine, guanethidine and methyldopa (PRICHARD and GILLAM, 1969; ZACHARIAS, 1969; PRICHARD et al., 1970b; ZACHARIAS et al., 1972). It is effective treatment for hypertension in pregnancy, reducing fetal mortality (ELIAHOU et al., 1978). When investigators have found less favourable responses of blood pressure to propranolol (HUMPHREYS and DELVIN, 1968; PATERSON and DOLLERY, 1966; RICHARDS, 1966; RICHARDSON et al., 1968; WAAL, 1966) the maximum doses used were less than the mean dose of 400–500 mg/day used by PRICHARD and GILLAM (1969), who, in addition (unlike the investigators mentioned above), used a diuretic in more than half of their patients. SEEDAT and REDDY (1971) using full dosage (up to 1920 mg/day) found only four of 13 Bantu patients were controlled by propranolol alone, but there was a better response in their Indian patients. ZACHARIAS et al. (1972) found a larger proportion of 311 patients achieved satisfactory blood pressure control than usually observed with other hypotensive drugs.

A formal within-patient, randomised comparison of bethanidine, methyldopa and propranolol (PRICHARD et al., 1976) confirms that the three drugs are of similar efficacy, but propranolol produces significantly less postural and exercise hypotension.

In severe and moderately severe hypertensives an average dose is 400–500 mg/day with about half of the patients needing a diuretic in addition. In a few instances other hypotensive agents may be required. A total of 1 g propranolol/day is not exceptional and we have used up to 4 g, but few patients only need a total of 40–80 mg/day. Initially propranolol was given three or four times a day, but twice (HANSSON et al., 1971a) or even once daily (WILSON et al., 1976a) is still effective. Doses may be increased until diastolic blood pressure supine and standing is in the range 80–100 mm Hg providing there be no clinical contra-indication and the standing pulse rate does not fall below 55 beats/min.

A considerable margin of safety with propranolol was demonstrated in a double-blind multi-dose-level trial of propranolol in angina pectoris (PRICHARD and GILLAM, 1971). The standing blood pressure of six mild hypertensive patients fell from a mean 115 mm Hg (154/96) to 102 mm Hg (135/85) ($p<0.005$) as the dose increased from 0 to an average of 320 mg daily; at double this dose (i.e. 640 mg daily), the standing blood pressure averaged 103 mm Hg (137/86).

Success with propranolol can often be correlated with dose; only too often the dose has been too low or inappropriately fixed so as to produce little or no effect (PRICHARD and GILLAM, 1969; ZACHARIAS, 1969).

Three points can be emphasised with reference to variation of dosage. First, dose requirements vary and fixed-dose trials, versus placebo or other drugs, may be less than optimal. Many trials in the literature were totally satisfactory but for the dose being set too low. Secondly, the variable dose requirement with propranolol is neither unique nor any greater than that seen with sympathetic inhibitory drugs such as guanethidine, bethanidine and methyldopa (PRICHARD and GILLAM, 1969). Finally, β-blocking drugs being new have been subject to careful pharmacokinetic studies and it appears that the principal reason, at least in the case of propranolol, is difference in absorption, which can vary over 20-fold (SHAND, 1976).

γ *Group III* Drugs of this group possess intrinsic sympathomimetic activity but no significant membrane activity.

Pindolol. Weight for weight, pindolol is the most potent β-adrenoceptor blocking drug in use, although this does not necessarily confer any advantage. A daily dose of 13 mg was approximately equivalent to propranolol (160 mg/day) or oxprenolol (200 mg/day) in a group of responsive hypertensive patients (WAAL-MANNING, 1970b); however, LAVER et al. (1974) found a 1:5 ratio for pindolol to propranolol.

Pindolol is an effective antihypertensive. FELTHAM et al. (1972) performed open and double-blind studies in 18 patients with between 15 and 80 mg/day. The maximum hypotensive effect in the double-blind phase occurred after 4 weeks, with less effect after 2 weeks' treatment. THORPE (1972) used 15–60 mg daily (average 26 mg) in an open study in 20 patients, and then in a between-subject comparison in 14 of the patients. Blood pressure on placebo ($n=8$) averaged 182/100 mm Hg; after 2 weeks of active treatment it was 150/92 mm Hg ($n=6$) and after 8 weeks of active treatment, 139/86 mm Hg. There was no later decline in blood pressure in the placebo group. MORGAN et al. (1972) obtained a good response in 45 of their 86 patients, and of those responding, 39 required 30 mg/day or less, the other ten between 30 and 50 mg, but increasing the dose to 80 mg/day did not affect the remainder. In four patients there was a rise in blood pressure with pindolol, a phenomenon observed by others (COLLINS and KING, 1972).

WAAL-MANNING and SIMPSON (1974) altered treatment from various hypotensive agents used with a diuretic to pindolol and a diuretic and got better control in 43 patients with fewer side-effects. The dose average was 15 mg/day and increases above 40–50 mg/day were of little or no value but a three-dose-level study in 24 patients taking up to 45 mg revealed a progressive increase in hypotensive effect to the highest dose level (KOLDSLAND, 1977).

In a double-blind cross-over study in 22 patients, pindolol (average 25 mg) produced a more consistent fall in blood pressure from placebo than alprenolol (mean 533 mg) (HARTIKAINEN and HEIKKILA, 1976). Pindolol (range 15–75 mg/day, mean 45 mg) was more effective (in an open study) than propranolol ($n=25$) (mean 760 mg/day) in 24 Indian and Bantu patients (SEEDAT et al., 1973). A more closely controlled double-blind variable-dose study in 35 patients (LAVER et al., 1974) compared pindolol (mean dose 58 mg/day) with propranolol (mean dose 289.3 mg/day); patients received a diuretic throughout. The blood pressures on the two drugs were similar: pindolol supine 138/92 mm Hg, standing 132/90 mm Hg; propranolol supine 137/90 mm Hg, standing 132/88 mm Hg. There was less postural effect than with previous treatment, which included methyldopa (mean daily dose 1.2 g) in 26 patients. It seems that pindolol may be given once daily (WILSON et al., 1976a).

δ) *Group IV* Beta-adrenoceptor blocking drugs of this group, e.g. sotalol (PRICHARD and BOAKES, 1974; VERNIORY et al., 1974) have no intrinsic sympathomimetic effect or significant membrane activity, but they are effective antihypertensive agents.

Sotalol. Propranolol and sotalol were equi-effective antihypertensive drugs (BERGLUND, 1977), but propranolol was twice as potent as sotalol. It seems to have about the same efficacy as methyldopa (PRICHARD and BOAKES, 1974; DOUGLAS-JONES, 1978). *Timolol* is effective (BROGDEN et al., 1974; LOHMOLLER and FROHLICH, 1975;

LUND-JOHANSEN, 1976a; CASTENFORS, 1977) and in mild hypertension most effect was seen with 20 mg daily, only a marginal further effect being achieved with a dose of 60 mg daily (SIMON et al., 1978). In 12 patients it was found that 30 mg timolol appeared equivalent to 120 mg propranolol (ALCOCER et al., 1975), and in a double-blind factorial trial (CHALMERS et al. 1976) there was an additive effect with timolol (10 mg thrice daily) and hydrochlorothiazide (50 mg once daily).

b) Division II: Cardioselective

All drugs in this division are effective antihypertensive drugs.

α) Group I These possess intrinsic sympathomimetic activity and membrane activity.

Acebutolol. Acebutolol has been found effective in hypertension (LETAC et al., 1974) with progressively increasing effects seen with 400 mg, 600 mg and 1,200 mg daily (HANSSON et al., 1977b).

β) Group III This group has intrinsic sympathomimetic action but no membrane action.

Practolol. The first in the group was practolol, which has an antihypertensive effect (LEISHMAN et al., 1970; PRICHARD et al., 1971) but unfortunately also serious adverse reactions involving the eye, skin and a sclerosing peritonitis. These have led to discontinuation of its use, except on an acute intravenous basis.

γ Group IV These have no intrinsic sympathomimetic activity or membrane activity.

Atenolol. Atenolol has been studied widely (HANSSON et al., 1975; LUND-JOHANSEN, 1976b; DOUGLAS-JONES and CRUICKSHANK, 1976; ZACHARIAS et al., 1977a; ZACHARIAS and COWEN, 1977; ZACHARIAS et al., 1977b) and is more effective than bendrofluazide (PETRIE et al., 1975; FAGARD et al., 1976). A comparative study of atenolol and other β-blocking drugs involved fixed doses; hence it is not possible to draw any conclusions on comparative efficacy. The drugs were also given once daily, which was inappropriate for some of the agents (WILCOX, 1978).

Metoprolol. Metoprolol (BENGTSSON et al., 1975; HANNSON et al., 1977a) at doses of 50 mg thrice daily ($n=15$) or 100 mg thrice daily ($n=8$) was equivalent in antihypertensive effect to propranolol 40 mg thrice daily and 80 mg thrice daily, respectively, in mild hypertensive women (BENGSTSSON, 1976). DAVIDSON et al. (1976) found metoprolol about 1.4 times as potent as propranolol. Others (BERGSTRAND et al., 1976) found metoprolol and methyldopa equi-effective in treatment of mild and moderate blood pressure.

Metoprolol once daily controlled blood pressure as effectively as a thrice-daily regime but fluctuations in plasma concentration were greater and there was less consistent control of exercise tachycardia (REYBROUCK et al., 1978).

c) Division III: Beta-Blocking Drugs with Alpha-Receptor Blocking Properties

Labetalol (RICHARDS, 1976), at present is the only available α- and β-blocking drug. It has been used in the treatment of hypertension (PRICHARD and BOAKES, 1976; BROWN et al., 1977) (see above).

4. Response of Blood Pressure to Physiological Stimuli During Treatment

a) With Inhibition of Sympathetic Supply to Alpha-Receptors

Despite differences between sympathetic inhibitory drugs such as guanethidine, debrisoquine or methyldopa (OATES et al., 1965; PRICHARD et al., 1968; HEFFERMAN et al., 1971), they all interfere with important cardiovascular homeostatic reflexes that are mediated largely by sympathetic constrictor fibres to α-adrenergic receptors.

There are therefore several important physiological factors that increase the hypotensive action of these sympathetic inhibitory drugs:

1) The tone in blood vessels is maintained by alteration in sympathetic vasoconstrictor activity, which rises on standing to counteract the hydrostatic effect of the weight of the increased column of blood. Sympathetic blocking drugs therefore produce a larger fall of blood pressure in the standing position when the need for sympathetic constriction is greater.

2) Although posture has the greatest single effect, increased demands come from muscle vessel dilatation after exercise, skin dilatation from a hot environment and splanchnic dilatation after a meal. These all compound falls in blood pressure when vasoconstriction that would otherwise occur is inhibited.

3) Obstruction to venous return as seen in straining at stool or in Valsalva's manoeuvre (more convenient for the laboratory) creates a need for vasoconstriction in order to maintain arterial pressure because there is reduced cardiac output secondary to reduced venous return to the heart. Excessive falls in blood pressure by blocking this response will be exaggerated if the inhibiting drug also results in constipation, as was the case when ganglion blocking drugs were used in the treatment of hypertension.

4) Any reduction of blood volume requires additional vasoconstriction to maintain blood pressure. Blood volume is reduced in the early hours of the day, particularly in hypertensives. This diurnal variation is probably responsible for the greater incidence of excessive hypotension on standing or after exercise in the early hours of the day.

The effect of these various physiological stresses is additive and clearly an excessive fall in blood pressure could occur in patients on treatment in the early hours of the day whilst performing exercise in the standing position, in a hot environment and after a good meal, e.g. 2 a.m. at a "dinner dance".

b) With Beta-Adrenoceptor Blockade

α) Blood Pressure Changes in Relation to Posture and Exercise. There is neither postural nor exercise hypotension when the blood pressure has been lowered by oral propranolol or other β-blocking drugs. Intra-arterial recordings of blood pressure confirm this for posture and either supine exercise (PRICHARD et al., 1970b) or erect exercise (PRICHARD et al., 1970c); the latter investigations, however, showed an increase in peripheral resistance on moving from the supine to a standing position. The rise in blood pressure on dynamic and static exercise is also lessened by β-blockade (SHINEBOURNE et al., 1967; NYBERG, 1977). Pindolol also in a multicentre open study lowered blood pressure from an average of 194/114 supine, 187/113 standing, to 158/97 and 154/97 mm Hg respectively (COLLINS and KING, 1972). The absence of exercise and postural effects with propranolol contrasts with those seen with sympathetic inhibitory drugs.

β) Effect of Increasing Environmental Temperature. Raising the temperature from 7° to 30° exaggerated postural and exercise hypotension in patients treated with bethanidine and guanethidine as a result of uncompensated vasodilatation in skin blood vessels. Repeat studies after propranolol showed that alterations in environmental temperature did not affect the response of blood pressure to posture and exercise (PRICHARD et al., 1970b)

γ) Action of Valsalva's Manoeuvre and the Blood Pressure Response to other Stresses. Intravenous propranolol (PRICHARD and GILLAM, 1966), pronethalol (PRICHARD, 1976) and practolol (unpublished observations) produce similar effects on reducing the overshoot after cessation of effort but without reducing vasoconstriction during it. Prolonged oral administration of propranolol does not inhibit vasoconstriction during the effort phase of Valsalva's manoeuvre, which contrasts with bethanidine, guanethidine and methyldopa (PRICHARD et al., 1970b). Propranolol may reduce rises in blood pressure during coitus (FOX, 1970), but it does not reduce the pressure response to pain, (NICOTERO et al., 1968) or cold water (GUAZZI et al., 1976). Rises in blood pressure from the stress of sorting ball bearings was reduced or abolished by 6 weeks' oral propranolol or metoprolol (LORIMER et al., 1976) but not by methyldopa, although this produced control of resting baseline blood pressure (DUNN et al., 1978). The rise in pressure in response to mental arithmetic was reduced by propranolol, 320 mg/day (GAZZI et al., 1976) but lower doses of propranolol, metoprolol or alprenolol reduced only peak pressures and not the overall rise from baseline values (NYBERG et al., 1977).

5. Use in Combination With Other Drugs

Diuretics have been used in combination with β-adrenoceptor blocking drugs since the earliest studies. Approximately equal numbers of patients received a diuretic in addition to propranolol as with previous therapy (PRICHARD and GILLAM, 1969). Subsequent experience with bethanidine, methyldopa and propranolol (PRICHARD et al., 1976) show that β-blocking drugs not only exert an additive antihypertensive effect but they probably antagonise the hypokalaemic effect of diuretics (CASTENFORS, 1977).

β-Adrenergic blocking drugs have also been used in combination with drugs which inhibit vasoconstrictor nerves, either at the endings or the receptor site, and also with vasodilators. They have also been used with drugs which directly relax vascular smooth muscle (PETTINGER and MITCHELL, 1976) such as hydrallazine, dihydrallazine and minoxidil. Minoxidil is reserved for the severe refractory hypertension frequently associated with advanced renal impairment, because it causes serious sodium and fluid retention, inexplicable hypertrichosis (GOTTLIEB et al., 1972; DORMOIS et al., 1975), and in large doses has produced lesions in the right atrium of dogs (DU CHARME et al., 1973).

Vasodilators produce reflex increases in heart rate and cardiac output (ABLAD, 1963; MONTGOMERY and DU CHARME, 1968; SANNERSTEDT et al., 1972) that are baroreceptor-mediated. Used alone in the treatment of hypertension relatively large doses are needed which cause an unacceptable tachycardia (dangerous in patients with embarrassed coronary circulation), sodium and fluid retention and side-effects such as headaches, nervousness and gastro-intestinal disturbances (GILMORE et al., 1970; HAMMER et al., 1971; KINCAID-SMITH, 1975). When used with a diuretic or drugs inhibiting reflex sympathetic activity, then lower doses are required and there is a reduction of side-effects. β-Adrenergic blocking agents also inhibit vasodilator-induced increases of plasma renin activity, which may be an important feature in the combined antihypertensive regime (PETTINGER and KEETON, 1975). In these combinations doses should be large enough to inhibit the reflex sympathetic activity caused by the vasodilator. ZACEST et al. (1972) achieved good control of supine and standing blood pressures in this manner in 17 of 23 patients without untoward reactions by giving a diuretic, propranolol 80–160 mg (mean 143 mg) daily and hydrallazine 40–400 mg (mean 225 mg). Chronic use of hydrallazine at this dose is unlikely to produce the "lupus phenomenon" (ZACEST, 1975). Alternatively, larger doses of β-blockers than are necessary to inhibit vasodilator side-effects can be useful (HANSSON et al., 1971 b). Successful results were seen in 17 patients with propranolol, mean 320 mg/day (maximum 640), and hydrallazine, mean 137 mg/day (maximum 200 mg). Similar doses of both drugs have also been used (IBSEN et al., 1978).

Other β-adrenergic blocking drugs used with hydrallazine or dihydrallazine have included oxprenolol, (AENISHÄNSLIN et al., 1972; TUCKMAN et al., 1972, 1973; SIITONEN et al., 1974; FREEMAN and KNIGHT, 1975), alprenolol (SANNERSTEDT et al., 1972), pindolol (PERSSON, 1975), practolol (DAHR, 1972) and atenolol (WILCOX and MITCHELL, 1977).

In severe and resistant hypertension, often associated with poor renal function, WILBURN et al. (1975) found mean doses of 475 mg propranolol, 33 mg minoxidil, and 578 mg frusemide daily to be effective. Other investigators have used smaller doses of propranolol with minoxidil, (GOTTLIEB et al., 1972; PETTINGER and MITCHELL, 1973; DORMOIS et al., 1975).

Prazosin alone lowers blood pressure but more so when administered with propranolol (STOKES and WEBER, 1974) and especially with large doses in patients with severe refractory hypertension (KINCAID-SMITH et al., 1973). In double-blind studies with a diuretic, β-blocking drugs and hydrallazine or prazosin, the vasodilators had equal hypertensive effect but prazosin caused fewer side-effects (KINCAID-SMITH, 1975). A major side-effect of this drug is acute hypotension, sometimes occurring within 3 h of the initial dose (MEEK et al., 1976). Symptoms suggestive of postural hypotension accompanied the addition of prazosin to a diuretic and either propranolol or oxprenolol or atenolol, but more prolonged use in doses of up to 15 mg/daily was not associated with postural or exercise hypotension (MARSHALL et al., 1977 b).

An α-adrenoceptor blocking drug (phenoxybenzamine) with propranolol causes a marked fall in blood pressure on standing (BEILEN and JUEL-JENSEN, 1972). There have been reports of the use of phentolamine in conjunction with β-receptor blocking agents. The duration of action of phentolamine is probably too short to be of much value (DAWSON et al., 1977), but some have found encouraging results (MAJID et al., 1974). Labetalol, which has α- and β-receptor blocking activity, is discussed above.

Combination of a β-adrenergic blocking drug such as propranolol with either methyldopa or a sympathetic inhibitor such as bethanidine has at least an additive effect or even a potentiating action, but there is a tendency for some postural and exercise hypotension which is absent on propranolol alone (DAY and PRICHARD, 1971;

PRICHARD, 1976). Similar additive effects are seen with oxprenolol and guanethidine (PEARSON et al., 1976) and atenolol and methyldopa (WEBSTER et al., 1977: WILSON et al., 1977).

6. Selection of Patients for Treatment

To predict a successful response to β-adrenergic blocking drugs is difficult. Renin levels may or may not be valuable (BUHLER et al., 1972, 1975) but it is found that older patients respond less well, as renin concentrations fall with age (BUHLER et al., 1975). There is no obvious correlation between cardiac output and response to β-blocking drugs (BIRKENHÄGER et al., 1971; TARAZI and DUSTAN, 1972; HANSSON et al., 1974); and none of age, blood volume (BIRKENHAGER et al., 1971; HANSSON et al., 1974), peripheral resistance, urinary adrenaline and noradrenaline (HANSSON et al., 1974; MEEKERS et al., 1975), aldosterone (HANSSON et al., 1974) and heart rate response to isoprenaline (HANSSON et al., 1974; SIMON et al., 1978) has any value in predicting response to β-blocking drugs. DISTLER et al. (1978), however, found a correlation between the ratio of exercise to resting plasma noradrenaline and response to atenolol.

7. Pressure Response

Sometimes blood pressure rises in hypertensive patients given β-adrenergic blocking drugs regardless of cardioselectivity, intrinsic sympathomimetic activity or membrane stabilising action. It was reported in the early work with acute administration of pronethalol (PRICHARD, 1964) in hypertension and more recently after atenolol (AMERY et al., 1976a; BLUM and ATSMON, 1977), oxprenolol (CROOK and RAFTERY, 1972), propranolol (DRAYER et al., 1976) and pindolol (WAAL-MANNING and SIMPSON, 1975; BJERLE et al., 1975).

Intrinsic sympathomimetic activity is unlikely to be the whole explanation, because it is seen with atenolol and propranolol, which do not possess significant intrinsic sympathomimetic activity. In fact, beta stimulation would generally be expected to produce a fall in peripheral resistance and therefore of blood pressure. It is just possible that stimulation of presynaptic β-receptors (ADLER-GRASCHINSKY and LANGER, 1975; STJARNE and BRUNDIN, 1975) could facilitate the release of noradrenaline and this cause a rise in blood pressure by α-receptor stimulation. Similarly the suggestion that blockade of peripheral β-receptors allows unopposed α-receptor activity is difficult to accept because the phenomenon is seen with the cardioselective agent atenolol. Fluid retention might be the explanation, since it can occur with all β-receptor blocking drugs and was seen with the patients on propranolol (DRAYER et al., 1978) and atenolol (AMERY et al., 1976b). The weights of patients showing pressor responses to pindolol were not given.

8. Conclusion

The value of β-adrenoceptor blocking drugs in the treatment of hypertension was demonstrated first with propranolol and subsequently with several other related substances. This is compatible with the mode of action being a function of β-adrenergic blockade and not some associated property. As with other potent antihypertensive drugs it is important to give proper attention to the dosage required for optimum results. These drugs are probably of similar potency to the adrenergic neuron inhibitor drugs and methyldopa, but have the advantage of neither postural nor exercise hypotension. Possible long-term benefits in reducing the manifestations of ischaemic heart disease are discussed below.

II. Angia Pectoris

1. Introduction

The sympathetic supply to the heart liberates noradrenaline which stimulates β-adrenoceptors on myocardial cells, and the resultant of several effects leads to an increase in cardiac work and myocardial oxygen consumption. Heart rate, isometric force and maximum velocity of shortening of ventricular muscle fibres increase (SONNENBLICK, 1962). Chemical energy release is increased from aerobic metabolism, and this can be estimated by the rise in myocardial oxygen consumption (SONNENBLICK et al., 1968). A high concentration of noradrenaline produces in addition a direct increase in myocardial metabolism – the "oxygen-wasting effect" (SARNOFF et al., 1965). However, myocardial-wall tension is a major determinant of cardiac oxygen consumption and this increases with a rise in intraventricular pressure and volume (Laplace's law); both these tend to decrease when cardiac contractility is enhanced by sympathetic nerve stimulation (SONNENBLICK and SKELTON, 1971). The net increase in myocardial demand for oxygen is normally balanced by an increase in coronary blood flow (LOMBARDO et al., 1953).

Angina pectoris apparently occurs when the demand for oxygen exceeds the supply, usually because coronary blood flow is restricted by coronary atherosclerosis under conditions requiring increased oxygen supply (KEEFER and RESNICK, 1928).

Sympathetic activity increases in conditions which precipitate attacks of angina, namely exercise, emotion, a cold environment and food, so that blockade of cardiac β-adrenoceptors might be expected to reduce the frequency of these attacks. It was on this basis that the development for clinical use was initially undertaken (BLACK and STEPHENSON, 1962).

While parasympathetic withdrawal is important in the tachycardia of exercise at low levels of activity, there is no doubt that sympathetic stimulation also plays a part in the tachycardia of exercise even at the low levels commonly achieved by patients with angina pectoris (BLACK and PRICHARD, 1973).

2. Mode of Action

There are four main factors – heart rate, ventricular systolic pressure, rate of rise of left ventricular pressure, i.e. the speed of left ventricular contraction, and the size of the left ventricle – that principally influence oxygen demand by the left ventricle (ROBINSON, 1971). Heart rate and systolic pressure seem the most important. ROBINSON (1967) showed that their product in any individual patient with angina pectoris tended to be about the same whether angina occurred spontaneously or was precipitated by exercise or stress such as mental arithmetic. β-Adrenergic blocking drugs reduce heart rate, thus reducing work done and allowing longer for diastolic filling. There is a reduction in the rise of blood pressure on exercise, the velocity of cardiac contraction

(SONNENBLICK et al., 1965; FURNIVAL et al., 1970; THADANI et al., 1973), and oxygen consumption at any given work load (WOLFSON and GORLIN, 1969). β-Blocking drugs also have other actions, e.g. metabolic effects, which may play a part in their antianginal action (TAYLOR, 1973).

Pronethalol (CHAMBERLAIN, 1966) and propranolol (SONNENBLICK et al., 1965) have both been found to increase left ventricular size in normal subjects and patients with ischaemic heart disease (CRAWFORD et al., 1975). CRAWFORD et al. (1975) found those patients with the largest hearts prior to propranolol showed the biggest increase after the administration of the drug. This action to some extent counterbalances the beneficial effects of β-adrenergic blocking drugs in angina.

It has been found in anaesthetised dogs that there is a reduction in coronary blood flow after propranolol (PARRATT and GRAYSON, 1966). Other work in dogs indicates that internal shunting occurs in the coronary circulation after β-adrenceptor blockade so that blood flow to an ischaemic area is maintained (PITT and CRAVEN, 1970), particularly in the subendocardial region (BECKER et al., 1971; MOIR, 1972; BERDEAUX et al., 1978). The change in regional blood flow could be important in reducing exercise-induced shifts of the ST segment observed after β-adrenoceptor inhibition (GIANELLY et al., 1967; PRICHARD et al., 1970a; SOWTON and SMITHEN, 1971; SANDLER and PISTEVOS, 1972; THADANI et al., 1973). Along with the reduction in myocardial oxygen consumption in man there is an associated decrease in coronary blood flow and an increase in calculated coronary vascular resistance (WOLFSON and GORLIN, 1969). Overall, the decrease in oxygen consumption can be seen as sufficient reason for the decrease in blood flow. Studies in man have shown no change in coronary venous oxygen saturation (LEWIS and BRINK, 1968; MENDEL and BRYNE-QUINN, 1966).

Whether the action of these drugs is simply a matter of producing the haemodynamic changes as outlined above or is more complicated, β-adrenergic blocking drugs, irrespective of whether or not they possess partial agonist properties or local anaesthetic activity (membrane stabilising action) or whether they produce general or selective blockade of β-adrenoceptors, have all produced some increase in acute working capacity before pain occurs. It appears that benefit therefore results from their common property, blockade of cardiac β-adrenoceptors (WILSON et al., 1969a; PRICHARD et al., 1970a; BOAKES and PRICHARD, 1973).

Propranolol, as generally used, is a racemic mixture of the dextrorotatory (+) and laevorotatory (−) isomers. Both isomers possess membrane stabilising activity, but only the (−) isomer has significant β-blocking activity (BARRETT, 1969). Similar results have been found in man (BENNET et al., 1970). The (+) isomer has been found to be ineffective in angina (WILSON et al., 1969a), even in doses of up to 80 mg intravenously (BOAKES and PRICHARD, 1973). Similarly the (+) isomer of alprenolol is ineffective in angina (BJORNTORP, 1968).

It has been found that glyceryl trinitrate relieves angina by decreasing the pressure-rate product, the figure obtained by multiplying systolic blood pressure by heart rate (ROBINSON, 1968), but if the work load is increased sufficiently to raise this product to the control level, pain still occurs. However, with β-blocking drugs, although exercise tolerance improves when pain occurs during acute exercise, the pressure-rate product has been found to be less than that reached prior to drug administration (BATTOCK et al., 1969; GIANELLY et al., 1967). The relative reduction in the pressure-rate product at the onset of pain occurred even though the level of sympathetic activity, estimated from the rise in plasma noradrenaline levels, was not reduced by the β-blocking drug (BATTOCK et al., 1969). BATTOCK et al. (1969) found that in their patients the product of systolic pressure and heart rate at the onset of pain was reduced by 30% of the control level during β-blockade. ALDERMAN et al. (1975) found a progressive reduction in the pressure-rate product as dosage (80, 160, 300 mg daily) of propranolol was increased.

The intravenous administration of β-blocking drugs that differed in their associated properties, namely propranolol (membrane stabilising action) oxprenolol (membrane stabilising and intrinsic sympathomimetic activity), practolol (intrinsic sympathomimetic activity and cardioselective blockade) and sotalol (minimal membrane stabilising action) depressed the pressure-rate product at the onset of pain to a similar extent (about 20%) in the same patients. (PRICHARD, 1971). Therefore in spite of increased exercise tolerance after β-adrenoceptor inhibition, patients exercise less than might be expected, probably because of an adverse effect of β-adrenoceptor blockade itself on the fourth factor mentioned above, left ventricular size. This means that in the ventricular wall there is increased tension, and therefore increased oxygen consumption at a given pressure (ROBINSON, 1971).

3. Effect

a) Division I: Non-selective

α) Group I Pronethalol, 300 mg orally, was found to produce an average increase of 44% in exercise tolerance (APTHORP et al., 1964). PRICHARD et al. (1970a) found that parenteral oxprenolol increased exercise tolerance by 26% in the first test and by 33% in the second. The intravenous (0.2 mg/kg) and acute oral administration (80 mg) of oxprenolol was found to increase acute exercise tolerance in a study by THADANI et al. (1973).

SEALEY et al. (1969) observed that intravenous alprenolol, 0.1 mg/kg, increased exercise tolerance by 29% ($p<0.02$) in ten patients with angina pectoris. The same group of workers performed acute exercise tests after random oral administration of alprenolol 50 mg and 100 mg and placebo (SEALEY et al., 1971). As a fourth treatment each patient received 200 mg. Total work increased by 9% after 50 mg (insignificant) 25% after 100 mg ($p<0.05$) and 17% after 200 mg (insignificant.

The effectiveness of β-blocking drugs in long-term treatment of angina was first demonstrated with pronethalol (FULTON and GREEN, 1963; PRICHARD et al., 1963; ROBINSON and PILKINGTON, 1963). The dosage required resulted in many side-effects, and its use was discontinued when it was found to produce tumours in mice (ALCOCK and BOND, 1964).

WILSON et al. (1969b) performed a variable-dose trial using 60–400 mg oxprenolol/day, with an adequate "run-in" period and 2 weeks on each treatment in 18 patients. This trial showed a very definite benefit from oxprenolol, 17 of the 18 patients having less angina on oxprenolol, and the remaining patient the same on placebo and oxprenolol. Less impressive results were obtained by BIANCHI et al. (1969) using a lower fixed dose, 40 mg four times a day, and SANDLER and PISTEVOS (1972) did not find any significant benefit in a short trial using 80 mg three times daily.

Some studies with alprenolol in doses of up to 400 mg/day have shown unconvincing results, perhaps illustrating the importance of the run-in period in angina trials.

On the other hand BJORNTORP (1967) performed a variable-dose trial, using between 200 and 400 mg alprenolol daily in 13 patients. This trial had an adequate run-in period, consisting of 2 weeks without treatment then 10 weeks during which dosage was gradually increased. There were eight patients who were finally satisfactory for comparative purposes. They had an average of ten attacks of angina weekly on alprenolol and 12.5 on placebo ($p<0.01$). AUBERT et al. (1970) used a less than optimum run-in period consisting of 4 weeks on placebo, but demonstrated a significant effect in 18 patients from a fixed dose of alprenolol, (100 mg four times daily) in terms of a reduced frequency of anginal attacks. HICKIE (1970) used an 8-week pretrial period in a large multicentre trial in 50 patients and showed a significant reduction in the number of anginal attacks (33%) and in glyceryl trinitrate consumption (32%) on alprenolol compared with placebo (p in both cases <0.005). BJORNTORP (1971) in nine patients showed that sustained release alprenolol (200 mg twice daily appeared as effective as the standard preparation, 100 mg four times a day. SOWTON and SMITHEN (1971) reported a fixed multidose study which is perhaps better regarded as separate studies of several dose levels, as the various dose levels were not given in random order. They used twice-daily doses of 100 mg, 200 mg and 400 mg alprenolol. Exercise tests at the end of each treatment period showed that compared with placebo, there was an increase in exercise tolerance of 21% from 200 mg/day ($p<0.02$), 17% from 400 mg/day ($p<0.05$) and 14% from 800 mg/day (not significant). Although this study shows that alprenolol is effective, the lack of random administration of increasing drug dosages means that no conclusion can be drawn about the presence or absence of a dose-response relationship (PRICHARD, 1974).

β Group II Intravenous propranolol, 5 mg, increased work performed by 40% in an open study involving 14 patients (GRANDJEAN et al., 1966) whilst PRICHARD et al. (1970a) reported that work increased by 32%–51% ($p<0.05$) in six patients given an average dose of 34 mg.

Oral Studies. There have been numerous studies that have demonstrated that propranolol is an effective anti-anginal drug. This has been demonstrated with fixed-dose trials (SRIVASTAVA et al., 1964; KEELAN, 1965; GINN and ORGAIN, 1966; NESTEL, 1966, GIANELLY et al., 1967; HARLEY and DAVIES, 1968; RABKIN et al., 1966; GRANT et al., 1966), fixed multidose trials (HEBB et al., 1968; MIZGALA et al., 1969), with most convincing results from variable dose level trials (WOLFSON et al., 1966; MILLER et al., 1975b; GILLAM and PRICHARD, 1965; AMSTERDAM et al., 1969).

In variable multidose trials each patient receives an individually adjusted dose, but in addition he receives a permutation on this individual dose. GILLAM and PRICHARD (1965) had used up to 400 mg daily, a dose considerably larger than that used in any other published reports with propranolol at that time. This raised the question: were these larger doses necessary for maximum benefit? GILLAM and PRICHARD (1966) described a trial where again an individually adjusted dose to maximum of 100 mg four times daily was used (average dose 304 mg daily); besides placebo, half-strength tablets (i.e. average dose 152 mg) were also given. Patients responded significantly better on full dose than on half dose. In a later trial in 16 patients, four different dose levels and placebo were used (PRICHARD and GILLAM, 1971). In the run-in period the dose of propranolol was found that resulted in a resting heart of 55–60 beats/min in the supine position, provided that side-effects did not intervene. Patients received from 80 to 1,380 mg/day, with an average of 417 mg. Identical tablets containing

40 mg, 20 mg, 10 mg and 5 mg propranolol and placebo were given for 2 weeks in random order so that after 10 weeks the patients had received each strength once. This 10-week cycle was repeated twice, a total of 30 weeks for the trial, each patient having received each treatment for 6 weeks. The average dosages were therefore 417 mg, 208 mg, 104 mg, 52 mg and zero.

There was a progressive reduction in the number of anginal attacks and in glyceryl trinitrate consumption as dosage increased. There were an average of 84.9 attacks of angina pain on placebo for the 6-week period, 67.2 on an average dose of 52 mg, 56.9 on 104 mg, 48.9 on 208 mg, and 37.8 attacks of pain for the 6-week period on an average dose of 417 mg/day. This dose-response study therefore showed a dose-dependent reduction of attacks of angina pectoris from propranolol.

γ *Group III* Pindolol produced a significant exercise tolerance in a study in 11 patients (STORSTEIN-SPILKER, 1970) but details of dosage were not given. Intravenous pindolol, 1 mg, increased exercise tolerance in five patients by 28% ($p<0.05$) compared with saline. Doses of 4 mg and 16 mg produced an increase in 47% ($p<0.01$) and 32% ($p<0.025$) respectively (BOAKES and PRICHARD, 1973). INPEA is also a member of the group, but has a low therapeutic ratio and a significant anti-anginal effect was not found when INPEA was given intravenously (PRICHARD, 1971).

Uncontrolled studies using oral pindolol have claimed benefit from pindolol in angina pectoris (YITITBASI and NALBANTGIL, 1970; ARAVANIS and MICHAELIDES, 1970). NAIR (1972), in a double-blind between-patient trial found that the 15 patients given pindolol, 10 mg daily, experienced fewer attacks of angina and had a lower glyceryl trinitrate consumption than an equal number of patients given placebo. SAINANI and MUKHERJEE (1972), in a similarly designed study involving 50 patients, found 40% less angina during treatment with pindolol, 10 mg (25 patients), than during placebo (25 patients; $p<0.05$).

δ *Group IV* Sotalol (average 50 mg) increased exercise tolerance by 33% after the first test, and by 45% after the second (PRICHARD et al., 1970a). Sotalol, 480 mg orally, increased exercise tolerance by 21% in five patients (ATKINS et al., 1971). TOUBES et al. (1970) briefly reported a fixed multidose level study in nine patients given 80, 160, 320, 640, and 1,280 mg sotalol/day. Unfortunately only 1 week on each dose level was used, but there was a significant reduction in glyceryl trinitrate consumption and patients had fewer and less severe angina attacks on sotalol ($p<0.05$). In a multicentre study sotalol up to a maximum of 480 mg/day resulted in an average of 5.1 attacks of angina a week. It was found superior to placebo, average 8.0 attacks a week (GOODING and BERMAN, 1974). BRAILOVSKY (1974) reported a very large multicentre trial of timolol in 307 patients. The average weekly angina attack rate on placebo was 8.9, on timolol 3.5 ($p<0.01$). The average dose of timolol was 30 mg, maximum 45 mg.

b) Division II: Cardioselective

Acute studies demonstrated practolol was an effective anti-anginal agent (ARESKOG and ADOLFSSON, 1969; COLTART, 1971; WILSON et al., 1969a; PRICHARD et al., 1970a). ROY et al. (1975) found that the increase in exercise tolerance after oral atenolol, 200 mg twice daily, of about 20% but the change was not statistically significant. ADOLFSSON et al. (1974) found 40 mg oral metoprolol in 17 patients produced a 42% increase in acute exercise tolerance ($p<0.01$).

Oral studies demonstrated that practolol was an effective anti-anginal agent (GEORGE et al., 1970; SOWTON et al., 1971), although some studies gave unconvincing results (SANDLER and CLAYTON, 1970).

However, severe sensitivity reactions have been reported with long-term administration of practolol, so that the drug is no longer being given as a prophylactic in angina. (RAFFERTY and DENMAN, 1973; FELIX et al., 1974; BROWN et al., 1974).

ROY et al. (1975) in a trial in 11 patients found atenolol was effective in significantly reducing the number of glyceryl trinitrate tablets consumed, at a dosage of 50 mg twice daily (average 9.2) and 200 mg twice daily (average 7.6) when compared with placebo (average 20.8). The attacks of angina also showed a significant reduction.

Tolamolol also appears to be an effective antianginal agent (JACKSON et al., 1975a) but this drug has been withdrawn because of long-term animal toxicity.

4. Comparison of Adrenergic Blocking Drugs

Acute exercise studies have found no significant difference between approximately equipotent β-blocking doses of propranolol, oxprenolol, practolol and sotalol (PRICHARD et al., 1970a) or between propranolol and pindolol (BOAKES and PRICHARD, 1973). THADANI et al. (1973) found no significant difference, in 16 patients, in the symptomatic, electrocardiographic and circulatory effects of oxprenolol, practolol and propranolol after intravenous and acute oral administration of dosage selected to give equal suppression of the exercise heart rate.

If two drugs are to be compared in a meaningful way it is desirable that they be given in optimum dosage. As the dosage of β-blocking drugs that can be tolerated varies considerably, a full comparison requires a variable-dose comparative trial.

a) Propranolol and Practolol

Other studies of acute tolerance have failed to reveal any difference between practolol and propranolol, after both intravenous (WILSON et al., 1969a) and oral administration (COLTART, 1971).

SANDLER and CLAYTON (1970) used a fixed dose of propranolol (320 mg daily) but variable doses of practolol, between 400 mg and an upper arbitrary limit of 1,200 mg a day. The 15 patients received each treatment for 4 weeks, but only the findings of the last 2 weeks were assessed. Propranolol produced a significant reduction ($p<0.05$) in attacks of angina (5.8 attacks a week compared with 8.3 on placebo) whereas practolol did not (9.1 attacks a week). Neither drug reduced glyceryl trinitrate consumption: both surprisingly produced an increase.

PRICHARD et al. (1971) reported a variable-dose comparative trial of practolol and propranolol. In this study average daily dosages of 766 mg and 95 mg propranolol and 1,004 mg practolol were used. Only two of the 14 patients received the upper arbitrary limit of practolol of 2,400 mg/day; side-effects limited dosage in the remainder. Four periods of 2 weeks were used for each treatment, i.e. a total of 8 weeks for each treatment. Propranolol was found significantly better than practolol in terms of amelioration of anginal attacks, glyceryl trinitrate consumption and well-being.

b) Propranolol and Alprenolol

HEATHERINGTON et al. (1973) compared multiple fixed doses of alprenolol (400–800 mg/day) and propranolol (160 mg–320 mg/day) and found an increase in exercise tolerance from both drugs compared with placebo, but no significant reduction in angina attacks or trinitrate consumption. Possible reasons for this have been discussed (PRICHARD, 1974).

c) Propranolol and Sotalol

Sotalol and propranolol have been compared in a variable-dose trial using a design similar to that of PRICHARD et al. (1971). Propranolol was found to be the more effective agent (HORN and PRICHARD, 1973). However, sotalol was significantly better than a low dose of propranolol.

d) Propranolol and Acebutolol

KHAMBATTA (1974) reported a study of acebutolol and propranolol, finding the former more effective. However, the dosage of propranolol used was very small, only 80 mg daily in 20 of the 25 patients, which is much below optimum. The comparison of either agent with placebo is not possible as placebo administration was not "blind".

5. Beta-Blocking Drugs and Other Anti-Anginal Agents

Single-blind acute exercise studies suggested a synergistic effect of propranolol and isosorbide (RUSSEK, 1968; BATTOCK et al., 1969). In a double-blind exercise study ADOLFSSON et al. (1972) found a combination of pindolol, 2 mg, and isosorbide, 5 mg, to be synergistic, total work on this combination (average 7,717 kpm) being significantly greater than that obtained with either pindolol, 2 mg (6,800 kpm), or isosorbide, 5 mg (6,043 kpm), alone. However, DAVIES et al. (1969) added oral isosorbide, 10 mg/day to propranolol, 40 mg/day, but did not find any further reduction of glyceryl trinitrate consumption. HANSEN et al. (1973) were not able to demonstrate any difference between alprenolol alone and alprenolol plus pentanitrol (PETN) in an acute exercise study.

AUBERT et al. (1970) found alprenolol (100 mg four times daily) was significantly better than pentaerythritol tetranitrate (30 mg four times daily), which was not different from placebo. KEYRILAINEN et al. (1973) reported alprenolol (100 mg four times daily) significantly better in terms of glyceryl trinitrate consumption and the severity of the anginal attacks on isosorbide (5 mg four times daily).

LIVESLEY et al. (1973) reported a comparative trial of fixed doses of propranolol and isosorbide dinitrate and two dose levels of verapamil. Patients had first 2 weeks on placebo, then 4 weeks on thrice-daily dosages of verapamil, 120 mg, isosorbide dinitrate, 20 mg, and placebo. The design of the trial could be criticised as treatments were not given in random order and the degree of blindness of the trial is in doubt (PRICHARD, 1974). Assessment of the final 2 weeks of each treatment period showed no significant difference between propranolol and the higher dose of verapamil. Propranolol treatment resulted in fewer anginal attacks than treatment with verapamil, 80 mg three times daily ($p < 0.05$), but these treatments did not differ significantly in terms of glyceryl trinitrate consumption or the response to an acute exercise test. Isosorbide was not significantly different from propranolol.

6. Withdrawal

It was reported that in a multidose study patients with angina pectoris experienced a higher incidence of chest pain when the first week of placebo was compared with the second week (PRICHARD and GILLAM, 1971), and more recently there have been reports that sudden cessation of propranolol may precipitate myocardial infarction. This could be due to unmasking of the progressive disease process, so that in the absence of β-blockade oxygen supply is not sufficient in some patients to meet even the requirements of the heart at rest (DIAZ et al., 1974). Another possibility is that chronic β-blocking therapy leads to an increase in endogenous sympathetic activity that is unmasked when the drug is stopped. It is relevant to note that one study in rats has found an increase in adrenal size and catecholamine concentration in rats given propranolol (KLINGE and ARO, 1971). Another conceivable cause is a reversal of the favourable rightward shift of the oxyhaemoglobin dissociation curve produced by propranolol, and a reversal of the reduced platelet aggregation produced by propranolol (MILLER et al., 1975a).

MILLER et al. (1975a) reported two ischaemic deaths, and four other serious reactions out of a total of 20 patients. These episodes occurred in out-patients who had received the drug for a period of 12 weeks. In contrast they had not observed any episodes in a "large number" of "symptomatic coronary patients" who had propranolol stopped abruptly prior to cardiac catheterisation, which might suggest that limitation of physical activity provided protection against withdrawal exacerbations of the disease. MYERS and WISENBERG (1977) reported that two patients experienced unstable angina with one fatal myocardial infarction 10 days later in a series of 53 anginal patients when propranolol was abruptly stopped in in-patients. A further survey of 55 patients who had propranolol stopped prior to cardiac catheterisation showed only one patient experienced any increase in pain (SHIROFF et al., 1978).

These facts should not be interpreted as being a contra-indication to the administration of β-blocking drugs in angina pectoris; overall there is good evidence that they reduce the incidence of myocardial infarction in ischaemic patients (see below). It does mean that β-blocking drugs should not normally be abruptly stopped, hence trial design will be influenced. An appropriate approach would be to administer two doses of the standard β-blocking drug and compare this with the agent under test, as indeed was the procedure used for ethical reasons in the trial reported of practolol and propranolol, thus avoiding any cessation of treatment (PRICHARD et al., 1971). Alternatively, the dose of β-blocking drug will have to be very cautiously reduced. In other than mildly affected patients, this should be under open conditions before it is attempted in a double-blind phase of a trial.

7. Regulation of Dose

There is evidence that the optimum dose varies between patients. It was shown with propranolol that greatest benefit is obtained with maximum tolerated dose (PRICHARD and GILLAM, 1971). It is improbable that other β-blocking drugs will differ in this respect. The dosage of propranolol may be commenced at 10 mg three or four times a day and increased as often as the patient is assessed until either the angina is controlled or the pulse rate is reduced to about 55 beats/min in the standing position, provided that this dosage does not cause troublesome side-effects. Previously we had used a supine rate of 55–60, but as this produces results still on the straight-line part of the dose-response curve (PRICHARD and GILLAM, 1971), the standing rate which represents a high state of sympathetic activity is a better guide. JACKSON et al. (1975b) found that the reliance on a supine rate of 55–60 could result in inadequate dosage, and in 15 of 21 patients previously considered unresponsive to β-blocking drugs they obtained improvement when dosage was increased to produce a maximum exercising heart rate of 100 beats/min or 100–125 beats/min that was unresponsive to further dose increments. Exercise which represents a high state of sympathetic activity is clearly a more sensitive guide to dosage and particularly so with β-blocking drugs with intrinsic sympathetic blocking activity. However, measuring the exercising heart rate is more cumbersome, so for ordinary use the standing rate is to be preferred, the use of exercising rate being reserved for the more refractory case. Alternatively dosage could be gradually arbitrarily increased until some minor side-effect prevented any further increment, an approach used to some degree in our first trial of propranolol in angina (GILLAM and PRICHARD, 1965).

An important source of the variation in dosage required in angina pectoris is the difference in plasma levels seen after an administration of propranolol (SHAND, 1976) which also occurs in ischaemic patients. ALDERMAN et al. (1975) observed a tenfold variation in plasma levels, although levels were measured over a range between 1½ and 3 h after the last dose. Additionally the actual serum concentration of propranolol required to produce maximum therapeutic response also varies considerably; a sixfold range has been found (PINE et al., 1975).

8. Value

If the contra-indications in asthma and cardiac insufficiency are observed and treatment is started at a low dosage, the use of these drugs is relatively safe. An effective prophylactic taken for angina will reduce the pain on exercise, anticipated or not, and reduce pain precipitated by other causes such as emotion. Although β-blockade may not totally relieve pain it does allow more pain-free exercise. It seems reasonable to use an effective prophylactic such as a β-blocking drug in any anginal patients who are experiencing regular attacks of pain. Glyceryl trinitrate can be used as usual; its hypotensive effect is not increased by propranolol (PRICHARD and GILLAM, 1971).

It has been suggested that some patients with angina pectoris do not respond to β-blocking drugs. This might occur in patients with poorly controlled heart failure (although these patients should not be so treated), as in these patients the disadvantageous increase in the size of the heart resulting from β-blockade may be greater than is usually seen. A larger heart requires a greater increase in wall tension for ejection, and an extra large increase in oxygen consumption from this source might outweigh the beneficial effects of β-blockade. However, at least this sequence is not invariable GILLAM and PRICHARD (1965) reported a patient who developed heart failure after 2 days on propranolol, 10 mg four times daily, but subsequently tolerated the drug (50 mg four times daily), after treatment with digitalis and diuretics. Later she once more became breathless on exertion, and this was relieved by reducing the propranolol dosage. However, a reduction in dosage was associated with increased angina pectoris. Her symptoms of heart failure and angina were inversely related to the dose of propranolol taken. A compromise of some breathlessness on exertion was acceptable for some relief of her angina.

The failure of chest pain to respond to β-blockade may be due to misdiagnosis. In one series there were 77% of failures on propranolol in "angina" patients without arteriographic changes, and 14% of failures in those with coronary arteriographic changes (AMSTERDAM et al., 1969).

A usual cause of so-called failure of angina pectoris to be improved by β-blockade is failure to use an adequate dose. Higher dosages with individual dosage adjustment are associated with a very low incidence of non-responders.

Lastly, there is the suggestion that long-term β-blockade improves prognosis. Angina pectoris appears to carry an overall annual mortality of about 3% (ZUKEL et al., 1969) or 4% (KANNEL and FEINLEIB, 1972). RUSSEK (1972) found that a regimen of propranolol, individually adjusted to produce a resting supine pulse of 55–60, plus sublingual isosorbide dinitrate resulted in a mortality of 1.25% per annum in 102 "good risk" patients, but 16% of 33 "poor risk" patients died (i.e. aged over 70 years, history of congestive heart failure, etc.). Others, however, have not found evidence to suggest an improvement in prognosis from long-term treatment with β-blocking drugs in angina pectoris (ZEFT et al., 1969).

In a series using concurrent controls, 91 patients treated with β-blockers (89% propranolol, 19% practolol and 7% oxprenolol) showed an infarction rate of 5.8% with a fatal infarct rate of 2.5% – significantly different from 126 patients not given β-blockers, who showed an annual infarction rate of 19.3% and a fatal infarction rate of 9.5% (LAMBERT, 1976).

There is evidence that medical treatment with propranolol may produce as good a result as surgical treatment. In a matched series of 40 patients (ARONOW and STEMMER, 1975), 3 months after operation there was a reduction in angina in the surgically treated group, but at 1 and 2 years no significant difference in angina, re-infarction rate or death rate was seen.

III. Cardiovascular Disease

1. Acute Myocardial Infarction

After the initial favourable report of SNOW (1966), investigators using propranolol for short-term administration after myocardial infarction failed to show any beneficial effect on mortality. Dosage, however, was rather low: 20 mg four times daily for 3 weeks (NORRIS et al., 1968), 20 mg four times daily for 4 weeks (BALCON et al., 1966), 10 mg four times daily for 2 weeks (CLAUSEN et al., 1966).

There is evidence that β-blocking drugs reduce the size of myocardial infarction. Studies in experimental animals suggest that β-adrenergic blocking drugs reduce the size of acute myocardial infarcts and that this is reflected in associated ST segment changes (MAROKO et al., 1971). It has been found that a greater histological reduction of infarct size by propranolol against coronary ligation in dogs, was obtained when it was given before and after ligation, compared with delaying administration for 3 h after ligation (RASMUSSEN et al., 1977). Blood flow after coronary ligation is not affected by propranolol and neither was myocardial creatine phosphokinase loss (PETER et al., 1978a).

It has been shown that various β-adrenergic blocking drugs reduce the ECG changes associated with ischaemia at rest and on exercise (PRICHARD et al., 1970a). PELIDES et al. (1972) using multiple precardial leads demonstrated that the acute administration of practolol reduces the degree and area of ST segment depression in patients with acute myocardial infarction. These observations have been confirmed (HJALMARSON et al., 1976). In addition, PETER et al. (1978b), found propranolol administered within 4 h of a transmural infarction significantly reduced cardiac enzymes. WAAGSTEIN and HJALMARSON (1976) found three cardioselective β-blocking agents, practolol, H 87/07 and metoprolol, reduced cardiac pain besides ST segment changes, after transmural myocardial infarction. Finally, MUELLER et al. (1974) demonstrated an improvement in myocardial metabolism following intravenous propranolol in infarction patients, as shown by an increased coronary sinus oxygen and increased lactate extraction.

Further evidence has been afforded by the observations of FOX et al. (1975). It was found that ischaemic patients matched for severity of pain, sex, age and previous cardiac history had significantly less severe ischaemic episodes if they were receiving β-adrenergic blocking drugs (a significantly lower incidence of final diagnosis of transmural infarct, and a higher incidence of coronary insufficiency) compared with those patients who were not on β-adrenergic blocking drugs.

2. Long-Term Cardioprotective Effect

There is evidence that the long-term administration of β-adrenergic blocking drugs may exert a cardioprotective effect. First, they reduce the tachycardia and arrhythmias of everyday stress, in pilots undergoing simulated flights (ELIASCH et al., 1967), in public speaking (TAGGART et al., 1973 a), in racing car driving (TAGGART and CARRUTHERS, 1972), in motor car driving (TAYLOR and MEERAN, 1973 a) and while travelling as a passenger in a car or by air (TAYLOR and MEERAN, 1973 b).

Although a number of the studies can be criticised on methodological grounds (FITZGERALD, 1976), investigations in postinfarction patients have suggested that there is a reduction in recurrence of myocardial infarction and/or sudden death in those patients given β-adrenergic blocking drugs (WILHELMSSON et al., 1974; AHLMARK et al., 1974; Multicentre TRIAL, 1975). A similar effect has been observed in patients with angina pectoris (LAMBERT, 1976).

This evidence, with the evidence for an effect in acute myocardial infarction, suggests that there is a cardioprotective effect in high-risk, i.e. post-myocardial-infarction patients. The use of other antihypertensives has not been associated with a reduction in incidence of myocardial infarction even though other complications of hypertension have been reduced. A recent study has suggested that propranolol-treated patients with hypertension have a lower incidence of myocardial infarction than those not given β-adrenergic blocking drugs (STEWART, 1976).

3. Vasculoprotective Effect

β-Adrenergic blocking drugs, other than merely lowering the blood pressure at rest or on exercise, have what could be termed an immediate vasculoprotective effect as they reduce the rate of rise of systolic pressure and therefore the force of the systolic pressure wave. However, they have a number of other actions that may be beneficial in inhibiting vascular degeneration.

β-Adrenergic blocking drugs do not effect the rise in catecholamines associated with various forms of stress; however, they abolish the rise in free fatty acids and triglycerides in response to racing car driving (TAGGART and CARRUTHERS, 1972; TAGGART et al., 1973 b), public speaking (TAGGART et al., 1973 a), and being a passenger in an airliner (CARRUTHERS et al., 1973). This action may be important in breaking a chain postulated for the effect of stress producing atheroma (CARRUTHERS, 1969; CARRUTHERS et al., 1973). Cholesterol levels are not affected in man, but experimentally the administration of propranolol to rabbits fed a high-cholesterol diet reduces the development of atheromatous lesions (WHITTINGTON-COLEMAN et al., 1973).

4. Blood

β-Adrenergic blocking drugs have been found to produce a number of changes in the blood. The clinical relevance of these findings remains to be defined but some of the effects have therapeutic potential. Propranolol, in relatively small dose, was found to return the abnormal sensitivity of platelets to aggregation by adenosine diphosphate in patients with angina pectoris to the level seen in normals (FRISHMAN et al., 1974) Platelet aggregation may be an important factor in sudden death in ischaemic patients (HAEREM, 1971).

It has been observed that alprenolol reduces blood viscosity (DINTENFASS and LAKE, 1976), this is likely to help blood flow, particularly in diseased vessels (DINTENFASS, 1977). Another observation that may be relevant in the effects of stress is that propranolol has been shown to reduce the rise in clotting factor VIII induced by adrenaline (INGRAM and JONES, 1966).

It was demonstrated in vitro that propranolol shifted the haemoglobin-oxygen dissociation curve to the right (PENDLETON et al., 1972). This was a non-specific effect as it was seen with the D isomer more effectively than the L form. The concentrations used were about 1,000 times those used therapeutically. However, similar findings were found in patients who had received first propranolol, four doses of 10 mg in 24 h (OSKI et al., 1972), but others obtained less impressive results after the acute administration of propranolol (BRAIN et al., 1974). More recently SCHRUMPF et al. (1977) demonstrated a rightward shift in the oxygen-haemoglobin dissociation curve in anginal patients who had received chronic oral treatment with propranolol.

OSKI et al. (1972) reported that 30% of red cell 2,3-diphosphoglycerate (DPG) was bound to cell membranes, and that propranolol released this binding and the released DPG combined with deoxyhaemoglobin and so produced the rightward shift in the dissociation curve. BRANN and NEWMAN (1973) could not, however, find evidence of any binding of DPG to the cell membrane. Another possible mechanism may be an effect on the cell membrane decreasing intracellular and so shifting the pH oxyhaemoglobin equilibrium curve to the right (AGOSTONI et al., 1973).

The decreased affinity of haemoglobin for oxygen allows an increased delivery of oxygen to the tissues which will be of value in ischaemic conditions. It will also help to offset the reduction in cardiac output and hence general reduction in blood flow associated with the administration of β-adrenergic blocking drugs.

5. Arrhythmias

At concentrations that inhibit the β-receptor, these drugs reduce the slope of sinus or ectopic pacemaker potentials, particularly when the slope has been increased by catecholamines (HOFFMAN and SINGER, 1967) or ouabain (CARMELIET and VERDONCK, 1967). The concentration of propranolol in vitro in isolated cardiac muscle to produce a membrane effect is 100–500 times that required to suppress cardiac arrhythmias (COLTART et al., 1971; SHAND, 1974, 1976), and thus the membrane-depressant properties of β-receptor antagonists are unlikely to be of relevance in the treatment of arrhythmias; in addition practolol is an effective anti-arrhythmic agent even though this drug has no membrane-depressant activity.

β-Receptor antagonists have been used in a wide variety of cardiac arrhythmias, and many supraventricular arrhythmias respond (SINGH and JEWITT, 1974). Sinus tachycardia (SCHAMROTH, 1966) and supraventricular ectopics due to digitalis intoxication are reduced by β-adrenergic blockade. β-Blocking drugs increase the refractory period of atrioventricular conduction tissue including re-entry circuits that appear to be responsible for many cases of paroxysmal supraventricular tachycardia (GOLDREYER, 1972). β-Adrenoceptor blocking drugs are useful in the treatment of paroxysmal supraventricular tachycardia (SCHAMROTH, 1966) and also for prophylaxis (GIANELLY et al., 1967), particularly in the Wolff-Parkinson-White syndrome (BURCHELL, 1973).

As β-adrenergic blocking drugs increase the refractory period of the atrioventricular node, they reduce the ventricular rate in atrial fibrillation without any effect on the fibrillation itself (GIBSON et al., 1968). Sinus rhythm is only occasionally restored in atrial fibrillation, although more often in atrial flutter (GIBSON and SOWTON, 1970). Their use in atrial fibrillation is limited, other than when it occurs with thyrotoxicosis. An infrequent use is to slow the ventricular rate when digitalis in maximum tolerated doses has failed to do so satisfactorily (STOCK, 1966) as the action of digitalis and β-blocking drugs on conduction tissue is additive.

Ventricular ectopics from a variety of causes are reduced by intravenous or short-term oral administration of β-blocking drugs (GIBSON and SOWTON, 1970) but whether β-blocking agents reduce the risk of sudden fatal arrhythmias in these patients is at present not known. There is evidence that patients having ventricular ectopics on their routine electrocardiograms have a higher incidence of sudden death (GOLDSTEIN and MOSS, 1972; ENGLAND, 1972). β-Adrenergic blocking drugs are not agents of first choice in acute attacks of ventricular tachycardia, unless the arrhythmias were precipitated by an excess of catecholamines, as in a phaeochromocytoma; since heart failure is readily precipitated, cardioversion is preferable. β-Blocking agents are of value, however, in the prophylaxis of attacks of paroxysmal ventricular tachycardia, particularly when the attacks have been produced by exercise (GIBSON and SOWTON, 1970). Intravenous β-blocking drugs have been used, usually combined with procainamide or lignocaine, in the prevention of recurrences of ventricular fibrillation following electrical defibrillation (SLOMAN et al., 1965; IKRAM, 1968).

It has been well known for a number of years that catecholamines result in arrhythmias in experimental myocardial infarction. Increased levels of adrenaline and noradrenaline have been found following myocardial infarction in man (SINGH and JEWITT, 1974). β-Blocking agents are useful administered acutely in the treatment of arrhythmias following infarction; perhaps practolol should be preferred (JEWITT and CROXON, 1971) as it produces less of a reduction in cardiac output, the long-term complications of practolol treatment not being a risk here. β-Blockers do not increase the reversion rate when given prior to DC shock in patients with atrial fibrillation, nor reduce relapse rate. However, sinus rhythm may be maintained for longer periods when they are given in combination with quinidine. β-Blocking drugs are useful in treating a wide variety of arrhythmias in anaesthesia (GIBSON et al., 1968) and in suppressing extra systoles in patients during artificial cardiac pacemaking (HARRIS, 1966). Digitalis-induced atrial and ventricular tachyarrhythmias respond well to β-blocking drugs (GIBSON and SOWTON, 1970).

All β-receptor blocking drugs seem to have comparable anti-arrhythmic properties regardless of the presence or absence of membrane-depressant activity. Thus propranolol, oxprenolol, pindolol and practolol, for instance, are likely to have similar anti-arrhythmic action in similar β-blocking doses. Any therapeutic superiority is likely to be related to side-effects associated with the different compounds (SINGH and JEWITT, 1974).

6. Congenital Heart Disease

Sympathetic stimulation with isoprenaline was observed to increase outflow tract obstruction in obstructive cardiomyopathy (BRAUNWALD and EBERT, 1962) and acute studies showed β-blockade reduced the pressure gradient across the obstruction induced by exercise and isoprenaline (COHEN et al., 1964; HARRISON et al., 1964). Most prolonged oral studies with propranolol have also demonstrated improvement of symptoms in most patients (CHERIAN et al., 1966; FLAMM et al., 1968; ADELMAN et al., 1970), but SLOMAN'S (1967) results in five cases were not impressive. β-Adrenergic blockade has little effect on obstruction at rest and propranolol was of limited value in patients with resting obstruction (ADELMAN et al., 1970). Likewise with practolol little reduction on left ventricular and diastolic pressure was found at rest, but on exercise there was a considerable reduction (WEBB-PEPLOE et al., 1971). In a comparative study both propranolol and practolol improved symptoms of hypertrophic cardiomyopathy but propranolol had a better anti-anginal effect (HUBNER et al., 1972). β-Adrenergic blocking drugs therefore are perhaps of some value in latent and labile obstruction of the outflow tract (FURBERG, 1974).

β-Blocking drugs have also been found to improve work performance and reduce left ventricular size in patients with advanced congestive cardiomyopathy (WAAGSTEIN et al., 1975).

7. Fallot's Tetralogy

Among the chief dangers to life in infants with Fallot's tetralogy are cyanotic attacks that are associated with a marked increase in the right-to-left shunt and drops in arterial oxygen saturation, because of increased infundibular obstruction. It has been suggested this obstruction might be due to excess circulatory noradrenaline (JOHNSON, 1961). β-Adrenergic blockade with pronethalol (HONEY et al., 1964) or propranolol (CUMMING, 1970) may reduce this obstruction. Propranolol may be of value in treating acute severe dyspnoeic attacks and prolonged oral treatment may postpone shunt surgery. ERIKSSON et al. (1969) selected ten of 65 patients with Fallot's tetralogy by therapeutic assessment that indicated less infundibular obstruction after propranolol. These ten patients over 9 months treatment had improved exercise tolerance and cyanotic attacks were prevented. These findings have been confirmed (MINHAS et al., 1976).

8. Other Cardiovascular Uses

Propranolol has also been used as part of the regime in the medical treatment of dissecting aneurysm of the aorta (McFarland et al., 1972). Not only does β-blockade lower the blood pressure, but it also reduces the rate of rise of systolic pressures, so reducing strain on the dissected aorta. On the other hand, unconvincing results have been found using propranolol to prevent dilatation of the aorta and dissection in Marfan's syndrome, although the dosage used was perhaps below optimum (Ose and McKusick, 1977). Preliminary results suggest that propranolol (40 mg qds) does not improve survival in cases of subarachnoid haemorrhage (Cameron and Haas, 1976). Subarachnoid haemorrhage is associated with prolonged cerebral artery spasm that may be the cause of considerable mortality and morbidity (Robertson, 1974). Boulin and Mohan (1977) found in vitro that contractions of the isolated human basilar artery induced by cerebrospinal fluid from patients with subarachnoid haemorrhage were reversed with high concentration of propranolol. This effect was not due to β-blockade, as the response was seen with the non-β-adrenoceptor-blocking (+) isomer.

IV. Hyperthyroidism

The clinical features of hyperthyroidism have been attributed to the potentiation of catecholamines by thyroxine (Harrison, 1964). Although more recent evidence suggests this is not true (Levey, 1971; Aoki et al., 1972; Spaulding and North, 1975), it has, however, been the basis of various attempts to block the sympathetic nervous system in the treatment of thyrotoxicosis. Initially, sympathectomy and sympatholytic drugs such as reserpine and guanethidine were used, but recently β-adrenergic receptor blocking drugs have been employed with success (Turner, 1974).

Propranolol reduces the peripheral manifestations of hyperthyroidism (Shanks et al., 1969; Nelson and McDevitt, 1975). It markedly reduces heart rate both at rest and on exercise (Howitt and Rowlands, 1966; McDevitt et al., 1968; Carruthers et al., 1974) and in some patients has resulted in actual fibrillation being converted to sinus rhythm (Parsons and Jewitt, 1967). There is a reduction in myocardial contractility and cardiac output (Howitt and Rowlands, 1966). The amplitude of tremor is reduced and the Achilles reflex time significantly prolonged by propranolol (Marsden et al., 1968). There is some evidence that the myopathic and neurological signs in hyperthyroidism may improve after propranolol (Pimstone et al., 1968; Kammer and Hamilton, 1974; Weinstein et al., 1975; Yeung and Tse, 1974; Rothberg et al., 1974). On the other hand, propranolol does not appear to reduce sweating (Allen et al., 1973) and no consistent effects of propranolol on the eye signs of thyrotoxicosis were found (Sneddon and Turner, 1966; Crombie and Lawson, 1968). The basal metabolic rate (Howitt and Rowlands, 1966; Pimstone and Joffe, 1970) and thyroid function tests (Hadden et al., 1969) are unaffected by propranolol. Glucose tolerance has been reported to deteriorate after propranolol (Horrower et al., 1977).

On the basis of their effects on resting heart rate in hyperthyroid patients, β-adrenergic receptor blocking drugs with intrinsic sympathomimetic activity have been shown to be less effective than drugs without this property and this has been claimed to be further evidence for potentiation of catecholamines in this disease (Turner, 1974). However, practolol has been shown to have more effect on exercise heart rate than on resting heart rate in hyperthyroid patients (CARRUTHERS et al., 1974) and the practice of assessing β-adrenergic receptor blocking drugs in hyperthyroidism by their effect on resting heart rate has been questioned. Also in a double-blind controlled trial of the effects of propranolol, 160 mg, and practolol, 480 mg daily, in hyperthyroid patients, practolol was found inferior to propranolol only in its effect on heart rate; practolol reduced heart rate by 17% and propranolol by 24% (NELSON and MCDEVITT, 1975).

Indications for the use of β-adrenergic receptor blocking drugs include the management of hyperthyroid crises (MACKIN et al., 1974). However, cases of thyrotoxic crisis have developed while patients were taking propranolol, although at a modest dose of 160 mg daily (ERIKSSON et al., 1977). β-Blocking drugs have been used in preoperative preparation for thyroidectomy (LEE et al., 1973; MICHIE et al., 1974) and during the period of onset of effect of antithyroid drugs (2–3 weeks for drug such as carbimazole) or of radio-iodine therapy (up to 3 months) (HADDEN et al., 1969; MONTGOMERY, 1975). Some have used β-blocking drugs as the only agent in the treatment of hyperthyroidism (PIMSTONE et al., 1968; MCLARTY et al., 1973; MONTGOMERY, 1975), with remission rates as high as 40% at 1 year (MONTGOMERY, 1975). However, it is generally believed that this form of treatment cannot be recommended except in patients intolerant of antithyroid drugs and in whom surgery or radio-iodine is not considered appropriate (TURNER, 1974). This is because it is impossible to select which patients will respond to propranolol alone; those who do not, remain thyrotoxic and may continue to lose weight. There have been reports of the use of propranolol in the treatment of neonatal and childhood thyrotoxicosis (SMITH and HOWARD, 1973; PEMBERTON et al., 1974; BUCKFIELD and DAVIS, 1966) and of hyperthyroidism in pregnancy (LANGER et al., 1974; BULLOCK et al., 1975).

V. Tremor

β-Adrenergic mechanisms are important in tremor from varying causes in normals, Parkinsonism, anxiety, hyperthyroidism, lithium toxicity and alcohol withdrawal (MCALLISTER et al., 1977). There is evidence that β-receptor antagonists reduce the tremor in each case while β-receptor stimulants aggravate the tremor.

Results in essential tremor have been inconsistent but propranolol has been found effective when proper attention was given to dosage (MCALLISTER et al., 1977). There is, however, some evidence that initial improvement may not always be maintained over long periods (MURRAY, 1976). Beta-blockade has also been reported as useful to suppress tremor in children following head injury (ELLISON, 1978).

VI. Psychotropic Uses

The first use of β-adrenergic blocking drugs in the psychiatric field was reported in 1966, but subsequently there has been an increase in interest and the number of applications (JEFFERSON, 1974; WHITLOCK and PRICE, 1974).

1. Anxiety

Anxiety state is manifest by a variable quantity of autonomic symptoms, which themselves can cause anxiety. Whether the awareness of bodily function or dysfunction is causative or this and the emotional changes have a common central origin is a matter for debate (WHITLOCK and PRICE, 1974).

GRANVILLE-GROSSMAN and TURNER (1966) found propranolol (20 mg qds) in a short-duration trial superior to placebo in relieving the autonomic symptoms of anxiety. This has been confirmed in single-blind studies (SUZMAN, 1971), while the D, i.e. non-β-blocking, isomer of propranolol was found ineffective (BONN and TURNER, 1971). Evidence that the benefit in anxiety was due to peripheral β-blockade was provided by the observation that practolol, which has low penetration of the brain (SCALES and COSGROVE, 1970), was also effective (BONN et al., 1972). Propranolol also is ineffective in relieving the central manifestations of anxiety (RAMSAY et al., 1973; TYRER and LADER, 1974a, b).

β-Adrenergic blocking drugs have also been tried in physiological anxiety. BREWER (1972) used a dose of propranolol (10–80 mg) to reduce the resting heart rate to between 55 and 65 and found a reduction in the feeling of nervousness prior to examinations, but again the central component of induced anxiety in normals is not affected (TYRER and LADER, 1974c). These drugs will, of course, reduce the tachycardia associated with stressful situations, e.g. public speaking (oxprenolol) (TAGGART et al., 1973a) and ski-jumping (oxprenolol) (IMHOF and BRUNNER, 1970).

β-Blocking drugs are therefore of value in relieving the somatic symptoms and any effect on psychic symptoms will be secondary. They are ineffective in patients with psychic anxiety, in contrast to the benzodiazepines (TYRER and LADER, 1974a).

2. Drug Dependence

There have been reports of the use of β-blocking drugs in the control of anxiety symptoms associated with alcohol withdrawal (CARLSSON and JOHANSON, 1971). In a double-blind controlled study in alcohol withdrawal, propranolol (40 mg qds) was found more effective than chlordiazepoxide (25 mg qds) and than a combination of the same dose of chlordiazepoxide and low-dose propranolol (10 mg qds) in reducing the tremor and possibly more effective in reducing the increased urinary catecholamine excretion (SELLERS et al., 1977). Other reports have not been so encouraging (GALLANT et al., 1973). There have also been reports of the reduction of anxiety symptoms associated with opiate withdrawal (HALLISTER and PRUSMACK, 1974) and LSD administration (LINKEN, 1971) by propranolol.

Some have noted a reduction in craving for addictive drugs: in two heroin addicts (GROSZ, 1972) and in a pethidine addict (LOWENSTEIN, 1973). It will be interesting to see if these findings are substantiated; one can only speculate on the mode of action: propranolol does not appear to influence morphine metabolism (BRUNK et al., 1974). Propranolol does not influence the subjective effects of cannabis (MORTZ et al., 1972) or amphetamine (JONSSON, 1972).

3. Psychosis

ATSMON et al. (1972) found propranolol improved patients with acute schizophrenia but had little effect in chronic care. They used an average dosage of 1,400 mg/day (400–4,200 mg/day) adjusted to achieve a drop in pulse rate 60–64/min; lower doses have been found ineffective (GARDOS et al., 1973). However, RACHENSPERGER et al.

(1974) used larger doses of oxprenolol (three cases) and propranolol (two cases) and only found marginal benefit. In contrast, YORKSTON et al. (1974) found all schizophrenic symptoms were relieved completely by propranolol in six of 14 patients who had been unresponsive to phenothiazines; one of the remaining patients had marked improvement, four moderate improvement. Relapse was seen in two patients who stopped their treatment. The dosage used was 500–3,500 mg/day, and toxic symptoms were minimised by gradual increase of dosage.

The use of propranolol in other psychoses has been reported. It has been found effective in controlling belligerence in seven patients with acute brain damage from various causes, stroke, closed head injury, and a gunshot wound (ELLIOTT, 1977). It was less effective in the manic phase of manic-depressive psychosis (STEINER et al., 1972) but more effective than chlorpromazine in postpartum psychosis (STEINER et al., 1973). These possible uses of β-blocking drugs await further evaluation.

4. Migraine

RABKIN et al. (1966) found that while treating patients with angina pectoris with propranolol, co-existent migraine was benefitted. This observation has been followed by a number of trials of the use of β-blocking drugs in this condition.

WEBER and REINMUTH (1972) using 80 mg propranolol/day found it was an effective prophylactic in migraine. A less convincing effect was seen with 60 mg daily (MALVEA et al., 1973), while LUDVIGSSON (1973) in a further double-blind study used 60 mg on children under 35 kg and 120 mg daily above 35 kg and found more impressive results, only two of 28 children not responding. WIDERØE and VIGANDER (1974) found propranolol, 160 mg daily, effective, all but two of the 49 patients showing some effect in an open study. A double-blind study was performed in 30 patients who responded well and there was a significant reduction in the monthly average of attacks of migraine from 1.7 to 0.4.

There is evidence that other β-adrenergic blocking drugs may be of value, open studies with pindolol have suggested it may be effective (ANTHONY et al., 1972) but a double-blind study with 15 mg or 7.5 mg pindolol daily failed to reveal a significant effect (SJAASTAD and STENSRUD, 1972).

It appears that β-blocking drugs may be a useful migraine prophylactic, but at the moment this is only reasonably established with propranolol. How they act is not clear (JOHNSON, 1978).

VII. Glaucoma

The acute systemic administration of the β-blocking drugs propranolol (PHILIPPS et al., 1967; COTE and DRANCE, 1968) and atenolol (MACDONALD et al., 1976, 1977) lowers intra-ocular tension. This also occurs after local administration with propranolol (MUSINI et al., 1971; VALE et al., 1972; BIETTI, 1972) and practolol (VALE and PHILLIPS, 1973; HAGEDOORN and TJOA, 1974). Prolonged oral administration of propranolol is also effective in reducing intra-ocular tension (COTE and DRANCE, 1968; PANDOLFI and OHRSTROM, 1974).

How exactly β-blocking drugs lower intra-ocular pressure is not clear but evidence suggests that it is a function of β-blockade and not of one of the associated properties

(PHILLIPS, 1976). Beta-blocking drugs, regardless of the presence or absence of associated properties, are effective and experiments in rabbits indicate the D isomer of propranolol is less effective than the racemic mixture (VALE and PHILLIPS, 1970).

VIII. Side-Effects

In the large series of 311 patients reported by ZACHARIAS et al. (1972) side-effects from propranolol in 55 patients were "tolerable" in seven dose-limiting, and in 26 patients the drug was stopped. It seems that the overall incidence of side-effects is probably at least no more than with other potent antihypertensive drugs (PRICHARD and GILLAM, 1969; ZACHARIAS et al., 1972; PRICHARD et al., 1976).

Two important untoward effects from β-adrenergic blocking drugs should be avoided with foresight in patient selection: heart failure and asthma. Patients in heart failure or patients with incipient left ventricular insufficiency (they may have no signs of heart failure on physical examination or chest X-ray) are critically dependent on sympathetic activity to the heart to maintain their cardiac output. Patients with left ventricular insufficiency should not be given a β-receptor blocking drug without prior administration of digitalis and diuretics. If these drugs alleviate the dyspnoea it is reasonable, with extra caution, to start the patient on a β-blocking drug. There have been reports that patients who have been put into failure by propranolol have been subsequently able to tolerate the drug after the administration of digoxin and a diuretic (GILLAM and PRICHARD, 1966; AMSTERDAM et al., 1969). If heart failure is uncontrolled, β-adrenergic blocking drugs should not be given. β-Adrenergic inhibitory drugs with intrinsic sympathomimetic stimulating action can also precipitate heart failure: alprenolol (LUND-LARSEN and SIVERTSSEN, 1969; LYON and NEVINS, 1971), INPEA (DEL BIANCO et al., 1966), oxprenolol (BIANCHI et al., 1969; FORREST, 1972) and pronethalol (APTHORP et al., 1964). There is no evidence that the direct membrane effect contributes significantly to heart failure (COLTART et al., 1971).

DUNER and PERNOW (1973) demonstrated that neither propranolol nor pindolol prevented the inotropic action of digitalis. CRAWFORD et al. (1975) have provided evidence to support the use of digoxin with propranolol. They found propranolol administration to a group of 20 patients with angina pectoris reduced the frequency of attacks, but in eight with evidence of abnormal left ventricular function there was a reduction in acute exercise tolerance after propranolol. However, the administration of digoxin abolished this reduction. The acute exercise tolerance in other patients without evidence of abnormal ventricular function was not improved with the addition of digoxin. Digoxin alone did not affect angina attack rate or acute exercise tolerance. Digoxin reduced the increased left heart dimension produced by propranolol, by 0.7 mm/m^2 in those with normal ventricular function, and by 1.6 mm/m^2 in those with abnormal ventricular function. The increased heart size after digoxin plus propranolol was not significantly different from that while on placebo, an increase of 0.5 mm/m^2 was seen in both groups.

Caution must be exercised with small doses, as the most dramatic change in the sympathetic environment of the heart takes place when treatment is commenced with a β-adrenergic receptor blocking drug, i.e. the small starting dose (PRICHARD, 1974). Reports of adverse reactions have confirmed the greatest danger of precipitating heart failure is at the start of treatment. In one study seven of eight patients suffered life-threatening adverse reactions due to impaired cardiac function, and they were receiving a very small dose of less than 40 mg propranolol/day (GREENBLATT and KOCH-WESER, 1974). A small percentage increase in dose levels entails less risk of suddenly precipitating heart failure than the first dose. We have given β-receptor blocking drugs to a total of over 300 patients, with dosage of up to 400 mg propranolol or sotalol daily; our only case of sudden cardiac decompensation was at the commencing dose of 10 mg propranolol four times daily.

Precipitate falls in blood pressure are rare after oral propranolol: they have been reported in patients with cardiomyopathy (BETT, 1968; TAYLOR, 1968). They have occurred after intravenous propranolol (STEPHEN, 1966) and rarely after oral and intravenous practolol (WISEMAN, 1971).

A common side-effect from β-adrenergic blocking drugs is coldness of the extremities, presumably as a result of peripheral vasoconstriction due to the reduced cardiac output and peripheral β-adrenergic blockade. It was reported in 25 of the series of 311 patients of ZACHARIAS et al. (1972), necessitating stopping propranolol in three patients.

MARSHALL et al. (1976) found symptoms of Raynaud's phenomenon were more common in patients receiving β-blockers than methyldopa. They suggested that this was less likely to occur in patients receiving a cardioselective agent. However, cardioselective agents can cause a serious reduction in peripheral flow and the exceptional case of gangrene has been reported (VALE and JEFFERYS, 1978).

There have been suggestions that intermittent claudication is worsened by β-adrenergic blocking drugs (RODGER et al., 1976) but a small controlled trial failed to reveal any adverse effect of even large doses of propranolol in claudication (REICHERT et al., 1975).

All non-selective β-adrenergic blocking drugs are likely to produce a significant increase in airway resistance in asthmatic subjects due to inhibition of sympathetic tone in bronchial smooth muscle (BEUMER, 1974). While cardioselective β-adrenergic blocking drugs appear superior to non-selective agents (DECALMER et al., 1978), even the cardioselective agents show only modest selectivity; a serious increase in airway resistance has been reported with practolol (WAAL-MANNING and SIMPSON, 1971).

PERKS et al. (1978) suggested that the cardioselective agent atenolol had less effect on airway resistance than oxprenolol in patients with chronic airway obstruction. In contrast, in normals, OH et al. (1978) found β-blocking agents with intrinsic sympathomimetic activity had less effect on airway resistance than the cardioselective agent metoprolol. However, the methodology of these studies has been criticised (MCDEVITT, 1978). There is other evidence that the non-selective β-blocking agent with intrinsic sympathomimetic activity has less effect on airway resistance than one without this associated property (BEUMER et al., 1978).

In normal subjects, inhibition of glucose mobilisation requires simultaneous blockade of α-receptors in the liver and β-receptors in muscle. Experiments in normals indicate β-blocking drugs without intrinsic sympathomimetic activity do not affect resting insulin or glucose levels or the fall of plasma glucose after insulin (EKBERG and HANSSON, 1977; SYVÄLAHTI et al., 1977). These agents with intrinsic sympathomimetic activity may cause a small elevation of blood glucose (SCHLIERF et al., 1973).

The rate of recovery of glucose levels after insulin hypoglycaemia is reduced and the increase of plasma glycerol inhibited as these depend in part on the reflex liberation of catecholamines in response to the hypoglycaemia and consequent β-adrenergic stimulation. Non-selective β-blocking drugs prolong insulin hypoglycaemia but selective agents probably do not (DEACON et al., 1977). There have been reports of diabetics treated with β-blockers experiencing prolonged hypoglycaemia (HESSE and PEDERSEN, 1973; WRAY and SUTCLIFFE, 1972).

A number of central nervous system side-effects occur as most β-adrenergic blocking drugs readily cross the blood-brain barrier. They include depression, often dose-related, confusion and blurring of vision, and visual hallucinations have been reported rarely. Troublesome dreams are not infrequent in patients taking large doses: vivid dreams occurred in 11 of the patients of ZACHARIAS et al. (1972). Dreams and insomnia can usually be controlled by taking the last dose no later than early evening, or even before, and also reducing the last dose if necessary. The occurrence of indigestion, often with some nausea, is a not uncommon side-effect which can often be avoided by taking the drug with meals (PRICHARD and GILLAM, 1969). Diarrhoea is unusual (ZACHARIAS et al., 1972), and constipation is more common than diarrhoea with practolol (WISEMAN, 1971). Skin rashes, purpura (with or without thrombocytopenia), paraesthesia and alopecia have been reported after propranolol.

One advantage of β-adrenergic blocking drugs is the lower incidence of nocturia that has been seen on propranolol than with other potent antihypertensive drugs (PRICHARD and GILLAM, 1969). Disturbances of sexual function are uncommon. There were no cases of impotence in the series of ZACHARIAS et al. (1972); of eight patients who had impotence on previous therapy, in two it was improved, in four it disappeared, while in the other two it was unchanged.

In recent years a number of severe sensitivity reactions have been reported with practolol, so that long-term use has ceased. These reactions have included a systemic lupus syndrome (RAFTERY and DENMAN, 1973). Antinuclear antibodies do not, however, appear to occur with β-blocking drugs other than practolol (WILSON et al., 1978).

Dry eyes and corneal ulceration has occurred from practolol (WRIGHT, 1975); it is doubtful that reactions occur to other β-blocking drugs. Practolol has been found to reduce tear lysozyme concentration, unlike other β-blocking drugs (MACKIE et al., 1977). Dry eyes, skin lesions, particularly a psoriasiform eruption which may occur from 3 weeks and up to 3 years (on average 10 months). (FELIX et al., 1974) and sclerosing peritonitis (BROWN et al., 1974) have occurred after starting practolol. An antibody binding to epithelial tissue has been demonstrated after practolol (AMOS et al., 1975).

Adverse reactions to β-adrenergic blocking drugs are uncommon except with practolol, particularly with correct patient selection, i.e. excluding cases of heart failure and asthma. It is soon after initiation of therapy that severe adverse reactions occur, even with small doses, but once therapy has been started gradual increase in dosage is not likely to be associated with precipitate adverse reactions.

IX. Conclusion

The β-adrenergic blocking drugs represent perhaps the most interesting and useful group of new drugs introduced in the last decade. Many uses have been discovered that were not predicted from the original animal pharmacology both within the area of cardiovascular disease, e.g. hypertension, and in other fields, e.g. psychiatric uses.

The place of β-adrenergic blocking drugs remains to be fully evaluated in a number of their indications, but they are well established as useful agents in a number of common conditions, notably hypertension and angina pectoris, with a more modest place in the treatment of arrhythmias.

Acknowledgements. We are most grateful to Mrs Jane MacKinnon for help in the preparation of this paper, and to Mrs MacKinnon and Miss J.C. Owens for the typing of the manuscript.

References

Abbs, E.T., Dodd, M.G.: The relation between the adrenergic neurone-blocking and noradrenaline-depleting actions of some guanidine derivatives. Br. J. Pharmacol. *51*, 237–247 (1974)
Ablad, B.: A study of the mechanism of the hemodynamic effects of hydralazine in man. Acta Pharmacol. Toxicol. [Suppl. 1] (kbh) *20*, 1–53 (1963)
Ablad, B., Ek, L., Johansson, B., Waldeck, B.: Inhibitory effect of propranolol on the vasoconstrictor response to sympathetic nerve stimulation. J. Pharm. Pharmacol. *22*, 627–628 (1970)
Abrams, W.B., Pocelinko, R., Klausner, M., Hanauer, L., Whitman, E.N.: Clinical pharmacological studies with debrisoquine sulfate, a new antihypertensive agent. J. New Drugs *4*, 268–283 (1964)
Adelman, A.G., Shah, P.M., Gramiak, R., Wigle, E.D.: Long-term propranolol therapy in muscular subaortic stenosis. Br. Heart J. *32*, 804–811 (1970)
Adi, F.C., Eze, C.J., Anwunah, A.: Comparison of debrisoquine and guanethidine in the treatment of hypertension. Br. Med. J. (1975) *1*, 482–485
Adler, S.: Methyldopa-induced decrease in mental activity. J. Am. Med. Assoc. *230*, 1428–1429 (1974)
Adler-Graschinsky, E., Langer, S.Z.: Possible role of a β-adrenoceptor in the regulation of noradrenaline release by nerve stimulation through a positive feed-back mechanism. Br. J. Pharmacol. *53*, 43–50 (1975)
Adolfsson, L., Areskog, N.H., Furberg, C., Granath, A., Zetterquist, S.: Synergistic effects of a new β-adrenergic blocker (pindolol) and isosorbide-dinitrate during exercise in patients with coronary insufficiency. Eur. J. Clin. Pharmacol. *5*, 37–40 (1972)
Adolfsson, L., Areskog, N.H., Furberg, C., Johnsson, G.: Effects of single doses of alprenolol and two cardioselective β-blockers (H 87/07 and H 93/26) on exercise-induced angina pectoris. Eur. J. Clin. Pharmacol. *7*, 111–118 (1974)
Aenishänslin, W., Pestalozzi-Kerpel, J., Dubach, U.C., Imhof, P.R., Turri, M.: Antihypertensive therapy with adrenergic beta-receptor blockers and vasodilators. Eur. J. Clin. Pharmacol. *4*, 177–181 (1972)
Agostoni, A., Berfasconi, C., Gerli, G.C., Luzzana, M., Rossi-Bernardi, L.: Oxygen affinity and electrolyte distribution of human blood: Changes induced by propranolol. Science *182*, 300–301 (1973)
Ahlmark, G., Saetre, H., Korsgren, M.: Reduction of sudden deaths after myocardial infarction. Lancet *1974 II*, 1563
Ahlquist, R.P.: A study of the adrenotropic receptors. Am. J. Physiol. *153*, 586–600 (1948)
Akhtar, N., Mikulic, E., Cohn, J.N., Chaudhry, M.H.: Hemodynamic effect of dobutamine in patients with severe heart failure. Am. J. Cardiol. *36*, 202–205 (1975)
Alcocer, L., Aspe, J., Gomez, E.A.: Anti-hypertensive effect of timolol, a new beta-blocking agent (Double-blind study). J. Int. Med. Res. *3*, 1–9 (1975)
Alcock, S.J., Bond, P.A.: Observations on the toxicity of alderlin (pronethalol) in laboratory animals. Proc. Eur. Soc. Study Drug Toxi. *4*, 30–39 (1964)
Alderman, E.L., Davies, R.O., Crowley, J.J., Lopes, M.G., Brooker, J.Z., Friedman, J.P., Graham, A.F., Matlof, H.J., Harrison, D.C.: Dose response effectiveness of propranolol for the treatment of angina pectoris. Circulation *51*, 964–975 (1975)
Allen, J.A., Lowe, D.C., Roddie, I.C., Wallace, W.F.M.: Studies on sweating in clinical and experimental thyrotoxicosis. Clin. Sci. Mol. Med. *45*, 765–773 (1973)

A. M. A. Committee on Hypertension: Drug treatment of ambulatory patients with hypertension. JAMA *225*, 1647–1653 (1972)
Amery, A., Deloof, W.: Cheese reaction during debrisoquine treatment. Lancet *1970 II*, 613
Amery, A., Verstraete, M., Bossaert, H., Verstreken, G.: Hypotensive action and side effects of clonidine – chlorthalidone and methyldopa – chlorthalidone in treatment of hypertension. Br. Med. J. (1970) *IV*, 392–395
Amery, A., Billiet, L., Boel, A., Fagard, R., Reybrouck, T., Willems, J.: Mechanism of hypotensive effect during beta adrenergic blockade in hypertensive patients. Hemodynamic and renin response to a new cardioselective agent; Tenormin or ICI 66082. Am. Heart J. *91*, 634–642 (1976a)
Amery, A., De Plaen, J.F., Fagard, R., Lijnen, P., Rebrouck, T.: The relationship between beta blockade, hyporeninaemic and hypotensive effect of two beta blocking agents. Postgrad. Med. J. [Suppl 4] *52*, 102–108 (1976b)
Aminu, J., D'Mello, A., Vere, D.W.: Interaction between debrisoquine and phenylephrine. Lancet *1970 II*, 935–936
Amory, D.W., Burnham, S.C., Cheney, F.W.: Comparison of the cardiopulmonary effects of subcutaneously administered epinephrine and terbutaline in patients with reversible airway obstruction. Chest *67*, 279–286 (1975)
Amos, H.E., Brigden, W.D., McKerron, R.A.. Untoward effects associated with practolol: Demonstration of antibody binding to epithelial tissue. Br. Med. J. (1975) *1*, 598–600
Amsterdam, E.A., Gorlin, R., Wolfson, S.: Evaluation of long-term use of propranolol in angina pectoris. JAMA *210*, 103–106 (1969)
Anavekar, S.N., Louis, W.J., Morgan, T.O., Doyle, A.E., Johnston, C.I.: The relationship of plasma levels of pindolol in hypertensive patients to effect on blood pressure, plasma-renin and plasma noradrenaline levels. Clin. Exp. Pharmacol. Physiol. *2*, 203–212 (1975)
Anderson, S.D., Rozea, P.J., Dolton, R., Lindsay, D.A.: Inhaled and oral bronchodilator therapy in exercise induced asthma. Aust. N. Zealand J. Med. *5*, 544–550 (1975)
Anderson, S.D., Seale, P.R., Bandler, L., Theobald, G., Lindsay, D.A.: Inhaled and oral salbutamol in exercise induced asthma. Am. Rev. Respir. Dis. *114*, 493–500 (1976)
Andersson, K.-E., Ingemarsson, I., Persson, C.G.A.: Relaxing effects of β-receptor stimulators in isolated gravid human myometrium. Life Sci. *13*, 335–344 (1973)
Andersson, K.-E., Bengtsson, L.P., Gustafason, I., Ingemarsson, I.: The relaxing effect of terbutaline on the human uterus during term labour. Am. J. Obstet. Gynaecol. *121*, 602–609 (1975a)
Andersson, K.-E., Bengtsson, L.P., Ingemarsson, I.: Terbutaline inhibition of midtrimester unterine activity induced by prostaglandin $F_{2\alpha}$ and hypertonic saline. Br. J. Obstet. Gynaecol. *82*, 745–749 (1975b)
Andersson, O., Berglund, G., Hansson, L.: Anti-hypertensive action, time of onset and effects on carbohydrate metabolism of labetalol. Br. J. Clin. Pharmacol. [Suppl.] *3*, 757–761 (1976)
Andy, J.J., Curry, C.L., Ali, N., Mehrotra, P.P.: Cardiovascular effects of dobutamine in severe congestive heart failure. Am. Heart J. *94*, 175–182 (1977)
Angel-James, J.E., Bobik, A.: Modification of blood pressure and aortic baroreceptor activity in propranolol-treated hypertensive rabbits (Proceedings). J. Physiol. *278*, 16P (1978)
Anthony, M., Lance, J.W., Somerville, B.: A comparative trial of pindolol, clonidine and carbemazapine in the interval therapy of migraine. Med. J. Aust. *59*, 1343–1346 (1972)
Anthracite, R.F., Vachon, L., Knapp, P.H.: Alpha-adrenergic receptors in the human lung. Psychosom. Med. *33*, 481–489 (1971)
Aoki, V.S., Wilson, W.R., Theilen, E.O.: Studies on the reputed augmentation of the cardiovascular effects of the catecholamines in patients with spontaneous hyperthyroidism. J. Pharmacol. Exp. Ther. *181*, 362–368 (1972)
Apperley, G.H., Daly, M.J., Levy, G.P.: Selectivity of beta adrenoceptor agonists and antagonists in bronchial, skeletal, vascular and cardiac muscle in the anaesthetised cat. Br. J. Pharmacol. *57*, 235–246 (1976)
Apthorp, G.H., Chamberlain, D.A., Hayward, G.W.: The effects of sympathectomy on the electrocardiogram and effort tolerance in angina pectoris. Br. Heart J. *26*, 218–226 (1964)
Aravanis, C., Michaelides, G.: Results of the use of a new beta-adrenergic blocker (LB46) in angina pectoris. Acta Cardiol. *25*, 501–509 (1970)

Areskog, N.H., Adolfsson, L.: Effects of a cardioselective beta-adrenergic blocker (ICI 50172) on exercise in angina pectoris. Br. Med. J. *1969 II*, 601–603
Aronow, W.S., Danahy, D.T.: Efficacy of trimazosin and prazosin therapy on cardiac and exercise performance in outpatients with chronic congestive heart failure. Am. J. Med. *65*, 155–160 (1978)
Aronow, W.S., Stemmer, E.A.: Two years follow-up of angina pectoris. Medical or surgical therapy. Ann. Intern. Med. *82*, 208–212 (1975)
As, A. van, Benjamin, C., Stern, J.D.: A new bronchodilator, hexoprenaline in obstructive pulmonary disease. Scand. J. Respir. Dis. *54*, 28–37 (1973)
Athanassiadis, D., Cranston, W.I., Juel-Jensen, B.E., Oliver, D.O.: Clinical observations on the effects of debrisoquine sulphate in patients with high blood pressure. Br. Med. J. *1966 II*, 732–735
Atkins, J.M., Blomqvist, G., Cohen, L.S., Mitchell, J.H., Mullins, C.B.: Serial exercise studies in ischaemic heart disease (I.H.D.). Effects of placebo and β-adrenergic blocking agents. Clin. Res. *19*, 62 (1971)
Atsmon, A., Blum, I., Steiner, M., Latz, A., Wijsenbeek, H.: Further studies with propranolol in psychotic patients. Psychopharmacologia *27*, 249–254 (1972)
Aubert, A., Nyberg, G., Slaastad, R., Tjeldflaat, L.: Prophylactic treatment of angina pectoris. A double-blind cross-over comparison of alprenolol and pentanitrol. Br. Med. J. *1970 I*, 203–206
Avery, G.S.: Salbutamol: a review. Drugs *1*, 274–302 (1971)
Aviado, D.M.: Toxicity of aerosols. J. Clin. Pharmacol. *15*, 86–104 (1975)
Awan, N.A., Miller, R.R., Miller, M.P., Specht, C., Vera, Z., Mason, D.T.: Clinical pharmacology and therapeutic application of prazosin in acute and chronic refractory congestive heart failure. Balanced systemic venous and arterial dilation improving pulmonary congestion and cardiac output. Am. J. Med. *65*, 146–154 (1978)
Ayres, S.M., Griesbach, S.J., Reimold, F., Evans, R.G.: Bronchial component in chronic obstructive lung disease. Am. J. Med. *57*, 183–191 (1974)
Baczko, A., Dabrowska, B., Wocial, B.: Ocena dzialania hipotensyjnego propranololu w leczeniu Nadcisnienia tetmizego. Pol. Arch. Med. Weun *38*, 397–402 (1967)
Bacon, C.J.: Nebulised salbutamol in treatment of acute asthma in children. Lancet *1978 I*, 158 (1978)
Baillie, P., Meehan, F.P., Tyack, A.J.: Treatment of premature labour with orciprenaline. Br. Med. J. (1970) *IV*, 154–155
Baker, S.B. de C., Foulkes, D.M.: Blood concentration of compounds in animal toxicity tests. In: Biological effects of drugs in relation to their plasma concentrations. Davies, D.S., Prichard, B.N.C. (eds.), pp. 41–50. London: MacMillan 1973
Balcon, R., Jewitt, D.E., Davies, J.P.H., Oram, S.: A controlled trial of propranolol in acute myocardial infarction. Lancet *1966 II*, 917–924
Barger, G., Dale, H.H.: Chemical structure and sympathomimetic action of amines. J. Physiol. *41*, 19–59 (1910)
Barnett, A.J., Cantor, S.: Observations of the hypotensive action of "catapres" in man (ST 155). Med. J. Aust. *1*, 87–91 (1968)
Barnett, A.J., Kalowski, S., Guest, C.: Labetalol compared with pindolol plus hydrallazine in the treatment of hypertension. A double-blind cross-over study. Med. J. Aust. *65*, 105–109 (1978)
Barrett, A.M.: A comparison of the effect of (±) propranolol and (+) propranolol in anaesthetised dogs: β-receptor blocking and haemodynamic action. J. Pharm. Pharmacol. *21*, 241–247 (1969)
Barrett, A.M., Nunn, B.: Adrenergic neurone blocking properties of (±) propranolol and (+) propranolol. J. Pharm. Pharmacol. *22*, 806–810 (1970)
Bateman, J.R.M., Clarke, S.W., Pines, A.: A two centre clinical comparison of oral reproterol and salbutamol in reversible airways obstruction. Clin. Trials J. *16*, 37–40 (1979)
Bath, J.C., Pickering, D., Turner, R.: Clinical experience with bethanidine in treatment of hypertension. Br. Med. J. (1967) *IV*, 519–521 (1967)
Battock, D.J., Alvarez, H., Chidsey, C.A.: Effects of propranolol and isosorbide dinitrate on exercise performance and adrenergic activity in patients with angina pectoris. Circulation *39*, 157–169 (1969)

Bauer, G.E., Croll, F.J.T., Goldrick, R.B., Jeremy, D., Raftos, J., Whyte, H.M., Young, A.A.: Guanethidine in treatment of hypertension. Br. Med. J. 1961 II, 410–415
Bauer, G.E., Hull, R.D., Stokes, G.S., Raftos, J.: The reversibility of side effects of guanethidine therapy. Med. J. Aust. *1*, 930–933 (1973)
Baum, T., Shropshire, A.T., Varner, L.L.: Contribution of the central nervous system to the action of several antihypertensive agents (methyldopa, hydrallazine and guanethidine). J. Pharmacol. Exp. Ther. *182*, 135–144 (1972)
Beale, J.P., Stephenson, N.C.: X-ray analysis of Th 1165 a and salbutamol. J. Pharm. Pharmacol. *24*, 277–80 (1972)
Beardshaw, J., Maclean, L., Chan-Yeung, M.: Comparison of the bronchodilator and cardiac effects of hydroxyphenylorciprenaline and orciprenaline. Chest *65*, 507–511 (1974)
Becker, L.C., Fortuin, N.H., Pitt, B.: Effect of ischaemia and antianginal drugs on the distribution of radioactive microspheres in the canine left ventricle. Circ. Res. *28*, 263–269 (1971)
Beilen, L.J., Juel-Jensen, B.E.: Alpha and beta adrenergic blockade in hypertension. Lancet *1972 I*, 979–982
Bellamy, D., Reed, J.W., Hutchison, D.C.S.: A double-blind study of the effects of salbutamol metered-dose aerosol on the resting and exercise pulmonary function of patients with emphysema. Thorax *33*, 680 (1978)
Bengtsson, C.: Comparison between alprenalol and chlorthalidone as antihypertensive agents. Acta Med. Scand. *191*, 433–439 (1972)
Bengtsson, C.: Comparison between metoprolol and propranolol as antihypertensive agents. Acta Med. Scand. *199*, 71–74 (1976)
Bengtsson, C., Johnsson, G., Regardh, C.G.: Plasma levels and effects of metoprolol on blood pressure and heart rate in hypertensive patients after acute dose and between two doses during long-term treatment. Clin. Pharmacol. Ther. *17*, 400–408 (1975)
Benjamin, C., As, A. van: Clinical trial of intravenous hexoprenaline in asthma. S. Afr. Med. J. *46*, 599–603 (1972)
Bennet, D., Balcon, R., Hoy, J., Sowton, E.: Haemodynamic effects of dextropranolol in acute myocardial infarction. Thorax *25*, 86–88 (1970)
Benraad, A.H., Schoenaker, A.H.: Thrombopenia after use of methyldopa. Lancet *1965 II*, 292
Berdeaux, A., Da Costa, C.P., Garnier, M., Boissier, J.-R., Giudicelli, J.-F.: Beta adrenergic blockade, regional left ventricular blood flow and ST-segment elevation in canine experimental myocardial ischemia. J. Pharmacol. Exp. Ther. *205*, 646–656 (1978)
Beregovich, J., Bianchi, C., Rubler, S., Lomnitz, E., Cagin, N., Levitt, B.: Dose-related hemodynamic and renal effects of dopamine in congestive heart failure. Am. Heart J. *87*, 550–557 (1974)
Beregovich, J., Bianchi, C., D'Angelo, R., Diaz, R., Rubler, S.: Hemodynamic effects of a new inotropic agent (dobutamine) in chronic heart failure. Br. Heart J. *37*, 629–634 (1975)
Berglund, G.: Antihypertensive effect of sotalol and propranolol: a double-blind cross-over study. Curr. Ther. Res. *21*, 21–27 (1977)
Bergman, J., Persson, H., Wetterlin, K.: Two new groups of selective stimulants of adrenergic receptors. Experientia *25*, 899–901 (1969)
Bergstrand, R.H., Vedin, J.A., Wilhelmsson, C.E., Berglund, G.: Comparative study of metoprolol and alpha-methyldopa in untreated essential hypertension. Eur. J. Clin. Pharmacol. *10*, 375–379 (1976)
Berkowitz, C., McKeever, L., Croke, R.P., Jacobs, W.R., Loeb, H.S., Gunnar, R.M.: Comparative responses to dobutamine and nitroprusside in patients with chronic low output cardiac failure. Circulation *56*, 918–924 (1977)
Bett, J.H.: Hypotension after oral propranolol. Lancet *1968 I*, 302
Beumer, H.M.: Adverse effects of β-adrenergic receptor blocking drugs on respiratory function. Drugs *7*, 130–138 (1974)
Beumer, H.M., Teirlinck, C., Wiseman, R.A.: Comparative investigation of the respiratory and cardiovascular effect of mepindolol, propranolol and pindolol in asthmatic patients. Int. J. Clin. Pharmacol. *16*, 249–253 (1978)
Bianchi, C., Lucchelli, P.E., Starcich, R.: Beta blockade and angina pectoris: a controlled multicentre clinical trial. Pharmacol. Clin. *1*, 161–167 (1969)
Bianco, S., Griffin, J.P., Kamburoff, P.L., Prime, F.J.: The effect of thymoxamine on histamine-induced bronchospasm in man. Br. J. Dis. Chest *66*, 27–32 (1972)

Bianco, S., Griffin, J.P., Kamburoff, P.L., Prime, F.J.: Prevention of exercise-induced asthma by indoramin. Br. Med. J. (1974) *4*, 18–20
Bibby, J.G., Higgs, S.A., Kent, A.P., Flint, A.P.F., Mitchell, M.D., Anderson, A.B.M., Turnbull, A.C.: Plasma steroid changes in pre-term labour in association with salbutamol infusion. Br. J. Obstet. Gynaecol. *85*, 425–430 (1978)
Bieniarz, J., Ivankovich, A., Scommegna, A.: Cardiac output during vitodrine treatment in premature labor. Am. J. Obstet. Gynaecol. *118*, 910–920 (1974)
Bietti, G.: Recent experimental, clinical and therapeutic research on the problems of intraocular pressure and glaucoma. Am. J. Ophthalmol. *73*, 475–500 (1972)
Birkenhäger, W.H., Krauss, X.H., Schalekamp, M.A.D.H., Kolsters, G., Kroon, B.J.M.: Antihypertensive effects of propranolol. Observations on predictability. Folia Med. Neerl. *14*, 67–71 (1971)
Bjerle, P., Jacobsson, K.A., Agert, G.: Paradoxical effect of pindolol. Br. Med. J. *4*, 284 (1975)
Bjorntorp, P.: The treatment of angina pectoris with a new beta-receptor blocking agent (H 56/28). Acta Med. Scand. *182*, 285–291 (1967)
Bjorntorp, P.: Treatment of angina pectoris with beta-adrenergic blockade. Mode of action. Acta Med. Scand. *184*, 259–262 (1968)
Bjorntorp, P.: Treatment of angina pectoris with beta-receptor blocking agents. Effect of long-term treatment with sustained release tablets. Acta Med. Scand. *189*, 299–301 (1971)
Black, J.W., Prichard, B.N.C.: Activation and blockade of β-adrenoceptors in common cardiac disorders. Br. Med. Bull. *29*, 163–167 (1973)
Black, J.W., Stephenson, J.S.: Pharmacology of a new adrenergic beta-receptor blocking compound (Nethalide). Lancet *1962 II*, 311–314
Blackhall, M.I., Dauth, M., Mahoney, M., O'Donnell, S.R.: Inhalation of fenoterol (Berotec) by asthmatic children. A clinical comparison with salbutamol, orciprenaline and isoprenaline. Med. J. Aust. *2*, 439–444 (1976)
Blackwell, E.W., Briant, R.H., Conolly, M.E., Davies, D.S., Dollery, C.T.: Metabolism of isoprenaline after aerosol and direct intrabronchial administration in man and dog. Br. J. Pharmacol. *50*, 587–591 (1974)
Blendis, L.M., Auld, R.B., Alexander, E.A., Levinsky, N.G.: Effect of renal beta and alpha-adrenergic stimulation on proximal sodium reabsorption in dogs. Clin. Sci. *43*, 569–576 (1972)
Bloom, D.S., Rosendorff, C., Kramer, R.: Clinical evaluation of prazosin as the sole agent for the treatment of hypertension. A double-blind cross-over study with methyldopa. Curr. Ther. Res. *18*, 144–150 (1975)
Bloomfield, P., Carmichael, J., Crompton, G.K.: Nebulised salbutamol in life-threatening asthma (Letter). Br. Med. J. (1979a) *I*, 1284–1285
Bloomfield, P., Carmichael, J., Petrie, G.R., Jewell, N.P., Crompton, G.K.: Comparison of salbutamol given intravenously and by intermittent positive pressure breathing in life-threatening asthma. Br. Med. J. (1979b) *I*, 848–850
Blum, I., Atsmon, A.: Hypertension complicating treatment with beta-adrenergic blocking drugs. Am. Heart J. *93*, 802–803 (1977)
Boakes, A.J., Prichard, B.N.C.: The effect of AH 5158, pindolol, propranolol and d-propranolol on acute exercise tolerance in angina pectoris. Br. J. Pharmacol. *47*, 673–674 (1973)
Boakes, A.J., Boeree, B.H., Prichard, B.N.C.: Dose response studies in oxprenolol, pindolol, practolol, propranolol and sotalol on tilt, valsalva's and exercise tachycardia. Naunyn-Schmeidebergs Arch. Pharmacol. *279*, R 42 (1973)
Boakes, A.J., Knight, E.J., Prichard, B.N.C.: Preliminary studies of the pharmacological effects of 5-(1-hydroxy-2-[(2-methyl-3-phenylpropyl) amino]-ethyl)-salicylamide (AH 5158) in man. Clin. Sci. *40*, 18–19 (1971)
Bock, K.D., Heimsoth, V., Merguet, P., Schonermat, J.: Klinische und klinischexperimentelle Untersuchungen mit einer neuen blutdrucksenkenden Substanz: Dichlorphenylaminoimidazolin. Dtsch. Med. Wochenschr. *91*, 1761–1770 (1966)
Bockaert, J., Tassin, J.P., Thiery, A.M., Glowinski, J., Premont, J.: Characteristics of dopamine and beta-adrenergic sensitive adenylate cyclases in the frontal cerebral cortex of the rat. Comparative effect of neuroleptics on frontal cortex and striatal dopamine sensitive adenyl cyclases. Brain Res. *122*, 71–86 (1977)

Bolli, P., Waal-Manning, H.J., Wood, A.J., Simpson, F.O.: Experience with labetalol in hypertension. Br. J. Clin. Pharmacol. [Suppl.] *3*, 765–771 (1976a)

Bolli, P., Wood, A.J., Simpson, F.O.: Effects of prazosin in patients with hypertension. Clin. Pharmacol. Ther. *20*, 138–141 (1976b)

Bonn, J.A., Turner, P.: D-propranolol and anxiety. Lancet *1971 I*, 1355–1356

Bonn, J.A., Turner, P., Hicks, D.C.: Beta-adrenergic receptor blockade with practolol in treatment of anxiety. Lancet *1972 I*, 814–815

Boulin, D.J., Mohan, J.: Effects of (+)- and (−)-propranolol on the responses of the isolated basilar artery to cerebrospinal fluid obtained from patients with subarachnoid haemorrhage and cerebral arterial spasm. Br. J. Clin. Pharmacol. *4*, 27–31 (1977)

Boura, A.L.A., Green, A.F.: Adrenergic neurone blockade and other acute effects caused by N-benzyl-N-'N''-dimethyl guanidine and its ortho-chloro derivative. Br. J. Pharmacol. *20*, 36–55 (1963)

Boura, A.L.A., Green, A.F.: Adrenergic neurone blocking agents. Ann. Rev. Pharmacol. *5*, 183–212 (1965)

Boura, A.L.A., Copp, F.C., Green, A.F., Hodson, H.F., Ruffell, G.K., Sim, M.F., Walton, E., Grivsky, E.M.: Adrenergic neurone-blocking agents related to choline 2,6-xylyl ether bromide (T.M. I O), bretylium and guanethidine. Nature *191*, 1312–1313 (1961)

Bowman, W.C., Nott, M.W.: Actions of sympathomimetic amines and their antagonists on skeletal muscle. Pharmacol. Rev. *21*, 27–72 (1969)

Bowman, W.C., Nott, M.W.: Actions of some sympathomimetic bronchodilator and β-adrenergic blocking drugs on contractions of cat soleus muscle. Br. J. Pharmacol. *38*, 37–49 (1970)

Bowman, W.C., Rodger, I.W.: Actions of the sympathomimetic bronchodilator rimiterol (R798), on the cardiovascular, respiratory and skeletal muscle systems of the anaesthetised cat. Br. J. Pharmacol. *45*, 574–583 (1972)

Boyd, G., Clark, C.J.: An evaluation of a controlled release aminophylline tablet (phyllocontin continus) as a concomitant therapy in patients receiving salbutamol. J. Int. Med. Res. [Suppl. 1] *7*, 34–35 (1979)

Brailovsky, D.: Timolol maleate (MK-950). A new beta-blocking agent for the prophylactic management of angina pectoris. A multicentre, multinational, cooperative trial. In: Beta-adrenergic blocking agents in the management of hypertension and angina pectoris. Magnani, B. (ed.), pp. 117–137. New York: Raven 1974

Brain, M.C., Caro, R.T., Kane, J., Lyonnais, J., Dollery, C.T.: Acute effects of varying doses of propranolol upon oxygen haemoglobin affinity in man. Br. J. Clin. Pharmacol. *1*, 67–70 (1974)

Brandon, M.L.: Long-term study comparing fenoterol and isoproterenol inhalation in asthmatic patients. Ann. Allergy *40*, 86–93 (1978)

Brann, E.G., Newman, D.J.: Oxygen affinity in red cells: inability to show membrane-bound 2,3-diphosphoglycerate. Science *179*, 593 (1973)

Braunwald, E., Ebert, P.A.: Hemodynamic alterations in idiopathic hypertrophic subaortic stenosis induced by sympathomimetic drugs. Am. J. Cardiol. *10*, 489–495 (1962)

Bravo, E.L., Tarazi, R.C., Dustan, H.P.: On the mechanism of suppressed plasma-renin activity during beta adrenergic blockade with propranolol. J. Lab. Clin. Med. *83*, 119–128 (1974)

Bravo, E.L., Tarazi, R.C., Dustan, H.P.: β-adrenergic blockade in diuretic-treated patients with essential hypertension. N. Engl. J. Med. *292*, 66–70 (1975)

Brecht, H.M., Banthien, F., Schoeppe, W.: Decrease in plasma noradrenaline levels following long-term treatment with pindolol in patients with essential hypertension. Klin. Wochenschr. *54*, 1095–1105 (1976)

Breckenridge, A., Dollery, C.T., Worlledge, S.M., Holborn, E.J., Johnson, G.D.: Positive direct coombs tests and antinuclear factor in patients treated with methyldopa. Lancet *1967 II*, 1265–1268 (1967)

Brettes, J.P., Renaud, R., Gandar, R.: A double-blind investigation into the effects of vitodrine on uterine blood flow during the third trimester of pregnancy. Am. J. Obstet. Gynecol. *124*, 164–168 (1976)

Brewer, C.: Beneficial effect of beta-adrenergic blockade on examination nerves. Lancet *1972 II*, 435

Briant, R.H., Reid, J.L.: Desmethylimipramine and the hypotensive action of clonidine in the rabbit. Br. J. Pharmacol. *46*, 563–564 (1972)
Briant, R.H., Reid, J.L., Dollery, C.T.: Interaction between clonidine and desipramine in man. Br. Med. J. *1973 I*, 522–523
Brittain, R.T.: A comparison of the pharmacology of salbutamol with that of isoprenaline orciprenaline and trimetoquinol. Postgrad. Med. J. [Suppl.] *47*, 11–16 (1971)
Brittain, R.T., Farmer, J.B., Jack, D.: Alpha-[(t-butylamino)methyl]-4-hydroxy-m-xylene-α-1,α-3 diol (AH 3365): a selective beta-adrenergic stimulant. Nature *219*, 862–863 (1968)
Brittain, R.T., Jack, D., Ritchie, A.C.: Recent beta-adrenoceptor stimulants. Adv. Drug Res. *5*, 197–253 (1970)
Brittain, R.T., Dean, C.M., Jack, D.: Sympathomimetic bronchodilator drugs. Pharmacol. Ther. Bull. *2*, 423–462 (1976)
Brod, J., Horbach, L., Just, H., Rosenthal, J., Nicolescu, R.: Acute effects of clonidine on central and peripheral haemodynamics and plasma renin activity. Eur. J. Clin. Pharmacol. *4*, 107–114 (1972)
Brogden, R.N., Speight, T.M., Avery, G.S.: Terbutaline: a preliminary report of its pharmacological properties and therapeutic efficacy in asthma. Drugs *6*, 324–332 (1973)
Brogden, R.N., Speight, T.M., Avery, G.S.: Timolol: a preliminary report of its pharmacological properties and therapeutic efficacy in angina and hypertension. Drugs *9*, 164–177 (1975)
Brodgen, R.N., Heel, R.C., Speight, T.M., Avery, G.S.: Prazosin: a review of its pharmacological properties and therapeutic efficacy in hypertension. Drugs *14*, 163–167 (1977)
Brooks, H.L., Stein, P.D., Matson, J.L., Hyland, J.W.: Dopamine-induced alterations in coronary hemodynamics in dogs. Circ. Res. *24*, 699–704 (1969)
Brown, J.J., Agabiti Rosei, E., Lever, A.F., Robertson, A.S., Robertson, J.I.S., Trust, P.M.: Emergency treatment of hypertension crisis following clonidine withdrawal. Br. Med. J. *1976 I*, 1341
Brown, J.J., Lever, A.F., Cumming, A.M.M., Robertson, J.I.S.: Labetalol in hypertension. Lancet *1977 I*, 1147
Brown, P., Baddeley, H., Read, A.E., Davies, J.D., McGarry, J.: Sclerosing peritonitis, an unusual reaction to a β-adrenergic blocking drug (practolol). Lancet *1974 II*, 1477–1481
Brunk, S.F., Delle, M., Wilson, W.R.: Effect of propranolol on morphine metabolism. Clin. Pharmacol. Ther. *16*, 1039–1044 (1974)
Buckfield, P.M., Davis, J.A.: β-adrenergic blockers in childhood thyrotoxicosis. Lancet *1966 I*, 1425
Buhler, F.R., Laragh, J.H., Baer, L., Vaughan, E.D., Brunner, H.R.: Propranolol inhibition of renin secretion. A specific approach to diagnosis and treatment of renin dependent hypertensive disease. N. Engl. J. Med. *287*, 1209–1214 (1972)
Buhler, F.R., Burkart, F., Lutold, F., Kung, M., Marbet, G., Pfisterer, M.: Antihypertensive beta blocking action as related to renin and age: a pharmacological tool to identify pathogenic mechanisms in essential hypertension. Am. J. Cardiol. *36*, 653–669 (1975)
Bullock, J.L., Harris, R.E., Young, R.: Treatment of thyrotoxicosis during pregnancy with propranolol. Am. J. Obstet. Gynecol. *121*, 242–245 (1975)
Burchell, H.B.: Management of tachycardia associated with Wolff-Parkinson White syndrome. In: Cardiac arrhythmias. Dreifus, L., Likoff, W. (eds.), p. 475. New York: Grune & Stratton 1973
Burden, A.C., Alexander, C.P.T.: Rebound hypertension after acute methyldopa withdrawal. Br. Med. J. *1976 I*, 1056–1057
Burnstock, G., Evans, B., Gannon, B.J., Heath, J.W., James, V.: A new method of destroying adrenergic nerves in adult animals using guanethidine. Br. J. Pharmacol. *43*, 295–301 (1971)
Bylund, D.B., Charness, M.E., Snyder, S.H.: Beta-adrenergic receptor labeling in intact animals with ^{125}I-hydroxybenzylpindolol. J. Pharmacol. Exp. Ther. *201*, 644–653 (1977)
Cambridge, D., Davey, M.J., Massingham, R.: The pharmacology of antihypertensive drugs with special reference to vasodilators, alpha-adrenergic blocking agents and prazosin. Med. J. Aust. [Suppl.] *2*, 2–6 (1977)
Cameron, M.M., Haas, R.H.: Adrenergic blockade in subarachroid haemorrhage. Acta Neurochir. (Wien) *34*, 261–264 (1976)

Camner, P., Strandberg, K., Philipson, K.: Increased mucociliary transport by adrenergic stimulation. Arch. Environ. Health *31*, 79–82 (1976)
Cannon, P.J., Whitlock, R.T., Morris, R.C., Angers, M., Laragh, J.H.: Effect of alpha-methyldopa in severe and malignant hypertension. JAMA *179*, 673–681 (1962)
Caplin, I., Haynes, J.T.: Complications of aerosol therapy in aerosol therapy in asthma. Ann. Allergy *27*, 65–69 (1969)
Carlsson, C., Johansson, T.: The psychological effects of propranolol in the abstinence phase of chronic alcoholics. Br. J. Psychiatry *119*, 605–606 (1971)
Carlsson, A., Lindqvist, M.: In vivo decarboxylation of α-methyldopa and α-methyl metatyrosine. Acta Physiol. Scand. *54*, 87–94 (1962)
Carmeliet, E., Verdonck, R.: Interaction between ouabain and butridine, a beta-adrenergic blocking substance on the heart. Eur. J. Pharmacol. *1*, 269–277 (1967)
Carney, I., Daly, M.J., Lightowler, J.E., Pickering, R.W.: The comparative pharmacology of WG 253 (rimiterol hydrobromide) a new bronchodilator. Arch. Int. Pharmacodyn. Ther. *194*, 334–345 (1971)
Carruthers, M., Taggart, P., Somerville, W.: Some effects of beta-blockade on the lipid response to certain acute emotions. In: New perspectives in beta blockade. Burley, D.M., Frier, Rondel, Taylor (eds.), pp. 307–311 Horsham: Ciba 1973
Carruthers, M.E.: Aggression and atheroma. Lancet *1969 II*, 1170–1171
Carruthers, S.G., Ghosal, A., McDevitt, D.G., Nelson, J.K., Shanks, R.G.: The assessment of β-adrenoceptor blocking drugs in hypertension. Br. J. Clin. Pharmacol. *1*, 93–98 (1974)
Carstairs, K.C., Breckenridge, A., Dollery, C.T., Worlledge, S.M.: Incidence of a positive direct Coombs test in patients on α-methyldopa. Lancet *1966 II*, 133–135
Castenfors, H.: Long-term effects of timolol and hydrochlorothiazide or hydrochlorothiazide and amiloride in essential hypertension. Eur. J. Clin. Pharmacol. *12*, 97–103 (1977)
Castenfors, J., Johnsson, H., Oro, L.: Effect of alprenolol on blood pressure and plasma renin activity in hypertensive patients. Acta Med. Scand. *193*, 189–195 (1973)
Chalmers, J., Horvath, J., Tiller, D., Bune, A.: Effects of timolol and hydrochlorothiazide on blood pressure and plasma renin activity. Double-blind factorial trial. Lancet *1976 II*, 328–331
Chamberlain, D.A.: Effects of β-adrenergic blockade on heart size. Am. J. Cardiol. *18*, 321–328 (1966)
Chamberlain, D.A., Howard, J.: Guanethidine and methyldopa: a haemodynamic study. Br. Heart J. *26*, 528–536 (1964)
Cherian, G., Brockington, I.M., Shah, P.M., Oakley, C.M., Goodwin, J.F.: Beta-adrenergic blockade in hypertrophic obstructive cardiomyopathy. Br. Med. J. *1966 I*, 895–898
Chervinsky, P.: A comparative evaluation of fenoterol and terbutaline in the treatment of asthma. Ann. Allergy *40*, 189–194 (1977)
Chervinsky, P., Chervinsky, G.: Metaproterenol tablets: their duration of effect by comparison with ephedrine. Curr. Ther. Res. *17*, 507–518 (1975)
Chidsey, C.A., Braunwald, E., Morrow, A.G.: Catecholamine excretion and cardiac stores of norepinephrine in congestive heart failure. Am. J. Med. *39*, 442–451 (1965)
Christoffel, K.K., Salafsky, I.: Fetal alcohol syndrome in dizygotic twins. J. Pediatr. *87*, 963–967 (1975)
Chrysant, S.G., Panayiotis, N., Adamopoulos, P.N., Nishiyama, K., Frohlich, E.D.: Hemodynamic effects of bethanidine: a new sympatholytic antihypertensive drug. Circulation [Suppl. III) *50*, 105 (1974)
Church, R.: Eczema provoked by methyldopa. Br. J. Dermatol. *91*, 373–378 (1974)
Clark, K.G.: Case history: Haemolysis and agranulocytosis complicating treatment with methyldopa. Br. Med. J. (1967) *IV*, 94
Clausen, J., Felsby, M., Jorgensen, F.S., Neilson, B.L., Roin, J., Strange, B.: Absence of prophylactic effect of propranolol in myocardial infarction. Lancet *1966 II*, 920–924
Cochrane, G.M., Clark, T.J.H.: A survey of asthma mortality in patients between the ages of 35 and 64 in the greater London hospitals in 1971. Thorax *30*, 300–305 (1975)
Cohen, A., Maxmen, J.S., Ragheb, M., Baleiron, H., Zaleski, E.J., Bing, R.J.: Effects of alpha-methyldopa on the myocardial blood flow, utilizing the coincidence counting method. J. Clin. Pharmacol. *7*, 77–83 (1967)

Cohen, J., Effat, H., Goodwin, J.F., Oakley, C.M., Steinger, R.E.: Hypertrophic obstructive cardiomyopathy. Br. Heart J. *26*, 16–32 (1964)
Cohn, J.N., Francoisa, J.A.: Vasodilator therapy of cardiac failure, Part I. N. Engl. J. Med. *297*, 27–31 (1977)
Cohn, J.N., Liptak, T.E., Freis, E.D.: Hemodynamic effects of guanethidine in man. Circ. Res. *12*, 298–307 (1963)
Collier, J.G., Dawnay, N.A.H., Nachev, C.H., Robinson, B.F.: Clinical investigations of an antagonist at α- and β-adrenoceptors – AH 5158A. Br. J. Pharmacol. *44*, 286–293 (1972)
Collier, J.G., Lorge, R.E., Robinson, B.F.: Comparison of effects of tolmesoxide (RX 71107), diazoxide, hydrallazine, prazosin, glyceryl trinitrate, and sodium nitroprusside on forearm arteries and dorsal hand veins of man. Br. J. Clin. Pharmacol. *5*, 35–44 (1978)
Collins, I.S., King, I.W.: Pindolol (visken, LB 46), a new treatment of hypertension. Report of a multicentre open study. Curr. Ther. Res. *14*, 185–194 (1972)
Collins, I.S., Pek, P.: Pharmacokinetics of prazosin, a new antihypertensive compound. Clin. Exp. Pharmacol. Physiol. *2*, 445–446 (1975)
Collins, J.M., McDevitt, D.G., Shanks, R.G., Swanton, J.G.: The cardio-toxicity of isoprenaline during hypoxia. Br. J. Pharmacol. *36*, 35–45 (1969)
Coltart, D.J.: Comparison of effects of propranolol and practolol on exercise tolerance in angina pectoris. Br. Heart J. *33*, 62–64 (1971)
Coltart, D.J., Gibson, D.G., Shand, D.G.: Plasma propranolol levels associated with suppression of ventricular ectopic beats. Br. Med. J. *1971 I*, 490–491
Conolly, M.E., Davies, D.S., Dollery, C.T., George, C.F.: Resistance to β-adrenoceptor stimulants (a possible explanation for the rise in asthma deaths). Br. J. Pharmacol. *43*, 389–402 (1971)
Conolly, M.E., Davies, D.S., Dollery, C.T., Morgan, C.D., Paterson, J.W., Sandler, M.: Metabolism of isoprenaline in dog and man. Br. J. Pharmacol. *46*, 458–472 (1972)
Constantine, J.W., McShane, W.K., Scriabine, A., Hess, H.J.: Analysis of the hypotensive action of prazosin. In: Hypertension: Mechanisms and management. Onesti, G., Kim, K.E., Moyer, J.H. (eds.), p. 449. New York: Grune & Stratton 1973
Conway, W.D., Minatoga, H., Lands, A.M., Skekosky, J.M.: Absorption and elimination profile of isoproterenol. III. The metabolic fate of dl isoproterenol-7-^{3}H in the dog. J. Pharmacol. Sci. *57*, 1135–1141 (1968)
Cooke, N.J., Kerr, J.A., Willey, R.F., Hoare, M.V., Grant, I.W.B., Crompton, G.K.: Response to rimiterol and salbutamol aerosols administered by intermittent postive-pressure ventilation. Br. Med. J. *1974 II*, 250–252
Coupar, I.M., Turner, P.: Relative potencies of some false transmitters on isolated human smooth muscle. Br. J. Pharmacol. *38*, 463–464P (1970)
Coté, G., Drance, S.M.: The effect of propranolol on human intraocular pressure. Can. J. Ophthalmol. *3*, 207–212 (1968)
Cranston, W.I., Brown, W.: Diurnal variation in plasma volume in normal and hypertensive subjects. Clin. Sci. *25*, 107–114 (1963)
Crawford, M.H., Le Winter, M.M., O'Rourke, R.A., Karliner, J.S., Ross, J.: Combined propranolol and dogoxin therapy in angina pectoris. Ann. Intern. Med. *83*, 449–455 (1975)
Crexells, C., Bourassa, M.C., Biron, P.: Effects of dopamine on myocardial metabolism in patients with ischaemic heart disease. Cardiovasc. Res. *7*, 438–445 (1973)
Crombie, A.L., Lawson, A.A.H.: Adrenergic blocking agents. A double-blind trial in the treatment of the eye signs of thyroid disorder. Br. J. Ophthalmol. *52*, 616–620 (1968)
Crook, B.R.H., Raftery, E.B.: Treatment of non-accelerated essential hypertension with oxprenolol. Circulation [Suppl. 11] *45*, 142 (1972)
Cullum, V.A., Farmer, J.B., Jack, D., Levy, G.P.: Salbutamol: a new selective β-adrenoceptor receptor stimulant. Br. J. Pharmacol. *35*, 141–151 (1969)
Cumming, G.R.: Propranolol in tetralogy of Fallot. Circulation *41*, 13–15 (1970)
DaCosta, J.L., Goh, B.K.: A comparative trial of subcutaneous terbutaline. Th 1165a and adrenaline in bronchial asthma. Med. J. Aust. *2*, 588–591 (1973)
Dahlstrom, A., Fuxe, K.: Evidence for the existence of monoamine containing neurones in the central nervous system 1. Acta Physiol. Scand. [Suppl. 232] *62*, 1–55 (1964)

Dahlstrom, A., Fuxe, K.: Evidence for the existence of monoamine containing neurones in the central nervous system 2. Acta Physiol. Scand. [Suppl. 247] *64*, 1–36 (1965)
Dahr, A.S.: Use of hydralazine and selective cardiac adrenergic blockade in therapy of essential hypertension. Circulation [Suppl. II] *142*, 45–46 (1972)
Dale, H.H.: On some physiological actions of ergot. J. Physiol. *34*, 163–206 (1906)
Dargie, H.J., Dollery, C.T., Daniel, J.: Labetalol in resistant hypertension. Br. J. Clin. Pharmacol. [Suppl.] *3*, 751–755 (1976)
Daubert, J.C., Gosse, P., Rio, M., Grall, J.Y., Bourdonnec, C., Pony, J.C., Gouffault, J.: Myocardiopathies en coeurs de grossesse. Role possibles des beta-mimetiques. Arch. Mal. Coeur *71*, 1283–1290 (1978)
Davidov, M., Kakaviatos, N., Finnerty, F.A. Jr.: The antihypertensive effects of an imidazoline compound. Clin. Pharmacol. Ther. *8*, 810–816 (1967)
Davidson, C., Thadani, U., Singleton, W., Taylor, S.H.: Comparison of antihypertensive activity of beta blocking drugs during chronic treatment. Br. Med. J. *1976 II*, 7–9
Davies, D.S.: Pharmacokinetics of inhaled substances. Postgrad. Med. J. [Suppl. 7] *51*, 69–75 (1975)
Davies, R.O., Mizgala, H.F., Khan, A.S.: Propranolol-isosorbide dinitrate: combined therapy in angina pectoris. Clin. Res. *17*, 635 (1969)
Dawson, A., Smith, I., Johnson, B.F.: The transient antihypertensive effect of phentolamine in patients receiving beta-blocker treatment. J. Int. Med. Res. *5*, 462–464 (1977)
Day, G.M., Prichard, B.N.C.: Hypotensive action from combination of propranolol and other hypotensive drugs. Br. J. Pharmacol. *41*, 408–409P (1971)
Day, M.D., Rand, M.J.: A hypothesis for the mode of action of α-methyldopa in relieving hypertension. J. Pharm. Pharmacol. *15*, 221–224 (1963)
Day, M.D., Rand, M.J.: Some observations on the pharmacology of α-methyldopa. Br. J. Pharmacol. Chemother. *22*, 72–86 (1964)
Day, M.D., Roach, A.G.: Cardiovascular effects of β-adrenoceptor blocking agents after intracerebroventricular administration in conscious normotensive cats. Clin. Exp. Pharmacol. Physiol. *1*, 333–339 (1974)
Day, M.D., Roach, A.G., Whiting, R.L.: The mechanism of the antihypertensive action of alpha-methyldopa in hypertensive rats. Eur. J. Pharmacol. *21*, 271–280 (1973)
Deacon, S.P., Karunanayake, A., Barnett, D.: Acebutolol, atenolol and propranolol and metabolic responses to acute hypoglycaemia in diabetics. Br. Med. J. *1977 II*, 1255–1257
Decalmer, P.B.S., Chatterjee, S.S., Cruickshank, J.M., Benson, M.K., Sterling, G.M.: Beta-blockers and asthma. Br. Heart J. *40*, 184–189 (1978)
De La Paz, A.G., Reyes, A.L., De Guia, R., Saldivar, C., Aquino, A., Saniel, E.G., Durante, M., Unson, L.: A new quinazoline derivative in the treatment of hypertension. A cooperative study in four medical centres in the Philippines. Philipp. J. Cardiol. *4*, 47 (1976)
Del Bianco, P.L., Bavazzano, A., Frianchi, G., Sicuteri, F.: Pharmacological and therapeutic effects of adrenergic beta blockade. Boll. Soc. Ital. Cardiol. *II*, 656–659 (1966)
Dent, R., Kellaway, G.S.M.: A pilot trial of labetalol (AH 5158A) a combined alpha and beta blocker in the treatment of hypertension. N. Z. Med. J. *86*, 213–215 (1977)
Dhainaut, J.-F., Boutonnet, G., Weber, S., Degeorges, M.: Responsabilité des beta-mimétiques prescrits au cours de la grossesse dans la genèse d'une cardiomyopathie du post partum? Nouv. Presse Med. *7*, 4058 (1978)
Diaz, R.G., Somberg, J., Freeman, E., Levitt, B.: Myocardial infarction after propranolol withdrawal. Am. Heart J. *88*, 257–258 (1974)
Dietzman, R.H., Lillehei, R.C.: The nature and treatment of shock. Br. J. Hosp. Med. *1*, 300–304 (1968)
Dintenfass, L.: Viscosity factors in hypertensive and cardiovascular diseases. Cardiovasc. Med. *2*, 337–354 (1977)
Dintenfass, L., Lake, B.: Beta blockers and blood viscosity. Lancet *1976 I*, 1026
Distler, A., Keim, H.J., Cordes, U., Philipp, T., Wolff, H.P.: Sympathetic responsiveness and antihypertensive effect of beta-receptor blockade in essential hypertension. Am. J. Med. *64*, 446–451 (1978)
Dollery, C.T., Harington, M.: Methyldopa in hypertension. Clinical and pharmacological studies. Lancet *1962 I*, 759–763

Dollery, C.T., Lewis, P.J.: Central hypotensive effect of propranolol. Postgrad. Med. J. [Suppl. 4] *52*, 116–120 (1976)
Dollery, C.T., Reid, J.L.: Central noradrenergic neurones and the cardiovascular actions of clonidine in the rabbit. Br. J. Pharmacol. *47*, 206–216 (1973)
Dollery, C.T., Emslie-Smith, D., Milne, M.D.: Clinical and pharmacological studies with guanethidine in the treatment of hypertension. Lancet *1960 II*, 381–387
Dollery, C.T., Emslie-Smith, D., Shillingford, J.P.: Haemodynamic effects of guanethidine. Lancet 1961 II, 331–334
Dollery, C.T., Harington, M., Hodge, J.V.: Haemodynamic studies with methyldopa. Effect on cardiac output and response to pressor amines. Br. Heart J. *25*, 670–676 (1963)
Dormois, J.C., Young, J.L., Nies, A.S.: Minoxidil in severe hypertension: value when conventional drugs have failed. Am. Heart J. *90*, 360–368 (1975)
Douglas-Jones, A.P.: Two antihypertensive regimens in family practice. Sotalol and methyldopa compared. Practitioner *220*, 804–808 (1978)
Douglas-Jones, A.P., Cruickshank, J.M.: Once daily dosing with atenolol in patients with mild or moderate hypertension. Br. Med. J. *1976 I*, 990–991
Doyle, A.E., Morley, A.: Studies on the absorption and excretion of (14C)-bethanidine in man. Br. J. Pharmacol. *24*, 701–704 (1965)
Drayer, J.I.M., Keim, H.J., Wever, M.A., Case, D.B., Laragh, J.H.: Unexpected pressor responses to propranolol in essential hypertension on interaction between renin, aldosterone, and sympathetic activity. Am. J. Med. *60*, 897–903 (1976)
Drayer, J.I.M., Weber, M.A., Longworth, D.L., Laragh, J.H.: The possible importance of aldosterone as well as renin in the long-term antihypertensive action of propranolol. Am. J. Med. *64*, 187–192 (1978)
Dubi, B., Studer, A., Scherrer, M.: Vergleich von inhalativ und ligual verabreichtem Isoprenalin (isoproteranol-aleudrin) bei Bronchialasthma. Schweiz. Med. Wochenschr. *104*, 1244–1250 (1974)
Du Charme, D.W., Freyburger, W.A., Graham, B.E., Carlson, R.G.: Pharmacologic properties of minoxidil. A new hypotensive agent. J. Pharmacol. Exp. Ther. *184*, 662–670 (1973)
Dulfano, M.J., Glass, P.: Evaluation of a new β_2-adrenergic receptor stimulant, terbutaline, in bronchial asthma. II. Oral comparison with ephedrine. Curr. Ther. Res. *15*, 150–157 (1973)
Duner, H., Pernow, B.: Haemodynamic effects of β-receptor blocking agents and digitalis in ischaemic coronary heart disease with angina pectoris. Acta Med. Scand. *194*, 517–523 (1973)
Dunlop, D., Shanks, R.G.: Inhibition of the carotid sinus reflex by the chronic administration of propranolol. Br. J. Pharmacol. *36*, 132–143 (1969)
Dunn, F.G., Melville, D.I., Jones, J.V., Lorimer, A.R., Lawrie, T.D.V.: Standardised stress and hypertension: comparison of effect of propranolol and methyldopa. Br. J. Clin. Pharmacol. *5*, 213–226 (1978)
Dunnill, M.S.: Pathology of asthma. In: Identification of asthma. Ciba Foundation Study Group No. 38. Porter, R., Brich, J. (eds.), pp. 35–46. Edinburgh, London: Churchill Livingstone 1971
Durairaj, S.K., Haywood, L.J.: Hemodynamic effect of dopamine in patients with resistant congestive heart failure. Clin. Pharmacol. Ther. *24*, 175–185 (1978)
Editorial: Deaths from asthma in young people. Br. Med. J. *1972 I*, 459
Editorial: Management of severe acute asthma. Br. Med. J. *1978 I*, 873–874
Edwards, R.C., Raftery, E.B.: Haemodynamic effects of long-term oral labetalol. Br. J. Clin. Pharmacol. [Suppl.] *3*, 733–736 (1976)
Ehrenkranz, R.A., Walker, A.M., Oakes, G.K., McLaughlin, M.K., Chez, R.A.: Effect of ritodrine infusion on uterine and umbilical flow in pregnant sheep. Am. J. Obstet. Gynecol. *126*, 343–349 (1976)
Eisenstadt, W.S., Nicholas, S.S.: The adverse effect of adrenergic aerosols in bronchial asthma. Ann. Allergy *27*, 283–288 (1969)
Ekberg, G., Hansson, B.-G.: Glucose tolerance and insulin release in hypertensive patients treated with the cardioselective β-receptor blocking agent metoprolol. Acta Med. Scand. *202*, 393–397 (1977)

Elegbelye, O.O., Williams, K.O., Femi-Pearse, D.: Comparison of the metabolic effects of salbutamol administered in a one minute bolus and a continuous infusion in patients with asthma. Isr. J. Med. Sci. *14*, 455–458 (1978)
Eliahou, H.E., Silverberg, D.S., Reisin, E., Romen, I., Mashiach, S., Serr, D.M.: Propranolol for the treatment of hypertension in pregnancy. Br. J. Obstet. Gynaecol. *85*, 431–436 (1978)
Eliasch, H., Rosen, A., Scott, H.M.: Systemic circulatory response to stress of simulated flight and to physical exercise before and after propranolol blockade. Br. Heart J. *29*, 671–683 (1967)
Elliot, F.A.: Propranolol for the control of belligerent behaviour following acute brain damage. Ann. Neurol. *1*, 489–491 (1977)
Elliott, W.C., Gorlin, R.: Isoproterenol in treatment of heart disease. JAMA *197*, 315–320 (1966)
Ellison, P.H.: Propranolol for severe post-head injury action tremor. Neurology (Minneap.) *28*, 197–199 (1978)
Engelhardt, G. von: Struktur-Wirkungsbeziehungen in einer Reihe von neuen Amino-Halogen substituierten Phenyl-amino-äthanolen. Arzneim. Forsch. *22*, 869–876 (1972)
England, R.A.: Treatment of ventricular arrhythmias in ambulatory patients. Med. Clin. North Am. *56*, 615–624 (1972)
Epstein, S.E., Braunwald, E.: The effect of beta adrenergic blockade on patterns of urinary sodium excretion. Studies in normal subjects and in patients with heart disease. Ann. Intern. Med. *65*, 20–27 (1966)
Eriksson, B.O., Thoren, C., Zetterquist, P.: Long-term treatment with propranolol in selected cases of Fallot's tetralogy. Br. Heart J. *31*, 37–44 (1969)
Eriksson, M., Rubenfield, S., Garber, A.J., Kohler, P.O.: Propranolol does not prevent thyroid storm. N. Engl. J. Med. *296*, 263–264 (1977)
Evans, M.E., Paterson, J.W., Shenfield, G.M., Thomas, N., Walker, S.R.: Proceedings: The pharmacokinetics of rimiterol in asthmatic subjects. Br. J. Pharmacol. *47*, 153–154P (1973a)
Evans, M.E., Walker, S.R., Brittain, R.T., Paterson, J.W.: The metabolism of salbutamol in man. Xenobiotica *3*, 113–120 (1973b)
Fagard, R., Amery, A., Deplaen, J.F., Lijnen, P., Missotten, A.: Plasma renin concentration and the hypotensive effect of bendrofluazide and of atenolol. Clin. Sci. Mol. Med. *51*, 215–217 (1976)
Fakuda, Y., Fujita, T., Shibuya, J., Albert, S.N.: The distribution between the intravascular and interstitial compartments of commonly utilised replacement fluids. Curr. Res. Anaesth. Analg. *48*, 831–838 (1969)
Farmer, J.B., Kennedy, I., Levy, G.P., Marshall, R.J.: Pharmacology of AH 5158; a drug which blocks both α- and β-adrenoceptors. Br. J. Pharmacol. *45*, 660–675 (1972)
Felix, R.H., Ive, F.A., Dahl, M.G.C.: Cutaneous and ocular reactions to practolol. Br. Med. J. *4*, 321–324 (1974)
Feltham, P.M., Watson, O.F., Peel, J.S., Dunlop, D.J., Turner, A.S.: Pindolol in hypertension: a double-blind trial. N. Z. Med. J. *76*, 167–171 (1972)
Fewings, J.D., Hodge, R.L., Scroop, G.C., Whelan, R.F.: The effect of bethanidine on the peripheral circulation in man. Br. J. Pharmacol. *23*, 115–122 (1964)
Finch, L.: The cardiovascular effects of intraventricular clonidine and BAY 1470 in conscious hypertensive cats. Br. J. Pharmacol. *52*, 333–338 (1974)
Finch, L.: The central hypotensive action of clonidine and BAY 1470 in cats and rats. Clin. Sci. Mol. Med. *48*, 273–276s (1975)
Finch, L., Haeusler, G.: Further evidence for a central hypotensive action of α-methyldopa in both the rat and cat. Br. J. Pharmacol. *47*, 217–228 (1973)
Fitzgerald, J.D.: Beta adrenergic blocking drugs. Present position and future developments. Acta Cardiol. (Brux.) [Suppl.] *151*, 199–216 (1972)
Fitzgerald, J.D.: The effect of β-adrenoceptor antagonists on the morbidity and mortality in cardiovascular disease. Postgrad. Med. J. *52*, 770–781 (1976)
Flamm, M.D., Harrison, D.C., Hancock, E.W.: Muscular subaortic stenosis. Prevention of outflow obstruction with propranolol. Circulation *38*, 846–858 (1968)

Fleisch, J.H., Titus, E.: The prevention of isoproterenol desensitization and isoproterenol reversal. J. Pharmacol. Exp. Ther. *181*, 425–433 (1972)
Formgren, H.: Clinical comparison of inhaled terbutaline and orciprenaline in asthmatic patients. Scand. J. Respir. Dis. *51*, 203–211 (1970)
Formgren, H.: Experiences of long-term treatment of asthma with terbutaline. A study on frequency of side effects and therapeutic effects. Acta Allergol. (Kbh.) *26*, 81–89 (1971)
Formgren, H.: The therapeutic value of oral long-term treatment with terbutaline (bricanyl) in asthma. A follow-up study of its efficacy and side effects. Scand. Respir. Dis. *56*, 321–328 (1975)
Forrest, W.A.: A total of 254 cases of angina pectoris treated with oxprenolol in hospital practice – a monitored release study. Br. J. Clin. Pract. *26*, 217–222 (1972)
Fournet, J.P., Dupard, M.C.: Trial of ventoline syrup in children. Med. Infant. *85*, 553–559 (1978)
Fournier, A., Hardin, J.M., Alexandre, J.M., Lombaert, M., Ronco, G., Bezoc, J.F., Desmet, G., Quichaud, J.: Anti-hypertensive effect of acebutolol: its relation to sympathetic nervous system responsiveness and to plasma renin and dopamine β-hydroxylase activities. Clin. Sci. Mol. Med. *51*, 477–480s (1976)
Fox, C.A.: Reduction in the rise of systolic blood pressure during human coitus by the β-adrenergic blocking agent, propranolol. J. Reprod. Fert. *22*, 587–590 (1970)
Fox, K.M., Chopra, M.P., Portal, R.W., Aber, C.P.: Long-term beta blockade: possible protection from myocardial infarction. Br. Med. J. *1975 I*, 117–119
Fraser, P.M., Speizer, F.E., Waters, S.D.M., Doll, R., Mann, N.M.: The circumstances preceding death from asthma in young people in 1968 to 1969. Br. J. Dis. Chest *65*, 71–84 (1971)
Fredholm, B.B., Lunell, N.O., Persson, B., Wager, J.: Actions of salbutamol in late pregnancy, plasma cyclic AMP, insulin and c-peptide, carbohydrate and lipid metabolism in diabetic and non-diabetic women. Diabetologia *14*, 235–242 (1978)
Freedman, B.J.: Trial of new bronchodilator, terbutaline, in asthma. Br. Med. J. *1971 I*, 633–636
Freedman, B.J.: Trial of a terbutaline aerosol in the treatment of asthma and a comparison of its effects with those of a salbutamol aerosol. Br. J. Dis. Chest *66*, 222–229 (1972)
Freeman, J.W., Knight, L.W.: Oxprenolol and hydralazine in the treatment of hypertension. Med. J. Aust. [Suppl. 1] *1*, 12–13 (1975)
Frick, M.H., Pörsti, P.: Combined alpha- and beta-adrenoceptor blockade with labetalol in hypertension. Br. Med. J. *1976 I*, 1046–1048
Frishman, W.H., Weksler, B., Christodoulou, J.P., Smithen, C., Killip, T.: Reversal of abnormal platelet aggregability and change in exercise tolerance in patients with angina pectoris following oral propranolol. Circulation *50*, 887–896 (1974)
Frohlich, E.D., Tarazi, R.C., Dustan, H.P., Page, I.H.: The paradox of beta adrenergic blockade in hypertension. Circulation *37*, 417–423 (1968)
Fügner, A.: An improved method for the study of reagin-mediated mast cell degranulation in rats. Experientia *29*, 708–710 (1973)
Fügner, A.: Inhibition of antigen-induced histamine release by β-adrenergic stimulants in vivo. Int. Arch. Allergy Appl. Immunol. *54*, 78–87 (1977)
Fulton, R.M., Green, K.G.: Effect of pronethalol in angina pectoris. Br. Med. J. *1963 II*, 1228–1229
Funahashi, A., Hamilton, L.H.: A study of a new bronchodilator, carbuterol. Am. Rev. Respir. Dis. *113*, 398–440 (1976)
Furberg, C., Michaelson, G.: Effect of aptin, a β-adrenergic blocking agent, in arterial hypertension. Acta Med. Scand. *186*, 447–450 (1969)
Furberg, G.D.: β-adrenergic receptor blocking drugs in hypertrophic obstructive cardiomyopathies, certain functional heart disorders and Fallot's tetralogy. Drugs *7*, 106–117 (1974)
Furhoff, A.K.: Adverse reactions with methyldopa – a decade's reports. Acta Med. Scand. *203*, 425–428 (1978)
Furnival, C.M., Linden, R.J., Snow, H.M.: Inotropic changes in the left ventricle: the effect of changes in heart rate, aortic pressure and end-diastolic pressure. J. Physiol. (Lond.) *211*, 359 (1970)
Furst, C.I.: The biochemistry of guanethidine. Adv. Drug Res. *4*, 133–161 (1967)

Gaddie, J., Legge, J.S., Petrie, G., Palmer, K.N.V.: The effect of an alpha-adrenergic receptor blocking drug on histamine sensitivity in bronchial asthma. Br. J. Dis. Chest *66*, 141–146 (1972)

Gallant, D.M., Swanson, W.C., Guerrero-Figueroa, R.: A controlled evaluation of propranolol in chronic alcoholic patients presenting with sympatomatology of anxiety and tension. J. Clin. Pharmacol. New Drugs *13*, 41 (1973)

Gandevia, B.: Pressurized sympathomimetic aerosols and their lack of relationship to asthma mortality in Australia. Med. J. Aust. *1*, 273–277 (1973)

Gardos, G., Cole, J.O., Orzack, M.H., Volicer, L.: Propranolol in treatment of resistant schizophrenics. Psychopharmacol. Bull. *9*, 43–44 (1973)

Garvey, H.L., Ram, N.: Comparative antihypertensive effects and tissue distribution of beta-adrenergic blocking drugs. J. Pharmacol. Exp. Ther. *194*, 220–233 (1975a)

Garvey, H.L., Ram, N.: Centrally induced hypotensive effect of β-adrenergic blocking drugs. Eur. J. Pharmacol. *33*, 283–294 (1975b)

Genest, J., Dornier, A., Boucher, R., Nowaczynski, W., Rojo-Ortega, J.M., Kuchel, O.: β-Adrenergic blocking agents and renin spectrum. In: New anti-hypertensive drugs. Scriabine, A., Sweet, C.S. (eds.), pp. 215–226 New York: Spectrum 1976

George, C.F., Nagle, R.E., Pentecost, B.L.: Practolol in treatment of angina pectoris. A double-blind study. Br. Med. J. *1970 II*, 402–404

Geumei, A., Miller, W.F., Paez, P.N., Gast, L.R.: Evaluation of a new oral β-adrenoceptor stimulant bronchodilator, terbutaline. Pharmacology *13*, 201–211 (1975)

Geumei, A.M., Miller, W.F., Miller, J., Gast, L.R.: Bronchodilator effect of a new oral β-adrenoreceptor stimulant, Th 1165a. A comparison with metoproterenol sulfate. Chest *70*, 460–465 (1976)

Geyskes, G.G., Boer, P., Dorhout Mees, E.J.: Clonidine withdrawal: mechanism and frequency of rebound hypertension. Br. J. Clin. Pharmacol. *7*, 55–62 (1979)

Ghose, R.R., Sampson, A.: Rapid onset of action of oral labetalol in severe hypertension. Curr. Med. Res. Opinion *5*, 147–151 (1977)

Gianelly, R.S., Goldman, R.H., Treister, B., Harrison, D.C.: Propranolol in patients with angina pectoris. Ann. Intern. Med. *67*, 1216–1225 (1967)

Gibson, D.G.: Pharmacodynamic properties of β-adrenergic blocking drugs in man. Drugs *7*, 8–38 (1974)

Gibson, D.G., Sowton, E.: The use of beta-adrenergic blocking drugs in dysrhythmias. Prog. Cardiovasc. Dis. *12*, 16–32 (1970)

Gibson, D.G., Balcon, R., Sowton, E.: The clinical use of ICI 50172 as an antidysrhythmic agent in patients with heart failure. Br. Med. J. (1968) *III*, 161–163

Gibson, D.G., Marshall, J.C., Lockey, E.: Assessment of proximal tubular sodium reabsorption during water diuresis in patients with heart disease. Br. Heart J. *32*, 399–405 (1970)

Gifford, R.W. Jr.: Clonidine in the management of mild hypertension in twenty-two patients. Cleveland Clin. Q. *36*, 173–182 (1969)

Gillam, P.M.S., Prichard, B.N.C.: Use of propranolol in angina pectoris. Br. Med. J. *1965 II*, 337–339 (1965)

Gillam, P.M.S., Prichard, B.N.C.: Propranolol in the therapy of angina pectoris. Am. J. Cardiol. *18*, 366–369 (1966)

Gillespie, T.A., Ambos, H.D., Sobel, B.E., Roberts, R.: Effects of dobutamine in patients with acute myocardial infarction. Am. J. Cardiol. *39*, 588–594 (1977)

Gilmore, E., Weil, J., Chidsey, C.: Treatment of essential hypertension with a new vasodilator in combination with beta-adrenergic blockade. N. Engl. J. Med. *282*, 521–527 (1970)

Ginn, W.M., Orgain, E.S.: Propranolol hydrochloride in the treatment of angina pectoris. JAMA *198*, 1214–1216 (1966)

Glass, P., Dulfano, M.J.: Evaluation of a new β_2-adrenergic receptor stimulant, terbutaline, in bronchial asthma. 1. Subcutaneous comparison with epinephrine. Curr. Ther. Res. *15*, 141–149 (1973)

Glontz, G.E., Saslaw, S.: Methyldopa fever. Arch. Intern. Med. *122*, 445–447 (1968)

Godfrey, S.: Childhood asthma. Br. J. Hosp. Med. *17*, 430–441 (1977)

Godfrey, S., König, P.: Inhibition of exercise induced asthma by different pharmacological pathways. Thorax *31*, 137–143 (1976)

Goldberg, A.D., Raftery, E.B.: Patterns of blood pressure during chronic administration of postganglionic sympathetic blocking drugs for hypertension. Lancet *1976 II*, 1052–1054
Goldberg, A.D., Raftery, E.B., Wilkinson, P.R.: The over-shoot phenomenon on withdrawal of clonidine therapy. Postgrad. Med. J. [Suppl. 7] *52*, 128–134 (1976)
Goldberg, L.I.: Cardiovascular and renal actions of dopamine: potential clinical applications. Pharmacol. Rev. *24*, 1–29 (1972)
Goldberg, L.I., Talley, R.C.: Current therapy of shock. Adv. Intern. Med. *17*, 363–378 (1971)
Goldberg, L.I., McDonald, R.H., Zimmerman, A.M.: Sodium diuresis produced by dopamine in patients with congestive heart failure. N. Engl. J. Med. *269*, 1060–1064 (1963)
Goldberg, L.I., Hseih, Y-Y., Resnekov, L.: Newer catecholamines for treatment of heart failure and shock. An update on dopamine and a first look at dobutamine. Prog. Cardiovasc. Dis. *19*, 327–340 (1977)
Goldberg, L.I., Kohli, J.D., Kotake, A.N., Volkman, P.H.: Characteristics of the vascular dopamine receptor; comparison with other receptors. Fed. Proc. *37*, 2396–2402 (1978)
Goldreyer, B.N.: Intracardiac electrocardiography in the analysis and understanding of cardiac arrhythmias. Ann. Intern. Med. *77*, 117–136 (1972)
Goldstein, S., Moss, A.J.: Sudden death and pre-hospital phase of acute myocardial infarction. Chest *61*, 600–602 (1972)
Gooding, P.G., Berman, E.: An evaluation of sotalol, a β-blocking agent, in patients with angina pectoris. Postgrad. Med. J. *50*, 734–736 (1974)
Gordon, R.D.: Effects of β-adrenoceptor blocking drugs on plasma volume, renin and aldosterone as components of their antihypertensive action. Drugs [Suppl. 1] *11*, 156–163 (1976)
Gottlieb, T.B., Katz, F.H., Chidsey, C.A.: Combined therapy with vasodilator drugs and beta adrenergic blockade in hypertension. A comparative study of minoxidil and hydralazine. Circulation *45*, 571–582 (1972)
Gould, L., Reddy, C.V.R., Kalanithi, P., Espina, L., Gomprecht, R.F.: Use of phentolamine in acute myocardial infarction. Am. Heart J. *88* (2), 144–148 (1974)
Graff-Lonnevig, V.: Double-blind trial with standard doses of fenoterol and salbutamol in asthmatic children. Acta Allergol. (Kbh.) *31*, 463–470 (1976)
Graham, R.M., Oates, H.F., Stoker, L.M., Stokes, G.S.: Alpha blocking action of the antihypertensive agent prazosin. J. Pharmacol. Exp. Ther. *201*, 747–752 (1977)
Grandjean, T., Hamer, N.J., Sowton, G.E., Melendz, L.: The effect of propranolol (inderal) on effort tolerance in angina pectoris. Cardiologica [Suppl. 2] *59*, 57–65 (1966)
Grant, R.H.E., Keelan, P., Kernohan, R.J., Leonard, J.C., Nancekieville, L., Sinclair, K.: Multicenter trial of propranolol in angina pectoris. Am. J. Cardiol. *18*, 361–365 (1966)
Granville-Grossman, K.L., Turner, P.: The effect of propranolol on anxiety. Lancet *1966 I*, 788–795
Greenblatt, D.J., Koch-Weser, J.: Adverse reactions to β-adrenergic receptor blocking drugs. A report from the Boston Collaborative Drug Surveillance Programme. Drugs *7*, 118–129 (1974)
Griffin, J.P., Turner, P.: Preliminary studies of a new bronchodilator (WG 253) in man. J. Clin. Pharmacol. *11*, 280–287 (1971)
Griffin, J.P., Williams, J.R.B., Maughan, E.: Studies in the human pharmacology and metabolism of rimiterol (pulmadil). Comparison with isoprenaline. Clin. Trials J. *10*, 13–17 (1973)
Grosz, H.J.: Narcotic withdrawal symptoms in heroin users treated with propranolol. Lancet *1972 II*, 564–565
Guazzi, M., Fiorentini, C., Polese, A., Olivari, M., Magrini, F.: Antihypertensive action of propranolol in man. Lack of evidence for a neural depressive effect. Clin. Pharmacol. Ther. *20*, 304–309 (1976)
Gunnar, R.M., Loeb, H.S., Pietras, R.J., Tobian, L.: Ineffectiveness of isoproterenol in shock due to acute myocardial infarction. JAMA *202*, 1124–1128 (1967)
Gunthner, W. Von: Experimental spirographic studies with 1-(3,5-dihydroxy-phenyl)-2-isopropyl aminoethanol sulphate as a therapeutic aerosol. Arzneim. Forsch. *12*, 1127–1129 (1962)
Gupta, S., Poddar, S.P., Nath, S.: Aerosolised bronchodilator therapy with and without IPPR in bronchial asthma – a comparative evaluation. Indian J. Chest Dis. *20*, 118–125 (1978)
Habersang, S. von, Klingler, K.H., Schlichtegroll, A. von: Struktur-Wirkungs-Beziehungen von bronchospasmolytisch wirksamen β-phenylathyl-amino-alkyl-xanthinen. Arzneim. Forsch. *27*, 14–21 (1977)

Hadden, D.R., Bell, T.K., McDevitt, D.G., Shanks, R.G., Montgomery, D.A.D., Weaver, J.A.: Propranolol and the utilisation of radioiodine by the human thyroid gland. Acta Endocrinol. (Kbh.) *61*, 393–399 (1969)

Haefely, W., Hurlimann, A., Thoenen, H.: Adrenergic transmitter changes and response to sympathetic nerve stimulation after differing pre-treatment with α-methyldopa. Br. J. Pharmacol. Chemother. *31*, 105–109 (1967)

Haerem, J.W.: Sudden coronary death: the occurrence of platelet aggregates in the epicardial arteries of man. Atherosclerosis *14*, 417 (1971)

Haeusler, G.: Clonidine-induced inhibition of sympathetic nerve activity: non indication for a central presynaptic or an indirect sympathomimetic mode of action. Naunyn-Schmiedebergs Arch. Pharmacol. *286*, 97–111 (1974)

Haeusler, G.: Cardiovascular regulation by central adrenergic mechanisms and its alteration of hypotensive drugs. Circ. Res. [Suppl. 1] *36*, 223–232 (1975)

Hagedoorn, A., Tjoa, S.T.: Practolol in the control of intraocular tension. Lancet *1974 I*, 733

Hamilton, M., Kopelman, H.: The treatment of severe hypertension with methyldopa. Br. Med. J. *1963 I*, 151–155

Hammer, J., Ulrych, M., Freis, E.D.: Hemodynamic and therapeutic effects of guancydine in hypertension. Clin. Pharmacol. Ther. *12*, 78–90 (1971)

Hansen, P.F., Rasmussen, P.A., Nyberg, G.: Alprenolol alone and in conjunction with pentanitrol in angina pectoris. Acta Med. Scand. *193*, 419–424 (1973)

Hansson, B.G., Hökfelt, B.: Prolonged treatment with penbutolol (HOE 893 d) in patients with moderate hypertension. I. Effects on blood pressure and pulse rate, catecholamines in blood and urine, plasma renin activity and urinary aldosterone under basal conditions and following exercise. Eur. J. Clin. Pharmacol. *9*, 9–19 (1975)

Hansson, B.G., Dymling, J.F., Hedeland, H., Hulthen, U.L.: Long-term treatment of moderate hypertension with the β_1-receptor blocking agent metoprolol. Eur. J. Clin. Pharmacol. *11*, 239–245 (1977 a)

Hansson, L.: Beta-adrenergic blockade in essential hypertension. Effects of propranolol on haemodynamic parameters and plasma renin activity. Acta Med. Scand. [Suppl.] *55*, 1–40 (1973)

Hansson, L., Hänel, B.: Labetalol, a new α- and β-adrenoceptor blocking agent in hypertension. Br. J. Clin. Pharmacol. [Suppl.] *3*, 763–764 (1976)

Hansson, L., Olander, R., Aberg, H.: Twice daily propranolol for the treatment of hypertension. Lancet *1971 a II*, 713

Hansson, L., Olander, R., Aberg, H., Malmcrona, R., Westerlund, A.: Treatment of hypertension with propranolol and hydralazine. Acta Med. Scand. *190*, 531–534 (1971 b)

Hansson, L., Pascual, A., Julius, S.: Comparison of guanadrel and guanethidine. Clin. Pharmacol. Ther. *14*, 204–208 (1973)

Hansson, L., Zweifler, A.J., Julius, S., Ellis, C.N.: Propranolol therapy in essential hypertension. Observations on predictability of therapeutic response. Int. J. Clin. Pharmacol. *10*, 79–89 (1974)

Hansson, L., Aberg, H., Karlberg, B.E., Westerlund, A.: Controlled study of atenolol in treatment of hypertension. Br. Med. J. *1975 I*, 367–370

Hansson, L., Berglund, G., Andersson, O., Holm, M.: Controlled trial of acebutolol in hypertension. Eur. J. Clin. Pharmacol. *12*, 89–92 (1977 b)

Harley, B.J.S., Davies, R.O.: Propranolol in the office treatment of angina pectoris. Can. Med. Assoc. J. *99*, 527–530 (1968)

Harris, A.: Long-term treatment of paroxysmal cardiac arrhythmias with propranolol. Am. J. Cardiol. *18*, 431–439 (1966)

Harrison, D.C., Chidsey, C.A., Braunwald, E.: Studies on the mechanism reaction of metaraminol (aramine). Ann. Intern. Med. *59*, 297–305 (1963)

Harrison, D.C., Braunwald, E., Glick, G., Mason, D.T., Chidsey, C.A.M., Ross, J. Jr.: Effects of β-adrenergic blockade on the circulation, with particular reference to observation in patients with hypertropic subaortic stenosis. Circulation *29*, 84–98 (1964)

Harrison, T.S.: Adrenal medullary and thyroid relationships. Physiol. Rev. *44*, 161–185 (1964)

Harrower, A.D.B., Nairn, I.M., Strong, J.A.: Effect of propranolol on glucose tolerance in hyperthyroidism. Postgrad. Med. J. *53*, 687–690 (1977)

Hartikainen, M., Heikkila, J.: Twice-daily pindolol and alprenolol in essential hypertension of moderate severity. Ann. Clin. Res. *8*, 85–92 (1976)
Hartley, D., Jack, D.: Selectivity of action in β-adrenoceptor stimulants. J. Appl. Chem. Biotechnol. *28*, 173–182 (1978)
Hastwell, G., Lambert, B.E.: The effect of oral salbutamol on serum potassium and blood sugar. Br. J. Obstet. Gynaecol. *85*, 767–769 (1978)
Hastwell, G.B., Halloway, C.P., Taylor, T.L.O.: A study of 208 patients in premature labour treated with orally administered salbutamol. Med. J. Aust. *1*, 465–469 (1978)
Hayes, J.M., Graham, R.M., O'Connell, B.P., Speers, E., Humphrey, T.J.: Effect of prazosin on plasma renin activity. Aust. N. Z. J. Med. *6*, 90 (1976)
Heatherington, D.J., Comerford, M.B., Nyberg, G., Besterman, E.M.M.: Comparison of two adrenergic beta-blocking agents, alprenolol and propranolol, in the treatment of angina pectoris. Br. Heart J. *35*, 320–333 (1973)
Hebb, A.R., Goodwin, T.F., Gunton, R.W.: A new beta-adrenergic blocking agent, propranolol, in the treatment of angina pectoris. Can. Med. Assoc. J. *98*, 246–251 (1968)
Heel, R.C., Brogden, R.N., Speight, T.M., Avery, G.S.: Fenoterol: A review of its pharmacological properties and therapeutic efficacy in asthma. Drugs *15*, 3–32 (1978)
Heffernan, A., Carty, A., O'Malley, K., Bugler, J.: A within patient comparison of debrisoquine and methyldopa in hypertension. Br. Med. J. *1971 I*, 75–78
Heise, A., Kroneberg, G.: α-sympathetic receptor stimulation in the brain and hypotensive activity of α-methyldopa. Eur. J. Pharmacol. *17*, 315–317 (1972)
Hemminki, E., Starfield, B.: Prevention and treatment of premature labour by drugs: review of controlled clinical trials. Br. J. Obstet. Gynaecol. *85*, 411–417 (1978)
Hendricks, C.H., Cibils, L.A., Pose, S.V., Eskes, T.K.A.B.: The pharmacologic control of excessive uterine activity with isoxsuprine. Am. J. Obstet. Gynecol. *82*, 1064–1078 (1961)
Henning, M.: Central sympathetic transmitters and hypertension. Clin. Sci. Mol. Med. *48*, 195–203 (1975)
Henning, M., Rubenson, A.: Evidence that the hypotensive action of methyldopa is mediated by the central actions of methylnoradrenaline. J. Pharm. Pharmacol. *23*, 407–411 (1971)
Henning, M., van Zwieten, P.A.: Central hypertensive effect of α-methyldopa. J. Pharm. Pharmacol. *20*, 409–417 (1968)
Herschfus, J.A., Bresnick, E., Levinson, L., Segal, M.S.: A new sympathomimetic amine (neosuprel) in the treatment of bronchial asthma. Ann. Allergy *9*, 769–773 (1951)
Hertting, G.: The fate of ^{3}H-isoproterenol in the rat. Biochem. Pharmacol. *13*, 1119–1128 (1964)
Herxheimer, H.: Dosage of ephedrine in bronchial and emphysema. Br. Med. J. *1946 I*, 350–352
Hesse, B., Pedersen, J.T.: Hypoglycaemia after propranolol in children. Acta Med. Scand. *193*, 551–552 (1973)
Hetzel, M.R., Clark, T.J.H.: Comparison of intravenous and aerosol salbutamol. Br. Med. J. *1976 II*, 919
Hetzel, M.R., Clark, T.J.H.: Comparison of salbutamol rotohaler with conventional pressurised aerosol. Clin. Allergy *7*, 563–568 (1977)
Hickie, J.B.: Alprenolol (aptin) in angina pectoris. A double-blind multicentre trial. Med. J. Aust. *2*, 268–272 (1970)
Hjalmarson, A., Waagstein, F., Waldenstrom, A.: Effects of cardioselective beta-blockers on chest pain, ECG and heart function in acute myocardial infarction. Br. Heart J. *38*, 530–531 (1976)
Hoefke, W., Warnke-Sachs, E.: Influence of desmethylimipramine on the hypotensive effect of clonidine. Arzneim. Forsch. *24*, 1046–1047 (1974)
Hoffman, B.F., Singer, D.H.: Appraisal of the effects of catecholamines on cardiac electrical activity. Ann. N.Y. Acad. Sci. *139*, 914–939 (1967)
Hollister, L.E., Prusmack, J.J.: Propranolol in withdrawal from opiates. Arch. Gen. Psychiatry *31*, 695–698 (1974)
Holloway, G.A., Frederickson, E.L.: Dobutamine, a new beta agonist. Anaesth. Analg. *53*, 616–622 (1974)
Holten, K.: Bronchodilator effect and effect on blood gases after subcutaneous injection and inhalation of terbutaline. Br. J. Dis. Chest *68*, 111–120 (1974)

Honey, M., Chamberlain, D.A., Howard, J.: The effect of β-sympathetic blockade on arterial oxygen saturation in Fallot's tetralogy. Circulation *30*, 501–510 (1964)
Hoobler, S.W., Sagastume, E.: Clonidine hydrochloride in the treatment of hypertension. Am. J. Cardiol. *28*, 67–73 (1971)
Hopkirk, J.A.C., Simpson, N.B., Fitzgerald, W.R.: Vomiting with clonidine withdrawal. Br. Med. J. (1975) *III*, 435
Horn, M.E., Prichard, B.N.C.: A variable dose comparative trials of propranolol and sotalol in angina pectoris. Br. Heart J. *35*, 555 (1973)
Horwitz, D., Fox, S.M., Goldberg, L.I.: Effects of dopamine in man. Circ. Res. *10*, 237–243 (1962)
Howitt, G., Rowlands, D.J.: Beta-sympathetic blockade in hyperthyrodism. Lancet *1966 II*, 628–631
Hua, A.S.P., Macdonald, I.M., Myers, J.B., Fang, P., Kincaid-Smith, P.: Studies with prazosin. A new effective hypotensive agent. II Two double-blind crossover studies comparing the effects of prazosin and hydrallazine. Med. J. Aust. *2*, 5–9 (1977)
Hubner, P., Ziady, G., Lane, G., Pridie, R., Scales, J.: Controlled clinical trial of β-adrenergic blockade in hypertrophic obstructive cardiomyopathy. Br. Heart J. *34*, 963 (1972)
Huhti, E.: Clinical comparison of terbutaline and isoprenaline administered by inhalation. A double-blind study. Ann. Clin. Res. *4*, 152–164 (1972)
Huhti, E., Poukkula, A.: Clinical comparison of fenoterol and albuterol administration by inhalation. Chest *73*, 348–351 (1978)
Hume, K.M., Gandevia, B.: Forced expiratory volume before and after isoprenaline. Thorax *12*, 276–278 (1957)
Humphreys, G.S., Delvin, D.G.: Ineffectiveness of propranolol in hypertensive Jamaicans. Br. Med. J. *1968 II*, 601–603
Hunyor, S.N., Hansson, L., Harrison, T.S., Hoobler, S.W.: Effects of clonidine withdrawal: possible mechanisms and suggestions for management. Br. Med. J. *1972 II*, 209–211
Hutchison, J.H.: Respiratory diseases. In: Practical paediatric problems, 4th ed., pp. 265–269. London: Lloyd-Luke 1975
Ibsen, H., Rasmussen, K., Aerenlund Jensen, H.: Aendringer i plasmavolumen, extracellulaervolumen og den glomerulaere filtrations-hastighed under kombinationsbehandling med propranolol og prazosin hos patienter med hypertension. Curr. Med. Res. Opinion *4*, (Suppl. 2), *4*, 83–88 (1977)
Ibsen, H., Rasmussen, Jensen, H.A., Leth, A.: Changes in plasma volume and extracellular volume after addition of hydrallazine to propranolol treatment in patients with hypertension. Acta Med. Scand. *203*, 419–423 (1978)
Ikram, H.: Propranolol in persistent ventricular fibrillation complicating acute myocardial infarction. Am. Heart J. *75*, 795–796 (1968)
Imhof, P., Brunner, H.: The treatment of functional heart disorders with beta-adrenergic blocking agents. Postgrad. Med. J. *46*, 96–101 (1970)
Ingemarsson, I.: Effect of terbutaline on premature labor. A double blind placebo controlled study. Am. J. Obstet. Gynecol. *125*, 520–524 (1976)
Ingenito, A.J., Barrett, J.P., Procita, L.: A centrally mediated peripheral hypotensive effect of α-methyldopa. J. Pharmacol. Exp. Ther. *175*, 593–599 (1970)
Ingram, G.I.C., Jones, R.V.: The rise in clotting factor VIII induced in man by adrenaline: effect of α- and β-blockers. J. Physiol. (Lond.) *187*, 447–454 (1966)
Inman, W.H.W., Adelstein, A.M.: Rise and fall of asthma mortality in England and Wales in relation to use of pressurised aerosols. Lancet *1969 II*, 279–285
Innes, I.R., Nickerson, M.: Norepinephrine, epinephrine and the sympathomimetic amines. In: The pharmacological basis of therapeutics, 5th ed. Goodman, L.S., Gilman, A. (eds.), pp. 477–513 (1975) New York: Macmillan
Irving, M.H., Britton, B.J., Wood, W.G., Padgham, C., Carruthers, M.: Effects of β-adrenergic blockade on plasma catecholamines in exercise. Nature *248*, 531–533 (1974)
Iversen, L.L.: Catecholamine uptake processes. Br. Med. Bull. *29*, 130–135 (1973)
Iwasawa, Y., Kiyomoto, A.: Studies on tetrahydroisoquinolines (THI). 1. Bronchodilator activity and structure-activity relationship. J. J. Pharmacol. *17*, 143–152 (1967)
Jackson, G., Atkinson, L., Oram, S.: Double-blind comparison of tolamolol, propranolol, practolol and placebo in the treatment of angina pectoris. Br. Med. J. (1975a) *I*, 708–712

Jackson, G., Atkinson, L., Oram, S.: Re-assessment of failed beta-blocker treatment in angina pectoris by peak-exercise heart rate measurements. Br. Med. J. (1975b) *III*, 616–618
Jackson, W.B.: Tolerance and side effects during long-term treatment of hypertension with debrisoquine. Aust. N. Z. J. Med. *2*, 357–365 (1972)
Jahre, J.A., Grace, W.J., Greenbaum, D.M., Sarg, M.J.: Medical approach to the hypotensive patient and the patient in shock. Clin. Manage. Crit. Care *4*, 577–587 (1975)
Janowsky, D.S., El-Yousef, M.K., Davis, J.M., Fann, W.E.: Antagonism of guanethidine by chlorpromazine. Am. J. Psychiatry *130*, 808–812 (1973)
Jefferson, J.W.: Beta-adrenergic receptor blocking drugs in psychiatry. Arch. Gen. Psychiatry *31*, 681–691 (1974)
Jennings, K., Parsons, V.: A study of labetalol in patients of European, West Indian and West African origin. Br. J. Clin. Pharmacol. [Suppl.] *3*, 773–775 (1976)
Jensen-Holm, J., Juul, P.: The effects of guanethidine pre- and post-ganglionic nerve division on the rat superior cervical ganglion: Cholinesterases and protein. Acta Pharmacol. Toxicol. *28*, 270–282 (1970)
Jewitt, D.E., Croxson, R.: Oractolol in the management of cardiac dysrhythmias following myocardial infarction and cardiac surgery. Postgrad. Med. J. [Suppl.] *47*, 25–29 (1971)
Johnson, A.M.: Norepinephrine and cyanotic attacks in Fallot's tetralogy. Br. Heart J. *23*, 197–202 (1961)
Johnson, E.S.: A basis for migraine therapy – the autonomic theory reappraised. Postgrad. Med. J. *54*, 231–242 (1978)
Johnson, J.W., Austin, K.L., Jones, G.S., Davis, G.H., King, T.M.: Efficacy of 17 alpha-hydroxyprogesterone caproate in the prevention of premature labor. N. Engl. J. Med. *293*, 675–680 (1975)
Johnson, P., Kitchin, A.H., Lowther, C.P., Turner, R.W.D.: Treatment of hypertension with methyldopa. Br. Med. J. *1966 I*, 133–137
Johnson, S.A., Gunnar, R.M.: Treatment of shock in myocardial infarction. JAMA *237*, 2106–2108 (1977)
Johnston, A.W., Prichard, B.N.C., Rosenheim, M.L.: The use of bethanidine in the treatment of hypertension. Lancet *1964 II*, 659–661
Jonsson, L.E.: Pharmacological blockade of amphetamine effects in amphetamine dependent subjects. Eur. J. Clin. Pharmacol. *4*, 206–211 (1972)
Julius, S., Pascual, A.V., Abbrecht, P.H., London, R.: Effect of beta-adrenergic blockade on plasma volume in human subjects. Proc. Soc. Exp. Biol. Med. *140*, 982–985 (1972)
Juul, P.: Effects of various antihypertensive guanidine derivatives on the adult rat superior cervical ganglion; histology, ultrastructure and cholinesterase histochemistry. Acta Pharmacol. Toxicol. (Kbh) *32*, 500–512 (1973)
Kakaviatos, N., Tuckman, J., Chupkovich, V., Finnerty, F.A. Jr.: Pressor and depressor of Ro5-3307/1 (Declinax). Am. J. Cardiol. *13*, 111–112 (1964)
Kaliner, M., Austen, K.F.: Immunologic release of chemical mediators from human tissues. Annu. Rev. Pharmacol. *15*, 177–189 (1975)
Kamburoff, P.L.: Bronchomotor tone and its modification by certain drugs. Postgrad. Med. J. *52*, 190–194 (1976)
Kammer, G.M., Hamilton, E.R.: Acute bulbar muscle dysfunction and hyperthyroidism: a study of four cases and review of the literature. Am. J. Med. *56*, 464–470 (1974)
Kane, J., Gregg, I., Richards, D.A.: A double-blind trial of labetalol. Br. J. Clin. Pharmacol. [Suppl.] *3*, 737–774 (1976)
Kannel, W.B., Feinleib, M.: Natural history of angina pectoris in the Framingham Study. Prognosis and survival. Am. J. Cardiol. *29*, 154–163 (1972)
Kardos, G.G.: Isoproterenol in the treatment of shock due to bacteraemia with gram-negative pathogens. N. Engl. J. Med. *274*, 868–873 (1966)
Karlberg, B., Hornkvist, P.E.: Propranolol in the treatment of hypertension. Opusc. Med. *16*, 296–299 (1971)
Kaumann, A.J., Birnbaumer, L.: Studies on receptor-mediated activation of adenylcyclases. J. Biol. Chem. *249*, 7874–7885 (1974)
Keefer, C., Resnick. W.: Angina pectoris. A syndrome caused by anoxemia of the myocardium. Arch. Intern. Med. *41*, 769–817 (1928)

Keelan, P.: Double-blind trial of propranolol (Inderal) in angina pectoris. Br. Med. J. *1965 I*, 897–898

Keighley, J.F.: Latrogenic asthma associated with adrenergic aerosols. Ann. Intern. Med. *65*, 985–995 (1966)

Kelliher, G.J., Buckley, J.P.: Central hypotensive activity of dl- and d-propranolol. J. Pharm. Sci. *59*, 1276–1280 (1970)

Kelly, D.T., Delgado, C.E., Taylor, D.R., Pitt, B., Ross, R.S.: Use of phentolamine in acute myocardial infarction associated with hypertension and left ventricular failure. Circulation *47*, 729–735 (1973)

Kelman, G.R.: Applied circulatory physiology, p. 188. London: Butterworths 1971

Kerr, J.W., Govindaraj, M., Patel, K.R.: Effect of alpha-receptor blocking drugs and disodium chromoglycate on histamine hypersensitivity in bronchial asthma. Br. Med. J. *1970 II*, 139–141

Kerstin, F., Follath, F., Moulds, R., Mucklow, J., McCloy, R., Sheares, J., Dollery, C.T.: A comparison of cardiovascular effects of dobutamine and isoprenaline after open heart surgery. Br. Heart J. *38*, 622–626 (1976,)

Keyrilainen, O., Nyberg, G., Uusitalo, A.J.: Effects of alprenolol and isosorbide dinitrate in angina pectoris. Acta Med. Scand. *193*, 281–292 (1973)

Khambatta, R.B.: Comparison of a new β-receptor blocking agent acebutolol (sectral) and propranolol. Clin. Trials J. [Suppl. 3] *11*, 59–67 (1974)

Khatri, I.M., Cohn, J.N.: Mechanism of exercise hypotension after sympathetic blockade. Am. J. Cardiol. *25*, 329–338 (1970)

Kincaid-Smith, P.: Vasodilators in the treatment of hypertension. Med. J. Aust. *1*, 7–9 (1975)

Kincaid-Smith, P., Fang, P., Laver, M.C.: A new look at the treatment of severe hypertension. Clin. Sci. Mol. Med. [Suppl. 1] *45*, 75–87S (1973)

Kincaid-Smith, P., MacDonald, I.M., Hua, A., Laver, M.C., Fang, P.: Changing concepts in the management of hypertension. Med. J. Aust. *1*, 327–332 (1975)

Kingsley, P.J., Littlejohns,. D.W., Prichard, B.N.C.: Isoprenaline-induced tachycardia in man. Br. J. Pharmacol. *46*, 539P (1972)

Kitchin, A.H., Turner, R.W.D.: Studies on debrisoquine sulphate. Br. Med. J. *1966 II*, 728–731

Klaustermeyer, W.B., Di Bernardo, R.L., Hale, F.C.: Intravenous isoproterenol: rationale for bronchial asthma. J. Allergy Clin. Immunol. *55*, 325–333 (1975)

Klevans, L.R., Kovacs, J.L., Kelly, R.: Central effect of beta adrenergic blocking agents on arterial blood pressure. J. Pharmacol. Exp. Ther. *196*, 389–395 (1976)

Klinge, E., Aro, S.: Effect of beta-adrenergic blocking compounds on tissue catecholamine levels. Eur. J. Immunol. *14*, 124–129 (1971)

Kobinger, W.: Über den Wirkungsmechanismus einer neuen antihypertensiven Substanz mit Imidazolinstruktur. Naunyn Schmiedebergs Arch. Pharmacol. *258*, 48–58 (1967)

Kobinger, W., Klupp, H.: Pharmacological and biochemical evidence for the activation of central alpha-adrenoceptors by clonidine and related compounds. In: Recent advances in hypertension. Milliez, P., Safar, M. (eds.), Vol. 1, pp. 53–56. Reims: Societe Alina 1975

Kobinger, W., Pichler, L.: Evidence for direct alpha-adrenoceptor stimulation of effector neurons in cardiovascular centers by clonidine. Eur. J. Pharmacol. *27*, 151–154 (1974)

Kobinger, W., Pichler, L.: Localization in the C.N.S. of adrenoceptors which facilitate a cardioinhibitory reflex. Naunyn Schmiedebergs Arch. Pharmacol. *286*, 371–377 (1975)

Kobinger, W., Walland, A.: Investigations into the mechanism of the hypotensive effect of 2-(2,6-dichlorophenylamino)-2-imidazoline hydrochloride. Eur. J. Pharmacol. *2*, 155–162 (1967)

Kobinger, W., Walland, A.: Involvement of adrenergic receptors in central vagus activity. Eur. J. Pharmacol. *16*, 120–122 (1971)

Koch, G.: Combined α- and β-adrenoceptor blockade with oral labetalol in hypertensive patients with reference to haemodynamic effects at rest and during exercise. Br. J. Clin. Pharmacol. [Suppl.] *3*, 729–732 (1976)

Koch, G.: Acute hemodynamic effects of alpha- and beta-receptor agent (AH 5158) on the systemic and pulmonary circulation at rest and during exercise in hypertensive patients. Am. Heart J. *93*, 585–591 (1977)

Koldsland, O.H.: The hypotensive action of pindolol (visken) at different dose levels. Curr. Ther. Res. *22*, 853–860 (1977)

Konzett, H.: Neue broncholytisch hochwirksame Körper der Adrenalinreihe. Naunyn Schmiedebergs Arch. Exp. Pathol. Pharmakol. *197*, 27–40 (1940)
Korner, P.I., Blombery, P.A., Bobik, A., Tonkin, A.M., Uther, J.B.: Valsalva vasoconstrictor reflex in human hypertension and after β-adrenoceptor blockade in conscious rabbits. Clin. Sci. Mol. Med. *51*, 365–368 (1976)
Koshy, M.C., Mickley, D., Bourgiognie, J., Blanfox, M.D.: Physiologic evaluation of a new antihypertensive agent: Prazosin HCl. Circulation *55*, 533–577 (1977)
Krasnow, N., Rolett, E.L., Yurchak, P.M., Hood, W.B., Gorlin, R.: Isoproterenol and cardiovascular performance. Am. J. Med. *37*, 514–525 (1964)
Kroneberg, G., Heise, A.: Evidence for an activation of central alpha-adrenoceptors as the cause of the central hypotensive effect of alpha-methyldopa and its metabolites. In: Recent advances in hypertension. Milliez, P., Safar, M. (eds.), Vol. 1, pp. 57–61. Reims: Societe Alina 1975
Lahdensuo, A., Alanko, K.: The efficacy, as modified by the circadian rhythm, of salbutamol administered by different routes. Scand. J. Respir. Dis. *57*, 231–238 (1976)
Lal, S., Savidge, R.S., Davies, D.M., Ali, M.M., Soni, V.: Intravenous salbutamol and cardiogenic shock. Lancet *1972 I*, 853–854 (1972)
Lal, S., Dash, C.H., Gribben, M.D.: An economical method of comparing inhaled bronchodilators in reversible diffuse airways obstruction. With special reference to a beta-2 stimulant – salmefamol. Thorax *29*, 317–322 (1974)
Lambert, D.M.D.: Effect of propranolol on mortality in patients with angina. Postgrad. Med. J. [Suppl. 4] *52*, 57–60 (1976)
Lancaster, R., Goodwin, T.J., Peart, W.S.: The effect of pindolol on plasma renin activity and blood pressure in hypertensive patients. Br. J. Clin. Pharmacol. *3*, 453–460 (1976)
Lands, A.M., Arnold, A., McAuliff, F.P., Luduena, F.P., Brown, T.G.: Differentiation of receptor systems activated by sympathomimetic amines. Nature *214*, 597–598 (1967)
Langer, S.Z.: Pre-synaptic regulation of catecholamine release. Biochem. Pharmacol. *23*, 1793–1800 (1974)
Langer, A., Hung, C.T., McAnulty, J.A., Harrigan, J.T., Washington, E.: Adrenergic blockade: a new approach to hyperthyroidism during pregnancy. Obstet. Gynaecol. *44*, 181–186 (1974)
Langley, J.N.: On the reactions of cells and of nerve-endings to certain poisons, chiefly as regards the reaction of striated muscles to nicotine and to curare. J. Physiol. (Lond.) *33*, 374–413 (1905)
Larsen, J.J., Hermansen, K.: Pharmacodynamics of a new selective β_2-adrenergic bronchodilator 3-(4-methoxy benzyl amino)-4-hydroxy-α-(tert-butylaminomethyl) benzyl alcohol HCl (QH25). Acta Pharmacol. Toxicol. (Kbh) *40*, 42–64 (1977)
Larsson, S., Svedmyr, N., Thiringer, G.: Lack of bronchial β-adrenoceptor resistance in asthmatics during long-term treatment with terbutaline. J. Allergy Clin. Immunol. *59*, 93–100 (1977)
Lauersen, N.H., Merkatz, I.R., Tejani, N., Wilson, K.H., Roberson, A., Mann, L.I., Fuchs, F.: Inhibition of premature labor: a multicenter comparison of ritodrine and ethanol. Am. J. Obstet. Gynecol. *127*, 837–845 (1977)
Laver, M.C., Fang, P., Kincaid-Smith, P.: Double blind comparison of two beta blocking drugs with previous therapy in the treatment of hypertension. Med. J. Aust. *1*, 174–176 (1974)
Laverty, R.: The mechanisms of action of some antihypertensive drugs. Br. Med. Bull. *29*, 152–157 (1973)
Lawford, P., Jones, B.J.M., Milledge, J.S.: Comparison of intravenous and nebulised salbutamol in the initial treatment of severe asthma. Br. Med. J. *1978 I*, 84
Lawson, D.H., Gloss, D., Jick, H.: Adverse reactions to methyldopa with particular reference to hypotension. Am. Heart J. *96*, 572–579 (1978)
Lee, T.C., Coffey, R.J., Mackin, J., Cobb, M., Routon, J., Canary, J.J.: The use of propranolol in the surgical treatment of thyrotoxic patients. Ann. Surg. *177*, 643–647 (1973)
Leegaard, J., Fjulsrud, S.: Terbutaline in children with asthma. Arch. Dis. Child. *48*, 229–232 (1973)
Lees, N.W.: The diagnosis and treatment of endotoxic shock. Anaesthesia *31*, 897–909 (1976)
Legge, J.S., Gaddie, J., Palmer, K.N.V.: Comparison of two oral selective β_2-adrenergic stimulant drugs in bronchial asthma. Br. Med. J. *1971 I*, 637–639

Leier, C.V., Webel, J., Bush, C.A.: The cardiovascular effects of the continuous infusion of dobutamine in patients with severe cardiac failure. Circulation *56*, 468–472 (1977)

Leier, C.V., Heban, P.T., Huss, P., Bush, C.A., Lewis, R.P.: Comparative systemic and regional haemodynamic effects of dopamine and dobutamine in patients with cardiomyopathic heart failure. Circulation *58*, 466–475 (1978)

Leifer, K.N., Wittig, H.J.: The $beta_2$ sympathomimetic aerosols in the treatment of asthma. Ann. Allergy *35*, 69–80 (1975)

Leishman, A.W., Matthews, H.L., Smith, A.J.: Guanethidine: Hypotensive drug with prolonged action. Lancet *1959 II*, 1044–1048

Leishman, A.W.D., Thirkettle, J.L., Allen, B.R., Dixon, R.A.: Controlled trial of oxprenolol and practolol in hypertension. Br. Med. J. (1970) *IV*, 342–344

Leitch, A.G., Hopkin, J.M., Ellis, D.A., Merchant, S., McHardy, G.J.R.: The effect of aerosol ipratropium bromide and salbutamol on exercise tolerance in chronic bronchitis. Thorax *33*, 711–713 (1978)

Lenney, W., Milner, A.D.: Recurrent wheezing in the pre-school child. Arch. Dis. Child. *53*, 468–473 (1978a)

Lenney, W., Milner, A.D.: At what age do bronchodilator drugs work? Arch. Dis. Child. *53*, 532–535 (1978b)

Lenney, W., Milner, A.D., Hiller, E.J.: Use of salbutamol powder in childhood asthma. Arch. Dis. Child. *53*, 958–961 (1978)

Leonetti, G., Mayer, G., Morganti, A., Terzoli, L., Zanchetti, A., Bianchetti, G., Disalle, E., Morselli, P.L., Chidsey, C.A.: Hypotensive and renin-suppressing activities of propranolol in hypertensive patients. Clin. Sci. Mol. Med. *48*, 491–499 (1975)

Leonetti, G., Terzoli, L., Morganti, A., Manfrin, M., Bianchini, C., Sala, C., Zanchetti, A.: Relation between the hypotensive and renin-suppressing activities of alpha-methyldopa in hypertensive patients. Am. J. Cardiol. *40*, 762–767 (1977)

Leopold, D., Handslip, P.: Additive interaction of aminophylline and salbutamol in asthma: an in vivo study using dose response curves. J. Int. Med. Res. [Supp. 1] *7*, 52–55 (1979)

Letac, B., Fillastre, J.P., Wolf, L.M.: The treatment of essential hypertension with acebutalol (sectral). Clin. Trials J. [Suppl. 3] *11*, 92–95 (1974)

Levey, G.S.: Catecholamine sensitivity, thyroid hormone and the heart: A re-evaluation. Am. J. Med. *50*, 413–420 (1971)

Levine, P.A., McGillavary, M., Klein, M.D., Faxon, D., Ryan, T.J.: Dopamine dose in cardiogenic shock. Circulation [Suppl. 11] *51–52*, 208 (1975)

Levine, R.J., Sjoerdsma, A.: Dissociation of the decarboxylase-inhibiting and norepinephrine-depleting effects of α-methyldopa, α-ethyldopa, 4-bromo, 3-hydroxybenzyloxyamine and related substances. J. Pharmacol. Exp. Ther. *146*, 42–47 (1964)

Levine, R.J., Strauch, B.S.: Hypertensive responses to methyldopa. N. Engl. J. Med. *275*, 946–948 (1966)

Lewis, C.M., Brink, A.J.: Beta-adrenergic blockade: haemodynamic and myocardial energy metabolism in patients with ischaemic heart disease. Am. J. Cardiol. *21*, 846–859 (1968)

Lewis, P.J., Haeusler, G.: Reduction in sympathetic nervous activity as a mechanism for hypotensive effect of propranolol. Nature *256*, 440 (1975)

Liggins, G.C., Vaughan, G.S.: Intravenous infusion of salbutamol in the management of premature labour. J. Obstet. Gynaecol. Br. Commonw. *80*, 29–32 (1973)

Light, R.W., Summer, W.R., Luchsinger, P.C.: Response of patients with chronic obstructive lung disease to the regular administration of nebulized isoproterenol. A double-blind crossover study. Chest *67*, 634–639 (1975)

Linken, A.: Propranolol for LSD-induced anxiety states. Lancet *1971 II*, 1039–1040

Lipshitz, J., Baillie, P.: Uterine and cardiovascular effects of $beta_2$ selective sympathomimetic drugs administered as an intravenous infusion. S. Afr. Med. J. *50*, 1973–1977 (1976)

Liu, D.T.Y., Blackwell, R.J.: The value of a scoring system in predicting outcome of pre-term labour and comparing the efficacy of treatment with aminophylline and salbutamol. Br. J. Obstet. Gynaecol. *85*, 418–424 (1978)

Livesley, B., Catley, P.F., Campbell, R.C., Oram, S.: Double-blind evaluation of verapamil, propranolol and isosorbide dinitrate against a placebo in the treatment of angina pectoris. Br. Med. J. *1973 I*, 375–378

Livett, B.G.: Histochemical visualisation of peripheral and central adrenergic neurones. Br. Med. Bull. *29*, 93–99 (1973)
Loeb, H.S., Khan, M., Klodnychy, M.Z., Sinno, M.Z., Towne, W.D., Gunnar, R.M.: Haemodynamic effects of dobutamine in man. Circ. Shock *2*, 29–35 (1975)
Loeb, H.S., Bredakis, J., Gunnar, R.M.: Superiority of dobutamine over dopamine for augmentation of cardiac output in patients with chronic low output cardiac failure. Circulation *55*, 375–381 (1977)
Lohmoller, G., Frohlich, E.D.: A comparison of timolol and propranolol in essential hypertension. Am. Heart J. *89*, 437–442 (1975)
Lombardo, T.A., Rose, L.R., Taeschler, M., Tuluy, S., Bing, R.J.: The effect of exercise on coronary blood flow, myocardial oxygen consumption and cardiac efficiency in man. Circulation *7*, 71–78 (1953)
Lorimer, A.R., Dunn, F.G., Jones, J.V., Clark, B., Lawrie, T.D.V.: Indications for beta-adrenoceptor blocking drugs in hypertension. Postgrad. Med. J. [Suppl. 4] *52*, 81–85 (1976)
Louis, W.J., Doyle, A.E., Anavekar, S.: Plasma norepinephrine levels in essential hypertension. N. Engl. J. Med. *288*, 599–601 (1973)
Louis, W.J., Brignell, M.J., McNeil, J.J., Christophidis, N., Vajda, F.J.E.: Labetalol in hypertension. Lancet *1978 I*, 452–453
Lowenstein, H.: Propranolol as a psychotropic agent. Lancet *1973 I*, 559–560
Lowther, C.P., Turner, R.W.D.: Guanethidine in the treatment of hypertension. Br. Med. J. *1963 II*, 776–781
Ludvigsson, J.: Propranolol in treatment of migraine in children. Lancet *1973 II*, 799
Lund-Johansen, P.: Haemodynamic changes in long-term α-methyldopa therapy of essential hypertension. Acta Med. Scand. *192*, 221–226 (1972)
Lund-Johansen, P.: Hemodynamic changes at rest and during exercise in long-term prazosin therapy of essential hypertension. In: Prazosin – Evaluation of a new hypertensive agent. Cotton, D.W.K. (ed.), pp. 43–53. Amsterdam: Excerpta Medica 1974
Lund-Johansen, P.: Hemodynamic long-term effects of timolol at rest and during exercise in essential hypertension. Acta Med. Scand. *199*, 263–267 (1976a)
Lund-Johansen, P.: Hemodynamic long-term effects of a new β-adrenoceptor blocking drug atenolol (ICI 66082) in essential hypertension. Br. J. Clin. Pharmacol. *3*, 445–451 (1976b)
Lund-Larsen, P.G., Sivertssen, E.: Hemodynamic effects of propranolol (inderal) and H 56/28 (aptin) in patients with acute myocardial infarction. A comparative study. Acta Med. Scand. *186*, 187–191 (1969)
Luria, M.H., Freis, E.D.: Treatment of hypertension with debrisoquin sulfate (Declinax). Curr. Ther. Res. *7*, 289–296 (1965)
Lyon, L.J., Nevins, M.A.: Alprenolol treatment of angina pectoris. JAMA *215*, 1669 (1971)
MacDonald, M.J., Cullen, P.M., Phillips, C.J.: Atenolol versus propranolol: a comparison of ocular hypotensive effect of an oral dose. Br. J. Ophthalmol. *60*, 789–791 (1976)
MacDonald, M.J., Gore, S.M., Cullen, P.M., Phillips, C.I.: Comparison of ocular hypotensive effects of acetazolamide and atenolol. Br. J. Ophthalmol. *61*, 345–348 (1977)
MacDougall, A.I., Addis, G.J., Mackay, N., Dymock, I.W., Turpie, A.G.G., Ballingall, D.L., MacLennan, W.J., Whiting, B., MacArthur, J.G.: Treatment of hypertension with clonidine. Br. Med. J. (1970) *III*, 440–442
Mackie, I.A., Seal, D.V., Pescod, J.M.: Beta-adrenergic receptor blocking drugs: tear lysozyme and immunological screening for adverse reaction. Br. J. Ophthalmol. *61*, 354–359 (1977)
Mackin, J.F., Canary, J.J., Pitman, C.S.: Thyroid storm and its management. N. Engl. J. Med. *291*, 1396–1398 (1974)
MacLean, L.D., Duff, J.H., Scott, H.M., Peretz, D.I.: Treatment of shock in man based on hemodynamic diagnosis. Surg. Gynecol. Obstet. *120*, 1–16 (1965)
Magnusson, G., Hansson, E.: Myocardial necrosis in the rat: a comparison between isoprenaline, orciprenaline, salbutamol and terbutaline. Cardiology *58*, 174–180 (1973)
Majid, P.A., Sharma, B., Taylor, S.H.: Phentolamine for vasodilator treatment of severe heart-failure. Lancet *1971 II*, 719–724
Majid, P.A., Meeran, M.K., Benaim, M.E., Sharma, B., Taylor, S.H.: Alpha and beta-adrenergic receptor blockade in the treatment of hypertension. Br. Heart J. *36*, 588–596 (1974)
Malmqvist, J., Oates, J.A.: Effects of adrenergic neuron-blocking guanidine derivatives on mitochondrial metabolism. Biochem. Pharmacol. *17*, 1845–1854 (1968)

Malta, E., Raper, C.: Non-catechol phenylethanolamines: agonistic and antagonistic actions on beta adrenoceptors in isolated tissues from guinea pig. Clin. Exp. Pharmacol. Physiol. *1*, 259–268 (1974)
Malvea, B.P., Gwon, N., Graham, J.R.: Propranolol prophylaxis of migraine. Headache *12*, 163–167 (1973)
Mándi, A., Galfóczy, G., Galambos, E.: Über die bronchodilatatorische Wirkung von Reproterol. Arzneim. Forsch. *27*, 60–63 (1977)
Maneksha, S.: A comparative assessment of three bronchodilator preparations in general practice. J. Int. Med. Res. [Suppl. 1] *7*, 62–66 (1979)
Marlin, G.E., Turner, P.: Comparison of the β_2-adrenoceptor selectivity of rimiterol, salbutamol and isoprenaline by the intravenous route in man. Br. J. Clin. Pharmacol. *2*, 41–48 (1975)
Maroko, P.R., Kjekshus, J.K., Sobel, B.E., Watanabe, T., Covell, J.W., Ross, J., Braunwald, E.: Factors influencing infarct size following experimental coronary artery occlusions. Circulation *43*, 67–82 (1971)
Marsden, C.D., Meadows, J.C.: The effect of adrenaline on the contraction of human muscle. J. Physiol. (Lond.) *207*, 429–448 (1970)
Marsden, C.D., Foley, T.H., Owen, D.A.L., McAllister, R.G.: Peripheral β-adrenergic receptors concerned with tremor. Clin. Sci. *33*, 53–65 (1967)
Marsden, C.D., Gimlette, T.M.D., McAllister, R.G., Owen, D.A.L., Miller, T.N.: Effect of β-adrenergic blockade on finger tremor and Achilles reflex time in anxious and thyrotoxic patients. Acta Endocrinol. (Kbh.) *57*, 353–362 (1968)
Marshall, A.J., Roberts, C.J.C., Barritt, D.W.: Raynaud's phenomenon as a side effect of betablockers in hypertension. Br. Med. J. *1976 I*, 1498–1499
Marshall, A.J., Barritt, D.W., Pocock, J., Heaton, S.T.: Evaluation of beta blockade, bendrofluazide and prazosin in severe hypertension. Lancet *1977a I*, 271–274
Marshall, I., Nasmyth, P.A., Russell, G.K., Shepperson, N.B.: Ergometrine: a presynaptic α-adrenoceptor agonist. Br. J. Clin. Pharmacol. *4*, 129 P (1977b)
Martin, L.E., Hopkins, R., Bland, R.: Metabolism of labetalol by animals and man. Br. J. Clin. Pharmacol. [Suppl.] *3*, 695–710 (1976)
Mason, D.T.: Afterload reduction and cardiac performance. Physiologic basis of systemic vasodilators as a new approach in treatment of congestive heart failure. Am. J. Med. *65*, 106–125 (1978)
Mason, D.T., Braunwald, E.: Effects of guanethidine, reserpine and methyldopa on reflex venous and arterial constriction in man. J. Clin. Invest. *43*, 1449–1463 (1964)
Massingham, R., Hayden, M.L.: A comparison of the effects of prazosin and hydrallazine on blood pressure, heart rate and plasma renin activity in conscious renal hypertensive dogs. Eur. J. Pharmacol. *30*, 121–124 (1975)
McAllister, R.G. Jr., Markesbery, W.R., Ware, R.W., Howell, S.M.: Suppression of essential tremor by propranolol: correlation of effect with drug plasma levels and intensity of beta-adrenergic blockade. Ann. Neurol. *1*, 160–166 (1977)
McDevitt, D.G.: β-adrenoceptor antagonists and respiratory function. Br. J. Clin. Pharmacol. *5*, 97–99 (1978)
McDevitt, D.G., Shanks, R.G., Hadden, D.R., Montgomery, D.A.D., Weaver, J.A.: The role of the thyroid in the control of heart-rate. Lancet *1968 I*, 998–1000
McDonald, R.H., Goldberg, L.I., McNay, J.L., Tuttle, E.P.: Effects of dopamine in man, augmenting of sodium excretion, glomerular filtration rate and renal plasma flow. J. Clin. Invest. *43*, 1116–1124 (1964)
McFarland, J., Willerson, J.T., Dinsmore, R.E., Austen, W.G., Buckley, M.J., Sanders, C.A., de Sanctis, R.W.: The medical treatment of dissecting aortic aneurysms. N. Engl. J. Med. *286*, 115–119 (1972)
McLarty, D.G., Brownlie, B.E., Alexander, W.D., Papapetrou, P.D., Horton, P.: Remission of thyrotoxicosis during treatment with propranolol. Br. Med. J. (1973) *II*, 332–334
McMartin, C., Simpson, P.: The absorption and metabolism of guanethidine in hypertensive patients requiring different doses of the drug. Clin. Pharmacol. Ther. *12*, 73–77 (1971)
McNay, J.L., McDonald, R.H., Goldberg, L.I.: Direct renal vasodilatation produced by dopamine in the dog. Circ. Res. *16*, 510–517 (1965)

Meek, D., Mamtora, H., Gabriel, R.: Acute hypertension following treatment with prazosin. Curr. Med. Res. Opinion *3*, 672–674 (1976)
Meekers, J., Missotten, A., Fagard, R., Demuynck, D., Harvengt, C., Pas, P., Billiet, L., Amery, A.: Predictive value of various parameters for the antihypertensive effect on the beta blocker ICI 66,082 (1). Arch. Int. Pharmacodyn. *213*, 294–306 (1975)
Mehta, J., Cohn, J.N.: Hemodynamic effects of labetalol, an alpha and beta adrenergic blocking agent, in hypertensive subjects. Circulation *55*, 370–375 (1977)
Mendel, D., Bryne-Quinn, E.: Effect of propranolol on pulse-rate, and coronary sinus and pulmonary artery oxygen-saturation in 4 patients undergoing cardiac catheterisation. Lancet *1966 II*, 1026
Mendlowitz, M., Naftchi, N., Gitlow, S.E., Wienreb, H.L., Wolf, R.L.: The effect of chlorothiazide and the congeners on the digital circulation in normotensive subjects and in patients with essential hypertension. Ann. N.Y. Acad. Sci. *88*, 964–974 (1960)
Mendlowitz, M., Naftchi, N.E., Wolf, R.L., Gitlow, S.E.: The effects of guanethidine and of alpha methyldopa on the digital circulation in hypertension. Am. Heart J. *69*, 731–739 (1965)
Merguet, P., Heimsoth, V., Murata, T., Bock, K.D.: Experimental study on the circulatory effects of 2-(2,6-dichlorophenylamino)-2-imidazoline hydrochloride in man. Pharmacol. Clin. *1*, 30–37 (1968)
Meyer, J.S., Sawada, T., Kitamura, A., Toyoda, M.: Cerebral blood flow after control of hypertension in stroke. Neurology (Minneap.) *18*, 772–781 (1968)
Michelakis, A.M., McAllister, R.G.: The effect of chronic adrenergic receptor blockade on plasma renin activity in man. J. Clin. Endocrinol. Metab. *34*, 386–394 (1972)
Michie, W., Hamer-Hodges, D.W., Pegg, C.A.S., Orr, F.G.G., Bewsher, P.D.: Beta blockade and partial thyroidectomy for thyrotoxicosis. Lancet *1974 I*, 1010–1011
Mikulic, E., Cohn, J.N., Franciosa, J.A.: Comparative hemodynamic effects of inotropic and vasodilator drugs in severe heart failure. Circulation *56*, 528–533 (1977)
Milledge, J.S., Morris, J.: A comparison of slow release salbutamol with slow release aminophylline in nocturnal asthma. J. Int. Med. Res. [Suppl. 1] *7*, 106–110 (1979)
Miller, R.R., Olson, H.G., Amsterdam, E.A., Mason, D.T.: Propranolol-withdrawal rebound phenomenon. Exacerbation of coronary events after abrupt cessation of antianginal therapy. N. Engl. J. Med. *293*, 416–418 (1975a)
Miller, R.R., Olson, H.G., Pratt, C.M., Amsterdam, E.A., Mason, D.T.: Efficacy of beta-adrenergic blockade in coronary heart disease. Propranolol in angina pectoris. Clin. Pharmacol. Ther. *18*, 598–605 (1975b)
Miller, J.: A comprehensive evaluation of metaproterenol, a new bronchodilator. J. Clin. Pharmacol. *7*, 34–40 (1967)
Miller, J., Wallace, D., Grieco, M.H., Frenkel, R., Larsen, K.: Double-blind trial of oral carbuterol in bronchial asthma. Ann. Allergy *39*, 12–17 (1977)
Minette, A.: Spirometric study of the bronchodilating effects of hydroxyphenyl orciprenaline (TH 1165a) in various forms in a group of 124 coal miners suffering from bronchospasm. Respiration *27*, 276–315 (1970)
Minette, A., Marcq, M., Gepts, L.: Carbuterol, fenoterol, orciprenaline, salbutamol and terbutaline per os in reversible obstructive chronic bronchitis. Bull. Eur. Physiopathol. Respir. *12*, 545–553 (1976)
Minhas, K., Elbl, F., Solinger, R., Ly, T.P., George, L., Fowler, J.F.R.: Effective role of propranolol in the management of tetralogy of Fallot. Circulation [Suppl. II] *54*, 72 (1976)
Mitchell, J.R., Cavanaugh, J.H., Arias, L., Oates, J.A.: Guanethidine and related agents 3. Antagonism of drugs which inhibit the norepinephrine pump in man. J. Clin. Invest. *49*, 1596–1604 (1970)
Mizgala, H.G., Khan, A.K., Davies, R.O.: Propranolol in the prophylactic treatment of angina pectoris. Can. Med. Assoc. J. *100*, 756–764 (1969)
Moe, R.A., Bates, H.M., Palkoski, Z.M., Banziger, R.: Cardiovascular effects of 3,4-Dihydro-2-(1H)-isoquinoline carboxamidine (declinax). Curr. Ther. Res. *6*, 299–318 (1964)
Mohammed, S., Hanenson, I.B., Magenheim, H.G., Gaffney, T.E.: The effects of alphamethyldopa on renal function in hypertensive patients. Am. Heart J. *76*, 21–27 (1968)
Moir, T.W.: Subendocardial distribution of coronary blood flow and the effect of antianginal drugs. Circ. Res. *30*, 621–627 (1972)

Montgomery, D.A.D.: Hyperthyroidism, results of treatment – an appraisal. Ulster Med. J. *44*, 73–87 (1975)
Montgomery, R., Du Charme, D.W.: Hemodynamic effects of chronic and acute changes in blood pressure (abstract). Fed. Proc. *27*, 758 (1968)
Montuschi, E., Pickens, P.T.: A clinical trial of two related adrenergic neurone-blocking agents – BW 392C60 and BW 467C60. Lancet *1962 II*, 897–901
Morgan, T.O., Louis, W.J., Dawborn, J.K., Doyle, A.E.: The use of pindolol (visken) in the treatment of hypertension. Med. J. Aust. *2*, 309–312 (1972)
Morgan, T.O., Roberts, R., Carney, S.L., Louis, W.J., Doyle, A.E.: Beta adrenergic receptor blocking drugs, hypertension and plasma renin. Br. J. Clin. Pharmacol. *2*, 159–164 (1975)
Mortz, R., Brown, D.J., Forney, R.B., Bright, T.P., Kiplinger, G.F., Rodda, B.E.: Propranolol antagonism of marihuana induced tachycardia. Life Sci. *11*, 999 (1972)
Mroczek, W.J., Finnerty, F.A. Jr.: Prazosin – a double-blind evaluation. In: Prazosin – Evaluation of a new antihypertensive agent, pp. 92–99 Cotton D.W.K. (ed.). Amsterdam: Excerpta Medica, 1974
Mroczek, W.J., Leibel, B.A., Finnerty, F.A. Jr.: Comparison of clonidine and methyldopa in hypertensive patients receiving diuretics. A doule-blind crossover study. Am. J. Cardiol. *29*, 712–717 (1972)
Mueller, H., Ayres, S.M., Gregory, J.J., Giannelli, S., Grace, W.J.: Hemodynamics, coronary blood flow and myocardial metabolism in coronary shock; response to l-norepinephrine and isoproterenol. J. Clin. Invest. *49*, 1885–1902 (1970)
Mueller, H.S., Ayres, S.M., Religa, A., Evans, R.G.: Propranolol in the treatment of acute myocardial infarction. Effect on myocardial oxygen and hemodynamics. Circulation *49*, 1078–1087 (1974)
Muir, A.L., Burton, J.L., Lawrie, D.M.: Circulatory effects at rest and exercise of clonidine; an imidazoline derivative with hypotensive properties. Lancet *1969 II*, 181–185
Multicentre International Study: Improvement in prognosis of myocardial infarction by long-term beta-adrenoceptor blockade using practolol. Br. Med. J. *3*, 735–740 (1975)
Mune, O., Norregaard, S.: Metaraminol (aramine) in the treatment of shock due to coronary occlusion. Nord. Med. *62*, 1255–1260 (1959)
Murray, T.J.: Long-term therapy of essential tremor with propranolol. Can. Med. Assoc. J. *115*, 892–894 (1976)
Musini, A., Fabbri, B., Bergamaschi, M., Mandelli, V., Shanks, R.G.: Comparison of the effect of propranolol, lignocaine and other drugs on normal and raised intraocular pressure in man. Am. J. Ophthalmol. *72*, 773–781 (1971)
Myers, M.G., Wisenberg, G.: Sudden withdrawal of propranolol in patients with angina pectoris. Chest *71*, 24–26 (1977)
Myers, M.G., Lewis, P.J., Reid, J.L., Dollery, C.T.: Brain concentration of propranolol in relation to hypotensive effect in the rabbit with observations on brain propranolol levels in man. J. Pharmacol. Exp. Ther. *192*, 327–335 (1975)
Nair, D.V.: A double-blind trial of visken, LB 46, in the treatment of angina pectoris. Indian Heart J. [Suppl. 1] *3*, 183–191 (1972)
Nash, C.W., Wolff, S.A., Ferguson, B.A.: Release of tritiated noradrenaline from perfused rat hearts by sympathomimetic amines. Can. J. Physiol. Pharmacol. *46*, 35–42 (1968)
Nayler, W.G., Price, J.M., Swann, J.B., McInnes, I., Race, D., Lowe, T.E.: Effect of the hypotensive drug ST 155 (catapres) on the heart and peripheral circulation. J. Pharmacol. Exp. Ther. *164*, 45–59 (1968)
Nelson, J.K., McDevitt, D.G.: Comparative trial of propranolol and practolol in hypertension. Br. J. Clin. Pharmacol. *2*, 411–416 (1975)
Nestel, P.J.: Evaluation of propranolol (inderal) in the treatment of angina pectoris. Med. J. Aust. *2*, 1274–1276 (1966)
Neville, A., Palmer, J.B.D., Gaddie, J., May, C.S., Palmer, K.N.V., Murchison, L.E.: Metabolic effects of salbutamol: comparison of aerosol and intravenous administration. Br. Med. J. *1977 I*, 413–414
Ng, J., Phelan, E.L., McGregor, D.D., Laverty, R., Smirk, H.: Properties of catapres, a new hypotensive drug: a preliminary report. N. Z. Med. J. *66*, 864–870 (1967)
Nicotero, J.A., Beamer, V., Moutsos, S.E., Shapiro, A.P.: Effects of propranolol on pressor responses to noxious stimuli in hypertensive patients. Am. J. Cardiol. *22*, 657–666 (1968)

Nielsen, I., Steiness, E., Hesse, B.: Acute and long-term salt depletion and β-blockade. Plasma renin activity response and its relation to blood pressure reduction in long-term treatment. Acta Med. Scand. *203*, 415–418 (1978)
Nies, A.S., McNeil, J.S., Schrier, R.W.: Mechanism of increased sodium reabsorption during propranolol administration. Circulation *44*, 596–604 (1971)
Nik-Akhtar, B., Rashed, M.A., Khakpour, M.: Effect of beta-adrenergic blocking agents (alprenolol and propranolol) in essential hypertension. Angiology *26*, 339–343 (1975)
Nilsson, H.T., Simonsson, B.G., Strom, B.: Fate of ^{3}H terbutaline sulphate administered to man as an aerosol. Eur. J. Clin. Pharmacol. *10*, 1–7 (1976)
Nogrady, S.G., Evans, W.V., Davies, B.H.: Reversibility of airways obstruction in bronchiectasis. Thorax *33*, 635–637 (1978)
Nolte, D., Galfoczy, G., Lode, H., Mandi, A., Mettys, H., Streseman, E.: Ergebnisse einer multizentrischen Prüfung des Bronchospasmolytikums Reproterol. Dtsch. Med. Wochenschr. *102*, 619–623 (1977)
Norris, R.M., Caughey, D.E., Scott, P.J.: Trial of propranolol in acute myocardial infarction. Br. Med. J. *1968 II*, 398–400
Novack, P.: The effect of guanethidine on renal, cerebral and cardiac hemodynamics. In: Hypertension, recent advances. The second Hahnemann symposium on hypertensive disease. Brest, A.N., Moyer, J.H. (eds.) pp. 444–448. Philadelphia: Lea & Febiger 1961
Nyberg, G.: Blood pressure and heart rate during sustained handgrip in hypertensive patients taking placebo, a non-selective β-blocker (propranolol) and a selective β-blocker (metoprolol). Curr. Ther. Res. *22*, 828–838 (1977)
Nyberg, G., Graham, R.M., Stokes, G.S.: The effect of mental arithmetic in normotensive and hypertensive subjects and its modification by β-adrenoceptor blockade. Br. J. Clin. Pharmacol. *4*, 469–474 (1977)
Oates, J.A., Gillespie, L., Udenfriend, S., Sjoerdsma, A.: Decarboxylase inhibition and blood pressure reduction by α-methyl -3,4-dihydroxy – DL phenylalamine. Science *131*, 1890–1891 (1960)
Oates, J.A., Seligmann, A.W., Clark, M.A., Rousseau, P., Lee, R.E.: The relative efficacy of guanethidine, methyldopa and pargyline as antihypertensive agents. N. Engl. J. Med. *273*, 729–734 (1965)
O'Donnell, T.V., Butler, G.M., Tocker, M.D.: A comparison of orciprenaline and salbutamol administered orally in 12 adult asthmatic patients. Postgrad. Med. J. [Suppl.] *47*, 115–118 (1971)
Offerhaus, L., van Zwieten, P.A.: Comparative studies on central factors contributing to the hypotensive action of propranolol, alprenolol and their enantiomers. Cardiovasc. Res. *8*, 488–495 (1974)
Oh, V.M., Kaye, C.M., Warrington, S.J., Taylor, E.A., Wadsworth, J.: Studies of cardioselectivity and partial agonist activity in beta adrenoceptor blockade comparing effect on heart rate and peak expiratory flow rate during exercise. Br. J. Clin. Pharmacol. *5*, 107–120 (1978)
Olsson, O.A.T.: The influence of some beta adrenergic stimulant compounds on intestinal motility in vitro and in vivo in mice. Acta Pharmacol. Toxicol. (Kbh) *31*, 33–42 (1972)
Olsson, O.A.T., Persson, C.G.A.: Relaxing potency of terbutaline and orciprenaline on rat uterus. J. Pharma. Pharmacol. *23*, 878–879 (1971)
Olsson, O.A.T., Persson, C.G.A., Persson, H., Sörenby, L.: Pharmacological properties of 1-(3′5′-diisobutyryloxy-phenyl)-2-(t-butylamino) ethanol hydrochloride (KWD 2058), a new sympathomimetic bronchodilator. Acta Pharmacol. Toxicol. (Kbh) *35*, 76–90 (1974)
Onesti, G., Brest, A.N., Novack, P., Kasparin, H., Moyer, J.H.: Pharmacodynamic effects of α-methyldopa in hypertensive subjects. Am. Heart J. *67*, 32–38 (1964)
Onesti, G., La Schiazza, D., Brest, A.N., Moyer, J.H.: Cardiac and renal hemodynamic effects of debrisoquine sulfate in hypertensive patients. Clin. Pharmacol. Ther. *7*, 17–20 (1966)
Onesti, G., Schwartz, A.B., Kim, K.E., Schwartz, C., Brest, A.N.: Pharmacodynamic effects of a new antihypertensive drug, catapres (ST 155). Circulation *39*, 219–228 (1969)
Onesti, G., Bock, K.D., Heimsoth, V., Kim, K.E., Merguet, P.: Clonidine, a new antihypertensive agent. Am. J. Cardiol. *28*, 74–83 (1971 a)
Onest, G., Schwartz, A.B., Kim, K.E., Paz-Martinez, V., Swartz, C.: Antihypertensive effect of clonidine. Circ. Res. [Suppl. 2] *28*, 53–69 (1971 b)

Onesti, G., Fernandes, M.A., Kim, K.E., Swartz, C.D.: Prazosin in the treatment of hypertension. Clin. Pharmacol. Ther. *15*, 216 (1974)
Ose, L., McKusick, V.A.: Prophylactic use of propranolol in the Marfon syndrome to prevent aortic dissection. Birth Defects *13*, 163–169 (1977)
Oski, F.A., Miller, L.D., Delivoria-Papadopoulus, M., Manchester, J.H., Shelburne, J.C.: Oxygen affinity in red cells: changes induced in vivo by propranolol. Science *175*, 1372–1373 (1972)
Owens, C.W.I.: Sustained released beta-blockade. Clin. Ther. *1*, 319–338 (1978)
Palmer, K.N.V.: Effect of bronchodilator drugs on arterial blood gas tensions in bronchial asthma. Postgrad. Med. J. [Suppl.] *47*, 75–77 (1971)
Palmer, K.N.V.: Muscle cramps and oral salbutamol (Letter). Br. Med. J. *1978 II*, 833
Palmer, K.N.V., Diament, M.L.: Effect of salbutamol on spirometry and blood gas tensions in bronchial asthma. Br. Med. J. *1969 I*, 31–32
Palmer, K.N.V., Legge, J.S., Hamilton, W.F.D., Diament, M.L.: Comparison of effect of salbutamol and isoprenaline on spirometry and blood gas tensions in bronchial asthma. Br. Med. J. *1970 II*, 23–24
Pandolfi, M., Ohrstrom, A.: Treatment of ocular hypertension with oral beta-adrenergic blocking agents. Acta Ophthalmol. *52*, 464–467 (1974)
Parker, S.S., Choo-Kang, Y.F.J., Cooper, E.J., Cameron, S.J., Grant, I.W.B.: Bronchodilator effect of oral salbutamol in asthmatics treated with corticosteroids. Br. Med. J. (1971) *IV*, 139–142
Parratt, J.R., Grayson, J.: Myocardial vascular reactivity after beta-adrenergic blockade. Lancet *1966 I*, 338–340
Parsons, V., Jewitt, D.: Beta-adrenergic blockade in the management of acute thyrotoxic crisis, tachycardia and arrhythmias. Postgrad. Med. J. *43*, 756–762 (1967)
Parving, H.H., Gyntelberg, F.: Albumin transcapillary escape rate and plasma volume during long-term beta-adrenergic blockade in essential hypertension. Scand. J. Clin. Lab. Invest. *32*, 105–110 (1973)
Patel, K.R.: The role of adrenoceptors in bronchial asthma. J. R. Coll. Physicians Lond. *13*, 165–170 (1979)
Paterson, J.W.: Human pharmacology: comparison of intravenous isoprenaline and salbutamol in asthmatic subjects. Postgrad. Med. J. [Suppl.] *47*, 38–39 (1971)
Paterson, J.W., Dollery, C.T.: Effect of propranolol in mild hypertension. Lancet *1966 II*, 1148–1150
Paterson, J.W., Conolly, M.E., Davies, D.S., Dollery, C.T.: Isoprenaline resistance and the use of pressurized aerosols in asthma. Lancet *1968 II*, 426–429
Paterson, J.W., Courtenay Evans, R.J., Prime, F.J.: Selectivity of bronchodilator action of salbutamol in asthmatic patients. Br. J. Dis. Chest *65*, 21–38 (1971)
Pearson, R.M., Bending, M.R., Bulpitt, C.J., George, C.F., Hole, D.R., Williams, F.M., Breckenridge, A.M.: Trial of combination of guanethidine and oxprenolol in hypertension. Br. Med. J. *1976 I*, 933–936
Pedersen, E.B., Kornerup, H.J.: Plasma renin concentration in essential hypertension during beta-adrenergic blockade and vasodilator therapy. Eur. J. Clin. Pharmacol. *12*, 93–96 (1977)
Pelides, L.J., Reid, D.S., Thomas, M., Shillingford, J.P.: Inhibition by β-blockade of the ST segment elevation after acute myocardial infarction in man. Cardiovasc. Res. *6*, 295–301 (1972)
Pemberton, P.J., McConnell, B., Shanks, R.G.: Neonatal thyrotoxicosis treated with propranolol. Case report. Arch. Dis. Child. *49*, 813–815 (1974)
Pendleton, R.G., Newman, D.J., Sherman, S.S., Brann, E.G., Maya, W.E.: Effect of propranolol upon the haemoglobin-oxygen dissociation curve. J. Pharmacol. Exp. Ther. *180*, 647–656 (1972)
Perks, W.H., Chatterjee, S.S., Croxson, R.S., Cruickshank, J.M.: Comparison of atenolol and oxprenolol in patients with angina or hypertension and co-existent chronic airways obstruction. Br. J. Clin. Pharmacol. *5*, 101–106 (1978)
Persson, H., Johnson, B.: A dual preparation technique for studying the differentiation of the effect of sympathomimetic agents on heart and tracheal muscle. Acta Med. Scand. [Suppl.] *512*, 21–24 (1970)

Persson, I.: Combination therapy of essential hypertension with pindolol (visken) and hydralazine. Eur. J. Clin. Pharmacol. *9*, 91–93 (1975)

Persson, K., Persson, K.: The metabolism of terbutaline in vitro by rat and human liver o-methyl transferase and momoamine oxidase. Xenobiotica *2*, 375–382 (1972)

Peter, T., Heng, M.K., Singh, B.N., Ambler, P., Nisbet, H., Elliott, R., Norris, R.M.: Failure of high doses of propranolol to reduce experimental myocardial ischaemic damage. Circulation *57*, 534–540 (1978a)

Peter, T., Norris, R.M., Clarke, E.D., Heng, M.K., Singh, B.N., Williams, B., Howell, D.R., Ambler, P.K.: Reduction of enzyme levels by propranolol after acute myocardial infarction. Circulation *57*, 1091–1095 (1978b)

Petri, J.C., Galloway, D.B., Webster, J., Simpson, W.T., Lewis, J.A.: Atenolol and bendrofluazide in hypertension. Br. Med. J. (1975) *III*, 133–135

Pettinger, W.A., Horst, W.A.: Qualifying metabolic effects of antihypertensive and other drugs at the sympathetic neuron level: Clinical and basic correlations. Ann. N. Y. Acad. Sci. *179*, 310–321 (1971)

Pettinger, W.A., Keeton, K.: Altered renin release and propranolol potentiation of vasodilatory drug hypotension. J. Clin. Invest. *55*, 236–243 (1975)

Pettinger, W.A., Mitchell, H.C.: Minoxidil – an alternative to nephrectomy for refractory hypertension. N. Engl. J. Med. *289*, 167–171 (1973)

Pettinger, W.A., Mitchell, H.C.: Additive effect of beta-adrenergic blockers in combination with vasodilators in lowering blood pressure. Aust. N. Z. Med. [Suppl. 3] *6*, 76–82 (1976)

Pettinger, W.A., Korn, A., Spiegel, H., Solomon, H.M., Pocelinko, R., Abrams, W.B.: Debrisoquin: a selective inhibitor of intraneuronal monoamine oxidase in man. Clin. Pharmacol. Ther. *10*, 667–674 (1969)

Phelan, P.D., Williams, H.E.: Studies of respiratory function in infants with recurrent asthmatic bronchitis. Aust. Paediatr. J. *5*, 187–196 (1969)

Phillips, C.I.: Beta-blockers in the treatment of chronic simple glaucoma. Br. Med. J. *1976 I*, 584

Phillips, C.I., Howitt, G., Rowlands, D.J.: Propranolol as ocular hypotensive agent. Br. J. Ophthalmol. *51*, 222–226 (1967)

Phillips, P.J., Vedig, A.E., Jones, P.L., Chapman, M.G., Collins, M., Edwards, J.B., Smeaton, T., Duncan, B.McL.: A comparison of the cardiovascular and metabolic effects of the β_2-adrenergic agonists salbutamol and rimiterol. Clin. Sci. Mol. Med. *55*, 18 P (1978)

Pickering, T.G., Gribbin, B., Petersen, E.S., Cunningham, D.J.C., Sleight, P.: Effects of autonomic blockade on the baroreflex in man at rest and during exercise. Circ. Res. *30*, 177–185 (1972)

Pimstone, B., Joffe, B.: The use and abuse of beta-adrenergic blockade in the surgery of hyperthyroidism. S. Afr. Med. J. *44*, 1059–1060 (1970)

Pimstone, N., Marine, N., Pimstone, B.: Beta-adrenergic blockade in thyrotoxic myopathy. Lancet *1968 II*, 1219–1220

Pine, M., Favrot, L., Smith, S., McDonald, K., Chidsey, C.A.: Correlation of plasma propranolol concentration with therapeutic response in patients with angina pectoris. Circulation *52*, 886–893 (1975)

Pines, A., Raafat, M., Taylor-Pearce, M.E., Hamad, F.: The effect of intravenous reproterol hydrochloride (bronchospasm). Clin. Trials J. *15*, 127–131 (1978)

Pitt, B., Craven, P.: Effect of propranolol on regional myocardial blood flow in acute ischaemia. Cardiovasc. Res. *4*, 176–179 (1970)

Poole-Wilson, P.A., Lewis, G., Angerpointer, T., Malcolm, A.D., Williams, B.T.: Haemodynamic effects of salbutamol and nitroprusside after cardiac surgery. Br. Heart J. *39*, 721–725 (1977)

Powles, A.C.P.: The bronchodilator effect of fenoterol (berotec). N. Z. Med. J. *81*, 249–251 (1975)

Prichard, B.N.C.: Hypotensive action of pronethalol. Br. Med. J. *1964 I*, 1227–1228

Prichard, B.N.C.: Aspects of the evaluation of antihypertensive drugs. In: Proceedings of the International Symposium on Clinical Pharmacology. pp. 193–208. Brussels: Royal Academies of Medicine of Belgium 1970

Prichard, B.N.C.: β-receptor antagonists in angina pectoris. Ann. Clin. Res. *3*, 344–352 (1971)

Prichard, B.N.C.: β-adrenergic receptor blocking drugs in angina pectoris. Drugs *7*, 55–84 (1974)
Prichard, B.N.C.: The combined effect of propranolol with bethanidine or methyldopa in hypertension. Adv. Clin. Pharmacol. *11*, 107–113 (1976)
Prichard, B.N.C., Boakes, A.J.: The use of sotalol in the treatment of hypertension. Excerpta Med. *4*, 7–24 (1974)
Prichard, B.N.C., Boakes, A.J.: Labetalol in long-term treatment of hypertension. Br. J. Clin. Pharmacol. *3*, 743–750 (1976)
Prichard, B.N.C., Boakes, A.J.: The use of beta-adrenoceptor blocking drugs in hypertension: a review. Curr. Med. Res. Opinion [Suppl. 5] *4*, 51–76 (1977)
Prichard, B.N.C., Gillam, P.M.S.: Use of propranolol (inderal) in the treatment of hypertension. Br. Med. J. *1964 II*, 725–727
Prichard, B.N.C., Gillam, P.M.S.: Propranolol in hypertension. Am. J. Cardiol. *18*, 387–391 (1966)
Prichard, B.N.C., Gillam, P.M.S.: Treatment of hypertension with propranolol. Br. Med. J. *1969 I*, 7–16
Prichard, B.N.C., Gillam, P.M.S.: Assessment of propranolol in angina pectoris. Clinical dose response curve and effect on electocardiogram at rest and on exercise. Br. Heart J. *33*, 473–480 (1971)
Prichard, B.N.C., Tuckman, J.: Management and mechanisms of drug treatment of hypertension. In: Hypertension, physiopathology and treatment. Genest, J. (ed.), pp. 1085–1117. Montreal: McGraw-Hill 1977
Prichard, B.N.C., Dickinson, C.J., Alleyne, G.A.O., Hurst, P., Hill, I.D., Rosenheim, M.L., Laurence, D.R.: Effect of pronethalol in angina pectoris. Br. Med. J. *1963 II*, 1226–1227
Prichard, B.N.C., Johnston, A.W., Hill, I.D., Rosenheim, M.L.: Bethanidine, guanethidine, and methyldopa in the treatment of hypertension; a within-patient comparison. Br. Med. J. *1968 I*, 135–144
Prichard, B.N.C., Aellig, W.H., Richardson, G.A.: The action of intravenous oxprenolol, practolol, propranolol and sotalol on acute exercise tolerance in angina pectoris: the effect on heart rate and the electrocardiogram. Postgrad. Med. J. [Suppl.] *46*, 77–85 (1970a)
Prichard, B.N.C., Gillam, P.M.S., Graham, B.R.: Beta receptor antagonism in hypertension; comparison with the effect of adrenergic neurone inhibition on cardiovascular responses. Int. J. Clin. Pharmacol. *4*, 131–140 (1970b)
Prichard, B.N.C., Shinebourne, E., Fleming, J., Hamer, J.: Haemodynamic studies in hypertensive patients on oral propranolol. Br. Heart J. *32*, 236–240 (1970c)
Prichard, B.N.C., Boakes, A.J., Day, G.M.: Practolol in the treatment of hypertension. Postgrad. Med. J. [Suppl.] *47*, 84–91 (1971)
Prichard, B.N.C., Thompson, F.O., Boakes, A.J., Jockes, A.M.: Some haemodynamic effects of compound AH 5158 compared with propranolol, propranolol plus hydrallazine, and diazoxide; the use of AH 5158 in the treatment of hypertension. Clin. Sci. Mol. Med. *48*, 97–100 (1975)
Prichard, B.N.C., Boakes, A.J., Graham, B.R.: A within-patient comparison of bethanidine, methyldopa and propranolol in the treatment of hypertension. Clin. Sci. Mol. Med. [Suppl. 3] *51*, 567–570 (1976)
Prichard, B.N.C., Boakes, A.J., Hernandez, R.: Long-term treatment of hypertension with labetalol. Br. J. Clin. Pharmacol. (1979, to be published)
Pugsley, D.J., Armstrong, B.K., Nassim, M.A., Beilin, L.J.: Controlled comparison of labetalol and propranolol in the management of severe hypertension. Br. J. Clin. Pharmacol. [Suppl.] *3*, 777–782 (1976)
Rabkin, R., Stables, D.P., Levin, N.W., Suzman, M.M.: The prophylactic value of propranolol in angina pectoris. Am. J. Cardiol. *18*, 370–383 (1966)
Rachensperger, W., Gaupp, R., Mattke, D.J., Schwartz, D., Stutte, K.H.: Behandlung von akuten schizophrenen Psychosen mit Beta-Receptoren-Blockern. Arch. Psychiatr. Nervenkr. *219*, 29–36 (1974)
Radford, M.: Effect of salbutamol in infants with wheezy bronchitis. Arch. Dis. Child. *50*, 535–538 (1975)
Raftery, E.B., Denman, A.M.: Systemic lupus erythematosus syndrome induced by practolol. Br. Med. J. *1973 II*, 452–455

Raftos, J., Bauer, G.E., Lewis, R.G., Stokes, G.S., Mitchell, A.S., Young, A.A., Machlachlan, I.: Clonidine in the treatment of severe hypertension; trial carried out in 1968–1972. Med. J. Aust. *1*, 786–793 (1973)

Ramsay, I., Greer, S., Bagley, C.: Propranolol in neurotic and thyrotoxic anxiety. Br. J. Psychiatry *122*, 555–560 (1973)

Rand, M.J., Wilson, J.: Mechanisms of the pressor and depressor actions of ST 155 (2(2,6-Dichlorophenylamino-)-2-imidazoline hydrochloride, (catapres). Eur. J. Pharmacol. *3*, 27–33 (1968)

Rasmussen, K., Jensen, H.A.E.: A crossover study between hydrallazine and prazosin. Clin. Sci. Mol. Med. *51*, 621–623 (1976)

Rasmussen, M.M., Reimer, K.A., Kloner, R.A., Jannings, R.B.: Infarct size reduction by propranolol before and after coronary ligation in dogs. Circulation *56*, 794–798 (1977)

Rehbinder, D.: The metabolism of clonidine: In: Catapres in hypertension. Conolly, M.E. (ed.), pp. 227–236. London: Butterworths 1970

Reichert, N., Shibolet, S., Adar, R., Gafni, J.: Controlled trial of propranolol in intermittent claudication. Clin. Pharmacol. Ther. *17*, 612–615 (1975)

Reid, J.L., Briant, R.H., Dollery, C.T.: Desmethylimipramine and the hypotensive action of clonidine in the rabbit. Life Sci. *12*, 459–467 (1973)

Reid, J.L., Jones, D.H., Dargie, H.J.: Plasma noradrenaline and hypertension. Postgrad. Med. J. [Suppl. 3] *53*, 40–42 (1977)

Reisman, R.E.: Asthma induced by adrenergic aerosols: J. Allergy *46*, 162–177 (1970)

Reiss, W., Rajagopalan, T.G., Imhof, P., Schmid, K., Keverle, H.: Metabolic studies on oxprenolol in animals and man by means of radio tracer techniques and GLC analysis. Postgrad. Med. J. [Suppl.] 32–43 (1970)

Reybrouck, T., Amery, A., Fagard, R., Jousten, P., Lijnen, P., Meulepas, E.: Beta-blockers: once or three times a day. Br. Med. J. *1978 I*, 1386–1388

Rice, A.J., Ferguson, R.K., Delle, M., Wilson, W.R.: Comparative beta blocking activities and effects on sodium excretion of sotalol and propranolol. Clin. Pharmacol. Ther. *II*, 567–573 (1970)

Richards, D.A.: Pharmacological effects of labetalol in man. Br. J. Clin. Pharmacol. *3*, 721–723 (1976)

Richards, D.A., Woodings, E.P., Stephens, M.D.B., Maconochie, J.G.: The effects of oral AH 5158, a combined α- and β-adrenoceptor antagonist, in healthy volunteers. Br. J. Clin. Pharmacol. *1*, 505–510 (1974)

Richards, D.A., Tuckman, J., Prichard, B.N.C.: Assessment of alpha and beta-adrenoceptor blocking action of labetalol. Br. J. Clin. Pharmacol. *3*, 849–855 (1976)

Richards, D.A., Maconochie, J.G., Bland, R.E., Hopkins, R., Woodings, E.P., Martin, L.E.: Relationship between plasma concentrations and pharmacological effects of labetalol. Eur. J. Clin. Pharmacol. *11*, 85–90 (1977a)

Richards, D.A., Prichard, B.N.C., Boakes, A.J., Tuckman, J., Knight, E.J.: Pharmacological basis for antihypertensive effects of intravenous labetalol. Br. Heart J. *39*, 99–106 (1977b)

Richards, D.A., Woodings, E.P., Maconochie, J.G.: Comparison of the effects of labetalol and propranolol in healthy men at rest and during exercise. Br. J. Clin. Pharmacol. *4*, 15–21 (1977c)

Richards, D.A., Prichard, B.N.C., Dobbs, R.J.: Adrenoceptor blockade of the circulatory responses to intravenous isoproterenol. Clin. Pharmacol. Ther. *24*, 264–273 (1978)

Richards, F.A.: Propranolol in hypertension. Am. J. Cardiol. *18*, 384–386 (1966)

Richardson, D.W., Wysso, E.M., Magee, J.H., Cavell, G.C.: Circulatory effects of guanethidine – Clinical, renal and cardiac responses to treatment with a novel antihypertensive agent. Circulation *22*, 184–190 (1960)

Richardson, D.W., Freund, J., Gear, A.S., Mauck, H.P., Preston, L.W.: Effect of propranolol on elevated arterial pressure. Circulation *37*, 534–542 (1968)

Richter, R.: Evaluation of success in treatment of threatening premature labor by betamimetic drugs. Am. J. Obstet. Gynecol. *127*, 482–486 (1977)

Riding, W.D., Dinda, P., Chatterjee, S.S.: The bronchodilator and cardiac effects of five pressure-packed aerosols in asthma. Br. J. Dis. Chest *64*, 37–45 (1970)

Robertson, J.T.: Cerebral arterial spasm. Current concepts. Clin. Neurosurg. *21*, 100–106 (1974)

Robie, N.W., Goldberg, L.I.: Comparative systemic and regional hemodynamic effects of dopamine and dobutamine. Am. Heart J. *90*, 340–345 (1975)

Robie, N.W., Nutter, D.O., Moody, C., McNay, J.L.: In vivo analysis of adrenergic receptor activity of dobutamine. Circ. Res. *34*, 663–671 (1974)

Robinson, B., Pilkington, T.: Effect of pronethalol in angina pectoris. Br. Med. J. *1963 II*, 1227–1228

Robinson, B.F.: Relation of heart rate and systolic blood pressure to the onset of pain in angina pectoris. Circulation, *35*, 1073–1083 (1967)

Robinson, B.F.: Mode of action of nitroglycerine in angina pectoris. Correlation between haemodynamic effects during exercise and provocation of pain. Br. Heart J. *30*, 295–302 (1968)

Robinson, B.F.: Mode of action of beta-antagonists in angina pectoris. Postgrad. Med. J. [Suppl.] *47*, 41–43 (1971)

Robson, R.D., Antonaccio, M.J.: Modification of baroreceptor function by clonidine: Evidence for an opposing action on baroreceptors of different location. In: Recent advances in hypertension. Milliez, P., Safar, M., (eds.), Vol. 2, pp. 37–47. Reims: Societe Alina, 1975

Roche: Data on renal excretion of debrisoquine and its metabolites. Reported by Roche Clinical Research Department. London: Roche 1975

Rodger, C.J., Sheldon, C.D., Lerski, R.A., Livingstone, W.R.: Intermittent claudication complicating beta-blockade. Br. Med. J. *1976 I*, 1125

Ronnov-Jessen, V., Hansen, J.: Blood volume and exchangeable sodium during treatment of hypertension with guanethidine and hydrochlorthiazide. Acta Med. Scand. *186*, 255–263 (1969)

Rosei, E.A., Brown, J.J., Lever, A.F., Robertson, A.S., Robertson, J.I.S., Trust, R.M.: Treatment of phaeochromocytoma and of clonidine withdrawal hypertension with labetalol. Br. J. Clin. Pharmacol. *3*, 809–815 (1976)

Rosenblum, R., Berkowitz, W.D., Lawson, D.: Effect of acute intravenous administration of isoproterenol on cardiorenal haemodynamics in man. Circulation *38*, 158–168 (1968)

Rosenblum, R., Tai, A.R., Lawson, D.: Dopamine in man: cardiorenal hemodynamics in normotensive patients with heart disease. J. Pharmacol. Exp. Ther. *183*, 256–263 (1972)

Rosendorff, C.: Prazosin: severe side-effects are dose-dependent. Br. Med. J. *3*, 508 (1976)

Ross, J. Jr.: Afterload mismatch and preload reserve: a conceptual framework for the analysis of ventricular function. Prog. Cardiovasc. Dis. *18*, 255–264 (1976)

Rothberg, M.P., Sherbert, R.T., Levey, G.S., Daroff, R.B.: Propranolol and hyperthyroidism. Reversal of upper motor neuron signs. JAMA *230*, 1017 (1974)

Rougier, M., Lahon, H.F.J., Clini, A.R.: Prazosin – a new antihypertensive agent. Br. J. Clin. Pract. *28*, 280–284 (1974)

Roy, P., Day, L., Sowton, E.: Effect of new β-adrenergic blocking agent, atenolol (tenormin) on pain frequency, trinitrin consumption and exercise ability. Br. Med. J. *3*, 195–197 (1975)

Ruffin, R.E., Fitzgerald, J.D., Rebuck, A.S.: A comparison of the bronchodilator activity of Sch 1000 and salbutamol. J. Allergy Clin. Immunol. 136–151 (1977)

Ruffin, R.E., Kenworthy, M.C., Newhouse, M.T.: Response of asthmatic patients to fenoterol inhalation, a method of quantifying the airway bronchodilator dose. Clin. Pharmacol. Ther. *23*, 338–345 (1978a)

Ruffin, R.E., Obminski, G., Newhouse, M.T.: Aerosol salbutamol administration by IPPB, lowest effective dose. Thorax *33*, 689–693 (1978b)

Russek, H.I.: Propranolol and isosorbide dinitrate synergism in angina pectoris. Am. J. Cardiol. *21*, 44–54 (1968)

Russek, H.I.: Prognosis in severe angina pectoris. Medical versus surgical therapy. Am. Heart J. *83*, 762–768 (1972)

Rutter, N., Milner, A.D., Hiler, E.J.: Effect of bronchodilators on respiratory resistance in infants and young children with bronchiolitis and wheezy bronchitis. Arch. Dis. Child. *50*, 719–722 (1975)

Sackner, M.A., Epstein, S., Wanner, A.: Effect of beta adrenergic agonists aerosolized by freon propellant on tracheal mucous velocity and cardiac output. Chest *69*, 593–598 (1976)

Sahay, J.N., Chatterjee, J.S.: A comparison of controlled release aminophylline (phyllocontin continus tablets) and sympathomimetic bronchodilators. J. Int. Med. Res. [Suppl. 1] *7*, 56–61 (1979)

Sainani, G.S., Mukherjee, A.K.: A double-blind trial of LB 46 (visken) in angina pectoris. Ind. Heart J. [Suppl. 1] *24*, 192–196 (1972)
Sakamoto, T., Yamada, T.: Hemodynamic effects of dobutamine in patients following open heart surgery. Circulation *55*, 525–533 (1977)
Saleeby, P.R., Ziskind, M.M.: Clinical study on carbuterol (SKF 40383). A new selective bronchodilator agent aerosol: double blind. Comparison with isoproterenol aerosol. Curr. Ther. Res. *17*, 225–233 (1975)
Salorinne, T., Stenius, B., Tukiainen, P., Poppius, H.: Double blind cross over comparison of clenbuterol tablets in asthmatic outpatients. Eur. J. Clin. Pharmacol. *8*, 189–195 (1975)
Sandler, G., Clayton, G.A.: Clinical evaluation of practolol, a new cardioselective β-blocking agent in angina pectoris. Br. Med. J. *1970 II*, 399–402
Sandler, G., Pistevos, A.: Clinical evaluation of oxprenalol in angina pectoris. Br. Heart J. *34*, 847–850 (1972)
Sannerstedt, R., Varnauskas, E., Werko, L.: Haemodynamic effects of methyldopa (aldomet) at rest and during exercise in patients with arterial hypertension. Acta Med. Scand. *171*, 75–82 (1962)
Sannerstedt, R., Stenberg, J., Vedin, A., Wilhelmsson, C., Werko, L.: Chronic beta-adrenergic blockade in arterial hypertension. Hemodynamic influences of di-hydrallazine and dynamic exercise and clinical effects of combined treatment. Am. J. Cardiol. *29*, 718–723 (1972)
Santa Cruz, R., Landa, J., Hirsch, J., Sackner, M.A.: Tracheal mucus velocity in normal man and patients with obstructive lung disease; effects of terbutaline. Am. Rev. Respir. Dis. *109*, 458–463 (1974)
Sarnoff, S.J., Gilmore, J.P., Weisfeldt, M.L., Daggett, W.M., Mansfield, P.B.: Influence of norepinephrine on myocardial oxygen consumption under controlled hemodynamic conditions. Am. J. Cardiol. *16*, 217–226 (1965)
Sattler, R.W., van Zwieten, P.A.: Acute hypotensive action of 2-(2,6 dichlorphenylamino-)-2-imidazoline hydrochloride (St 155) after infusion into the cats vertebral artery. Eur. J. Pharmacol. *2*, 9–13 (1967)
Scales, B., Cosgrove, M.B.: The metabolism and distribution of the selective beta blocking agent practolol. J. Pharmacol. Exp. Ther. *175*, 338–347 (1970)
Schamroth, L.: Immediate effects of intravenous propranolol on various cardiac arrhythmias. Am. J. Cardiol. *18*, 438–443 (1966)
Schindl, R. von: Bodyplethysmographische und blutgasanalytische klinisch experimentelle Untersuchungen mit dem neuen Bronchospasmolyticum Hexoprenalin. Arzneim. Forsch. *20*, 1755–1763 (1970)
Schlierf, G., Papenberg, J., Raetzer, H.: The effect of 1-(Indol-4-yl-oxy)-3-isopropylamino-propan-2-ol (LB-46, visken) on carbohydrate and lipid metabolism. Eur. J. Clin. Pharmacol. *5*, 154–157 (1973)
Schmitt, H.: On some unexplained effects of clonidine. In: Recent advances in hypertension. Milliez, P., Safar (eds.), vol. 2, pp. 63–72. Reims: Societe Alina 1975
Schmitt, H., Schmitt, H., Boissier, J.R., Guidicelli, J.F.: Centrally mediated decrease in sympathetic tone induced by 2-(2,6 Dichlorphenylamino-)-2-imidazoline hydrochloride (St 155, catapresan). Eur. J. Pharmacol. *2*, 147–148 (1967)
Schmitt, H., Schmitt, H., Fenard, S.: Evidence for an alpha-sympathomimetic component in the effect of catapresan on vasomotor centres: Antagonism by piperoxane. Eur. J. Pharmacol. *14*, 98–100 (1971)
Schnaper, H.W., Oberman, A.: Double-blind studies of the clinical effectiveness of prazosin. Postgrad. Med. [Suppl.] *58*, 81–87 (1975)
Scholtysik, G., Salzmann, R.: Interaction between antidepressant and centrally acting antihypertensive drugs. Naunyn Schmiedebergs Arch. Pharmacol. *279*, 23 (1973)
Schumann, A., Herxheimer, H.: The bronchodilator action of salbutamol in asthmatics. Postgrad. Med. J. [Suppl.] *47*, 92–99 (1971)
Schwitter, E., Fevrier, D., Bachofen, H.: Die Inhalation von B-Stimulatoren. Wirkung des im Oropharynx und des im Bronchialbaum angelagerten Anteils des Inhalats. Schweiz. Med. Wochenschr. *105*, 497–499 (1975)
Scott, D.B., Buckley, F.P., Drummond, G.B., Littlewood, D.G., Macrae, W.R.: Cardiovascular effects of labetalol during halothane anaesthesia. Br. J. Clin. Pharmacol. *3*, 817–821 (1976)

Scrumpf, J.D., Sheps, D.S., Wolfson, S., Aronson, A.L., Cohen, L.S.: Altered hemoglobin-oxygen affinity with long-term propranolol therapy in patients with coronary artery disease. Am. J. Cardiol. *40*, 76–82 (1977)

Seale, J.P., Anderson, S.D., Lindsay, D.A.: A comparison of oral theophylline and oral salbutamol in exercise induced asthma. Aust. N. Z. J. Med. *7*, 270–274 (1977)

Sealey, B.J., Liljedal, J., Ablad, B., Nyberg, G.: The effects of intravenous alprenalol on exercise tolerance in patients with angina pectoris. Pharmacol. Clin. *2*, 46–50 (1969)

Sealey, B.J., Liljedal, J., Nyberg, G., Ablad, B.: Acute effects of oral alprenalol on exercise tolerance in patients with angina pectoris. A dose response study. Br. Heart J. *33*, 481–488 (1971)

Sedenberg-Olsen, P., Ibsen, H.: Plasma volume and extracellular fluid volume during long term treatment with propranolol in essential hypertension. Clin. Sci. *43*, 165–170 (1972)

Seedat, Y.K., Reddy, J.: Propranolol in the South African non-white hypertensive patient. S. Afr. Med. J. *45*, 284–285 (1971)

Seedat, Y.K., Vawda, E.I., Mitha, S., Ramasar, R.: Clonidine. Lancet *1969 II*, 591

Seedat, Y.K., Stewart-Wynne, E.G., Reddy, J., Randeree, M.: Experiences with beta-adrenergic blocking drugs in hypertension. S. Afr. Med. J. *47*, 259 (1973)

Sellers, E.M., Zilm, D.H., Degani, N.C.: Comparative efficacy of propranolol and chlordiazepoxide in alcohol withdrawal. J. Stud. Alcohol *38*, 2096–2108 (1977)

Seppälä, M., Räihä, N.C.R., Tamminen, V.: Ethanol elimination in a mother and her premature twins. Lancet *1971 I*, 1188–1189

Shand, D.G.: Pharmacokinetic properties of β-adrenergic receptor blocking drugs. Drugs *7*, 39–47 (1974)

Shand, D.G.: The pharmacokinetics of propranolol: a review. Postgrad. Med. J. [Suppl. 4] *52*, 22–25 (1976)

Shanks, R.G., Hadden, D.R., Lowe, D.C., McDevitt, D.G., Montgomery, D.A.D.: Controlled trial of propranolol in thyrotoxicosis. Lancet *1969 I*, 993–994

Sharma, B., Goodwin, J.F.: Beneficial effect of salbutamol on cardiac function in severe congestive cardiomyopathy. Circulation *58*, 449–460 (1978)

Shaw, J., Hunyor, S.N., Korner, P.I.: The peripheral circulatory effects of clonidine and their role in the production of arterial hypotension. Eur. J. Pharmacol. *14*, 101–111 (1971)

Shenfield, G.M., Paterson, J.W.: Clinical assessment of bronchodilators drugs delivered by aerosol. Thorax *28*, 124–128 (1973)

Shenfield, G.M., Evans, M.E., Walker, S.R., Paterson, J.W.: The fate of nebulised salbutamol (albuterol) administered by intermittent positive pressure respiration to asthmatic patients. Am. Rev. Respir. Dis. *108*, 501–505 (1973)

Shinebourne, E., Fleming, J., Hamer, J.: Effects of beta-adrenergic blockade during exercise in hypertensive and ischaemic heart disease. Lancet *1967 II*, 1217–1220

Shiroff, R.A., Mathis, J., Zelis, R., Schneck, D.W., Babb, J.D., Leaman, D.M., Hayes, A.H.: Propranolol rebound – A retrospective study. Am. J. Cardiol. *41*, 778–780 (1978)

Siitonen, L., Janne, J., Keyrilainen, O., Koskinen, P., Leskinen, O., Pitkajarvi, T., Reinikainen, M.: Hydralazine and beta-adrenergic blockade in the treatment of hypertension. Ann. Clin. Res. *6*, 341–346 (1974)

Silverman, M., Konig, P., Godfrey, S.: The use of serial exercise tests to assess the efficacy and duration of action of drugs for asthma. Thorax *28*, 574–578 (1973)

Simi, W.W., Miller, W.C.: Clinical investigation of fenoterol, a new bronchodilator in asthma. J. Allergy Clin. Immunol. *59*, 178–181 (1977)

Simon, G., Kiowski, W., Julius, S.: Antihypertensive and β-adrenoceptor antagonist action of timolol. Clin. Pharmacol. Ther. *23*, 152–157 (1978a)

Simon, P., Lecruibier, Y., Jouvent, R., Puech, A.J., Allilaire, J.F., Wildöcher, D.: Experimental and clinical evidence of the antidepressant effect of a beta-adrenergic stimulant. Psychol. Med. *8*, 335–338 (1978b)

Simonsson, B.G., Stiksa, J., Ström, B.: Double-blind trial with increasing doses of salbutamol and terbutaline aerosols in patients with reversible airways obstruction. Acta Med. Scand. *192*, 371–376 (1972a)

Simonsson, B.G., Svedmyr, N., Skoogh, B.-E., Andersson, R., Bergh, N.P.: In vivo and in vitro studies on alpha-receptors in human airways; potentiation with bacterial endotoxin. Scand. J. Respir. Dis. *53*, 227–236 (1972b)

Simonsson, B.G., Svedenblad, H., Ström, B.: Bronchodilatory and circulatory effects of two doses of a B-2 agonist (terbutaline) inhaled with IPPB in patients with reversible airways obstruction. Scand. J. Respir. Dis. *57*, 252–258 (1976)

Simpson, F.O.: Beta-adrenergic blocking drugs in hypertension. Drugs *7*, 85–105 (1974)

Simpson, F.O., Bolli, P., Wood, A.J.: Use of prazosin at the Dunedin Hypertension Clinic: Controlled and open studies and pharmacokinetic observations. Med. J. Aust. [Suppl.] *2*, 17–22 (1977)

Sims, B.A.: Investigation of salbutamol tolerance. Br. J. Clin. Pharmacol. *1*, 291–294 (1974)

Sims, C.D., Chamberlain, G.V.P., Boyd, I.E., Lewis, P.J.: A comparison of salbutamol and ethanol in the treatment of pre-term labour. Br. J. Obstet. Gynaecol. *85*, 761–766 (1978)

Singh, B.N., Jewitt, D.E.: Beta-adrenergic receptor blocking drugs in cardiac arrhythmias. Drugs *7*, 426–461 (1974)

Singh, B.N., Till, M.R., Kelly, D.T.: The effects of oxprenolol (trasicor, Ciba 39089-Ba) on patterns of urinary sodium excretion in man. Am. J. Cardiol. *27*, 372–375 (1971)

Sinha, J.N., Tangri, K.K., Bhargrava, K.P., Schmitt, H.: Central sites of sympatho-inhibitory effects of clonidine and l-dopa. In: Recent advances in hypertension. Milliez, P., Safar, M., (eds.), Vol. 1, pp. 97–109. Reims: Societe Alina 1975

Sjaastad, O., Stensrud, P.: Clinical trial of a beta receptor blocking agent (LB 46) in migraine prophylaxis. Acta Neurol. Scand. *48*, 124–128 (1972)

Skinner, C., Gaddie, J., Palmer, K.N.V.: Comparison of intravenous AH 5158 (ibidomide) and propranolol in asthma. Br. Med. J. *1975 II*, 59–61

Sloman, G.: Propranolol in management of muscular subaortic stenosis. Br. Heart J. *29*, 783–787 (1967)

Sloman, G., Robinson, J.S., McLean, K.: Propranolol (inderal) in persistent ventricular fibrillation. Br. Med. J. *1965 I*, 895–896

Smet, G., Hoobler, S.W., Sanbar, S., Julius, S.: Clinical observations on a new antihypertensive drug 2-(2,6-dichlorphenylamine)-2-imidazoline hydrochloride. Am. Heart J. *77*, 473–478 (1969)

Smirk, H.: The hypotensive action of B.W. 467C60. Lancet *1963a I*, 743–746

Smirk, H.: Hypotensive action of methyldopa. Br. Med. J. *1963b I*, 146–151

Smith, A.D.: Mechanisms involved in the release of noradrenaline from sympathetic nerves. Br. Med. Bull. *29*, 123–129 (1973)

Smith, C.S., Howard, N.J.: Propranolol in the treatment of neonatal thyrotoxicosis. J. Pediatr. *83*, 1046–1048 (1973)

Smith, H.J., Oriol, A., Morch, J., McGregor, M.: Hemodynamic studies in cardiogenic shock. Treatment with isoproterenol and metaraminol. Circulation *35*, 1084–1091 (1967)

Smith, I.S., Fernandes, M., Kim, K.E., Swartz, C., Onesti, G.: A three-phase clinical evaluation of prazosin. Postgrad. Med. [Suppl.] *58*, 53–60 (1975)

Smith, R.N., Davies, H.J.: Long-term use of salbutamol inhaler in general practice. Practitioner *210*, 425–428 (1973)

Smith, S.K., Thompson, D.: The effect of intravenous salbutamol upon plasma and urinary potassium during premature labour. Br. J. Obstet. Gynaecol. *84*, 344–347 (1977)

Sneddon, J.M., Turner, P.: Adrenergic blockade and the eye signs of thyrotoxicosis. Lancet *1966 II*, 525–526

Snow, P.J.D.: Treatment of acute myocardial infarction with propranolol. Am. J. Cardiol. *18*, 458–462 (1966)

Sonnenblick, E.H.: Implications of muscle mechanics of the heart. Fed. Proc. *21*, 975–990 (1962)

Sonnenblick, E.H., Skelton, C.L.: Myocardial energetics: basic principles and clinical implications. N. Engl. J. Med. *285*, 668–675 (1971)

Sonnenblick, E.H., Braunwald, E., Williams, J.F., Glick, G.: Effects of exercise in myocardial force-velocity relations in intact unanaesthetised man: relative roles in change in heart rate, sympathetic activity and ventricular dimensions. J. Clin. Invest. *44*, 2051–2062 (1965)

Sonnenblick, E.H., Ross, J., Braunwald, E.: Oxygen consumption of the heart. Newer concepts of its multifactorial determination. Am. J. Cardiol. *22*, 328–336 (1968)

Sorenby, L.: Inhibition of the antigen-induced release of histamine from guinea-pig lung by terbutaline. Acta Pharmacol. Toxicol. (Kbh) *34*, 267–272 (1974)

Sorenby, L.: The beta-adrenoceptors of the lung mediating inhibition of antigen-induced histamine release. Eur. J. Pharmacol. *30*, 140–147 (1975)
Sotaniemi, E.A., Hokkanen, O.T., Ahokas, J.T., Pelkonen, R.O., Ahlqvist, J.: Hepatic injury and drug metabolism in patients with alpha-methyldopa-induced liver damage. Eur. J. Clin. Pharmacol. *12*, 429–435 (1977)
Sowton, E., Smithen, C.: Double-blind three-dose trial of oral alprenalol in angina pectoris. Br. Heart J. *33*, 601–606 (1971)
Sowton, E., Smithen, C., Leaver, D., Barr, I.: Effect of practolol on exercise tolerance in patients with angina pectoris. Am. J. Med. *51*, 63–70 (1971)
Spaulding, S.W., Noth, R.H.: Thyroid-catecholamine interactions. Med. Clin. North Am. *59*, 1123–1131 (1975)
Spector, G.L., Gross, G., Schultz, L., Sisco, C., Farr, R.S.: Idiosyncratic bronchoconstriction following isoproterenol. Clin. Res. *23*, 352 A (1975)
Speizer, F.E., Doll, R., Heaf, P.: Observations on recent increase in mortality from asthma. Br. Med. J. *1968 I*, 335–339
Srivastava, S.C., Dewar, H.A., Newell, D.J.: Double-blind trial of propranolol (inderal) in angina of effort. Br. Med. J. *1964 II*, 724–725
Starke, K., Montel, H.: Involvement of alpha-receptors in clonidine-induced inhibition of transmitter release from central monoamine neurones. Neuropharmacology *12*, 1073–1080 (1973)
Steen, S.N., Smith, R., Kuo, J., Ziment, I., Beall, G.N.: Effect of fenoterol on airway conductance in asthmatic patients. IRCS J. Med. Sci. *3*, 591 (1975)
Steen, S.N., Smith, R., Kuo, J., Ziment, I., Beall, G.N.: Comparison of the bronchodilator effects of aerosol fenoterol and isoproterenol. Chest *72*, 724–730 (1977)
Steiner, M., Blum, I., Wijsenbeek, H., Atsmon, A.: Results of the treatment of psychoses with propranolol. Kupat-Holim Yearb. b. 2, 201–209 (1972)
Steiner, M., Latz, A., Blum, I., Atsom, A., Wijsenbeek, H.: Propranolol versus chlorpromazine in the treatment of psychoses associated with childbearing. Psychiatr. Neurol. Neurochir. *76*, 421–426 (1973)
Stemple, D.R., Griffin, J.C., Kernoff, R.S., Harrison, D.C.: Metabolic and electrophysiologic effect of nitroprusside and dopamine in experimental acute myocardial infarction. Clin. Res. *24*, 141 A (1976)
Stephen, S.A.: Unwanted effects of propranolol. Am. J. Cardiol. *18*, 463–468 (1966)
Stephens, J., Ead, H., Spurrell, R.: Haemodynamic effects of dobutamine with special reference to myocardial blood flow. A comparison with dopamine and isoprenaline. Br. Heart J. *42*, 43–50 (1979)
Stern, S., Hoffman, P.M., Braun, K.: Cardiovascular responses to carotid and vertebral artery infusions of propranolol. Cardiovasc. Res. *5*, 425–430 (1971)
Stewart, I.McD.G.: Compared incidence of first myocardial infarction in hypertensive patients under treatment containing propranolol or excluding β-receptor blockade. Clin. Sci. Mol. Med. *51*, 509s-511s (1976)
Stjärne, L., Brundin, J.: Dual adrenoceptor-mediated control of noradrenaline secretion from human vasoconstrictor nerves: Facilitation by β-receptors and inhibition by α-receptors. Acta Physiol. Scand. *94*, 139–141 (1975)
Stock, J.P.P.: Beta-adrenergic blocking drugs in the clinical management of cardiac arrhythmias. Am. J. Cardiol. *18*, 438–444 (1966)
Stokes, G.S., Weber, M.A.: Prazosin: Preliminary report and comparative studies with other anti-hypertensive agents. Br. Med. J. *1974 II*, 298–300
Stokes, G.S., Weber, M.A., Thornell, I.R.: Beta-blockers and plasma renin activity in hypertension. Br. Med. J. *1974 I*, 60–62
Stokes, G.S., Gain, J.M., Mahony, J.F., Stewart, J.H., Raftos, J.: Long-term use of prazosin in combination or alone for treating hypertension. Med. J. Aust. [Suppl.] *2*, 13–16 (1977 a)
Stokes, G.S., Graham, R.M., Gain, J.M., Davis, P.R.: Influence of dosage and dietary sodium on the first-dose effects of prazosin. Br. Med. J. *1977 b I*, 1507–1508
Stoner, J.D., Bolen, J.L., Harrison, D.C.: Comparison of dobutamine and dopamine in treatment of severe heart failure. Br. Heart J. *39*, 536–539 (1977)
Storstein-Spilker, L.: The influence of the β-receptor blocking agent LB-46, isosorbide-dinitrate and their combination on the exercise ECG. Cardiovasc. Res. 4, 298 (1970)

Strauss, F.G., Franklin, S.S., Lewin, A.J., Maxwell, M.H.: Withdrawal of antihypertensive therapy: hypertensive crisis in renovascular hypertension. JAMA *238*, 1734–1736 (1977)
Stumpe, K.O., Kolloch, R., Vetter, H., Gramann, W., Krück, F., Ressel, Ch., Higuchi, M.: Acute and long-term studies of the mechanism of action of beta-blocking drugs in lowering blood pressure. Am. J. Med. *60*, 853–865 (1976)
Suzman, M.M.: The use of beta-adrenergic blockade with propranolol in anxiety syndromes. Postgrad. Med. J. [Suppl.] *47*, 104 (1971)
Svedmyr, N., Malmberg, R., Thiringer, G.: The effect of a new adrenergic B_2-receptor-stimulating agent (rimiterol, R798) in patients with chronic obstructive lung disease. Scand. J. Respir. Dis. *53*, 302–313 (1972)
Svedmyr, N., Larsson, S., Thiringer, G. (Letter) Studies of resistance to long acting adrenergic beta-stimulators in asthmatic patients. Br. Med. J. *1974 II*, 668–669
Svedmyr, N.L., Larsson, S.A., Thiringer, G.: Development of "resistance" in beta-adrenergic receptors of asthmatic patients. Chest *69*, 479–483 (1976)
Syvälahti, E., Lammintausta, R., Iisalo, E., Kanto, J.: Cardioselective (metoprolol) and non-selective (propranolol) beta-blockade and glucose homoeostasis. Ann. Clin. Res. *9*, 292–295 (1977)
Tabori, D.V., Čonkić, B., Todić, V., Mijatović, M., Mirković, S., Zečević, D., Camprag, D.: Die bronchodilatatorische Wirkung von Reproterol bei Patienten mit Asthma bronchiale und obstruktiver Bronchitis. Arzneim. Forsch. *27*, 55–60 (1977)
Taggart, P., Carruthers, M.: Suppression by oxprenolol of adrenergic response to stress. Lancet *1972 II*, 256–258
Taggart, P., Carruthers, M., Somerville, W.: Electrocardiogram, plasma catecholamines and lipids and their modification by oxprenolol when speaking before an audience. Lancet *1973a II*, 341–346
Taggart, P., Carruthers, M., Somerville, W.: Intense emotional stress: effect of oxprenolol on the electrocardiogram, plasma catecholamines and lipids. In: New perspectives in beta blockade. Burley, D.M., Frier, Rondel and Taylor (eds.), pp. 287–290. Horsham: Ciba 1973b
Takeshita, A., Tanaka, S., Nakamura, M.: Effects of propranolol on baroreflex sensitivity in borderline hypertension. Cardiovasc. Res. *12*, 148–151 (1978)
Talbot, S., Smith, A.J.: Factors predisposing to postural hypotensive symptoms in the treatment of high blood pressure. Br. Heart J. *37*, 1059–1063 (1975)
Talbot, S., O'Malley, B.C., Bing, R.F.: Debrisoquine, guanethidine and bethanidine in hypertension. Br. Med. J. *1975 II*, 278
Talley, R.C., Goldberg, L.I., Johnson, C.E., McNay, J.L.: A haemodynamic comparison of dopamine and isoproterenol in patients in shock. Circulation *39*, 361–378 (1969)
Tamby Raja, R.L.: Prevention of pre-term delivery in twins – a neurohormonal approach. In: Twin research: Clinical studies. Alan, R. (ed.), pp. 117–121. New York: Liss 1978
Tarazi, R.C., Dustan, H.P.: Beta-adrenergic blockade in hypertension. Practical and theoretical implications of long term haemodynamic variations. Am. J. Cardiol. *29*, 633–640 (1972)
Tarazi, R.C., Frohlich, E.D., Dustan, H.P.: Plasma volume changes with long-term beta adrenergic blockade. Am. Heart J. *82*, 770–776 (1971)
Tarazi, R.C., Ibrahim, M.M., Dustan, H.P., Ferrario, C.M.: Cardiac factors in hypertension. Circ. Res. [Suppl. 1] *34*, 213–221 (1974)
Tarazi, R.C., Dustan, H.P., Bravo, E.L.: Haemodynamic effects of propranolol in hypertension: a review. Postgrad. Med. J. [Suppl. 4] *52*, 92–100 (1976)
Taylor, J.A.: Hypotension after oral propranolol. Lancet *1968 I*, 532–533
Taylor, J.A., Twomey, T.M., von Wittenau, M.S.: The metabolic fate of prazosin. Xenobiotica *7*, 357–364 (1977)
Taylor, S.H.: Mechanism of action of adrenergic beta-receptor antagonists in angina pectoris. In: New perspectives in beta-blockade. Burley, D.M., Frier, J.H., Rondel, R.K., Taylor, S.H., (eds.), pp. 107–127. Horsham: Ciba 1973
Taylor, S.H., Meeran, M.K.: Different effects of adrenergic beta-receptor blockade on heart rate response to mental stress, catecholamines and exercise. Br. Heart J. *4*, 257–259 (1973a)
Taylor, S.H., Meeran, M.K.: The cardiovascular response to some environmental stresses and their modification by oxprenolol. In: New perspectives in beta blockade. Burley, D.M., Frier, J.H., Rondel, R.K., Taylor, S.H., (eds.), pp. 293–306. Horsham: Ciba 1973b

Taylor, S.H., Sutherland, G.R., Hutchison, D.C., Langford-Kidd, B.S., Robertson, P.C., Kennelly, B.M., Donald, K.W.: The effects of intravenous guanethidine on the systemic and pulmonary circulation in man. Am. Heart J. *63*, 239–264 (1962)

Taylor, W.F., Heimlich, E.M., Strick, L., Busser, R.S.: Ephedrine and theophylline in asthmatic children: quantitative observations on the combination and ephedrine tachyphylaxis. Ann. Allergy *23*, 437–440 (1965)

Tewari, S.N., Grant, R.H.E.: Propranolol in hypertension. Postgrad. Med. J. *44*, 509–512 (1968)

Thadani, U., Sharma, B., Meeran, M.K., Majid, P.A., Whitaker, W., Taylor, S.H.: Comparison of adrenergic beta-receptor antagonists in angina pectoris. Br. Med. J. *1973 I*, 138–142

Thiringer, G., Bergh, N.P., Svedmyr, N.: A comparative study of the effects of isoetharine and some other adrenergic beta stimulators in chronic obstructive airways disease. Scand. J. Res. Dis. *52*, 183–191 (1971)

Thiringer, G., Svedmyr, N.: Comparison of infused and inhaled terbutaline in patients with asthma. Scand. J. Respir. Dis. *57*, 17–24 (1976)

Thomas, D.J.B., Dove, A.F., Alberti, K.G.M.M.: Metabolic effects of salbutamol infusion during premature labour. Br. J. Obstet. Gynaecol. *84*, 497–499 (1977)

Thompson, F.D., Joekes, A.M., Hussein, M.M.: Labetalol used as a hypotensive agent in the presence of renal disease. Kidney Int. *11*, 287 (1977)

Thorpe, P.: A controlled study of pindolol (visken) on hypertension. Med. J. Aust. *2*, 306–309 (1972)

Tibblin, G., Ablad, B.: Anti-hypertensive therapy with alprenolol, a beta-adrenergic receptor antagonist. Acta Med. Scand. *186*, 451–458 (1969)

Timmis, A.D., Strak, S.K., Chamberlain, D.A.: Haemodynamic effects of salbutamol in patients with acute myocardiol infarction and severe left ventricular dysfunction. Br. Med. J. II, 1101–1103 (1979)

Toghill, P.J., Smith, P.G., Benton, P., Brown, R.C., Matthews, H.L.: Methyldopa liver damage. Br. Med. J. *3*, 545–548 (1974)

Toubes, D.B., Ferguson, R.K., Rice, A.J., Aoki, V.S., Funk, D.C., Wilson, W.R.: β-adrenergic blockade vs. placebo in angina pectoris. Clin. Res. *18*, 345 (1970)

Trautlein, J., Allegra, J., Gillin, M.: A long-term study of low-dose aerolised terbutaline sulphate. J. Clin. Pharmacol. *16*, 361–366 (1976)

Trinker, F.R.: The significance of the relative potencies of noradrenaline and α-methyl-noradrenaline for the mode of action of α-methyldopa. J. Pharm. Pharmacol. *23*, 306–308 (1971)

Trust, P.M., Rosei, E.A., Brown, J.J., Fraser, R., Lever, A.F., Morton, J.J., Robertson, J.I.S.: Effect on blood pressure, angiotensin II and aldosterone concentrations during treatment of severe hypertension with intravenous labetalol: comparison with propranolol. Br. J. Clin. Pharmacol. *3*, 799–803 (1976)

Tuckman, J., Shillingford, J.P.: The effect of different degrees of tilt on cardiac output, heart rate and blood pressure in normal man. Br. Heart J. *28*, 32–39 (1966)

Tuckman, J., Slater, S.R.: Differences of cardiac output changes with progressive tilting in normotensive and hypertensive man (abstract). Circulation [Suppl. III] *29*, 171 (1964)

Tuckman, J., Slater, S.R., Kupfer, S.: Comparison of blood volume increases in the legs and change of cardiac output in normotensive and hypertensive man. Fed. Proc. *25*, 267 (1966)

Tuckman, J. Reich. T., Lyon, A.F., Goodman, B., Mendlowitz, M., Jacobson, J.H.: Electrical stimulation of the sinus nerves in hypertensive patients. Hypertension *16*, 23–38 (1968)

Tuckman, J., Martin, R., Hodler, J.: Hypertoniebehandlung mit hohen Dosen von Oxprenolol, allein oder in Kombination mit dem Vasodilator Dihydrallazine. Helv. Med. Acta *36*, 243–244 (1972)

Tuckman, J., Messerli, F., Hodler, J.: Treatment of hypertension with large doses of the beta-adrenergic blocking drug oxprenolol alone and in combination with the vasodilator dihydralazine. Clin. Sci. Mol. Med. *45*, 159–161 (1973)

Turner, A.S.: Prazosin in hypertension. Br. Med. J. *1976 II*, 1257–1258

Turner, A.S., Watson, O.F., Brocklehurst, J.E.: Prazosin in hypertension. Clinical studies with special reference to initiation of therapy. Med. J. Aust. [Suppl. 2] *2*, 33–37 (1977)

Turner, P.: β-adrenergic receptor blocking drugs in hyperthyroidism. Drugs *7*, 48–54 (1974)

Tuttle, R.R.: The inotropic and chronotropic effects of dobutamine and isoproterenol on cat atria and papillary muscles at different temperatures. Fed. Proc. *33*, 503 (1974)
Tuttle, R.R., Mills, J.: Dobutamine: development of a new catecholamine to selectively increase cardiac contractility. Circ. Res. *36*, 185–196 (1975)
Tuttle, R.R., Pollock, D.G., Todd, G., Tust, R.: Dobutamine: containment of myocardial infarction size by a new inotropic agent (abstract). Circulation [Suppl. 4] *48*, 132 (1973)
Tuttle, R.R., Hillman, C.C., Toomey, R.E.: Differential β-adrenergic sensitivity of atrial and ventricular tissue assessed by chronotropic, inotropic and cyclic AMP responses to isoprenaline and dobutamine. Cardiovasc. Res. *10*, 452–458 (1976)
Tweel, H.K.: Th 1165a, a new bronchodilator: clinical comparative evaluation with metaproterenol. Ann. Allergy *29*, 142–147 (1971)
Tyrer, P.J., Lader, M.H.: Response to propranolol and diazepam in somatic and psychic anxiety. Br. Med. J. *1974a II*, 14–16 (1974a)
Tyrer, P.J., Lader, M.H.: Physiological response to propranolol and diazepam in chronic anxiety. Br. J. Clin. Pharmacol. *1*, 387–390 (1974b)
Tyrer, P.J., Lader, M.H.: Physiological and psychological effects of $\pm$ propranolol, + propranolol and diazepam in induced anxiety. Br. J. Clin. Pharmacol. *1*, 379–385 (1974c)
Ulrych, M., Frohlich, E.D., Dustan, H.P., Page, I.H.: Immediate haemodynamic effects of beta-adrenergic blockade with propranolol in normotensive and hypertensive man. Circulation *37*, 411–416 (1968)
Vale, J.A., Jefferys, D.B.: Peripheral gangrene complicating beta-blockade. Lancet *1978 I*, 1216
Vale, J., Phillips, C.I.: Effect of DL- and D-propranolol on ocular tension in rabbits and patients. Exp. Eye Res. *9*, 902–908 (1970)
Vale, J., Phillips, C.I.: Practolol (eraldin) eye drops as an ocular hypotensive agent. Br. J. Ophthalmol. *57*, 210–214 (1973)
Vale, J., Gibbs, A.C.C., Phillips, C.I.: Topical propranolol and ocular tension in the human. Br. J. Ophthalmol. *56*, 770–775 (1972)
Van Metre, T.E.: Adverse effects of inhalation of excessive amounts of nebulised isoproterenol in status asthmaticus. J. Allergy *43*,, 101–113 (1969)
Van Zwieten, P.A., Pauer, M., van Spanning, H.W., de Langen, C.: Interaction between centrally acting hypotensive drugs and tricyclic anti-depressants. Arch. Int. Pharmacodyn. *214*, 12–30 (1975)
Vargas-Garcia, C., Macedo-Garcia, J., Ahued, R.A., Favela, L.E.: Terbutalina un nuevo uteroinhibidor. Ginecol. Obstet. Mex. *36*, 75–79 (1974)
Vatner, S.F., McRitchie, R.J., Braunwald, E.: Effects of dobutamine on left ventricular performance, coronary dynamics and distribution of cardiac output in conscious dogs. J. Clin. Invest. *53*, 1265–1273 (1974)
Vaughan-Williams, E.M., Raine, A.E.G.: Effect of prolonged beta-receptor blockade on dry weight and electrophysiological responses of rabbit hearts. Lancet *1974 II*, 1048–1049
Vaughan-Williams, E.M., Tasgal, J., Raine, A.E.G.: Morphometric changes in rabbit ventricular myocardium produced by long-term beta-adrenoceptor blockade. Lancet *1977 II*, 850–852
Verbesselt, R., Mullie, A., Tjandramaga, T.B., de Schepper, P.J., Dessain, P.: The effect of food intake on the plasma kinetics and toleration of prazosin. Acta Ther. *2*, 27 (1976)
Verniory, A., Staroukine, M., Telerman, M., Delwiche, F.: Effect of sotalol on arterial pressure and renin-angiotensin system in hypertensive patients. Excerpta Med. *4*, 36–45 (1974)
Villareal, H., Exaire, J.E., Rubio, V., Davila, H.: Effect of guanethidine and bretylium tosylate on systemic and renal hemodynamics in essential hypertension. Am. J. Cardiol. *14*, 633–640 (1964)
Von Ehringer, H.: Die Wirkung von 2-(2,6 Dichlorophenylamino)-2-Imidazolin-Hydrochlorid auf die Extremitätendurchblutung, den Blutdruck und die Venenkapazität bei Normotonikern. Arzneim. Forsch. *16*, 1165–1169 (1966)
Von Hoefke, W., Kobinger, W.: Pharmakologische Wirkungen des 2-(2,6-Dichloro-phenylamino)-2-Imidazolin-Hydrochlorids einer neuen, antihypertensiven Substanz. Arzneim. Forsch. *66*, 1038–1050 (1966)
Vorburger, C.: Discussion In: Catapres in hypertension. Conolly, M.E. (ed.), p. 215. London: Butterworths 1970

Waagstein, F., Hjalmarson, A.C.: Double-blind study of the effect of cardioselective beta-blockade on chest pain in acute myocardial infarction. Acta Med. Scand. [Suppl.] *587*, 201–208 (1976)

Waagstein, F., Hjalmarson, A., Varnauskas, E., Wallentin, I.: Effect of chronic beta-adrenergic receptor blockade in congestive cardiomyopathy. Br. Heart J. *31*, 1022–1036 (1975)

Waal, H.L.: Hypotensive action in propranolol. Clin. Pharmacol. Ther. *7*, 588–598 (1966)

Waal-Manning, H.J.: Lack of effect of D-propranolol on blood pressure and pulse rate in hypertensive patients. Proc. Univ. Otago Med. Sch. *48*, 80–81 (1970a)

Waal-Manning, H.J.: Comparative studies on the hypotensive effects of beta-adrenergic receptor blockade. In: Symposium on beta-adrenergic receptor blocking drugs. Simpson, F.O. (ed.), p. 64. Auckland: Ciba 1970b

Waal-Manning, H.J.: The antihypertensive action of several β-adrenoreceptor blocking drugs. N. Z. Med. J. *83*, 223–226 (1976)

Waal-Manning, H.J., Simpson, F.O.: Practolol treatment in asthmatics. Lancet *1971 II*, 1264–1265

Waal-Manning, H.J., Simpson, F.O.: Pindolol: A comparison with other antihypertensive drugs and a double blind placebo trial. N. Z. Med. J. *80*, 151–157 (1974)

Waal-Manning, H.J., Simpson, F.O.: Paradoxical effect of pindolol. Br. Med. J. *1975 III*,155–156

Walinsky, P., Chatterjee, K., Forrester, J., Parmley, J.J., Swan, J.C.: Enhanced left ventricular performance with phentolamine in acute myocardial infarction. Am. J. Cardiol. *33*, 37–41 (1974)

Walker, S.R., Evans, M.E., Richards, A.J., Paterson, J.W.: The clinical pharmacology of oral and inhaled salbutamol. Clin. Pharmacol. Ther. *13*, 861–867 (1972)

Walsh, J.A., Hyman, C., Maronde, R.F.: Venous distensibility in essential hypertension. Cardiovasc. Res. *3*, 338–349 (1969)

Walters, W.A.W., Wood, C.: A trial of oral ritodrine for the prevention of premature labour. Br. J. Obstet. Gynaecol. *84*, 26–30 (1977)

Warrell, D.A., Robertson, D.G., Newton Howes, J., Conolly, M.E., Paterson, J.W., Beilin, L.J., Dollery, C.T.: Comparison of cardiorespiratory effects of isoprenaline and salbutamol in patients with bronchial asthma. Br. Med. J. *1970 I*, 65–70

Wasserman, M.A., Levy, B.: Cardiovascular and bronchomotor responses to selective beta adrenergic receptor agonists in the anaesthetised dog. J. Pharmacol. Exp. Ther. *189*, 445–455 (1974)

Watson, J., Richens, A.: The effects of salbutamol and terbutaline on physiological tremor, bronchial tone and heart rate. Br. J. Clin. Pharmacol. *1*,, 223–227 (1974)

Webb-Peploe, M.M., Oakley, C.M., Croxon, R.S., Goodwin, J.F.: Cardioselective beta-adrenergic blockade in hypertrophic obstructive cardiomyopathy. Postgrad. Med. J. [Suppl.] *47*, 93–96 (1971)

Weber, R.B., Reinmuth, O.M.: The treatment of migraine with propranolol. Neurology (Minneap.) *22*, 366–369 (1972)

Webster, J., Jeffers, T.A., Galloway, D.B.: Atenolol, methyldopa and chlorthalidone in moderate hypertension. Br. Med. J. *1977 I*, 76–78

Weinstein, R., Schwartzman, R., Levey, G.S.: Propranolol reversal of bulbar dysfunction and proximal myopathy in hyperthyroidism. Ann. Intern. Med. *82*, 540–541 (1975)

Werner, U., Starke, K., Schumann, H.J.: Actions of clonidine and 2-(2-methyl-6-ethyl-cyclohexylamino-)-2-oxazoline on postganglionic autonomic nerves. Arch. Int. Pharmacodyn. *195*, 282–290 (1972)

Wesselius, de Casparis, A., Thiery, M., Yo le Sian, A., Baumgarten, K., Brosens, I., Gamisans, O., Stolk, J.G., Vivier, W.: Results of double-blind, multicentre study with ritodrine in premature labour. Br. Med. J. *1971 III*,144–147

Whitlock, F.A., Price, J.: Use of β-adrenergic receptor blocking drugs in psychiatry. Drugs *8*, 109–124 (1974)

Whitsett, T.L., Chrysant, S.G., Dillard, B.L., Anton, A.H.: Abrupt cessation of clonidine administration: a prospective study. Am. J. Cardiol. *41*, 1285–1290 (1978)

Whittington-Coleman, P.J., Carrier, O., Douglas, B.H.: The effects of propranolol on cholesterol-induced atheromatous lesions. Atherosclerosis *18*, 337–345 (1973)

Widerøe, T.E., Vigander, T.: Propranolol in the treatment of migraine. Br. Med. J. *2*, 699–701 (1974)

Wilburn, R.L., Blaufuss, A., Bennett, C.M.: Long-term treatment of severe hypertension with minoxidil, propranolol and furosemide. Circulation *52*, 706–713 (1975)

Wilcox, R.G.: Randomised study of six beta-blockers and a thiazide diuretic in essential hypertension. Br. Med. J. *1978 II*, 383–385

Wilcox, R.G., Mitchell, J.R.A.: Contribution of atenolol, bendrofluazide and hydrallazine to the management of severe hypertension. Br. Med. J. *1977 II*, 547–550

Wildholz, U., Bachofen, H., Scherrer, M.: Inhalation of beta stimulants: Dose response relationship. Lung *154*, 273–282 (1978)

Wilhelmsson, C., Vedin, J.A., Wilhelmsen, L., Tibblin, G., Werko, L.: Reduction of sudden deaths after myocardial infarction by treatment with alprenolol. Lancet *1974 II*, 1157–1160

Williams, S., Seaton, A.: Intravenous or inhaled salbutamol in severe acute asthma. Thorax *32*, 555–558 (1977)

Williams, S.J., Parish, R.W., Seaton, A.: Comparison of intravenous aminophylline and salbutamol in severe asthma. Br. Med. J. *1975 IV*, 685

Wilson, A.F., Novey, H.S., Cloninger, P., Davis, J., White, D.: Cardiopulmonary effects of long term bronchodilator administration. J. Allergy Clin. Immunol. *58*, 204–212 (1976b)

Wilson, A.G., Brooke, O.G., Lloyd, H.F., Robinson, B.F.: Mechanism of action of beta-adrenergic receptor blocking agents in angina pectoris; comparison of action of propranolol with dexpropranolol and practolol. Br. Med. J. *1969a IV*, 399–401

Wilson, C., Scott, M.E., Abdel-Mohsen, A.: Atenolol and methyldopa in the treatment of hypertension. Postgrad. Med. J. [Suppl. 3] *53*, 123–127 (1977)

Wilson, D.F., Watson, O.F., Peel, J.S., Turner, A.S.: Trasicor in angina pectoris: a double-blind trial. Br. Med. J. *1969b II*, 155–157

Wilson, J.D., Bullock, J.Y., Sutherland, D.C., Main, C., O'Brien, K.P.: Antinuclear antibodies in patients receiving non-practolol beta-blocker. Br. Med. J. *1978 I*, 14–16

Wilson, M., Morgan, G., Morgan, T.: The effect on blood pressure of β-adrenoceptor blocking drugs administered once daily and their duration of action when therapy is ceased. Br. J. Clin. Pharmacol. *3*, 857–861 (1976a)

Winer, N., Chokshi, D.S., Yoon, M.S., Freedman, A.D.: Adrenergic receptor mediation of renin secretion. J. Clin. Endocrinol. Metab. *29*, 1168–1175 (1969)

Wing, L.M.H., Reid, J.L., Davies, D.S., Dargie, H.J., Dollery, C.T.: Apparent resistence to hypotensive effect of clonidine. Br. Med. J. *1977 I*, 136–138

Wiseman, R.A.: Practolol-accumulated data on unwanted effects. Postgrad. Med. J. [Suppl.] *47*, 68–71 (1971)

Wolfson, S., Gorlin, R.: Cardiovascular pharmacology of propranolol in man. Circulation *40*, 501–511 (1969)

Wolfson, S., Heinle, R.A., Herman, M.N., Kemp, H.G., Sullivan, J.M., Gorlin, R.: Propranolol in angina pectoris. Am. J. Cardiol. *18*, 345–353 (1966)

Wood, A.J., Bolli, B., Simpson, F.O.: Prazosin in normal subjects: plasma levels, blood pressure and heart rate. Br. J. Clin. Pharmacol. *3*, 199–201 (1976)

Wood, D.W., Downe, J.J., Scheinkopf, H., Lecks, H.I.: Intravenous isoproterenol in the management of respiratory failure in childhood status asthmaticus. J. Allergy Clin. Immunol. *50*, 75–81 (1972)

Wood, R.E., Wanner, A., Hirsch, J., Farrell, P.M.: Tracheal mucociliary transport in patients with cystic fibrosis and its stimulation by terbutaline. Am. Rev. Respir. Dis. *111*, 733–738 (1975)

Worlledge, S.M., Carstairs, K.C., Dacie, J.V.: Autoimmune haemolytic anaemia associated with α-methyldopa therapy. Lancet *1966 II*, 135–139

Wray, R., Sutcliffe, S.B.J.: Propranolol induced hypoglycaemia and myocardial infarction. Br. Med. J. *1972 II*, 592

Wright, P.: Untoward effects associated with practolol administration: oculomucocutaneous syndrome. Br. Med. J. *1975 I*, 595–598

Wyse, S.D., Gibson, D.G., Branthwaite, M.A.: Haemodynamic effects of salbutamol in patients needing circulatory support after open heart surgery. Br. Med. J. *1974 III*, 502–503

Yacoub, M.H., Boyland, E.: Cardiovascular effects of intravenous salbutamol after open heart operations. Lancet *1973 I*, 1260–1261
Yeung, R.T.T., Tse, T.F.: Thyrotoxic peuodic paralysis. Effect of propranolol. Am. J. Med. *57*, 584–590 (1974)
Yititbasi, O., Nalbantgil, I.: Essai d'un nouveau beta-bloquer, le LB 46, dans le traitement de l'angine de poitrine. Praxis *59*, 1218–1221 (1970)
Yorkston, N.J., Zaki, S.A., Malik, M.K.U., Morrison, R.C., Harvard, C.W.H.: Propranolol in the control of schizophrenic symptoms. Br. Med. J. *1974 IV*, 633–635
Zacest, R.: The clinical pharmacology of hypotensive vasodilator drugs. Med. J. Aust. [Suppl. 1] 4–7 (1975)
Zacest, R., Gilmore, E., Koch-Weser, J.: Treatment of essential hypertension with combined vasodilation and beta-adrenergic blockade. N. Engl. J. Med. *286*, 617–622 (1972)
Zacharias, F.J.: Treatment of hypertension with propranolol. Br. Med. J. *1969 I*, 712
Zacharias, F.J., Cowen, K.J.: Controlled trial of propranolol in hypertension. Br. Med. J. *1970 I*, 471–474
Zacharias, F.J., Cowen, K.J.: Comparison of propranolol and atenolol in hypertension. Postgrad. Med. J. [Suppl. 3] *53*, 111–113 (1977)
Zacharias, F.J., Cowen, K.J., Vickers, J., Wall, B.G.: Propranolol in hypertension. A study of long-term therapy. 1964–1970. Am. Heart J. *83*, 755–761 (1972)
Zacharias, F.J., Cowen, K.J., Cuthbertson, P.J.R., Johnson, T.B.W., Prestt, J., Thompson, J., Vickers, J., Simpson, W.T., Tuson, R.: Atenolol in hypertension: a study of long term therapy. Postgrad. Med. J. [Suppl. 3] *53*, 102–110 (1977a)
Zacharias, F.J., Hayes, P.J., Cruickshank, J.M.: Atenolol in hypertension: a double blind comparison of the response to three different doses. Postgrad. Med. J. [Suppl. 3] *53*, 114–115 (1977b)
Zaimis, E.: Vasopressor drugs and catecholamines. Anaesthiology *29*, 732–762 (1968)
Zaimis, E., Hanington, E.: A possible pharmacological approach to migraine. Lancet *1969 II*, 298–300
Zeft, H.J., Patterson, S.D., Orgain, E.S.: Propranolol in the long term treatment of angina pectoris. Ann. Intern. Med. *70*, 1082 (1969)
Zlatnik, F.J., Fuchs, F.: A controlled study of ethanol in premature labor. Am. J. Obstet. Gynecol. *112*, 610–612 (1972)
Zukel, W.J., Cohen, B.M., Mattingly, T.W., Hrubec, Z.: Survival following first diagnosis of coronary artery disease. Am. Heart J. *78*, 159–170 (1969)
Zweifler, A.J., Esler, M.: Dissociation of fall in blood pressure, renin activity and heart rate during propranolol therapy. Circulation [Suppl. II] *54*, 87 (1976)

Author Index

Page numbers *in italics* refer to bibliography

Subject Index

Handbook of Experimental Pharmacology

Continuation of "Handbuch der experimentellen Pharmakologie"

Volume 10
Die Pharmakologie anorganischer Anionen

Volume 11
Lobelin und Lobelia-alkaloide

Volume 12
Morphin und morphinähnlich wirkende Verbindungen

Volume 14: Part 1
The Adrenocortical Hormones I

Part 2
The Adrenocortical Hormones II

Part 3
The Adrenocortical Hormones III

Volume 16
Erzeugung von Krankheitszustände durch das Experiment/Experimental Production of Diseases

Part 1
Blut (In Vorbereitung)

Part 2
Atemwege

Part 3
Heart and Circulation

Part 4
Niere, Nierenbecken, Blase

Part 5
Liver

Part 6
Schilddrüse
(In Vorbereitung)

Part 7
Zentralnervensystem

Part 8
Stütz- und Hartgewebe

Part 9
Infektionen I

Part 10
Infektionen II

Part 11A
Infektionen III

Part 11B
Infektionen IV

Part 12
Tumoren I

Part 13
Tumoren II

Part 14
Tumoren III
(In Vorbereitung)

Part 15
Kohlenhydratstoffwechsel, Fieber/ Carbohydrate Metabolism, Fever

Volume 17
Ions alcalino-terreux

Part 1
Systèmes isolés

Part 2
Organismes entiers

Volume 18
Histamine and Anti-Histaminics

Part 1
Histamine. Its Chemistry, Metabolism and Physiological and Pharmacological Actions

Part 2
Histamine II and Anti-Histaminics

Volume 19
5-Hydroxytryptamine and Related Indolealkylamines

Volume 20: Part 1
Pharmacology of Flourides I

Part 2
Pharmacology of Fluorides II

Volume 21
Beryllium

Volume 22: Part 1
Die Gestagene I

Part 2
Die Gestagene II

Volume 23
Neurohypophysical Hormones and Similar Polypeptides

Volume 24
Diuretica

Springer-Verlag
Berlin
Heidelberg
New York

Handbook of Experimental Pharmacology

Continuation of "Handbuch der experimentellen Pharmakologie"

Volume 25
Bradykinin, Kallidin and Kallikrein

Volume 26
H. Fischer: **Vergleichende Pharmakologie von Überträgersubstanzen in tiersystematischer Darstellung**

Volume 27
Anticoagulantien

Volume 28: Part 1
Concepts in Biochemical Pharmacology I

Part 3
Concepts in Biochemical Pharmacology III

Volume 29
Oral wirksame Antidiabetika

Volume 30
Modern Inhalation Anestetics

Volume 32: Part 1
Insulin I

Part 2
Insulin II

Volume 34
Secretin, Cholecystokinin, Pancreozymin and Gastrin

Volume 35: Part 1
H. E. Voss, G. Oertel:
Androgene I

Part 2
Androgens II and Antiandrogens/ Androgene II und Antiandrogene

Volume 36
Uranium – Plutonium – Transplutonic Elements

Volume 37
Angiotensin

Volume 38: Part 1
Antineoplastic and Immunosuppressive Agents I

Part 2
Antineoplastic and Immunosuppressive Agents II

Volume 39
Antihypertensive Agents

Volume 40
Organic Nitrates

Volume 41
Hypolipidemic Agents

Volume 42
Neuromuscular Junction

Volume 43
Anabolic-Androgenic Steroids

Volume 44
Heme and Hemoproteins

Volume 45: Part 1
Drug Addiction I

Part 2
Drug Addiction II

Volume 46
Fibrinoltics and Antifibrinolytics

Volume 47
Kinetics of Drug Action

Volume 48
Arthropod Venoms

Volume 49
Ergot Alkaloids and Related Compounds

Volume 50: Part 1
Inflammation

Part 2
Anti-Inflammatory Drugs

Volume 51
Uric Acid

Volume 52
Snake Venoms

Volume 53
Ganglionic Transmission

Springer-Verlag
Berlin
Heidelberg
New York

GPSR Compliance

The European Union's (EU) General Product Safety Regulation (GPSR) is a set of rules that requires consumer products to be safe and our obligations to ensure this.

If you have any concerns about our products, you can contact us on ProductSafety@springernature.com

In case Publisher is established outside the EU, the EU authorized representative is:

Springer Nature Customer Service Center GmbH
Europaplatz 3
69115 Heidelberg, Germany

Batch number: 10838053

Printed by Printforce, the Netherlands